PASS CCRN®!

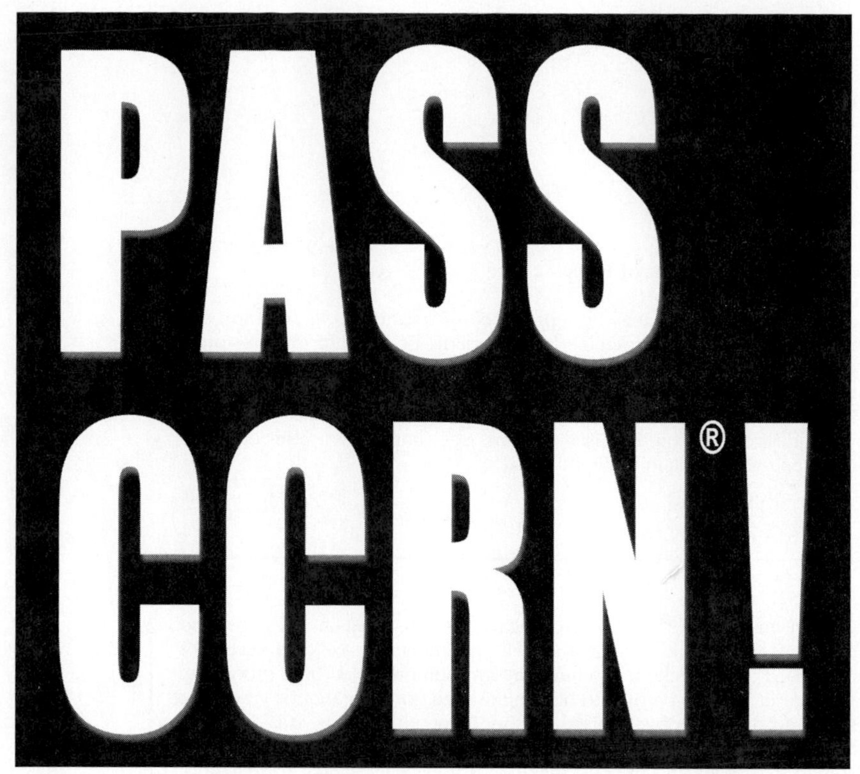

Third Edition

ROBIN DONOHOE DENNISON
DNP, RN, CCNS
Critical Care Consultant
Lexington, Kentucky

with 260 illustrations

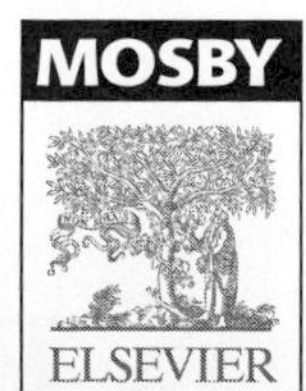

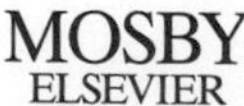

11830 Westline Industrial Drive
St. Louis, Missouri 63146

PASS CCRN®! ISBN: 978-0-323-02592-8
Copyright © 2007 by Mosby, Inc., an imprint of Elsevier Inc.

All rights reserved. No part of this publication may be reproduced or transmitted in any form or by any means, electronic or mechanical, including photocopying, recording, or any information storage and retrieval system, without permission in writing from the publisher.
Permissions may be sought directly from Elsevier's Health Sciences Rights Department in Philadelphia, PA, USA: phone: (+1) 215 239 3804, fax: (+1) 215 239 3805, e-mail: healthpermissions@elsevier.com. You may also complete your request on-line via the Elsevier homepage (http://www.elsevier.com), by selecting 'Customer Support' and then 'Obtaining Permissions'.

Notice

Knowledge and best practice in this field are constantly changing. As new research and experience broaden our knowledge, changes in practice, treatment and drug therapy may become necessary or appropriate. Readers are advised to check the most current information provided (i) on procedures featured or (ii) by the manufacturer of each product to be administered, to verify the recommended dose or formula, the method and duration of administration, and contraindications. It is the responsibility of the practitioner, relying on their own experience and knowledge of the patient, to make diagnoses, to determine dosages and the best treatment for each individual patient, and to take all appropriate safety precautions. To the fullest extent of the law, neither the Publisher nor the Authors assume any liability for any injury and/or damage to persons or property arising out of or related to any use of the material contained in this book.

The Publisher

Previous editions copyrighted 2000 and 1996.

ISBN: 978-0-323-02592-8

Publisher: Barbara Nelson Cullen
Senior Developmental Editor: Jennifer Ehlers
Publishing Services Manager: John Rogers
Senior Project Managers: Doug Turner, Helen Hudlin
Designer: Kim Denando

Working together to grow libraries in developing countries

www.elsevier.com | www.bookaid.org | www.sabre.org

ELSEVIER BOOK AID International Sabre Foundation

Printed in the United States of America.
Last digit is the print number: 9 8 7 6 5 4 3

This third edition is dedicated to all the nurses
who have attended my CCRN® reviews
throughout the United States
and helped me refine the content and the process
for preparing for the CCRN® examination.

EXPERT CONTENT REVIEWERS for this Edition

Anne Wojner, PhD, RN, CCRN, FAAN
Health Outcomes Institute
Fountain Hills, Arizona
Neurologic

Theresa Loan, PhD, RN
Associate Professor
Eastern Kentucky University
Richmond, Kentucky;
Former Clinical Nurse Specialist
Nutrition Support Service
University of Kentucky Medical Center
Lexington, Kentucky
Nutrition

Darlene M. Legge, RN, BSN, CCRN
Team Leader
Electrophysiology/Pacing/Noninvasive
Cardiac and Vascular Departments
Baylor Heart and Vascular Hospital
Dallas, Texas
Pacemakers

Karen S. March, PhD, RN, CCRN, APRN-BC
Associate Professor of Nursing
York College of Pennsylvania
York, Pennsylvania
Pharmacology

CONTRIBUTORS

Contributors to First Edition

Betty Nash Blevins, RN, MSN, CCRN, CS
Susan Carver, RN, BSN
Frank Hicks, RN, MSN, CCRN
Wendy M. Johnson, RN, CCRN
Paul Langlois, RN, PhD, CCRN
Julie Mueller, RN, MS, CCRN
Paulette Rollant, RN, PhD, CCRN
Gial Tagney, RN, MSN, CCRN, CEN, CFRN
Ann M. Walthall, Illustrator

Contributors to Second Edition

Janice Dobbins Andrews, RN, MSN
Betty Nash Blevins, RN, MSN, CCRN, CS
Kimberly A. Litton, RN, MS, CS, CCRN
Leanna R. Miller, RN, MN, CCRN, CEN, APRN
Julie Gottemoller Mueller, RN, MS, CCRN
Connie O'Daniel, RN, MSN, CCRN
Toni E. Simpson King, RN, BSN
Linda Weld, MSN, CCRN

PREFACE

Welcome to *Pass CCRN®!* And congratulations—you have chosen the most up-to-date, comprehensive review of critical care nursing available on the market today. If you are a registered nurse planning to take the CCRN® examination for certified critical care practice offered by the American Association of Critical Care Nurses (AACN) Certification Corporation, this book is the tool that you need to prepare for the examination with confidence.

Information in this text is organized according to the latest CCRN® examination blueprint, which is summarized inside the front cover for quick reference. This test plan, issued by the AACN Certification Corporation, identifies the content areas tested and the percentage of the examination devoted to each. Only content included in the test blueprint is covered in this book, eliminating extraneous information that can be distracting. The book also offers an array of learning activities to help you understand and retain key concepts. In fact, more than 1,000 additional multiple-choice questions are provided on the CD that accompanies this book so that you can practice your test-taking skills in a format that simulates the examination itself.

I have written this book for nurses who are preparing to take the CCRN® examination. Having taught exam-preparation seminars for the last 20 years has helped me learn what information will best equip nurses to sit for the examination and has familiarized me with the strengths and weaknesses of current exam-preparation books on the market. My goal is to provide a pertinent content review, fun but challenging learning activities, realistic practice questions, and comprehensive mock examinations that reflect the content and complexity of the CCRN® examination.

Content Review

Pass CCRN®! follows a succinct outline format that makes the information easy to read, understand, and remember. Illustrations and tables further explicate and clarify content, highlight key concepts, and enhance written explanations.

This edition of *Pass CCRN®!* offers significantly revised content throughout the book along with a new chapter on critical care pharmacology and new sections in the following important areas:

- Anemias
- Pulmonary hypertension
- Intraabdominal hypertension and compartment syndrome
- Gastrointestinal surgery
- Pain management
- Evidence-based practice
- Spiritual aspects of care, including principles of caring for the bereaved
- Generational diversity

Coverage of each body system begins with a brief review of anatomy and physiology. This refresher lays the foundation for introducing more complex topics in the areas of assessment, intervention, and evaluation. Assessment includes health history, physical examination, diagnostic studies, and system-specific assessment methods. For example, the cardiovascular chapter discusses hemodynamic monitoring and electrocardiography, the pulmonary chapter covers interpretation of arterial blood gases, and the neurology chapter presents intracranial pressure monitoring.

Pathologic conditions listed on the CCRN® blueprint are included in the content review. Each condition is first defined, followed by separate sections that explore Etiology, Pathophysiology, Nursing Diagnoses, Clinical Presentation, and Collaborative Management, including medical and nursing management. Finally, relevant legal and ethical issues are explored in sections on Professional Caring and Ethical Practice.

Learning Activities

Sometimes we learn best when information is organized and accessed in unfamiliar ways—that's the principle at work behind the diverse learning activities in this book. Every chapter features a range of question styles, including matching, fill-in-the-blank, comparison, and crossword puzzles, to test comprehension and improve recall for readers with a variety of learning styles.

You won't be asked to complete a crossword puzzle or a matching exercise when you take the CCRN® examination of course, but doing so helps you learn and retain an astonishing amount of information. It also makes your study sessions more enjoyable, encouraging you to stick to the timetable that you have set for yourself. I hope that working through these activities, many of which are new to this edition of the book, will be a pleasurable way to review terminology, anatomy and physiology, and pharmacology.

Review CD

Another great way to study is to use the enclosed CD. It contains more than 1,000 review questions written in a format that represents the actual CCRN® examination. The questions have been thoroughly updated to reflect the percentages set forth for each content area on the most recent test blueprint and current practice.

The CD offers two modes: a quiz mode in which practice questions are arranged by body system and a test mode that offers realistic practice CCRN® examinations. The quiz mode allows you to select topic areas in which you need additional review and create quizzes that target those areas. The practice-test mode, on the other hand, replicates the actual CCRN® exam as closely as possible. This timed mode draws questions from all content areas in the number and proportion called for in the latest CCRN® exam blueprint. The program will reshuffle the questions randomly (but retaining the correct percentages in each content area) to create as many practice tests as you like. Both modes are self-scoring. An autolaunch feature makes the CD easy to use even if you are technologically inexperienced.

Instant rationales are given to explain which answer is correct and why it is the best answer among the possible choices. Test-taking strategy tips are provided as appropriate to show you how to think through the questions if you are not sure of the content. Both of these features will boost your confidence and make you a better test taker on the important day of the CCRN® examination. Analyzing your performance on several practice exams will help you focus your final preparation on your weakest areas.

Other Helpful Features

Appendix A is a table of nursing diagnoses commonly used in critical care. In addition to the diagnoses themselves, the table includes defining characteristics, nursing interventions, and expected outcomes. Appendix B is a list of abbreviations used in this book and common in critical care. Each term is always spelled out in the text the first time it is used, but this appendix will help you identify abbreviations later if you don't remember them. Appendix C lists laboratory studies important in the care of critically ill adults, including the normal range of values for each. I recommend that you study this list just before taking the exam. Appendix D is a list of formulae commonly used in the evaluation of critically ill patients.

This book is not a comprehensive critical care textbook, nor is it intended to be. Instead, I've focused selectively on the information likely to be covered on the CCRN® examination. I believe *Pass CCRN®!* is the only book you need to prepare for the examination, but if you would like an additional text to strengthen your knowledge of particular areas, I recommend *Thelan's Critical Care Nursing: Diagnosis and Management*, by Linda D. Urden et al., published by Elsevier.

Critical care nursing has never been more exciting. For those of us who thrive on this challenge, keeping up with new research and clinical developments is a continual test of our mettle. CCRN® certification is a prestigious credential for those of us who specialize in critical care nursing. I am confident that, if you study this book and use the enclosed CD to practice your test-taking skills, you will pass the examination.

I would love to hear from you about your success with the examination, how this book helped you, and how you feel it could be even more useful. E-mail me at rddennison@aol.com or write to me at the following address:

Robin Donohoe Dennison, DNP, RN, CCNS
c/o Nursing Editorial
Elsevier
11830 Westline Industrial Drive
St. Louis, MO 63146

I believe that this book will be your most valuable resource in preparing for the CCRN® examination. Good luck!

Robin Donohoe Dennison

ACKNOWLEDGMENTS

I thank all of the reviewers and item writers for previous editions and the expert reviewers for this edition.

Thanks to Barbara Cullen for her continuing belief in me and this book. Also, I have been blessed with two wonderful developmental editors, Melissa Martin and Julie Vitale, for this edition. I appreciate your patience and your encouragement throughout this process.

Joe Lawler reworked and polished the questions on the CD-ROM. Writing good test questions is a special talent, and I appreciate his skill.

Finally, I thank my husband and the love of my life, R. Russell Dennison, Jr., for his patience through my recent doctoral studies and this third edition. I am truly blessed.

CONTENTS

The Critical Care Certification Examination

CHAPTER 1

Certification

Definition

Process by which a nongovernmental agency (e.g., American Association of Critical-Care Nurses [AACN]) validates an individual nurse's qualification and knowledge for practice in a defined functional or clinical area of nursing; this validation is based on predetermined standards of practice (AACN, 2005b)

Purpose

Certification has been advocated as one method of assurance of competence.

1. Competence is the "the application of knowledge and the interpersonal, decision-making, and psychomotor skills expected for the nurse's practice role, within the context of public health, welfare, and safety" (National Council of State Boards of Nursing, 1996, p. 5).
2. Continued competence refers to the maintenance of adequate knowledge and skills for safe, ongoing practice that occurs after the initial demonstration of competence at the time of licensure (National Council of State Boards of Nursing, 1996).

Benefits of Achieving Critical Care Registered Nurse (CCRN®) Certification

1. For the nurse
   a. Self-satisfaction and validation of your knowledge and clinical judgment in your chosen nursing specialty
   b. Motivation to update and maintain your knowledge base
   c. Career mobility: National certification is as prestigious in one state as another
   d. Clinical advancement and promotion
      (1) CCRN® certification is a clinical credential, and you must maintain a clinical practice to maintain your certification.
      (2) Most critical care unit nurse managers encourage their nursing staff to become certified.
      (3) Certification often is recommended or required for promotion up a clinical career ladder.
   e. Financial remuneration
      (1) Some hospitals offer a bonus for CCRN® certification.
      (2) Some hospitals offer an hourly differential for CCRN® certification.
      (3) Some hospitals prefer certified nurses for clinical or administrative promotion.
      (4) Many hospitals reimburse the nurse for the expense of taking the test if the nurse attains a passing score.
   f. Continued practice in critical care: Some hospitals require CCRN® certification to continue to practice in critical care settings.
2. Other stakeholders: patients and their families, employers

The Synergy Model

The Synergy Model serves as the organizing framework for the certification examinations offered by the AACN Certification Corporation (AACN, 2005a; Figure 1-1).

Definition of Synergy

"An evolving phenomenon that occurs when individuals work together in mutually enhancing ways toward a common goal" (Curley, 1998)

Core Concept (AACN, 2005a)

The needs or characteristics of patients and families influence and drive the characteristics or competencies of nurses.

1. Nursing practice should be based on the needs of the patient and family.
2. Patients with more complex needs require nurses with advanced knowledge and skills.
3. The desired result is optimal outcomes for the patient, the nurse, and the system.

Assumptions (AACN, 2005a)

1. Patients are biologic, psychological, social, and spiritual entities who present at a particular developmental stage.
2. The patient, family, and community contribute to providing a context for the nurse-patient relationship.

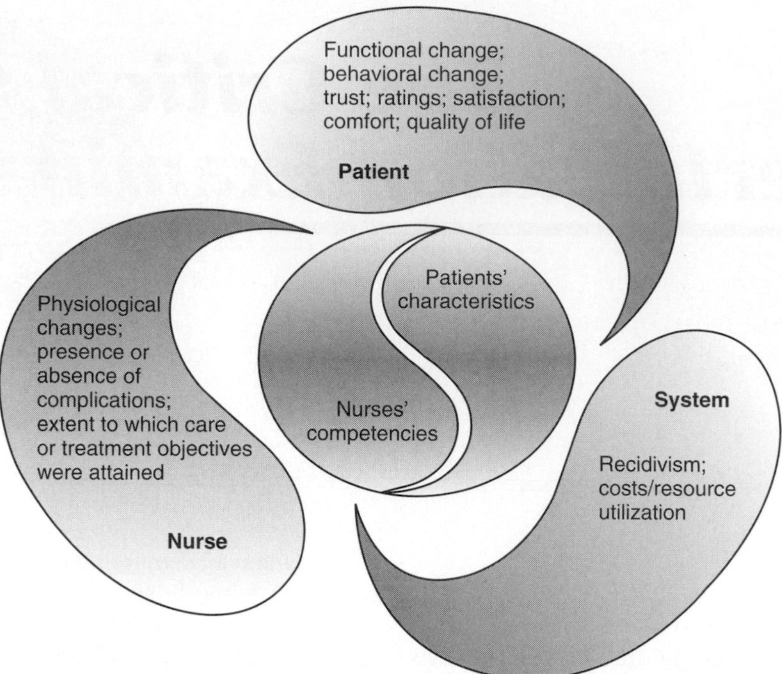

Figure 1-1 The synergy model delineates three outcome levels: those derived from the patient, the nurse, and the health care system. (From Curley, M.A.Q. [1998]. Patient-nurse synergy: Optimizing patients' outcomes. *American Journal of Critical Care,* 7[1], 64-72.)

3. Patients can be described by a number of characteristics.
4. Nurses can be described in a number of dimensions.
5. A goal of nursing is to restore a patient to an optimal level of wellness as defined by the patient.

Patient Characteristics (AACN, 2005a)

1. Resiliency: the capacity to return to a restorative level of functioning using compensatory coping mechanisms; the ability to bounce back quickly after an insult
2. Vulnerability: susceptibility to actual or potential stressors that may affect patient outcomes adversely
3. Stability: the ability to maintain a steady state equilibrium
4. Complexity: the intricate entanglement of two or more systems (e.g., body, family, and therapies)
5. Resource availability: extent of resources (e.g., technical, fiscal, personal, psychological, and social)
6. Participation in care: extent to which the patient and family engage in aspects of care
7. Participation in decision making: extent to which the patient and family engage in decision making
8. Predictability: a summative characteristic that allows one to expect a certain trajectory of illness

Nurse Characteristics (AACN, 2005a)

1. Clinical judgment: clinical reasoning, which includes clinical decision making, critical thinking, and a global grasp of the situation, coupled with nursing skills acquired through a process of integrating formal and experiential knowledge
2. Advocacy/moral agency: working on another's behalf and representing the concerns of the patient, family, and community; serving as a moral agent in identifying and helping to resolve ethical and clinical concerns within the clinical setting
3. Caring practices: the constellation of nursing activities that are responsive to the uniqueness of the patient and family and that create a compassionate and therapeutic environment, with the aim of promoting comfort and preventing suffering
4. Collaboration: working with others in a way that promotes and encourages each person's contributions toward achieving optimal and realistic patient goals; collaboration involves intradisciplinary and interdisciplinary work with all colleagues
5. Systems thinking: the body of knowledge and tools that allow the nurse to appreciate the care environment from a perspective that recognizes the holistic interrelationship that exists within and across health care systems
6. Response to diversity: the sensitivity to recognize, appreciate, and incorporate differences into the provision of care
7. Clinical inquiry or innovator/evaluator: the ongoing process of questioning and evaluating practice, providing informed practice, and innovating through research and experiential learning
8. Facilitator of learning of patient/family educator: the ability to facilitate patient and family learning

What Is Tested

Although this model serves as the theoretical model for the CCRN® examination, you are not tested regarding knowledge of the synergy model or terminology; you are tested on application of the model.

The Adult Examinations Offered by the AACN Certification Corporation

Requirements to Take the Examinations (AACN, 2005a)

1. Current unrestricted registered nurse (RN) license in the United States or in any of its territories that use the NCLEX® for RN licensure
2. Clinical practice in critical care (or progressive care for the progressive care certified nurse [PCCN®] examination): 1750 hours within the previous 2-year period with 875 of the hours accrued in the most recent year preceding application to take the examination
3. Bachelor of science in nursing (BSN) is not a requirement. Although the American Nurses Credentialing Corporation does require a BSN to sit for its certification examinations, the AACN Certification Corporation is not a member of the American Nurses Credentialing Corporation and does not require a BSN to sit for the CCRN® examination.
4. To obtain an application
   a. Call AACN at (800) 899-2226.
   b. Visit the AACN Certification Corporation at *http://www.certcorp.org*
5. After completion of the application process, you will receive approval to take the exam by mail; you must schedule testing within the next 90 days.

Testing

1. Computer-based testing is available most weekdays year-round, but a pencil-and-paper version is available only once a year at the location of the AACN National Teaching Institute.
2. Requirements on the day of the exam
   a. Entrance ticket that was mailed when application was approved
   b. Two pieces of identification, one of which must have a current photograph
   c. Timely arrival: If you arrive more than 15 minutes late, you will not be admitted.
3. The computerized form of the test is administered by Applied Measurement Professionals at their testing centers nationwide.
   a. Instructions are given at the beginning of the examination; do take the time to read the instructions carefully.
   b. A simple function calculator is permitted.
   c. Scrap paper is provided.

Cognitive Levels of Questions

1. Knowledge questions require you to remember previously learned information.
2. Comprehension questions require you to understand the information.
3. Application questions require you to use information.
4. Analysis questions require you to break down information into its component parts and to recognize commonalities, differences, and interrelationships.
5. Synthesis questions require you to put parts of information together to form a new conclusion.
6. Evaluation questions require you to judge the value of information.
7. Questions on the examinations are distributed across these cognitive levels.

Distribution of Questions Related to the Nursing Process

All phases of nursing process are included on the examination.

Passing Score

1. The passing score for these examinations is approximately 70%.
2. About two thirds of nurses taking the CCRN® examination for the first time pass the exam; nurses retaking the test for recertification have a higher passing rate.
   a. No data are available regarding the passing rate for the PCCN® examination at this time.

The CCRN® Examination

1. Basic information about the CCRN® examination
   a. Critical care is considered to be at the more acute end of the critical care continuum.
      (1) Patients in critical care
         (a) Are unstable and have complex needs
         (b) Require intense resources such as staffing, monitoring, and supplies
            (i) Frequently require invasive hemodynamic monitoring, intravenous medication titration, and mechanical ventilation
         (c) Require persistent nursing vigilance
   b. The test is designed to evaluate your understanding of the common body of knowledge needed to function effectively in a critical care setting.
      (1) The test consists of 150 multiple-choice questions to be completed within 3 hours; 25 of these items are not scored but are test items for the development of future exams.
      (2) The questions relate to patient problems unique to critical care and to nationally recognized practice with the focus being on clinical decision making rather than memorization and recall.
   c. Blueprint for the CCRN® examination (Table 1-1)
      (1) The blueprint identifies the categories tested and the percentage of questions in each category.
      (2) The blueprint is based on a Role Delineation/CCRN® Validation Study conducted by the AACN in 2003; in essence, this study identified tasks, knowledge, and experiences required of an RN practicing in a critical care setting and what should be on the examination.

(3) The blueprint identifies what percentage of questions is in each area and what disease entities are on the examination.
(a) NOTE: This book includes only content and disease entities that are on the blueprint and the examination. Although it may be important to understand myxedema coma, it is not on the blueprint, not on the examination, and not in this book. Focus on what is on the blueprint and the examination.

The PCCN® Examination (AACN, 2005c)

1. Basic information about the PCCN® examination
   a. Progressive care is considered to be at the less acute end of the critical care continuum.
      (1) Patients in progressive care
         (a) Are moderately stable or stable with a high potential for becoming unstable
         (b) Require moderate resources
            (i) Central venous pressure monitoring may be required, but arterial catheters and pulmonary arterial catheters are not typical with these patients.
            (ii) Frequent intravenous medication titration is not typical with these patients.
            (iii) Chronic mechanical ventilation is not uncommon, but frequent mechanical ventilator changes are not typical with these patients.
         (c) Require intermittent nursing vigilance
      (2) Refers collectively to units described as intermediate care units, direct observation units, step-down units, telemetry units, and transitional care units
   b. The test is designed to evaluate your understanding of the common body of knowledge needed to function effectively in a progressive care setting.
      (1) The test consists of 125 multiple-choice questions to be completed within 2½ hours; 25 of these items are not scored but are test items for the development of future exams.
      (2) The questions relate to patient problems unique to progressive care and to nationally recognized practice with the focus being on clinical decision making rather than memorization and recall.
   c. Blueprint for the PCCN® examination (Table 1-2)
      (1) The blueprint identifies what percentage of questions is in each area and what disease entities are on the examination.

Table 1-1 Blueprint for the CCRN® Examination Indicating Distribution of Questions on Each Section

Category Tested	Percent of Questions
Clinical Judgment	**80%**
Cardiovascular	32%
Pulmonary	17%
Multisystem	8%
Gastrointestinal	6%
Neurology	5%
Renal	5%
Endocrine	4%
Hematology/immunology	3%
Professional Caring and Ethical Practice	**20%**
Advocacy/moral agency	4%
Caring practices	4%
Collaboration	4%
Systems thinking	2%
Response to diversity	2%
Clinical inquiry	2%
Facilitatory of learning	2%

From American Association of Critical-Care Nurses. (2005). *AACN Certification Corporation*. Retrieved October 23, 2005, from http://www.aacn.org/pdfLibra.NSF/Files/CertExamHandbook/$file/CertExamHandbook.pdf

Table 1-2 Blueprint for the PCCN® Examination Indicating Distribution of Questions on Each Section

Category Tested	Percent of Questions
Clinical Judgment	**80%**
Cardiovascular	37%
Pulmonary	13%
Multisystem	6%
Renal	6%
Gastrointestinal	5%
Hematology/immunology	5%
Neurology	4%
Endocrine	4%
Professional Caring and Ethical Practice	**20%**
Caring practices	4%
Collaboration	4%
Facilitatory of learning	4%
Advocacy/moral agency	2%
Systems thinking	2%
Response to diversity	2%
Clinical inquiry	2%

From American Association of Critical-Care Nurses. (2005). *AACN Certification Corporation*. Retrieved October 23, 2005, from http://www.aacn.org/pdfLibra.NSF/Files/CertExamHandbook/$file/CertExamHandbook.pdf

Contact Information

For more specific information about these examinations, the application and application process, and the testing process, visit *http://www.aacn.org* or call the AACN at (800) 899-2226.

Preparation to Improve Performance on These Examinations

Be Positive!

1. Avoid negative self-talk; "I'll never pass this exam" can be a self-fulfilling prophecy because you begin to believe it.
2. Practice positive self-talk.
   a. Write down some affirmations (positive statements) related to your preparation and performance on this examination. Box 1-1 lists suggested affirmations.
   b. Say these and other affirmations that you have written over and over again throughout your preparation time; say them like you believe them, and you will!
   c. Record your affirmations on audiotape and play them often; play them in the car, while you walk or do dishes, or any other time when you can listen and repeat them.

Schedule the Examination

1. Complete the application and send it to the AACN.
2. The AACN will send you an authorization letter indicating that you meet the requirements to take the examination, along with instructions on how to schedule the examination.
   a. Call the testing service to schedule your examination date and time; you must schedule the examination within 90 days of the date printed on your authorization letter.
   b. This flexibility in scheduling allows you to avoid scheduling conflicts between the examination and major life events such as a family wedding, graduation, or birth.
   c. Schedule the time of the examination according to when you do your best thinking or are most productive: Schedule for morning if you are a lark or afternoon if you are an owl.
3. DO SCHEDULE THE EXAM so that you have a target date; you can reschedule up to 4 business days before the scheduled test day if something comes up that interferes with your ability to complete the examination on the scheduled day.

BOX 1-1 Affirmations

I am a knowledgeable critical care nurse.
I understand the information important for this examination.
I am an excellent test taker.
I feel prepared for this exam.
I will pass this exam.

Prepare for the Test

1. Establish a realistic schedule for your preparation; 1- to 2-hour time slots are probably the most helpful.
   a. Study examination content: Plan to review a system per evening, day, or weekend, depending on how much time you have left before the examination.
      (1) Set priorities.
         (a) Study your weak areas first.
         (b) Study the large-percentage content areas even if you feel confident about them: you should feel especially confident about cardiac, pulmonary, and multisystem content because these three areas constitute 57% of the examination.
      (2) Review content using this review book.
         (a) Highlight areas about which you do not feel confident; you may need to refer to more comprehensive critical care texts or articles when you need additional clarification.
         (b) Complete the learning activities at the end of each chapter to consolidate your knowledge by looking at the information in another way.
      (3) Practice using your test-taking skills by doing practice questions.
         (a) In addition to looking at the answer, read the rationale; remember that the question may not be written exactly the same as the practice question, but the concept may be on the examination.
         (b) If you still do not understand why you missed the question, refer back to the section in this book or a critical care text to understand why the correct answer is better than your answer.
         (c) In addition to looking at the answer and the rationale, read the test-taking strategy; this information will help you identify how to approach a similar question to which you do not know the answer.
         (d) Analyze why you missed a question. Consider the following:
            (i) Did you not know the content? Study this content again.
            (ii) Did you misread the question? Slow down and read the question more thoroughly.
            (iii) Did you misread the options? Slow down and read all of the options and select the best one.
            (iv) Did you miss an important element such as age, diagnosis, or parameter? Again, slow down and read the question carefully; mentally highlight the critical points in the case study that you feel are important.

(v) Did you read into the question?
a) Do not assume information that is not given; take the question at face value.
b) Do not assume that the question is intended to trick you. There are no trick questions on the practice exam questions on the CD-ROM with this book or on the CCRN® or PCCN® examinations.

(4) Study in a quiet place with minimal distractions.
(a) Avoid getting too comfortable; sit upright at a desk or table so that you can spread out your study materials.
(b) Reading, repeating, and writing are methods that improve remembering.
(c) Use margins to write down memory joggers or additional thoughts.

2. If you like study groups, organize a study group of nurses who also are preparing for the CCRN® or PCCN® examination.
   a. Include only members who will fulfill their obligation to participate.
   b. Establish guidelines for the group.
      (1) When will you meet?
      (2) What will you do at the meetings?
         (a) A selected member may present essential content related to his or her specific area of interest.
         (b) Members may collect resource materials related to the specified content area and may distribute them to fellow members.
         (c) Members may discuss review questions related to the specified content area.
      (3) What are the group members' expectations?
3. Create memory joggers.
   a. Almost everyone knows "On Old Olympus' Towering Tops A Fin And German Viewed Some Hops" to remember the 12 cranial nerves; establish others that help you identify things that you have trouble remembering.
4. Remember case study links: for example, you remember a patient with a triglyceride level greater than 2000 mg/dL who developed acute pancreatitis and then acute respiratory distress syndrome helps you remember that a major risk factor for acute pancreatitis is hypertriglyceridemia and that a major complication of acute pancreatitis is acute respiratory distress syndrome.

Take a Practice Test

Take a practice test 1 week before the examination; use this test to identify weak areas for final study time.

1. Analyze which categories (systems) are your weakest and strongest.
2. Analyze which cognitive level question is the most difficult for you.
3. Analyze which component of the nursing process is most difficult for you.

Final Preparations

1. Do not cram the night before the examination; cramming usually just decreases your self-confidence and increases your anxiety.
2. Go to bed at your usual time; if you go to bed early, you probably will not go to sleep anyway and will just worry about the test.
3. Do not consume alcohol or other sedating drugs the night before or the day of the examination.
4. Choose comfortable clothes that allow layering so you can remove or add clothing in response to the room temperature; wear bright colors (e.g., yellow, red, hot pink, or orange) to project a more optimistic image.
5. Take a watch and a sweater; do not forget your glasses if you wear them.
6. Eat a healthful but light meal before the examination; avoid simple carbohydrates such as a doughnut or Danish pastry.
7. Be sure to take two forms of identification, with one of them being government-issued photo identification that contains a signature.
8. Plan to arrive 15 minutes before your scheduled appointment; if you arrive later than 15 minutes after the scheduled testing time, you will not be admitted.

Performance During the Examination

Control of Anxiety

1. Remember that some anxiety increases your performance; panic does not.
2. Feeling adequately prepared decreases anxiety; take the time to prepare for this examination, including practicing your test-taking strategies.
3. Use visualization: see yourself receiving your passing score.
4. Use deep breathing and/or progressive muscle relaxation.
   a. Deep breathing is performed by putting your hand below your costal margin and breathing deeply enough to raise your hand; focus on your breathing instead of anything else.
      (1) Use this method at anytime during the examination when you feel frustrated or stressed.
   b. Progressive muscle relaxation is performed by contracting a group of muscles and then relaxing it: leg, leg, arm, arm, back, face.
      (1) Use this techniques in the car before you go in to take the examination and at anytime during the examination that you feel tense.
5. Use meditation or prayer depending on your religious beliefs. These techniques are also helpful in verbalizing your goals and desires.

Test-Taking Skills

1. Reading questions thoroughly
   a. Mentally highlight key points as you read the question.
      (1) Age and gender of the patient
      (2) Setting: prehospital, emergency, critical care, progressive care, home care
      (3) Medical diagnosis and other coexisting diagnoses
      (4) Time frame in relation to admission, trauma, surgery, pain, visitation
   b. Look for key words such as *except, least, most, never, always, initially, first, last, early, late, indicated, contraindicated, priority,* and *best.*
   c. Make sure that you understand what the question really is; answer *the* question, not just *a* question.
   d. Read all the options and the stem.
   e. After you read the stem, answer the question without looking at the options. If your answer is there, it is probably right; however, still go ahead and read all options. There may be one better than your answer.
2. Choosing the correct answer
   a. Assumptions
      (1) Do not assume information that is not given; the only assumption is an ideal situation unless the question indicates otherwise.
      (2) All important information is included.
         (a) Do not read into the question such as "maybe she's a diabetic" or "maybe he has COPD"; if information is important to the question, it will be included.
      (3) Included information is probably important.
         (a) Extraneous information usually is not included, so if the case study or question gives you information that you feel is extraneous or superfluous, ask yourself why this information was given and how it is important to this situation.
   b. Answer questions according to national standards of care and national guidelines rather than regional, local, or specific physician's practices.
   c. Select options that are therapeutic based on evidence and show respect and acceptance for the patient and the family; eliminate options that are based on tradition rather than science and options that are inappropriate, disrespectful, or punitive.
   d. Repetition of a word or a synonym of the word in the stem and an option may help you to identify the correct answer.
   e. If more than one option appears correct, look for the most comprehensive option.
3. Answering priority questions
   a. Priority one is always whatever must be done to prevent death; always follow the ABC order: airway, then breathing, and finally circulation.
   b. Priority two is whatever must be done to prevent disability or serious complication; consider this D for disability.
   c. Priority three is pain or discomfort; if nothing in the case study or question could cause death or disability, consider pain to be the priority.
   d. Actual problems always take precedence over potential problems; for example, actual hypoxemia takes precedence over potential oxygen toxicity.
   e. If there are two potential problems, the priority is the one that is more likely to cause death or disability.
4. Answering questions where the answers have multiple answers (also referred to as *multiple/multiples*).
   a. If the option has more than one answer (such as *x* and *y* or even *w, x, y,* and *z*), both or all of the answers must be correct for the option to be correct.
   b. Elimination works well with this type of question; if there is one answer in the option that is incorrect, eliminate that option.
5. Guessing
   a. Do not leave any question blank; unanswered questions are counted as incorrect, so you should never not answer a question even if you must guess.
   b. You are not penalized for guessing, but guess only as a last resort.
   c. First, eliminate any choices that you can; it is better to guess between two choices than to guess between four.
      (1) Eliminate clearly wrong answers.
      (2) Eliminate any response that has no relationship to the question.
      (3) Eliminate similar options that say essentially the same thing, for they cannot both be correct.
      (4) *All, always, never, none,* or *only* options are *usually* incorrect.
   d. If you cannot even eliminate to two, then look for the option that is different from the others; for example:
      (1) Three antibiotics and an antifungal, choose the antifungal option.
      (2) Three beta-blockers and a calcium channel blocker, choose the calcium channel blocker.
      (3) Three specific and one comprehensive option, choose the comprehensive option.
   e. Bookmark questions that you feel unsure of and to which you want to go back. At the end of the test, the computer allows you to go back to these marked items and review them before unmarking them and continuing to the end of the examination.
6. Changing answers
   a. It may be helpful to change answers in a different color when doing a practice test; then evaluate how many you changed from wrong to right and how many you changed from right to wrong.
   b. If you change more from wrong to right, you most likely miss questions because you do not

read them thoroughly, so when you realize that you misread a question, then by all means change your answer.
   c. If you change more from right to wrong, do not change your initial answer (unless you realize in this case that you have misread the question), for first impressions tend to be correct more often.
7. Answering math questions
   a. Math questions are usually drug calculations such as dopamine in micrograms per kilogram per minute but could be other critical care calculations.
   b. You are allowed to use a simple function calculator, and you are provided with scratch paper and pencil.
   c. Recheck your math if you have time.
8. Maintaining concentration
   a. Write down things such as formulas, normal values, and toxic levels that you are afraid that you might forget on your scratch paper before you do the first question.
   b. Change your process of reading the case study, the question, and the options.
      (1) Read the options in reverse order from option d to option a. Use this action especially when you suspect that option a or b is the correct option.
      (2) Make this change every 25 to 50 questions OR
         (a) When you are physically tired, mentally anxious, or lose your concentration abilities
         (b) When you come to the easier or the more difficult questions
   c. Rephrase the question rather than rereading the same question over and over.
   d. Use three slow, deep breaths to regroup and get refocused at any time.
   e. Sign out and go to the restroom and splash water on your face if you are losing your ability to concentration, but remember that the clock does not stop during this time, so consider this if you are a slow test taker.
9. Budgeting your time.
   a. If you are a slow test taker, you may run short on time, but more likely you will run out of mental energy because concentration for a 2- to 3-hour period is difficult.
   b. You should try to be at least halfway through the examination in 75 minutes for the CCRN® examination and in 60 minutes for the PCCN® examination; this halfway point will leave you some time to recheck your math and go back to the marked items.
   c. One helpful technique to save time is to read the question (at end of case study) and then go back and read the case study. Because we frequently read the case study, then the question at the end of the case study, and then reread the case study, this technique saves you time because you know what you are looking for in the case study.
   d. Do not be distressed by persons finishing before you; we all take examinations at different speeds, and the others may not even be taking the AACN Certification Corporation examinations, since several exams often are given at the same place and same time.

Reasons for Failing the Examination

Knowledge Deficit

1. Prepare to take the examination even if you feel that you are an experienced critical care nurse, since we all have our chosen areas of interest and our weak areas.
2. Use this book to review the content for the examination, and complete the learning activities at the end of each chapter.
3. Take a practice examination 1 week before the examination to identify your weak areas; use your final study time to focus on those weak areas.

Testing Errors

1. Practice using your test-taking skills with the questions on the CD-ROM included with this book, and pay close attention to the rationale and the test-taking strategy included with each question.
2. Use the learned test-taking strategies during the CCRN® examination.

Test Anxiety and Negative Thinking

Believe in your ability to pass the exam, and control your anxiety with prayer, meditation, deep breathing, and/or progressive relaxation.

Test Results

You will be given your test results at the completion of computerized testing and within 6 to 8 weeks by mail for pencil-and-paper testing.

Congratulate Yourself on Having the Initiative to Take the Examination

If You Pass, Flaunt It!

1. You should display your credential on your hospital name badge.
2. You should proudly write it after *RN* when you sign your name; CCRN® and PCCN® are not written with periods; so, for example, you should write it as *Your Name, RN, CCRN.*

3. Encourage others to become certified; offer to tutor, mentor, and share study materials to assist your colleagues to become certified too.

If You Fail, Try Again!

1. The fear of the unknown is now gone.
2. You know clearly what your weak areas are from the score breakdown that was given to you as you left the testing site.
3. Prepare by focusing on your weak areas, and then reapply to take the test again.
4. You can do it!

Maintaining Your CCRN® Certification

Certification

For a 3-year period

Recertification

Achieved by providing evidence of continued practice (432 hours over the 3-year period with 144 of those hours accrued in the year before recertification) and retaking the examination or submitting the appropriate information about your continuing education and professional activities for review for renewal.

LEARNING ACTIVITIES

1. Why do you want to take this examination?

____
____
____
____

2. List your top five life priorities for the next year. Is CCRN® (or PCCN®) certification on this list? What is the ranking for CCRN® (or PCCN®) certification?

First ______________________________
Second ______________________________
Third ______________________________
Fourth ______________________________
Fifth ______________________________

3. Prioritize this list from 1 (least comfortable) to 9 (most comfortable). Use this list to schedule your preparation with 1 being first and 9 being last.

Knowledge area	Comfort level
Cardiovascular	
Pulmonary	
Multisystem	
Neurology	
Gastrointestinal	
Renal	
Endocrine	
Hematology/immunology	
Professional caring and ethical practice	

4. Describe your plan to prepare for the CCRN® (or PCCN®) examination.

____
____
____
____

5. List three new test-taking strategies that you have learned from this chapter and will use while taking the CCRN® (or PCCN®) examination.

A. ______________________________
B. ______________________________
C. ______________________________

References

American Association of Critical-Care Nurses. (2005a). *AACN Certification Corporation.* Retrieved October 23, 2005, from http://www.aacn.org/pdfLibra.NSF/Files/CertExamHandbook/$file/CertExamHandbook.pdf

American Association of Critical-Care Nurses. (2005b). *General information regarding certification: Definition of certification.* Retrieved October 23, 2005, from http://www.aacn.org/certcorp/certcorp.nsf/vwdoc/BasicCertInfo?opendocument#Definition%20of

American Association of Critical-Care Nurses. (2005c). *PCCN—Certification for progressive care nurses.* Retrieved October 23, 2005, from http://www.aacn.org/certcorp/certcorp.nsf/vwdoc/PCCN?opendocument

Curley, M. A. Q. (1998). Patient-nurse synergy: Optimizing patients' outcomes. *American Journal of Critical Care, 7*(1), 64-72.

National Council of State Boards of Nursing. (1996). *Assuring competence.* Retrieved May 20, 2002, from http://www.ncsbn.org/public/resources/ncsbn_competence_two.htm

Bibliography

American Association for Critical-Care Nurses & AACN Certification Corporation. (2003). Safeguarding the patient and the profession: The value of critical care nurse certification. *American Journal of Critical Care, 12*(2), 154-164.

Beitz, J. (1997). Unleashing the power of memory: The mighty mnemonic. *Nurse Educator, 22*(2), 25-29.

Berke, W. J., & Ecklund, M. M. (2003). Keep pace with step-down care. *Critical Care Nurse, 23*(1), 56-58.

Gage, M. (1998). From independence to interdependence: Creating synergistic healthcare teams. *Journal of Nursing Administration, 28*(4), 17-26.

Gloe, D. (1999). Study habits and test-taking tips. *Dermatology Nursing, 11*(6), 439-443, 447-449.

Hansten, R., & Washburn, M. (2000). Facilitating critical thinking. *Journal of Nurses in Staff Development, 16*(1), 23-30.

Kaplow, R. (2002). Applying the synergy model to nursing education. *Critical Care Nurse, 22*(3), 77-81.

Kerfoot, K. (2002). The leader as synergist. *Critical Care Nurse, 22*(2), 126-129.

Markey, D. W. (2001). Applying the synergy model: Clinical strategies. *Critical Care Nurse, 21*(3), 72-76.

Muenzen, P. M., Greenberg, S., & Pirro, K. A. (2004). *Final report of a comprehensive study of critical care nursing practice.* New York: Professional Examination Service Department of Research and Development.

Mullen, J. E. (2002). The synergy model as a framework for nursing rounds. *Critical Care Nurse, 22*(6), 66-68.

Nugent, P. M., & Vitale, B. A. (2000). *Test success: Test-taking techniques for beginning nursing students* (3rd ed.). Philadelphia: F. A. Davis Company.

Pope, B. B. (2002). The synergy match-up. *Nursing Management, 33*(5), 38-41.

Rollant, P. D. (1999). *Soar to success: Do your best on nursing tests!* St. Louis, MO: Mosby.

Sides, M. B., & Korchek, N. (1998). *Nurse's guide to successful test-taking* (3rd ed.). Philadelphia: J. B. Lippincott Company.

The Cardiovascular System: Physiology and Assessment

CHAPTER 2

Selected Concepts in Anatomy and Physiology

General Information about the Cardiovascular System

1. The cardiovascular system is a continuous, fluid-filled elastic circuit with a pump.
2. The cardiovascular system provides communication between all body parts through transportation of oxygen, nutrients, hormones, water, enzymes, vitamins, minerals, buffers, leukocytes, antibodies, and wastes; these functions maintain dynamic equilibrium to maintain homeostasis.
3. The cardiovascular system consists of the heart and vascular system.

The Heart

1. Bioelectrically driven, muscular, four-chamber organ that provides forward propulsion of blood into the vascular system
2. Size of a closed fist: usually approximately 9 cm wide and 12 cm long; weighs approximately 4 g/kg of ideal body weight
3. Lies in the mediastinum between the sternum (anterior) and the spine (posterior) with two thirds of the heart to the left of the midline and one third of the heart to the right of the midline (Figure 2-1)
4. Shaped like a blunt cone
   a. Apex
      (1) Inferior, anterior, and to the left
      (2) Normally at fifth left intercostal space at the midclavicular line
      (3) On the upper surface of the diaphragm
   b. Base
      (1) Superior, posterior, and to the right
      (2) Normally at level of second intercostal space
5. Layers of the cardiac wall (Figure 2-2)
   a. Pericardium: maintains the heart in a stationary position
      (1) Fibrous
         (a) Loose-fitting, white fibrous layer
         (b) Acts as a barrier against infection and neoplastic invasion
      (2) Serous
         (a) Parietal layer: lines inner surface of fibrous pericardium
         (b) Visceral layer: lines the surface of the heart; synonymous with epicardium
      (3) Pericardial space
         (a) Located between the parietal and visceral layers of the serous pericardium
         (b) Contains 10 to 30 mL of lubricating fluid
            (i) Protects the heart against friction and erosion
            (ii) Provides a well-lubricated sac in which the heart moves during contraction
   b. Epicardium: synonymous with visceral layer of serous pericardium
   c. Myocardium
      (1) Largest portion of the cardiac wall
      (2) Consists of the following:
         (a) Specialized conduction fibers
         (b) Interlacing cardiac muscle fibers
   d. Endocardium
      (1) Consists of the following:
         (a) Connective tissue
         (b) Elastic fibers
         (c) Endothelial cells
            (i) Form a smooth surface for blood contact
            (ii) Deter clot formation
      (2) Contiguous with the lining of the great vessels
      (3) Lines the heart chambers and valves
6. Cardiac skeleton
   a. Composed of continuous dense connective tissue
   b. Located at the base of the heart and in the interventricular septum
   c. Serves as the point of origin and insertion for cardiac muscle fibers
   d. Supports the heart valves; includes the four valve rings (annuli)
7. Cardiac chambers (Figure 2-3)
   a. Atria
      (1) Located posterior, superior, and to the right of the corresponding ventricles

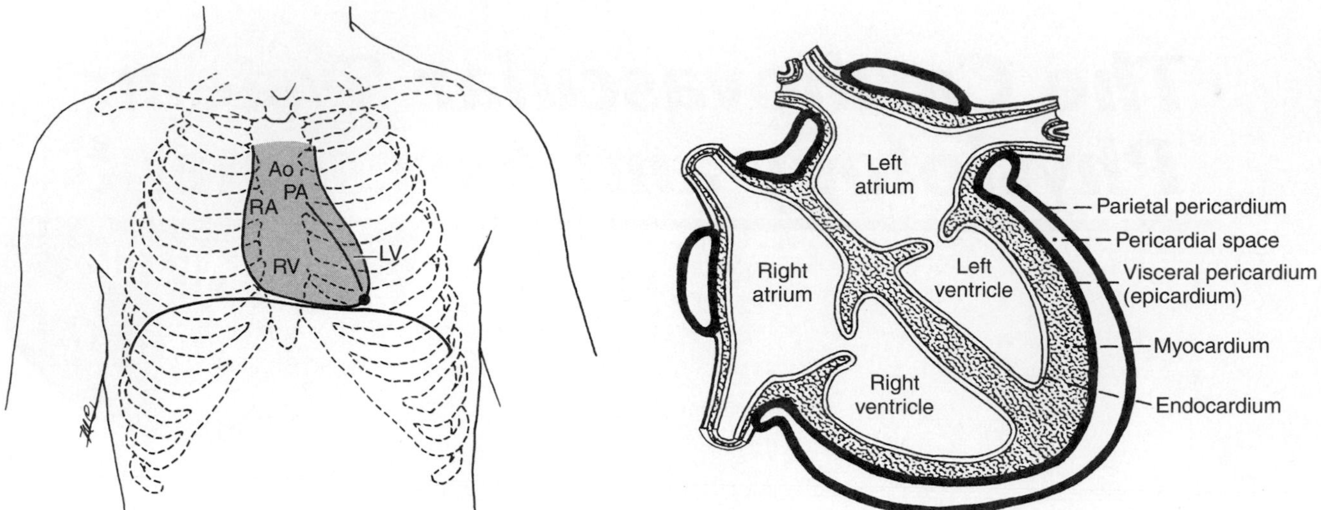

Figure 2-1 Location and orientation of the heart within the thorax. *Ao,* Aorta; *PA,* pulmonary artery; *RA,* right atrium; *RV,* right ventricle; *LV,* left ventricle. (From Price, S., & Wilson, L. [1996]. *Pathophysiology: Clinical concepts of disease processes* [5th ed.]. St. Louis: Mosby-Year Book.)

Figure 2-2 Layers of the cardiac wall. (From Copstead, L. [1995]. *Perspectives on pathophysiology.* Philadelphia: W. B. Saunders.)

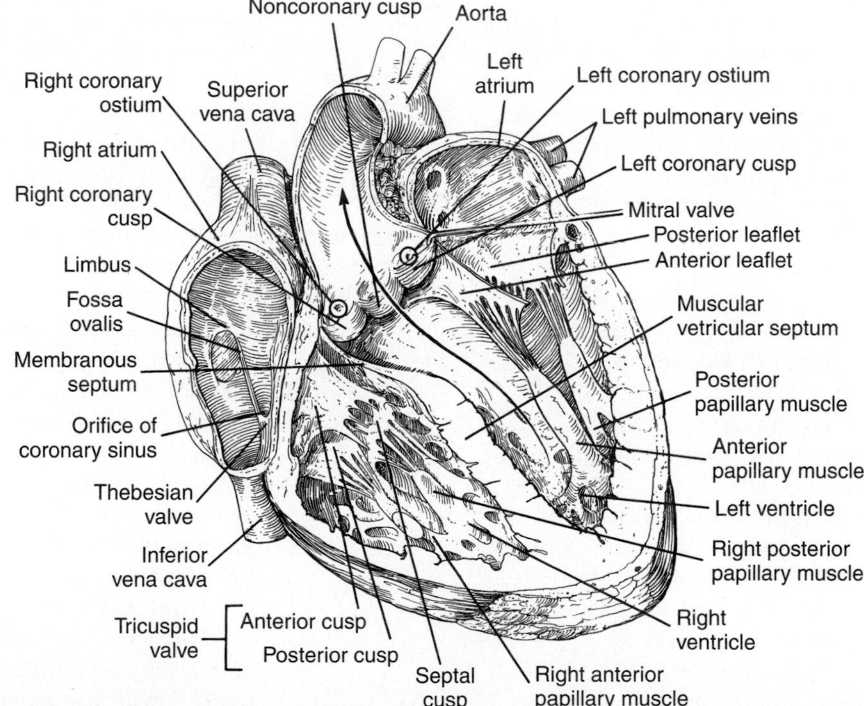

Figure 2-3 Interior of the heart showing cardiac chambers (pulmonary artery removed for visualization). (From Seifert, P. C. [1994]. *Mosby's perioperative nursing series: Cardiac surgery.* St. Louis: Mosby.)

(2) Contain the interatrial septum to divide left and right atria

(3) Contain the trabeculae to divide atria and ventricles

(4) Thin-walled, low-pressure chambers
   (a) Right: 2 mm thick, 2 to 6 mm Hg pressure
   (b) Left: 3 mm thick, 6 to 12 mm Hg pressure

(5) Act as reservoirs and booster pumps for the ventricles
   (a) Passive ventricular filling: 70% to 75% of ventricular filling is passive as blood falls through the atrium into the ventricle
   (b) Active ventricular filling: 25% to 30% of ventricular filling is active as the atrium contracts at the end of ventricular diastole

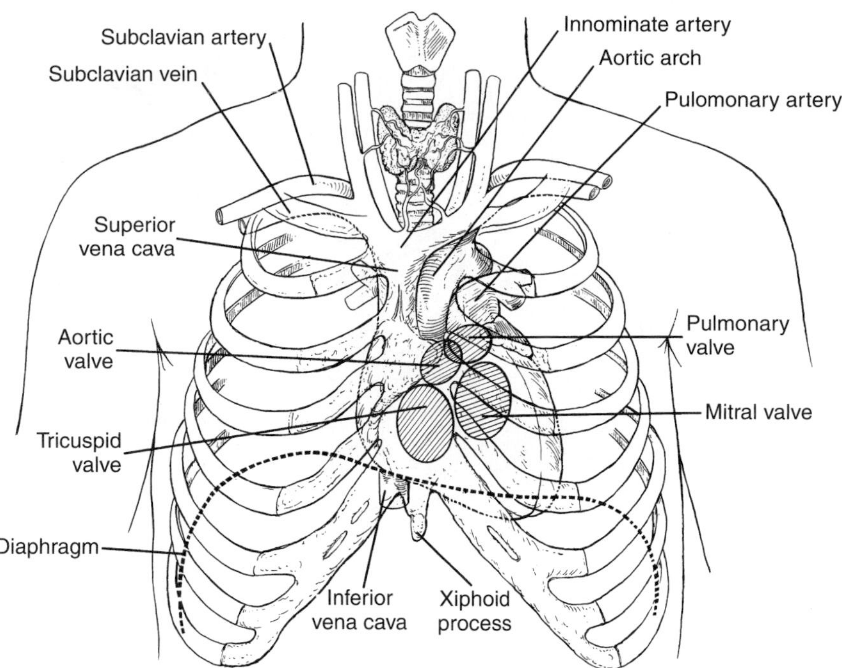

Figure 2-4 Position of the cardiac valves. (From Seifert, P. C. [1994]. *Mosby's perioperative nursing series: Cardiac surgery*. St. Louis: Mosby.)

(6) Right atria
 (a) Inflow tracts
  (i) Superior vena cava
  (ii) Inferior vena cava
  (iii) Coronary sinus
  (iv) Thebesian veins
 (b) Outflow tract: through the tricuspid valve to right ventricle
(7) Left atria
 (a) Inflow tracts: four pulmonary veins (only case of veins carrying oxygenated blood)
 (b) Outflow tract: through the mitral valve to left ventricle

b. Ventricles
(1) Located anterior, inferior, and to the left of the corresponding atria
(2) Contain the interventricular septum to divide the left and right ventricles
(3) Contain the trabeculae to divide atria and ventricles
(4) Act as pumps receiving blood from the atria and pumping blood into the great vessels
(5) Right ventricle
 (a) Thin-walled: 3 to 5 mm
 (b) Low-pressure pump: normally approximately 25/5 mm Hg
 (c) Inflow tract
  (i) Right atria via the tricuspid valve
  (ii) Thebesian veins
 (d) Outflow tract: pulmonary artery (only case of artery carrying deoxygenated blood)
(6) Left ventricle
 (a) Thick-walled: 8 to 15 mm
 (b) High-pressure: normally approximately 120/5 mm Hg
 (c) Inflow tract
  (i) Left atria via the mitral valve
  (ii) Thebesian veins
 (d) Outflow tract: aorta

8. Cardiac valves (Figure 2-4)
a. Purpose: maintain unidirectional flow
(1) Permit antegrade flow: narrowing of the valvular orifice preventing normal antegrade flow is referred to as *stenosis*
(2) Prevent retrograde flow: inadequate closure of the valvular orifice allowing retrograde flow is referred to as *regurgitance*, *incompetence*, or *insufficiency*

b. Atrioventricular valves: tricuspid and mitral valves
(1) Valves are located between atria and ventricles.
 (a) Tricuspid valve is between right atria and right ventricle.
 (b) Mitral valve is between left atria and left ventricle.
(2) Consist of annulus (fibrous supporting ring), cusps (two for mitral, three for tricuspid), and papillary muscles, which attach to valve cusps by chordae tendineae (Figure 2-5); the cusps are joined for 0.5 to 1 cm at the annulus (referred to as a *commissure*)
(3) Open passively during diastole
(4) Close when papillary muscles contract
(5) Cause the first heart sound, S_1, when they close; two components of S_1: M_1 (mitral valve component) and T_1 (tricuspic valve component)

c. Semilunar valves: aortic and pulmonic valves
(1) Located between ventricles and great vessels
 (a) Pulmonic valve is located between the right ventricle and the pulmonary artery.
 (b) Aortic valve is located between the left ventricle and the aorta.

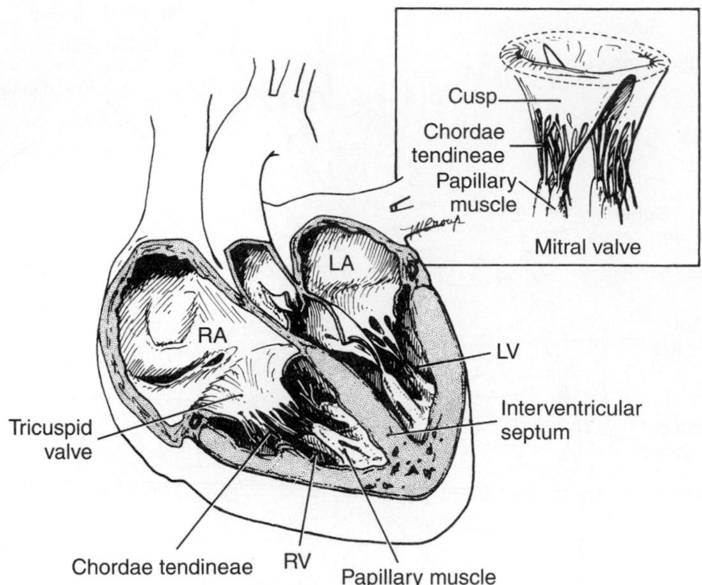

Figure 2-5 Atrioventricular valve. *LA,* Left atrium; *LV,* left ventricle; *RV,* right ventricle; *RA,* right atrium. (From Price, S. A., & Wilson, L. M. [1996] *Pathophysiology: Clinical concepts of disease processes* [5th ed.]. St. Louis: Mosby.)

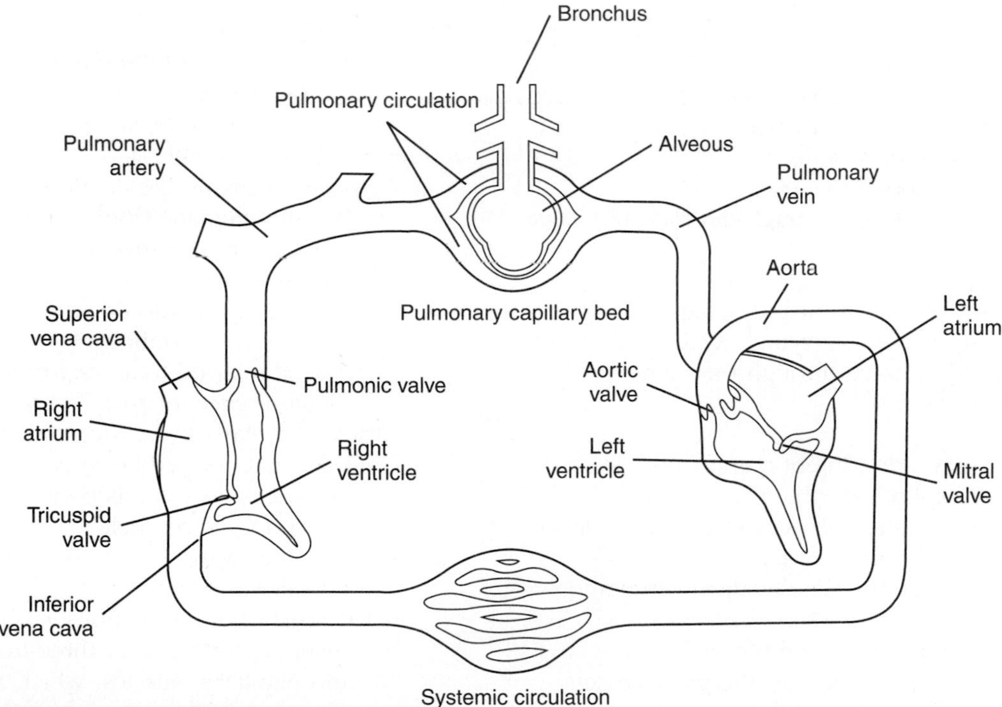

Figure 2-6 Pathway of blood through the heart and the vascular system. (Courtesy Edwards Lifesciences, Irvine, CA.)

(2) Consist of annulus and three cusps
(3) Function by pressure gradients
(4) Cause the second heart sound, S_2, when they close; two components of S_2: A_2 (aortic valve component) and P_2 (pulmonic valve component)

9. Pathway of blood through the heart and the vascular system: venae cavae (superior and inferior) → right atrium → tricuspid valve → right ventricle → pulmonic valve → pulmonary artery → pulmonary capillary bed → pulmonary veins → left atrium → mitral valve → left ventricle → aortic valve → aorta → arteries → arterioles → capillaries → venules → veins → venae cavae (Figure 2-6)
10. Coronary vasculature
    a. Coronary arteries are the first branch off the aorta, immediately outside the aortic valve.
    b. Coronary arteries lie on the epicardium, but branches penetrate through to the myocardium and subendocardium.

c. The myocardium receives 5% of cardiac output and extracts 65% to 80% of oxygen in the blood even at basal rate.
   (1) Blood flow through the coronary arteries is determined almost entirely by local autoregulation in response to the metabolic needs of the myocardium.
   (2) Myocardial blood flow is increased by dilation of the coronary arteries.

d. Coronary artery perfusion
   (1) Effect of cardiac cycle
      (a) The left ventricle is perfused primarily during diastole because of compression of musculature around intramuscular vessels during systole.
      (b) The right ventricle is perfused throughout the cardiac cycle, but perfusion is greater during diastole.
   (2) Effect of aortic pressure
      (a) The pressure in the aorta immediately outside the aortic valve (referred to as *aortic root pressure*) is significant in coronary artery filling pressure.
      (b) Coronary artery perfusion pressure is equal to the diastolic blood pressure minus the pulmonary artery occlusive pressure (previously known as *pulmonary artery wedge pressure* or *pulmonary capillary wedge pressure*); normal coronary artery perfusion pressure is 60 to 80 mm Hg.
   (3) Myocardial oxygen consumption (Figure 2-7)
      (a) Determinants of myocardial oxygen demand include the following:
         (i) Heart rate
         (ii) Preload
         (iii) Afterload
         (iv) Contractility
      (b) Determinants of myocardial oxygen supply include the following:
         (i) Patent arteries
         (ii) Diastolic pressure
         (iii) Diastolic time
         (iv) Oxygen extraction
            a) Hemoglobin concentration
            b) Arterial oxygen saturation
      (c) Imbalances between supply and demand cause ischemia; prolonged imbalance causes infarction.

e. Coronary arteries and distribution (Figure 2-8)
   (1) Left coronary artery before bifurcation is referred to as the *left main coronary artery;* the left main coronary artery divides into left anterior descending and left circumflex arteries.
      (a) Left anterior descending coronary artery supplies the following:
         (i) Anterior left ventricle
         (ii) Anterior two thirds of the interventricular septum
         (iii) Apex of left ventricle
         (iv) Bundle of His and bundle branches

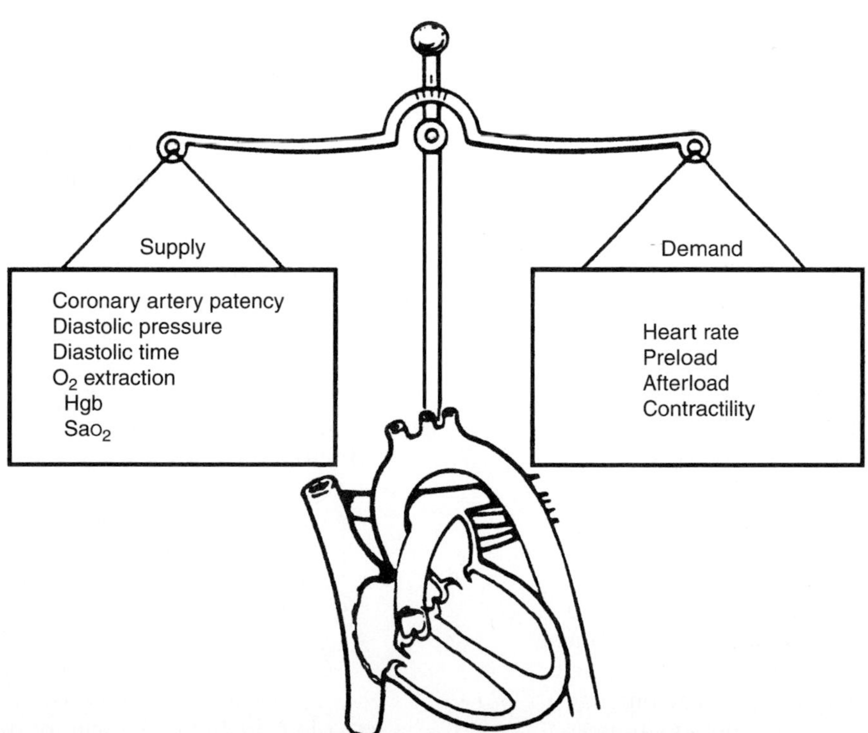

Figure 2-7 Factors influencing myocardial oxygen supply and demand. *Hgb,* Hemoglobin concentration; *Sao_2,* arterial oxygen saturation. (Courtesy Edwards Lifesciences, Irvine, CA.)

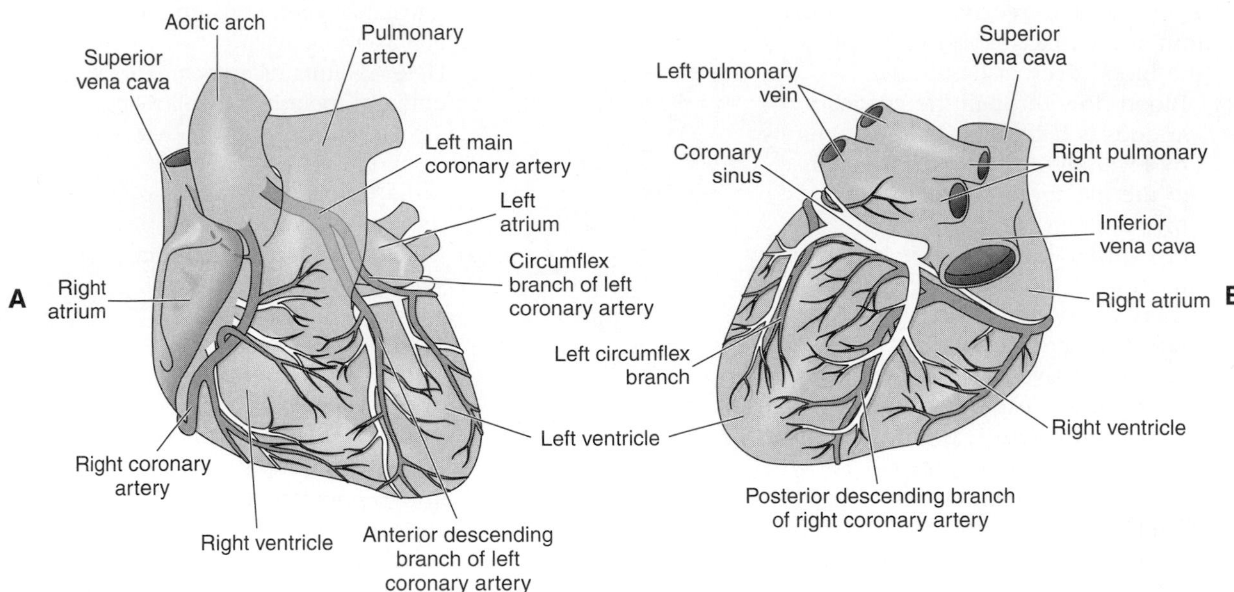

Figure 2-8 The coronary circulation. **A,** Anterior surface. **B,** Posterior surface. (From Hatchett, R., & Thompson, D. [Eds.]. [2002]. *Cardiac nursing: A comprehensive guide.* Edinburgh: Churchill Livingstone.)

(b) Left circumflex coronary artery supplies the following:
(i) Left atrium
(ii) Sinoatrial node in 45% of hearts
(iii) Atrioventricular node in 10% of hearts
(iv) Obtuse marginal branch supplies the following:
a) Lateral left ventricle
b) Posterior left ventricle

(2) Right coronary artery supplies the following:
(a) Right atrium
(b) Sinoatrial node in 55% of hearts
(c) Left posterior hemibundle (dual blood supply: left anterior descending and right coronary artery)
(d) Atrioventricular node in 90% of hearts
(e) Marginal branch supplies:
(i) Lateral right ventricle
(ii) Inferior right ventricle
(f) In right coronary artery–dominant hearts (approximately 80% of hearts), a branch of right coronary artery referred to as the *posterior descending artery* supplies the following:
(i) Anterior right ventricle
(ii) Inferior wall of left ventricle
(iii) Posterior left ventricle
(iv) Posterior one third of septum

(3) Collateral circulation
(a) Circulation consists of interarterial vessels that connect, or anastomose, with each other
(b) Factors that foster development of collateral flow include anemia, hypoxemia, and arteriosclerosis (gradual occlusion).

f. Coronary veins
(1) Most coronary veins empty into the coronary sinus, which empties into the right atrium.
(2) The thebesian veins drain some of venous blood from myocardium directly into the right atrium, right ventricle, and left ventricle rather than through the coronary sinus; this venous blood emptying directly into the left ventricle accounts for a normal physiologic shunt because it slightly decreases oxygen saturation.

g. Lymph vessels
(1) Main cardiac channel empties into the pretracheal node and then into the right lymphatic duct.
(2) Drainage system is facilitated by cardiac contraction.

11. Electrophysiology and the conduction system
a. Types of cardiac cells
(1) Pacemaker cells
(2) Electrical conducting cells
(3) Myocardial muscle cells

b. Properties of cardiac cells
(1) Automaticity: ability of the certain cardiac cells to initiate impulses regularly and spontaneously
(2) Excitability: ability of the cardiac cells to respond to a stimulus
(3) Conductivity: ability of cardiac cells to respond to a cardiac impulse by transmitting the impulse along cell membranes
(4) Contractility: ability of the cardiac cells to respond to an impulse by muscle contraction

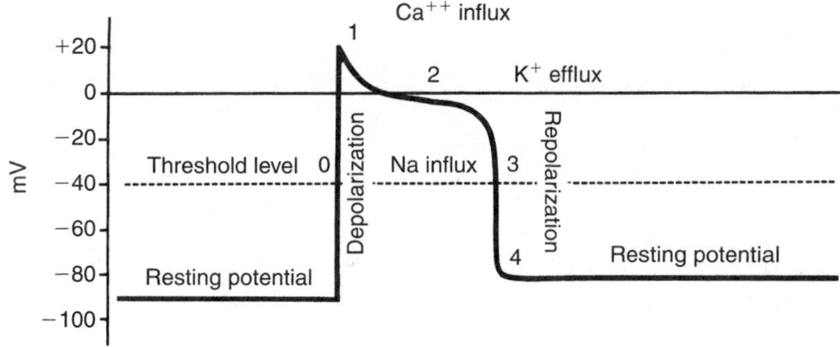

Figure 2-9 Action potential of a myocardial cell. (From Urden, L. D., Stacy, K. M., & Lough, M. E. [2005]. *Thelan's critical care nursing: Diagnosis and management* [5th ed.]. St. Louis: Mosby.)

c. Action potential of myocardial cells (Figure 2-9)
   (1) Phase 4: resting membrane potential
      (a) This phase coincides with isoelectric line between T wave and QRS complex.
      (b) Electrical charge within the cell is −80 to −95 mV.
      (c) Negativity is maintained by the sodium-potassium pump.
         (i) An active transport system requires energy to pump sodium out of the cell and potassium into the cell.
         (ii) When cellular energy (adenosine triphosphate) supplies are low, such as during shock, this resting membrane potential cannot be maintained and irritability occurs.
   (2) Phase 0: rapid depolarization of the cell
      (a) This phase coincides with QRS complex.
      (b) It occurs when a stimulus is applied to the cell.
      (c) Cell membrane permeability to sodium increases significantly so that sodium rushes into the cell (influx) and potassium begins to move out (efflux).
      (d) If the stimulus is strong enough to reach a critical level known as the *threshold potential* (−60 to −70 mV), then the cell responds entirely and depolarization occurs.
      (e) This phase is referred to as the *sodium* (or *fast*) channel.
      (f) Class I antidysrhythmic agents (e.g., procainamide and lidocaine) block the influx of sodium into the cell, thereby preventing the achievement of threshold potential and depolarization.
   (3) Phase 1: brief, partial repolarization
      (a) Sodium channels close
      (b) Potassium efflux continues
      (c) Chloride influx occurs
   (4) Phase 2: slowing of the repolarization causing a plateau
      (a) This phase coincides with ST segment.
      (b) Calcium influx keeps the cell isoelectric but still depolarized as potassium efflux occurs at approximately the same rate.
      (c) This plateau allows a more sustained contraction.
      (d) This phase is referred to as *calcium* (or *slow*) channel.
      (e) Class IV antidysrhythmics (calcium channel blockers [e.g., verapamil and diltiazem]) block the movement of calcium and prolong repolarization and refractoriness.
   (5) Phase 3: sudden acceleration in the rate of repolarization
      (a) Potassium movement accelerates during this phase; potassium efflux occurs at the beginning of phase 3 to exceed the influx of calcium and potassium influx occurs at the end of phase 3.
      (b) Repolarization is completed.
      (c) Class III antidysrhythmics (e.g., amiodarone, ibutilide, and dofetilide) block the movement of potassium during this phase and prolong refractoriness.
   (6) Phase 4: resting membrane potential
d. Action potential of pacemaker cells (Figure 2-10)
   (1) Pacemaker cells have the property of automaticity.
   (2) They demonstrate slow diastolic depolarization because of a time-dependent leak of sodium into the cell.
   (3) When enough sodium has entered the cell that threshold potential is reached, spontaneous depolarization occurs.
   (4) Rate of diastolic depolarization determines intrinsic rate of pacemakers.
      (a) Sinoatrial node: 60 to 100 times per minute
      (b) Atrioventricular junction: 40 to 60 times per minute
      (c) Purkinje fibers: 20 to 40 times per minute
e. Refractoriness (Figure 2-11)
   (1) Absolute refractory period
      (a) No matter how strong the impulse is, the cell cannot be depolarized during this period.
      (b) This period correlates with the time from phase 0 to mid-phase 3 on the action potential and from the QRS complex to the peak of the T wave on the electrocardiogram.

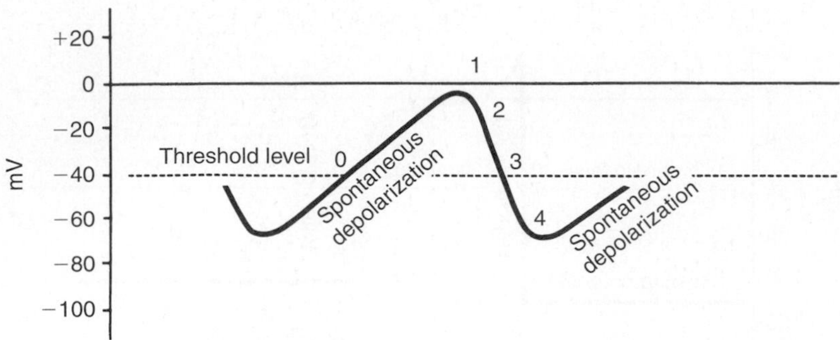

Figure 2-10 Action potential of a pacemaker cell. (From Urden, L. D., Stacy, K. M., & Lough, M. E. [2006]. *Thelan's critical care nursing: Diagnosis and management* [5th ed.]. St. Louis: Mosby.)

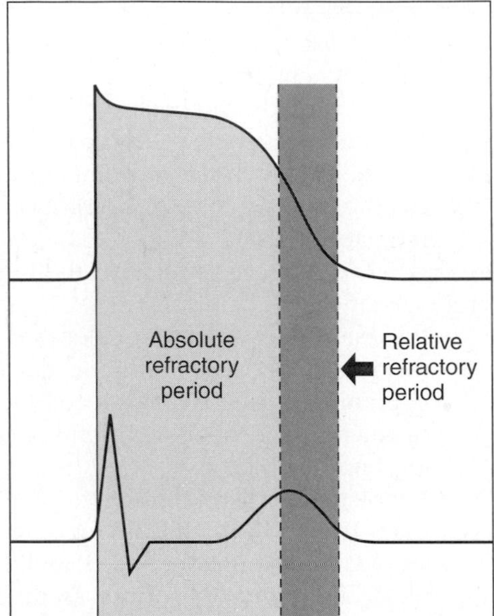

Figure 2-11 Absolute and relative refractory periods correlated with the myocardial cell action potential and with electrocardiogram tracing. (From Urden, L. D., Stacy, K. M., & Lough, M. E. [2006]. *Thelan's critical care nursing: Diagnosis and management* [5th ed.]. St. Louis: Mosby.)

(2) Relative refractory period
   (a) If the impulse is strong enough, the cell may respond but may respond abnormally (e.g., R-on-T may cause ventricular tachycardia or ventricular fibrillation).
   (b) This period correlates with late phase 3 of the action potential and the descending limb of the T wave on the electrocardiogram.

(3) Effective refractory period: the absolute refractory period plus the relative refractory period

f. Conduction system (Figure 2-12)
   (1) Sinoatrial node
      (a) Functions as the natural pacemaker of the heart because it has the fastest intrinsic rate (60 to 100 times per minute)
      (b) Located in the right atrial wall near opening of superior vena cava
   (2) Internodal pathways
      (a) Three pathways between sinoatrial node and atrioventricular node
         (i) Anterior tract (Bachmann's)
         (ii) Middle tract (Wenckebach's)
         (iii) Posterior tract (Thorel's)
   (3) Bachmann's bundle (interatrial pathway): pathway that takes the impulse from right atrium to left atrium
   (4) Atrioventricular node
      (a) Located at the base of right atrium at top of interventricular septum
      (b) Accounts for the physiologic delay of 0.08 to 0.12 second to allow the atria to depolarize completely, contract, and finish filling the ventricles before the ventricles are stimulated
      (c) Contains no pacemaker cells; primary function is to slow down the impulse
   (5) Atrioventricular junction
      (a) Tissue surrounding atrioventricular node and bundle of His that contains pacemaker cells
      (b) Functions as a secondary pacemaker with intrinsic rate of 40 to 60 times per minute
   (6) Bundle of His
      (a) First portion of interventricular conduction system
   (7) Bundle branches
      (a) Right bundle branch takes the impulse to the right ventricular myocardium
      (b) Left bundle branch divides into three hemibundles
         (i) Septal hemibundle depolarizes the interventricular septum in a left-to-right direction.
         (ii) Anterior hemibundle depolarizes the anterior and superior left ventricle.
         (iii) Posterior hemibundle depolarizes the posterior and inferior left ventricle.
         (iv) Hemiblocks
            a) Block of the septal hemibundle does not cause a clinically identifiable situation.

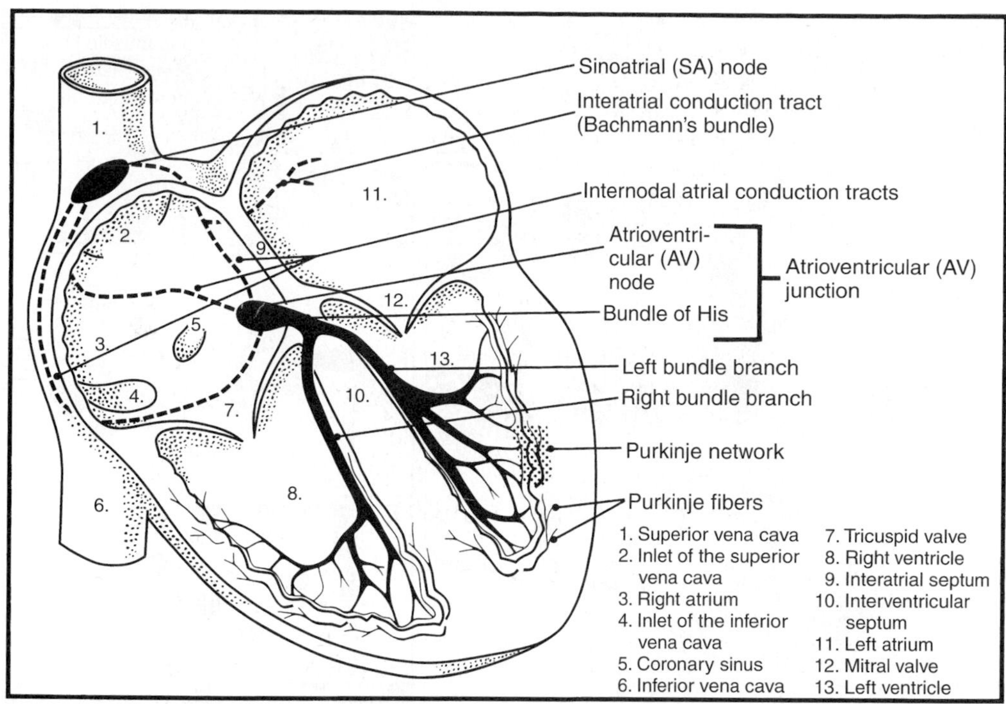

Figure 2-12 The conduction system. (From Huszar, R. J. [1994]. *Basic dysrhythmias: Interpretation and management* [2nd ed.]. St. Louis: Mosby.)

b) The posterior hemibundle is thicker than the anterior hemibundle and has a dual blood supply and so is less susceptible to block than the anterior hemibundle.

c) These three major branches (right bundle branch, left anterior hemibundle, left posterior hemibundle) are referred to as *fascicles* as in unifascicular, bifascicular, and trifascicular block.

(8) Purkinje fiber system

(a) Takes the impulse from the bundle branches through the wall of the ventricles to subendocardial layers

(b) Acts as a final tertiary pacemaker if upper pacemakers fail at the inherent rate of 20 to 40 times per minute

(9) Intercalated disks separate adjacent myocardial cells to allow rapid cell-to-cell transmission of electrical impulses and almost simultaneous activation and contraction of myocardial cells; this capability of the myocardium to respond as if it were one muscle is referred to as a *functional syncytium*.

g. Depolarization of cardiac chambers occurs from endocardium to epicardium.

h. Repolarization of cardiac chambers occurs from epicardium to endocardium.

12. Muscle mechanics

a. Cardiac muscle is similar to skeletal muscle except for the following:

(1) Cardiac muscle has more mitochondria than skeletal muscle; cardiac muscle has greater adenosine triphosphate requirements because of the high energy requirements of the repetitive muscular action of the heart.

(2) Cardiac muscle remains contracted 150 to 300 times longer than skeletal muscle.

(3) Cardiac muscle forms a functional syncytium.

(a) Intercalated disks lie between myocardial cells; they offer low electrical impedance, allowing electrical stimuli to pass with ease from cell to cell.

(b) Stimulation of any muscle fiber results in stimulation of the entire muscle mass (all-or-none response).

(c) The heart acts as if it were one muscle (i.e., functional syncytium)

b. Cardiac muscle ultrastructure (Figure 2-13)

(1) A sarcomere is the basic contractile unit of the myocardium.

(a) The sarcomere measures between 1.6 and 2.2 μm; it contains a centrally placed nucleus surrounded by intracellular protein fluid called *sarcoplasm*, which is surrounded by a membrane called a *sarcolemma*.

(b) The sarcomere is composed of two sets of overlapping myofilaments, including the thick myosin myofilament and the thin actin myofilament.

(c) Troponin and tropomyosin are regulatory proteins in the sarcomere that form a troponin-tropomyosin complex to cover the myosin binding sites and inhibit cross bridging of actin and myosin when in the muscle is in a resting state.

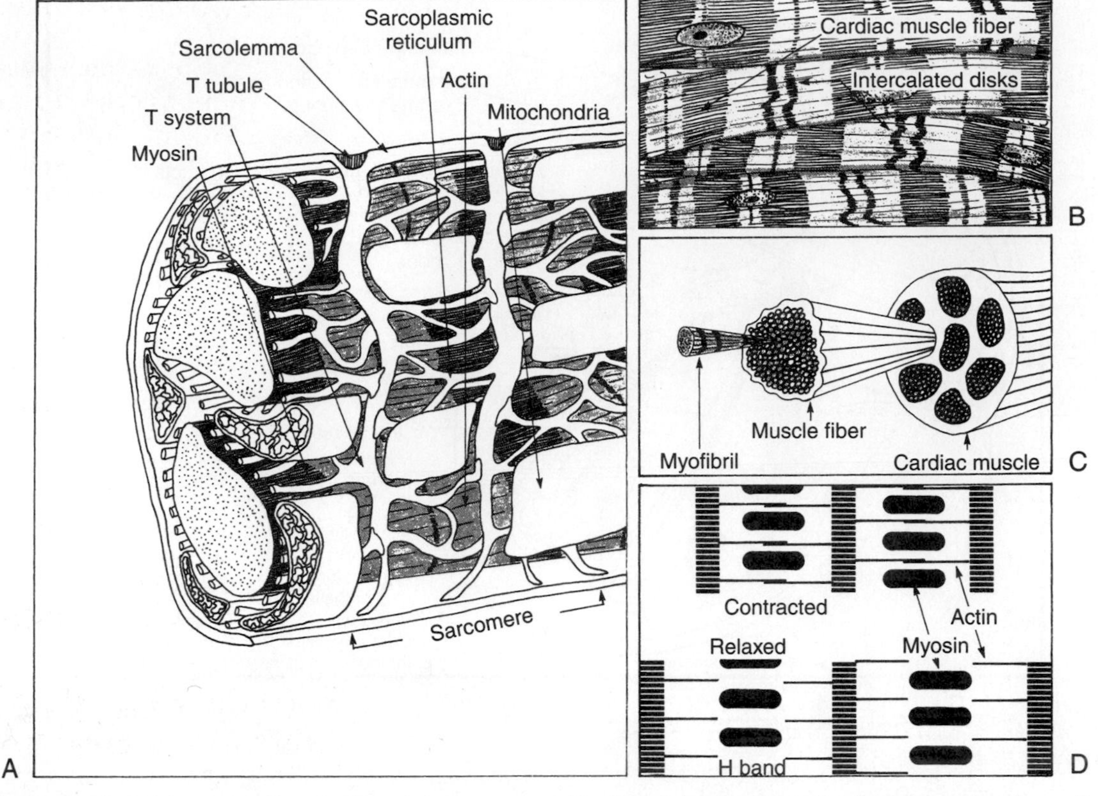

Figure 2-13 Cardiac muscle. **A,** The ultrastructure. **B,** Intercalated disks lie between muscle cells. **C,** Myofibrils form muscle fibers, which form cardiac muscle. **D,** Actin and myosin are myofilaments, which interlace in the presence of calcium to cause muscle contraction and shortening. (From Guzzetta, C. E., & Dossey, B. M. [1992]. *Cardiovascular nursing: Holistic practice*. St. Louis: Mosby.)

(d) The sarcoplasmic reticulum, a continuation of the sarcolemma, penetrates the cell to form a complex tubular (T tubule) system surrounding each fibril.
(e) Calcium is stored in the sarcoplasmic reticulum and is necessary for the cross bridging of actin and myosin.

c. Excitation-contraction process
(1) The wave of depolarization spreads through conduction system to myocardial muscle cell.
(2) The action potential reaches the sarcolemma, and the T tubules transmit the action potential from sarcolemma to interior of the cell.
(3) Calcium enters the cell during phase 2 of the action potential through calcium channels in the sarcolemma and the T tubules; more calcium is released from intracellular stores in the sarcoplasmic reticulum.
(4) Calcium binds with troponin to move the troponin and tropomyosin out of the way of the myosin binding sites.
(5) Actin and myosin myofilaments interact to form cross bridges that slide these overlapping myofilaments past one another.
(6) Shortening of the sarcomere occurs.
(7) Multiple sarcomere shortenings, muscle contraction, and ejection of blood from chamber occur.
(8) Calcium is pumped back into the sarcoplasmic reticulum, which dissociates actin-myosin cross bridges; without the antagonist effect of calcium, troponin and tropomyosin form a troponin-tropomyosin complex that inhibits the cross bridging of actin and myosin.
(9) Muscle relaxation occurs.

13. Cardiac cycle (Figure 2-14)
a. Systole
(1) Isovolumetric contraction: subphase 1
(a) Contraction increases pressure in the ventricle, but there is no change in volume because the atrioventricular valves are closed and the semilunar valves have not yet opened.
(b) Ventricular pressure must exceed the pressure in the great vessel to open the semilunar valve.
(c) This subphase accounts for two thirds of oxygen consumption of the ventricle.
(d) This subphase follows the QRS complex.
(2) Maximal ejection: subphase 2
(a) When the pressure in the ventricle exceeds the pressure in the great vessel, the semilunar valve opens and blood is ejected rapidly into the great vessel.

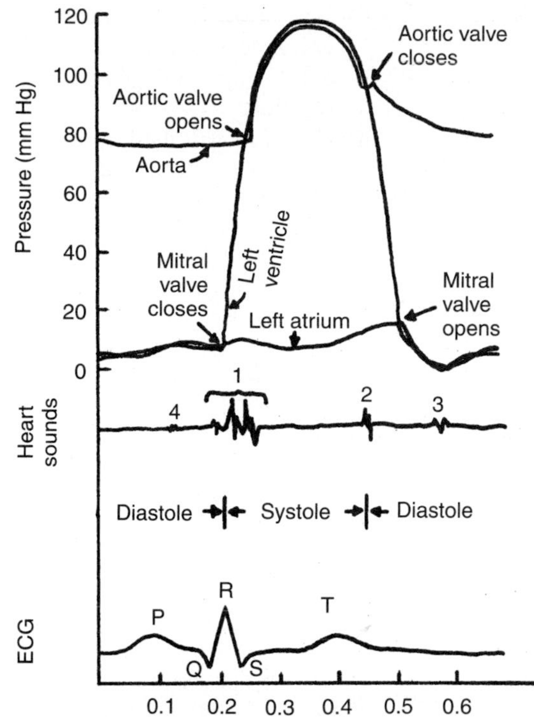

Figure 2-14 Wenger diagram demonstrates the cardiac cycle, showing electrocardiographic events, heart sounds, and pressure curves. (From Wenger, N., et al. [1980]. *Cardiology for nurses*. St. Louis: McGraw-Hill.)

(b) Aortic and pulmonary artery pressures increase rapidly, and ventricular volume decreases sharply.
(c) This subphase occurs during the ST segment.

(3) Reduced ejection (also referred to as *protodiastole*): subphase 3
(a) Blood is ejected slowly from the ventricle to the great vessel.
(b) Ventricular pressure and volume decrease.
(c) When the pressure in the great vessel is greater than the pressure in the ventricle, the semilunar valve closes and systole ends.
(d) This subphase occurs during the T wave.

b. Diastole

(1) Isovolumetric relaxation: subphase 1
(a) Relaxation occurs and ventricular pressure decreases, but volume does not change because the semilunar valves have closed and the atrioventricular valves have not yet opened.
(b) This subphase occurs after the T wave.

(2) Rapid filling: subphase 2
(a) During this phase, the atrioventricular valves open and blood rushes into the ventricles.
(b) Atrial and ventricular pressures decrease, and ventricular volume increases.
(c) Ventricular pressure is less than atrial pressure.
(d) This subphase occurs during the TP interval.

(3) Reduced filling (also referred to as *diastasis*): subphase 3
(a) Atrial and ventricular pressures slowly increase, and ventricular volumes increase with slow filling of ventricles.
(b) Coronary artery blood flow is optimal.
(c) This subphase occurs during the TP interval.

(4) Atrial contraction: subphase 4
(a) This subphase is also referred to as the *atrial kick*.
(b) Atrial contraction accounts for 15% to 30% of diastolic filling volume, may be up to 50% when left ventricular filling is impeded (e.g., mitral stenosis).
(c) Atrial pressure decreases, and ventricular volume and pressure increase.
(d) This subphase occurs after P wave.

14. Regulation of cardiac function

a. Intrinsic control of the heart

(1) Determinants of cardiac output (Figure 2-15 and Table 2-1)

(a) Heart rate

(i) Definition: number of times per minute that the ventricles contract

(ii) Evaluation
a) Count the number of pulses palpable in 1 minute; the radial, brachial, femoral, or carotid pulses are most often used.
b) If the apical rate is auscultated with a stethoscope or the electrocardiogram monitor is used to evaluate the heart rate, a palpable pulse with each audible heart sound or QRS complex must be confirmed.

(iii) Effect of heart rate on cardiac output
a) If heart rate is less than 50 or greater than 150 beats/min, cardiac output often falls and the tendency to dysrhythmias increases.

(iv) Effect of heart rate on myocardial oxygen consumption
a) Although an increase in heart rate may increase cardiac output, an increase in heart rate greater than 120 beats/min tends to increase myocardial oxygen demand more than the increase in coronary blood flow, potentially causing ischemia, especially in patients with coronary artery disease.

(v) Table 2-1 describes factors affecting heart rate.

(b) Preload

(i) Definition: the stretch on the myofibrils at the end of diastole
a) The degree of myofibril stretch is affected by the ventricular volume.

b) Although preload is a volume concept, it traditionally has been evaluated by the pressure in the ventricle at the end of diastole.
   i) The relationship between volume and pressure is affected by the compliance of the ventricle.
   ii) In a normally compliant ventricle, a linear relationship exists between volume and pressure.
   iii) In a noncompliant ventricle, a disproportionate increase in pressure occurs with changes in volume; this is referred to as *diastolic dysfunction*.

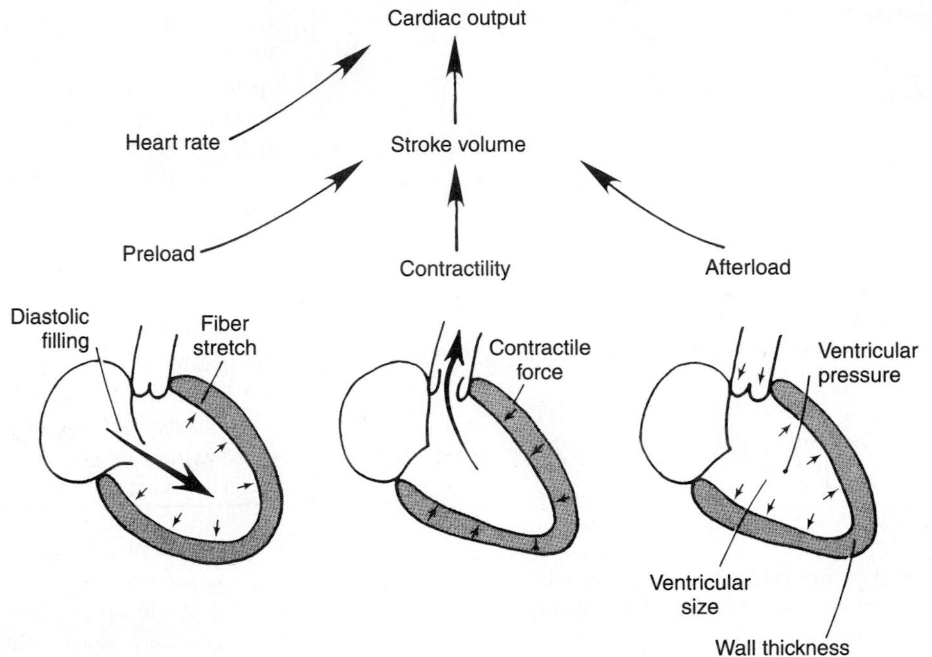

Figure 2-15 Determinants of cardiac output. (From Price, S. A., & Wilson, L. M. [1996]. *Pathophysiology: Clinical concepts of disease processes* [5th ed.]. St Louis: Mosby.)

Table 2-1 Determinants of Cardiac Output

Parameter	Conditions		Treatments	
	Increased	Decreased	To increase	To decrease
Heart rate: evaluated by palpation of pulse	Sympathetic nervous system (SNS) stimulation (e.g., exercise, fever, infection, pain, anxiety, hypovolemia or hypervolemia, and most physiologic or psychological stressors)	• Peripheral nervous system (vagal) stimulation (e.g., Valsalva maneuver, coughing, suctioning, vomiting, and carotid stimulation) • Conduction abnormalities (e.g., sinus blocks second or third-degree atrioventricular blocks) caused by ischemia, infarction, or inflammation • Drug effects (e.g., beta-blockers and digoxin)	• Treatment of cause (e.g., reperfusion therapies for myocardial infarction and antiemetics for vomiting) • Parasympatholytic drugs (e.g., atropine) • Sympathomimetic drugs (e.g., epinephrine) Pacemaker	• Treatment of cause (e.g., antipyretics for fever, analgesics for pain, and anxiolytics for anxiety) • Cardiac glycosides (e.g., digoxin) • Beta-blockers (e.g., propranolol and esmolol) • Calcium channel blockers (e.g., verapamil and diltiazem) • Other antidysrhythmic drugs dependent on rhythm • Vagal maneuvers • Overdrive pacemaker • Ablation • Cardioversion or defibrillation

Table 2-1 Determinants of Cardiac Output—cont'd

Parameter	Conditions		Treatments	
	Increased	Decreased	To increase	To decrease
Afterload: evaluated by calculation of SVR and SVRI (left ventricle) and PVR and PVRI (right ventricle)	• Vasoconstriction as from SNS stimulation or vasopressors • Hypertension • Aortic valve disease • Hypercoagulability • Pulmonary hypertension (right ventricle)	• Hypotension • Vasodilation (e.g., vasogenic shock such as septic shock, neurogenic shock, or anaphylactic shock)	• Adjustment of vasodilator dosage • Vasopressors (e.g., phenylephrine, norepinephrine, dopamine, and vasopressin)	• Arterial vasodilators (e.g., nitroprusside, nitroglycerin greater than 1 mcg/kg/min, hydralazine, calcium channel blockers [e.g., nifedipine], alpha-blockers [e.g., phentolamine and labetalol]) • Angiotensin-converting enzyme (ACE) inhibitors [e.g., captopril and enalapril] or angiotensin receptor blockers (e.g., losartan and valsartan) • Phosphodiesterase inhibitors (e.g., milrinone) • Intraaortic balloon pump • Right ventricle specifically: oxygen; pulmonary vasodilators (e.g., aminophylline and nitric oxide)
Preload: evaluated by pulmonary artery occlusive pressure (left ventricle) and right atrial pressure (right ventricle) or RVEDV if a right ejection fraction (REF) catheter is used	• Heart failure • Hypervolemia • Bradydysrhythmias	• Hypovolemia • Excessive vasodilation (e.g., vasogenic shock) • Increased intrathoracic pressure • Cardiac tamponade • Right ventricular failure or infarction (decreases preload for the left ventricle) • Tachydysrhythmias • Loss of atrial contraction (e.g., atrial fibrillation)	• Adjustment of vasodilator dosage • Isotonic crystalloids (e.g., normal [0.9%] saline or lactated Ringer's solution) • Colloids (e.g., albumin, plasma protein fraction, dextran, hetastarch) • Blood and/or blood products	• Diuretics (e.g., furosemide) • Venous vasodilators (e.g., nitroglycerin, morphine sulfate, nitroprusside, calcium channel blockers [e.g., nifedipine]) • ACE inhibitors (e.g., captopril and enalapril) or angiotensin receptor blockers (e.g., losartan and valsartan), • Nesiritide (Natrecor)
Contractility: evaluated by calculation of stroke volume and LVSWI (left ventricle) and RVSWI (right ventricle)	• SNS stimulation (see heart rate for selected factors that stimulate SNS) • Sympathomimetic drugs (e.g., epinephrine)	• Myocardial ischemia or infarction • Cardiomyopathy • Hypoxemia • Acidosis • Drug adverse effects (e.g., barbiturates, anesthetics, beta-blockers, calcium channel blockers, and most antidysrhythmic drugs)	• Cardiac glycosides (e.g., digoxin) • Sympathomimetics (e.g., dobutamine, and dopamine at medium [~5 mcg/kg/min] dose) • Phosphodiesterase inhibitors (e.g., milrinone) • Glucagon	• Beta-blockers (e.g., propranolol and metoprolol) • Calcium channel blockers (e.g., diltiazem and verapamil)

LVSWI, Left ventricular stroke work index; *PVR,* pulmonary vascular resistance; *PVRI,* pulmonary vascular resistance index; *RVEDV,* right ventricular end-diastolic volume; *RVSWI,* right ventricular stroke work index; *SVR,* systemic vascular resistance; *SVRI,* systemic vascular resistance index.

iv) Some causes of noncompliance of the ventricle include myocardial ischemia or infarction, ventricular hypertrophy, hypertrophic cardiomyopathy, restrictive pericarditis, and cardiac tamponade.

c) Right ventricular volumetric monitoring allows more accurate evaluation of preload through the evaluation of right ventricular volumes rather than pressure and evaluation of right ventricular ejection fraction.

(ii) Evaluation

a) Invasive: atrial pressure correlates to end-diastolic pressure for the respective ventricle

i) Right ventricular preload correlates to central venous pressure or right atrial pressure if no tricuspid valve disease

ii) Left ventricular preload correlates to pulmonary artery occlusive pressure or left atrial pressure if no mitral valve disease

iii) Right ventricular end-diastolic volume (requires right ejection fraction catheter)

b) Noninvasive evaluation

i) Right ventricle: Jugular venous distention, hepatomegaly, and peripheral edema indicate high right ventricular preload; flat neck veins when the patient is flat and oliguria indicate low right ventricular preload.

ii) Left ventricle: S_3, crackles, and dyspnea indicate high left ventricular preload; clinical indications of hypoperfusion (Table 2-2) indicate low left ventricular preload.

iii) Effect of preload on stroke volume and cardiac output

- Starling's Law of the Heart and the Frank-Starling mechanism: Within physiologic limits, the greater the stretch on the myofibrils, the greater the force of the subsequent contraction (Figure 2-16).
- Understretching and overstretching of the myofibrils results in a less than optimal contraction.

iv) Effect of preload on myocardial oxygen consumption: As preload increases, myocardial oxygen consumption increases.

v) Table 2-1 describes factors affecting preload.

(c) Afterload

(i) Definition: the pressure against which the ventricle must pump to open the semilunar valve; affected by vascular resistance, ventricular diameter, and the mass and viscosity of blood

(ii) Evaluation

a) Invasive: calculated parameter

i) Right ventricular afterload correlates to pulmonary vascular resistance and pulmonary vascular resistance index

ii) Left ventricular afterload correlates to systemic vascular resistance and systemic vascular resistance index

b) Noninvasive

i) Right ventricle: Loud P_2 and high pulmonary artery diastolic pressure indicate high right ventricular afterload; low pulmonary artery diastolic pressure indicates low right ventricular afterload.

Table 2-2 Clinical Indications of Hypoperfusion

Normal	Subclinical Hypoperfusion	Clinical Hypoperfusion	Shock
Cardiac index 2.5-4 L/min/m^2	Cardiac index 2.2-2.5 L/min/m^2	Cardiac index 2-2.2 L/min/m^2	Cardiac index less than 2 L/min/m^2
Normal	• No clinical indications of hypoperfusion, though an expert nurse may detect subtle changes in the patient. • Hypoperfusion at this stage is detected by hemodynamic monitoring.	• Tachycardia • Narrowed pulse pressure • Tachypnea • Cool skin • Oliguria • Diminished bowel sounds • Restlessness → confusion	• Dysrhythmias • Hypotension • Tachypnea • Cold, clammy skin • Anuria • Absent bowel sounds • Lethargy → coma

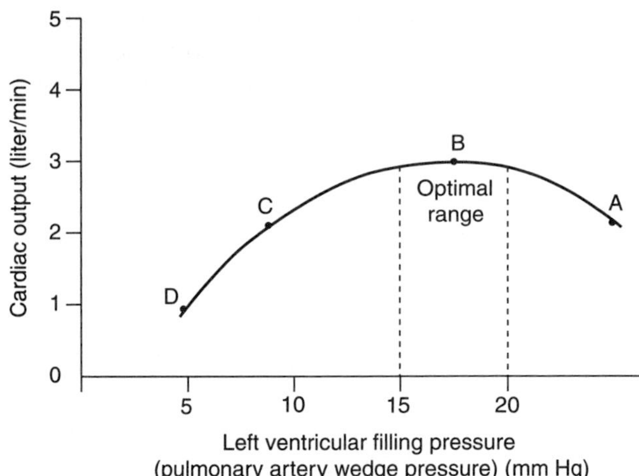

Figure 2-16 Relationship between pulmonary artery occlusive pressure and cardiac output. *A,* Overstretched myofibrils resulting in decreased contractility and cardiac output. *B,* Optimally stretched myofibrils resulting in optimally stretched myofibrils and optimal cardiac output. *C,* Normal stretched myofibrils resulting in normal (but suboptimal) cardiac output. *D,* Understretched myofibrils resulting in decreased contractility and cardiac output.

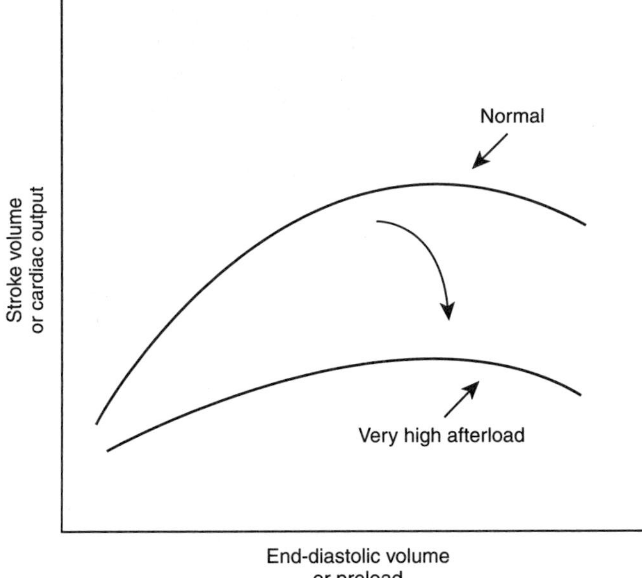

Figure 2-17 Relationship between afterload and stroke volume. (From Hicks, G. H. [2000]. *Cardiopulmonary anatomy and physiology.* Philadelphia: W. B. Saunders.)

ii) Left ventricle: Loud A_2, cool, pale extremities, and high systemic arterial diastolic pressure indicate high left ventricular afterload; low systemic arterial diastolic pressure indicates low left ventricular afterload.

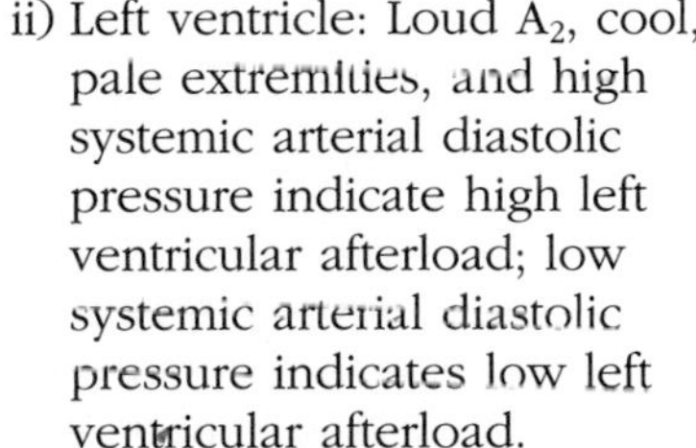

iii) Effect of afterload on stroke volume and cardiac output (Figure 2-17)

iv) Effect of afterload on myocardial oxygen consumption: As afterload increases, myocardial oxygen consumption increases.

v) Table 2-1 describes factors affecting afterload.

(d) Contractility

(i) Definition: contractile force of the heart independent of preload and afterload

a) Laplace's law states that the amount of contractile force generated within a chamber depends on the radius of the chamber and the thickness of its walls; therefore, the smaller the radius and the thicker the wall, the greater the force of contraction.

b) Contractility also is affected significantly by endogenous catecholamines (e.g., epinephrine).

(ii) Evaluation

a) Invasive: calculated parameters

i) Right ventricle contractility correlates to right ventricular stroke work index

ii) Left ventricular contractility correlates to left ventricular stroke work index

iii) Ejection fraction by right ejection fraction catheter

b) Noninvasive indicators of decreased contractility

i) Clinical indicators of hypoperfusion (Table 2-2)

ii) Diminished heart sounds

iii) Ejection fraction by multiple gated acquisition scan or Doppler echocardiogram

(iii) Effect of contractility on stroke volume and cardiac output (Figure 2-18)

(iv) Effect of contractility on myocardial oxygen consumption: As contractility increases, myocardial oxygen consumption increases.

(v) Table 2-1 describes factors affecting contractility.

b. Extrinsic control of the heart

(1) Neurologic control of the heart

(a) Autonomic nervous system

(i) Terms used to describe cardiac effects

a) Chronotropic: effect on heart rate

b) Inotropic: effect on contractility

c) Dromotropic: effect on conductivity

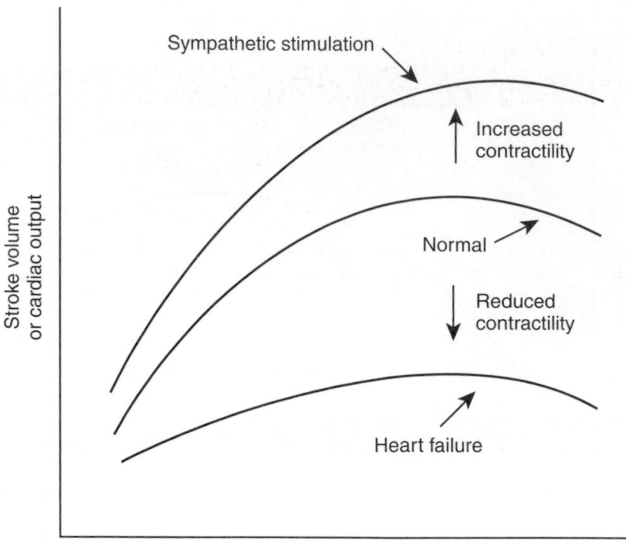

Figure 2-18 Relationship between contractility and stroke volume. (From Hicks, G. H. [2000]. *Cardiopulmonary anatomy and physiology*. Philadelphia: W. B. Saunders.)

(ii) Sympathetic nervous system
  a) This branch is referred to as *fight or flight*.
  b) Sympathetic nervous system is innervated by physiologic or psychological stress.
  c) It causes positive chronotropic, inotropic, and dromotropic effects.
  d) Sympathetic nervous system receptors and effects are listed in Table 2-3.
  e) Sympathomimetic drugs frequently are used in critical care to augment these effects, especially after the patient's endogenous supplies are depleted; these drugs vary in their receptor stimulation and the potency of the stimulation (Table 2-4)

(b) Parasympathetic (vagal) nervous system
  (i) This branch maintains steady state.
  (ii) The parasympathetic nervous system causes negative chronotropic, inotropic, and dromotropic effects.
  (iii) Though the cardiovascular effects of the parasympathetic nervous system are generally undesirable in critical care, they may decrease myocardial oxygen consumption by up to 50%.
  (iv) Parasympatholytic (or vagolytic) agents (e.g., atropine) block these effects.

(c) Chemoreceptors
  (i) Chemoreceptors are located in carotid and aortic bodies.
  (ii) They are sensitive to changes in Pa_{O_2}, Pa_{CO_2}, and pH.
  (iii) Hypoxia, hypercapnia, and acidosis cause changes in heart rate and ventilatory rate.

(d) Baroreceptor reflex
  (i) Baroreceptors are located in the carotid sinus and aortic arch.
  (ii) They are sensitive to arterial pressure.
  (iii) Increased blood pressure causes vagal stimulation, resulting in decrease in heart rate and contractility.

(e) Bainbridge reflex
  (i) Accelerator receptors are located in the right atrium.
  (ii) These receptors are sensitive to right atrial pressure.
  (iii) Increased right atrial pressure causes increase in heart rate.

(f) Respiratory reflex
  (i) Inspiration decreases intrathoracic pressure, which increases venous return to the right side of the heart, which causes the Bainbridge reflex. When the increased venous return reaches the left side of the heart, left ventricular cardiac output increases, which increases arterial blood pressure and decreases the heart rate through stimulation of baroreceptors.
  (ii) This process is at least partly responsible for sinus dysrhythmia; an interaction between the respiratory and cardiac centers in the medulla also contributes.

c. The endocrine function of the heart
  (1) Atrial natriuretic peptide (ANP)
    (a) Produced and stored by specialized atrial muscle cells
    (b) Triggers for ANP release
      (i) Primary cause of ANP release is increased atrial stretch.
      (ii) Other causes of ANP release include acute increase in intravascular volume, exercise, and endogenous or exogenous vasopressors.
    (c) Actions and effects: important regulator of blood volume and blood pressure
      (i) Inhibits sodium transport in the collecting ducts of the kidney, resulting in increased urine output
      (ii) Acts as an antagonist to angiotensin II, epinephrine, and endothelin, resulting in decrease in heart rate and vasodilation
      (iii) Diminishes the renin-angiotensin-aldosterone system, resulting in sodium and water excretion
      (iv) Decreases proliferation of cardiac fibroblasts and smooth muscle cells, resulting in the prevention of ventricular remodeling

Table 2-3 Sympathetic Nervous System (Adrenergic) Receptors and Effects

Receptor	Location of Receptors	Effects Receptors
Alpha	Vessels	Vasoconstriction of most vessels, especially the arterioles
$Beta_1$	Heart	Increase in heart rate (chronotropic effect), contractility (inotropic effect), and conductivity (dromotropic effect)
$Beta_2$	Bronchial and vascular smooth muscle	Bronchodilation, vasodilation
Dopaminergic	Renal and mesenteric artery bed	Dilation of renal and mesenteric arteries

Table 2-4 Sympathomimetic Agents and Receptor Stimulation

Drug	Alpha	$Beta_1$	$Beta_2$
Phenylephrine	++++	0	0
Norepinephrine	++++	++	0
Epinephrine	++++	++++	++
Dopamine	++ less than 5 mcg/kg/min; +++ more than 10 mcg/kg/min	++++ less than 10 mcg/kg/min	+
Dobutamine	+	++++	++
Isoproterenol	0	++++	++++

(2) Brain natriuretic peptide (BNP)
(a) First discovered in animal brain tissue (hence the name), but it is produced by ventricular muscle tissue
(b) Triggers for BNP release: increased intravascular volume
(c) Actions and effects: similar to atrial natriuretic peptide with dilation of arteries and veins
(d) Measurement of BNP is being used as a diagnostic study for diagnosis of heart failure and as a therapeutic pharmacologic agent (i.e., nesiritide [Natrecor]) for heart failure
(3) C-type natriuretic peptide
(a) Lowest concentration of circulating plasma natriuretic peptides; distributed predominantly in the central nervous system, kidneys, and endothelial cells
(b) Actions and effects: marked vasodilatory effects but no natriuretic effect
(4) Endothelin
(a) Potent vasoconstrictive peptides produced by endothelial cells
(b) Causes an increase in renin, aldosterone, antidiuretic hormone, and sympathetic nervous system effects to increase in systemic vascular resistance

Vascular System

1. Function: supply blood, nutrients, hormones to the tissues and remove metabolic wastes from the tissues
2. Resistance to flow
   a. Poiseuille's formula states that resistance depends on the following:
      (1) The length of the vessel
      (2) The radius of the vessel
      (3) The viscosity of the blood
   b. Blood flow through the body also is influenced by neurologic stimulation affecting vascular tone and features that cause turbulence within the vascular lumen, such bifurcations or protrusions from the vessel wall into the vessel lumen (e.g., atherosclerosis)
3. Components of the vascular system (Figure 2-19)
   a. Arteries
      (1) The arteries are the delivery system that distributes and regulates the amount of oxygenated blood flow to various tissue beds.
      (2) Arteries are able to stretch during systole and recoil during diastole.
      (3) The arterial system is a high-pressure circuit.
      (4) The layers of the arterial wall consist of the following (Figure 2-20):
         (a) Intima: thin lining of endothelium and a small amount of elastic tissue; decreases resistance to flow and minimizes the chance of platelet aggregation
         (b) Media: smooth muscle and elastic tissue; changes the lumen diameter as needed
         (c) Adventitia: connective tissue; strengthens and shapes the vessels

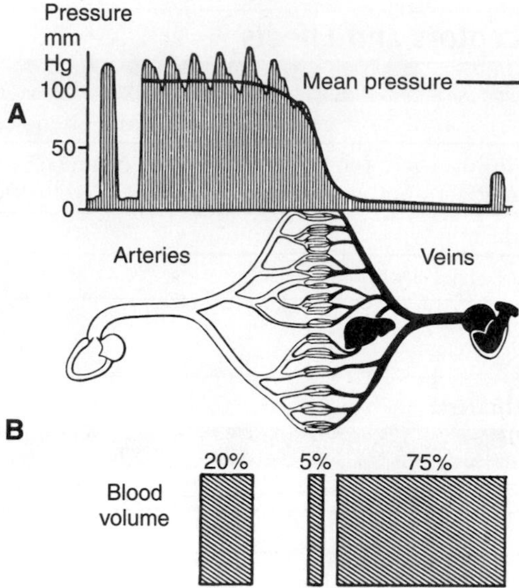

Figure 2-19 Components of the vascular system. **A,** Mean pressure in components of vascular system. **B,** Volume in components of vascular system. (Reprinted with permission from Rushmer, R. [1976]. *Cardiovascular dynamics* [4th ed.]. Philadelphia: W. B. Saunders.)

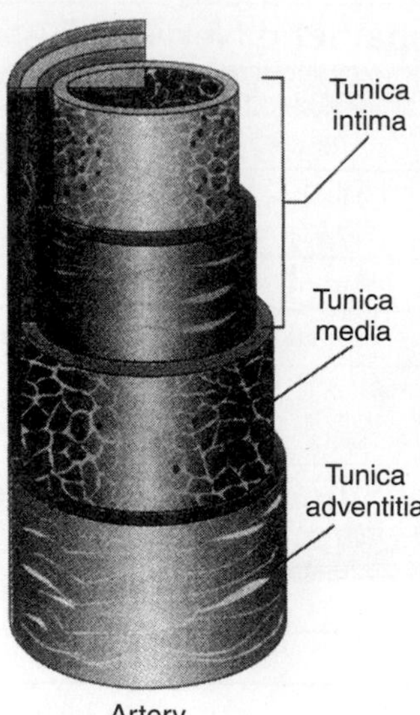

Figure 2-20 Layers of the arterial wall. (From Copstead, L. [1995]. *Perspectives on pathophysiology*. Philadelphia: W. B. Saunders.)

b. Arterioles
   (1) Arterioles are vital to the maintenance of blood pressure and systemic vascular resistance.
   (2) Arterioles may lead to any of the following:
      (a) Capillaries
      (b) Metarterioles
      (c) Precapillary sphincters that control blood flow into capillary bed

c. Capillaries
   (1) The capillary bed is the nutrient bed where exchange of gases, nutrients, and metabolites takes place by the process of diffusion.
   (2) Capillaries contain no smooth muscle.
   (3) The diameter of the capillary depends on changes in precapillary and postcapillary tone.
   (4) Capillary dynamics are influenced by four pressures (Figure 2-21).
      (a) Hydrostatic pressures push.
         (i) Capillary hydrostatic pressure pushes fluid out of the capillary and into interstitium.
         (ii) Interstitial hydrostatic pressure pushes fluid out of interstitium and into the capillary.
      (b) Colloidal oncotic pressures pull.
         (i) Capillary colloidal oncotic pressure pulls and holds fluid in the capillary.
         (ii) Interstitial colloidal oncotic pressure pulls and holds fluid in the interstitium.
      (c) Pressures pushing fluid out of the capillary dominate at the arterial end; pressures pushing fluid back into the capillary dominate at the venous end.
      (d) Edema is caused by an imbalance in these pressures or an increase in capillary permeability; *third spacing* is a term used to describe fluid accumulation in any space that is not intravascular or intracellular (e.g., interstitial edema, ascites, pleural effusion, pericardial effusion, and into the lumen of the intestine)
         (i) Heart failure: Peripheral edema is caused by venous congestion and excessive capillary hydrostatic pressure at the venous end.
         (ii) Protein malnutrition or liver disease: A decrease in plasma proteins decreases capillary colloidal oncotic pressure and allows excessive fluid to leak out of the capillary.

d. Veins
   (1) The venous system is the return system that brings deoxygenated blood back to the heart and lungs.
   (2) Veins act as a reservoir; the venous system holds 65% to 70% of the total blood volume.
   (3) The venous pump sends blood back to the right side of the heart; the skeletal muscles contract, compress veins, and propel blood toward the heart.
   (4) Valves in the veins prevent retrograde blood flow.

4. Blood pressure
   a. Regulation
      (1) Autonomic nervous system
      (2) Renin-angiotensin-aldosterone system (Figure 2-22)

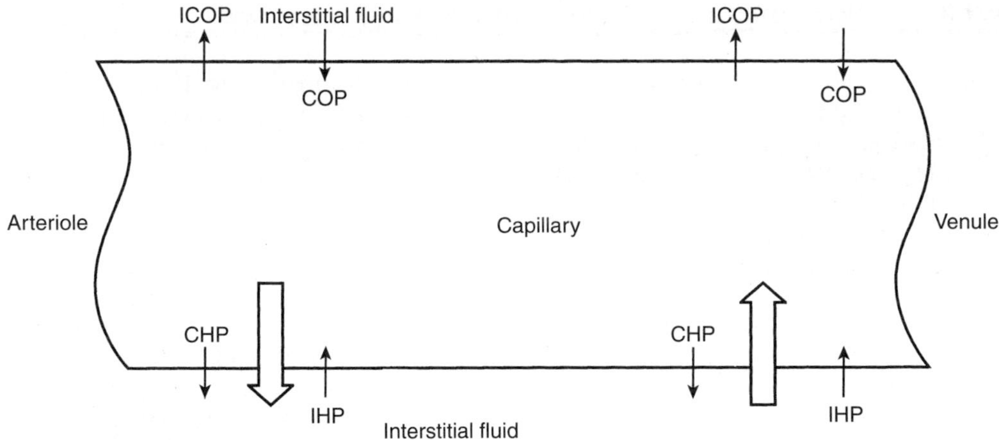

Figure 2-21 Capillary dynamics. Forces out of the capillary dominate at the arteriole end, whereas forces back into the capillary dominate at the venule end. *CHP,* Capillary hydrostatic pressure; *COP,* colloidal oncotic pressure; *ICOP,* interstitial colloidal oncotic pressure; *IHP,* interstitial hydrostatic pressure.

ANGIOTENSINOGEN
(produced by the liver and in the blood)

RENIN
(released by the juxtaglomerular apparatus of the kidney in response to hypoperfusion of the kidney [e.g., hypovolemia, hypotension, renovascular disease], sympathetic nervous system stimulation, hyponatremia)

ANGIOTENSIN I

ANGIOTENSIN-CONVERTING ENZYME
(produced by the lung and this conversion occurs as blood circulates through the lung)

ANGIOTENSIN II

VASOCONSTRICTION

ALDOSTERONE
(released from adrenal cortex)

Increase in SVR (afterload) and BP

SODIUM AND WATER RETENTION
(by the renal tubules)

Increase in blood volume (preload) and BP

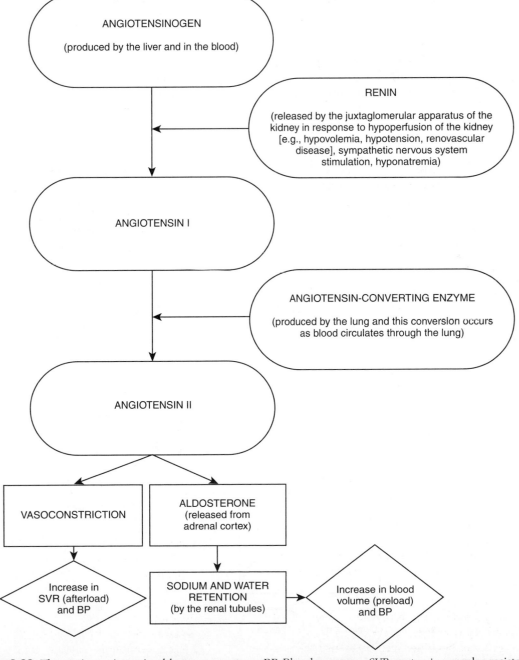

Figure 2-22 The renin-angiotensin-aldosterone system. *BP,* Blood pressure; *SVR,* systemic vascular resistance.

(a) Renin is secreted by the kidney in response to the following:
(i) Decreased blood pressure stimulating stretch receptors in juxtaglomerular cells
(ii) Sympathetic nervous system stimulation
(iii) Hyponatremia
(b) Renin stimulates the conversion of angiotensinogen to angiotensin I.
(c) Angiotensin I is converted to angiotensin II by angiotensin-converting enzyme as the blood travels through the lung.
(d) Angiotensin II causes vasoconstriction and secretion of aldosterone.
(e) Vasoconstriction and sodium and water retention increase blood pressure and decrease renin secretion.
(3) Capillary fluid shifts: especially from interstitial to intravascular
(4) Local control mechanisms

b. Factors affecting arterial blood pressure (Figure 2-23)

c. Pulse pressure (Figure 2-24)
(1) The difference between systolic and diastolic pressures
(2) Affected by stroke volume and arterial elastance

d. Mean arterial pressure (see Figure 2-24)
(1) The average pressure in the aorta and its major branches during cardiac cycle
(2) Calculated by either of the following formulae, where *BP* is blood pressure:
(a) [BP systolic + (BP diastolic × 2)] ÷ 3
(b) BP diastolic + (pulse pressure ÷ 3)
(3) Normal: 70 to 105 mm Hg
(4) Affected by cardiac output and systemic vascular resistance

5. Control and regulation of peripheral blood flow

a. Local control mechanisms
(1) Autoregulation is the ability of the tissues to control blood flow. Vasodilation is caused by hypoxia, hypercapnia, acidosis.
(2) Precapillary sphincters, which precede every capillary bed, relax and permit more blood flow when oxygen tension falls; they constrict and restrict blood flow when oxygen tension rises.

b. Autonomic nervous system
(1) Increased sympathetic nervous system stimulation: vasoconstriction
(a) Maintains arterial pressure
(b) Decreases vascular capacitance, increasing venous return to the heart and preload
(2) Decreased sympathetic nervous system stimulation: vasodilation

c. Baroreceptors
(1) Increase in blood pressure or blood volume results in the following:
(a) Decreased heart rate and contractility
(b) Peripheral vasodilation
(c) Decrease in systemic vascular resistance and blood pressure
(2) Decrease in blood pressure or blood volume results in the following:
(a) Increased heart rate and contractility
(b) Peripheral vasoconstriction
(c) Increase in systemic vascular resistance and blood pressure

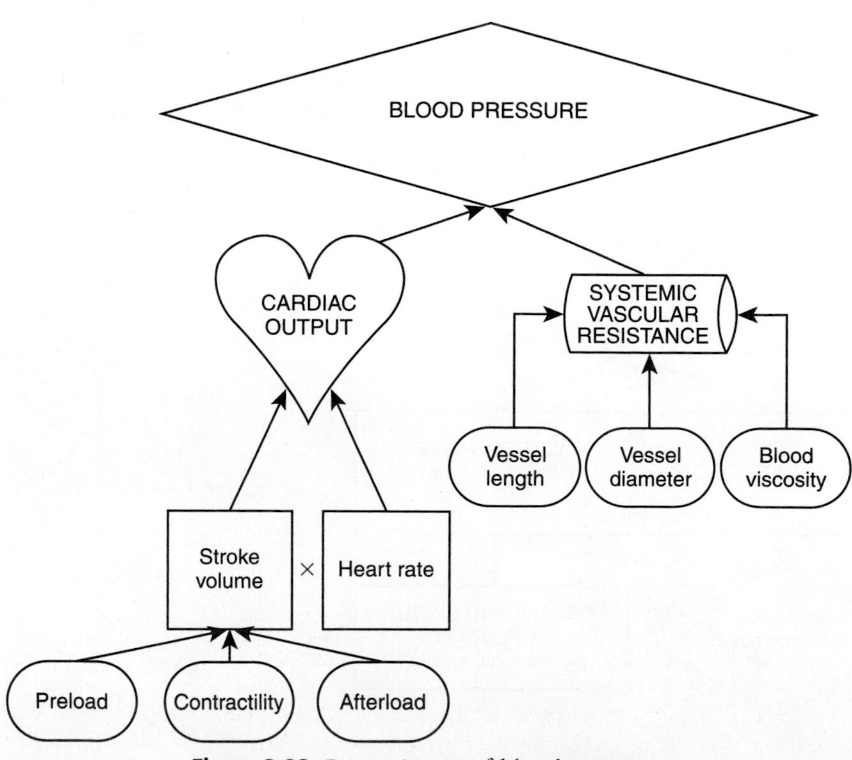

Figure 2-23 Determinants of blood pressure.

d. Vasomotor center in medulla
  (1) Vasoconstrictor area causes the following:
    (a) Increase in heart rate, cardiac output, blood pressure
    (b) Venoconstriction, which decreases vascular capacitance, thus increasing venous return to the heart, preload, and blood pressure
  (2) Vasodepressor area causes the following:
    (a) Decrease in heart rate, cardiac output, blood pressure
    (b) Venodilation, which increases vascular capacitance, thus decreasing venous return to the heart, preload, and blood pressure

Oxygen Delivery to the Tissue (Do_2)/ Oxygen Consumption by the Tissues (Vo_2) (Figure 2-25)

1. Parameters used to evaluate the balance between oxygen supply and oxygen consumption
   a. Oxygen delivery to the tissues (Do_2/Do_2I)

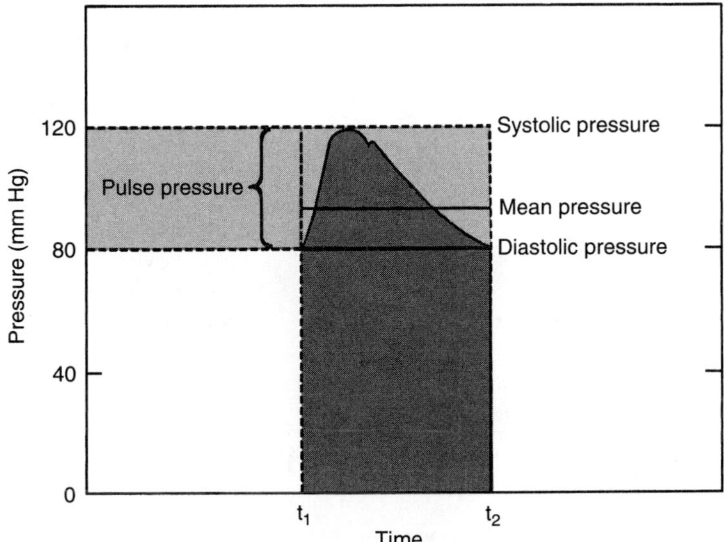

Figure 2-24 Blood pressure, pulse pressure (difference between systolic and diastolic pressures), and mean arterial pressure (calculated or measured average pressure). (Modified from Berne, R. M., & Levy, M. N. [1997]. *Cardiovascular physiology* [7th ed.]. St. Louis: Mosby.)

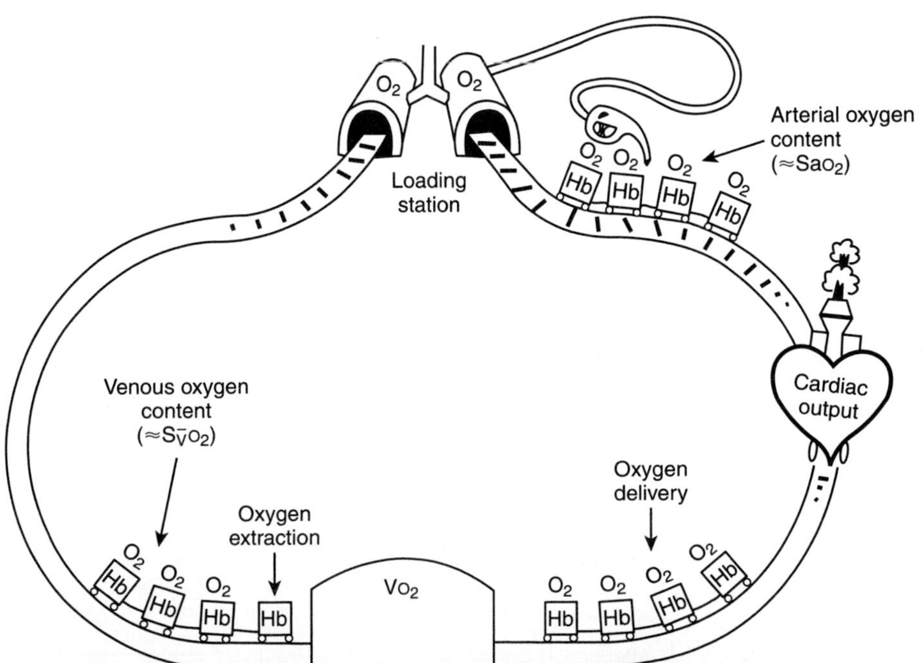

Figure 2-25 Schematic demonstrating oxygen delivery/oxygen consumption (Do_2/Vo_2). (From *Understanding continuous mixed venous oxygen saturation monitoring with the Swan Ganz TD System*. Baxter Healthcare Corporation, Edwards Critical Care.)

(1) Do_2 (Figure 2-26)
(a) Product of cardiac output and arterial oxygen content
(i) Cardiac output is a product of heart rate and stroke volume; stroke volume is affected by preload, afterload, and contractility.
(ii) Arterial oxygen content is a product of hemoglobin and arterial saturation.
(b) Formula: CO × Hgb × Sao_2 × 13.4, where *CO* is cardiac output, *Hgb* is hemoglobin saturation, and *Sao_2* is arterial oxygen saturation
(i) Cardiac output in liters/minute
(ii) Hemoglobin in grams/deciliter
(iii) Saturation as a decimal (e.g., 95% is 0.95)
(c) Normal Do_2: 900 to 1100 mL/min (~1000 mL/min)
(2) Do_2I: Do_2 divided by body surface area so as to consider body size
(a) Formula: CI × Hgb × Sao_2 × 13.4, where *CI* is cardiac index
(i) Cardiac index in liters/minute/meter squared
(ii) Hemoglobin in grams/deciliter
(iii) Saturation as a decimal (e.g., 95% is 0.95)
(b) Normal: 550 to 650 mL/min/m^2 (~600 mL/min/m^2)
(3) Examples of situations that decrease Do_2/Do_2I
(a) Decrease in Sao_2 (e.g., acute respiratory failure, decrease in the inspired oxygen level such as smoke inhalation, or decrease in barometric pressure such as high altitudes)
(b) Decrease in hemoglobin (e.g., anemia or hemorrhage)
(c) Decrease in cardiac output (e.g., heart failure or hypovolemia)

b. Oxygen consumption by the tissues (Vo_2/Vo_2I)
(1) Vo_2: volume of oxygen consumed by the tissues each minute
(a) Determined by comparing the oxygen content in the arterial blood to the oxygen content in the mixed venous blood (e.g., drawn from the distal tip of pulmonary artery catheter)
(b) Formula: CO × Hgb × 13.4 × (Sao_2 − Svo_2), where *Svo_2* is venous oxygen saturation
(c) Normal Vo_2: 200 to 300 mL/min (~250 mL/min)
(2) Vo_2I: Vo_2 divided by body surface area so as to consider body size
(a) Formula: CI × Hgb × 13.4 × (Sao_2 − Svo_2)
(b) Normal: 110 to 160 mL/min/m^2 (~150 mL/min/m^2)
(3) Examples of situations that increase Vo_2/Vo_2I
(a) Having a dressing change
(b) Being bathed
(c) Being repositioned
(d) Having a visitor
(e) Being weighed on a sling scale
(f) Having a physical examination
(g) Agitation
(h) Shivering
(i) Fever
(j) Increased work of breathing
(k) Severe infection
(l) Burns

c. Oxygen extraction ratio (O_2ER)
(1) Evaluation of the amount of oxygen that is extracted from the arterial blood as it passes through the capillaries; ratio of the difference between the content of oxygen in the arterial blood and the content of oxygen in venous blood to the content of oxygen in the arterial blood
(2) Formula: (Cao_2 − Cvo_2) ÷ Cao_2, where *Cao_2* is arterial oxygen content and *Cvo_2* is venous oxygen content
(3) Normal: 22% to 30% (~25%)

d. Oxygen extraction index (O_2EI)
(1) Estimation of oxygen extraction ratio calculated using only saturations
(2) Formula: (Sao_2 − Svo_2) ÷ Sao_2
(3) Normal: 20% to 27% (~25%)

e. Oxygen reserve in venous blood
(1) Determined by measuring the oxygen saturation in mixed venous blood in the pulmonary artery (i.e., Svo_2)

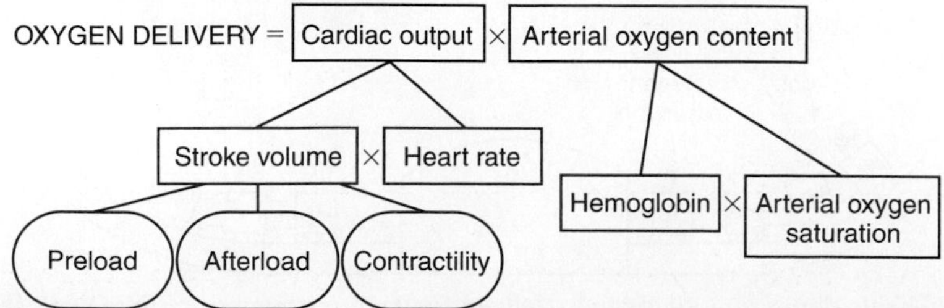

Figure 2-26 Determinants of oxygen delivery. (From Daily, E. K., & Schroeder, J. S. [1994]. *Techniques in bedside hemodynamic monitoring*. St. Louis: Mosby.)

(2) Normal: 60% to 80% (~75%)
(3) Note that normal Sao_2 is ~99% and Svo_2 is ~75% (the tissues used ~25%); note that normal Cao_2 is ~20 mL/dL and Cvo_2 is ~15 mL/dL (the tissues used ~25%); note that normal Do_2 is ~1000 mL/min and Vo_2 is ~250 mL/min (the tissues used ~25%); there is normally ~75% oxygen reserve

f. Serum arterial lactate level
(1) Lactic acidosis is the result of anaerobic metabolism, and an elevated serum arterial lactate level indicates a tissue oxygen deficit.
(2) Normal serum arterial lactate level: less than 1 mmol/L

2. Physiologic compensation for increased demand for oxygen at the cellular level
a. Increase in cardiac output
b. Redistribution of blood flow by recruiting underperfused capillary beds
c. Increased oxygen extraction by the cells

3. Critical Do_2 point (Figure 2-27)
a. A critical level of oxygen delivery exists where oxygen delivery and consumption are interdependent.
b. When the critical oxygen delivery point is exceeded, oxygen consumption is dependent on oxygen delivery, and oxygen deficit, anaerobic metabolism, and lactic acidosis will occur.
(1) If Svo_2 improves with increase in Do_2, oxygen delivery and consumption are independent.
(2) If Svo_2 does not improve with increase in Do_2, oxygen consumption is dependent on oxygen delivery.
c. Therapeutic efforts to decrease Vo_2 and increase Do_2 may be used, although the effects of superoptimization of Do_2 greater than 1000 mL/min on mortality, morbidity, length of hospital stay, and hospital costs are still unclear.

Cardiovascular Assessment

Interview

1. Chief complaint: identifies why the patient is seeking help and the duration of the problem
2. Symptoms related to cardiac disorders
a. Chest pain: may also be identified as indigestion, burning, discomfort, tightness, pressure in midchest, epigastrium, or left arm (Table 2-5 describes differentiation of chest pain)
(1) PQRST format for describing complaint
(a) P
(i) Provocation: What provokes or worsens the pain?
(ii) Palliation: What relieves the pain? (also include what was used but did not relieve pain)
(b) Q
(i) Quality: What does the pain feel like?
(c) R
(i) Region: Where is the pain?
(ii) Radiation: If the pain radiates, to what area does the pain radiate?
(d) S
(i) Severity: How severe is the pain?
a) Pain scale: The most frequently used scale in adults is the 1-to-10 scale with 1 being negligible and 10 being the worst imaginable.

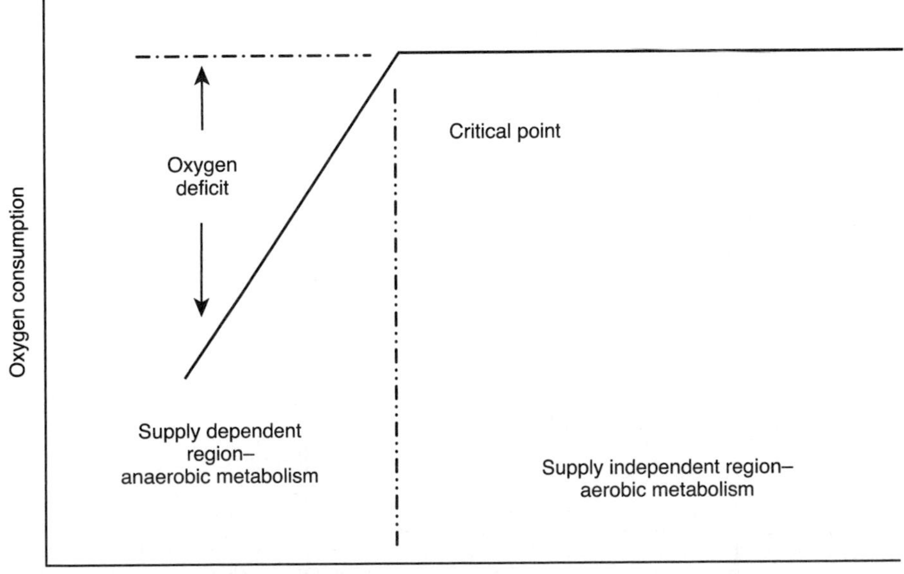

Figure 2-27 Critical oxygen delivery point. A critical level of oxygen delivery exists whereby oxygen delivery and consumption are independent. Once this critical oxygen delivery point is exceeded, oxygen consumption becomes dependent on oxygen delivery. (From Dantzker, D. R., & Scharf, S. M. [1998]. *Cardiopulmonary critical care*. Philadelphia: W. B. Saunders.)

Table 2-5 Differentiation of Chest Pain

Cause	Provocation	Palliation	Quality	Region/Radiation	Severity	Timing	Associated Signs/Symptoms
Angina pectoris	• Exercise • Exertion • Exposure to cold • Emotional stress • Eating • Smoking	• Rest • Oxygen • Nitroglycerin • Calcium channel blocker (e.g., nifedipine)	• Heaviness or pressure • Tightness • Squeezing • Dull ache • Burning • Not always described as pain but as discomfort	• Substernal • May be diffuse and vague • May radiate to arms, neck, jaw, back, upper abdomen	• Mild to severe	• Gradual or sudden onset • Duration: usually 1-4 minutes but may be 5-15 minutes	• Tachycardia, tachypnea • Dyspnea • Nausea, vomiting • Diaphoresis • Weakness • Anxiety • May have ST-T wave changes with pain
Acute myocardial infarction	• No specific precipitator • Lifestyle change and stress • Usually occurs within 3 hours of awakening	• Narcotics • Reperfusion by fibrinolytic or percutaneous coronary intervention (e.g., angioplasty, atherectomy) • No relief with rest and/or nitroglycerin	• As for angina • Heaviness or pressure • May show Levine's sign (clenched fist over sternum)	• As for angina	• No symptoms to severe • Absence of pain is common in patients with diabetes mellitus and in older adults	• Sudden onset • Duration: >30 minutes; usually 1-2 hours	• As for angina • Tachycardia, tachypnea • Dyspnea • Feeling of impending doom • S_4 • ECG changes: T wave inversion, ST segment elevation, eventually Q waves
Dissecting aortic aneurysm	• Peripheral vascular disease • Marfan syndrome • Aortitis • Hypertension and/or hypertensive crisis • Chest trauma	• Narcotics • Surgery • No relief with rest and/or nitroglycerin	• Tearing • Ripping	• Anterior chest • Radiation to shoulders, neck, back, abdomen	• Severe	• Sudden onset • Worse at onset • Duration: hours to days	• Tachycardia, tachypnea • Dysphagia • Confusion • Diaphoresis • Syncope • Dyspnea • Anxiety • Unilateral absence of pulse; BP differences between sides • Motor/sensory changes • Murmur of aortic regurgitation

Pericarditis	• Myocardial infarction • Cardiac surgery • Trauma • Infections • Uremia • Lupus erythematosus	• Nonsteroidal antiinflammatory agents (e.g., ibuprofen; indomethacin) • Sitting up and leaning forward	• Sharp • Stabbing • Knifelike • Worsened by inspiration, coughing, movement, recumbent position	• Precordial • Substernal • Radiation to neck, shoulders, arms, back	• Mild to severe	• Sudden onset • Duration: days	• Tachycardia, tachypnea • Fever • Dyspnea • Pericardial friction rub • Leukocytosis • Diffuse concave ST segment
Pulmonary embolism	• Venous stasis (e.g., immobility, pelvic surgery, atrial fibrillation) • Hypercoagulability (e.g., oral contraceptives, malignancy, polycythemia) • Injury to vessel wall (e.g., IVs, vascular surgery)	• Narcotics • High Fowler's position • Splinting of chest	• Sharp • Knifelike • Shooting • Deep ache • Pressure • Worsened by deep inspiration or coughing	• Substernal or lateral chest • Radiation to shoulder or neck	• Mild to severe	• Sudden onset • Duration: minutes to hours	• Tachycardia, tachypnea • Dyspnea • Pallor or cyanosis • Cough • Anxiety, feeling of impending doom • Sinus tachycardia or atrial dysrhythmias • Accentuated P_2 • Right-sided S_4, possible right-sided S_3 • If RVF: JVD • If pulmonary infarction: pleural friction rub, hemoptysis, fever

BP, Blood pressure; *ECG*, electrocardiagram; *NTG*, *SG*, fourth heart sound; *JVD*, Jugular venous distention; *P_2*, pulmonic component of second sound; *RVF*, right ventricular failure.

Continued

Table 2-5 Differentiation of Chest Pain—cont'd

Cause	Provocation	Palliation	Quality	Region/Radiation	Severity	Timing	Associated Signs/Symptoms
Pneumothorax	• Congenital bleb • Emphysematous bullous • Large tidal volumes or PEEP on mechanical ventilator • Chest trauma • Exacerbated by coughing, exertion, or Valsalva maneuver	• Narcotics • Insertion of chest tube	• Tearing • Sharp • Worsened by breathing	• Lateral chest • May radiate to shoulder, back, arms	• Mild to severe	• Sudden onset • Duration: hours to days	• Tachypnea • Tachycardia • Dyspnea • Anxiety • JVD • Hyperresonance to percussion of affected side • Diminished breath sounds on affected side • Subcutaneous emphysema may be seen • Tracheal deviation may be seen, especially with tension pneumothorax
Pleuropulmonary (e.g., pleurisy)	• Respiratory infection • Aspiration	• Narcotics • Relief with sitting up	• Sharp • Worsened by coughing, inspiration, or movement	• Lateral chest • May radiate to shoulder, neck	• Moderate	• Gradual onset • Duration: days to weeks	• Tachypnea • Tachycardia • Dyspnea • Fever • Productive cough • Pleural friction rub
Gastrointestinal chest pain	• Cold liquids • Food intake, especially spicy foods, acidic foods or foods high in fat • Alcohol • Caffeine • Stress • Smoking • Exercise	• Sitting up • Antacids • Esophageal spasm (may be relieved by nitroglycerin)	• "Heartburn" • Dull, burning • Squeezing • Worsened by eating or supine position	• Retrosternal or lower substernal • Upper abdomen • Midline • May radiate to left arm, neck, jaw, upper abdomen, back, shoulder	• Mild to moderate	• Gradual or sudden onset • Duration: minutes to days	• Dyspnea • Diaphoresis • Anxiety • Dysphagia • Eructation • Vomiting

Musculoskeletal chest pain	• Neck or arm strain • Movement • Coughing • Deep breathing • CPR	• Rest • Heat • Nonsteroidal antiinflammatory agents (e.g. aspirin, ibuprofen)	• Soreness • Stabbing or sticking sensation • Tenderness • Worsened with inspiration and movement	• Localized to one side of chest	• Mild to moderate	• Gradual or sudden onset • Duration: weeks	• Tachypnea • Splinting respirations • Localized tenderness over site of pain
Psychosomatic chest pain	• Stress • Fatigue	• Rest • Anxiolytics	• Dull ache • Sharp • Stabbing • Superficial	• Precordium • Localized; frequently on left side • No radiation	• Mild to moderate	• Gradual or sudden onset • Duration: minutes to days	• Hyperpnea • Dyspnea • Palpitations • Dry mouth • Dizziness • Tingling of hands, mouth • Fatigue • Frequent sighing

CPR, Cardiopulmonary resuscitation, *PEEP*, positive end-expiratory pressure; *RVF*, right ventricular failure; *JVD*, jugular vein distention.

(e) T
(i) Timing: Is the pain intermittent or continuous? What is the relationship to other events or activities?

b. Dyspnea
(1) Shortness of breath or "breathlessness"
(2) Exertional dyspnea
(3) Orthopnea: Patient is unable to lie flat because of dyspnea.
(4) Paroxysmal nocturnal dyspnea: Patient awakens with a feeling of suffocation 1 to 2 hours after going to sleep; if accompanied by wheezing, may be called *cardiac asthma*.

c. Cough: Cardiac cough usually occurs at night and is precipitated by supine position, exertion, or by turning to one side.
d. Hemoptysis: may be related to pulmonary edema.
e. Palpitations: unpleasant awareness of the heartbeat when at rest; may be described as skipping, pounding, thumping sensation; associated with premature beats or other dysrhythmia
f. Syncope
(1) Effort syncope: transient loss of consciousness that occurs shortly after heavy activity is started; may be associated with aortic or subaortic stenosis
(2) Stokes-Adams attack: dramatic loss of consciousness; related to heart block or dysrhythmia
(3) Pacemaker syncope: syncope caused by malfunction or failure of an artificial pacemaker
(4) Hypersensitive carotid sinus syncope: syncope caused by pressure applied on a carotid sinus body of a patient with atherosclerotic and hypersensitive carotid arteries

g. Headache: may be related to hypertension
h. Ascites: may be related to right ventricular failure
i. Abdominal pain: may be related to right ventricular failure
j. Edema or weight gain: frequently related to right ventricular failure; also described as bloated feeling, swelling, tightening of clothing, tightening of shoes, marks left from constricting garments
k. Fatigue or weakness: may be related to right ventricular failure
l. Nocturia: may be related to heart failure
m. Diaphoresis: may be related to sympathetic nervous system stimulation or infection
n. Unexplained joint pain: may be related to rheumatic fever
o. Intermittent claudication: hip, thigh, or calf pain that occurs with exercise and ceases with rest; indicative of peripheral arterial disease
p. Peripheral skin changes: decrease in hair distribution, skin color changes, skin ulcerations that will not heal, or a thin, shiny appearance to the skin may indicate peripheral vascular disease
q. Calf tenderness: may be related to thrombophlebitis; may be accompanied by red, warm skin over vein
r. Varicose veins: dilated, sometimes painful, veins

3. History of present illness: use PQRST format
a. Provocation, palliation
b. Quality, quantity
c. Region, radiation
d. Severity
e. Timing
f. Associated symptoms

4. Medical history
a. Past illnesses
(1) Coronary artery disease
(a) Angina
(b) Myocardial infarction
(2) Cerebrovascular disease: transient ischemic attacks or cerebral infarction (stroke)
(3) Dysrhythmias
(4) Hypertension
(5) Hyperlipidemia
(6) Peripheral vascular disease
(7) Rheumatic fever or rheumatic heart disease
(8) Murmur or known valvular heart disease
(9) Pulmonary disease (e.g., asthma or chronic obstructive pulmonary disease)
(10) Pulmonary embolism
(11) Connective tissue disorders
(12) Endocrine disorders especially diabetes mellitus
(13) Kidney disease
(14) Alcoholism
(15) Anemia
(16) Bleeding disorders

b. Past chest trauma: History of recent trauma is important to differentiate myocardial infarction from myocardial contusion; recent chest trauma would serve as a contraindication for fibrinolytics
c. Past surgical procedures
(1) Cardiac surgery: Identify whether coronary artery bypass grafting, valve replacement, or other type of cardiac surgery has been done.
(2) Percutaneous coronary intervention (PCI) procedures: angioplasty; atherectomy; stent placement; valvuloplasty
(3) Pacemaker insertion

d. Allergies and type of reaction
e. Past diagnostic studies (e.g., stress electrocardiogram, cardiac catheterization, and echocardiogram)

5. Family history
a. Coronary artery disease (CAD)
b. Cerebrovascular disease
c. Congenital heart defects
d. Sudden cardiac death
e. Peripheral vascular disease
f. Hypertension
g. Diabetes mellitus
h. Hyperlipidemia
i. Kidney disease
j. Bleeding disorders

6. Social history
   a. Relationship with spouse or significant other; family structure
   b. Occupation
   c. Educational level
   d. Usual activity level and ability to perform activities of daily living
   e. Stress level and usual coping mechanisms
   f. Personality type
      (1) Type A: sense of time urgency; hostility; aggression; ambition; competitiveness; impatience; frustration
      (2) Type B: none of the above qualities
   g. Recreational habits
   h. Exercise habits
   i. Dietary habits
   j. Caffeine intake
   k. Tobacco use: recorded as pack-years (number of packs per day times the number of years he or she has been smoking)
   l. Alcohol use: recorded as alcoholic beverages consumed per month, week, or day
   m. Toxin exposure
   n. Travel
7. Medication history
   a. Prescribed drug, dose, frequency, time of last dose
   b. Nonprescribed drugs
      (1) Over-the-counter drugs including herbal supplements
      (2) Substance abuse (e.g., cocaine and amphetamines)
   c. Patient's understanding of drug actions and side effects
   d. Drugs causing potential problems for patients with cardiovascular disease
      (1) Sinus or cold remedies: may contain ephedrine and increase blood pressure
      (2) Over-the-counter weight reduction agents: may contain ephedrine
      (3) Aspirin: prolongs blood clotting
      (4) Tricyclic antidepressants: may cause dysrhythmias (e.g., torsades de pointes)
      (5) Phenytoin: may cause dysrhythmias
      (6) Phenothiazines: may cause dysrhythmias, hypotension
      (7) Oral contraceptives: may predispose to embolus, thrombosis
      (8) Doxorubicin (Adriamycin): may cause cardiomyopathy
      (9) Lithium: may cause dysrhythmias
      (10) Corticosteroids: causes sodium and fluid retention and exacerbate heart failure
      (11) Theophylline preparations: cause tachycardia and may cause dysrhythmias
      (12) Cardiac stimulant (e.g., cocaine): cause tachycardia and may cause dysrhythmias and coronary artery spasm

Landmarks (Figure 2-28)

1. Anatomical
   a. Clavicle
   b. Sternum
   c. Ribs
   d. Intercostal spaces
   e. Angle of Louis
   f. Xiphoid process
   g. Costal margin
   h. Costal angle
2. Imaginary
   a. Midsternal line
   b. Midclavicular line
   c. Anterior axillary line
   d. Midaxillary line
   e. Posterior axillary line
   f. Scapular line
   g. Midspinal line
3. Location of heart
   a. Between the sternum and spinal column
   b. Lies between second intercostal space and fifth intercostal space
   c. Apex normally at fifth left intercostal space at midclavicular line

Inspection and Palpation

1. Vital signs
   a. Blood pressure: sitting; lying; standing
      (1) Reduction of up to 15 mm Hg in systolic and 5 mm Hg in diastolic blood pressure when standing is normal; greater reduction indicates orthostatic changes.
         (a) To assess for orthostatic changes, assist the patient to a standing position, wait 2 to 3 minutes, and then repeat measurement of blood pressure and heart rate.
      (2) Variation of up to 15 mm Hg between arms is normal.
      (3) Blood pressure in lower extremities is expected to be 10 mm Hg higher than in upper extremities.
      (4) Narrowed pulse pressure frequently indicates vasoconstriction as occurs with innervation of sympathetic nervous system (e.g., hypovolemic shock); widened pulse pressure frequently indicates excessive vasodilation as occurs with excessive vasodilatory mediator release (e.g., septic shock).
   b. Heart rate
      (1) Monitor rhythm if electrocardiogram monitor is available.
      (2) Tachycardia frequently indicates innervation of sympathetic nervous system.
   c. Respiratory (ventilatory) rate: Tachypnea frequently indicates innervation of sympathetic nervous system.
   d. Temperature: Fever may indicate inflammatory or infectious process (e.g., myocardial infarction, pericarditis, or endocarditis)
   e. Height
   f. Weight

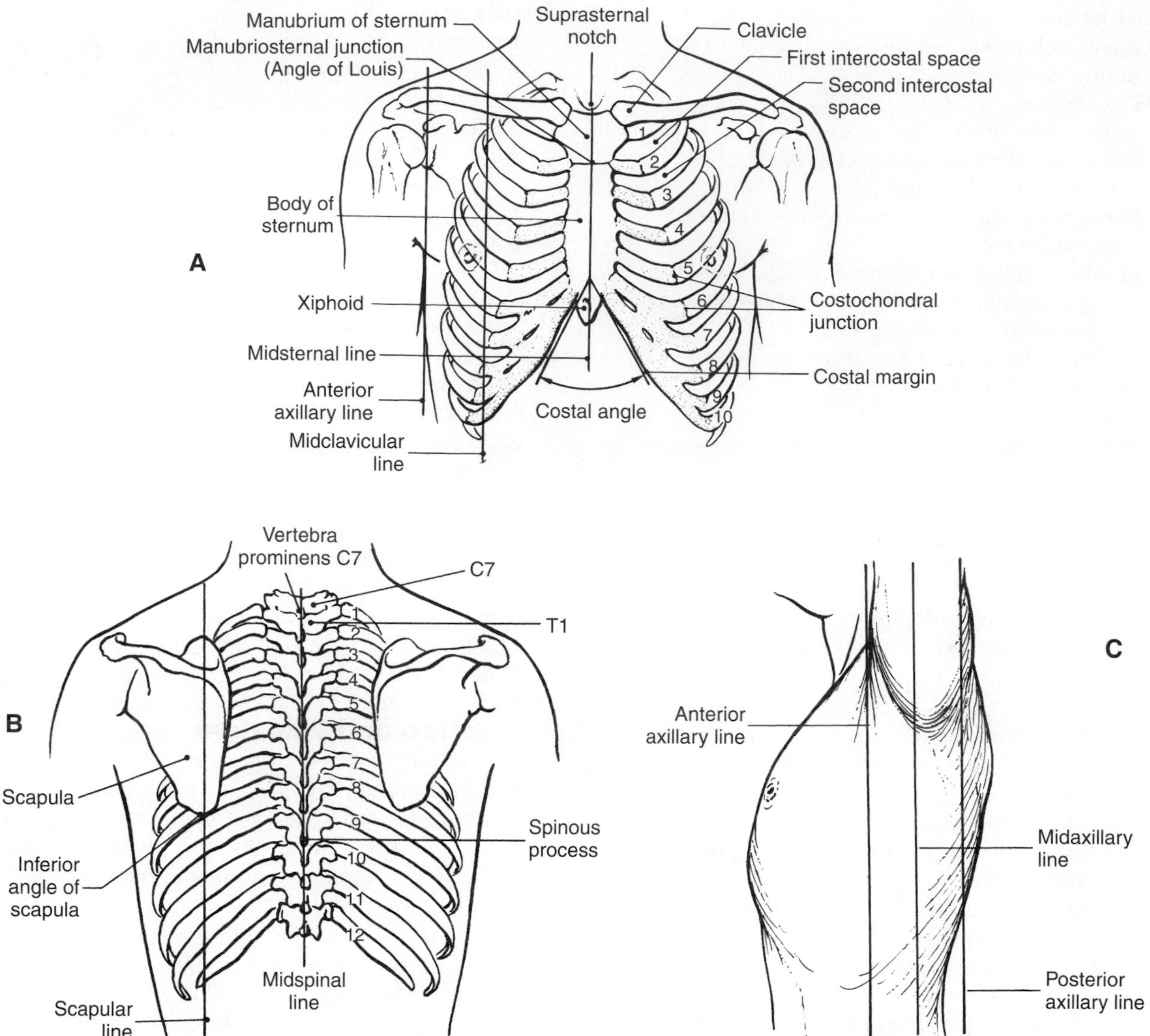

Figure 2-28 Landmarks of the thorax. **A,** Anterior. **B,** Posterior. **C,** Lateral. (From Barkauskas, V. [1994]. *Health and physical assessment.* St Louis: Mosby.)

2. General survey
   a. Apparent health status: consistency of apparent age and chronologic age
   b. Level of consciousness
   c. Gross deformity
   d. Nutritional status
   e. Stature/posture
   f. Gait
3. Skin and appendages
   a. Color
      (1) Pallor: may be indication of anemia, sympathetic nervous system innervation, or sympathomimetic agents (e.g., phenylephrine [Neo-Synephrine], norepinephrine [Levophed], or dopamine [Intropin])
      (2) Cyanosis
         (a) Peripheral (or cold) cyanosis is seen on fingertips and toes and is associated with peripheral hypoperfusion or vasoconstriction.
         (b) Central (or warm) cyanosis is seen on lips, tongue, and mucous membranes and is associated with 5 g/dL of deoxygenated hemoglobin
            (i) Central cyanosis may be late or impossible sign of hypoxemia in anemic patients.
            (ii) Central cyanosis may be a relatively early sign of hypoxemia in polycythemic patients; patients with chronic bronchitis are nicknamed *blue bloaters: blue* because of chronic hypoxemia and *bloaters* because of chronic right ventricular failure.
         (c) In dark skinned patients, cyanosis appears as an ashen color.
      (3) Ruddiness: related to polycythemia or hypercapnia
   b. Moisture: diaphoresis; dryness

c. Temperature: Cold skin may be related to hypoperfusion.
d. Turgor: Decrease in skin turgor, also referred to as *tenting,* are related to interstitial dehydration.
e. Edema
  (1) Edema indicates increase in interstitial fluid of 30% above normal.
  (2) Note the location of the edema.
    (a) Facial
      (i) Allergies: profound facial edema in anaphylaxis
      (ii) Steroids: exogenous (e.g., prednisone) or endogenous (e.g., Cushing's syndrome)
      (iii) Renal disease (e.g., nephrotic syndrome)
    (b) Dependent edema: right ventricular failure
    (c) Generalized edema (anasarca): end-stage heart failure; end-stage renal failure; severe hypoproteinemia
  (3) Degree of pitting
    (a) Grade 1+ = 0 to ¼ inch
    (b) Grade 2+ = ¼ to ½ inch
    (c) Grade 3+ = ½ to 1 inch
    (d) Grade 4+ = greater than 1 inch
f. Lesions
  (1) Arterial disease may cause ulcers at toes or points of trauma
  (2) Venous disease may cause ulcers at sides of ankles

4. Fingertips and nailbeds
  a. Color: bluish nailbeds with peripheral cyanosis
  b. Clubbing
    (1) Loss of normal angle between base of nail and skin; clubbing present if angle is greater than 180 degrees
    (2) Indicative of chronic hypoxia
  c. Splinter hemorrhages
    (1) Red to black linear streaks under nailbed that run from base to tip of nail
    (2) May indicate bacterial endocarditis
  d. Osler's nodes:
    (1) Painful red subcutaneous nodules on fingertips
    (2) May indicate embolization in infective endocarditis

5. Head and neck
  a. Face
    (1) Facial expression
    (2) Facial flushing: episodic facial flushing may indicate pheochromocytoma
  b. Head bobbing up and down with each heartbeat
    (1) Referred to as *de Musset's sign*
    (2) Indicates aortic aneurysm or regurgitation
  c. Eyes
    (1) Xanthoma palpebrarum (also called *xanthelasma*)
      (a) Benign, fatty, fibrous, yellowish plaque, nodule, or tumor on the eyelids
      (b) Associated with hyperlipidemia
    (2) Corneal arcus
      (a) Light-colored ring surrounding the iris
      (b) May be normal finding in elderly patient (called *arcus senilis*)
      (c) Abnormal in younger patient; associated with hyperlipidemia
    (3) Exophthalmos: may be seen in advanced heart failure with pulmonary hypertension
  d. Ears
    (1) Diagonal bilateral earlobe creases (referred to as *McCarty's sign*): may indicate coronary artery disease if seen in individuals under 45 years of age
  e. Neck
    (1) Jugular venous distention
      (a) To evaluate jugular venous distention (Figure 2-29)
        (i) Place patient in a 45-degree angle.
        (ii) Identify the sternal angle: raised notch that is created where the manubrium and the body of the sternum join; also called *manubriosternal junction* or *angle of Louis.*
        (iii) Measure height of neck vein distention above the level of the sternal angle.
        (iv) Normal height of neck vein distention is 1 to 2 cm above the sternal angle.
      (b) Neck vein distention of greater than 2 cm above the sternal angle is indicative of any of the following:
        (i) Right ventricular failure
        (ii) Hypervolemia
        (iii) Tension pneumothorax
        (iv) Cardiac tamponade

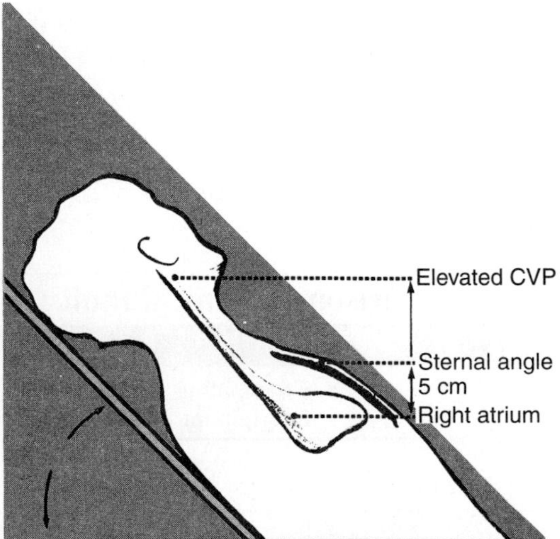

Figure 2-29 Jugular venous distention and estimation of central venous pressure *(CVP).* Assess jugular venous distention with patient in 45-degree angle. Determine height of jugular venous distention above the sternal angle. Add 5 cm to this measurement to estimate central venous pressure in centimeters of water pressure. (From Guzzetta, C. E., & Dossey, B. M. [1992]. *Cardiovascular nursing: Holistic practice.* St. Louis: Mosby.)

(c) To estimate central venous pressure
(i) Add 5 cm to the height of neck vein distention
(ii) Normal central venous pressure (in centimeters of water): 3 to 8
(d) To evaluate hepatojugular (or abdominojugular) reflux
(i) Apply pressure over right upper quadrant.
(ii) Evaluate increase in neck vein distention.
(iii) Increase in neck vein distention greater than 3 cm is indicative of hepatojugular reflux and right ventricular failure.

6. Precordium: inspect and palpate entire precordium
a. Point of maximal impulse or apical impulse
(1) Frequently visible and usually palpable; may not be palpable in patients with obesity, muscular chest wall, or an increased anterior-posterior diameter
(2) Location
(a) Normal location of the point of maximal impulse is at the fifth left intercostal space at the midclavicular line
(b) Lateral displacement is associated with any of the following:
(i) Left ventricular dilation (e.g., aortic or mitral insufficiency)
(ii) Upward displacement of the diaphragm (e.g., pregnancy or ascites)
(iii) Right to left mediastinal shift (e.g., right pleural effusion or tension pneumothorax)
(iv) Left ventricular hypertrophy or failure
(c) Medial displacement may occur with any of the following:
(i) Downward displacement of the diaphragm (e.g., chronic obstructive pulmonary disease)
(ii) Left to right mediastinal shift (e.g., left pleural effusion or tension pneumothorax)
(3) Intensity
(a) Normal intensity is only a light tap.
(b) Failure may cause increase the intensity and cause a heave.
(4) Size
(a) Normal size is approximately 1 to 2 cm.
(b) The size is more diffuse with ventricular aneurysm.
b. Heave
(1) Lifting of the chest wall is indicative of failure.
(2) Left ventricular heave felt at or near the apex.
(3) Right ventricular heave (or lift) felt at or near the sternum.
c. Thrill
(1) Palpable vibration associated with murmur or bruit
(2) Felt where the murmur is heard the loudest or at location of bruit

7. Abdomen
a. Aortic pulsation
(1) Normally visible, especially during expiration
(2) Normally palpable at midline or slightly to left of midline; feel for lateral expansion that might be indicative of aneurysm

8. Extremities
a. Arterial versus venous disease (Table 2-6)
b. Temperature
(1) Coolness or coldness may indicate decreased blood flow caused by hypoperfusion or vasoconstriction.
(2) Excessive warmth may indicate hyperthyroidism or fever.
c. Peripheral pulses
(1) Location (Figure 2-30)
(a) Carotid: Palpate only lower half and never palpate both carotid arteries simultaneously.
(b) Brachial
(c) Radial
(d) Ulnar
(e) Femoral
(f) Popliteal
(g) Posterior tibialis
(h) Dorsalis pedis

Table 2-6 Comparison of Clinical Indications of Arterial and Venous Peripheral Vascular Disease

	Arterial	Venous
Pain	• Excruciating in acute occlusion • Intermittent claudication in chronic occlusion	• Crampy pain • Homan's sign in thrombophlebitis
Pulses	• Diminished or absent	• Normal (but may be difficult to palpate because of edema)
Color	• Pale	• Normal or ruddy
Temperature	• Cool or cold	• Warm
Edema	• Absent	• Present; may be severe
Skin changes	• Thin, shiny, atrophic skin • Loss of hair • Thickened toenails	• Brown pigmentation at ankles
Ulcerations	• At toes or points of trauma	• At sides of ankles

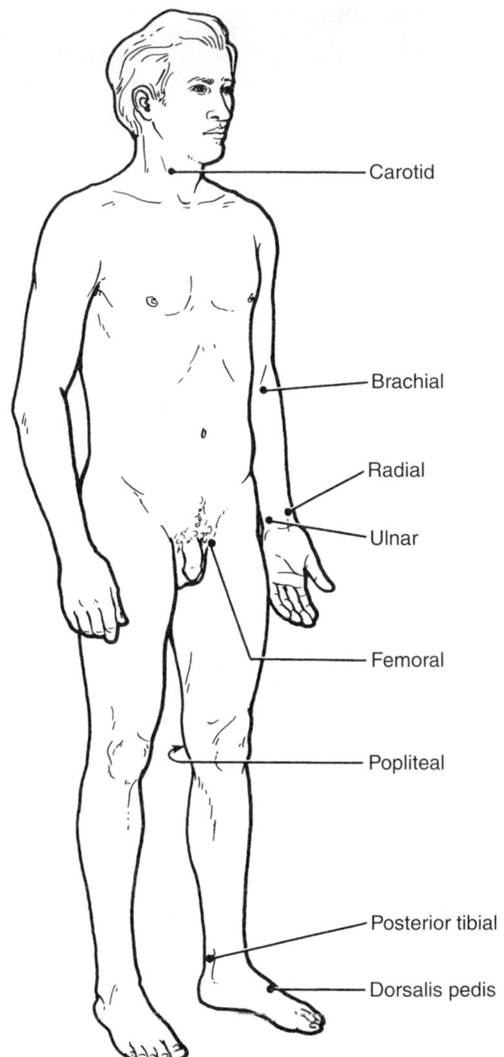

Figure 2-30 Locations of peripheral pulses. (From Lewis, S. M., & Collier, I. C. [1992]. *Medical-surgical nursing: Assessment and management of clinical problems* [3rd ed.]. St. Louis: Mosby.)

ARTERIAL PULSE ABNORMALITIES

Type	Description
Pulsus magnus	Pulse is readily palpable, not easily obliterated by fingers, and does not fade Pulse is felt as a brisk impact; can occur with or without increased pulse pressure
Pulsus parvus	Pulse is difficult to feel, easily obliterated by the fingers, and may fade out Pulse is slow to rise, has a sustained summit, and falls slowly If both weak and variable in amplitude, pulse is termed "thready"
Pulsus alterans	Pulses have large amplitude beats followed by pulses of small amplitude Rhythm remains normal
Pulsus paradoxus	Pattern is exaggerated (greater than 10 mm Hg) during inspiration, and amplitude is increased during expiration Heart rate and rhythm are unchanged Inspiration Expiration Inspiration
Pulsus bisferiens (double-peaked)	Best felt by palpating carotid artery Two systolic peaks occur in disorders that cause rapid left ventricular ejection of large stroke volume with wide pulse pressure
Water-hammer, collapsing	Pulse has greater amplitude than normal pulse Pulse marked by rapid rise to a narrow summit followed by a sudden descent

Figure 2-31 Pulse contour. (Modified from Cannobio, M. M. [1990]. *Cardiovascular disorders*. St. Louis: Mosby.)

(2) Rate and rhythm
(3) Amplitude
 (a) 0 = not palpable
 (b) 1+ = weak and thready, easily obliterated
 (c) 2+ = normal, not easily obliterated
 (d) 3+ = full and bounding, cannot be obliterated
(4) Capillary refill rate
 (a) Color should return to blanched area within 3 seconds; delay beyond 3 seconds indicates hypoperfusion.
(5) Apical-radial pulse deficit
 (a) Performed by two nurses using one watch
 (b) Deficit (radial pulse rate less than apical rate) indicative of dysrhythmia (e.g., atrial fibrillation or ventricular ectopy)
(6) Pulse contour (Figure 2-31)
 (a) Pulsus magnus
  (i) Strong, bounding pulses with rapid upstroke and downstroke
  (ii) Characteristic of any of the following:
   a) Hypertension
   b) Thyrotoxicosis
   c) Aortic insufficiency
   d) Patent ductus arteriosus
   e) Arteriovenous fistula
 (b) Pulsus parvus
  (i) Small, weak pulse
  (ii) Characteristic of any of the following:
   a) Aortic stenosis: also pulsus tardus (late)
   b) Mitral stenosis
   c) Constrictive pericarditis
   d) Cardiac tamponade

(c) Pulsus alternans
(i) Alternating pulse waves, every other beat being weaker than the preceding one
(ii) Characteristic of left ventricular failure
(d) Pulsus paradoxus
(i) Pulsus paradoxus is an exaggeration of normal physiologic response to inspiration
a) The normal decrease in blood pressure during inspiration is 10 mm Hg or less.
b) Blood pressure drop of more than 10 mm Hg during inspiration is pulsus paradoxus.
(ii) Pulsus paradoxus may be characteristic of any of the following conditions:
a) Pericardial effusion
b) Constrictive pericarditis
c) Cardiac tamponade
d) Severe lung disease
e) Advanced heart failure
f) Hemorrhagic shock
(e) Pulsus bisferiens
(i) Two pulses palpated during systole with second slightly weaker than the first
(ii) Characteristic of any of the following:
a) Hypertrophic cardiomyopathy
b) Constrictive cardiomyopathy
c) Aortic stenosis or regurgitation
(f) Water-hammer (or *Corrigan's*) pulse
(i) Increased pulse pressure with a rapid upstroke and downstroke and shortened peak
(ii) Characteristic of aortic regurgitation
d. Homans' sign
(1) Identified by dorsiflexing the foot with the knee slightly bent
(2) Homans' sign is present if the patient has pain in the calf with this action
(3) Suggestive of thrombophlebitis
e. Petechiae or ecchymosis
f. Varicose veins
g. Neurovascular assessment
(1) Assess neurovascular status in all of the following situations:
(a) After cardiac catheterization
(b) After percutaneous coronary intervention (e.g., angioplasty, atherectomy, or valvuloplasty)
(c) When the patient has intraaortic balloon pump catheter in place
(d) When the patient has a fracture of an extremity (to monitor for compartment syndrome)
(e) When the patient has a circumferential burn of an extremity

BOX 2-1 Clinical Manifestations of Acute Arterial Occlusion

Pain
Pallor
Pulselessness
Paresthesia
Paralysis
Polar (cold)

Note: These six *P*s are your format for neurovascular assessment.

(2) Monitor for clinical indications of acute arterial occlusion: six *P*s (Box 2-1)
h. Clinical indications of hypoperfusion (Table 2-2); because hypoperfusion is progressive, the earlier these changes are identified, the more appropriate the management and the chances for successfully reversing these changes

Auscultation

1. Qualities of a good stethoscope
a. Snug-fitting earplugs to eliminate extraneous sounds
b. Tubing
(1) Two tubings are preferable for high-frequency sounds.
(2) Tubing should be not longer than 12 to 15 inches.
c. Chest piece
(1) Diaphragm
(a) Used for high-pitched sounds (e.g., S_1, S_2, splits of S_1 and S_2, pericardial friction rubs, and most murmurs)
(b) Held firmly against skin
(2) Bell
(a) Used for low-pitched sounds (e.g., S_3, S_4, and murmurs of atrioventricular valve stenosis)
(b) Held only tightly enough against skin to create a seal
2. Auscultatory areas (Figure 2-32)
a. Mitral: fifth left intercostal space at midclavicular line
b. Tricuspid: fifth left intercostal space at left sternal border
c. Erb's point: third left intercostal space at left sternal border
d. Pulmonic: second left intercostal space at left sternal border
e. Aortic: second right intercostal space at right sternal border
3. Method of cardiac auscultation
a. Ensure a quiet room by turning off television and radio and asking others to be quiet.
b. Listen to all four auscultatory area with bell and diaphragm.
c. Concentrate on one cardiac event at a time: S_1; S_2; systole; diastole.

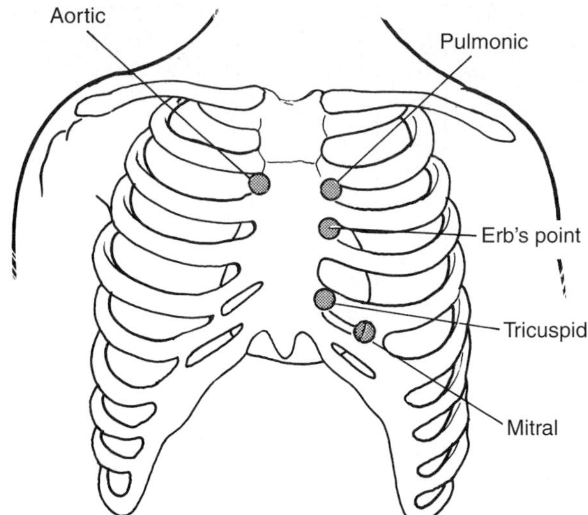

Figure 2-32 Cardiac auscultatory areas. (From Price, S. A., & Wilson, L. M. [1994]. *Pathophysiology: Clinical concepts of disease processes* [4th ed.]. St. Louis: Mosby.)

4. Heart sounds
 a. Rules to consider
  (1) Heart events of the left side precede heart events of the right side (i.e., the mitral component [M_1] precedes the tricuspid component [T_1] of S_1, and the aortic component [A_2] precedes the pulmonic component [P_2] of S_2).
  (2) Heart events of the left side are normally louder than heart events of the right side (i.e., M_1 is the loudest component of S_1, and A_2 is the loudest component of S_2).
  (3) Heart events of the left side are normally loudest during expiration, and heart events of the right side are normally loudest during inspiration.
 b. S_1
  (1) Caused by closure of the atrioventricular valves: mitral and tricuspid
  (2) Marks the end of diastole and the beginning of systole
  (3) Loudest at the apex
  (4) Note if single sound or split
  (5) Note any increase in intensity (closing snap)
 c. S_2
  (1) Caused by closure of the semilunar valves: aortic and pulmonic
  (2) Marks the end of systole and the beginning of diastole
  (3) Loudest at the base
  (4) Note if single sound or split
  (5) Note any increase in intensity
 d. Splits
  (1) Split S_1
   (a) Both components (M_1 and T_1) of S_1 can be heard.
   (b) A split S_1 is heard best at the tricuspid area.
   (c) A narrowly split S_1 may be normal.
   (d) A split S_1 is more often abnormal than normal and is associated with any of the following:
    (i) Right bundle branch block
    (ii) Left ventricular (epicardial) pacemaker
    (iii) Left ventricular ectopy
  (2) Split S_2
   (a) Both components (A_2 and P_2) of S_2 can be heard.
   (b) A split S_2 is heard best at the pulmonic area.
   (c) Inspiratory only split of S_2 is normal.
    (i) Called a *physiologic split of S_2*
    (ii) Normal and frequently heard in individuals under 50 years of age
    (iii) Split only during inspiration
    (iv) Caused by changes in intrathoracic pressure related to ventilation; increased venous return to right ventricle and decreased venous return to left ventricle delay pulmonic valve closure (P_2)
   (d) Expiratory split of S_2 is abnormal
    (i) Increased splitting during inspiration (split on expiration but split more during inspiration); associated with any of the following:
     a) Right bundle branch block
     b) Left ventricular ectopy
     c) Left ventricular (epicardial) pacemaker
     d) Severe mitral regurgitation
     e) Pulmonary stenosis
     f) Pulmonary hypertension
     g) Ventricular septal defect
    (ii) Fixed splitting (split the same on inspiration and expiration); associated with atrial septal defect
    (iii) Paradoxical split (split on expiration but not on inspiration); associated with any of the following:
     a) Left bundle branch block
     b) Right ventricular (endocardial) pacemaker
     c) Right ventricular ectopy
     d) Severe aortic stenosis or regurgitation
     e) Patent ductus arteriosus
 e. Extra heart sounds (Table 2-7 is a summary of extra heart sounds)
  (1) S_3
   (a) Also called a *ventricular gallop*
   (b) Dull, low-pitched sound occurring early in diastole after S_2; may sound like "Ken-tuc-ky" with the "ky" being the S_3
   (c) Caused by rapid rush of blood into a dilated ventricle; considered abnormal in patients over 30 years of age

Table 2-7 Extra Sounds

Sound	Cause	Timing	Location	Pitch	Position	Respiratory Effect
S_3 (also called *ventricular gallop*)	Rapid ventricular filling into dilated ventricle	Early diastole (rapid filling phase of diastole)	Mitral if LV; tricuspid if RV	Low	Heard best in left lateral position	LV S_3 increases with expiration; RV S_3 increases with inspiration
S_4 (also called *atrial gallop*)	Atrial contraction into noncompliant ventricle	Late diastole (atrial contraction phase of diastole)	Mitral area if LV; tricuspid area if RV	Low	Heard best in left lateral position	LV S_4 increased with expiration; RV S_4 increased with inspiration
Quadruple rhythm	All four heart sounds are heard	S_3 heard in early diastole, and S_4 heard in late diastole	Apex	Low	Heard best in left lateral position	As for S_3, S_4
Summation gallop	S_1, S_2 heard along with merged S_3 and S_4; occurs with tachycardia	Mid-diastole	Apex	Low	Heard best in left lateral position	As for S_3, S_4
Pericardial friction rub	Inflammation of the pericardium	Systolic, early diastolic, and late diastolic components	Lower left sternal border	High	Heard best with patient leaning forward	Heard best if patient holds breath after expiration
Pericardial knock	Constriction of the pericardium	Early diastole	Lower left sternal border	Low	Heard best with patient leaning forward or in left lateral position	Heard best if patient holds breath after expiration
Ejection click	Opening of defective semilunar valve	Early systole	Aortic or pulmonic	High	Heard best with patient leaning forward	Aortic: not affected by respiratory phase Pulmonic: increased with expiration
Midsystolic click	Prolapse of mitral valve leaflet	Mid-systole	Mitral	High	Heard best in left lateral position	Increased with expiration
Opening snap	Abrupt recoil of stenotic atrioventricular valve	Early diastole	Mitral	High	Heard best in left lateral position	Mitral: increased with expiration Tricuspid: increased with inspiration
Mediastinal crunch	Pneumomediastinum; heart movements displacing air that is present in the mediastinum	Random	Apex or lower left sternal border	High	Heard best in left lateral position	Increased with inspiration

LV, Left ventricle; *RV*, right ventricle; S_1, first heart sound; S_2, second heart sound; S_3, third heart sound; S_4, fourth heart sound.

(d) Heard best with bell, with the patient lying on the left side
(i) Left-sided S_3
a) Heard best at apex
b) Heard best during expiration
(ii) Right-sided S_3
a) Heard best at sternum
b) Heard best during inspiration
(e) Associated primarily with failure
(f) Also may be associated with any of the following:
(i) Fluid overload
(ii) Cardiomyopathy
(iii) Ventricular septal defect or patent ductus arteriosus
(iv) Mitral or tricuspid regurgitation
(2) S_4
(a) Also called an *atrial gallop*
(b) Dull, low-pitched sound occurring late in diastole before S_1; may sound like "Ten-nes-see" with the "Ten" being the S_4
(c) Caused by atrial contraction of blood into a noncompliant ventricle; abnormal in adults
(d) Heard best with bell with patient lying on the left side
(i) Left-sided S_4: heard best at apex
(ii) Right-sided S_4: heard best at sternum
(e) Associated with any of the following:
(i) Myocardial ischemia or infarction
(ii) Hypertension
a) Systemic: left-sided S_4
b) Pulmonary: right-sided S_4
(iii) Ventricular hypertrophy
(iv) Atrioventricular blocks
(v) Severe aortic or pulmonic stenosis
(3) Quadruple rhythm: all four heart sounds heard
(4) Summation gallop
(a) All four heart sounds with tachycardia
(b) Merging of S_3 and S_4 causes a louder middiastolic sound
(5) Pericardial friction rub
(a) High-pitched "to-and-fro" scratchy sound; usually triphasic including systolic, early diastolic, and late diastolic components
(b) Heard best at the fourth/fifth intercostal space at lower left sternal border with patient leaning forward
(c) Differentiate between pericardial and pleural friction rubs: ask the patient to hold his or her breath; if the rub persists, it is a pericardial friction rub
(d) Caused by inflammation of the pericardium; commonly heard after myocardial infarction or cardiac surgery
(6) Pericardial knock
(a) Loud, early diastolic sound heard best at lower left sternal border
(b) Caused by constrictive pericarditis
(7) Snaps
(a) Opening snap
(i) Short, high-pitched sound heard early in diastole at third/fourth left intercostal space at left sternal border; earlier, sharper, higher pitched than S_3
(ii) Caused by either of the following:
a) Opening of stenotic atrioventricular valve; usually precedes a diastolic murmur
b) Increased flow (e.g., ventricular septal defect or patent ductus arteriosus)
(b) Closing snap
(i) Really a loud S_1
(ii) Caused by closure of atrioventricular valve
(8) Clicks: high-pitched sounds heard during systole
(a) Aortic ejection click
(i) High-pitched sound heard early in systole over aortic area to apex; may precede systolic ejection murmur
(ii) Caused by aortic valve disease or dilated aorta (e.g., aortic aneurysm or coarctation)
(b) Pulmonic ejection click
(i) High-pitched sound heard early in systole over pulmonic area
(ii) Caused by pulmonic valve disease, pulmonary embolism, pulmonary hypertension, hyperthyroidism
(c) Midsystolic click
(i) High-pitched sound heard best at apex or lower left sternal border
(ii) May occur alone or before a late systolic murmur
(iii) Caused by mitral valve prolapse or mitral regurgitation
(d) Prosthetic valve click: metallic click caused by opening and closing of prosthetic valve
(9) Mediastinal crunch
(a) Crunching sound heard best at apex or along left sternal border in left lateral position
(b) Caused by air in mediastinum

f. Murmurs
(1) Causes of turbulence (referred to as a *murmur* if intracardiac or referred to as a *bruit* if extracardiac) (Figure 2-33)
(a) Increased flow across a normal valve (e.g., flow murmur)
(i) Also may be called *functional* (as opposed to structural); always soft (not louder than grade II/VI) and systolic (but never holosystolic)
(ii) Caused by any of the following:
(a) Hyperthermia
(b) Anemia
(c) Pregnancy
(d) Hyperthyroidism

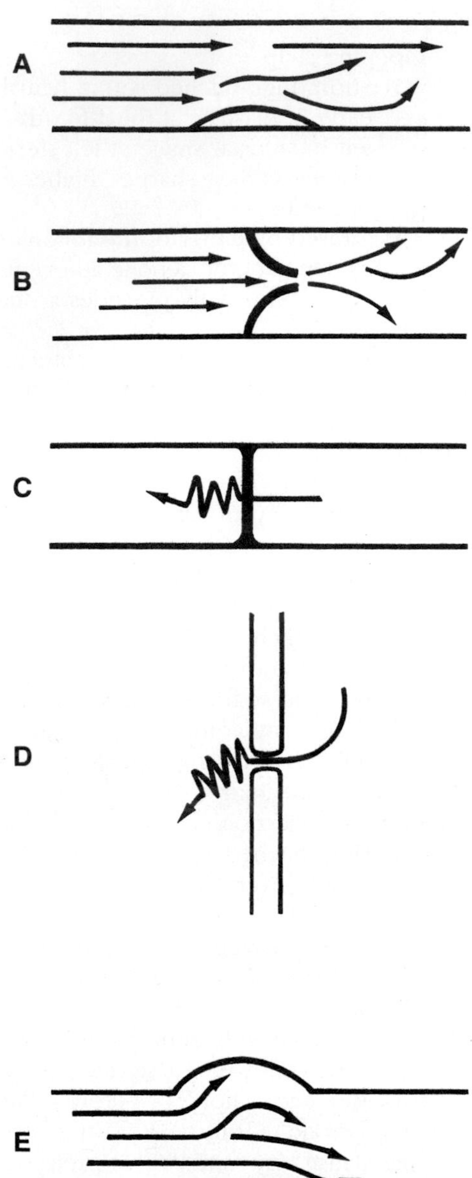

Figure 2-33 Causes of turbulence. **A,** Increased flow across a normal valve. **B,** Forward flow through a stenotic valve. **C,** Backward flow through an incompetent valve. **D,** Flow through a septal defect or an atrioventricular fistula. **E,** Flow into a dilated chamber or a portion of a vessel. (From Thompson, D. A. [1981]. *Cardiovascular assessment.* St. Louis: Mosby.)

(b) Forward flow through a stenotic valve
(c) Backward flow through a regurgitant (also called *insufficient* or *incompetent*) valve
(d) Flow through an atrioventricular fistula or septal defect
(e) Flow into a dilated chamber or a portion of a vessel

(2) Description
(a) Timing
(i) Systolic
a) Holosystolic: atrioventricular regurgitation or ventricular septal defect
b) Ejection (midsystolic): semilunar stenosis
c) Late: papillary muscle dysfunction, mitral valve prolapse, hypertrophic cardiomyopathy (previously called *idiopathic hypertrophic subaortic stenosis*)
(ii) Diastolic
a) Early diastolic: semilunar regurgitation
b) Middiastolic or late diastolic: atrioventricular stenosis
(b) Location: place at which the murmur is loudest
(c) Radiation: direction in which the murmur radiates
(d) Intensity: Levine scale
(i) Grade I/VI: barely audible, difficult to detect
(ii) Grade II/VI: clearly audible but quiet
(iii) Grade III/VI: moderately loud, without a thrill
(iv) Grade IV/VI: loud; with or without a thrill
(v) Grade V/VI: very loud, thrill present, audible with stethoscope partially off the chest
(vi) Grade VI/VI: loudest possible, thrill present, audible with stethoscope off the chest
(e) Configuration
(i) Crescendo: gets louder
(ii) Decrescendo: gets softer
(iii) Crescendo-decrescendo: louder then softer
(iv) Plateau: even intensity throughout
(f) Pitch
(i) High pitched (heard best with diaphragm)
a) Mitral and tricuspid regurgitation
b) Aortic and pulmonic stenosis
c) Aortic and pulmonic regurgitation
(ii) Low pitched (heard best with bell): mitral and tricuspid stenosis
(g) Quality
(i) Soft
(ii) Harsh
(iii) Blowing
(iv) Musical
(v) Rumbling
(vi) Rough

(3) Table 2-8 describes common murmurs.

5. Vascular sound
a. Bruit
(1) Turbulent sound
(2) May be heard over carotid arteries, aorta, and renal, iliac, and femoral arteries
(3) Associated with plaque or aneurysm

Table 2-8 Common Murmurs

Timing	Location	Radiation	Intensity	Configuration	Pitch	Quality	Condition
Holosystolic	Mitral	Toward left axilla	I-V/VI	Plateau	High	Blowing, harsh, or musical	Mitral regurgitation
Holosystolic	Tricuspid	Along right sternal border toward apex if radiates	I-V/VI	Plateau	High	Blowing, harsh, or musical	Tricuspid regurgitation
Holosystolic	3-4 intercostal space at lower sternal border	Radiates widely throughout precordium	Varies	Plateau	High	Harsh	Ventricular septal rupture or defect
Midsystolic (systolic ejection murmur)	Aortic	Toward right side of neck	Varies	Crescendo-decrescendo	Medium to high	Harsh	Aortic stenosis
Midsystolic (systolic ejection murmur)	Pulmonic	No radiation or toward left side of neck	III-IV/VI	Crescendo-decrescendo	Medium to high	Harsh	Pulmonic stenosis
Early diastole	Aortic or Erb's point	Toward apex	I-VI/VI	Decrescendo	High	Blowing	Aortic regurgitation
Early diastole	Pulmonic	Toward apex if radiates	Varies	Decrescendo	High	Blowing	Pulmonic regurgitation
Mid to late diastole	Mitral	Usually none	I-II/VI	Crescendo	Low	Rumbling	Mitral stenosis
Mid to late diastole	Tricuspid	Usually none; may radiate to apex or xiphoid	Varies	Decrescendo	Low	Rumbling	Tricuspid stenosis

ICS, Intercostal space.

b. Doppler pulse
   (1) A Doppler stethoscope is used to identify presence of pulse if the pulse is not palpable and may be used to confirm that the pulse palpated is the patient's and not the nurse's.
c. Doppler pressure
   (1) A Doppler stethoscope is used to measure the blood pressure distal to vascular lesions or surgery.
   (2) Apply sphygmomanometer on the calf or below the graft site and inflate to a pressure above the patient's systolic brachial pressure; allow pressure to decrease, and note pressure when pulse is audible again; note posterior tibial pressure and dorsalis pedis pressures.
   (3) Use the best pressure (posterior tibial or dorsalis pedis) to calculate the ankle-brachial index (ABI).
      (a) Divide the systolic pressure from the leg by the brachial systolic pressure (ankle/brachial) to calculate the ankle-brachial index.
      (b) Evaluation
         (i) Unreliable: greater than 1; consider using toe/brachial index described subsequently
         (ii) Normal: 0.95 to 1
         (iii) Mildly abnormal: 0.95 to 0.75
         (iv) Claudicant: 0.75 to 0.5
         (v) Ischemic: 0.5 to 0.25
         (vi) Severe ischemia: less than 0.25
         (vii) Clinically significant: decrease of 0.15 or more
      (c) Some recommend toe/brachial index using the systolic pressure of the great toe and dividing it by the brachial systolic pressure; normal and abnormal values are the same as for ankle-brachial index.

Diagnostic Studies

1. Serum chemistries
   a. Sodium: normal 136 to 145 mEq/L
   b. Potassium: normal 3.5 to 5.5 mEq/L
   c. Chloride: normal 96 to 106 mEq/L
   d. Calcium: normal 8.5 to 10.5 mg/dL
   e. Phosphorus: normal 3 to 4.5 mg/dL
   f. Magnesium: normal 1.5 to 2.2 mEq/L or 1.8 to 2.4 mg/dL
   g. Glucose: normal 70 to 110 mg/dL
   h. Blood urea nitrogen: normal 5 to 20 mg/dL
   i. Creatinine: normal 0.7 to 1.5 mg/dL
   j. Enzymes
      (1) Total creatine kinase: normal 55 to 170 units/L for males; 30 to 135 units/L for females
      (2) Creatine-kinase, myocardial bound: 0% of total creatine kinase
      (3) L-lactate dehydrogenase: 90 to 200 units/L
      (4) L-lactate dehydrogenase-1: 17% to 25% of total L-lactate dehydrogenase
   k. Muscle proteins
      (1) Myoglobin: normal less than 110 ng/mL
      (2) Troponin I: normal less than 1.5 ng/mL
      (3) Troponin T: normal less than 0.1 ng/mL
   l. Lipid profile
      (1) Cholesterol: normal 150 to 200 mg/dL
      (2) Triglycerides: normal 40 to 150 mg/dL
      (3) Lipoprotein-cholesterol fractionation
         (a) High-density lipoprotein: normal 29 to 77 mg/dL
         (b) Low-density lipoprotein: normal 62 to 130 mg/dL
   m. Homocysteine: normal less than 15 μmol/L
   n. C-reactive protein: normal less than 1 mg/dL
   o. Brain-type natruretic peptide: normal less than 100 pg/mL
      (1) Heart failure
         (a) Mild: 100 to 300 pg/mL
         (b) Moderate: 300 to 700 pg/mL
         (c) Severe: more than 700 pg/mL
      (2) Also may be earlier indicator of acute myocardial infarction than either creatine kinase (myocardial bound) or troponin I
2. Arterial blood gases
   a. pH: normal 7.35 to 7.45
   b. $Paco_2$: normal 35 to 45 mm Hg
   c. Hco_3: normal 22 to 26 mM
   d. Pao_2: normal 80 to 100 mm Hg
   e. Sao_2: greater than 95%
   f. Arterial lactate: less than 1 mmol/L
3. Hematology
   a. Hematocrit: normal 40% to 52% for males; 35% to 47% for females
   b. Hemoglobin: normal 13 to 18 g/dL for males; 12 to 16 g/dL for females
   c. White blood cells: normal 3500 to 11,000 cells/mm^3
   d. Erythrocyte sedimentation rate: normal up to 15 mm/hr for males; up to 20 mm/hr for females
4. Clotting profile
   a. Prothrombin time: normal 12 to 15 seconds; therapeutic 1.5 to 2.5 times normal
   b. Partial thromboplastin time: normal 60 to 90 seconds; therapeutic 1.5 to 2.5 times normal
   c. Activated partial thromboplastin time: normal 25 to 38 seconds; therapeutic 1.5 to 2.5 times normal
   d. Activated clotting time: normal 70 to 120 seconds; therapeutic 150 to 190 seconds
   e. Thrombin time: normal 10 to 15 seconds
   f. Bleeding time: normal 1 to 9½ minutes
   g. International normalized ratio: normal less than 2
      (1) Therapeutic range for atrial fibrillation: 1.5 to 2.5
      (2) Therapeutic range for deep vein thrombosis or pulmonary embolus: 2 to 3
      (3) Therapeutic range for prosthetic valves: 2.5 to 3.5
   h. Platelets: normal 150,000 to 400,000 cells/mm^3
5. Urine
   a. Glucose: normal negative
   b. Ketones: normal negative
   c. Specific gravity: 1.005 to 1.03
   d. Osmolality: 50 to 1200 mOsm/L
6. Other diagnostic studies (Table 2-9)

Table 2-9 Cardiovascular Diagnostic Studies

Study	Evaluates	Comments
Aortography	• Aortic valve insufficiency • Aneurysms or dissection of ascending aorta • Coarctation of the aorta • Injuries to the aorta and major branches	• Contrast medium used: Check for allergy to iodine, shellfish, dye; ensure hydration following procedure. • Monitor for clinical indications of anaphylaxis (e.g., flushing, urticaria, and stridor). • Monitor puncture site.
Cardiac biopsy	• Effect of cardiotoxic drugs • Evidence of cardiac transplant rejection • Inflammatory heart disease • Tumors • Cardiomyopathy	• Observe closely for signs of cardiac perforation and/or cardiac tamponade.
Cardiac catheterization and coronary angiography	• Severity of coronary artery stenosis • Cardiac muscle function • Pressures within the heart • Cardiac output and ejection fraction • Blood gas analysis within chambers • Allows angioplasty, atherectomy, intracoronary stents, or lasers to reduce coronary artery obstruction	• Before test: ◦ Check for allergy to iodine, shellfish, dye (contrast medium used). • After the test: ◦ Ensure hydration following procedure (contrast medium used). ◦ Keep extremity in which catheter was placed immobilized in a straight position for 6-12 hours. ◦ Monitor arterial puncture point for hemorrhage or hematoma. ◦ Monitor neurovascular status of affected limb. ◦ Note complaints of back pain and vital sign changes (may indicate retroperitoneal hemorrhage).
Chest radiography	• Cardiac size and shape • Presence of pulmonary congestion or pleural effusions • Presence of thoracic aneurysm or calcification of the aorta • Position of pulmonary artery and cardiac catheter, pacemaker, or wires	• Inquire about possibility of pregnancy.
Computed tomography	• Left ventricular wall motion • Cardiac tumors • Myocardial infarction • Pericardial effusion • Aortic aneurysm • Aortic dissection	• Examination may be done with or without contrast medium. • If contrast medium used, check for allergy to iodine, shellfish, dye, and ensure hydration following procedure.
Digital subtraction angiography	• Vascular disease and degree of occlusion	• Contrast medium used: Check for allergy to iodine, shellfish, dye; ensure hydration following procedure. • Monitor for clinical indications of anaphylaxis (e.g., flushing, urticaria, and stridor). • Monitor puncture site.
Doppler ultrasonography Duplex ultrasonography	• Vascular disease and degree of occlusion	
Echocardiography • M-mode: single ultrasound beam • Two-dimensional: planar ultrasound beam; wider view of heart and structures • Doppler: addition of Doppler to demonstrate flow of blood through the heart	• Chamber size and wall thickness • Valve functioning ◦ Papillary muscle functioning ◦ Prosthetic valve functioning • Ventricular wall motion abnormalities • Intracardiac masses • Presence of pericardial fluid • Intracardiac pressures (Doppler) • Ejection fraction and cardiac output (Doppler) • Valve gradients (Doppler)	• Transesophageal echocardiography is particularly better if patient is obese, has chronic obstructive pulmonary disease, chest wall deformity, chest trauma, or thick chest dressings. • Monitor for methemoglobinemia if local anesthetic (e.g., Cetacaine) is used.

Continued

Table 2-9 Cardiovascular Diagnostic Studies—cont'd

Study	Evaluates	Comments
• Color flow: Doppler blood flow superimposed on two-dimensional echocardiogram • Stress echocardiography: images before, during, and after exercise or pharmacologic stress • Transesophageal echocardiography: transducer placed in esophagus	• Intracardiac shunts (Doppler) • Thoracic aneurysm (transesophageal)	
Electrocardiography	• Dysrhythmias • Conduction defects including intraventricular blocks • Electrolyte imbalance • Drug toxicity • Myocardial ischemia, injury, infarction • Chamber hypertrophy	• List what drugs the patient is receiving on request of electrocardiogram. • Be alert to electrical safety hazards.
Electrophysiologic studies	• Dysrhythmias under controlled circumstances • Best therapy for control of dysrhythmia: drug, required dosage of therapy; pacemaker; catheter ablation	• Patients may have near-death experience during electrophysiologic studies; encourage expression of fears, concerns, anxieties. • Monitor puncture site.
Holter monitor	• Suspected dysrhythmias over 24-hour period • Pacemaker function • Silent ischemia	• Instruct patient regarding importance of diary-keeping.
Intravascular ultrasound	• Coronary artery size and patency • Structure of vessel wall • Coronary artery stent position and patency • Aorta and presence of aneurysm, aneurysm dissections	• As for cardiac catheterization
Magnetic resonance imaging	• Three-dimensional view of the heart • Anatomy and structure of the heart and great vessels including cardiomyopathy; congenital defect; masses; aneurysm • Changes in chemistry of tissues before structural changes occur	• Test does not involve radiation or dyes. • Test cannot be used in patients with any implanted metallic device, including pacemakers, implantable defibrillators, metallic heart valves, or intracranial aneurysm clips.
Multiple-gated acquisition scan (radionuclide angiography)	• Ventricular size and ventricular wall motion • Cardiac output, cardiac index, end-systolic volume, end-diastolic volume, and ejection fraction • Intracardiac shunts	• Assure patient that amount of radioactive material is minimal.
Pericardiocentesis and pericardial fluid analysis	• Presence of blood, pus, pathogens, or malignancy • Also used for emergency relief of cardiac tamponade	• Observe closely for signs of cardiac tamponade.
Peripheral angiography	• Atherosclerotic plaques, occlusion, aneurysms, or traumatic injury	• Before test: ◦ Contrast medium is used—check for allergy to iodine, shellfish, or dye. • After the test: ◦ Contrast medium is used—ensure hydration after procedure.

Table 2-9 Cardiovascular Diagnostic Studies—cont'd

Study	Evaluates	Comments
		○ Keep extremity in which catheter was placed immobilized in a straight position for 6-12 hours. Monitor arterial puncture point for hemorrhage or hematoma. ○ Monitor neurovascular status of affected limb. ○ Monitor for indications of systemic emboli.
Phonocardiography	• Extra heart sounds and murmurs in relation to the cardiac cycle and electrocardiogram	• Rarely used today
Plethysmography: arterial or venous	*Arterial* • Patency of peripheral arteries and presence of occlusive vascular disease *Venous* • Patency of peripheral venous system and presence of deep vein thrombosis	• Test requires one normal extremity because one extremity is compared to the other.
Positron emission tomography (cardiac PET scan)	• Severity of coronary artery stenosis • Collateral circulation • Patency of bypass grafts • Size and location of infarcted tissue	• Assure patient that amount of radioactive material is minimal.
Signal-averaged electrocardiogram	• Presence of late electrical potentials that may be responsible for malignant ventricular dysrhythmias; may be performed before and after ablation	• Patient must lie still for 10 minutes.
Stress electrocardiography	• Persons with high risk for coronary artery disease, patients with known coronary artery disease, or postsurgical patients for ischemia with exercise or pharmacologic agents (e.g. adenosine, dipyridamole, or dobutamine) • Exercise-induced dysrhythmias	• One millimeter or greater transient ST segment depression 80 msec after the J point is suggestive of coronary artery disease. • Monitor closely for exercise-induced hypotension or ventricular dysrhythmias.
Technetium-99 pyrophosphate scan	• Size, location of acute myocardial infarction (infarcted areas show increased uptake of radioactivity [hot spots] 1-7 days after myocardial infarction)	• Assure patient that amount of radioactive material is minimal. • Peak accuracy is obtained at 12-48 hours after initial symptoms.
Thallium stress electrocardiography	• Myocardial ischemia during exercise (ischemic areas show decreased uptake of radioactivity [cold spots])	• Assure patient that amount of radioactive material is minimal.
Thallium-201 scan	• Myocardial ischemia (ischemic areas show decreased uptake of radioactivity [cold spots])	• Assure patient that amount of radioactive material is minimal.
Vectorcardiography	• Chamber hypertrophy • Bundle branch blocks and hemiblocks • Myocardial ischemia or infarction	• As for electrocardiography
Venography (ascending contrast phlebography)	• Deep leg veins • Presence of deep vein thrombosis • Competence of deep vein valves • May be used to locate suitable vein for arterial bypass graft	• Contrast medium used: Check for allergy to iodine, shellfish, dye; ensure hydration after procedure. • Monitor for clinical indications of anaphylaxis (e.g., flushing, urticaria, and stridor). • Monitor puncture site.
Ventriculography	• Ventricular wall motion • Wall thickness • Ventricular aneurysm • Mitral valve motion • Left ventricular end-diastolic volume, end-systolic volume, stroke volume, ejection fraction • Intracardiac shunt	• Contrast medium used: Check for allergy to iodine, shellfish, dye; ensure hydration after procedure. • Monitor for clinical indications of anaphylaxis (e.g., flushing, urticaria, and stridor). • Monitor puncture site.

Electrocardiography

General Information

1. The electrocardiograph measures and records the electrical activity of the heart by measuring electrical potential at the skin surface. The electrocardiogram is a recording of that activity.
2. An electrocardiogram is used to detect or demonstrate any of the following:
   a. Rhythm disturbances
   b. Conduction defects
   c. Electrolyte imbalances
   d. Drug effects and toxicity
   e. Chamber enlargement or hypertrophy
   f. Myocardial ischemia, injury, or infarction
3. Electrocardiogram paper (Figure 2-34)
   a. Horizontal axis measures time
      (1) Each small (1 mm) box is equal to 0.04 second.
      (2) Each large (5 mm) box is equal to 0.2 second.
      (3) Small marks at the top of the paper identify 3-second intervals.
   b. Vertical axis measures voltage.
      (1) Useful only if standardized, as on multiple-lead electrocardiogram; rhythm strips generally are not standardized because the size (i.e., gain) can be changed
      (2) If standardized
         (a) Each small (1 mm) box is equal to 0.1 mV.
         (b) Each large (5 mm) box is equal to 0.5 mV.
4. Rule of electrical flow
   a. Impulses traveling toward the positive pole of a lead cause a positive deflection.
   b. Impulses traveling toward the negative (or away from the positive) pole of a lead cause a negative deflection.

Rhythm Strip Analysis

1. Monitoring electrode placement (Figure 2-35)
   a. Lead II: positive at apex; negative under right clavicle; ground usually placed under left clavicle
      (1) Advantages
         (a) Upright P and QRS waves
         (b) Normal appearance
      (2) Disadvantage: ectopy and aberrancy look alike
   b. MCL_1: positive at fourth intercostal space at right sternal border; negative under left clavicle; ground usually placed under right clavicle
      (1) Advantages
         (a) Better differentiation of ectopy from aberrancy
         (b) Differentiation of left bundle branch block from right bundle branch block
         (c) Differentiation of left ventricular ectopy from right ventricular ectopy
      (2) Disadvantages
         (a) Diphasic P wave
         (b) Negative QRS complex
   c. MCL_6: positive at fifth intercostal space at left midaxillary line has some advantages; also may be used in differentiation of ectopy from aberrancy

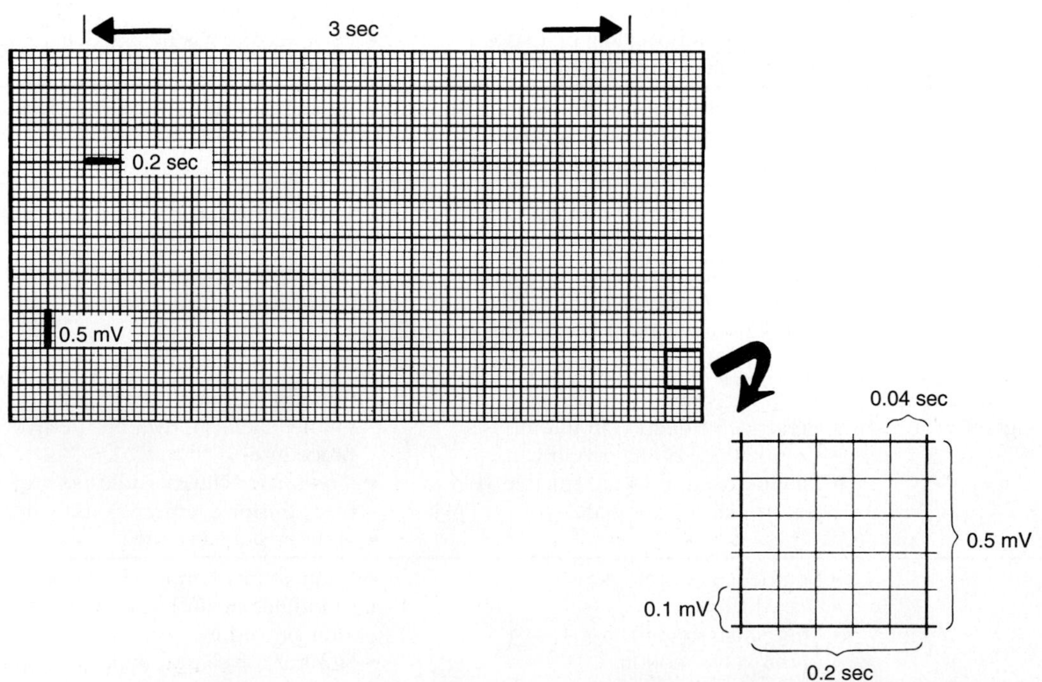

Figure 2-34 Electrocardiogram paper: Horizontal axis represents time with each small block equal to 0.04 second and each large block equal to 0.20 second with 3-second intervals marked off at top of paper; vertical axis represents voltage when standardized with each small block equal to 0.1 mV and each large block equal to 0.5 mV. (From Kinney, M. R., Packa, D. R., & Dunbar, S. B. [1993]. *AACN's clinical reference for critical-care nursing* [3rd ed.]. St. Louis: Mosby.)

A

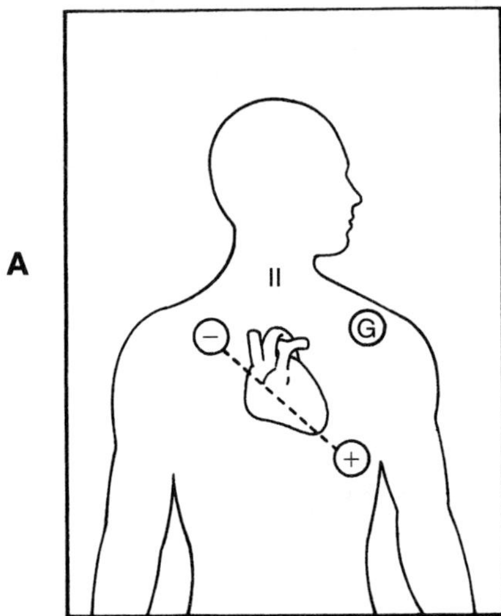

B

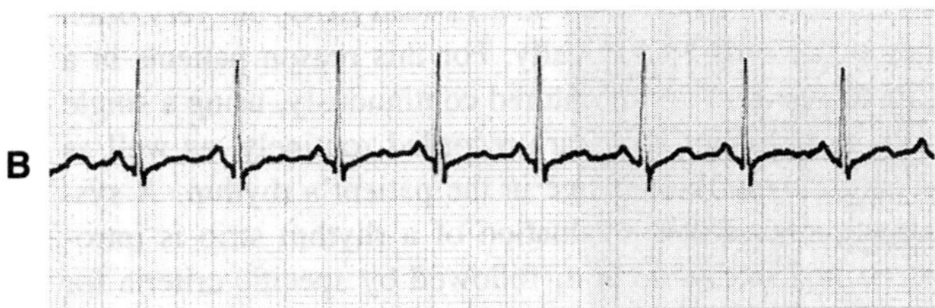

C

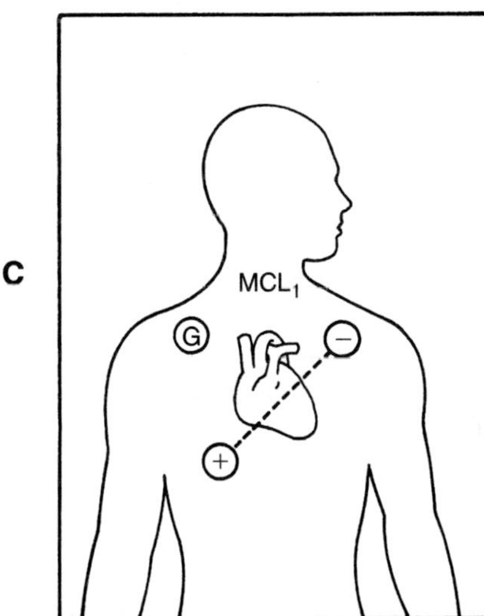

D

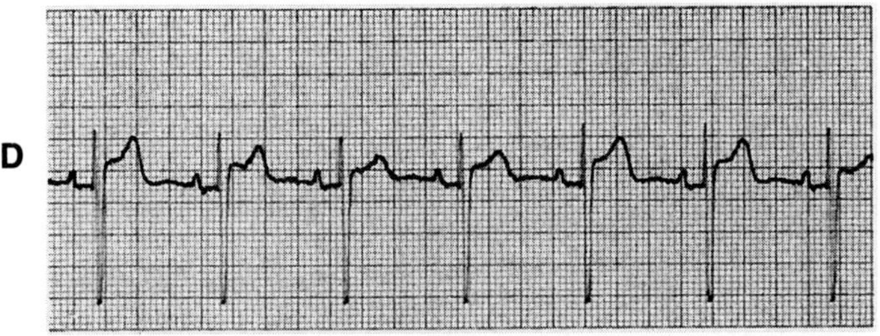

Figure 2-35 Monitoring leads. **A,** Electrode placement for lead II. **B,** Representation of appearance of electrocardiogram in lead II. **C,** Electrode placement for MCL_1. **D,** Representation of appearance of electrocardiogram in MCL_1. (From Urden, L. D., Lough, M. E., & Stacy, K. M. [1995]. *Priorities in critical care nursing.* St. Louis: Mosby.)

2. Components of a single cardiac cycle (Figure 2-36)
   a. P wave
      (1) Represents atrial depolarization
      (2) First deflection from the isoelectric line
      (3) Normal P wave: no more than 2.5 mm tall and no more than 0.11 second wide
   b. PR segment
      (1) Represents the delay in atrioventricular node
      (2) Isoelectric line between P wave and QRS complex
   c. PR interval
      (1) Represents atrial depolarization plus delay in atrioventricular node
      (2) Measured from beginning of P wave to beginning of QRS complex
      (3) Normal PR interval: 0.12 to 0.20 second
   d. Q wave: the first negative wave after the P wave but before the R wave
   e. R wave: the first positive wave after the P wave
   f. S wave: the negative wave after the R wave
   g. QRS complex
      (1) Represents ventricular depolarization
      (2) May have one, two, or all three: Q, R, S
      (3) Measured from beginning of the first wave of complex to the end of last wave of complex
      (4) Normal QRS interval: 0.06 to 0.11 second
      (5) Normal QRS amplitude: less than 30 mm in chest leads
   h. ST segment
      (1) Represents the time during which the ventricles have depolarized completely and the beginning of repolarization
      (2) Located between the QRS complex and the beginning of the T wave
      (3) Normal: isoelectric at baseline
   i. J point
      (1) The angle at which the QRS complex ends and the ST segment begins
      (2) The J point deviates from the isoelectric line if the ST segment is elevated or depressed
   j. T wave
      (1) Represents ventricular repolarization
      (2) Wave after the QRS complex; may be positive or negative
      (3) Normal T wave: less than 5 mm in limb leads and less than 10 mm in chest lead
   k. U wave
      (1) May represent repolarization of the Purkinje fibers
      (2) Small wave after the T wave; often not seen because of its low voltage
      (3) Normal U wave: less than or equal to 1 mm
   l. QT interval
      (1) Represents time of ventricular depolarization and repolarization
      (2) Measured from first wave of QRS complex to the end of the T wave

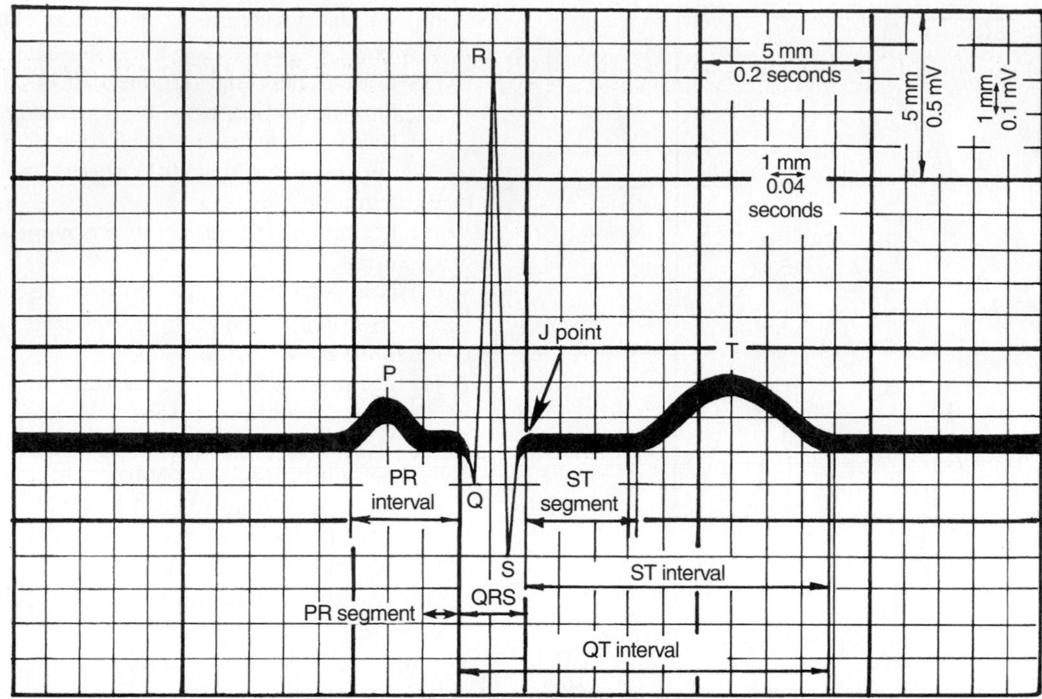

Figure 2-36 Components of a single cardiac cycle. (From Seidel, J. C. [1986]. *The Methodist Hospital: Basic electrocardiography—A modular approach.* St. Louis: Mosby.)

(3) Normal QT interval based on heart rate; the slower the heart rate, the longer the normal QT interval, and the faster the heart rate, the shorter the normal QT interval
(a) For heart rates between 60 to 100 beats/min, the normal QT interval is less than half of the RR interval.
(4) To correct for changes in heart rate (especially for heart rates not between 60 to 100 beats/min), calculate the QTc.
(a) Formula: QT divided by the square root of the R-R interval
(b) Normal QTc: 0.32 to 0.44

3. Steps in analysis of a rhythm strip (Table 2-10)
4. Criteria for basic dysrhythmias and blocks (Table 2-11)
a. The pacemaker rule: The fastest rate will control the heart.
(1) This is usually the sinoatrial node unless an irritable focus (e.g., atrial, junctional, or ventricular) is faster; this is called *irritability*.
(2) If an upper pacemaker (e.g., sinoatrial node) fails, it is up to lower pacemakers (e.g., junctional or ventricular) to assume control: this is called *escape*.
5. Electrocardiogram changes in electrolyte imbalance
a. Hypokalemia
(1) If 3 mEq/L or less
(a) Flat T wave with prominent U wave
(b) T wave and U wave of approximately same amplitude
(c) ST segment flattening and/or depression
(2) If 2 mEq/L or less
(a) U wave taller than T wave
(b) Prolongation of QT interval
(c) ST segment depression
(3) If 1 mEq/L or less
(a) U wave fuses with T wave
b. Hyperkalemia
(1) If greater than 5.5 mEq/L
(a) Tall, narrow, peaked T waves
(b) QRS complex widens
(c) P wave widens and becomes shallow
(2) If 6.5 mEq/L or greater: QRS complex widens more
(3) If 8 mEq/L or greater
(a) Wide QRS complex merged with T wave
(b) P wave barely visible
(4) If 12 mEq/L or greater: P wave disappears
c. Hypocalcemia
(1) Prolonged QT interval
(2) Prolonged ST segment
d. Hypercalcemia
(1) Shortened QT interval
(2) Shortened ST segment
e. Hypomagnesemia
(1) Prolonged QT interval
(2) Broad, flattened T wave
f. Hypermagnesemia
(1) PR interval and QT interval prolonged
(2) Prolonged QRS complex
6. Drug effects on the electrocardiogram
a. Digitalis
(1) Scooping of ST-T wave (known as *digitalis effect*)

Table 2-10 Rhythm Strip Analysis

Component	Assesment
Regularity (rhythm)	• Is it regular? • Is it irregular? • Are there any patterns to the irregularity? • Are there any ectopic beats; if so, are they early (premature) or are they late (escape)? • Is regularity of P waves and QRS complexes the same? (If there is only one P wave for each • QRS complex, only one regularity needs to be recorded.)
Rate	• *Methods* ◦ Count dark lines between P waves or QRS complexes as 300, 150, 100, 75, 60, 50, 43, 38, 33, 30. ◦ Count number of QRS complexes in a 6-second strip and multiple by 10. ◦ Use a rate ruler. • Are atrial and ventricular rates the same? (If there is only one P wave for each QRS complex, only one rate needs to be recorded.)
P waves	• Are the P waves regular? • Is there one P wave for every QRS complex? • Is there a P wave in front of the QRS complex or behind it? • Is the P wave normal and upright in lead II? • Are there more P waves than QRS complexes? • Do all P waves look alike? • Are irregular P waves associated with ectopic beats? If so, are they early (premature) or late (escape)?
PR intervals	• Is PR interval measurement within normal range? (Normal interval is 0.12-0.20 second.) • Are all PR intervals constant? • If PR interval varies, is there a pattern to the changing measurements?
QRS complexes	• Is QRS complex measurement within normal limits? (Normal interval is 0.06-0.11 second.) • Are all QRS complexes of equal duration? • Do all QRS complexes look alike? • Are unusual QRS complexes associated with ectopic beats? If so, are they early (premature) or late (escape)?
QT interval	• Is the QT measurement within normal limits? (Measured QT is less than half of previous R-R interval or QTc of 0.32-0.44.)
Patient presentation	• Is the patient symptomatic? • Are there clinical indications of hypoperfusion such as hypotension, syncope, or chest pain?

(2) Shortened QT interval
(3) PR interval may be prolonged

b. Type IA antidysrhythmic drugs (e.g., procainamide, quinidine, and disopyramide)
(1) QT interval prolongation
(2) T wave flattening

Multiple-Lead Electrocardiogram Analysis

1. Electrocardiogram leads (Figure 2-37)

a. Limb leads: frontal plane
(1) Lead I: positive at left arm; negative at right arm
(2) Lead II: positive at foot; negative at right arm
(3) Lead III: positive at foot; negative at left arm
(4) Lead aVR: unipolar right arm
(5) Lead aVL: unipolar left arm
(6) Lead aVF: unipolar foot

b. Chest leads: horizontal plane
(1) Lead V_1: fourth intercostal space at right sternal border
(2) Lead V_2: fourth intercostal space at left sternal border
(3) Lead V_3: halfway between V_2 and V_4
(4) Lead V_4: fifth intercostal space at left midclavicular line
(5) Lead V_5: fifth intercostal space at left anterior axillary line
(6) Lead V_6: fifth intercostal space at left midaxillary line
(7) The R wave gets taller across the precordium from V_1 to V_6 (referred to as *normal progression of the R wave across the precordium*); the S wave gets smaller across the precordium (V_1 to V_6).
(8) Conditions associated with poor R wave progression across the precordium include the following:
(a) Anterior myocardial infarction
(b) Left bundle branch block
(c) Emphysema
(9) Conditions associated with low voltage across the precordium include the following:
(a) Emphysema
(b) Pericardial effusion
(c) Myocardial infarction
(d) Obesity

Text continued on p. 62

Table 2-11 Criteria for Basic Dysrhythmias and Blocks

Rhythm	Rate	Regularity	P Waves	PR Interval	QRS Complex Duration
Normal sinus rhythm	60-100 beats/min	Atrial and ventricular rhythms regular	Normal	0.12-0.20 second and constant	Less than 0.12 second
Sinus bradycardia	Less than 60 beats/min	Atrial and ventricular rhythms regular	Normal	0.12-0.20 second and constant	Less than 0.12 second
Sinus tachycardia	Greater than 100 beats/min (usually 100-160 beats/min)	Atrial and ventricular rhythms regular	Normal	0.12-0.20 second and constant	Less than 0.12 second
Sinus dysrhythmia	Usually 60-100 beats/min but may be slower or faster	Atrial and ventricular rhythms regularly irregular; rate increases with inspiration (so R-R interval shortens) and decreases with expiration (so R-R interval lengthens); difference between shortest and longest R-R interval is less than 0.12 second	Normal	0.12-0.20 second and usually constant; may vary slightly with rate variation	Less than 0.12 second
Sinus block (sinus exit block)	Dependent on underlying rhythm	Atrial and ventricular rhythms regular with an irregularity; R-R interval at block measures an exact multiple of the normal R-R interval	One or more entire cardiac cycle is absent; P wave absent during block	None during block	QRS complex absent during block
Sinus arrest	Dependent on underlying rhythm	Atrial and ventricular rhythms regular with an irregularity (a pause); R-R interval at pause measures more or less than an exact multiple of the normal R-R interval	Indefinite period of time without an entire cardiac cycle; P wave absent during arrest	None during arrest	QRS complex absent during arrest
Premature atrial contractions	Dependent on underlying rhythm	Dependent on underlying rhythm; premature atrial complex interrupts underlying rhythm	P wave of this early beat differs from sinus P; the ectopic P wave is early and may be flattened, notched, or lost in preceding T wave	Usually 0.12-0.20 second but may be greater than 0.20 second	Less than 0.12 second
Wandering atrial pacemaker	Usually 60-100 beats/min	Atrial and ventricular rhythms usually slightly irregular	P waves look different beat to beat; at least three different-looking P waves	0.12-0.20 second and may vary	Less than 0.12 second

Supraventricular tachycardia*	Greater than 100 beats/min; usually 150-250 beats/min	Atrial and ventricular rhythms regular	P waves are impossible to distinguish; may be lost in QRS complex or preceding T wave	Cannot measure	Less than 0.12 second
Atrial tachycardia	150-250 beats/min	Atrial and ventricular rhythms regular	P wave differs from sinus P; may merge with preceding T wave	0.12-0.20 second	Less than 0.12 second
Multifocal atrial tachycardia (also called *chaotic atrial rhythm*)	Usually 100-150 beats/min	Atrial and ventricular rhythms usually slightly irregular	P waves look different beat to beat; at least three different-looking P waves	0.12-0.20 second and may vary	Less than 0.12 second
Atrial flutter	Atrial rate approximately 300 beats/min; ventricular rate varies with conduction through the atrioventricular node; 2:1 atrial flutter has a ventricular rate of approximately 150 beats/min; 4:1 atrial flutter has a ventricular rate of approximately 75 beats/min	Atrial flutter waves regular; ventricular rhythm (response) usually regular	No true P waves; flutter waves have characteristic sawtooth appearance	No true P waves	Less than 0.12 second
Atrial fibrillation	Atrial rate greater than 350 beats/min; ventricular rate varies greatly depending on conduction through atrioventricular node	Atrial fibrillatory waves irregular; ventricular rhythm irregularly irregular	No true P waves; fibrillatory waves manifested by quivering baseline	No true P waves	Less than 0.12 second
Premature junctional contraction	Dependent on underlying rhythm	Dependent on underlying rhythm; premature junctional contraction interrupts underlying rhythm	P wave if visible will be inverted; may be in front of, in, or after the QRS complex	Can be measured only if P wave is in front of QRS complex; PR interval will be less than 0.12 second if measurable	Less than 0.12 second
Junctional escape rhythm	40-60 beats/min	Atrial and ventricular rhythms regular	If visible, P wave inverted; may be in front of, in, or after the QRS complex	Can be measured only if P wave is in front of QRS complex; PR interval will be less than 0.12 second if measurable	Less than 0.12 second

*Supraventricular tachycardia refers to any narrow QRS complex tachycardia the focus of which cannot be identified definitely; the term should be used only when a more definitive diagnosis cannot be made.

Continued

Table 2-11 Criteria for Basic Dysrhythmias and Blocks—cont'd

Rhythm	Rate	Regularity	P Waves	PR Interval	QRS Complex Duration
Accelerated junctional rhythm	60-100 beats/min	Atrial and ventricular rhythms regular	If visible, P wave inverted; may be in front of, in, or after the QRS complex	Can be measured only if P wave is in front of QRS complex; PR interval will be less than 0.12 second if measurable	Less than 0.12 second
Junctional tachycardia	Greater than 100 beats/min; usually 100-180 beats/min	Atrial and ventricular rhythms regular	If visible, P wave inverted; may be in front of, in, or after the QRS complex	Can be measured only if P wave is in front of QRS complex; PR interval will be less than 0.12 second if measurable	Less than 0.12 second
First-degree atrioventricular nodal block	Dependent on underlying rhythm	Dependent on underlying rhythm	P wave normal	Greater than 0.20 second	Less than 0.12 second
Second-degree atrioventricular nodal block Mobitz I[†] (Wenckebach)	Atrial rate dependent on underlying rhythm; ventricular rate dependent on conduction ratio; atrial rate greater than ventricular rate	Atrial rhythm regular, ventricular rhythm irregular (P-P interval is regular, but R-R interval is irregular); groupings identifiable between P waves that were not conducted	P waves normal, but some P waves not followed by a QRS complex	Normal PR interval progressively lengthens until a P wave is not followed by a QRS complex; entire cycle begins again with normal PR interval	Less than 0.12 second
Second-degree atrioventricular nodal block Mobitz II[†]	Atrial rate dependent on underlying rhythm; ventricular rate dependent on conduction ratio but usually less than 60 beats/min; atrial rate greater than ventricular rate	Atrial rhythm regular, ventricular rhythm regular or irregular depending on whether conduction ratio varies or is constant; P-P interval regular, but some R-R intervals may be twice normal length	P waves normal, but there are P waves not followed by a QRS complex without preceding progressive lengthening	Usually 0.12-0.20 second of conducted P waves but may be longer; constant for each conducted QRS complex	0.12 second or longer
Third-degree (or complete) atrioventricular block	Atrial rate dependent on underlying rhythm; ventricular rate dependent on focus of escape rhythm (40-60 beats/min if escape focus is junctional, 20-40 beats/min if escape focus is ventricular)	Atrial rhythm regular, ventricular rhythm usually regular; P-P interval regular; R-R interval usually regular	Normal but P waves not followed by (associated with) QRS complex	No consistent PR interval; no relationship between the P waves and the QRS complexes	Less than 0.12 second if escape focus is junctional; 0.12 second or longer if escape focus is ventricular

Left bundle branch block	Dependent on underlying rhythm	Dependent on underlying rhythm	P wave normal	0.12-0.20 second as long as no coexisting atrioventricular nodal block	0.12 second or longer; QRS complex is negative in V_1
Right bundle branch block	Dependent on underlying rhythm	Dependent on underlying rhythm	P wave normal	0.12-0.20 second as long as no coexisting atrioventricular nodal block	0.12 second or longer; QRS complex is positive in V_1
Premature ventricular contraction	Dependent on underlying rhythm	Dependent on underlying rhythm; premature ventricular contraction interrupts underlying rhythm	No associated P wave	No associated P wave; cannot measure PR interval	0.12 second or longer; QRS complex of premature ventricular contraction looks different from normal QRS complexes
Monomorphic ventricular tachycardia	100-250 beats/min Ventricular tachycardia is usually ~150 beats/min; ventricular tachycardia at 200-250 beats/min may be called ***ventricular flutter***	Ventricular rhythm usually regular; if dissociated P waves are identifiable, atrial rhythm regular	No associated P waves but may have dissociated P waves scattered through the rhythm	No associated P waves; cannot measure PR interval	0.12 second or longer; QRS complex of ventricular tachycardia looks different from normal QRS complexes
Polymorphic ventricular tachycardia (torsades de pointes)	150-250 beats/min	Ventricular rhythm may be regular	None	None	0.12 second or longer with QRS complex that seems to twist around a center line; gradual alteration in the amplitude and direction of the QRS complex
Ventricular fibrillation	None	Irregular; chaotic baseline	None	None	None
Idioventricular rhythm	20-40 beats/min	Ventricular rhythm usually regular; no atrial activity	None	None	0.12 second or longer
Accelerated idioventricular rhythm	40-100 beats/min	Ventricular rhythm usually regular; no atrial activity	None	None	0.12 second or longer
Asystole	None	No atrial or ventricular activity	None	None	None

†A 2:1 block is a second-degree block but may be type I or type II; the QRS complex width may be helpful in differentiating between the two. If the QRS complex is of normal width, it is probably type I; if the QRS complex is 0.12 second or greater, it is probably type II.

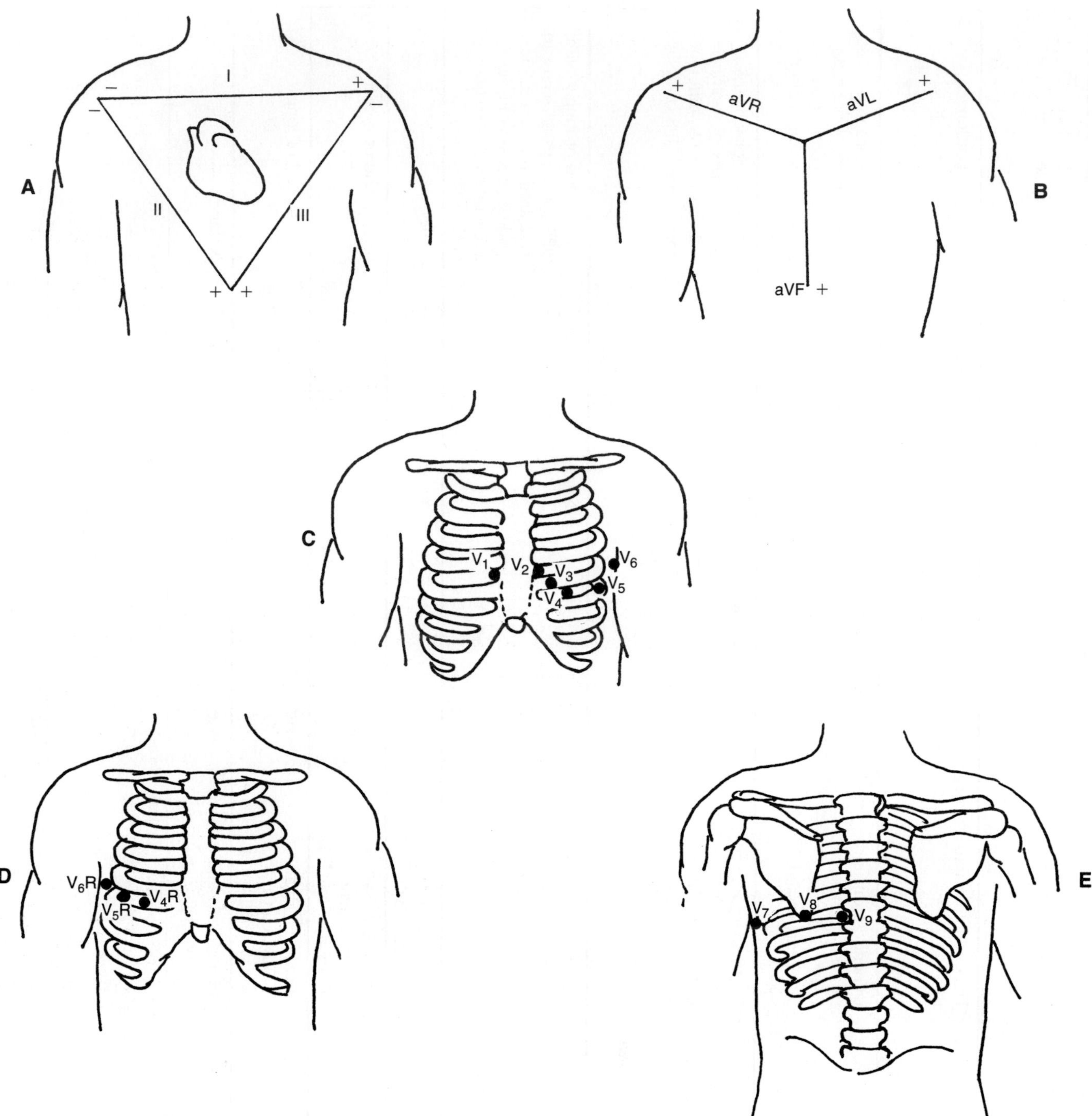

Figure 2-37 Electrocardiogram leads. **A,** Bipolar limb leads: I, II, III. **B,** Unipolar limb leads: aVR, aVL, aVF. **C,** Standard chest leads: V_1 to V_6. **D,** Right ventricular leads: V_4R to V_6R. **E,** Posterior leads: V_7 to V_9.

c. Specialty leads
  (1) Posterior leads
    (a) Lead V_7: fifth intercostal space at left posterior axillary line
    (b) Lead V_8: halfway between V_7 and V_8
    (c) Lead V_9: fifth intercostal space next to vertebral column
  (2) Right ventricular leads
    (a) Lead V_4R: fifth intercostal space at right midclavicular line
    (b) Lead V_5R: fifth intercostal space at right anterior axillary line
    (c) Lead V_6R: fifth intercostal space at right midaxillary line
    (d) The standard 12 leads plus V_4R to V_6R and V_7 to V_9 make the 18 leads of an 18-lead electrocardiogram
    (e) Right ventricular leads routinely performed on patients with electrocardiogram indicators of inferior myocardial infarction (33% to 50% of patients with inferior myocardial infarction have concurrent right ventricular infarction)

2. Mean QRS axis
   a. Represents the average direction of ventricular depolarization
   b. Described on a 360-degree circle
      (1) Normal axis
         (a) Downward and to the left (0 to 90 degrees)
         (b) Caused by the normal direction of depolarization from superior to inferior and the larger muscle mass of the left ventricle
      (2) Left axis deviation
         (a) Upward and to the left (0 to −90 degrees)
         (b) May be caused by any of the following:
            (i) Normal variant: only considered abnormal if more negative than −30 degrees
            (ii) Left ventricular hypertrophy
            (iii) Left anterior hemiblock
            (iv) Septal or inferior myocardial infarction
            (v) Ventricular pacemaker
            (vi) Mechanical shift of heart to more horizontal: ascites; pregnancy; abdominal tumor
      (3) Right axis deviation
         (a) Downward and to the right (+90 to ±180 degrees)
         (b) May be caused by any of the following:
            (i) Normal variant: only considered abnormal if more positive than +110 degrees
            (ii) Right ventricular hypertrophy
            (iii) Pulmonary embolism
            (iv) Left posterior hemiblock
            (v) Lateral myocardial infarction
            (vi) Dextrocardia
      (4) Indeterminate axis
         (a) Upward and to the right (−90 to ±180)
         (b) Though this axis deviation frequently is referred to as "no-man's land" or extreme right axis deviation, it could be extreme right axis deviation or extreme left axis deviation; therefore indeterminate is more appropriate.
         (c) May be caused by any of the following:
            (i) Ventricular tachycardia
            (ii) Ventricular pacing
            (iii) Multiple infarctions
            (iv) Hyperkalemia
            (v) Severe right ventricular hypertrophy (e.g., severe pulmonary disease)
   c. Quadrant method (Figure 2-38)
      (1) Determine which quadrant in which the mean QRS axis is located by using the direction of the QRS complex in leads II and aVF.
         (a) Lead I
            (i) Positive pole is at the left arm and negative pole is at the right arm.
            (ii) If the mean QRS axis is to the left, there will be a predominantly positive QRS complex in lead I.
            (iii) If the mean QRS axis is to the right, there will be a predominantly negative QRS complex in lead I.
         (b) Lead aVF
            (i) Positive pole is at the foot.
            (ii) If the mean QRS axis is downward, there will be a predominantly positive QRS complex in lead aVF.
            (iii) If the mean QRS axis is upward, there will be a predominantly negative QRS complex in lead aVF.
      (2) If QRS complex is positive in I and positive in aVF, mean QRS axis is normal (0 to +90).
      (3) If QRS complex is positive in I and negative in aVF, a left axis deviation exists (0 to −90).
      (4) If QRS complex is negative in I and positive in aVF, a right axis deviation exists (+90 to ±180)
      (5) If QRS complex is negative in I and negative in aVF, an indeterminate axis deviation exists (−90 to ±180)

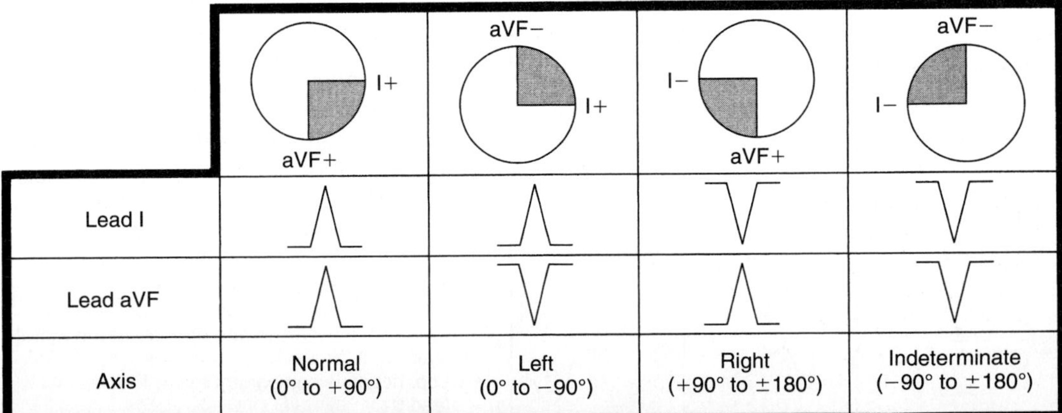

Figure 2-38 Quadrant method of axis determination. (Modified from Kinney, M. R., Packa, D. R., & Dunbar, S. B. [1998]. *AACN's clinical reference for critical-care nursing* [4th ed.]. St. Louis: Mosby.)

3. Bundle branch blocks (Figure 2-39)
   a. Block of either bundle branch causes a delay in the conduction through the ventricles and a prolongation of the QRS interval; branching (commonly referred to as "rabbit ears") or slurring of the QRS complex also usually occurs, indicating that the two ventricles are depolarized out of synchronization.
   b. Left bundle branch block is a bifascicular block (loss of both major hemibundles) and is manifested by the following:
      (1) QRS complex of 0.12 second or more
      (2) QRS complex that is positive in V_6 and negative in V_1
   c. Right bundle branch block is a unifascicular block and is manifested by the following:
      (1) QRS complex of 0.12 second or more
      (2) QRS complex that is positive in V_1 and negative in V_6
4. Chamber enlargement and/or hypertrophy
   a. Atrial enlargement is manifested by changes in the P wave; the two best P wave leads are lead II and lead V_1 (Figure 2-40).
      (1) In lead II: Look for tall or wide P waves.
      (2) In lead V_1 or MCL_1: The first half of the normally diphasic P wave represents the right atrium, and the second half of the normally diphasic P wave represents the left atrium. Look for a more dominant initial or terminal phase of the diphasic P wave in V_1 or MCL_1.
   b. Right atrial enlargement is manifested by the following electrocardiogram changes:
      (1) Tall (greater than 2.5 mm), peaked P wave in II
      (2) Larger initial phase of the diphasic P wave normally seen in V_1

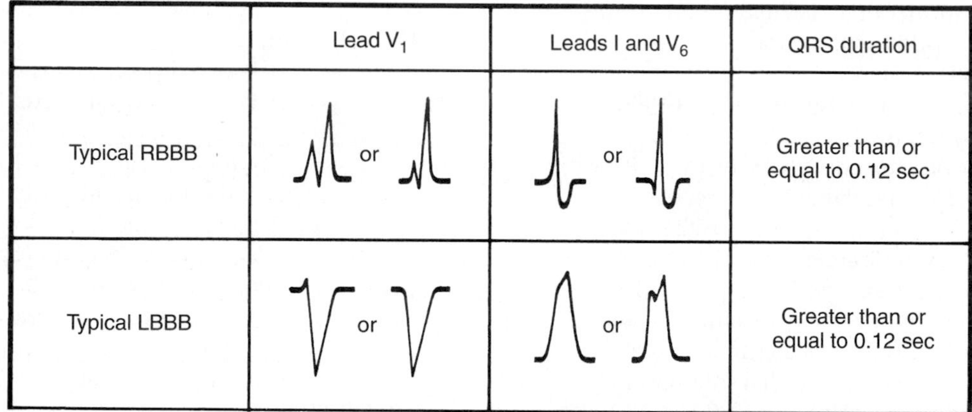

Figure 2-39 Bundle branch blocks. *LBBB,* Left bundle branch block; *RBBB,* right bundle branch block. (Modified from Grauer, K. [1992]. *Practical guide to ECG interpretation*. St. Louis: Mosby.)

Condition	P wave appearance Lead II	Lead V_1	Mnemonic features
Normal sinus rhythm (NSR)		or	• The P should be upright in lead II if there is sinus rhythm • The P may be upright, negative or biphasic in lead V_1 with sinus rhythm
RAE (=**P** **P**ulmonale)	2.50		• **P**rominent (greater than or equal to 2.5 mm tall) **p**eaked P waves in the **p**ulmonary leads (II, III, and aVF)
LAE (=**P** **M**itrale)	0.12	or	• **M**-shaped, widened (greater than or equal to 0.12 sec) P waves in one or more of the **m**itral leads (I, II, or aVL) • Deep, negative component to the P wave in lead V_1

Figure 2-40 Atrial enlargement. *LAE,* Left atrial enlargement; *RAE,* right atrial enlargement. (From Grauer, K. [1998]. *A practical guide to ECG interpretation* [2nd ed.]. St. Louis: Mosby.)

c. Left atrial enlargement is manifested by the following electrocardiogram changes:
   (1) Wide (greater than or equal to 0.12 second), notched P wave in II
   (2) Larger terminal phase of the diphasic P wave normally seen in V_1
d. Ventricular hypertrophy is manifested by changes in the QRS complex; look at changes in the precordial leads for ventricular hypertrophy.
e. Right ventricular hypertrophy causes a change in the usual left ventricular dominance across the precordial leads (Figure 2-41).
   (1) QRS amplitude: R wave larger than S wave in V_1 and V_2; S wave larger than R wave in V_5 and V_6 (indicative of change from the normal dominance of the left ventricle to dominance of right ventricle).
   (2) Right axis deviation: QRS complex is negative in I; QRS complex is positive in aVF.
   (3) Right atrial enlargement may be evident.
   (4) ST-T wave changes in V_1 and V_2 are indicative of right ventricular strain.

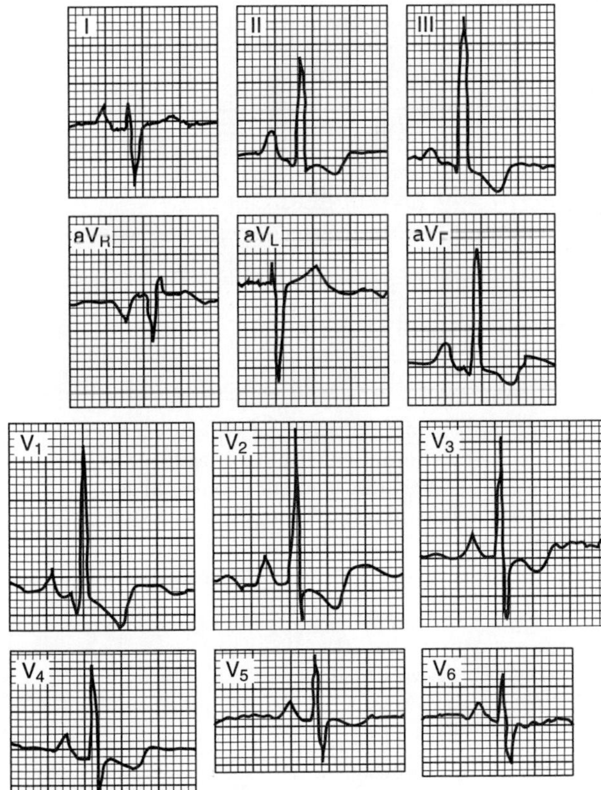

Figure 2-41 Right ventricular hypertrophy with right atrial enlargement. Note tall, peaked P waves in lead II with dominant initial component of the P wave in V_1 as evidence of right atrial enlargement. Note dominant R wave in V_1 and reverse progression of the R wave across the precordium along with right axis deviation and right ventricular strain (ST segment depression and asymmetrical T wave inversion in V_1 and V_2) as evidence of right ventricular hypertrophy. (From Conover, M. B. [2003]. *Understanding electrocardiography* [8th ed.]. St. Louis: Mosby.)

f. Left ventricular hypertrophy causes an exaggeration of the usual left ventricular dominance across the precordial leads (Figure 2-42).
   (1) QRS amplitude
      (a) Deepest S wave in V_1 or V_2 plus tallest R wave in V_5 or V_6 greater than or equal to 35 mm
      (b) R wave in lead aVL greater than or equal to 12 mm
   (2) Left axis deviation: QRS complex is positive in I; QRS complex negative in aVF.
   (3) Left atrial enlargement may be evident.
   (4) ST-T wave changes in V_5 and V_6 are indicative of left ventricular strain.

5. Myocardial ischemia, injury, infarction
   a. Electrocardiogram indicators (Figure 2-43)
      (1) Ischemia is manifested by T waves changes; these are the earliest changes in the evolution of myocardial infarction.
         (a) Indicative change: symmetrically inverted T waves in leads facing the ischemic area
         (b) Reciprocal change: tall T waves in leads opposite the ischemic area
      (2) Injury is manifested by ST segment changes; these are intermediate changes in the evolution of myocardial infarction.
         (a) Indicative change: ST segment elevation in leads facing the injured area
         (b) Reciprocal change: ST segment depression in leads opposite the injured area
      (3) Infarction is manifested by Q waves changes; these are the latest changes in the evolution of myocardial infarction.
         (a) Indicative change: pathologic Q waves (0.04 second wide and/or one fourth the height of the R wave) in leads facing the necrotic area
         (b) Reciprocal change: tall R waves in leads opposite the necrotic area
         (c) Q waves
            (i) Are normal in many leads; to be pathologic (i.e., indicative of infarction), they must be 0.4 second wide and one fourth the height of the R wave
            (ii) Take up to 24 hours to develop
            (iii) Relate to mass loss of myocardium
            (iv) Prevented by successful reperfusion therapies (e.g., fibrinolytic drugs and percutaneous coronary intervention)
      (4) Some conditions may make electrocardiogram diagnosis of myocardial infarction difficult by changing the morphology of the QRS complex, the ST segment, and/or the T waves. Some examples include the following:
         (a) Unstable angina (e.g., Wellens syndrome)
         (b) Ventricular pacemakers

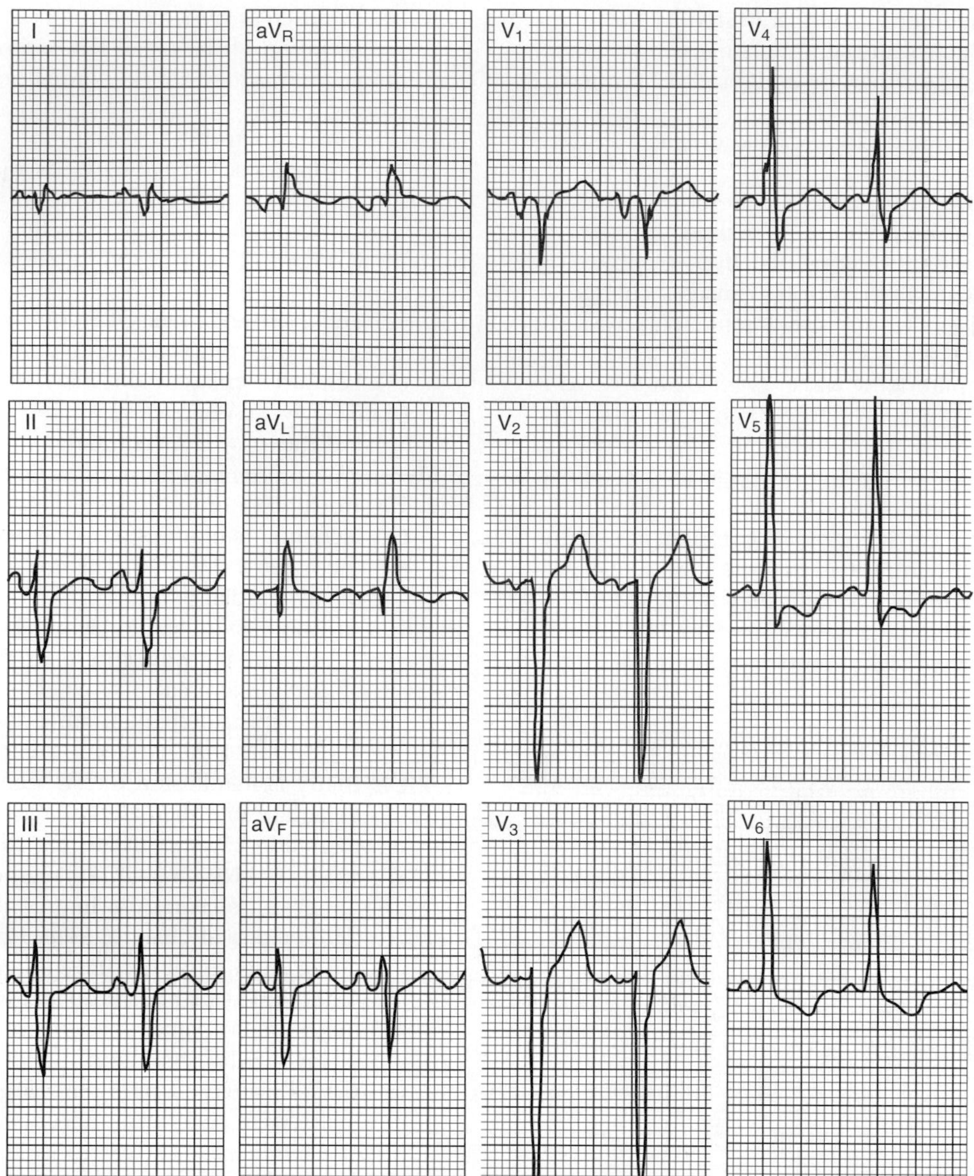

Figure 2-42 Left ventricular hypertrophy with left atrial enlargement. Note wide, notched P waves in lead II with dominant terminal component of the P wave in V_1 as evidence of left atrial enlargement. Note deep S wave in V_2 and tall R wave in V_5 with left axis deviation and left ventricular strain (ST segment depression and asymmetrical T wave inversion in V_5 and V_6) as evidence of left ventricular hypertrophy. (From Conover, M. B. [2003]. *Understanding electrocardiography* [8th ed.]. St. Louis: Mosby.)

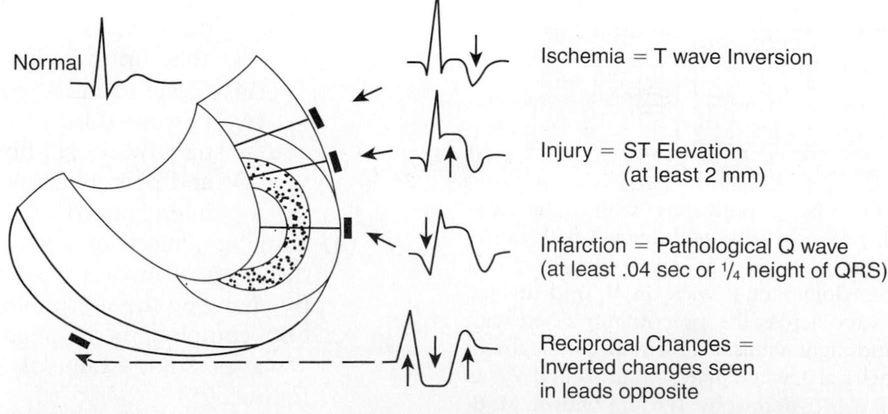

Figure 2-43 Electrocardiogram indicators of ischemia, injury, infarction, and reciprocal changes. (From Harvey, M. [2000]. *Study guide to core curriculum for critical care nursing* [3rd ed.]. Philadelphia: Saunders.)

(c) Left bundle branch block: chance of acute myocardial infarction is more likely if the following are present:
(i) New onset
(ii) ST segment depression of 1 mm in leads V_1 and V_2
(iii) ST segment elevation of more than 5 mm
(d) Ventricular hypertrophy
(e) Wolff-Parkinson-White syndrome
(f) Pericarditis
(g) Hypothermia
(h) Hemorrhagic stroke
(i) Electrolyte imbalances

b. Location (Table 2-12)
(1) Anterior left ventricle: indicative changes in V_3 and V_4 (possibly V_2)
(2) Septal: indicative changes in V_1 and V_2
(3) Lateral left ventricle indicative changes in I, aVL, and/or V_5 and V_6
(a) Leads I and aVL are considered high lateral leads.
(b) Leads V_5 and V_6 are considered low lateral leads.
(4) Inferior left ventricle: indicative changes in II, III, and aVF
(5) Posterior left ventricle
(a) Reciprocal changes in V_1 and V_2
(b) Indicative changes in V_7, V_8, or V_9
(i) Leads V_8 and V_9 are the most significant.
(6) Right ventricular: Indicative changes in V_4R, V_5R, V_6R; V_4R are the most significant.

c. Determination of age of myocardial infarction (Table 2-13)

6. Electrocardiogram changes in angina
a. Variant (also referred to as *Prinzmetal's* or *vasospastic*) angina
(1) Angina at rest caused by spasm of the coronary artery or arteries
(2) Manifested by ST segment elevation with pain
b. Wellens syndrome (Figure 2-44)
(1) Group of signs that is associated with occlusion of proximal left anterior descending artery and high risk of sudden cardiac death in a patient with unstable angina
(a) Symmetrical, deeply inverted T waves in V_2 and V_3 that persist even when the patient is pain free
(b) Little or no ST segment elevation
(c) Little or no enzyme elevation
(d) No development of Q waves or loss of precordial R waves
(2) Cardiac catheterization with percutaneous coronary intervention is indicated.

Table 2-12 Electrocardiogram Lead Correlation with Myocardial Infarction Locations*

Location	Leads	Coronary Artery Affected
Anterior	(V_2), V_3, V_4	LAD
Septal	V_1, V_2	LAD
Anteroseptal	V_1, V_2, V_3, (V_4)	LAD
Lateral	I, aVL (high lateral), V_5, V_6 (low lateral)	LCA
Anterolateral	V_3, V_4, V_5, V_6, (I, aVL)	LCA
Inferior	II, III, aVF	RCA
Right ventricle	V_4R, V_5R, V_6R may be transient	RCA
Posterior	V_7, V_8, V_9 or reciprocal in V_1, V_2, V_3	RCA and/or LCA

LAD, Left anterior descending artery; *LCA,* left circumflex artery; *RCA,* right coronary artery.
*Changes also may be seen in leads in parentheses.

Table 2-13 Determination of Age of Myocardial Infarction

Description	Electrocardiographic Characteristics	Time from Onset of Pain
Hyperacute	• ST segment elevation • Tombstone-shape T waves or T wave inversion	Minutes to hours
Acute	• ST segment elevation • T wave inversion • Pathologic Q waves	Hours to days
Recent	• T wave inversion • Pathologic Q waves	Weeks to months
Old	• Pathologic Q waves	After several months

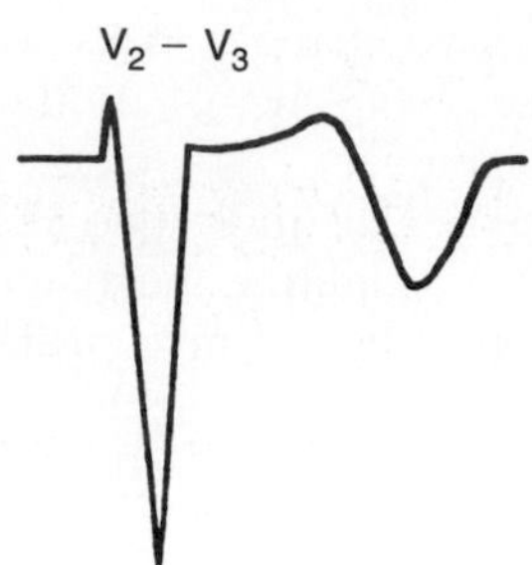

Figure 2-44 Wellens syndrome. (From Conover, M. [2003]. *Understanding electrocardiography.* [8th ed.]. St. Louis: Mosby-Year Book.)

7. Electrocardiogram changes in pericarditis
   a. ST segment normal in V_1 and aVR, but all other leads show ST segment elevation
   b. Depression of PR interval in limb leads and leads (V_5, V_6) of left side of chest
   c. Decrease in QRS complex voltage if pericardial effusion present
8. Electrocardiogram changes in myocardial trauma (e.g., myocardial contusion)
   a. Nonspecific ST and T wave changes; infarction pattern if necrosis
   b. High risk of dysrhythmias and atrioventricular nodal blocks

ST Segment Monitoring

1. Continuous monitoring of ST segment for changes associated with ischemia because the ischemia may not cause chest pain (referred to as *silent ischemia*)
2. Indications
   a. Acute coronary syndrome
   b. Myocardial infarction
   c. Following percutaneous coronary intervention: optional depending on clinical indications such as chest pain and dysrhythmias
   d. During and following cardiac surgery
   e. During and following noncardiac surgery in patients at risk of myocardial ischemia
3. Lead choice
   a. Choose a lead that best demonstrates ST changes during ischemia, evolving myocardial infarction, or at the time of balloon occlusion during percutaneous coronary intervention (referred to as the patient's *ischemic fingerprint*)
   b. If information regarding the ischemic fingerprint is not available, use lead III and V_3.
4. Note significant changes in the ST segment: ST segment elevation or depression of at least 1 mm for at least 60 seconds is considered significant.
   a. ST segment elevation represents more severe, usually transmural, ischemia.
   b. ST segment depression represents less severe, usually subendocardial, ischemia or reciprocal changes of ischemia.
   c. Other causes of ST segment deviation include electrolyte imbalances, pericarditis, hypothermia, ventricular aneurysm, hypothyroidism, hyperventilation, pulmonary infarction, and drugs such as digoxin.

Hemodynamic Monitoring

Definitions (Table 2-14 for Formulae and Normals)

1. Cardiac output: the amount of blood ejected by the ventricle in 1 minute
2. Cardiac index: the cardiac output indexed for differences in body size by dividing by body surface area
3. Stroke volume: the amount of blood ejected by the ventricle with each contraction; also defined as the difference between the end-diastolic volume and the end-systolic volume
4. Stroke index: the stroke volume indexed for differences in body size by dividing by body surface area
5. Ejection fraction: percentage of blood in the ventricle that is ejected during systole; normal is 55% to 75%
6. Afterload: the pressure against which the ventricle must pump; the pressure required to open the semilunar valve
   a. Right ventricular afterload is evaluated by pulmonary vascular resistance and pulmonary vascular resistance index.
   b. Left ventricular afterload is evaluated by systemic vascular resistance and systemic vascular resistance index.
7. Preload: the volume of blood in the ventricle at the end of diastole (end-diastolic pressure); determines the stretch on the myofibrils and the subsequent force of the next contraction (according to Starling's Law of the Heart)
   a. Though preload is a volume concept, atrial pressures commonly are used to evaluate preload.
      (1) Atrial pressure correlates to the end-diastolic pressure for the respective ventricle and, therefore, to the preload for the respective ventricle when ventricular compliance and atrioventricular valve function is normal.
         (a) Right ventricular end-diastolic pressure and preload are evaluated by right atrial pressure.
         (b) Left ventricular end-diastolic pressure and preload are evaluated indirectly by pulmonary artery occlusive pressure or directly by left atrial pressure
   b. Right ventricular volumetric monitoring allows measurement of right ventricular systolic volume, right ventricular end-diastolic volume, and right ventricular ejection fraction, which are a more accurate reflection of preload especially in patients with decreased ventricular compliance.
8. Hemodynamic monitoring: the monitoring of blood flow generally through the use of invasive catheters

Table 2-14 Hemodynamic Parameters, Methods of Measurement or Calculation, and Normal Values

Parameter	Method of Measurement or Calculation	Normal
Heart rate (HR)	Measured as follows: Count rate at apex or number of R waves by electrocardiogram monitor	60-100 beats/min
Mean arterial pressure (MAP)	Calculated as follows: [BP systolic + (BP diastolic × 2)] ÷ 3, where *BP* is blood pressure Systolic and diastolic pressures can be obtained directly (arterial line) or indirectly (auscultated using a sphygmomanometer)	70-105 mm Hg (Normal systolic BP is 90-140 mm Hg; normal diastolic BP is 60-90 mm Hg)
Cardiac output (CO)	Measured as follows: Usually by thermodilution technique	4-8 L/min
Cardiac index (CI)	Calculated as follows: CO ÷ BSA, where *BSA* is body surface area	2.5-4 L/min/m^2
Stroke volume (SV)	Calculated as follows: CO ÷ HR	60-120 mL/beat
Stroke index (SI)	Calculated as follows: SV ÷ BSA	30-65 mL/m^2/beat
Right atrial pressure (RAP)	Measured as follows: At the proximal port of the pulmonary artery catheter; this port is located in the right atrium	2-6 mm Hg 3-8 cm H_2O
Pulmonary artery pressure	Measured as follows: At the distal port of the pulmonary artery catheter with the balloon deflated; the tip is located in a pulmonary arteriole	Systolic: 15-30 mm Hg Diastolic: 5-15 mm Hg Mean (PAm): 10-20 mm Hg
Pulmonary artery occlusive pressure (PAOP)	Measured as follows: At the distal port of the pulmonary artery catheter with the balloon inflated; because pressures on the right side of the heart are blocked by the inflated balloon, PAOP indirectly reflects left atrial pressure, left ventricular end-diastolic pressure, and left ventricular preload	8-12 mm Hg (NOTE: Though 8-12 mm Hg is normal, many patients require a higher pressure [as high as 15-20 mm Hg] to achieve optimal stretch on the myofibrils and optimal preload.)
Systemic vascular resistance	Calculated as follows: [(MAP − RAP) × 80] ÷ CO	900-1400 dynes/sec/cm^{-5}
Systemic vascular resistance index	Calculated as follows: [(MAP − RAP) × 80] ÷ CI	1700-2600 dynes/sec/cm^{-5}/m^2
Pulmonary vascular resistance	Calculated as follows: [(PAm − PAOP) × 80] ÷ CO	100-250 dynes/sec/cm^{-5}
Pulmonary vascular resistance index	Calculated as follows: [(PAm − PAOP) × 80] ÷ CI	225-315 dynes/sec/cm^{-5}/m^2
Left ventricular stroke work index	Calculated as follows: [SI × (MAP − PAOP)] × 0.0136	45-65 g • m/m^2
Right ventricular stroke work index	Calculated as follows: [SI × (PAm − RAP)] × 0.0136	5-12 g • m/m^2
Coronary artery perfusion pressure	Calculated as follows: Diastolic BP − PAOP	60-80 mm Hg
Right ventricular end-diastolic volume (RVEDV)	Measured as follows: By thermodilution method with right ejection fraction (REF) pulmonary artery catheter	100-160 mL
Right ventricular end-diastolic volume index	Calculated as follows: RVEDV ÷ BSA	60-100 mL/m^2

Continued

Table 2-14 Hemodynamic Parameters, Methods of Measurement or Calculation, and Normal Values—cont'd

Parameter	Method of Measurement or Calculation	Normal
Right ventricular end-systolic volume (RVESV)	Measured as follows: By thermodilution method with REF pulmonary artery catheter	50-100 mL
Right ventricular end-systolic volume index	Calculated as follows: RVESV ÷ BSA	30-60 mL/m^2
Right ventricular ejection fraction	Measured as follows: By thermodilution method with REF pulmonary artery catheter	40%-60%
Arterial oxygen saturation (Sao_2)	Measured as follows: By pulse oximetry or by arterial blood gas analysis	95%-100%
Venous oxygen saturation (Svo_2)	Measured as follows: By Svo_2 port of a fiberoptic oximetric pulmonary artery catheter or by mixed venous blood gas analysis	60%-80%
Arterial oxygen content (Cao_2)	Calculated as follows: $1.34 \times Hgb \times Sao_2$, where *Hgb* is the concentration of hemoglobin	18-20 mL/dL
Venous oxygen content (Cvo_2)	Calculated as follows: $1.34 \times Hgb \times Svo_2$	12-16 mL/dL
Oxygen delivery	Calculated as follows: $CO \times Cao_2 \times 10$	900-1100 mL/min
Oxygen delivery index	Calculated as follows: $CI \times Cao_2 \times 10$	550-650 mL/min/m^2
Oxygen consumption	Calculated as follows: $CO \times Hgb \times 13.4 \times (Sao_2 - Svo_2)$	200-300 mL/min
Oxygen consumption index	Calculated as follows: $CI \times Hgb \times 13.4 \times (Sao_2 - Svo_2)$	110-160 mL/min/m^2
Oxygen extraction ratio	Calculated as follows: $(Cao_2 - Cvo_2)/Cao_2$	22%-30%
Oxygen extraction index	Calculated as follows: $(Sao_2 - Svo_2)/Sao_2$	20%-27%

General Information Regarding Hemodynamic Monitoring

1. Uses
   a. Measure hemodynamic parameters pressures and record waveforms
      (1) Arterial catheter: systemic arterial blood pressure including systolic, diastolic, and mean
      (2) Central venous pressure catheter: central venous pressure measured as a mean
      (3) Pulmonary artery catheter
         (a) Right atrial pressure is measured as a mean.
         (b) Pulmonary artery pressures include systolic, diastolic, and mean pressures.
         (c) Pulmonary artery occlusive pressure is measured as a mean as an indirect reflection of left atrial pressure.
         (d) Cardiac output usually is measured by thermodilution technique.
         (e) Specialized catheters also allow the evaluation of the following:
            (i) Oxygen saturation of mixed venous blood
            (ii) Right ejection fraction: right ventricular end-systolic volume, right ventricular end-diastolic volume, right ventricular stroke volume, and right ventricular ejection fraction
   b. Obtain blood samples
      (1) Arterial catheter
         (a) Intermittent arterial samples for arterial blood gases and serum arterial lactate
         (b) Continuous intraarterial blood gas monitoring allows measurement of pH, Pao_2, $Paco_2$ through the use of fiberoptic and electrochemical sensors in an intraarterial catheter.

(2) Central venous catheter: venous
(3) Pulmonary artery catheter
(a) Right atrial (proximal port): venous
(b) Pulmonary artery (distal port): mixed venous
c. Provide central venous access for administration of fluids or drugs
(1) Central venous catheter: usually triple lumen
(2) Pulmonary artery catheter
(a) Right atrial (proximal) port
(b) Pulmonary artery (distal) port: heparinized flush solution only to ensure patency; not to be used for fluid or drug administration
(c) VIP catheters: provide an extra right atrial port
d. Perform intracardiac pacing via specialized pulmonary artery catheter
2. Common indications for hemodynamic monitoring
a. Shock of any cause
b. Myocardial infarction especially with the following:
(1) Acute left or right ventricular failure
(2) Refractory pain
(3) Significant hypotension or hypertension
(4) Right ventricular infarction
(5) Mechanical complications (e.g., papillary muscle rupture or rupture of interventricular septum)
c. Postcardiac surgery
d. Acute right ventricular failure (e.g., after pulmonary embolism)
e. Severe valvular disease
f. Cardiac tamponade
g. Pulmonary edema of uncertain cause: used to differentiate between cardiac and noncardiac pulmonary edema
h. Pulmonary hypertension
i. Acute respiratory failure (e.g., acute respiratory distress syndrome)
j. Need for evaluation of fluid status to guide fluid resuscitation (e.g., burns, multiple trauma, and complex surgical procedures especially in patients with preexisting cardiopulmonary disease)
k. Need for evaluation of hemodynamic response to potent pharmacologic agents (e.g., hypertensive crisis treated with nitroprusside)
3. Controversies regarding invasive hemodynamic monitoring
a. Which patients actually benefit from invasive hemodynamic monitoring (i.e., benefits outweigh risks) is unclear
b. An institutional and human tendency is to "routinize" technology (Benner, 2003) such as invasive monitoring.
c. A retrospective, observation study (i.e., no controls of confounding variables) showed an association between invasive monitoring and an increase in mortality (Connor et al., 1996).
d. Studies suggest that nurses' and physicians' knowledge regarding hemodynamic waveforms and data interpretation is limited.
e. Interrater variability and lack of reproducibility continue to be problematic in evaluating values.
f. Research efforts to link hemodynamic monitoring with improvement in outcomes continue.
4. Components of a pressure monitoring system (Figure 2-45)
a. Physiologic signal: intravascular pressure carried to the transducer by a catheter (inserted into the cardiovascular circuit) and fluid-filled tubing
(1) Static pressure is produced by the volume of blood in the vascular system at zero flow.
(2) Dynamic pressure is produced by the heart and is equal to flow multiplied by resistance.
(3) Hydrostatic pressure is related to the density of the fluid, gravity, and the height of the column of blood between the heart and the vessels.
(a) "Zeroing" the pressure monitoring system by leveling the air-fluid interface of the transducer at the phlebostatic axis (which correlates to the atrial level), turning the stopcock to open the system to air, and ensuring that the digital display and the graphic representation indicate zero corrected for the hydrostatic gradient.
b. Transducer: converts the mechanical signal to an electrical signal
c. Monitor
(1) Amplifier: device that increases the magnitude of the electrical signal and filters out electrical interference
(2) Oscilloscope: device that displays the resultant signal as a pressure waveform and as a numerical value on a meter or a digital display
(3) Recorder: device that records the pressure waveform on paper for analysis

Hemodynamic Parameters

1. Arterial and ventricular pressures measured as systolic/diastolic and atrial pressures measured as a mean
2. Systemic arterial blood pressure
a. Pressure in a systemic artery; reflects systemic arterial blood pressure
b. Blood pressure equals cardiac output multiplied by systemic vascular resistance; changes in blood pressure are due to a change in cardiac output or in systemic vascular resistance
c. Measured by a catheter in a peripheral artery or the second lumen of an intraaortic balloon catheter (central aortic arterial line)
(1) Radial artery site is the preferred peripheral site because of collateral circulation provided by ulnar artery.
(a) Allen's test must be performed before any radial artery puncture to assess patency of radial-ulnar arch; this test is performed by compressing the radial and ulnar arteries to blanch the hand; upon releasing the ulnar artery, evaluate the time until return of color; if longer than 7 seconds, this radial artery should not be punctured (for arterial blood gases or for radial artery cannulation).

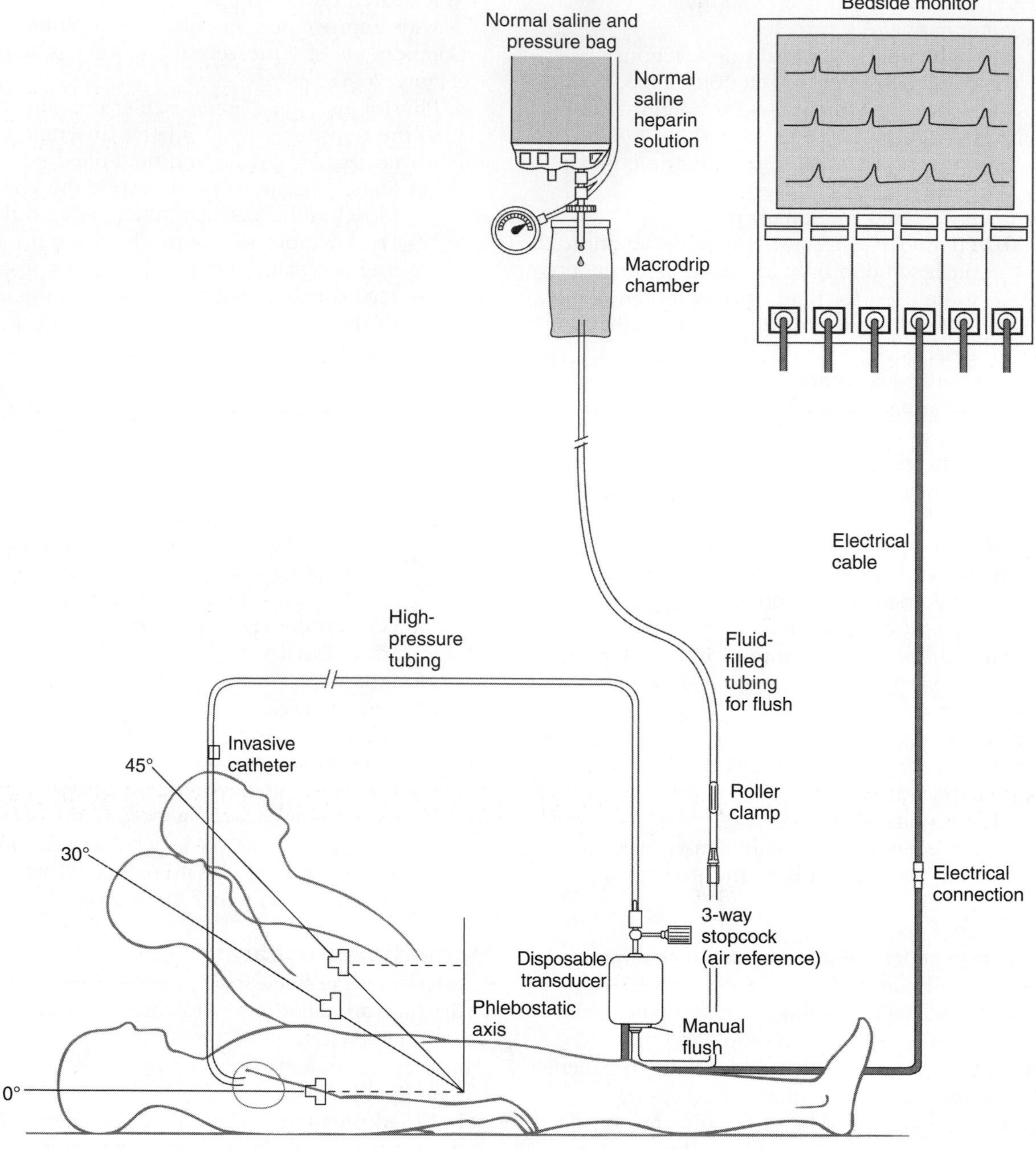

Figure 2-45 Components of a pressure monitoring system. (From Urden, L.D., Stacy, K.M., & Lough, M.E. [2005]. *Thelan's critical care nursing: Diagnosis and management* [5th ed.]. St. Louis: Mosby.)

(2) Neurovascular assessment of the limb distal to any arterial line is essential; thrombosis or embolization may cause acute arterial occlusion and loss of limb.

d. Systolic arterial pressure: maximal pressure with which the blood is ejected from the left ventricle

e. Diastolic arterial pressure: reflects the rapidity of flow of the ejected blood through the arterial system and the elasticity of the vessel

(1) Diastolic pressure is expected to be higher (and pulse pressure be narrowed) if there is endogenous catecholamine release or the patient is receiving sympathomimetic agents (e.g., epinephrine, dopamine [Intropin], or norepinephrine [Levophed])

(2) Diastolic pressure is expected to be lower (and pulse pressure be widened) if there are excessive vasodilatory mediators (e.g., septic shock or anaphylactic shock).

f. Mean arterial pressure: average pressure occurring in the aorta and its major branches during the cardiac cycle; mean arterial pressure of at least 60 mm Hg is necessary to perfuse the vital organs

g. Normal pressure values
   (1) Systolic: 90 to 140 mm Hg
   (2) Diastolic: 60 to 90 mm Hg
   (3) Mean: 70 to 105 mm Hg
h. Normal waveform (Figure 2-24)
i. Causes of abnormal pressures (Table 2-15)
   (1) Arterial catheter versus cuff pressures
      (a) Arterial catheters are a direct measurement and therefore are more accurate (assuming proper zeroing, leveling, and dynamic response), especially in shock states, severe hypertension, vasoconstriction, and obesity.
         (i) Indirect blood pressure measurements including auscultation and oscillometric methods tend to underestimate systolic pressure and overestimate diastolic pressure.
         (ii) Mean arterial pressures tend to be the same even in these situations and are a more consistent evaluation of perfusion pressure.
      (b) Expect radial artery catheters to show a pressure slightly higher (~10 mm Hg) than brachial cuff measurement because the radial artery is smaller than the brachial artery.
      (c) If there is a significant variation between pressure measured by arterial catheter and pressure auscultated using a sphygmomanometer other than in the situations previously listed, do the following:
         (i) Check the pressure monitoring system for air bubbles, occlusions, and positioning of catheter against wall of artery.
         (ii) Ensure that the air-fluid interface of the transducer is level with the phlebostatic axis.
         (iii) Ensure adequate damping of the pressure monitoring system.

3. Right atrial pressure
   a. Pressure in the right atrium
   b. Reflects venous return to right side of the heart; also, reflects right ventricular end-diastolic pressure and preload as long as right ventricular compliance and tricuspid valve function are normal

Table 2-15 Causes of Abnormal Hemodynamic Pressures

Parameter	Increased	Decreased
Systemic arterial blood pressure *Normal:* • *Systolic: 90-140 mm Hg* • *Diastolic: 60-90 mm Hg* • *Mean: 70-105 mm Hg*	• Increase in systemic vascular resistance (e.g., hypertension or sympathetic nervous system innervation) • Increase in cardiac output (e.g., hyperthyroidism)	• Decrease in systemic vascular resistance (e.g., sepsis or anaphylaxis) • Decrease in cardiac output (e.g., myocardial infarction or tachydysrhythmias)
Right atrial pressure *Normal:* • *2-6 mm Hg* • *3-8 cm H_2O*	• Hypervolemia • Tricuspid valve dysfunction: stenosis or regurgitation • Right ventricular failure or infarction • Ventricular septal defect with left-to-right shunt • Pulmonic stenosis • Pulmonary hypertension ○ Active: hypoxemic pulmonary vasoconstriction (Pao_2 less than 60 mm Hg) – Pulmonary embolism – Chronic obstructive pulmonary disease – Acute respiratory distress syndrome ○ Passive: mitral valve dysfunction (stenosis or regurgitation) • Positive pressure ventilation • Constrictive pericarditis • Cardiac tamponade • Chronic left ventricular failure (right atrial pressure would be a late indication of left ventricular failure)	• Hypovolemia • Vasodilation ○ Venous vasodilators (e.g., nitroglycerin and morphine) ○ Endogenous systemic vasodilation (e.g., septic shock, anaphylactic shock, or neurogenic shock)
Right ventricular pressure *Normal:* • *Systolic: 15-30 mm Hg* • *End-diastolic: 0 to 8 mm Hg*	• Right ventricular failure or infarction • Ventricular septal defect with left-to-right shunt • Pulmonary hypertension • Mitral valve dysfunction: stenosis or regurgitation • Constrictive pericarditis • Cardiac tamponade • Chronic left ventricular failure	• Hypovolemia • Excessive vasodilation (e.g., vasodilators, septic shock, anaphylactic shock, or neurogenic shock)

Continued

Table 2-15 **Causes of Abnormal Hemodynamic Pressures—cont'd**

Parameter	Increased	Decreased
Pulmonary artery pressure *Normal:* • *Systolic: 15 to 30 mm Hg* • *Diastolic: 5 to 15 mm Hg* • *Mean: 10 to 20 mm Hg*	• Hypervolemia • Ventricular septal defect with left-to-right shunt • Pulmonary hypertension • Positive pressure ventilation • Mitral valve dysfunction: stenosis or regurgitation • Constrictive pericarditis • Cardiac tamponade • Left ventricular failure	• Hypovolemia • Excessive vasodilation (e.g., vasodilators, septic shock, anaphylactic shock, or neurogenic shock)
Pulmonary artery occlusive pressure *Normal:* • *8 to 12 mm Hg*	• Positive pressure ventilation especially with positive end-expiratory pressure (PEEP) • Hypervolemia • Mitral valve dysfunction: stenosis or regurgitation • Constrictive pericarditis • Cardiac tamponade • Left ventricular failure • Severe aortic stenosis	• Hypovolemia • Excessive vasodilation (e.g., vasodilators, septic shock, anaphylactic shock, or neurogenic shock)
Cardiac output and cardiac index *Normal:* • *CO 4-8 L/min* • *CI 2.5-4 L/min*	• Sympathetic nervous system innervation (endogenous catecholamines [e.g., stress and exercise]) • Exogenous catecholamines (e.g., epinephrine, isoproterenol, dobutamine, and dopamine) • Other positive inotropes (e.g., digitalis and amrinone) • Infection, early sepsis • Hyperthyroidism • Anemia	• Decreased contractility (e.g., myocardial infarction, cardiomyopathy, and beta-blockers) • Increased afterload (e.g., systemic or pulmonary hypertension, aortic or pulmonic stenosis, or polycythemia) • Alteration in preload: excessively increased (e.g., hypervolemia or heart failure) or decreased (e.g., hypovolemia, cardiac tamponade, or mitral or tricuspid valve disease) • Significantly increased or decreased heart rate (e.g., bradydysrhythmias or tachydysrhythmias)
Venous oxygen saturation *Normal:* *60%-80%*	• Increased oxygen supply and delivery ∘ Increased arterial oxygen saturation (Sa_{O_2}); (e.g., increased fraction of inspired oxygen [Fi_{O_2}], continuous positive airway pressure [CPAP], or PEEP) ∘ Increase in cardiac output/cardiac index (e.g., inotropes, intraaortic balloon pump, ventricular assist device, decrease in excessive afterload, hyperdynamic [i.e., early] stage of septic shock) ∘ Increased hemoglobin (e.g., blood administration) • Decreased oxygen demand ∘ Anesthesia and/or analgesics ∘ Muscle paralysis or sedation ∘ Hypothermia ∘ Sleep ∘ Hypothyroidism ∘ Beta-blockers • Decreased oxygen extraction at tissue level ∘ Early sepsis ∘ Cyanide toxicity • Shift of oxyhemoglobin dissociation curve to the left (e.g., alkalosis, hypothermia, decreased levels of -2,3 diphosphoglycerate) • Ventricular defect with left-to-right intracardiac shunt (e.g., ventricular septal defect or rupture) • Technical problems ∘ Pulmonary artery catheter in occluded position ∘ Deposits of fibrin on the tip of the catheter	• Decreased oxygen supply and delivery ∘ Decrease in Sa_{O_2} (e.g., decreased Fi_{O_2}, CPAP, or PEEP, suctioning, acute respiratory failure, or pulmonary edema) ∘ Decrease in cardiac output/cardiac index (e.g., shock, heart failure, hypovolemia, dysrhythmias, excessive CPAP or PEEP, negative inotropes, or excessive afterload) ∘ Decrease in hemoglobin (e.g., anemia or hemorrhage) or abnormal hemoglobin (e.g., methemoglobinemia or sickle cell anemia) • Increased metabolic needs (e.g., seizures, shivering, restlessness, pain, hyperthermia, increased work of breathing, increased metabolic rate, or exertion [e.g., turning, bathing, or active range of motion]) • Shift of oxyhemoglobin dissociation curve to the right (e.g., acidosis or hyperthermia)

c. Measured through catheter in superior vena cava (central venous pressure) or at the proximal port of pulmonary artery catheter (right atrial pressure)
   (1) Insertion of a central venous pressure catheter or pulmonary artery catheter
      (a) Catheterization is preceded by insertion of a venous introducer into the internal jugular, subclavian, basilic, or femoral vein. The right internal jugular vein is the preferred site because the risk of pneumothorax is reduced by the use of the internal jugular vein.
      (b) The catheter then is threaded through the introducer into place with the central venous pressure catheter tip in the superior vena cava and the pulmonary artery catheter tip in a pulmonary arteriole in the dependent area (West zone 3), though the right atrial pressure is measured from the proximal port that is in the right atrium.
   (2) Though these parameters (central venous pressure and right atrial pressure) are not actually the same, they are the same in practicality and frequently are used interchangeably.
   (3) Central venous pressure may be measured by a water manometer in centimeters of water or by a transducer in millimeters of mercury.
   (4) Right atrial pressure from the proximal port of the pulmonary artery catheter generally is measured by a transducer in millimeters of mercury.
   (5) To convert values, remember that 1 mm Hg is equal to 1.36 cm H_2O.
d. Normal pressure value: 2 to 6 mm Hg (or 3 to 8 cm H_2O)
e. Causes of abnormal pressures (Table 2-15)
f. Normal waveform (Figure 2-46)

4. Right ventricular pressure
   a. Pressure in the right ventricle
   b. Measured only during insertion of the pulmonary artery catheter as the distal tip of the pulmonary artery catheter is floated through the right ventricle
   c. Normal pressure values
      (1) Systolic: 15 to 30 mm Hg
      (2) End-diastolic: 0 to 8 mm Hg
   d. Causes of abnormal pressures (Table 2-15)
   e. Normal waveform (Figure 2-47)
5. Pulmonary artery pressure
   a. Pressure in the pulmonary artery with the balloon *deflated*

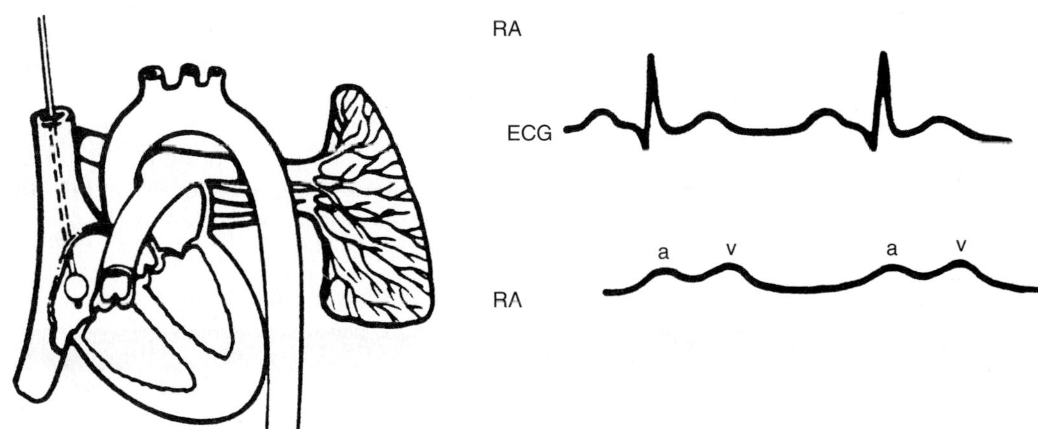

Figure 2-46 Right atrial waveform. (Courtesy Baxter Healthcare, Irvine, CA.)

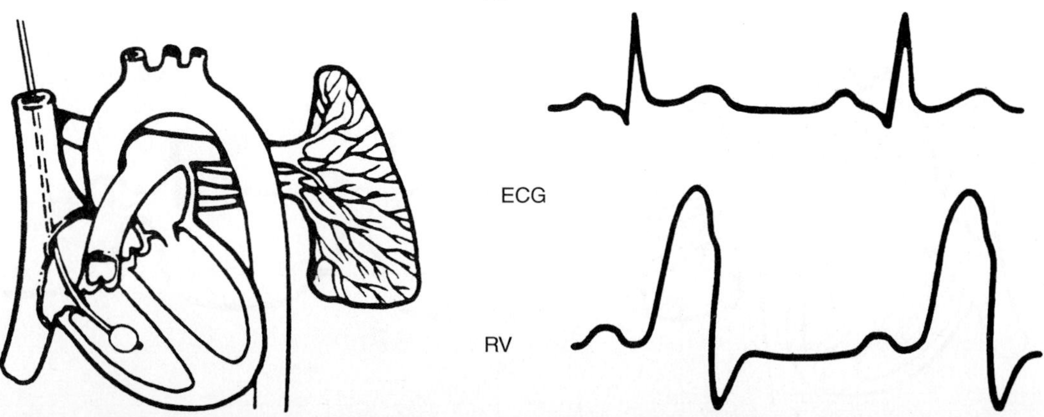

Figure 2-47 Right ventricular waveform. (Courtesy Baxter Healthcare, Irvine, CA.)

b. Measured from the distal tip of the pulmonary artery catheter with balloon *deflated*
 (1) Pulmonary artery systolic pressure: pressure in the pulmonary artery during right ventricular systole
 (2) Pulmonary artery end-diastolic pressure: pressure in the pulmonary artery at the end of right ventricular diastole; reflects left atrial pressure in the absence of pulmonary disease and left ventricular end-diastolic pressure in the absence of pulmonary disease and mitral valve dysfunction
c. Normal pressure values (Box 2-2)
 (1) Systolic: 15 to 30 mm Hg
 (2) Diastolic: 5 to 15 mm Hg
 (3) Mean: 10 to 20 mm Hg
d. Causes of abnormal pressures (Table 2-15)
e. Causes for lack of correlation between pulmonary artery end-diastolic pressure and pulmonary artery occlusive pressure (pulmonary artery end-diastolic pressure normally is 2 to 5 mm Hg greater than pulmonary artery occlusive pressure)
 (1) Pulmonary artery end-diastolic pressure more than 5 mm Hg greater than pulmonary artery occlusive pressure is caused by any of the following:
  (a) Tachycardias greater than 125 beats/min
  (b) Pulmonary hypertension
   (i) Active: hypoxemic pulmonary vasoconstriction with Pa_{O_2} less than 60 mm Hg (e.g., acute respiratory distress syndrome, chronic obstructive pulmonary disease, or pulmonary embolus)
   (ii) Passive: mitral valve dysfunction (stenosis or regurgitation)
 (2) Pulmonary artery occlusive pressure greater than pulmonary artery end-diastolic pressure is caused by any of the following:
  (a) Pulmonary artery end-diastolic pressure artificially low or pulmonary artery occlusive pressure artificially high
  (b) Mitral regurgitation with mean of pulmonary artery occlusive pressure used rather than the *a* wave amplitude (because mitral regurgitation causes large *v* waves on the pulmonary artery occlusive pressure waveform, it increases the pulmonary artery occlusive pressure if the mean is used; use the *a* wave measurement when there are large *v* waves)
  (c) Forceful atrial contraction
f. Normal waveform (Figure 2-48)
g. Changes in waveform (Table 2-16)
 (1) Fling (also referred to as *whip*) (Figure 2-49)
 (2) Dampened (Figure 2-50)

6. Pulmonary artery occlusive pressure (also referred to as *pulmonary capillary wedge pressure* or *pulmonary artery wedge pressure*)
 a. Pressure in the pulmonary artery with the balloon *inflated;* reflects pressure from the left atrium in the absence of pulmonary hypertension
 b. Measured from the distal tip of the pulmonary artery catheter with the balloon *inflated;* the balloon blocks pressures of the right side of the heart from the distal tip; left atrial pressure reflects left ventricular end-diastolic pressure and left ventricular preload in the absence of mitral valve disease or left atrial tumor

BOX 2-2 Hemodynamic Parameters Reflect Status of Cardiac Pressures

Right atrial pressure (RAP) = Right side of the heart
Pulmonary artery end-diastolic pressure (PAd) = Pulmonary vascular bed
Pulmonary artery occlusive pressure (PAOP) = Left side of the heart

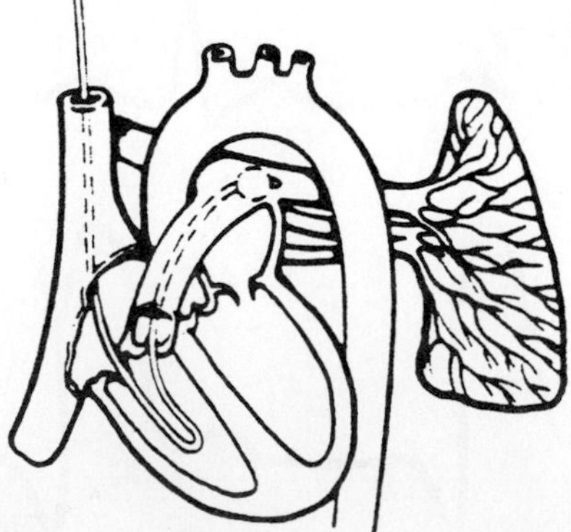

Figure 2-48 Pulmonary artery waveform. (Courtesy Baxter Healthcare, Irvine, CA.)

Table 2-16 Hemodynamic Waveform Abnormalities

Abnormality	Cause	Implications/Treatment
Pulmonary Artery Pressure Waveform		
Fling (or whip) (Figure 2-49)	• Excessive catheter length in right atrium or right ventricle • Catheter tip is located near the pulmonic valve	• Turn patient to left side to see if catheter will float out into pulmonary artery. • Monitor closely for indications that the catheter has flipped back into right ventricle. ◦ Loss of dicrotic notch is characteristic of an arterial waveform. ◦ Decrease in diastolic pressure to close to 0 mm Hg ◦ Ventricular ectopy: premature ventricular contractions, possible ventricular tachycardia • Inflate balloon to increase the chance that it will float distally back into position. • Catheter needs to be repositioned distally for fling or if catheter is in right ventricle.
Damped (Figure 2-50)	• Air bubbles within the pressure monitoring system • Catheter occlusion (e.g., fibrin at the tip of the catheter or catheter tip against the wall of the vessel) • Spontaneous occluded position	• Check the system for bubbles or blood; check that stopcocks are positioned correctly and that stopcocks are covered with dead-end stopcock port covers (no holes). • Try to aspirate the catheter; DO NOT FLUSH since catheter may be in wedge position; if a clot is aspirated, discard and flush catheter. • If still damped, ask patient to take deep breaths, cough, and turn to side; if still in spontaneous occluded position, catheter needs to be repositioned proximally.
Pulmonary Artery Occlusive Pressure Waveform		
Large *a* waves	• Mitral stenosis • Severe aortic stenosis • Hypertension • Atrioventricular block with atrioventricular asynchrony	
Large *v* waves	• Mitral regurgitation • Ventricular septal defect	• NOTE: ***In patients with large v waves:*** ◦ The mean pulmonary artery occlusive pressure (PAOP) may be higher than diastolic pulmonary artery pressure; do not use mean as the pressure value for PAOP. ◦ Use the measurement of the *a* wave for the pressure value for PAOP because the mitral valve is open during the *a* wave (atrial contraction) and this value has better correlation with left ventricular end-diastolic pressure.
Large *a* and *v* waves (looks like M)	• Cardiac tamponade • Constrictive pericarditis • Hypervolemia • Left ventricular failure	

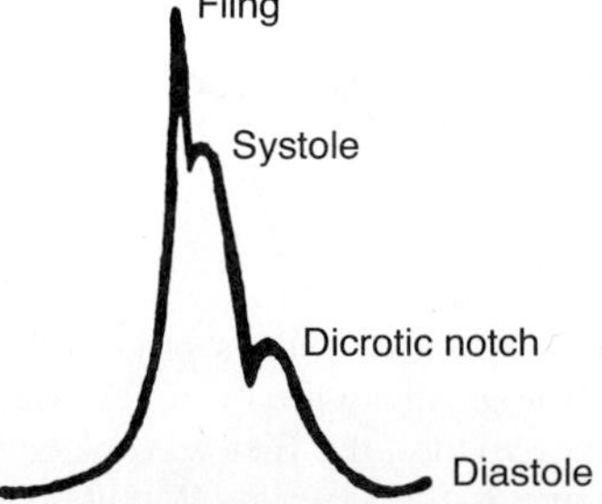

Figure 2-49 Pulmonary artery waveform: catheter fling.

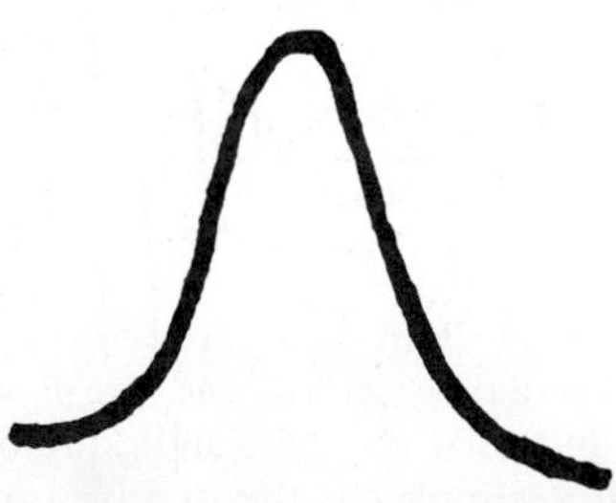

Figure 2-50 Pulmonary artery waveform: damped waveform.

c. Normal pressure value: 8 to 12 mm Hg (measured as a mean); remember that some patients require a pulmonary artery occlusive pressure as high as 15 to 20 mm Hg for optimal preload
d. Causes of abnormal pressures (Table 2-15)
e. Normal waveform (Figure 2-51)
   (1) The *a* wave correlates with atrial contraction: it is the first wave seen after the QRS complex using dual channel recording.
   (2) The *v* wave correlates with ventricular contraction: it is the first wave after the T wave using dual channel recording.
f. Changes in waveform (Table 2-16)
   (1) Large *a* waves
   (2) Large *v* waves
   (3) Large *a* waves and large *v* waves

7. Left atrial pressure
   a. Pressure in the left atrium; reflects left ventricular end-diastolic pressure and left ventricular preload in the absence of mitral valve disease or left atrial tumor
   b. Measured by a catheter placed directly in the left atrium, usually placed during cardiac surgery
   c. A pulmonary artery catheter usually used to measure pulmonary artery occlusive pressure as an indirect reflection of left atrial pressure because of the risk of complications related to direct left atrial catheter (e.g., air embolism or cardiac tamponade)
   d. Normals and waveforms as for pulmonary artery occlusive pressure
8. Cardiac output
   a. Amount of blood ejected by the ventricle each minute
   b. Invasive monitoring by thermodilution technique
      (1) Intermittent: method
         (a) A known volume of a known temperature solution is injected into an unknown volume of blood at a known temperature.
         (b) The injectate solution (usually normal saline) is injected into the proximal lumen (right atrium) of the pulmonary artery catheter.
         (c) The injectate mixes with the blood.
         (d) The temperature change is sensed downstream at the thermistor located 4 cm from the distal tip of the pulmonary artery catheter.
         (e) The amount of the unknown volume of blood is deduced from the amount of change in temperature.
         (f) Calculate the average of three measurements that are within 10% of a median value.
      (2) Continuous (referred to as *continuous cardiac output*)
         (a) Method
            (i) A thermal filament in the right ventricle creates a signal by warming the blood as it flows past.
            (ii) The thermistor at the distal tip measures the temperature of the blood downstream.
            (iii) The computer produces a thermodilution curve and calculates the cardiac output.
            (iv) The cardiac output is updated approximately every 5 minutes.
         (b) Advantages over intermittent method
            (i) More accurate especially in patients with low output states
            (ii) Continuously updated
            (iii) Decreases required nursing time
            (iv) Eliminates interrater reliability caused by variability in injectate volume, rate of injection, and selection or elimination of values for averaging
            (v) Reduces risks of contamination and fluid overload
         (c) Disadvantage: catheter cost is greater than the cost of conventional catheter

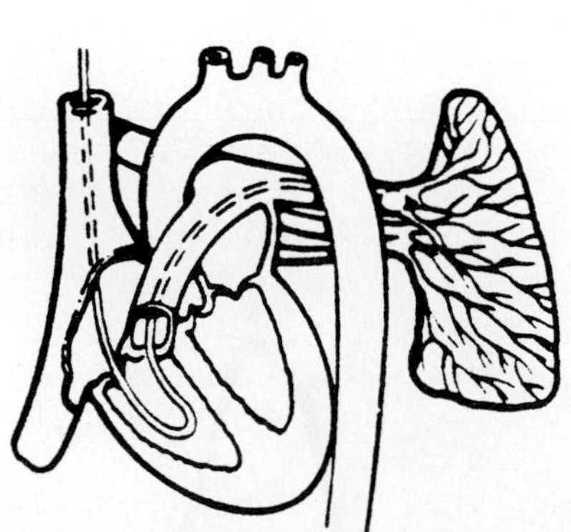

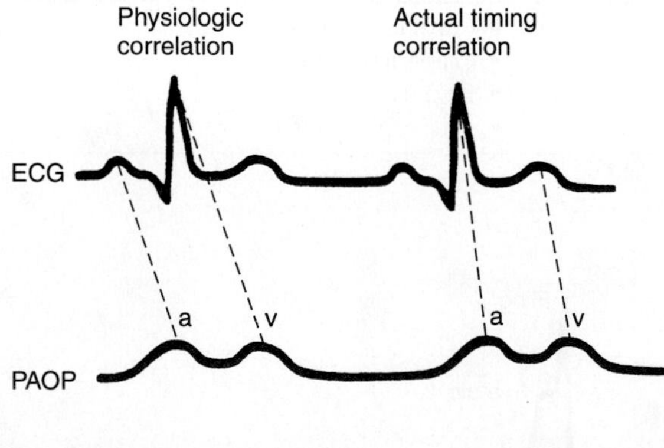

Figure 2-51 Pulmonary artery occlusive pressure waveform. Though the *a* wave correlates physiologically to atrial depolarization and the P wave and the *v* wave correlate physiologically with the QRS complex and ventricular depolarization, tubing and catheter cause a time delay. In actuality, the first wave seen after the QRS complex is the *a* wave, and the first wave seen after the T wave is the *v* wave. (Modified from illustration courtesy Baxter Healthcare, Irvine, CA.)

c. Noninvasive measurement by bioimpedance
   (1) Uses thoracic electrical bioimpedance technology
      (a) Impedance (Z): resistance to flow of electrical current
   (2) Method
      (a) Four dual sensors are placed on each side of the neck and thorax.
      (b) A low-amplitude, high-frequency electrical signal is emitted from the outer sensors through the thorax.
      (c) Blood is an excellent conductive medium, and electricity follows the path of least resistance, and the aorta is the largest, most distensible, blood-filled vessel in the thoracic cavity.
      (d) Aortic blood flow is tracked readily by this method.
   (3) Allows continuous measurement of the following parameters
      (a) Composite parameters
         (i) Cardiac output
         (ii) Cardiac index
         (iii) Stroke volume
      (b) Thoracic fluid status
         (i) Base thoracic impedance (Zo): normal 20 to 30 ohms for males and 25 to 35 ohms for females
      (c) Afterload
         (i) Systemic vascular resistance: normal 900 to 1400 dynes/sec/cm^{-5}
      (d) Contractility
         (i) Change in impedance over time (dZ/dt): normal 0.8 to 2.5 ohms/sec
         (ii) Acceleration contractility index (ACI): normal 2 to 5 ohms/sec
         (iii) Left cardiac work index (LCWI): normal 3 to 5 kg/min/m^2
         (iv) Preejection period: normal 0.05 to 0.12 second
         (v) Ventricular ejection time: normal 0.25 to 0.35 second
      (e) Change in impedance divided by change in time (dZ/dt)
   (4) Causes no risk or discomfort to the patient, but the patient must be supine, recumbent, and quiet
   (5) Contraindicated in patients with impedance-driven pacemakers that calculate minute ventilation to regulate the pacemaker rate because the impedance current may cause the pacemaker rate to accelerate

d. Noninvasive measurement by transesophageal Doppler ultrasonography
   (1) Uses Doppler ultrasound technology
   (2) Method
      (a) Ultrasound probe, similar to an orogastric tube, is placed in the esophagus to the level of the third intercostal space and is oriented to the descending thoracic aorta.
      (b) Image displayed represents changes in blood flow in the descending thoracic aorta with each systolic cycle.
   (3) Allows measurement or calculation of cardiac output and index, stroke volume and index, systemic vascular resistance and index, flow time corrected for heart rate, peak velocity of blood during systole, stroke distance, minute distance, and mean acceleration
      (a) Preload: flow time corrected (FTc)
      (b) Contractility: peak velocity (PV)
      (c) Afterload: velocity and flow time

e. Normal value: cardiac output, 4 to 8 L/min; cardiac index, 2.5 to 4 L/min

f. Causes of abnormal parameters (Table 2-15)

9. Mixed venous oxygen saturation
   a. Oxygen saturation of the blood as it returns to the lung for reoxygenation
      (1) Represents the average of the venous oxygen saturations of all organs and tissues
      (2) Provides a global perspective of how well the body's demand for oxygen is met by the amount of oxygen supplied
   b. Measurement
      (1) Blood gas analysis of blood drawn from the distal lumen of the pulmonary artery catheter
      (2) Fiberoptic oximetric pulmonary artery catheter
         (a) Perform calibration as indicated.
            (i) In vitro before the catheter is inserted
            (ii) In vivo every 24 hours
         (b) Monitor the signal quality indicator to ensure reliability.
         (c) Note that accuracy may be affected by hematocrit, catheter position, blood temperature, or pH.
   c. Normal venous oxygen saturation: 60% to 80%
      (1) Affected by changes in oxygen delivery and/or oxygen consumption
   d. Causes of abnormal parameter (Table 2-15)

10. Central venous oxygen saturation ($Scvo_2$)
   a. Oxygen saturation of the blood in the superior vena cava
      (1) Measure serves as a surrogate for venous oxygen saturation before pulmonary artery catheterization is performed or when pulmonary artery catheter placement is not possible, such as when admission to a critical care unit is not possible or not yet necessary
      (2) Though the $Scvo_2$ consistently overestimates the venous oxygen saturation (by around 5% to 15%) under shock conditions, there is a close correlation between the two parameters.
   b. Measurement
      (1) Blood gas analysis of blood drawn from a catheter in the superior vena cava or right atrium

(2) Fiberoptic oximetric central venous catheter with the tip in the superior vena cava or right atrium

c. Normal $Scvo_2$: greater than 70%

(1) Affected by changes in oxygen delivery and/or oxygen consumption

d. Causes of abnormal parameter as for venous oxygen saturation

11. Right ventricular parameters

a. Measured with special right ejection fraction (REF) pulmonary artery catheter

b. Normal values for right ventricular parameters (Table 2-14)

12. Oxygenation parameters

a. Calculated parameters

b. Normal values for oxygenation parameters (Table 2-14)

13. Gastric tonometry

a. Detects regional alterations in tissue perfusion based on the concept that the splanchnic circulation is the first body system to be affected by inadequate perfusion

b. Method

(1) A vented nasogastric tube with a tonometer balloon located a few inches from the distal tip of the catheter is placed into the stomach; a three-way stopcock is at the proximal end of the tonometer port.

(2) The tonometer balloon is filled with saline and is permeable to carbon dioxide.

(3) After a period of equilibration, saline samples taken from the balloon are analyzed for carbon dioxide to reflect the $Pico_2$ (intramucosal carbon dioxide) at the same time that arterial blood is drawn for bicarbonate level.

(4) The intramucosal pH (pHi) then is calculated; a low pHi (less than 7.20) indicates perfusion abnormality.

c. Trends are monitored and interventions evaluated by changes in pHi.

14. Sublingual capnography

a. Detects regional alterations in tissue perfusion; developed to overcome limitations and difficulties of gastric tonometry

b. Method: A sensor is placed under the patient's tongue and is held in place for 60 to 90 seconds.

c. Increases in $P_{sl}CO_2$ correlates with decreases in arterial blood pressure and cardiac index and an increase in serum lactate.

Measurement, Interpretation, and Safe Use of Hemodynamic Monitoring for Clinical Decision Making

1. Maximize accuracy, reproducibility, reliability of measured parameters

a. The transducer must be leveled and balanced to zero (i.e., *zeroed*) with each head of bed position change and/or at least every 12 hours.

(1) Level the air-fluid interface of the transducer to the phlebostatic axis at the time of setup, anytime the head of bed is changed, anytime that the transducer and monitoring cable are disconnected, or at any time the accuracy of the pressure readings is questionable.

(a) The air-fluid interface (also referred to as the *air reference port*) of the transducer needs to be leveled with the phlebostatic axis to ensure accuracy of measurement; the phlebostatic axis correlates with the right atrium and is at the fourth intercostal space and midway between the sternum anterior and the spine posterior (Figure 2-52).

(i) Mark the phlebostatic axis on the patient's chest so that clinicians are consistent.

(ii) Be aware of the clinical importance of having the air-fluid interface level with the phlebostatic axis.

a) If transducer too high, readings will be too low.

b) If transducer too low, readings will be too high.

(b) Though the patient should be supine, there is no need to put the head of bed flat to take pressure measurements as long as the head of bed is elevated no more than 60 degrees and the air-fluid interface is at the level of the phlebostatic axis (Figure 2-52).

(c) Patients should be supine; lateral positions may affect pressure readings and cardiac output measurements.

(2) Balance to zero at the time of setup, anytime the head of bed is changed, anytime that the transducer and monitoring cable are disconnected, or at any time the accuracy of the pressure readings is questionable.

(a) Zero referencing the transducer requires closing the transducer to the patient, opening of the stopcock closest to the transducer to air, and ensuring that the monitor and the recorder read 0 ± 1 mm Hg.

(b) This negates the force exerted by the atmosphere so that only cardiovascular pressures are sensed, measured, and recorded.

b. Ensure accurate calibration

(1) Calibration ensures the accuracy of a quantitative measuring instrument.

(2) Transducer calibration

(a) To calibrate a transduce, a known pressure (e.g., using a sphygmomanometer) is exerted on the transducer to see that the monitor measures and displays it correctly.

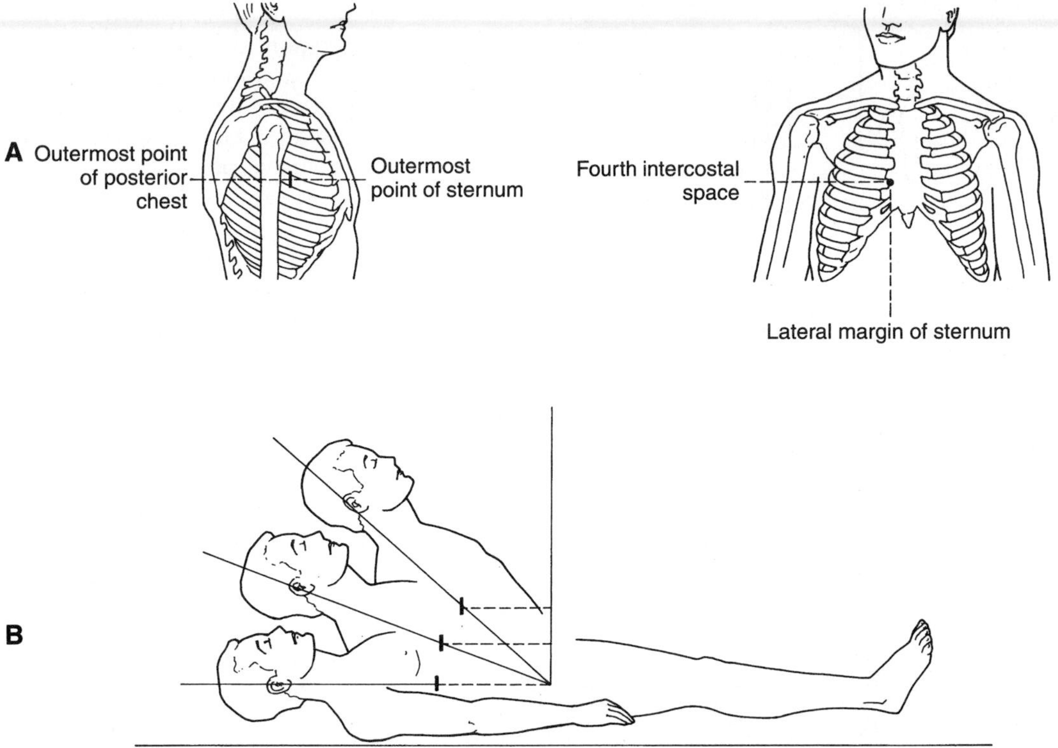

Figure 2-52 Phlebostatic axis. **A,** Location of phlebostatic axis. **B,** Note that the measurements are accurate with head of bed elevated up to 45 degrees as long as the air-fluid interface is level with the phlebostatic axis. (From Flynn, J. B. M., & Bruce, N. P. [1993]. *Introduction to critical care skills*. St. Louis: Mosby.)

(b) Reusable transducers require calibration before use, whereas disposable transducers are precalibrated and only require calibration if the accuracy of the measurements is questionable.

(3) Monitor calibration
- (a) Some monitors require calibration.
- (b) Consult the operating manual for specific instructions for the monitor in use.

(4) Oximetry calibration
- (a) Venous oxygen saturation oximeters require calibration with the oxygen saturation measured from blood drawn from the distal port of the pulmonary artery catheter (frequently referred to as *mixed venous oxygen saturation*).
- (b) This calibration is done in vitro before catheter insertion and in vivo daily and anytime that the fiberoptics may have been damaged, the oximeter module is disconnected from the fiberoptic pulmonary artery catheter, or the venous oxygen saturation values are questionable.

c. Ensure adequate damping using the square wave test (also referred to as *dynamic response test* or *frequency response test*) (Figure 2-53) on initial pressure monitoring setup, at least every 12 hours, when the system has been opened (e.g., zeroing, drawing blood, or changing tubing), whenever the waveform appears distorted or damped, or at any time the accuracy of the pressure readings is questionable.

(1) Fast-flush the system causing the waveform to square off at the top of the screen.

(2) Analyze the waveform after the flush.
- (a) One or two oscillations indicate an optimally damped system.
- (b) No peaks should be more than 1 mm apart, and the second peak should be less than one third the height of the first peak.

(3) Overdamping
- (a) Evidence: no oscillations after the square wave
- (b) Potential effects on pressure readings: underestimation of systolic and overestimation of diastolic pressures
- (c) Treatment
  - (i) Check for occlusion (e.g., kinks and clots) or air in system.
  - (ii) Ensure that noncompliant tubing is in place between the catheter and the transducer.
  - (iii) Ensure tight-fitting connections.

(4) Underdamping
- (a) Evidence: more that two oscillations after square wave or more than one to two blocks between bounces
- (b) Potential effects on pressure readings: overestimation of systolic and underestimation of diastolic pressures

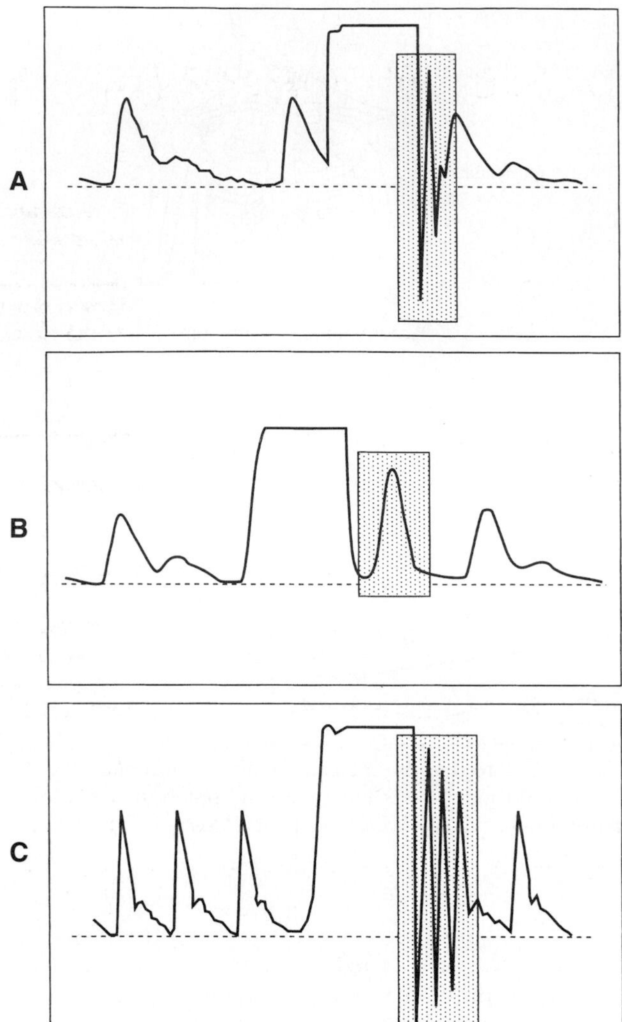

Figure 2-53 Square wave test using the fast-flush valve. **A,** Normal test and accurate waveform. **B,** Overdamped. **C,** Underdamped.

(c) Treatment
   (i) Restrict catheter and tubing length to 4 feet maximum.
   (ii) Add a damping device to absorb unwanted frequency vibration or turn a stopcock slightly.

d. Obtain chest radiograph after insertion of central venous pressure or pulmonary artery catheter to ensure proper positioning of the catheter.
   (1) The tip of a central venous pressure catheter is positioned in the superior vena cava.
   (2) The tip of a pulmonary artery catheter is positioned in a pulmonary arteriole in lung zone 3.
      (a) When the catheter tip of the pulmonary artery catheter is inserted in lung regions in which alveolar pressure exceeds venous pressure (zones 1 and 2), pulmonary artery occlusive pressure will not accurately represent left atrial pressure; also positive end-expiratory pressure in a patient who is hypovolemic or has noncompliant lungs can convert a zone 3 into a zone 1 or 2, causing discrepancies between pulmonary artery occlusive pressure and left atrial pressure.
      (b) An ideally positioned pulmonary artery catheter will occlude the pulmonary arteriole and show a pulmonary artery occlusive pressure waveform when between 1.25 and 1.5 mL of air has been used to inflate the 1.5 mL capacity balloon.
         (i) When a pulmonary artery occlusive pressure waveform is seen when less than 1.25 mL has been injected into the 1.5 mL capacity balloon, the catheter is too distal and prone to cause arteriolar occlusion without balloon inflation (referred to as *spontaneous wedge*).
         (ii) When the balloon is inflated to obtain a pulmonary artery occlusive pressure measurement, the nurse must observe the monitor and stop injecting air into the balloon as soon as the pulmonary artery waveform converts to a pulmonary artery occlusive pressure waveform to avoid overwedging and potentially fatal pulmonary artery rupture.

e. Analyze the graphic recording with simultaneous electrocardiogram as the most reliable means of measuring hemodynamic pressure at end expiration (Figure 2-54).
   (1) Graphic method is more reliable than digital or cursor methods.
   (2) Pressure readings obtained at end expiration minimize the effects of intrathoracic pressure changes because intrathoracic pressures are closest to atmospheric pressure at the end of expiration.
      (a) Spontaneously breathing patient: Expiration is positive (high point of fluctuation).
      (b) Positive pressure mechanically ventilated patient: Expiration is neutral (low point of fluctuation).
      (c) Remember: ventilator valley, patient peak

f. Ensure accuracy of thermodilution cardiac output measurements
   (1) Use continuous cardiac output technology if possible.
   (2) If intermittent methodology is used, do the following:
      (a) Room temperature injectates for cardiac output determination by thermodilution are adequate as long as a 12° F difference exists between blood temperature and injectate temperature. Keep injectate solution and tubing away from direct sunlight and heat lamps.

A

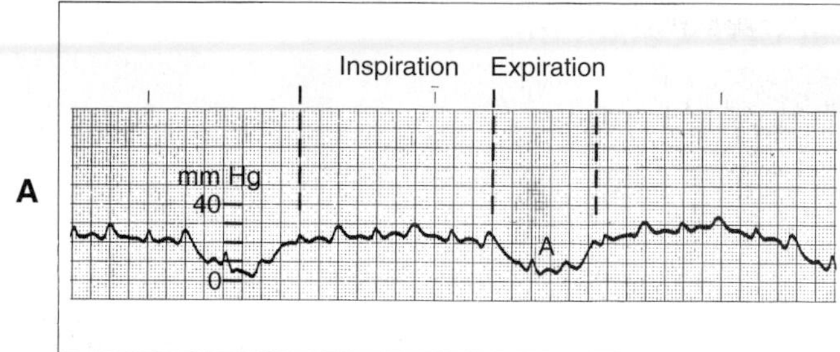

B

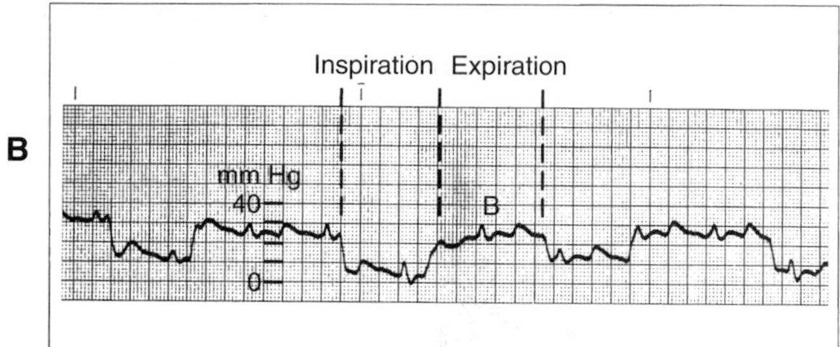

Figure 2-54 Hemodynamic measurements are done at end expiration. **A,** When a patient is receiving positive pressure mechanical ventilation, inspiration is positive and expiration is neutral. Readings should be done at the valley. Remember ventilation-valley. **B,** When a patient is breathing spontaneously, inspiration is negative and expiration is positive. Readings should be done at the peak. Remember patient-peak. (Reprinted with permission from Schermer, L. [1998]. Physiologic and technical variables affecting hemodynamic measurements. *Critical Care Nurse, 8*[2], 33-40.)

(b) Iced injectates may be used in low or high cardiac output states or if the cardiac output value obtained using room temperature is suspected to be inaccurate.
(c) Cardiac output injectate must be injected within 4 seconds.

(3) Enter the appropriate computation constant into the cardiac output computer or monitor for calculation of cardiac output; catheter size and type and volume and temperature of injectate determine the computation constant.

2. Ensure patency of the catheter by maintaining a heparinized flush system unless contraindicated.
   a. Usual heparin concentration is 1 unit of heparin per 1 mL of flush solution.
      (1) Heparin is contraindicated in patients with a history of heparin-induced thrombosis and thrombocytopenia (also referred to as *heparin-associated thrombosis* and *thrombocytopenia* or *white clot syndrome*).
   b. Intermittent flush devices deliver 3 to 5 mL/hr as long as the pressure bag is maintained at 300 mm Hg.
3. Correlate numerical value of the parameter with the patient's clinical presentation.
   a. Hemodynamic parameter changes may precede clinical presentation changes (e.g., subclinical hypoperfusion).
   b. Hemodynamic parameter changes may reflect inaccurate measurements; take care to be consistent in measuring techniques.
   c. Note trends of change of measured parameters over time and in response to therapeutic interventions.
   d. Notify the physician of significant changes from patient's normal values.
      (1) Pulmonary artery systolic more than 4 to 7 mm Hg
      (2) Pulmonary artery diastolic more than 4 to 7 mm Hg
      (3) Pulmonary artery occlusive pressure more than 4 mm Hg
4. Use hemodynamic parameters in clinical decision making.
   a. Determination of best positive end-expiratory pressure (PEEP): positive end-expiratory pressure that will give the best Pa_{O_2} and arterial oxygen saturation without causing a drop in cardiac output and cardiac index.
   b. Determination of best pulmonary artery occlusive pressure or optimal point on Starling's curve.
      (1) Determine the pulmonary artery occlusive pressure that will give the best stroke volume and cardiac output without producing pulmonary edema
      (2) Right ventricular end-diastolic volume may be a more valid parameter to monitor in evaluation of best stretch and filling volumes.
         (a) The main issue is: Does pressure truly reflect volume?
         (b) Pressure is not a reflection of volume in patients with poor ventricular compliance.
         (c) These measurements require a special right ejection fraction pulmonary artery catheter.
   c. Determination of true pulmonary artery occlusive pressure with patients on PEEP (especially important if patient is on high levels of PEEP)
      (1) Convert centimeters of water measurement of positive end-expiratory pressure to millimeters of mercury by dividing by 1.36.
      (2) Subtract one half of the positive end-expiratory pressure (in millimeters of mercury) from the measured pulmonary artery occlusive pressure to get a "true" pulmonary artery occlusive pressure when evaluating fluid status and filling volumes.
      (3) This is of questionable clinical value, for trends rather than absolute pressure measurements are of the most clinical significance.
   d. Use the patient's clinical presentation and hemodynamic parameters to detect physiologic alterations and responses to therapy (Table 2-17).
      (1) Use indexes to evaluate parameters (e.g., cardiac index versus cardiac output).

Table 2-17 **Hemodynamic Profiles for Selected Critical Care Conditions**

Condition	Clinical Presentation	Hemodynamic Presentation
Cardiogenic shock	• Tachycardia, hypotension, tachypnea • S_3 • Crackles • Dyspnea • Jugular vein distention • Hepatomegaly • Peripheral edema • Oliguria	• RAP, PAP, PAOP elevated • SVR, SVRI increased • LVSWI decreased • CO/CI decreased • $Sa{O_2}$, $Sv{O_2}$ decreased • $D{O_2}$ decreased
Hypovolemic shock	• Flat neck veins • Tachycardia, hypotension, tachypnea • Oliguria	• RAP, PAP, PAOP decreased • SVR, SVRI increased • CO/CI decreased • $Sv{O_2}$ decreased • $D{O_2}$ decreased
Anaphylactic shock	• Hypotension, tachypnea • Tachycardia • Angioedema • Warmth, erythema, pruritus, hives • Wheezing, stridor	• RAP, PAP, PAOP decreased • SVR, SVRI decreased • CO/CI decreased • $Sv{O_2}$ decreased • $D{O_2}$ decreased
Neurogenic shock	• Hypotension, tachypnea • Bradycardia • Warm, dry, flushed skin • Hypothermia • Neurologic deficit	• RAP, PAP, PAOP decreased • SVR, SVRI decreased • CO/CI decreased • $Sv{O_2}$ decreased • $D{O_2}$ decreased
Septic shock (early) (late as in hypovolemic shock)	• Tachycardia, hypotension, tachypnea • Hyperthermia • Irritability, confusion • Warm, moist, flushed skin	• RAP, PAP, PAOP decreased • SVR, SVRI decreased • CO/CI increased • $Sv{O_2}$ increased • $D{O_2}$ increased • $V{O_2}$ decreased
Pulmonary hypertension (chronic obstructive pulmonary disease, pulmonary embolism, mitral valve disease, hypoxemia)	• Tachycardia • Jugular vein distention may occur • Dyspnea	• RAP may be elevated • PVR greater than 250 dynes/sec/cm^{-5} • PAm greater than 20 mm Hg • PAd more than 5 mm Hg greater than PAOP • $Sa{O_2}$, $Sv{O_2}$ decreased
Cardiac pulmonary edema	• Tachycardia • Dyspnea • Crackles • S_3	• RAP, PAP, PAOP elevated • PVR, PVRI elevated • SVR, SVRI elevated • CO/CI decreased • $Sa{O_2}$, $Sv{O_2}$ decreased • $D{O_2}$ decreased
Noncardiac pulmonary edema (e.g., acute respiratory distress syndrome)	• Dyspnea • Crackles • Evidence of decreased lung compliance (e.g., increased work of breathing if patient spontaneously breathing, increased peak and plateau pressures if patient is being mechanically ventilated)	• PAP elevated, PAOP normal • PVR, PVRI elevated • $Sa{O_2}$, $Sv{O_2}$ decreased • $D{O_2}$ decreased

Table 2-17 Hemodynamic Profiles for Selected Critical Care Conditions—cont'd

Condition	Clinical Presentation	Hemodynamic Presentation
Cardiac tamponade	• "Fullness" in chest • Tachycardia, hypotension, tachypnea • Muffled heart sounds • Jugular vein distention • Electrical alternans	• RAP, PAP, PAOP elevated • Equalization of intracardiac pressures; RAP, PAd, PAOP elevated within a 5 mm Hg variation • Large *a* and *v* waves (M) on PAOP waveform • Pulsus paradoxus (drop in blood pressure more than 10 mm Hg during inspiration) • CO/CI decreased • Svo_2 decreased • Do_2 decreased
Papillary muscle rupture (acute mitral regurgitation)	• Tachycardia, hypotension, tachypnea • Dyspnea • Crackles • S_3 • New holosystolic murmur at apex	• RAP, PAP, PAOP elevated • Large *v* waves on PAOP waveform • CO/CI decreased • Sao_2, Svo_2 decreased • Do_2 decreased
Rupture of ventricular septum	• Tachycardia, hypotension, tachypnea • New holosystolic murmur at lower left sternal border	• RAP, PAP elevated • Large *v* waves on PAOP waveform • Increased Svo_2 (or mixed venous oxygen saturation) • Increased oxygen gradient (oxygen step-up) between blood drawn from proximal port (right atrial) and distal port (pulmonary artery) • Inaccurate cardiac output measurement: because cardiac output measurement by thermodilution is actually a right ventricular cardiac output, measured cardiac output will be high, but the cardiac output from the left ventricle is actually low. • Do_2 decreased
Left ventricular myocardial infarction	• Chest pain • S_4 at apex • Electrocardiogram changes of LVMI	• RAP, PAP, PAOP may be increased • LVSWI may be decreased • CO/CI may be decreased
Right ventricular myocardial infarction	• Chest pain • S_4 at sternum • Distended jugular neck veins • Clear lungs • Electrocardiogram changes of RVMI	• RAP may be elevated • PAP, PAOP may be decreased • RVSWI may be decreased • CO/CI may be decreased

CO/CI, Cardiac output/cardiac index; *Do_2,* oxygen delivery; *LVSWI,* left ventricular stroke work index; *PAd,* pulmonary artery pressure, diastolic; *PAm,* pulmonary artery pressure, mean; *PAOP,* pulmonary artery occlusive pressure; *PAP,* pulmonary artery pressure; *PVR,* pulmonary vascular resistance; *PVRI,* pulmonary vascular resistance index; *RAP,* right atrial pressure; *RVSWI,* right ventricular stroke work index; *S_3,* third heart sound; *S_4,* fourth heart sound; *Sao_2,* arterial oxygen saturation; *Svo_2,* venous oxygen saturation; *SVR,* systemic vascular resistance; *SVRI,* systemic vascular resistance index; *Vo_2,* oxygen consumption.

(2) Use therapeutic manipulations (e.g., drug administration and titration, fluid therapy, and intraaortic balloon pump) to optimize cardiac output and vital organ perfusion while minimizing myocardial oxygen consumption (Figure 2-55)

5. Prevent, detect, and assist in management of complications of hemodynamic monitoring (Table 2-18).

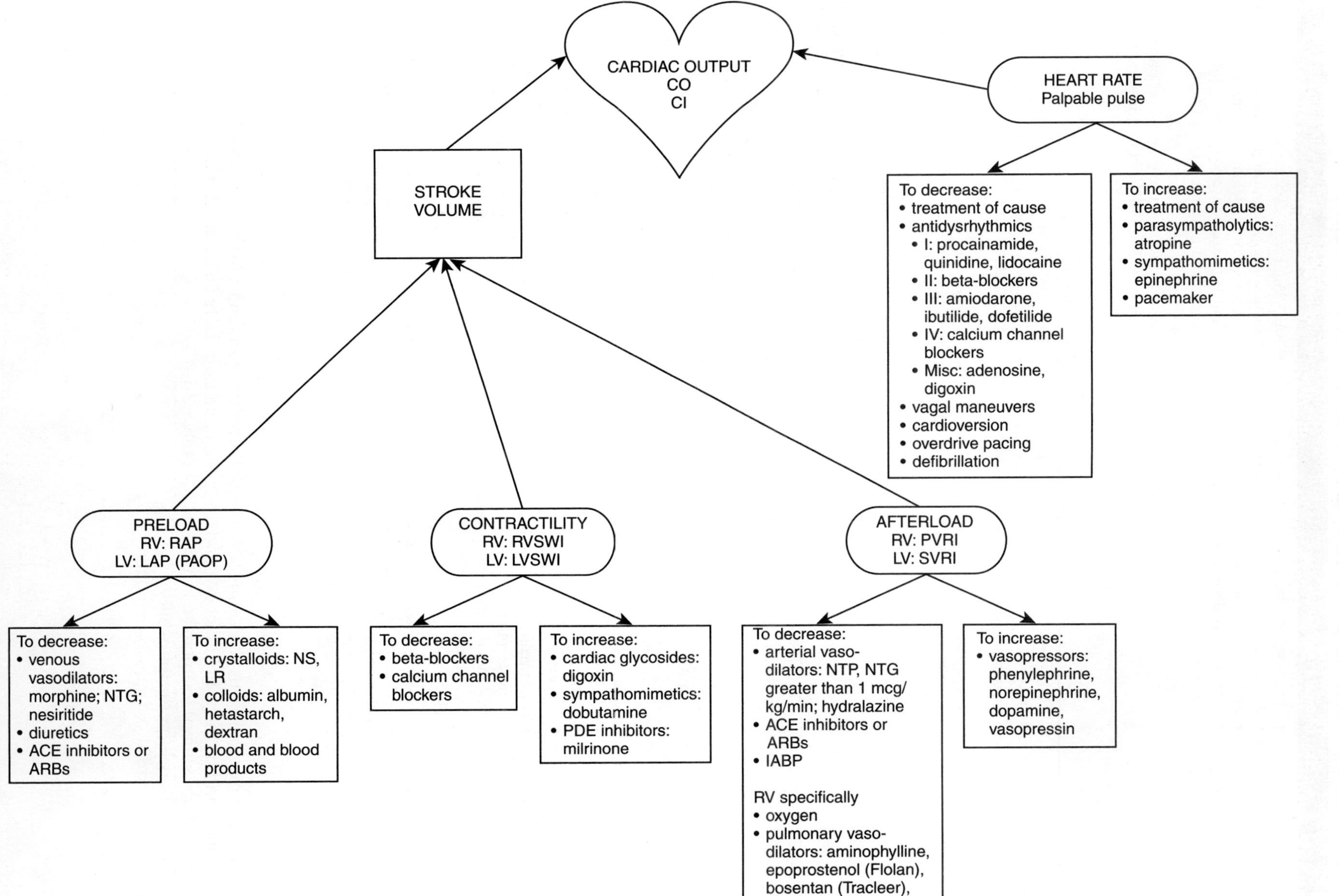

Figure 2-55 Therapeutic manipulations to optimize cardiac output and vital organ perfusion and/or to minimize myocardial oxygen consumption. *ACE,* angiotensin-converting enzyme; *ARB,* angiotensin receptor blocker; *CI,* cardiac index; *CO,* cardiac output; *IABP,* intraaortic balloon pump; *LAP,* left atrial pressure; *LR,* lactated Ringer's solution; *LV,* left ventricle; *LVSWI,* left ventricular stroke work index; *NS,* normal saline; *NTG,* nitroglycerin; *NTP,* nitroprusside; *PAOP,* pulmonary artery occlusive pressure; *PDE,* phosphodiesterase; *PVRI,* pulmonary vascular resistance index; *RAP,* right atrial pressure; *RV,* right ventricle; *RVSWI,* right ventricular stroke work index; *SVRI,* systemic vascular resistance index.

Table 2-18 Complications of Hemodynamic Monitoring

Complications	Prevention/Detection/Treatment
Air emboli	• Use Trendelenburg's position for insertion of deep vein catheters. • Place sterile gloved finger over needle hub with any disconnection during insertion to prevent air emboli. • Aspirated air from flush solution bag to avoid air embolus with inadvertent emptying of flush solution bag. • Flush all lumens with saline before insertion of catheters. • Monitor the pressure monitoring system for air bubbles. • Use only Luer-Lok connections. • Have the patient hold his or her breath during catheter-tubing disconnects (e.g., tubing changes or removal of deep vein catheters). • If air embolus is suspected, turn patient to left side with head down (i.e., Durant's maneuver) and administer oxygen.
Arterial puncture (during venous cannulation)	• Hold pressure for at least 5-10 minutes; a longer time may be required for patients who are taking anticoagulants or patients who have received fibrinolytics.
Balloon rupture	• Test the balloon before insertion by inflating the balloon and holding it in a basin of sterile saline and watching for bubbling. • Store catheters away from sunlight and heat. • Limit the length of time that catheter is left in (ideally less than 72 hours). • Limit the number of times the balloon is inflated to only when indicated (balloons are expected to last about 72 inflations); use diastolic pulmonary artery pressure as a reflection of LVEDP in patients without pulmonary hypertension. • Do not overinflate balloon; stop injecting air as soon as the PAOP waveform is seen. • Do not aspirate air from the balloon; allow passive deflation and reattach the empty syringe to the balloon port. • This complication is particularly dangerous in right-to-left shunt (e.g., neonates); adults shunt left-to-right. • Indications that the balloon has ruptured include inability to obtain PAOP waveform and absence of resistance during inflation. • If balloon rupture has occurred, label balloon lumen accordingly so that others do not continue to try to inflate balloon; use diastolic pulmonary artery pressure as a reflection of LVEDP in patients without pulmonary hypertension; if a PAOP is required, a new pulmonary artery catheter must be inserted.
Clotting and catheter occlusion	• Maintain heparinized normal saline drip with an intermittent flush device. • Monitor for any change in waveform (e.g., damping).

Dysrhythmias: usually ventricular dysrhythmias or right bundle branch block	• Have emergency equipment (including transcutaneous pacemaker) available during insertion.
	• Inflate balloon to capacity (e.g., 1.5 mL) when the catheter is in the right atrium during insertion so that the balloon cushions the catheter tip.
	• Observe the electrocardiogram monitor closely during insertion.
	• Ensure that the catheter has been sutured in place to decrease risk of movement.
	• Assess pulmonary artery pressure waveform for indications that the catheter has flipped back into right ventricle.
	  ◦ Request catheter repositioning for catheter fling or right ventricular waveform.
	  ◦ If right ventricular waveform is noted, inflate balloon to capacity (e.g., 1.5 mL) to cushion the catheter tip.
	  ◦ Turn patient to left side to encourage distal migration of catheter back into pulmonary artery.
	  ◦ Deflate balloon after successful repositioning back into the pulmonary artery.
	• Observe the electrocardiogram monitor closely during removal of the pulmonary artery catheter; remove the catheter in a smooth continuous movement with balloon deflated.

Emboli	• Aspirate if you suspect a small clot, rather than flush.
Exsanguination	• Use only Luer-Lok connections • Maintain alarms in ON position; pressure alarms are usually set 10 to 20 mm Hg above and below the patient's normal.
Fluid overload	• Limit the number of fast flushes. • Use 5 mL instead of 10 mL for cardiac outputs when indicated, or use continuous cardiac output, which requires no fluid boluses for determination of cardiac output. • Limit the frequency of cardiac outputs to every 4 hours unless required more often.

LVEDP, Left ventricular end-diastolic pressure; *PAOP,* pulmonary artery occlusive pressure.

Continued

Table 2-18 Complications of Hemodynamic Monitoring—cont'd

Complications	Prevention/Detection/Treatment
Hematoma	• Maintain pressure for 5-10 minutes with single-thickness pressure dressing after catheter removal; a longer time may be required for patients who are taking anticoagulants or patients who have received fibrinolytics.
Hypothermia	• Use room temperature injectate. • Apply blankets and radiant heaters as needed.
Infection	• Encourage percutaneous catheter insertion (results in a much lower incidence of infection than does cutdown). • Change the flush solution bag whenever it is empty or every 72-96 hours or according to your hospital protocol. • Change the tubing every 72-96 hours or according to your hospital protocol. • Dress and inspect the site using sterile technique every 72-96 hours or according to your hospital protocol. • Avoid clear semipermeable dressings in patients with oily skin. • Use normal saline rather than 5% dextrose in water for the heparinized flush solution. • Flush well after drawing blood samples; do not allow dried blood to stay in stopcock ports or tubing. • Limit the number of stopcocks in the pressure monitoring system. • Replace all vented stopcock covers with nonvented "deadend" caps. • Use strict sterile technique with blood sampling and cardiac outputs. • Encourage use of catheter sleeve over pulmonary artery catheter to allow for sterile catheter manipulation. • Limit the length of time that catheter is left in place (ideally less than 72-96 hours). • Monitor for clinical indications of infection at catheter insertion site: redness, warmth, induration, purulent drainage, and pain at insertion site. • Monitor for clinical indications of catheter sepsis: fever, chills, leukocytosis, positive blood culture and/or catheter culture.
Microshock	• Recognize that this risk is due to elimination of the skin as a protection from microshock in patients with intracardiac catheters. • Ensure that all electrical equipment is properly functioning and grounded. • Do not touch the patient and a piece of electrical equipment at the same time.
Nerve palsy	• Maintain limbs in functional position (e.g., do not keep the wrist hyperextended).
Pneumothorax, hemothorax, chylothorax during insertion	• Have chest radiograph taken after central vein catheter cannulation. • Assist with insertion of chest tube if pneumothorax (air in pleural space), hemothorax (blood in pleural space), or chylothorax (lymph fluid in pleural space) occurs.
Pulmonary artery rupture	• Recognize patients at high risk: elderly patients; patients with pulmonary hypertension; patient receiving anticoagulant, fibrinolytic, or platelet aggregation inhibitor therapy; hypothermic patients. • Inflate balloon with only enough air to cause PAOP waveform; do not overinflate and limit inflation time to a maximum of 15 seconds, for prolonged inflation and excessive balloon volume put too much tension on the vessel wall. • Monitor patient for hemoptysis, dyspnea, and hypotension as indications of pulmonary artery rupture. • If rupture of the pulmonary artery does occur, increase the fraction of inspired oxygen, suction fluids from the airway, position the patient with the affected lung down, assist with intubation with double-lumen endotracheal tube, use positive end-expiratory pressure or pulmonary artery catheter balloon inflation for tamponade effect as prescribed, monitor vital signs and oxygenation levels closely for changes, and prepare the patient for surgery if requested.
Pulmonary infarction	• Inflate balloon only long enough for graphic recording. • Continuously monitor pulmonary artery pressure so that if catheter advances into PAOP position, it will be noted and the catheter will be repositioned. • Request proximal repositioning if it takes less than 1.25 mL to achieve occluded position, because this indicates that the catheter is positioned too distal and spontaneously may occlude the pulmonary arteriole (commonly referred to as *spontaneous wedge*) and cause ischemia and infarction. • Monitor for chest pain, dyspnea, and decreased arterial oxygen saturation as an indication of pulmonary infarction.

Table 2-18 Complications of Hemodynamic Monitoring—cont'd

Complications	Prevention/Detection/Treatment

Thrombosis	• Maintain heparinized normal saline drip with intermittent flush device; keep pressure bag at 300 mm Hg.
	• Limit the length of time that catheter is left in place (ideally less than 72 hours).
	• Prevent trauma to the intima by skillful catheter insertion.
	• To prevent/detect arterial thrombosis with arterial catheters.
	  ○ Select the site with collateral flow (e.g., radial artery).
	  ○ Use the smallest catheter feasible (e.g., 20 gauge for radial artery cannulation).
	  ○ Perform neurovascular assessment hourly to detect acute arterial occlusion promptly.
	• If arterial occlusion occurs, assist with intraarterial fibrinolytic or embolectomy.

LEARNING ACTIVITIES

NOTE: Remember that you will not see questions like these on the CCRN® examination but that these activities allow you to approach the content from a different perspective to remember it better. Multiple-choice questions (like those on the CCRN® examination) are on the CD-ROM.

1. **DIRECTIONS:** Complete the following crossword puzzle dealing with cardiovascular anatomy and physiology.

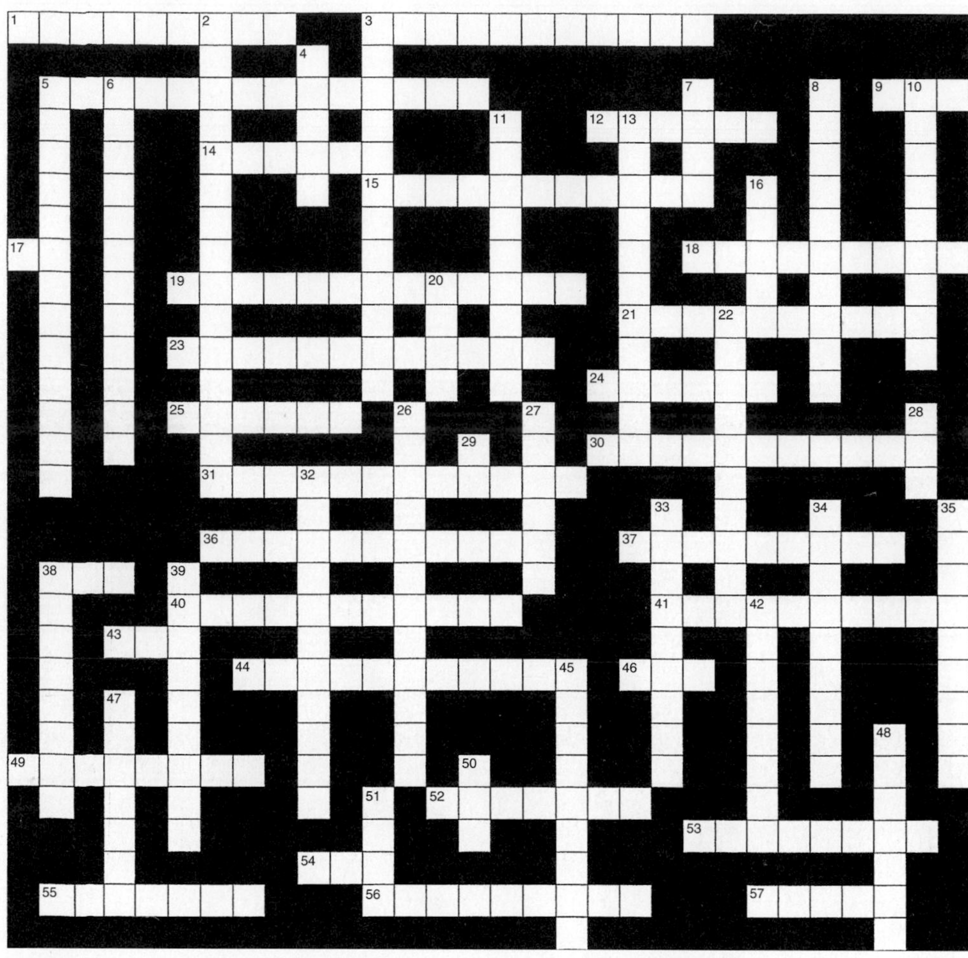

ACROSS

1. The valve between the right atrium and the right ventricle
3. A mineralocorticoid secreted by the adrenal cortex that causes renal retention of sodium and water
5. Receptors located in the carotid and aortic bodies sensitive to PaO_2, $PaCO_2$, and pH
9. The measured parameter used to evaluate right ventricular preload (abbreviation)
12. The type of vessel that leads away from the heart
14. Phase 1 of the action potential may be referred to as the ___ channel
15. A potent endogenous vasoconstrictor
17. The ___ node is the natural pacemaker of the heart (abbreviation)
18. A lower chamber of the heart
19. Pressure receptors
21. The outermost layer of the artery
23. The effect on heart rate
24. The valve between the left ventricle and the aorta
25. An upper chamber of the heart
30. The branch of the autonomic nervous system referred to as the fight-or-flight system
31. The ability of the cardiac cells to respond to a cardiac impulse by transmitting the impulse along the cell membrane
36. The innermost layer of the heart, contiguous with the heart valves
37. The type of vessel that provides oxygen and nutrients to the tissues
38. The calculated parameter used to evaluate right ventricular afterload (abbreviation)
40. The type of pressure that pushes fluid out of the capillary
41. The change in pressure related to change in volume

43. The calculated parameter used to evaluate left ventricular afterload
44. Contains fibrous and serous layers
46. The coronary artery that supplies blood to the right atrium, right ventricle, and the inferior left ventricle (abbrev)
49. The relaxation phase of the cardiac cycle
52. Phase 2 of the action potential may be referred to as the ___ channel
53. The ___ fraction is the percentage of blood that was in the ventricle at the beginning of systole that was pumped out during systole
54. Hormone secreted by the ventricle in response to increased intravascular volume (abbreviation)
55. The stretch on the myofibrils
56. Phase 3 of the action potential may be referred to as the ___ channel
57. The calculated parameter used to evaluate left ventricular contractility (abbreviation)

DOWN

2. The branch of the autonomic nervous sytem that maintains a steady state
3. The ability of the cardiac cells to initiate impulses regularly and spontaneously
4. The middle layer of the artery
5. The ability of the cardiac cells to respond to a stimulus by muscle contraction
6. The ability of the cardiac cells to respond to a stimulus
7. The type of vessel that leads back to the heart
8. The middle (muscle) layer of the heart
10. The pressure against which the ventricle must pump
11. The effect on contractility
13. The reflex responsible for the increase in heart rate during inspiration
16. The substance secreted by the kidney in response to hypotension
20. The measured parameter used to evaluate left ventricular preload (abbreviation)
22. The outermost layer of the heart
26. Disks that lie between myocardial cells to allow rapid transmission of the wave of depolarization through the heart
27. The innermost layer of the artery
28. The coronary artery that supplies blood to the left atrium and the lateral left ventricle (abbreviation)
29. The ___ node slows the impulse down so that the atria can complete their contraction phase before the ventricles are stimulated to contract (abbreviation)
32. The effect on conductivity
33. The branches of the interventricular conduction system are referred to as ___
34. The muscles that contract to close the mitral and tricuspid valves
35. The absolute refractory period plus the relative refractory period is referred to as the ___ refractory period
38. The valve between the right ventricle and the pulmonary artery
39. The ___ potential must be met for depolarization to occur
42. Fibers that transmit the cardiac impulse throughout the ventricular layer
45. A cardiac muscle fiber
47. The contraction phase of the cardiac cycle
48. The type of pressure that pulls fluid into the capillary
50. The coronary artery that supplies blood to the anterior left ventricle and the anterior two thirds of the septum (abbreviation)
51. Diastolic blood pressure minus pulmonary artery occlusive pressure (abbreviation)

2. **DIRECTIONS:** Identify the coronary artery that usually supplies the following structures. Identify the coronary artery as LAD (left anterior descending artery), LCA (left circumflex artery), or RCA (right coronary artery).

Structure	Coronary artery
Anterior left ventricle	
Atrioventricular node	
Bundle branches	
Inferior left ventricle	
Lateral left ventricle	
Left atrium	
Posterior left ventricle	
Right atrium	
Right ventricle	
Sinoatrial node	
Septum	

3. **DIRECTIONS:** Identify the determinants of myocardial oxygen supply and myocardial oxygen demand.

Myocardial oxygen supply	Myocardial oxygen demand

4. **DIRECTIONS:** Identify the primary factor(s) affected in each condition and the primary effect(s) of each treatment. Indicate increase or decrease of heart rate, preload, afterload, or contractility by appropriate arrows (↑ or ↓).

NOTE: Sympathetic nervous system responses may be seen in any of these conditions, but they are secondary, not primary.

Conditions				
Aortic stenosis	___ Heart rate	___ Preload	___ Afterload	___ Contractility
Bradydysrhythmias	___ Heart rate	___ Preload	___ Afterload	___ Contractility
Cardiac tamponade	___ Heart rate	___ Preload	___ Afterload	___ Contractility
Cardiogenic shock	___ Heart rate	___ Preload	___ Afterload	___ Contractility
Cardiomyopathy	___ Heart rate	___ Preload	___ Afterload	___ Contractility
Heart failure	___ Heart rate	___ Preload	___ Afterload	___ Contractility
Hypertension	___ Heart rate	___ Preload	___ Afterload	___ Contractility
Hypovolemia	___ Heart rate	___ Preload	___ Afterload	___ Contractility
Left ventricular myocardial infarction	___ Heart rate	___ Preload	___ Afterload	___ Contractility
Neurogenic shock	___ Heart rate	___ Preload	___ Afterload	___ Contractility
Pulmonary hypertension	___ Heart rate	___ Preload	___ Afterload	___ Contractility
Right ventricular myocardial infarction	___ Heart rate	___ Preload	___ Afterload	___ Contractility
Septic shock—early	___ Heart rate	___ Preload	___ Afterload	___ Contractility
Septic shock—late	___ Heart rate	___ Preload	___ Afterload	___ Contractility
Tachydysrhythmias	___ Heart rate	___ Preload	___ Afterload	___ Contractility
Treatments				
Aminophylline	___ Heart rate	___ Preload	___ Afterload	___ Contractility
Digoxin (Lanoxin)	___ Heart rate	___ Preload	___ Afterload	___ Contractility
Dobutamine (Dobutrex)	___ Heart rate	___ Preload	___ Afterload	___ Contractility
Dopamine (3-5 mcg/kg/min)	___ Heart rate	___ Preload	___ Afterload	___ Contractility
Dopamine (5-10 mcg/kg/minute)	___ Heart rate	___ Preload	___ Afterload	___ Contractility
Dopamine (more than 10 mcg/kg/min)	___ Heart rate	___ Preload	___ Afterload	___ Contractility
Fluid challenge	___ Heart rate	___ Preload	___ Afterload	___ Contractility
Furosemide (Lasix)	___ Heart rate	___ Preload	___ Afterload	___ Contractility
Intraaortic balloon pump	___ Heart rate	___ Preload	___ Afterload	___ Contractility
Isoproterenol (Isuprel)	___ Heart rate	___ Preload	___ Afterload	___ Contractility
Milrinone (Primacor)	___ Heart rate	___ Preload	___ Afterload	___ Contractility
Nesiritide (Natrecor)	___ Heart rate	___ Preload	___ Afterload	___ Contractility
Nitroglycerin	___ Heart rate	___ Preload	___ Afterload	___ Contractility
Nitroprusside (Nipride)	___ Heart rate	___ Preload	___ Afterload	___ Contractility
Phenylephrine (Neo-Synephrine)	___ Heart rate	___ Preload	___ Afterload	___ Contractility
Propranolol (Inderal)	___ Heart rate	___ Preload	___ Afterload	___ Contractility
Vasopressin (Pitressin)	___ Heart rate	___ Preload	___ Afterload	___ Contractility

5. **DIRECTIONS:** Match the receptor of the sympathetic nervous system with its physiologic effect.

___ Alpha a. Increase in heart rate, contractility, conductivity
___ $Beta_1$ b. Dilation of the renal and mesenteric arteries
___ $Beta_2$ c. Vasoconstriction
___ Dopaminergic d. Vasodilation, bronchodilation

6. **DIRECTIONS:** Identify which of these sympathomimetic (adrenergic) drugs cause the most powerful stimulation of each of these receptors.

___ Alpha a. Albuterol (Proventil)
___ $Beta_1$ b. Fenoldopam (Corlopam)
___ $Beta_2$ c. Phenylephrine (Neo-Synephrine)
___ Dopaminergic d. Dobutamine (Dobutrex)

7. **DIRECTIONS:** Identify the formula for each of these parameters.

Parameter	Formula
a. Cardiac output	
b. Stroke index	
c. Blood pressure	
d. Coronary artery perfusion pressure	
e. Mean arterial pressure	
f. Systemic vascular resistance	
g. Delivery of oxygen to the tissues	

8. DIRECTIONS: Identify possible causes of the following heart sounds.

Heart sound	Possible causes
S_1	
S_2	
Physiologic split of S_2	
Paradoxical split of S_2	
Fixed, wide split of S_2	
S_3	
S_4	
Pericardial friction rub	
Midsystolic click	
Holosystolic murmur	
Systolic ejection murmur	
Early diastolic murmur	
Mid to late diastolic murmur	

9. DIRECTIONS: Complete the following table describing common murmurs.

Condition	Timing	Location	Pitch
Mitral regurgitation			
Mitral stenosis			
Aortic regurgitation			
Aortic stenosis			
Mitral valve prolapse			
Papillary muscle dysfunction or rupture			
Ventricular septal defect or rupture			

10. DIRECTIONS: Match the dysrhythmia to the appropriate characteristic.

___ 1. Normal sinus rhythm
___ 2. Sinus bradycardia
___ 3. Sinus tachycardia
___ 4. Premature atrial contraction
___ 5. Atrial fibrillation
___ 6. Atrial flutter
___ 7. Supraventricular tachycardia
___ 8. Premature junctional contraction
___ 9. Junctional escape rhythm
___ 10. Accelerated junctional rhythm
___ 11. Junctional tachycardia
___ 12. Premature ventricular complex
___ 13. Accelerated idioventricular rhythm
___ 14. Ventricular tachycardia
___ 15. Ventricular fibrillation
___ 16. Asystole
___ 17. First-degree atrioventricular block
___ 18. Second-degree atrioventricular block, type I
___ 19. Second-degree atrioventricular block, type II
___ 20. Third-degree atrioventricular block

a. PR interval greater than 0.20 second
b. Early P wave that looks different from other P waves followed by normal QRS complex
c. Sawtooth waves on baseline, no clearly identifiable P waves, normal QRS complex
d. QRS complex is early, greater than 0.12 second, with T wave in opposite direction of QRS complex
e. Regular rhythm, normal P waves, normal QRS complexes, rate less than 60 beats/min
f. Quivering baseline, irregularly irregular occurring QRS complexes.
g. QRS complex is early with inverted P wave immediately (less than 0.12 second) before the QRS complex, in the the QRS complex
h. Regular rhythm with rate of 40 to 60 beats/min with narrow QRS complex with inverted P wave immediately (less than 0.12 second) before the QRS complex, in the QRS complex, or immediately after the QRS complex
i. Flat line, no QRS complexes
j. Regular rhythm, normal P waves, normal QRS complexes, rate greater than 100 beats/min
k. Regular rhythm, normal P waves, normal QRS complexes, rate 60 to 100 beats/min
l. Progressive PR interval lengthening until a P wave is not followed by a QRS complex
m. Regular rhythm with rate of 60 to 100 beats/min with narrow QRS complex with inverted P wave immediately (less than 0.12 second) before the QRS complex, in the QRS complex, or immediately after the QRS complex
n. Wide QRS complex (greater than 0.12 second) rhythm with rate of 40 to 100 beats/min.
o. Regular rhythm with rate of greater than 100 beats/min with narrow QRS complex with inverted P wave immediately (less than 0.12 second) before the QRS complex, in the QRS complex, or immediately after the QRS complex
p. Regular rhythm with rate with rate 150 to 250 beats/min without clearly discernible P waves with narrow QRS complex
q. P wave not followed by QRS complex without preceding progression of PR interval
r. No relationship between P waves and QRS complexes; escape rhythm established by atrioventricular junction or ventricle
s. Irregular baseline, absence of QRS complexes
t. Wide QRS complex (greater than 0.12 second) rhythm with rate greater than 100 beats/min

11. DIRECTIONS: Analyze the following electrocardiogram rhythm strips. All strips are 6 seconds.

a.

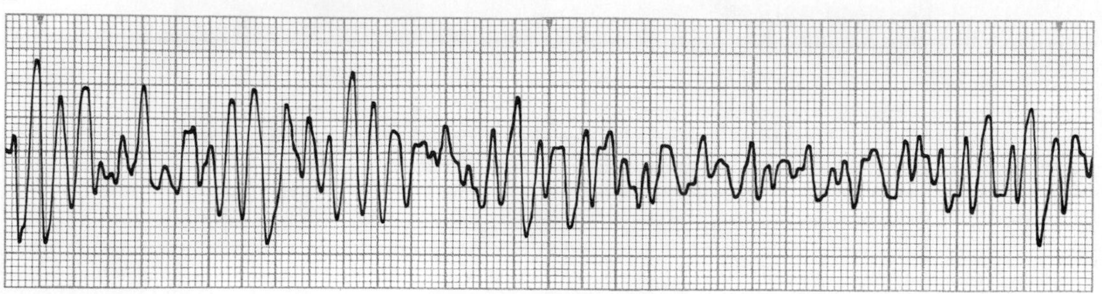

Interpretation ________________________________

b.

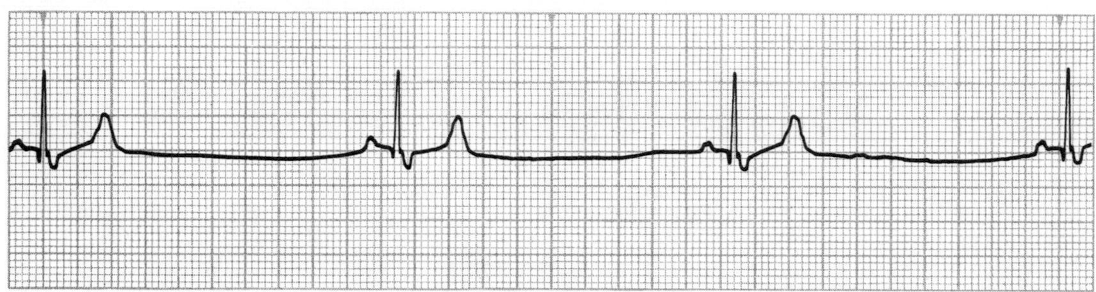

Interpretation ________________________________

c.

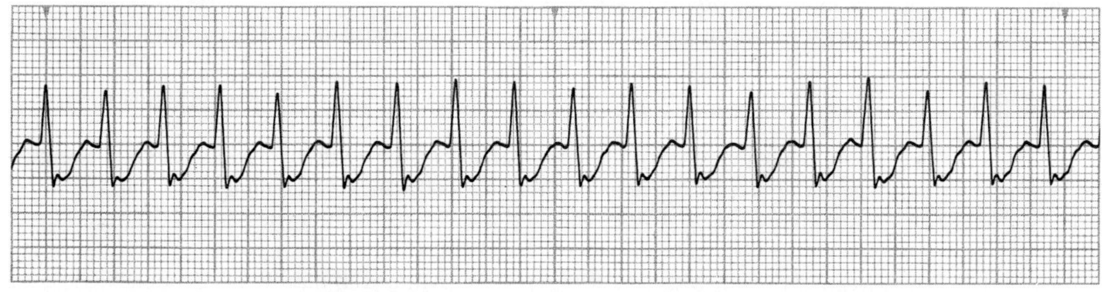

Interpretation ________________________________

d.

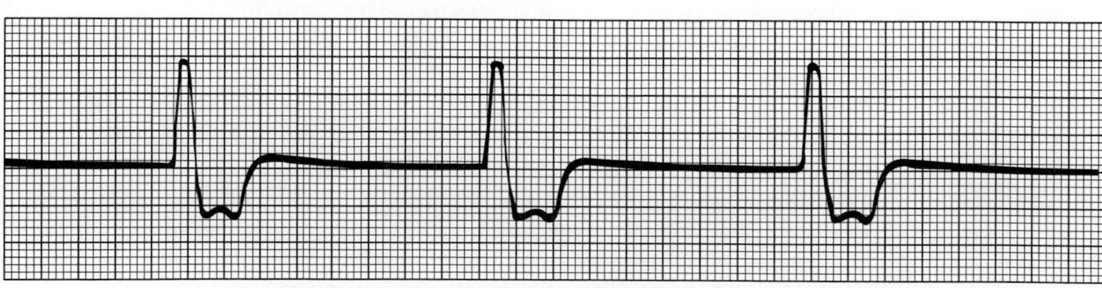

Interpretation ________________________________

e.

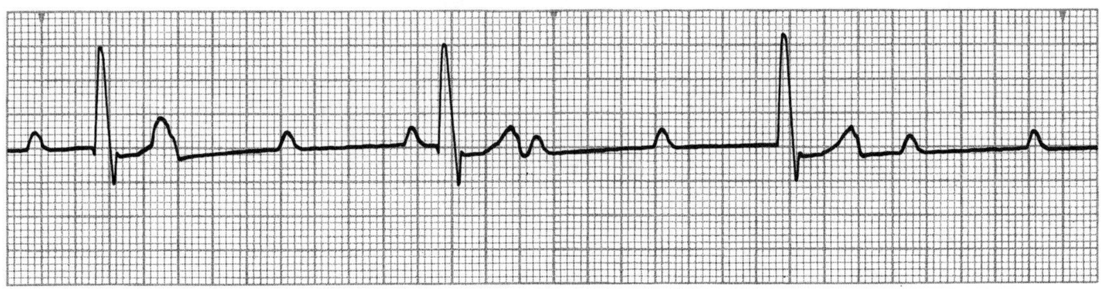

Interpretation ______________________________

f.

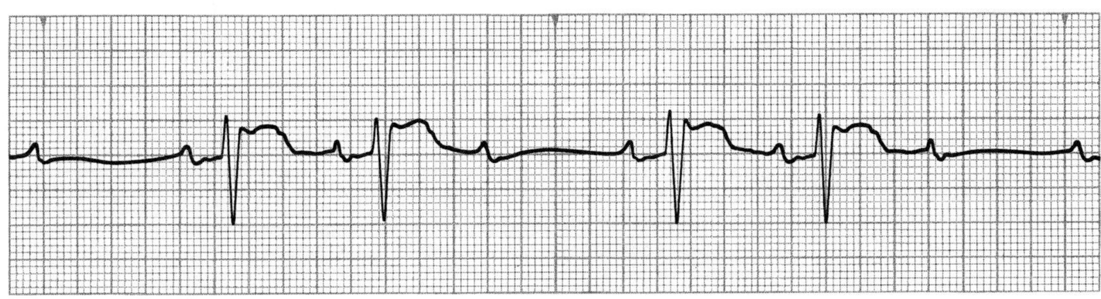

Interpretation ______________________________

g.

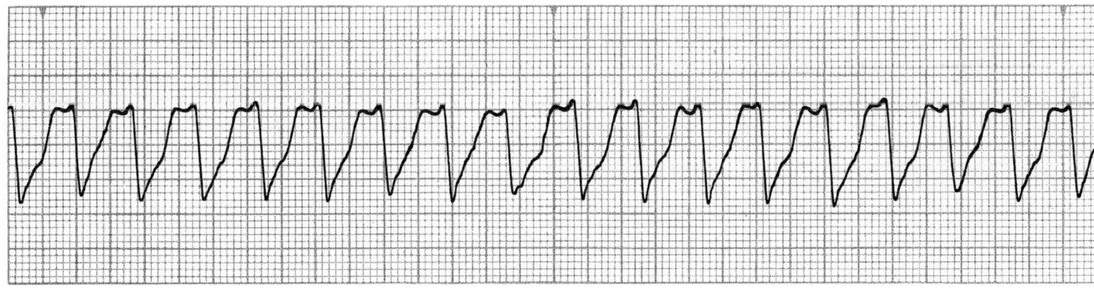

Interpretation ______________________________

h.

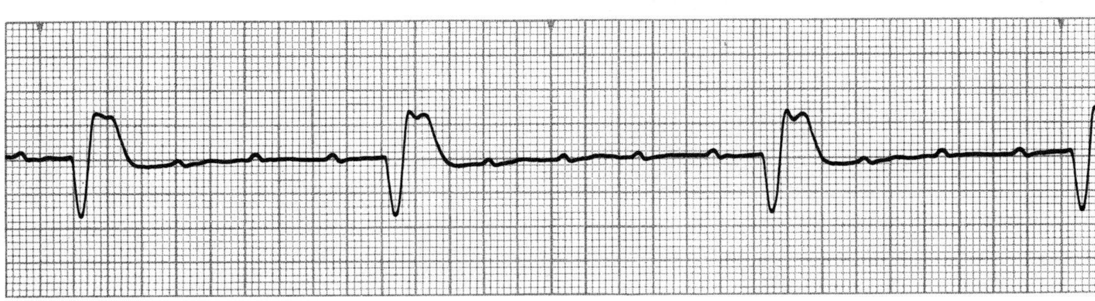

Interpretation ______________________________

i.

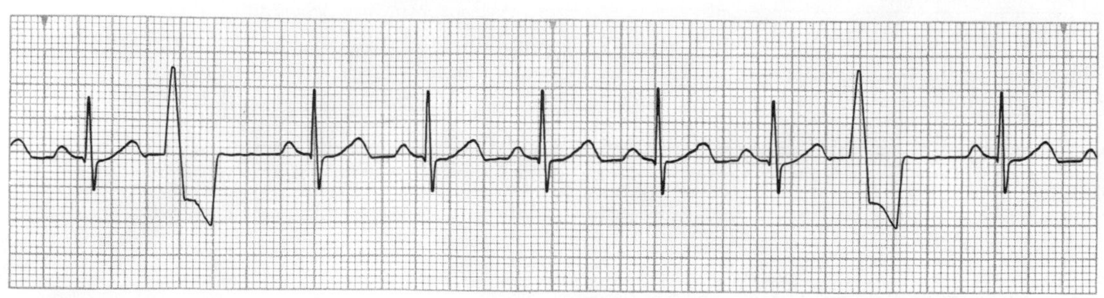

Interpretation ____________________

12. **Directions:** Identify the major diagnostic features of the following electrocardiogram abnormalities.

Condition	Electrocardiogram diagnostic features
Acute myocardial infarction	
Hypercalcemia	
Hyperkalemia	
Hypocalcemia	
Hypokalemia	
Left atrial enlargement	
Left bundle branch block	
Left ventricular hypertrophy	
Pericarditis	
Variant angina	
Right atrial enlargement	
Right bundle branch block	
Right ventricular hypertrophy	
Wellens syndrome	

13. **Directions:** Complete the following table by identifying which cardiac wall the following lead groupings evaluate.

Lead groupings	Cardiac wall
II, III, aVF	
V_4R	
I, aVL	
V_1, V_2	
V_3, V_4	
V_5, V_6	
V_8, V_9	

14. Directions: Analyze the following 12-lead electrocardiograms for left or right bundle branch block.

a.

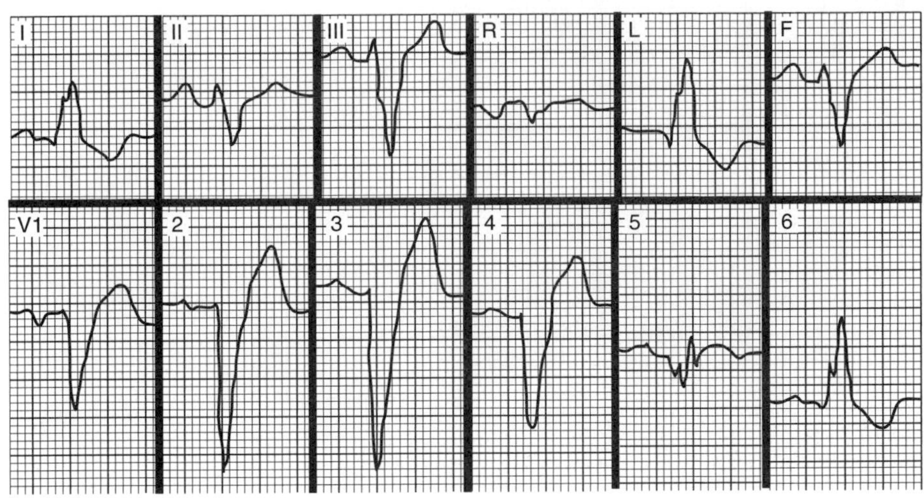

Interpretation ______________________________

b.

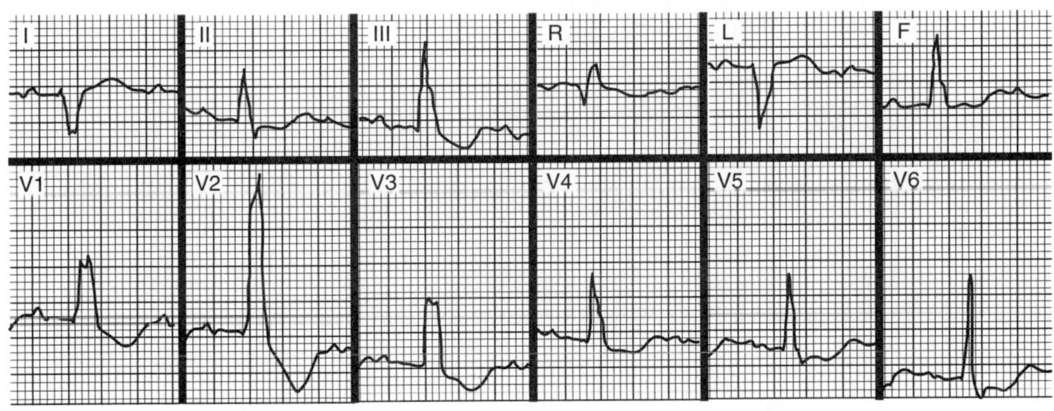

Interpretation ______________________________

15. Directions: Analyze the following 12-lead electrocardiograms for atrial enlargement or ventricular hypertrophy.

a.

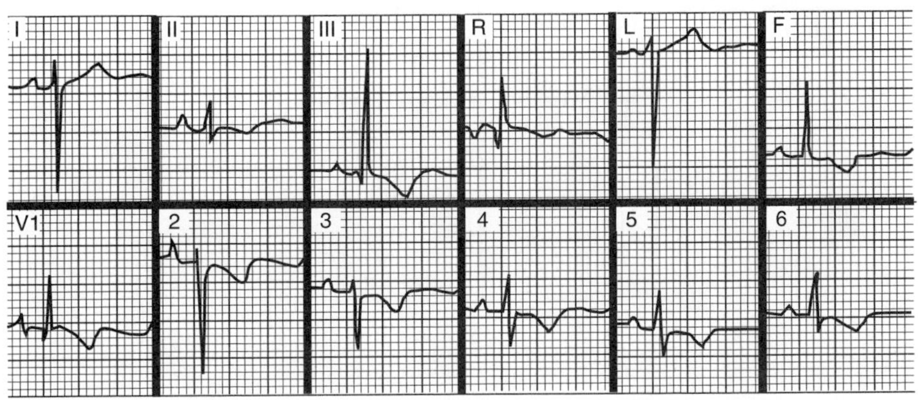

Interpretation ______________________________

b.

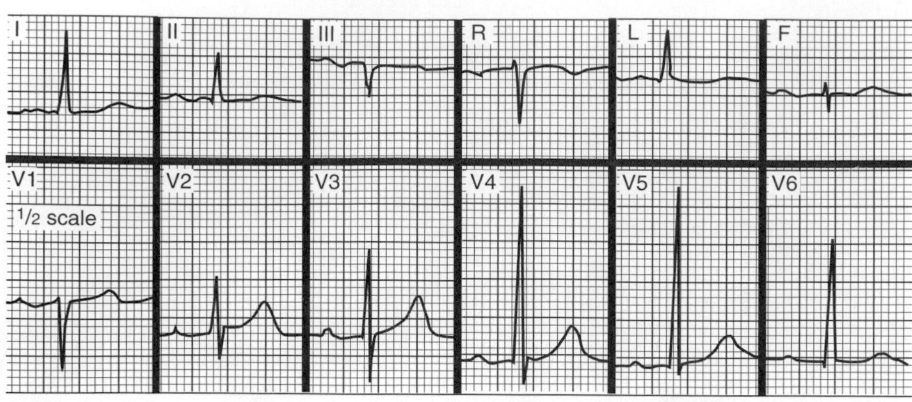

Interpretation ______________________________

16. Directions: Analyze the following 12-lead electrocardiograms from patients with acute chest pain for indications of myocardial infarction. Identify location and age of myocardial infarction if present.

a.

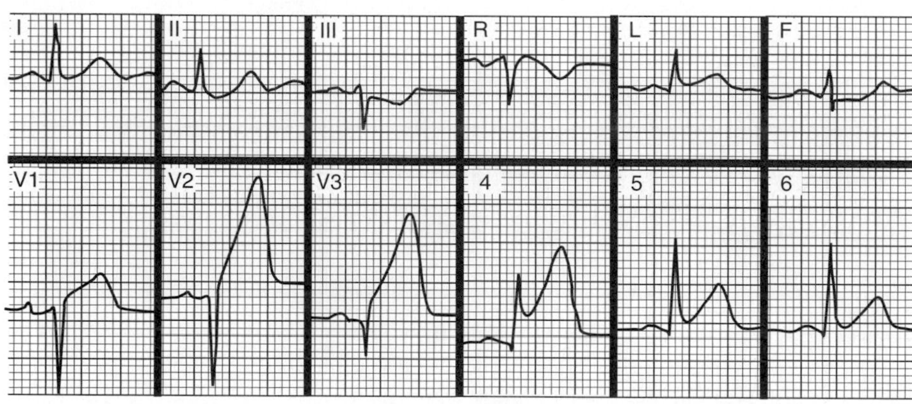

Interpretation ______________________________

b.

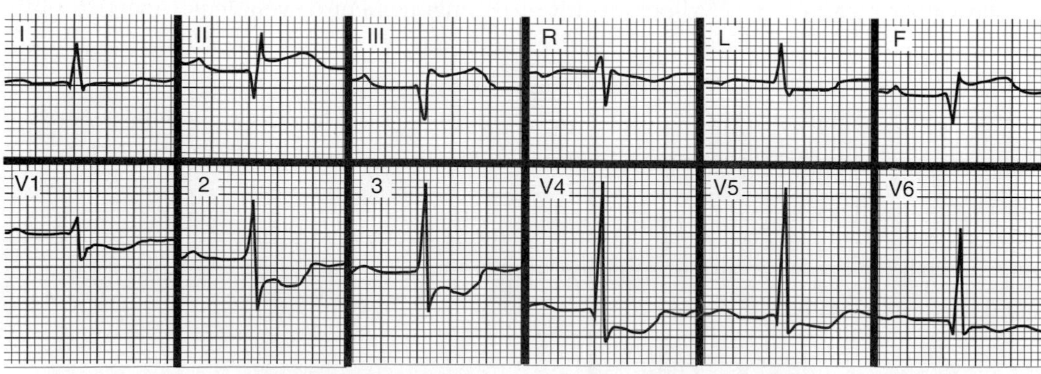

Interpretation ______________________________

17. DIRECTIONS: Complete the following crossword puzzle dealing with hemodynamic monitoring.

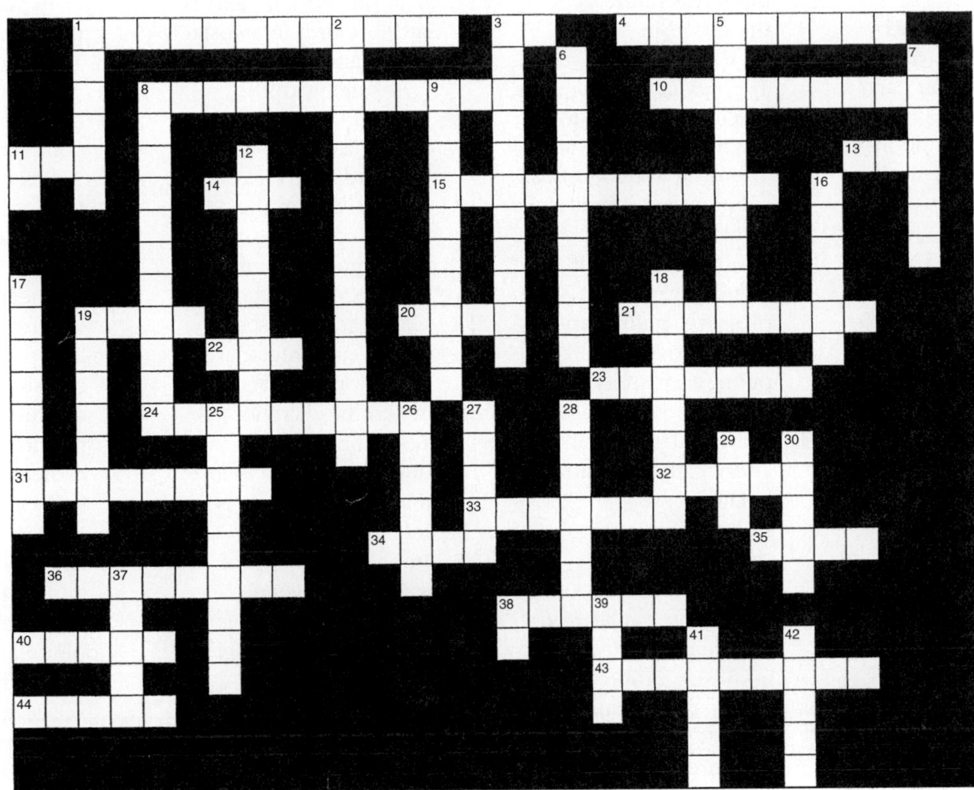

Across

1. ___ of pressures is an indication of cardiac tamponade
3. The amount of blood ejected by the heart in 1 minute (abbreviation)
4. The v wave of the pulmonary artery occlusive pressure waveform represents contraction of the ___
8. Pulmonary ___ is evidenced by pulmonary vascular resistance greater than 250 dynes/sec/cm^{-5}, pulmonary artery mean greater than 20 mm Hg, and difference between pulmonary artery end-diastolic pressure and pulmonary artery occlusive pressure greater than 5 mm Hg
10. To ___ a pulmonary artery catheter is to use more air than is required to cause a pulmonary artery occlusive pressure waveform
11. The pressure in the superior vena cava (abbreviation)
13. The derived parameter calculated by using height and weight; used in calculation of indexed parameters (abbreviation)
14. The parameter that is measured from the proximal port of the pulmonary artery catheter (abbreviation)
15. Zeroing the transducer negates the effect of ___ pressure
19. ___ will increase pulmonary artery pressure and pulmonary artery occlusive pressure by increasing intrathoracic pressures (abbreviation)
20. In ___ calibration of a venous oxygen saturation catheter is done with the catheter inside the body
21. The ___ notch of the pulmonary artery waveform represents closure of the pulmonic valve
22. The average blood pressure over time (abbreviation)
23. Svo_2 is a reflection of oxygen ___
24. Represents the pressure required to open the semilunar valve
31. The original brand name of pulmonary artery catheter (two words)
32. The air-fluid interface of the transducer must be ___ with the phlebostatic axis
33. Using more air than required to cause a pulmonary artery occlusive pressure waveform may cause pulmonary artery ___ manifested by massive hemoptysis
34. To ___ the transducer the stopcock closest to the transducer is opened to air and the baseline on the monitor and the numeric value is adjusted
35. Diastolic blood pressure minus pulmonary artery occlusive pressure determines ___ (abbreviation)
36. Do_2 is an abbreviation for oxygen ___
38. Oxygen ___ is when the oxygen saturation in the pulmonary artery is higher than in the right atrium; indication

of ventricular septal rupture

40. An intermittent ___ device maintains patency of a catheter by delivering a minimal amount of solution each hour
43. Inflation of the balloon at the distal tip of the pulmonary artery catheter causes ___ and blocks right heart pressures to allow measurement of left heart pressure
44. Pressures in the ___ are measured as a mean

DOWN

1. Indications of pulmonary artery catheter migration back into the right ventricle includes loss of dicrotic notch, decrease in diastolic pressure, and ___
2. Technique for measuring cardiac output
3. Vo_2 is an abbreviation for oxygen ___
5. The lumen of the pulmonary artery catheter that measures the temperature of the blood in the pulmonary artery
6. The device that converts mechanical signal to an electrical signal
7. The drug added to flush solution to prevent catheter occlusion
8. The major cause of a decrease in right atrial pressure, pulmonary artery pressure, and pulmonary artery occlusive pressure
9. Leaving the pulmonary artery catheter balloon inflated or a spontaneous wedge may cause pulmonary ___
11. The amount of blood ejected by the heart in 1 minute and indexed to body size (abbreviation)
12. To ___ a transducer a known amount of pressure is exerted on the transducer to see that the pressure is measured correctly
16. The most likely cause of an above normal venous oxygen saturation
17. The phlebostatic axis is at the fourth intercostal space and ___ and correlates with the right atrium
18. The relaxation phase of the cardiac cycle
19. The stretch on the myofibrils that determines the force of the next contraction
25. Gastric ___ is used to detect early regional perfusion defect
26. When the dicrotic notch on the pulmonary artery waveform is lost and the amplitude is lessened
27. In ___ calibration of a venous oxygen saturation catheter is done with the catheter outside the body
28. The contraction phase of the cardiac cycle
29. The calculated parameter indicative of left ventricular afterload (abbreviation)
30. ___ nerve palsy occurs when the wrist in maintained in hyperextended position
37. The calculated parameter indicative of left ventricular contractility and indexed to body size (abbreviation)
38. The amount of blood ejected from the heart each beat (abbreviation)
39. The parameter measured from the distal tip of the pulmonary artery catheter with the balloon inflated; indirectly measures left atrial pressure (abbreviation)
41. Excessive artifact on the pulmonary artery waveform caused by excessive movement of the catheter
42. Venous oxygen saturation may be evaluated by drawing a ___ venous blood gas

18. DIRECTIONS: Match the pathologic condition with its hemodynamic profile.

___ Cardiac tamponade	a. ↑RAP, ↓ PAOP, ↓ CO/CI, Svo_2, Do_2
___ Noncardiac pulmonary edema	b. ↑PAP and PAOP, ↑Svo_2, large *v* waves on PAOP waveform, falsely ↑CO/CI, new systolic murmur at lower left sternal border
___ Cardiac pulmonary edema	c. ↑PAP and PAOP, large *v* waves on PAOP waveform, new systolic murmur at apex
___ Rupture of interventricular septum	d. PAd, PVR, PAm are ↑, and the difference between PAd and PAOP is greater than 5 mm Hg
___ Pulmonary hypertension	e. ↓ RAP, PAP, PAOP, ↑SVR, ↓ CO/CI, Svo_2, Do_2
___ Papillary muscle rupture	f. ↑RAP, PAP, PAOP, ↑SVR, ↓ Sao_2, Svo_2, Do_2
___ Right ventricular myocardial infarction	g. ↑PAP and PAOP, crackles, ↓ Sao_2, Svo_2, Do_2
___ Cardiogenic shock	h. ↑PAP, normal or decreased PAOP, crackles, ↓ Sao_2, Svo_2, Do_2
___ Hypovolemic shock	i. RAP, PAd, and PAOP are ↑and within 5 mm Hg of one another, large *a* waves and large *v* waves on PAOP waveform, ↓ CO/CI, Svo_2, Do_2

CO/CI, Cardiac output/cardiac index; *Do_2,* oxygen delivery; *PAd,* diastolic pulmonary artery pressure; *PAm,* mean pulmonary artery pressure; *PAOP,* pulmonary artery occlusive pressure; *PAP,* pulmonary artery presssure; *PVR,* pulmonary vascular resistance; *RAP,* right atrial pressure; *Sao_2,* arterial oxygen saturation; *Svo_2,* venous oxygen saturation; *SVR,* systemic vascular resistance.

19. Directions: Identify whether the parameters in these case studies are decreased, normal, or increased. Discuss implications and treatment goals.

A. Patient A is a 44-year-old man who was transported to the emergency department after having chest pain for 6 hours. He had ST segment elevation from V_2 to V_6. He also has a history of two previous myocardial infarctions and the electrocardiogram shows a previous inferior myocardial infarction. The next day, Q waves are noted from V_2 to V_6 (indicating extensive anterior myocardial infarction) despite fibrinolytic therapy administered in the emergency department. He is now hypotensive with an S_3 audible at his cardiac apex and crackles audible in his lung bases. Urine output has been marginal for the last 2 hours. The physician inserts a pulmonary artery catheter to allow better evaluation of current status as well as response to therapy. His body surface area is 1.7 m^2.

Parameter	↑, ↓, or Normal	Parameter	↑, ↓, or Normal
BP: 88/70 mm Hg		SV: 23 mL/beat	
MAP: 76 mm Hg		SI: 14 mL/m^2/beat	
HR: 128 beats/min		SVR: 1813 $dynes/sec/cm^{-5}$	
RA: 8 mm Hg		SVRI: 3022 $dynes/sec/cm^{-5}$	
PA: 42/26 mm Hg		PVR: 240 $dynes/sec/cm^{-5}$	
PAm: 31 mm Hg		PVRI: 400 $dynes/sec/cm^{-5}$	
PAOP: 22 mm Hg		LVSWI: 10.3 $g \cdot m/m^2$	
CO: 3 L/min		RVSWI: 2.7 $g \cdot m/m^2$	
CI: 1.8 $L/min/m^2$		Svo_2: 51%	
Sao_2: 88% on 5 L/min via nasal cannula		Do_2I: 318 $mL/min/m^2$	

BP, Blood pressure; *CI,* cardiac index; *CO,* cardiac output; *Do_2I,* oxygen delivery index; *HR,* heart rate; *LVSWI,* left ventricular stroke work index; *MAP,* mean arterial pressure; *PA,* pulmonary artery pressure; *PAm,* mean pulmonary artery pressure; *PAOP,* pulmonary artery occlusive pressure; *PVR,* pulmonary vascular resistance; *PVRI,* pulmonary vascular resistance index; *RA,* right atrial pressure; *RVSWI,* right ventricular stroke work index; *Sao_2,* arterial oxygen saturation; *SI,* stroke index; *SV,* stroke volume; *Svo_2,* venous oxygen saturation; *SVR,* systemic vascular resistance; *SVRI,* systemic vascular resistance index.

Implications and treatment goals:

B. Patient B is a 52-year-old being admitted to the critical care unit after surgery for repair of hemothorax after a gunshot wound. The postanesthesia care unit nurse gives you a report of massive blood loss before surgery and estimated blood loss in the operating room was 1 L. He has had 5 L of lactated Ringer's solution and two units of packed red blood cells. Medical history includes myocardial infarction 5 years ago and angioplasty 2 years ago for intractable angina. A pulmonary artery catheter was inserted before surgery to evaluate fluid status and cardiac function and to aid in fluid resuscitation. Body surface area is 1.9 m^2.

Parameter	↑, ↓, or Normal	Parameter	↑, ↓, or Normal
BP: 92/70 mm Hg		SV: 24 mL/beat	
MAP: 77 mm Hg		SI: 13 mL/m^2/beat	
H: 122 beats/min		SVR: 2097 dynes/sec/cm^{-5}	
RA: 1 mm Hg		SVRI: 4053 dynes/sec/cm^{-5}	
PA: 20/6 mm Hg		PVR: 221 dynes/sec/cm^{-5}	
PAm: 11 mm Hg		PVRI: 427 dynes/sec/cm^{-5}	
PAOP: 3 mm Hg		LVSWI: 13.1 g • m/m^2	
CO: 2.9 L/min		RVSWI: 1.8 g • m/m^2	
CI: 1.5 L/min/m^2		Svo_2: 50%	
Sao_2: 98% on 5 L/min via nasal cannula		Do_2I: 138 mL/min/m^2	
Hgb: 7 g/dL			

BP, Blood pressure; *CI,* cardiac index; *CO,* cardiac output; *Do_2I,* oxygen delivery index; *Hgb,* hemoglobin concentration; *HR,* heart rate; *LVSWI,* left ventricular stroke work index; *MAP,* mean arterial pressure; *PA,* pulmonary artery pressure; *PAm,* mean pulmonary artery pressure; *PAOP,* pulmonary artery occlusive pressure; *PVR,* pulmonary vascular resistance; *PVRI,* pulmonary vascular resistance index; *RA,* right atrial pressure; *RVSWI,* right ventricular stroke work index; *Sao_2,* arterial oxygen saturation; *SI,* stroke index; *SV,* stroke volume; *Svo_2,* venous oxygen saturation; *SVR,* systemic vascular resistance; *SVRI,* systemic vascular resistance index.

Implications and treatment goals:

____

____

____

____

____

____

____

____

LEARNING ACTIVITIES ANSWERS

1.

- 1 TRICUSPID
- 2 PARASYMPATHETIC
- 3 ALDOSTERONE
- 3 AUTOMATICITY
- 4 MEDIA
- 5 CHEMORECEPTORS
- 5 CONTRACTILITY
- 6 EXCITABILITY
- 7 VEIN
- 8 MYOCARDIUM
- 9 RAP
- 10 AFTERLOAD
- 11 INOTROPIC
- 12 ARTERY
- 13 RESPIRATORY
- 14 SODIUM
- 15 ANGIOTENSIN
- 16 RENIN
- 17 SA
- 18 VENTRICLE
- 19 BARORECEPTORS
- 20 PAOP
- 21 ADVENTITIA
- 21 EPICARDIUM
- 23 CHRONOTROPIC
- 24 AORTIC
- 25 ATRIUM
- 26 INTERCALATED
- 27 INTIMA
- 28 LCA
- 29 AV
- 30 SYMPATHETIC
- 31 CONDUCTIVITY
- 32 DROMOTROPIC
- 33 FASCICLES
- 34 PAPILLARY
- 35 EFFECTIVE
- 36 ENDOCARDIUM
- 37 CAPILLARY
- 38 PVR
- 38 PULMONIC
- 39 THRESHOLD
- 40 HYDROSTATIC
- 41 COMPLIANCE
- 42 PURKINJE
- 43 SVR
- 44 PERICARDIUM
- 45 MYOFIBRIL
- 46 RCA
- 47 SYSTOLE
- 48 ONCOTIC
- 49 DIASTOLE
- 50 LAD
- 51 CAD
- 52 CALCIUM
- 53 EJECTION
- 54 BNP
- 55 PRELOAD
- 56 POTASSIUM
- 57 LVSWI

2.

Structure	Coronary artery
Anterior left ventricle	LAD
Atrioventricular node	Most commonly RCA; less commonly LCA
Bundle branches	LAD
Inferior left ventricle	RCA
Lateral left ventricle	LCA
Left atrium	LCA
Posterior left ventricle	Most commonly RCA; less commonly LCA
Right atrium	RCA
Right ventricle	RCA
Sinoatrial node	Most commonly RCA; less commonly LCA
Septum	LAD

3.

Myocardial oxygen supply	Myocardial oxygen demand
Coronary artery patency	Heart rate
Diastolic pressure	Preload
Diastolic time	Afterload
Oxygen extraction: hemoglobin; SaO_2	Contractility

4. Remember that you were asked to identify primary effects. If you gave answers other than these, perhaps you were thinking of the secondary effects, especially those mediated by the sympathetic nervous system.

Conditions				
Aortic stenosis	___ Heart rate	___ Preload	↑ LV Afterload	___ Contractility
Bradydysrhythmias	↓ Heart rate	↑ Preload	___ Afterload	___ Contractility
Cardiac tamponade	___ Heart rate	↓ Preload	___ Afterload	___ Contractility
Cardiogenic shock	___ Heart rate	↑ Preload	↑Afterload	↓ Contractility
Cardiomyopathy	___ Heart rate	___ Preload	___ Afterload	↓ Contractility
Heart failure	___ Heart rate	↑ Preload	↑ Afterload	↓ Contractility
Hypertension	___ Heart rate	___ Preload	↑ LV Afterload	___ Contractility
Hypovolemia	___ Heart rate	↓ Preload	___ Afterload	___ Contractility
Left ventricular myocardial infarction	___ Heart rate	___ Preload	___ Afterload	↓ Contractility
Neurogenic shock	↓ Heart rate	↓ Preload	↓ Afterload	___ Contractility
Pulmonary hypertension	___ Heart rate	___ Preload	↑RV Afterload	___ Contractility
Right ventricular myocardial infarction	___ Heart rate	↑RV Preload ↓ LV Preload	___ Afterload	↓ Contractility
Septic shock—early	___ Heart rate	↓ Preload	↓ Afterload	___ Contractility
Septic shock—late	___ Heart rate	___ Preload	↑ Afterload	___ Contractility
Tachydysrhythmias	↑ Heart rate	↓ Preload	___ Afterload	___ Contractility
Treatments				
Aminophylline	___ Heart rate	___ Preload	↓ RV Afterload	___ Contractility
Digoxin (Lanoxin)	↓ Heart rate	___ Preload	___Afterload	↑ Contractility
Dobutamine (Dobutrex)	___ Heart rate	↓ Preload	↓ Afterload	↑ Contractility
Dopamine (3-5 mcg/kg/min)	↑ Heart rate	___ Preload	___ Afterload	↑ Contractility
Dopamine (5-10 mcg/kg/min)	↑ Heart rate	___ Preload	↑ Afterload	↑ Contractility
Dopamine (more than 10 mcg/kg/min)	↑ Heart rate	___ Preload	↑ Afterload	___ Contractility
Fluid challenge	___ Heart rate	↑ Preload	___ Afterload	___ Contractility
Furosemide (Lasix)	___ Heart rate	↓ Preload	↓ RV Afterload	___ Contractility
Intraaortic balloon pump	___ Heart rate	___ Preload	↓ Afterload	___ Contractility
Isoproterenol (Isuprel)	↑ Heart rate	↓ Preload	↓ Afterload	↑ Contractility
Milrinone (Primacor)	___ Heart rate	↓ Preload	↓ Afterload	↑ Contractility
Nesiritide (Natrecor)	___ Heart rate	↓ Preload	↓ Afterload	___ Contractility
Nitroglycerin	___ Heart rate	↓ Preload	* Afterload	___ Contractility
Nitroprusside (Nipride)	___ Heart rate	↓ Preload	↓ Afterload	___ Contractility
Phenylephrine (Neo-Synephrine)	___ Heart rate	___ Preload	↑ Afterload	___ Contractility
Propranolol (Inderal)	↓ Heart rate	___ Preload	___ Afterload	↓ Contractility
Vasopressin (Pitressin)	___ Heart rate	___ Preload	↑ Afterload	___ Contractility

LV, Left ventricular; *RV*, right ventricular.
*Nitroglycerin will decrease afterload if dosage is greater than 1 mcg/kg/min or approximately 70 mcg/min in a 70-kg patient.

5.

Alpha	c.	Vasoconstriction
$Beta_1$	a.	Increase in heart rate, contractility, conductivity
$Beta_2$	d.	Vasodilation, bronchodilation
Dopaminergic	b.	Dilation of the renal and mesenteric arteries

6.

Alpha	c.	Phenylephrine (Neo-Synephrine)
$Beta_1$	d.	Dobutamine (Dobutrex)
$Beta_2$	a.	Albuterol (Proventil)
Dopaminergic	b.	Fenoldopam (Corlopam)

7.

Parameter	**Formula**
a. Cardiac output	Heart rate × Stroke volume
b. Stroke index	Cardiac index ÷ Heart rate
c. Blood pressure (BP)	Cardiac output × Systemic vascular resistance
d. Coronary artery perfusion pressure	Diastolic BP – Pulmonary artery occlusive pressure
e. Mean arterial pressure	[BP systolic + (BP diastolic × 2)] ÷ 3
f. Systemic vascular resistance	[(Mean arterial pressure – Right atrial pressure) × 80] ÷ Cardiac output
g. Delivery of oxygen to the tissues	Hemoglobin saturation × Arterial oxygen saturation × Cardiac output × 13.4

8.

Heart sound	Possible causes
S_1	Closure of mitral and tricuspid valves
S_2	Closure of aortic and pulmonic valves
Physiologic split of S_2	Changes in intrathoracic pressure created by ventilation
Paradoxical split of S_2	Left bundle branch block; right ventricular pacemaker or ectopy; severe aortic valve disease; patent ductus arteriosus
Fixed, wide split of S_2	Atrial septal defect; acute pulmonary hypertension; pulmonic stenosis
S_3	Heart failure; fluid overload; cardiomyopathy; ventricular septal defect; patent ductus arteriosus
S_4	Myocardial ischemia or infarction; hypertension; ventricular hypertrophy; atrioventricular block; severe aortic or pulmonic stenosis
Pericardial friction rub	Pericarditis
Midsystolic click	Mitral valve prolapse; mitral regurgitation
Holosystolic murmur	Mitral regurgitation; tricuspid stenosis; ventricular septal defect
Systolic ejection murmur	Aortic stenosis; pulmonic stenosis
Early diastolic murmur	Aortic regurgitation; pulmonic regurgitation
Mid to late diastolic murmur	Mitral stenosis; tricuspid stenosis

9.

Condition	Timing	Location	Pitch
Mitral regurgitation	Systolic	Mitral (apex)	High
Mitral stenosis	Diastolic	Mitral (apex)	Low
Aortic regurgitation	Diastolic	Aortic (base)	High
Aortic stenosis	Systolic	Aortic (base)	High
Mitral valve prolapse	Systolic	Mitral (apex)	High
Papillary muscle dysfunction or rupture	Late systolic after midsystolic click	Mitral (apex)	High
Ventricular septal defect or rupture	Systolic	Lower left sternal border	High

10.

k 1. Normal sinus rhythm
e 2. Sinus bradycardia
j 3. Sinus tachycardia
b 4. Premature atrial contraction
f 5. Atrial fibrillation
c 6. Atrial flutter
p 7. Supraventricular tachycardia
g 8. Premature junctional contraction
h 9. Junctional escape rhythm
m 10. Accelerated junctional rhythm
o 11. Junctional tachycardia
d 12. Premature ventricular complex
n 13. Accelerated idioventricular rhythm
t 14. Ventricular tachycardia
s 15. Ventricular fibrillation
i 16. Asystole
a 17. First-degree atrioventricular block
l 18. Second-degree atrioventricular block, type I
q 19. Second-degree atrioventricular block, type II
r 20. Third-degree atrioventricular block

11. a. Ventricular fibrillation

b. Sinus bradycardia with wide QRS complex (assess for bundle branch block on 12-lead electrocardiogram)

c. Supraventricular tachycardia; this is a regular narrow QRS complex tachycardia with no discernible P waves; the P waves could be hidden in the QRS complex or T wave, so there is no way to identify where above the ventricle the rhythm originates, but the rate of 180 beats/min suggests an atrial origin

d. Idioventricular (escape) rhythm

e. Underlying sinus rhythm (atrial rate is 90 beats/min); there is a third-degree atrioventricular block with a ventricular escape rhythm (ventricular rate is 35 beats/min)

f. Underlying rhythm is sinus rhythm (atrial rate is 80 beats/min); there is a second-degree Mobitz I (Wenckebach) atrioventricular block present; conduction ratio is 3:2, and ventricular rate is 40 to 50 beats/min

g. Ventricular tachycardia (monomorphic)

h. Underlying rhythm is sinus tachycardia (atrial rate is 145 beats/min); there is a second-degree Mobitz II block present; conduction ratio is variable, but the PR interval of the conducted P wave is consistent

i. Sinus rhythm with two unifocal premature ventricular contractions

12.

Condition	Electrocardiogram diagnostic features
Acute myocardial infarction	Q waves at least 0.04 second wide and/or one fourth the height of the R wave along with ST segment elevation and symmetrically inverted T waves
Hypercalcemia	Shortened QT interval, shortened ST segment
Hyperkalemia	Tall peaked T waves, widening of QRS complex, atrial asystole
Hypocalcemia	Prolonged QT interval, prolonged ST segment
Hypokalemia	Flat T waves, prominent U wave, ST segment depression
Left atrial enlargement	Wide (greater than 0.11 second), notched P wave in lead II, dominant terminal component of P wave in V_1
Left bundle branch block	Wide (0.12 second or more) QRS complex, which is below the baseline in V_1
Left ventricular hypertrophy	Increased QRS complex amplitude, left axis deviation, ST-T wave changes in V_5 and V_6
Pericarditis	Diffuse ST segment elevation
Variant angina	ST segment elevation with pain
Right atrial enlargement	Tall (greater than 2.5 mm) peaked P wave in lead II, dominant initial component of P wave in V_1
Right bundle branch block	Wide (0.12 second or more) QRS complex, which is above the baseline in V_1
Right ventricular hypertrophy	R wave larger than S wave in V_1 and V_2; S wave larger than R wave in V_5 and V_6; right axis deviation; ST-T wave changes in V_1 and V_2
Wellens syndrome	Symmetrically, deeply inverted T waves in V_2 and V_3 with little or no ST segment elevation

13.

Lead groupings	Cardiac wall
II, III, aVF	Inferior
V_4R	Right ventricular
I, aVL	Lateral (high)
V_1, V_2	Septal
V_3, V_4	Anterior
V_5, V_6	Lateral (low)
V_8, V_9	Posterior

14. a. Left bundle branch block: Note the indicative changes of bundle branch block in V_6 (left ventricular lead) and that the wide QRS complex is totally below the isoelectric line in V_1.

b. Right bundle branch block: Note the indicative changes of bundle branch block in V_1 (right ventricular lead) and that the wide QRS complex is totally above the isoelectric line in V_1.

15. a. Right axis deviation: Note the negative QRS complex in I and positive QRS complex in aVF. Right atrial enlargement: Note the tall, peaked P wave in lead II and dominant initial component of the P wave in V_1. Right ventricular hypertrophy: Note the dominant R wave in V_1 along with right axis deviation, right atrial enlargement, and strain pattern.

b. Normal axis: Note the positive QRS complex in I and isoelectric QRS complex in aVF. Left atrial enlargement: Note the wide, notched P wave in lead II. Left ventricular hypertrophy: Note the deep S wave (must be doubled because the voltage was halved when the electrocardiogram was recorded) in V_1 and tall R wave in V_5. To check for voltage criteria, add the S wave in V_1 or V_2 and the R wave in V_5 or V_6. Because the sum is greater than 35 mm (40 in this case), voltage criteria for left ventricular hypertrophy is met.

16. a. Normal axis: Note the positive QRS complex in I and positive QRS complex in aVL. ST segment elevation is noted from V_1 to V_6. Pathologic Q waves are noted in V_2 and V_3. There is a small R wave in V_1, so the negative wave in that lead is an S wave. This electrocardiogram shows evidence of hyperacute anterior myocardial infarction with injury extending to the septal and lateral walls.

b. Left axis deviation: Note the positive QRS complex in I and negative QRS complex in aVF. ST segment elevation and pathologic Q waves noted in II, III, and aVF are indicative of acute inferior myocardial infarction. Reciprocal changes in the V leads (ST segment depression from V_1 to V_5) suggests concurrent posterior wall infarction.

17.

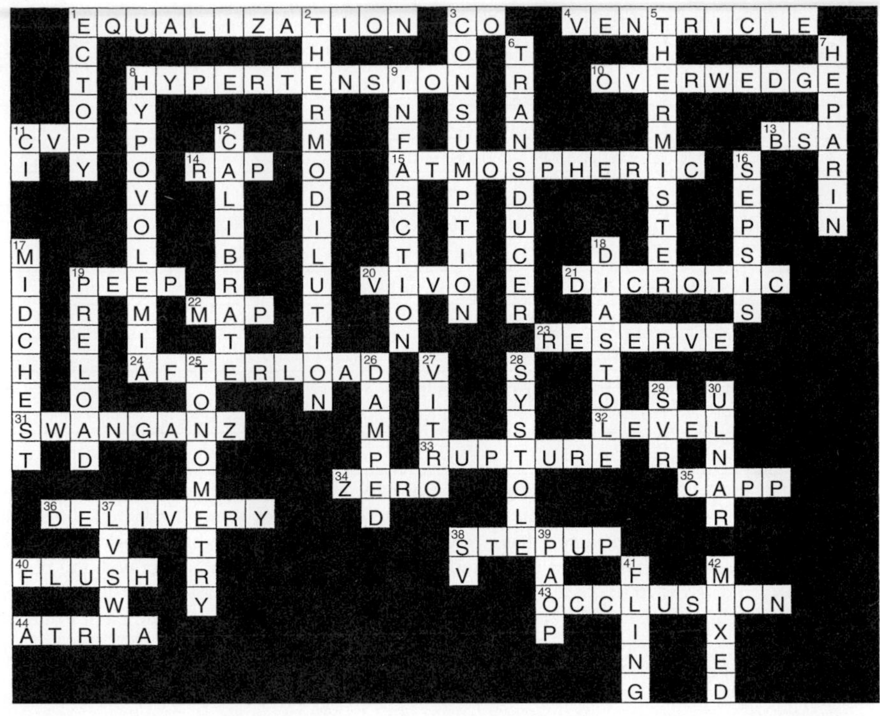

18.

Cardiac tamponade	i.	RAP, PAd, and PAOP are ↑ and within 5 mm Hg of one another, large *a* and large *v* waves on PAOP waveform, ↓ CO/CI, Svo_2, Do_2
Noncardiac pulmonary edema	h.	↑ PAP, normal or decreased PAOP, crackles, ↓ Sao_2, Svo_2, Do_2
Cardiac pulmonary edema	g.	↑ PAP and PAOP, crackles, ↓ Sao_2, Svo_2, Do_2
Rupture of interventricular septum	b.	↑ PAP and PAOP, ↑ Svo_2, large *v* waves on PAOP waveform, falsely ↑ CO/CI, new systolic murmur at lower left sternal border
Pulmonary hypertension	d.	PAd, PVR, PAm are ↑, and the difference between PAd and PAOP is greater than 5 mm Hg
Papillary muscle rupture	c.	↑ PAP and PAOP, large *v* waves on PAOP waveform, new systolic murmur at apex
Right ventricular myocardial infarction	a.	↑ RAP, ↓ PAOP, ↓ CO/CI, Svo_2, Do_2
Cardiogenic shock	f.	↑ RAP, PAP, PAOP, ↑ SVR, ↓ Sao_2, Svo_2, Do_2
Hypovolemic shock	e.	↓ RAP, PAP, PAOP, ↑ SVR, ↓ CO/CI, Svo_2, Do_2

19.

A.

Parameter	↑, ↓, or Normal	Parameter	↑, ↓, or Normal
BP: 88/70 mm Hg	↓	SV: 23 mL/beat	↓
MAP: 76 mm Hg	↓	SI: 14 mL/m²/beat	↓
HR: 128 beats/min	↑	SVR: 1813 dynes/sec/cm^{-5}	↑
RAP: 8 mm Hg	↑	SVRI: 3022 dynes/sec/cm^{-5}	↑
PAP: 42/26 mm Hg	↑	PVR: 240 dynes/sec/cm^{-5}	Normal
PAm: 31 mm Hg	↑	PVRI: 400 dynes/sec/cm^{-5}	Normal
PAOP: 22 mm Hg	↑	LVSWI: 10.3 g • m/m²	↓
CO: 3 L/min	↓	RVSWI: 2.7 g • m/m²	↓
CI: 1.8 L/min/m²	↓	Svo_2: 51%	↓
Sao_2: 88%	↓	Do_2I: 318 mL/min/m²	↓

Discussion: Patient A is in cardiogenic shock as evidenced by the low cardiac index, increased pulmonary artery occlusive pressure and right atrial pressure, and the increase in systemic vascular resistance and systemic vascular resistance index. Myocardial oxygen demand is being increased by the increased heart rate, increased preload (note pulmonary artery occlusive pressure and right atrial pressure), and increased afterload (note systemic vascular resistance). Treatment priorities at this time are to increase contractility (dobutamine), decrease preload (dobutamine will affect preload to some degree but careful intravenous titration of nitroglycerin or the administration of furosemide may be required), and decrease afterload (intraaortic balloon pump would be used because the degree of hypotension is such that even careful titration of an arterial vasodilator such as nitroprusside likely would drop the mean arterial pressure to below 60 mm Hg, which is required to perfuse vital organs).

B.

Parameter	↑, ↓, or Normal	Parameter	↑, ↓, or Normal
BP: 92/70 mm Hg	Low normal	SV: 24 mL/beat	↓
MAP: 77 mm Hg	Normal	SI: 13 mL/m^2/beat	↓
HR: 122 beats/min	↓	SVR: 2097 $dynes/sec/cm^{-5}$	↑
RAP: 1 mm Hg	↓	SVRI: 4053 $dynes/sec/cm^{-5}$	↑
PAP: 20/6 mm Hg	↓	PVR: 221 $dynes/sec/cm^{-5}$	Normal
PAm: 11 mm Hg	↓	PVRI: 427 $dynes/sec/cm^{-5}$	Normal
PAOP: 3 mm Hg	↓	LVSWI: 13.1 $g \cdot m/m^2$	↓
CO: 2.9 L/min	↓	RVSWI: 1.8 $g \cdot m/m^2$	↓
CI: 1.5 $L/min/m^2$	↓	Svo_2: 50%	↓
Sao_2: 95% on 5 L/min via nasal cannula	Normal with supplemental oxygen	Do_2I: 134 $mL/min/m^2$	↓
Hgb: 7 g/dL	↓		

Discussion: Patient B is in hypovolemic shock as evidenced by the low cardiac index with low pulmonary artery occlusive pressure and right atrial pressure. Heart rate and systemic vascular resistance and systemic vascular resistance index are elevated because of sympathetic nervous system stimulation. The current treatment priority is to replace blood volume because surgery has been accomplished to stop the blood loss. Considering that the primary fluid loss was blood, blood replacement in the form of whole blood or packed red blood cells is required along with the normal saline as a primary crystalloid. Hemoglobin is critical for oxygen delivery to the tissues, and the patient's history of coronary artery disease accentuates this need. Notice how profound the oxygen delivery is reduced because the hemoglobin and the cardiac output are insufficient to deliver oxygen to the tissues adequately.

References

Benner, P. (2003). Beware of technologic imperatives and commercial interests that prevent best practices! *American Journal of Critical Care, 12*(5), 469-471.

Connors, A. F., Speroff, T., Dawson, N. V., Thomas, C., Harrell, F. E., Wagner, D., et al. (1996). The effectiveness of right heart catheterization in the initial care of critically ill patients. *Journal of American Medical Association*, 276(11), 889-897.

Bibliography

Adams, K. L. (2004). Hemodynamic assessment: The physiologic basis for turning data into clinical information. *AACN Clinical Issues, 15*(4), 534-546.

Adams-Hamoda, M. G., Caldwell, M. A., Stoots, N. A., & Drew, B. J. (2003). Factors to consider when analyzing 12-lead electrocardiograms for evidence of acute myocardial ischemia. *American Journal of Critical Care, 12*(1), 9-18.

Aehlert, B. (2002). *ECGs made easy* (2nd ed.). St. Louis, MO: Mosby.

Ahrens, T. A., & Schallom, L. (2001). Comparison of pulmonary artery and central venous pressure waveform measurements via digital and graphic measurement methods. *Heart and Lung, 30*(1), 26-38.

Albert, N. M., Hail, M. D., Li, J., & Young, J. B. (2004). Equivalence of the bioimpedance and thermodilution methods in measuring cardiac output in hospitalized patients with advanced, decompensated chronic heart failure. *American Journal of Critical Care, 13*(6), 469-479.

American Association for Critical-Care Nurses. (2004). *Practice Alert: Pulmonary artery pressure measurement.* Retrieved December 21, 2006, from http://www.aacn.org//AACN/practiceAlert.nsf/Files/PAPMonitoring4-7-04/$file/PAPMonitoring.pdf

Attin, M. (2001). Electrophysiology study: A comprehensive review. *American Journal of Critical Care, 10*(4), 260.

Bally, K., Campbell, D., Chesnick, K., & Tranmer, J. E. (2003). Effects of patient-controlled music therapy during coronary angiography on procedural pain and anxiety distress syndrome. *Critical Care Nurse, 23*(2), 50-58.

Bassan, R., Potsch, A., Maisel, A., Tura, B., Villacorta, H., Nogueira, M. V., et al. (2005). B-type natriuretic peptide: A novel early blood marker of acute myocardial infarction in patients with chest pain and no ST-segment elevation. *European Heart Journal, 26*(3), 234-240.

Berry, B. E., & Pinard, A. E. (2002). Assessing tissue oxygenation. *Critical Care Nurse, 22*(3), 22-42.

Carr, M. W., & Grey, M. L. (2002). Magnetic resonance imaging: Overview, risks, and safety measures. *American Journal of Nursing, 102*(12), 26-33.

Chernecky, C., Alichnie, M. C., Garrett, K., George-Gay, B., Hodges, R. K., & Terry, C. (2002). *ECGs and the heart.* Philadelphia: W. B. Saunders.

Collins, A. S. (2001). More than a pump: The endocrine functions of the heart. *American Journal of Critical Care, 10*(2), 94-96.

Connaughton, M. (2001). *Evidence-based coronary care.* London: Churchill Livinstone.

Connors, A. F., Speroff, T., Dawson, N. V., Thomas, C., Harrell, F. E., Wagner, D., et al. (1996). The effectiveness of right heart catheterization in the initial care of critically ill patients. *Journal of American Medical Association*, 276(11), 889-897.

Conover, M. B. (2003). *Understanding electrocardiography* (8th ed.). St. Louis, MO: Mosby.

Daily, E. K. (2001). Hemodynamic waveform analysis. *Journal of Cardiovascular Nursing, 15*(2), 6-22, 87-88.

Darovic, G. (2002). *Hemodynamic monitoring: Invasive and noninvasive clinical application* (3rd ed.). Philadelphia: W. B. Saunders.

Darty, S. N., Thomas, M. S., Neagle, C. M., Link, K. M., Wesley-Farrington, D., & Hundley, W. G. (2002). Cardiovascular magnetic resonance imaging. *American Journal of Nursing, 102*(12), 34-39.

Drew, B. J. (2002). Celebrating the 100th birthday of the electrocardiogram: Lessons learned from research in cardiac monitoring. *American Journal of Critical Care, 11*(4), 378-388.

Futterman, L., & Lemberg, L. (2002). Novel markers in the acute coronary syndrome: BNP, IL-6, PAPP-A. *American Journal of Critical Care, 11*(2), 168-172.

Geiter Jr., H. B. (2002). Understanding axis deviation. *Nursing 2002, 32*(10), 32cc31-32cc34.

Geiter Jr., H. B. (2003). Understanding bundle-branch block. *Nursing 2003, 23*(4), 32cc31-32cc36.

George, E., & Tasota, F. J. (2003). Predicting heart disease with C-reactive protein. *Nursing 2003, 33*(5), 70-71.

Hatchett, R., & Thompson, D. (Eds.). (2002). *Cardiac nursing: A comprehensive guide.* Edinburgh: Churchill Livingstone.

Huszar, R. J. (2002). *Basic dysrhythmias: Interpretation and management* (3rd ed.). St. Louis, MO: Mosby.

Iregui, M., Prentice, D., Sherman, G., Schallom, L., Sona, C., & Kollef, M. H. (2003). Physician's estimates of cardiac index and intravascular volume based on clinical assessment versus transesophageal Doppler measurements obtained by critical care nurses. *American Journal of Critical Care, 12*(4), 336-342.

Jesurum, J. (2004). Svo_2 monitoring. *Critical Care Nurse, 24*(4), 73-76.

Johnson, K. L. (2004). Diagnostic measures to evaluate oxygenation in critically ill adults. *AACN Clinical Issues, 15*(4), 506-524.

Jowett, N. I., & Thompson, D. R. (2003). *Comprehensive cardiac care.* London: Baillicre Tindall.

Leeper, B. (2003). Monitoring right ventricular volumes: A paradigm shift. *AACN Clinical Issues, 14*(2), 208-219.

McAvoy, J. (2004). Case studies of ST-segment elevation before and after percutaneous coronary intervention. *Critical Care Nurse, 24*(6), 32-39.

Mehta, M. (2003). Assessing cardiovascular status. *Nursing 2003, 33*(1), 56-58.

Nagell, K. D., & Nagell, R. (2003). *A case-based approach to ECG interpretation.* St. Louis, MO: MosbyJems.

Pagana, K. D., & Pagana, T. J. (2003). *Mosby's diagnostic and laboratory test reference* (6th ed.). St. Louis, MO: Mosby.

Peacock IV, W. F. (2002). The B-type natriuretic peptide assay: A rapid test for heart failure. *Cleveland Clinic Journal of Medicine, 69*(3), 243-256.

Perloff, J. K. (2000). *Physical examination of the heart and circulation* (3rd ed.). Philadelphia: W. B. Saunders.

Peterson, D. A. (2001). Plunging into preload and afterload. *Dimensions of Critical Care Nursing, 20*(3), 32-36.

Price, S. A., & Wilson, L. M. (2003). *Pathophysiology: Clinical concepts of disease processes.* St. Louis, MO: Mosby.

Quaal, S. J. (2001). Improving the accuracy of pulmonary artery catheter measurements. *Journal of Cardiovascular Nursing, 15*(2), 71-82.

Rice, W. (2000). A comparison of hydrostatic leveling methods in invasive pressure monitoring. *Critical Care Nurse, 20*(6), 20.

Saul, L., & Shatzer, M. (2003). B-type natriuretic peptide testing for detection of heart failure. *Critical Care Nursing Quarterly, 26*(1), 35-39.

Sole, M. L., Klein, D. G., & Moseley, M. J. (2005). *Introduction to critical care nursing* (4th ed.). Philadelphia: Elsevier Saunders.

Thomas, S. A., Liehr, P., DeKeyser, F., Frazier, L., & Friedmann, E. (2002). A review of nursing research on blood pressure. *Journal of Nursing Scholarship, 34*(4), 313-321.

Urden, L., Stacy, K., & Lough, M. (2002). *Thelan's critical care nursing: Diagnosis and management* (4th ed.). St. Louis, MO: Mosby.

Wadas, T. M. (2005). The implantable hemodynamic monitoring system. *Critical Care Nurse, 25*(5), 14-27.

Wallach, S. G. (2004). Cannulation injury of the radial artery: Diagnosis and treatment algorithm. *American Journal of Critical Care, 13*(4), 315-319.

Wiegand, D. L.-M. J., & Carlson, K. K. (2005). *AACN procedure manual for critical care* (5 ed.). Philadelphia: W. B. Saunders.

Wigginton, M. (2001). Expanded ECGs: Easy as V_4, V_5, V_6. Use these techniques to get a wider view of myocardial damage. *Nursing 2001, 31*(1), 50.

Woods, S., Froelicher, E. S. S., & Motzer, S. U. (2000). *Cardiac nursing* (4th ed.). Philadelphia: Lippincott.

The Cardiovascular System: Pathologic Conditions

CHAPTER 3

Cardiopulmonary Arrest

Definition

A sudden cessation of the cardiac output and effective circulation; cardiac arrest is followed by ventilatory cessation

Etiology

1. Dysrhythmias
2. Electrical shock
3. Drowning
4. Asphyxiation
5. Trauma
6. Hypothermia
7. Terminal phases of a chronic illness (cardiopulmonary resuscitation [CPR] may not be attempted on this patient according to advanced directives and "do not resuscitate" [DNR] orders)

Pathophysiology

1. Cardiac arrest ceases delivery of oxygen and removal of carbon dioxide, causing tissue hypoxia and metabolic (i.e., lactic) acidosis.
2. Ventilatory arrest causes hypercapnia, respiratory acidosis, and hypoxemia.
3. Eventually the cerebral cortex is damaged irreversibly, and severe neurologic deficit or biologic death occurs.

Clinical Presentation

1. Loss of consciousness
2. Absence of breathing; agonal breathing may be a precursor to cardiopulmonary arrest
3. Absence of central pulses
4. Absence of auscultated or palpated blood pressure (BP)
5. Anoxic seizures may occur
6. Urinary and bowel incontinence may occur
7. Electrocardiogram (ECG)
   a. Most commonly ventricular fibrillation (VF)
   b. Less commonly ventricular tachycardia (VT)
   c. Rarely asystole
   d. Cardiopulmonary arrest with a stable electrical rhythm (referred to as *pulseless electrical activity* [PEA])

Nursing Diagnoses (see Appendix A)

1. Ineffective Myocardial Tissue Perfusion related to absence of cardiac output
2. Ineffective Cerebral Tissue Perfusion related to absence of cardiac output
3. Risk for Injury related to cardiopulmonary resuscitation, intubation, invasive catheter insertion
4. Impaired Gas Exchange related to absence of ventilation
5. Interrupted Family Processes related to sudden change in health status and potential for death
6. Anxiety related to near-death experience, sudden change in health status, and potential for death

Collaborative Management

1. Initiate CPR (Table 3-1).
2. Provide basic life support (BLS) as recommended by current American Heart Association (AHA) guidelines (Figure 3-1).
   a. Responsiveness: Establish unresponsiveness, and then call for the resuscitation team.
   b. Airway and ventilation
      (1) Open airway using head tilt–chin lift maneuver; use jaw thrust maneuver if you suspect cervical spine injury.
      (2) Evaluate ventilation by looking of the rise and fall of the chest, listening and feeling for airflow for no more than 10 seconds.
         (a) If the patient is adequately breathing, position patient on the left side in recovery position.
         (b) If the patient is not breathing or breathing inadequately, provide ventilation by delivering two breaths (each over 1 second) of 500 to 600 mL by any of the following methods:
            (i) Mouth to mask ventilation
            (ii) Manual resuscitation bag-valve-mask secured over nose and mouth
            (iii) Manual resuscitation bag to endotracheal (ET) tube or tracheostomy tube if already in place

Table 3-1 Primary and Secondary Survey in Cardiopulmonary Arrest

	Primary Survey	Secondary Survey
Focus	CPR and defibrillation	Assessment and treatment
A	Open the airway.	Use invasive airways.
B	Deliver ventilations.	Assess for adequate oxygenation and ventilation.
C	Perform chest compressions.	Establish IV access, diagnose rhythm disturbances, and administer drugs.
D	Defibrillate.	Diagnosis: Search for and treat reversible causes.

Modified from American Heart Association & International Liaison Committee on Resuscitation. (2000). Guidelines 2000 for cardiopulmonary resuscitation and emergency cardiovascular care: an internation consensus on science. *Circulation, 102*(Suppl.), I1-I384.
CPR, Cardiopulmonary resuscitation; *IV,* intravenous.

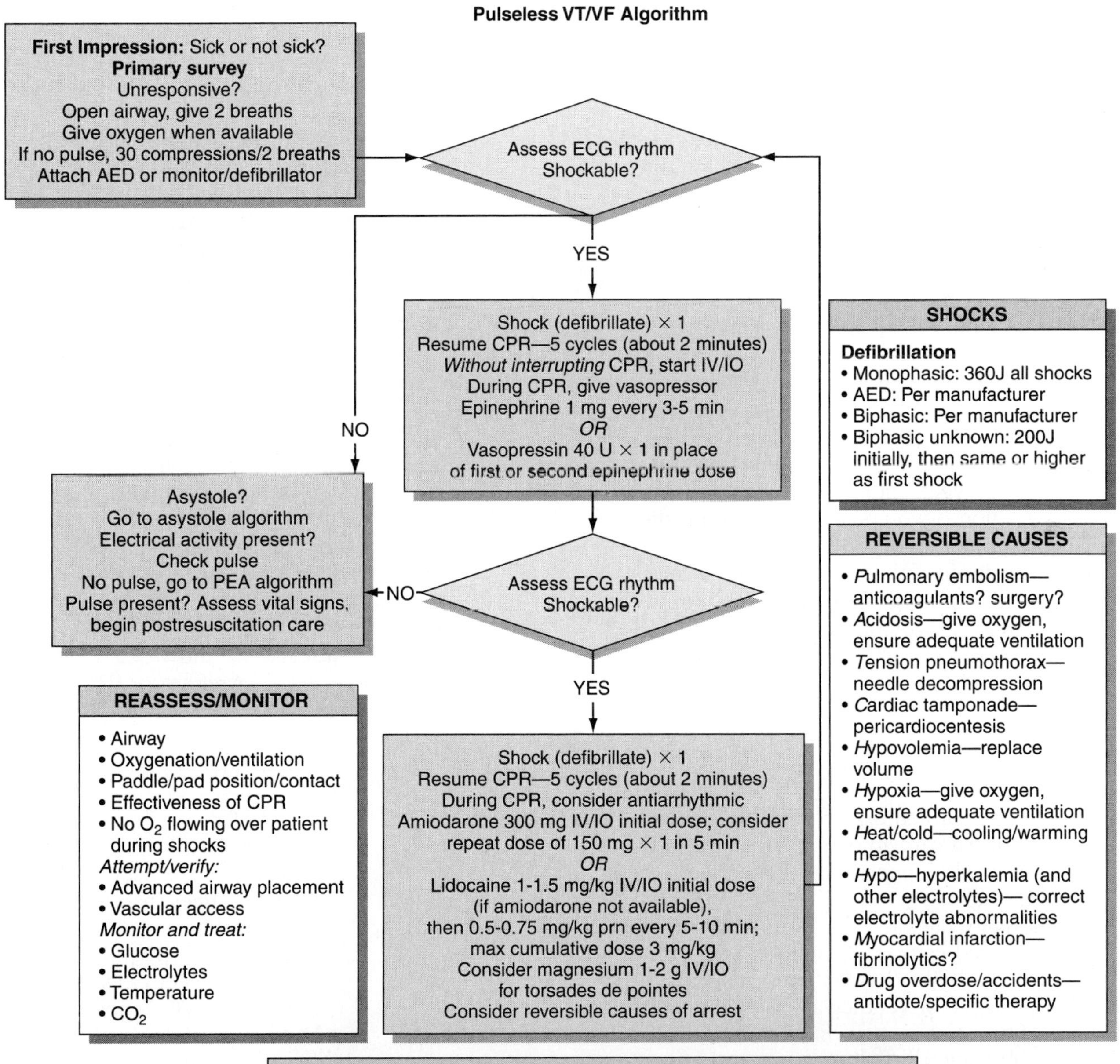

Figure 3-1 Pulseless Ventricular Tachycardia/Ventricular Fibrillation Algorithm. (From Aehlert, B. [2007]: *ACLS Study Guide* [3rd ed.], St. Louis: Mosby.)

(c) Note that each rescue breath does make the chest rise.
(i) If the chest does not rise when the first breath is delivered, perform the head tilt–chin lift maneuver again before repeating the attempt to deliver the breath.
(d) Maintain ventilator rate of 12 to 15 breaths/min; hyperventilation is associated with poor survival rates.

c. Circulation
(1) Assess for signs of circulation (e.g., adequate breathing, coughing, movement, and carotid pulse) for no more than 10 seconds.
(2) If there is no pulse, deliver compressions.
(a) Place heel of one hand over the lower half of sternum; place the other hand over the first hand.
(b) Compress the sternum at a depth of $1\frac{1}{2}$ to 2 inches at a rate of 100 compressions per minute.
(i) New guidelines emphasize that the provider push hard and fast, allowing the chest to recoil completely after each compression.
(c) Limit interruptions in chest compressions.
(i) Brief pauses for ventilations are indicated for bag-valve-mask ventilation.
(ii) Once an advanced airway (e.g., ET tube, laryngeal mask airway [LMA], or Combitube) is in place, maintain compressions without pauses for ventilation.

d. Coordination of compressions and ventilation
(1) Maintain a ratio of 30 compressions to two ventilations if there is only one rescuer.
(2) Maintain a ratio of five compressions to one ventilation if there are two rescuers.
(a) Allow $1\frac{1}{2}$- to 2-second pause for ventilation after five compressions if the patient is not intubated; this pause is not recommended if the patient is intubated.

e. Considerations
(1) CPR performed expertly provides only 20% of normal cardiac output, but most of this goes to the upper body, including the heart and brain.
(2) Mortality rates increase despite prompt CPR if advanced cardiac life support (ACLS) is delayed beyond 12 minutes.
(3) Resistance of ventricular dysrhythmias to defibrillation occurs over time; prompt defibrillation is critical to survival.

3. Provide advanced cardiac life support (ACLS) as recommended by current AHA guidelines.
a. Use ACLS algorithms to provide assistance with decision making in a cardiopulmonary arrest (Figures 3-2 to 3-4).
b. Identification and treatment of the cause of cardiac arrest is especially important in treatment of PEA.
c. Use electrical therapies to change an abnormal cardiac rhythm to a normal one.
(1) Principle: By delivering a shock of sufficient strength, a critical mass of myocardium is depolarized simultaneously, allowing emergence of a dominant normal rhythm.
(2) Precordial thump
(a) Note that the current AHA guidelines provide no recommendation for or against the use of a precordial thump for ACLS providers because there are no prospective studies evaluating efficacy.
(b) Uses
(i) For witnessed VF or pulseless VT only if a defibrillator is not immediately available; do not allow delivery of a precordial thump to delay defibrillation
(ii) For VT with a pulse only if a defibrillator and pacemaker are readily available as deterioration to VF or asystole may occur
(iii) For use only early for ventricular dysrhythmias; precordial thump delivers minimal voltage (approximately 25 J), so it is only likely to be effective if the duration of the ventricular dysrhythmia is short
(c) Method: Solitary thump with the heel of the hand is delivered to the midsternum from a height of 8 to 12 inches.
(3) Defibrillation: defibrillation should be performed for VF or pulseless VT within 3 minutes.
(a) Uses
(i) Pulseless VT and VF
(ii) Unstable or refractory VT with a pulse
(iii) Also useful in asystole in which the rhythm is unclear and could be fine VF
(b) Biphasic defibrillation
(i) Advantages
a) Offers equal or better efficacy at lower energies than traditional monophasic waveform defibrillators: 200 J is safe and has equal or greater efficiency for terminating VF compared with higher-energy monophasic shock
b) Less risk of myocardial injury and skin burns
(ii) Technology first used with automatic implantable cardioverter-defibrillators (AICDs) and automatic external defibrillators (AEDs)

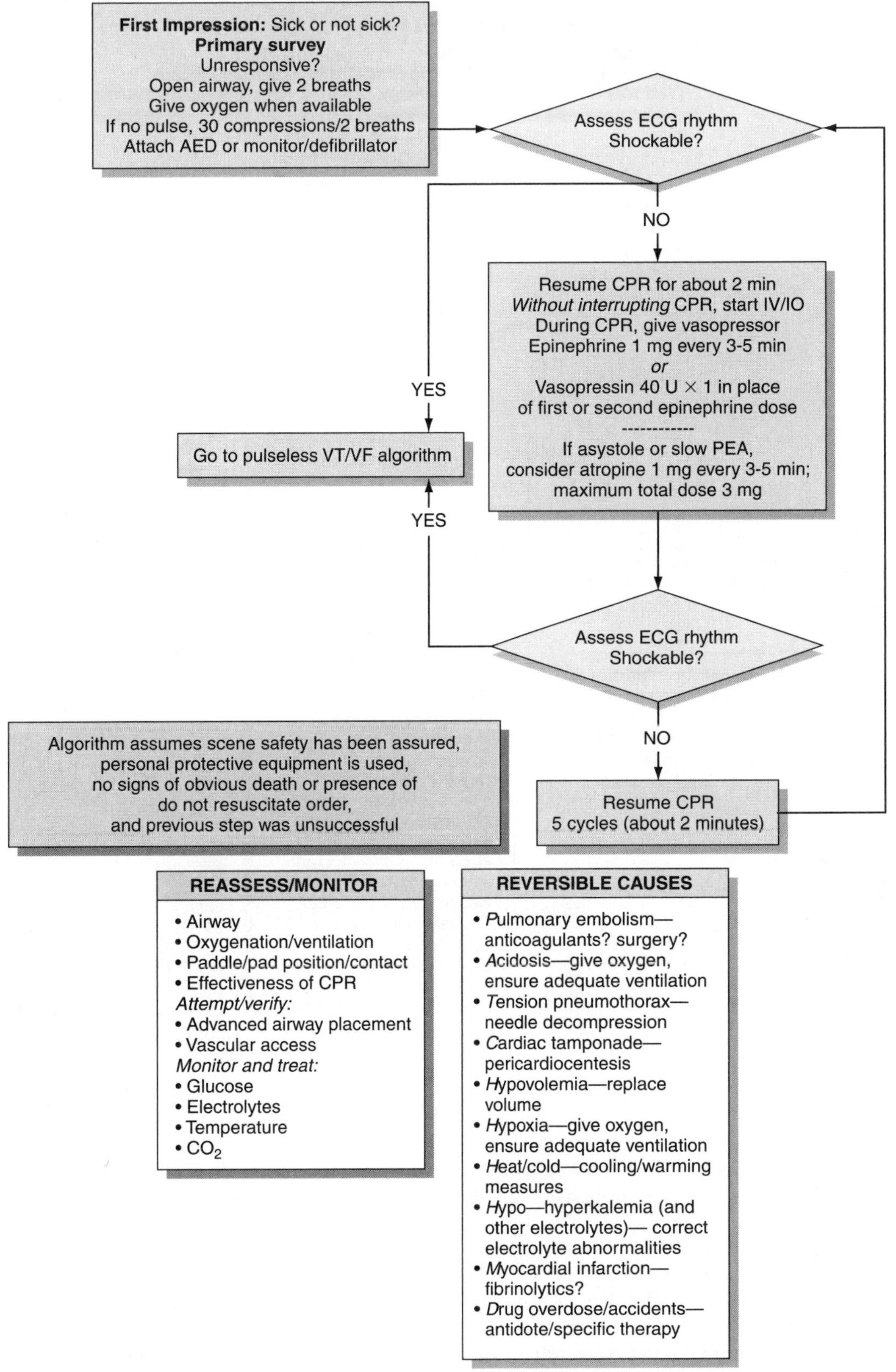

Figure 3-2 Asystole/Pulseless Electrical Activity Algorithm (From Aehlert, B. [2007]: *ACLS Study Guide* [3rd ed.], St. Louis: Mosby.)

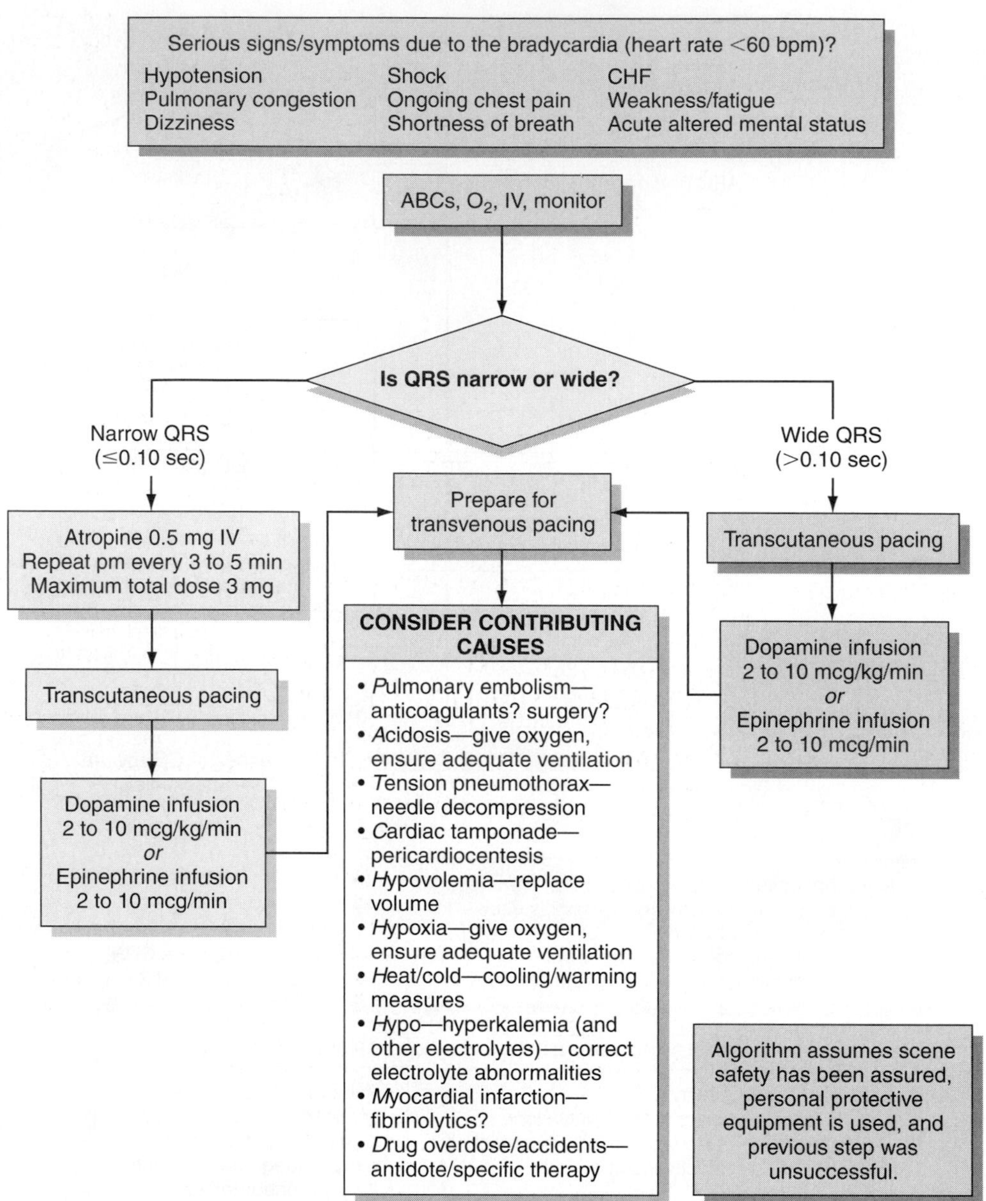

Symptomatic Bradycardia
Serious signs/symptoms due to the bradycardia (heart rate <60 bpm)?
Hypotension
Pulmonary congestion
Dizziness
Shock
Ongoing chest pain
Shortness of breath
CHF
Weakness/fatigue
Acute altered mental status
ABCs, O2, IV, monitor
Is QRS narrow or wide?
Narrow QRS
(≤0.10 sec)
Wide QRS
(>0.10 sec)
Atropine 0.5 mg IV
Repeat pm every 3 to 5 min
Maximum total dose 3 mg
Transcutaneous pacing
Dopamine infusion
2 to 10 mcg/kg/min
or
Epinephrine infusion
2 to 10 mcg/min
Prepare for
transvenous pacing
CONSIDER CONTRIBUTING CAUSES
• Pulmonary embolism—anticoagulants? surgery?
• Acidosis—give oxygen, ensure adequate ventilation
• Tension pneumothorax—needle decompression
• Cardiac tamponade—pericardiocentesis
• Hypovolemia—replace volume
• Hypoxia—give oxygen, ensure adequate ventilation
• Heat/cold—cooling/warming measures
• Hypo—hyperkalemia (and other electrolytes)— correct electrolyte abnormalities
• Myocardial infarction—fibrinolytics?
• Drug overdose/accidents—antidote/specific therapy
Transcutaneous pacing
Dopamine infusion
2 to 10 mcg/kg/min
or
Epinephrine infusion
2 to 10 mcg/min
Algorithm assumes scene safety has been assured, personal protective equipment is used, and previous step was unsuccessful.

Figure 3-3 Symptomatic Bradycardia Algorithm (From Aehlert, B. [2007]: *ACLS Study Guide* [3rd ed.], St. Louis: Mosby.)

a) In the first phase, the current moves from one paddle to the other (as in monophasic defibrillation).
b) In the second phase, the current reverses direction.

(iii) Physiologic mechanism is not fully understood.

(c) Method for manual defibrillation
(i) Check pulse: make sure that VF pattern is not merely artifact caused by loose ECG electrode.
(ii) Remove any foil-lined patches from the patient's chest (e.g., nitroglycerin patches) because they may cause arcing and patient burns.
(iii) Turn defibrillator on, and make sure that the synchronizer switch is off so that charge is delivered as soon as buttons are pushed; most defibrillators automatically reset to nonsynchronized mode so you can immediately defibrillate if VF occurs after cardioversion.
(iv) Apply defibrillation pads to chest for paddle placement or apply conductive jelly to paddles.
a) Anterior: Place one paddle to the right of the sternum below the right clavicle and the other paddle lateral to the apex in the left midaxillary line.

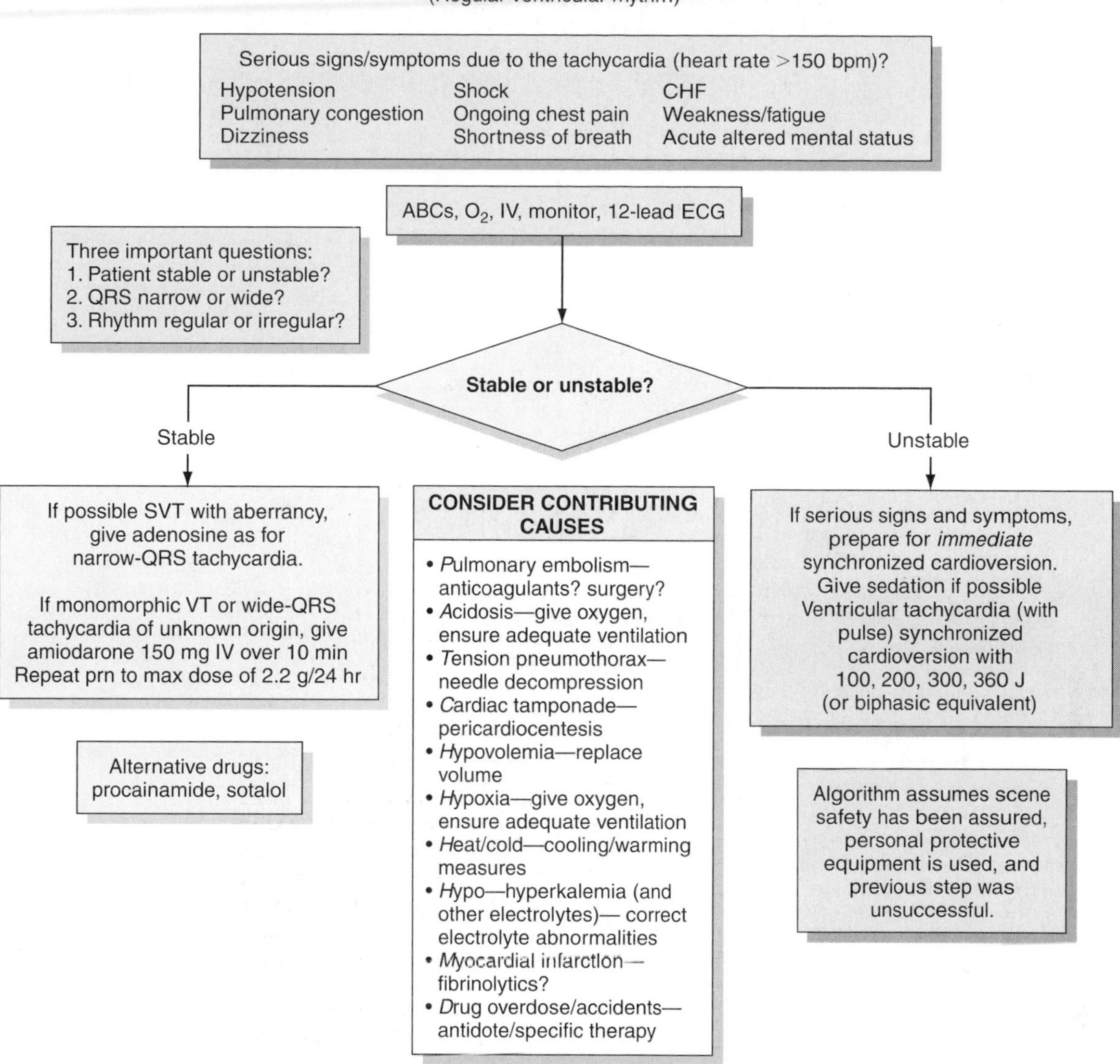

Wide-QRS Tachycardia
(Regular ventricular rhythm)
Serious signs/symptoms due to the tachycardia (heart rate >150 bpm)?
Hypotension
Pulmonary congestion
Dizziness
Shock
Ongoing chest pain
Shortness of breath
CHF
Weakness/fatigue
Acute altered mental status
ABCs, O2, IV, monitor, 12-lead ECG
Three important questions:
1. Patient stable or unstable?
2. QRS narrow or wide?
3. Rhythm regular or irregular?
Stable or unstable?
Stable
Unstable
If possible SVT with aberrancy, give adenosine as for narrow-QRS tachycardia.
If monomorphic VT or wide-QRS tachycardia of unknown origin, give amiodarone 150 mg IV over 10 min Repeat prn to max dose of 2.2 g/24 hr
Alternative drugs: procainamide, sotalol
CONSIDER CONTRIBUTING CAUSES
• Pulmonary embolism—anticoagulants? surgery?
• Acidosis—give oxygen, ensure adequate ventilation
• Tension pneumothorax—needle decompression
• Cardiac tamponade—pericardiocentesis
• Hypovolemia—replace volume
• Hypoxia—give oxygen, ensure adequate ventilation
• Heat/cold—cooling/warming measures
• Hypo—hyperkalemia (and other electrolytes)— correct electrolyte abnormalities
• Myocardial infarction—fibrinolytics?
• Drug overdose/accidents—antidote/specific therapy
If serious signs and symptoms, prepare for immediate synchronized cardioversion. Give sedation if possible Ventricular tachycardia (with pulse) synchronized cardioversion with 100, 200, 300, 360 J (or biphasic equivalent)
Algorithm assumes scene safety has been assured, personal protective equipment is used, and previous step was unsuccessful.

Figure 3-4A Wide-QRS Tachycardia Algorithm (From Aehlert, B. [2007]: *ACLS Study Guide* [3rd ed.], St. Louis: Mosby.)

b) Anterior-posterior: Place the anterior paddle over the apex and the posterior paddle below the right scapula; this paddle placement may be better for obese patients, patients with hyperinflated lungs (e.g., chronic obstructive pulmonary disease [COPD]), and for patients with an AICD.

c) Pacemakers
   i) In patients with permanent pacemakers, the paddles should not be placed within 5 to 10 cm of the pulse generator.
   ii) Turn temporary pacemaker pulse generator off during defibrillation.

(v) Charge to appropriate voltage for defibrillation.
   a) Biphasic: 150 to 200 J for a biphasic truncated exponential waveform or 120 J for a rectilinear biphasic waveform
   b) Monophasic: 360 J

(vi) Apply paddles to defibrillation pads or jellied paddles to chest using firm (~25 pounds) pressure.

(vii) Say the word *clear* and ensure that no one is touching the patient or the bed.

(viii) Press both discharge buttons simultaneously.

(ix) Resume CPR beginning with chest compressions; note that current guidelines recommend only one shock before resuming CPR.

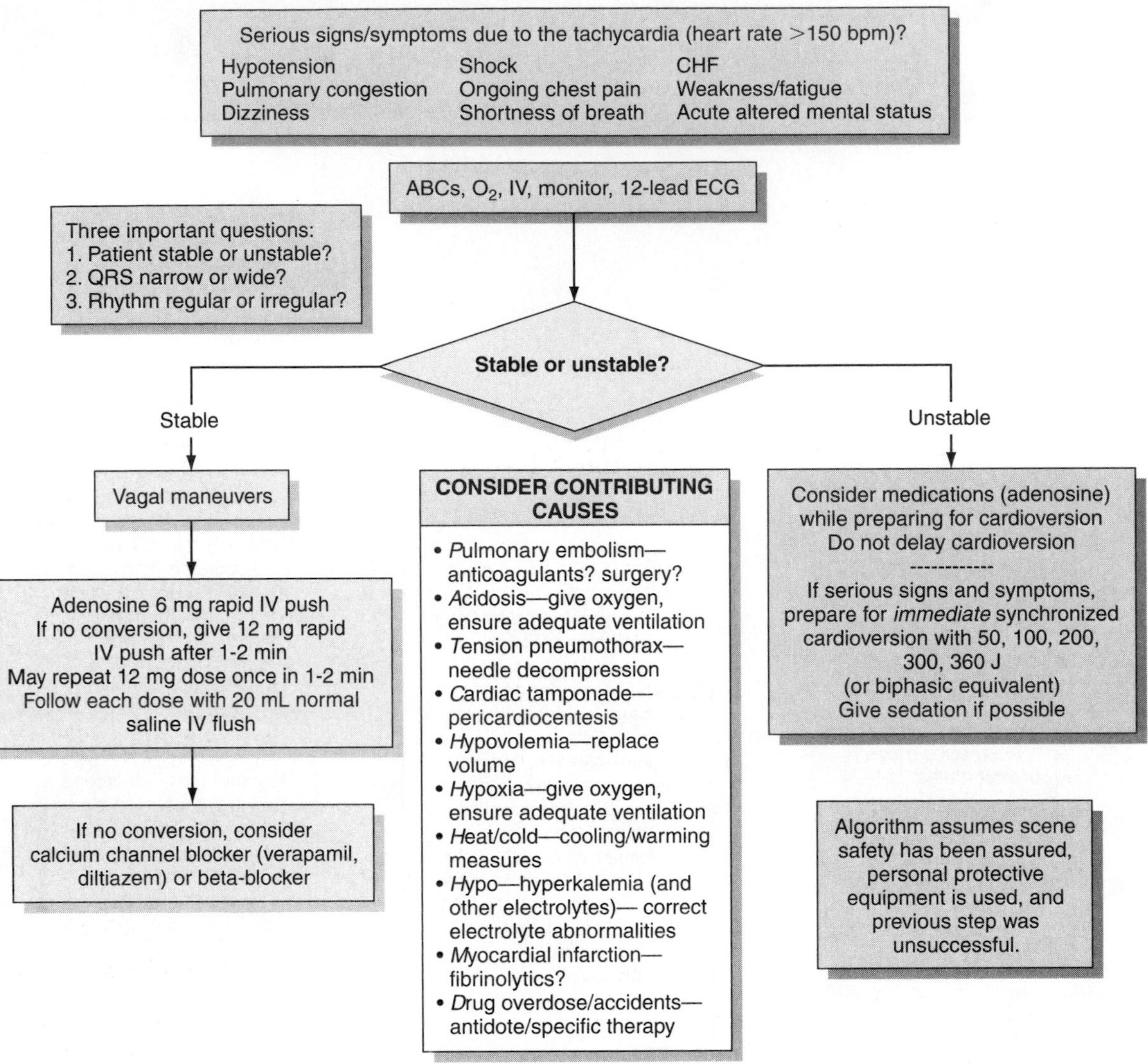
Narrow-QRS Tachycardia
(Regular ventricular rhythm)
Serious signs/symptoms due to the tachycardia (heart rate >150 bpm)?
Hypotension
Shock
CHF
Pulmonary congestion
Ongoing chest pain
Weakness/fatigue
Dizziness
Shortness of breath
Acute altered mental status
ABCs, O2, IV, monitor, 12-lead ECG
Three important questions:
1. Patient stable or unstable?
2. QRS narrow or wide?
3. Rhythm regular or irregular?
Stable or unstable?
Stable
Unstable
Vagal maneuvers
Adenosine 6 mg rapid IV push
If no conversion, give 12 mg rapid IV push after 1-2 min
May repeat 12 mg dose once in 1-2 min
Follow each dose with 20 mL normal saline IV flush
If no conversion, consider calcium channel blocker (verapamil, diltiazem) or beta-blocker
CONSIDER CONTRIBUTING CAUSES
• Pulmonary embolism—anticoagulants? surgery?
• Acidosis—give oxygen, ensure adequate ventilation
• Tension pneumothorax—needle decompression
• Cardiac tamponade—pericardiocentesis
• Hypovolemia—replace volume
• Hypoxia—give oxygen, ensure adequate ventilation
• Heat/cold—cooling/warming measures
• Hypo—hyperkalemia (and other electrolytes)— correct electrolyte abnormalities
• Myocardial infarction—fibrinolytics?
• Drug overdose/accidents—antidote/specific therapy
Consider medications (adenosine) while preparing for cardioversion
Do not delay cardioversion
If serious signs and symptoms, prepare for immediate synchronized cardioversion with 50, 100, 200, 300, 360 J
(or biphasic equivalent)
Give sedation if possible
Algorithm assumes scene safety has been assured, personal protective equipment is used, and previous step was unsuccessful.

Figure 3-4B Narrow-QRS Tachycardia Algorithm (From Aehlert, B. [2007]: *ACLS Study Guide* [3rd ed.], St. Louis: Mosby.)

(x) Recheck rhythm after five cycles (~2 minutes).
  a) If rhythm and pulse are restored, administer antidysrhythmic drug therapy.
  b) If rhythm and pulse are not restored, continue with appropriate algorithm.

(d) Method for using a semiautomatic external defibrillator
  (i) Attach the device to the patient: put one pad to the right of the sternum below the right clavicle, and place the other pad lateral to the apex in the left midaxillary line.
  (ii) Turn the device on.
  (iii) Ensure that the patient is completely still and that no one is touching the patient.
  (iv) Press the analyze button. The device will signal *stand clear* and perform a 3-second analysis.
  (v) If VT or VF is detected, the AED will charge to 200 J (biphasic) and display a "shock indicated" message.
  (vi) Call *clear* and ensure that no one is touching the patient.
  (vii) Press the shock button to deliver the shock if it was indicated.
  (viii) If rhythm and pulse are restored, administer antidysrhythmic drug therapy.
  (ix) If rhythm and pulse are not restored, continue CPR and appropriate algorithm.

(e) Successful defibrillation is less likely if any of following present:
  (i) Hypoxia
  (ii) Severe acidosis

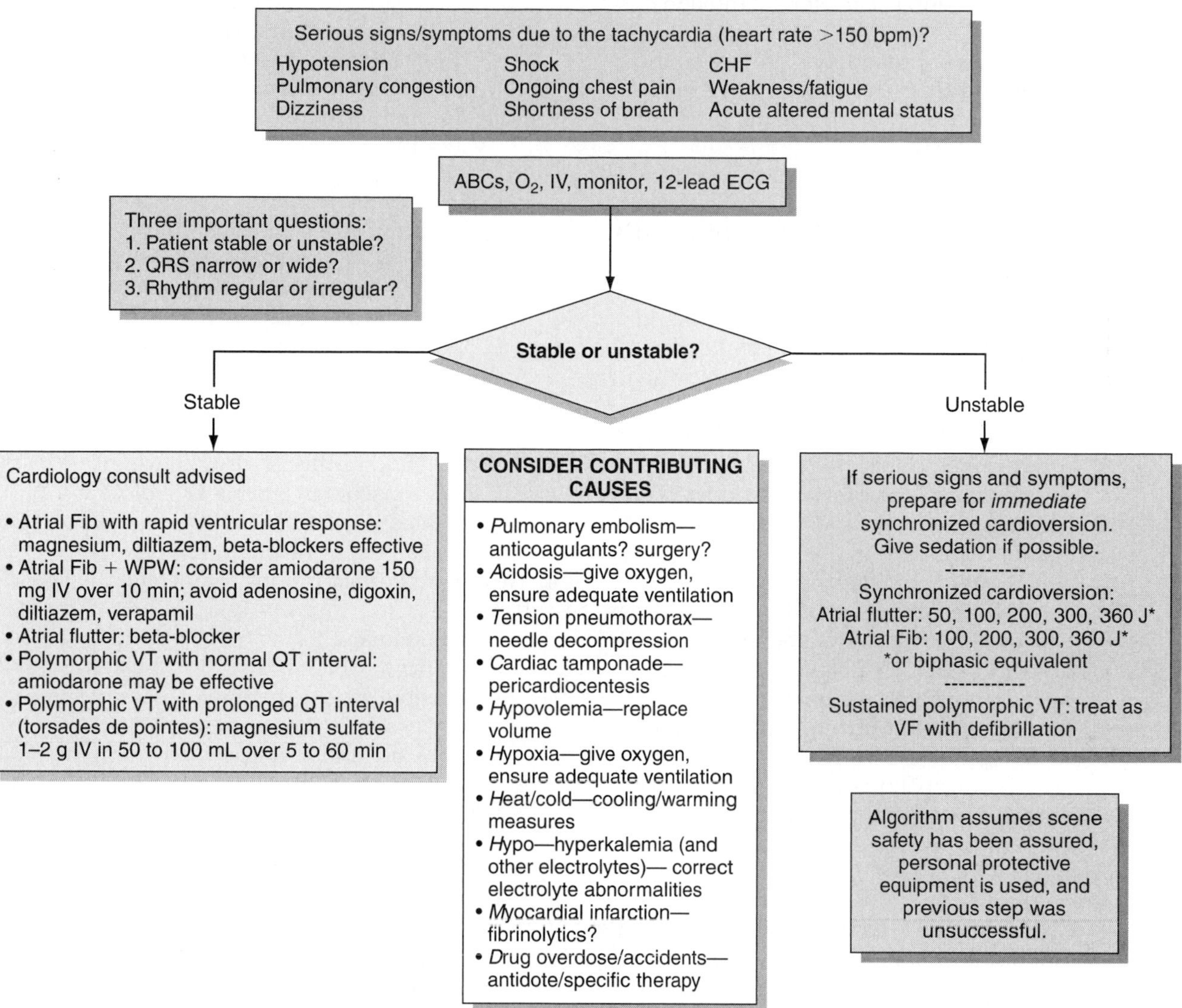
Irregular Tachycardia
Serious signs/symptoms due to the tachycardia (heart rate >150 bpm)?
Hypotension
Shock
CHF
Pulmonary congestion
Ongoing chest pain
Weakness/fatigue
Dizziness
Shortness of breath
Acute altered mental status
ABCs, O_2, IV, monitor, 12-lead ECG
Three important questions:
1. Patient stable or unstable?
2. QRS narrow or wide?
3. Rhythm regular or irregular?
Stable or unstable?
Stable
Unstable
Cardiology consult advised
• Atrial Fib with rapid ventricular response: magnesium, diltiazem, beta-blockers effective
• Atrial Fib + WPW: consider amiodarone 150 mg IV over 10 min; avoid adenosine, digoxin, diltiazem, verapamil
• Atrial flutter: beta-blocker
• Polymorphic VT with normal QT interval: amiodarone may be effective
• Polymorphic VT with prolonged QT interval (torsades de pointes): magnesium sulfate 1–2 g IV in 50 to 100 mL over 5 to 60 min
CONSIDER CONTRIBUTING CAUSES
• Pulmonary embolism—anticoagulants? surgery?
• Acidosis—give oxygen, ensure adequate ventilation
• Tension pneumothorax—needle decompression
• Cardiac tamponade—pericardiocentesis
• Hypovolemia—replace volume
• Hypoxia—give oxygen, ensure adequate ventilation
• Heat/cold—cooling/warming measures
• Hypo—hyperkalemia (and other electrolytes)— correct electrolyte abnormalities
• Myocardial infarction—fibrinolytics?
• Drug overdose/accidents—antidote/specific therapy
If serious signs and symptoms, prepare for *immediate* synchronized cardioversion. Give sedation if possible.

Synchronized cardioversion:
Atrial flutter: 50, 100, 200, 300, 360 J*
Atrial Fib: 100, 200, 300, 360 J*
*or biphasic equivalent

Sustained polymorphic VT: treat as VF with defibrillation
Algorithm assumes scene safety has been assured, personal protective equipment is used, and previous step was unsuccessful.

Figure 3-4C Irregular Tachycardia Algorithm (From Aehlert, B. [2007]: *ACLS Study Guide* [3rd ed.], St. Louis: Mosby.)

(iii) Alkalosis
(iv) Local ionic imbalance
(v) Ischemia
(vi) Long VF duration

(f) Complications
(i) Dysrhythmias: asystole; bradycardia; atrioventricular (AV) blocks; VF
(ii) Hypotension
(iii) Myocardial damage
(iv) Pulmonary edema
(v) Emboli
(vi) Muscle pain
(vii) Skin burns

(4) Temporary pacemaker: for patients who have problem with impulse formation and/or conduction
(a) Transcutaneous pacemaker
(i) Large surface skin electrodes applied anterior and posterior
a) Posterior: positive electrode applied between spine and left scapula at level of heart
b) Anterior: negative electrode applied at left fourth intercostal space at midclavicular line
(ii) May be painful for patient and should be replaced by transvenous lead as soon as possible
(b) Transvenous pacemaker
(i) Lead is threaded into the apex of the right ventricle via subclavian or internal jugular vein.

d. Intravenous (IV) access
(1) Establish patency of existing central or peripheral IV or heparin lock; if a central vein catheter is in place when the arrest occurs, use it to administer drugs during the resuscitation.

(2) Antecubital or external jugular veins are preferred if a venous catheter or additional venous catheters must be established.
(a) Peak drug concentrations are lower and circulation times are longer when drugs are administered by peripheral sites compared with central sites.
(b) If peripheral venous access is used for resuscitation drugs, administer bolus drugs rapidly, follow with a 20 mL saline, and elevate the extremity for 10 to 20 seconds.
(3) Central vein cannulation may be performed.
(a) The major disadvantage of central vein cannulation during cardiopulmonary arrest is the need to stop CPR.
(i) Internal jugular and subclavian sites requires cessation of CPR.
(ii) Femoral vein cannulation does not require cessation of CPR.
(b) Another consideration is that unsuccessful central vein cannulation may contraindicate the use of fibrinolytic drugs and increase the risk of the use of glycoprotein (GP) IIb/IIIa agents (e.g., abciximab [ReoPro], eptifibatide [Integrilin], or tirofiban [Aggrastat]) and anticoagulants.
(4) Distal wrist and hand veins and distal saphenous veins in the legs are the least favorable sites for drug administration during CPR.

e. ET intubation
(1) Attempt as soon as feasible, but defibrillation and administration of epinephrine are first and second priorities.
(2) Hyperventilation with 100% oxygen should precede any intubation attempt.
(3) Stop CPR no more than 30 seconds to allow ET intubation by a skilled clinician.
(4) Confirm ET tube placement by listening for equal bilateral breath sounds along with esophageal detector device, end-tidal carbon dioxide indicator, or capnography; chest x-ray is obtained after the patient is stabilized.
(5) Advantages of ET intubation include reduction of the risk of vomiting and aspiration and provision of a relative airway seal.
(6) If IV route cannot be established but ET tube placement has been achieved, some emergency drugs can be given via the ET tube; however, the IV route is preferred.
(a) Epinephrine, lidocaine, atropine, naloxone, and vasopressin may be administered via the ET tube.
(b) ET administration of drugs requires adjusting the dose to 2 to 2.5 times the usual dose and diluting the drug with isotonic saline to make a total volume of at least 10 mL; follow with several quick insufflations with the manual resuscitation bag.
(7) Two alternative airway techniques are placed orally and are inserted past the hypopharynx but not into the trachea.
(a) LMA
(b) Esophageal-tracheal Combitube (ETC)

f. Oxygen therapy
(1) Administer 100% oxygen during cardiopulmonary arrest with a bag-valve-mask; a reservoir bag or tubing attached to the bag-valve-mask is required to achieve as high a concentration of oxygen as possible.
(2) Remember that there is no contraindication to 100% oxygen during cardiopulmonary arrest.

g. IV fluids: Use normal saline to maintain adequate preload and to mix IV drug infusions.

h. Use pharmacologic agents as indicated in algorithms (Figures 3-2 to 3-4); specific drug information is available in Chapter 13.

4. Treat hypothermia if body temperature is less than 95° F (35° C).
a. Initial treatment
(1) Perform CPR.
(2) Defibrillate for the initial series of three shocks for VF or pulseless VT.
(3) Intubate and ventilate with warm, humidified oxygen.
(4) Obtain IV access, and administer warmed saline intravenously.
b. If core temperature is less than 86° F (30° C)
(1) Continue CPR but withhold IV medications.
(2) Continue with warm inspired oxygen and warm IV fluids.
(3) Also, peritoneal lavage with warm saline, extracorporeal rewarming, and esophageal rewarming tubes may be used.
c. If core temperature is greater than 86° F (30° C)
(1) Continue CPR and administer medications intravenously, but space longer than usual ACLS intervals.
(2) Repeat defibrillation for pulseless VT or VF as core temperature rises above 95° F

5. Consider cerebral resuscitation principles.
a. Avoid administration of calcium, which has been shown to cause cerebral vessel spasm.
b. Avoid administration of dextrose in water: use isotonic normal saline rather than D_5W. The dextrose in D_5W is metabolized quickly to leave only hypotonic water; this contributes to hypoosmolality and potentially cerebral edema.
c. Use other interventions to improve brain outcome as prescribed.
(1) Positioning: Elevate head of bed 30 degrees; avoid neck flexion or rotation; avoid hip flexion.
(2) Adequate ventilation: Maintain $Paco_2$ at ~35 mm Hg to prevent dilation of cerebral vessels.
(3) Hyperoxemia: Maintain Pao_2 greater than 100 mm Hg for a few hours after CPR.

(4) Increased cerebral perfusion pressure: Maintain brief mild hypertension with mean arterial pressure (MAP) 110 to 130 mm Hg for 1 to 5 minutes (contraindicated in neurologic trauma), and then MAP 90 to 100 mm Hg.
(5) Induced hypothermia may be considered if the patient is unresponsive but with an adequate BP following resuscitation.
 (a) Maintain body temperature between 32° to 34° C for 12 to 24 hours along with drugs to sedate and prevent shivering.
 (b) Rewarm patient gradually over 8 hours.
(6) Brain hypothermia: Apply cooled saline packs to head.
(7) Pharmacologic agents
 (a) Osmotic agents (e.g., mannitol [Osmitrol]) to increase cortical circulation and reduce cerebral edema
 (b) Calcium channel blockers (e.g., nimodipine [Nimotop]) to prevent cerebral vasospasm
 (c) Anticonvulsants (e.g., phenytoin [Dilantin]) to prevent seizures
 (d) Muscle paralytics (e.g., pancuronium [Pavulon]) to decrease cerebral oxygen requirements
 (e) Steroids (e.g., methylprednisolone [Solu-Medrol]) to reduce cerebral edema

6. Monitor for complications of CPR
 a. Fracture of sternum or ribs
 b. Hemothorax
 c. Pneumothorax
 d. Laceration of abdominal viscera especially the liver
 e. Myocardial contusion
 f. Cardiac rupture
7. Provide postresuscitation care

Psychosocial Consideration Related to Cardiopulmonary Arrest

1. The patient
 a. During the resuscitation
  (1) Touch the patient's hand and talk to the patient during the resuscitation efforts.
  (2) Maintain the patient's modesty and dignity during the resuscitation efforts with drapes, curtains, and doors; ensure that all team members are respectful of the patient.
 b. After the resuscitation
  (1) Patients frequently (~40%) have near-death experience during cardiac arrest but are frequently reluctant to discuss it.
   (a) As the patient regains consciousness, assure patient that he or she is not alone; reorient the patient to person, place, and time.
   (b) Consider asking the patient if he or she remembers anything that occurred during the time his or her heart was stopped.
 c. If the resuscitation efforts are unsuccessful, provide respectful and culturally sensitive care of the body.
2. The family
 a. Need for information
  (1) If the patient's condition has been worsening, inform the family of the worsening condition.
  (2) If the cardiopulmonary arrest was sudden, inform the family about what has happened, what is being done, and an estimate of how long it may be before more information will be available.
   (a) If information must be conveyed by telephone, tell the family that the situation is serious but do not tell of a death by telephone.
 b. Need for privacy
  (1) Escort the family to a family conference room where they can grieve apart from other visitors, but do not leave them alone.
  (2) Ask whether someone, such as a religious leader or a family member or friend, can be called; offer to call someone from pastoral services or have a social worker or a volunteer to be there with them.
  (3) Allow the family to "tell their story," but do not give inappropriate reassurance.
  (4) Be honest; do not give inappropriate reassurance but be hopeful, warm, and caring.
 c. Family presence during cardiopulmonary arrest is being advocated today as part of holistic care.
  (1) Adhere to the family's wishes if these do not conflict with the wishes of the patient.
  (2) Give consideration to the family members' coping abilities.
  (3) If a family member (generally limited to one member) desires to be present during resuscitation efforts:
   (a) Prepare the family member for what to expect.
   (b) Drape the patient appropriately.
   (c) Set limits before entering the room; explain where they may stand and whether they may touch the patient, such as hold the patient's hand.
   (d) If the patient is not responding to resuscitation efforts and death is imminent, allow the family member time to talk to the patient.
   (e) If the code team asks the family member to leave, escort the person out, and make sure that someone stays with that person.
 d. If resuscitation efforts are successful, allow family visitation as soon as possible.
 e. If resuscitation efforts are not successful:
  (1) The physician usually informs the family of the patient's death.
  (2) Express your sympathy.
  (3) Answer whatever questions the family asks.
  (4) Ask the family members whether they desire to see the body, and prepare them for what they will see.

(5) Prepare the body for visitation by discarding trash and removing clutter; remove the ET tube if legally acceptable (i.e., not a coroner's case), and remove any blood from the face and hands.
(6) Place several chairs close to the body, and escort the family to the bedside; stay with them.

3. Other patients
   a. Screen the patient being resuscitated from other patients.
   b. Make sure that other patients are being cared for during resuscitation efforts on one of the patients.
   c. After the resuscitation, patients frequently ask about what happened; be honest but respect to the patient's right to privacy.
4. The staff
   a. Constructively critical multidisciplinary review of the resuscitation efforts aids in quality improvement, team building, and stress reduction.
      (1) Performance of the team as a team: Identification of poor performance of an individual member should not occur in a group setting.
      (2) Adequacy of supplies and equipment
   b. Counseling services should be available for staff.

Dysrhythmias and Blocks

Definitions

1. Dysrhythmia: any cardiac rhythm other than sinus rhythm at a normal rate
2. Block: failure of an intrinsic impulse to be conducted through the conduction system

Etiology

1. General
   a. Congenital
      (1) Long QT syndrome
      (2) Accessory pathways
      (3) Brugada syndrome
         (a) More common in Southeast Asians and Japanese
         (b) ST segment elevation in leads V_1 and V_2 are commonly associated with right bundle branch block (RBBB)
         (c) Sudden cardiac death may occur as a result of polymorphic VT and VF
   b. Myocardial ischemia or infarction
   c. Hypoxemia/hypoxia
   d. Electrolyte imbalance
   e. Acid-base imbalance
   f. Sympathetic nervous system stimulation via endogenous catecholamines or sympathomimetic drugs (e.g., epinephrine, isoproterenol, or dopamine)
   g. Drug effects or toxicity
      (1) "Holiday heart" syndrome caused by excessive alcohol consumption; this binge drinking may cause acute dysrhythmias, usually a supraventricular tachycardia (SVT)
2. Table 3-2 describes etiology of each dysrhythmia

Pathophysiology: Arrhythmogenic Mechanisms

1. Problems with impulse formation
   a. Altered automaticity
      (1) Enhanced automaticity
         (a) Abnormal condition of latent pacemaker cells in which their firing rate is increased beyond their inherent rate (even nonpacemaker cells may depolarize spontaneously)
         (b) Resting membrane potential is less negative or threshold potential is lower, increasing the chance of depolarization
         (c) Caused by any of the following:
            (i) Hypoxia
            (ii) Hypercapnia
            (iii) Ischemia, infarction
            (iv) Hypokalemia, hypocalcemia
            (v) Catecholamines
            (vi) Hyperthermia
            (vii) Digitalis toxicity
            (viii) Stretching of the heart muscle
         (d) Cause of most atrial, junctional, and ventricular ectopic beats and most VTs
      (2) Depressed automaticity
         (a) Resting membrane potential is more negative or threshold potential is higher, decreasing the chance of depolarization
         (b) Caused by any of the following:
            (i) Vagal stimulation
            (ii) Hyperkalemia, hypercalcemia
            (iii) Decreased catecholamines
            (iv) Hypothermia
            (v) Beta-blockers
         (c) Cause of bradycardia or blocks
   b. Triggered activity
      (1) Repetitive ectopic firing is caused by afterdepolarizations; an afterdepolarization is an abnormal electrical impulse that occurs during or after repolarization of an action potential.
      (2) If an afterdepolarization is strong enough to reach threshold, a triggered beat occurs.
      (3) This activity is not self-generating but depends on the preceding beat.
      (4) They may be early or late.
         (a) Early: occur when the QT interval is prolonged
            (i) Caused by prolongation of repolarization and effective refractory period
            (ii) Example: torsades de pointes
         (b) Delayed: the result of elevated intracellular calcium
            (i) Caused by any of the following:
               a) Electrolyte imbalances
               b) Catecholamines
            (ii) Example: tachycardias of digitalis toxicity

Text continued on p. 128

Table 3-2 Basic Dysrhythmia and Block Management

Rhythm	Etiology	Significance	Treatment
General	• Hypoxia • Ischemia • Electrolyte imbalance • Acid-base imbalance • Drug effect or toxicity	• Depends on patient's clinical presentation • Monitor for clinical manifestations of hypoperfusion	• Treat cause: ◦ Correct ischemia if possible ◦ Correct hypoxemia and hypoxia ◦ Correct electrolyte imbalance ◦ Correct acid-base imbalance ◦ Correct drug toxicity • Provide general emergency management for any symptomatic patient: ◦ Oxygen ◦ IV access ◦ Multiple lead ECG if rhythm interpretation is required or if ischemia is suspected
Sinus bradycardia	• Athletic heart • Sleep • Vagal stimulation • Myocardial ischemia or infarction ◦ Inferior or posterior MI • Fibrodegenerative changes of the SA node (e.g., sick sinus syndrome) • Increased intracranial pressure • Hypothermia • Hypothyroidism • Cervical or mediastinal tumor • Drug effect: digitalis; beta-blockers; calcium channel blockers; opiates	• Depends on rate • If too slow, cardiac output decreases: ◦ Clinical manifestations of hypoperfusion may include hypotension, syncope, chest pain, or HF ◦ Escape beats (atrial, junctional, or ventricular) may occur	• None if asymptomatic • If clinical manifestations of hypoperfusion occur: ◦ Atropine ◦ Transcutaneous pacemaker
Sinus tachycardia	• Stress, fear, anxiety, pain, anger • Exercise • Hypovolemia or hypervolemia • Shock • Hypoxia • Fever • Anemia • Hyperthyroidism • Inflammatory heart disease • Myocardial ischemic or infarction ◦ Anterior MI • Fibrodegenerative changes (e.g., sick sinus syndrome) • HF • Pulmonary embolism • Drug effect: epinephrine, isoproterenol; dopamine; atropine; caffeine; nicotine; amphetamines; cocaine; alcohol; aminophylline	• Usually not significant except in patients with heart disease; then it may cause angina, MI, HF, or shock	• Treat cause: ◦ Anxiolytics for anxiety ◦ Analgesics for pain ◦ Antipyretics for fever ◦ Fluids for hypovolemia ◦ Treatment of HF ◦ Avoidance of stimulants • Usually does not require other treatment, but the following also may be used: ◦ Sedation and/or beta-blocker may be used to decrease or block the effects of catecholamines ◦ Diltiazem
Sinus dysrhythmia	• Normal; variation in sympathetic and parasympathetic stimulation during ventilation • In older patient, may indicate sick sinus syndrome • Digitalis toxicity	• Normal variation • May be seen in digitalis toxicity	• None • Discontinue digitalis if toxicity is cause

Continued

Table 3-2 Basic Dysrhythmia and Block Management—cont'd

Rhythm	Etiology	Significance	Treatment
Sinus block (sinus exit block)	• Fibrodegenerative changes of the sinus node (e.g., sick sinus syndrome) • Ischemia of SA node (e.g., MI) • Vagal stimulation • Inflammatory heart disease (e.g.,myocarditis) • Drug toxicity: digitalis	• Depends on frequency and duration of pauses • If patient loses consciousness (Stokes-Adams attacks), this is significant and requires treatment	• Discontinue digitalis if toxicity is cause • Atropine • Pacemaker if frequent pauses, long pauses, or if patient is having Stokes-Adams attacks
Sinus arrest	• Fibrodegenerative changes (e.g., sick sinus syndrome) • Ischemia of SA node (e.g., MI) • Vagal stimulation • Electrolyte imbalance: potassium, magnesium • Drug toxicity: digitalis	• Depends on frequency and duration of pauses • If patient loses consciousness (Stokes-Adams attacks), very significant and requires treatment	• Discontinue digitalis if toxicity is cause • Atropine • Pacemaker if frequent pauses, long (more than 3-second) pauses, or if patient is having Stokes-Adams attacks
Premature atrial contractions	• Increased sympathetic stimulation: stress, fear, anxiety, pain • Exercise • Inflammatory heart disease (e.g., myocarditis) • Myocardial ischemia • Valvular heart disease (e.g., mitral stenosis or mitral valve prolapse) • HF • Electrolyte imbalance • Hypoxia • Drug effect: caffeine; nicotine; alcohol • Drug toxicity: digitalis	• Usually benign but may precede atrial tachycardia, flutter, or fibrillation • Considered significant if more than six contractions per minute	• Treat the cause • Usually no treatment necessary; but if frequent, treatment may include digitalis, quinidine, propranolol, beta-blockers, calcium channel blockers, or anxiolytic drugs
Wandering atrial pacemaker	• Vagal stimulation • Sinus bradycardia • Digitalis toxicity	• May represent multiple atrial escape beats	• Usually none needed • Discontinue digitalis if toxicity is suspected • Atropine may be used to increase slow sinus rate
Atrial tachycardia (Paroxysmal atrial tachycardia refers to the sudden interruption of sinus rhythm by a rapid ectopic focus—starts and ends abruptly)	• Increased sympathetic stimulation: stress, fear, anxiety, pain • Exercise • Inflammatory heart disease (e.g., myocarditis) • Myocardial ischemia or infarction • Hypoxia • Hyperthyroidism • Valvular heart disease (e.g., mitral valve prolapse) • COPD • Wolff-Parkinson-White syndrome • Drug effect: caffeine; nicotine; alcohol • Drug toxicity: digitalis (frequently PAT with block)	• Patient may experience palpitations and clinical manifestations of hypoperfusion (e.g., hypotension, syncope, chest pain, and HF) because diastolic filling time and preload are greatly reduced • Myocardial oxygen consumption is increased, and myocardial oxygen supply is decreased, so myocardial ischemia may occur or worsen	• Depends on patient's tolerance, cause, and history of previous attacks • Discontinue digitalis if toxicity is suspected • Initial treatment: vagal stimulation; adenosine; if the rhythm persists, continue with the following: ◦ If considered reentrant (PSVT) and normal LV function: beta-blocker, calcium channel blocker, digoxin (if not the cause), cardioversion, procainamide, amiodarone, sotalol, flecainide, or propafenone ◦ If considered reentrant (PSVT) and abnormal LV function: digoxin (if not the cause), amiodarone, diltiazem

Table 3-2 Basic Dysrhythmia and Block Management—cont'd

Rhythm	Etiology	Significance	Treatment
			◦ For nonreentrant AT with normal LV function: calcium channel blocker, beta-blocker, amiodarone, digoxin, flecainide, propafenone ◦ For nonreentrant AT with abnormal left ventricular function: amiodarone, diltiazem, digoxin • Other considerations: ◦ Right atrial pacing ◦ Ablation may be indicated for recurrent AV nodal reentrant tachycardia. • NOTE: If associated with WPW syndrome, do not use adenosine, beta-blockers, calcium channel blockers, or digoxin; preferred agent is amiodarone
Multifocal atrial tachycardia (may also be called *chaotic atrial rhythm*)	• Pulmonary hypertension (e.g., COPD, pulmonary embolism) • Digitalis toxicity • Valvular heart disease • HF • Electrolyte imbalance: hypokalemia, hypomagnesemia • Drug toxicity: digitalis	• Demonstrates atrial irritability that may lead to atrial tachycardia, flutter, or fibrillation	• Treat cause: electrolyte replacement • Discontinue digitalis if toxicity is suspected • Normal left ventricular function: calcium channel blocker, beta-blocker, amiodarone, digoxin, flecainide, propafenone • Abnormal left ventricular function: amiodarone, diltiazem, digoxin
Atrial fibrillation	• HF • Cardiomyopathy • Myocardial ischemia or infarction ◦ Especially anterior myocardial infarction • Valvular heart disease (e.g., mitral stenosis or mitral regurgitation) • Hyperthyroidism inflammatory heart disease (e.g., pericarditis) • Hypertension • After cardiotomy • Pulmonary hypertension (e.g., COPD or pulmonary embolism) • WPW syndrome • Drug effect: alcohol	• No effective atrial contraction, so loss of atrial kick • Mural thrombi formation predisposes to emboli. • Significance varies greatly on rate: may cause clinical manifestations of hypoperfusion (e.g., hypotension, syncope, chest pain, or HF)	• Rate control ◦ Normal LV function: beta-blocker or calcium channel blocker for rate control at rest and during exercise; digoxin as a second-line drug (only controls rate at rest) ◦ Abnormal LV function: digoxin, diltiazem, or amiodarone • Though no additional treatment is required acutely, if rate is controlled (between 60 and 100 beats/min), it is desirable actually to convert the AF to NSR if possible to reduce the risk of stroke and increase ventricular diastolic filling volume and cardiac output (considered rhythm control and maintenance) ◦ Normal LV function with duration less than 48 hours: cardioversion or amiodarone, ibutilide, dofetilide, procainamide, disopyramide, flecainide, propafenone, sotalol ◦ Abnormal LV function of less than 48-hour duration: cardioversion or amiodarone

Continued

Table 3-2 Basic Dysrhythmia and Block Management—cont'd

Rhythm	Etiology	Significance	Treatment
			◦ Duration longer than 48 hours or unknown duration: anticoagulation followed by cardioversion • If slow ventricular response rate, atropine or pacemaker may be needed ◦ Consider digitalis as cause of slow ventricular response rate; withhold digitalis if cause • NOTE: If associated with WPW syndrome: do NOT use adenosine, beta-blockers, calcium channel blockers, or digoxin; preferred agent is amiodarone • Other nonacute considerations: ◦ Implantable atrial defibrillator ◦ Ablation or maze procedure may be performed • Long-term anticoagulation is needed for chronic AF to prevent mural thrombi and risk for embolic stroke; desirable INR is 2 to 3
Atrial flutter	• HF • Myocardial ischemia or infarction • Valvular heart disease • Inflammatory heart disease (e.g., pericarditis) • Hypertension • After cardiotomy • Pulmonary hypertension (e.g., COPD or pulmonary embolism) • Hyperthyroidism • Drug effect: alcohol • Drug toxicity: digitalis	• Atrial contraction not effective • Significance varies greatly depending on rate • If rate is rapid, may cause clinical manifestations of hypoperfusion (e.g., hypotension, syncope, chest pain, or HF) because diastolic filling time and preload are greatly reduced	• As for AF • Anticoagulation may be prescribed for atrial flutter, but the risk of mural thrombi and stroke is considered lower than for atrial fibrillation
Premature junctional contraction	• Myocardial ischemia or infarction ◦ Especially inferior MI • HF • Valvular heart disease • Hypoxia • Drug effect: nicotine; caffeine; alcohol • Drug toxicity: digitalis • Also etiology as for PACs	• Usually benign but may predispose to junctional tachycardia if frequent	• Usually none necessary • Discontinue digitalis if toxicity is cause • Sedation • Beta-blockers
Junctional escape rhythm	• Vagal stimulation • SA block • Complete AV block • Myocardial ischemia or infarction • Valvular heart disease • Hypoxia • After cardiotomy • Drug toxicity: digitalis	• Protects patient from asystole • Do not suppress	• Treat failure of sinus node • Atropine • Pacemaker may be needed • Discontinue digitalis if digitalis toxicity is cause

Table 3-2 **Basic Dysrhythmia and Block Management—cont'd**

Rhythm	Etiology	Significance	Treatment
Accelerated junctional rhythm	• Vagal stimulation • SA block • Complete AV block • Myocardial ischemia or infarction • Reperfusion of myocardium • Hypoxia • Inflammatory heart disease (e.g., myocarditis) • After cardiotomy • Drug toxicity: digitalis	• Protects patient from asystole • Do not suppress	• Treat failure of sinus node • Discontinue digitalis if digitalis toxicity is cause
Junctional tachycardia	• Myocardial ischemia or infarction • Reperfusion of myocardium • Inflammatory heart disease • After cardiotomy • Drug toxicity: digitalis	• Usually stops spontaneously and usually is tolerated well	• Treat cause • Discontinue digitalis if digitalis toxicity is cause • Vagal stimulation • Adenosine • Amiodarone • Beta-blockers or calcium channel blockers if normal LV function
First-degree AV nodal block	• Normal variation • Myocardial ischemia or infarction • Conduction system fibrosis • Inflammatory heart disease (e.g., myocarditis) • Vagal stimulation • After cardiotomy • Myocardial contusion • Hyperkalemia • Drug toxicity: digitalis; beta-blockers; calcium channel blockers	• Relatively benign but may progress to second- or third- degree block	• Observe closely for progression of block • Discontinue digitalis if digitalis toxicity is cause
Second-degree AV nodal block Mobitz I (Wenckebach)	• Myocardial ischemia or infarction ○ Inferior or posterior MI • Conduction system fibrosis • Inflammatory heart disease • After cardiotomy • Myocardial contusion • Drug toxicity: digitalis; beta-blockers; calcium channel blockers	• Block is at AV node • Occurs more often in inferior MI (lesion of right coronary artery) • Relatively benign: usually transient, and does not usually progress to complete heart block	• Usually does not require treatment • Monitor for progression of block • Discontinue digitalis if digitalis toxicity is cause • Atropine may be used if rate is slow and patient is symptomatic
Second-degree AV nodal block Mobitz II	• Myocardial ischemia or infarction ○ Anterior MI • Hypertension • Valvular heart disease • Conduction system fibrosis • Inflammatory heart disease (e.g., myocarditis) • After cardiotomy • Myocardial contusion	• Block is at bundle of His, which accounts for the slight widening of the QRS complex • Occurs more often in anterior MI (lesion of left anterior descending coronary artery) • Ominous, for it often progresses to CHB	• Atropine may be used but is not usually helpful • Prophylactic use of pacemaker
Third-degree (or complete) AV block	• Myocardial ischemia or infarction • Conduction system fibrosis • Inflammatory heart disease • After cardiotomy • Myocardial contusion • Hypoxia	• If no escape rhythm is established, the patient has ventricular asystole	• Observe for clinical manifestations of hypoperfusion if inferior MI with junctional escape rhythm • Atropine may be used but is usually not helpful

Continued

Table 3-2 Basic Dysrhythmia and Block Management—cont'd

Rhythm	Etiology	Significance	Treatment
	• Electrolyte imbalance: potassium • Drug toxicity: digitalis		• Pacemaker especially if: ◦ Anterior MI ◦ Inferior MI with ventricular escape rhythm
Left bundle branch block (LBBB)	• Myocardial ischemia or infarction ◦ Anterior MI • Fibrodegenerative changes • After cardiotomy	• Bifascicular block considered more serious than RBBB especially in presence of acute MI • Monitor this patient closely during pulmonary artery catheter insertion because trifascicular block may occur	• New LBBB in acute MI may be treated with prophylactic pacemaker, especially if an atrioventricular nodal block is also present
Right bundle branch block (RBBB)	• Myocardial ischemia or infarction ◦ Anterior or inferior MI • Fibrodegenerative changes • After cardiotomy • Pulmonary artery catheter insertion • Acute pulmonary embolism	• None; cardiac output is not affected by delayed ventricular depolarization (wide QRS complex)	• Monitor closely for development of LBBB
Premature ventricular contraction (PVC)	• Increased sympathetic nervous system stimulation (e.g, endogenous catecholamines or sympathomimetic drugs [e.g., epinephrine, isoproterenol, or dopamine]) • Myocardial ischemia or infarction • Reperfusion of myocardium • HF • Ventricular aneurysm • Cardiomyopathy • Hypoxia • Acidosis • Electrolyte imbalance: potassium; calcium; magnesium • Drug toxicity: digitalis; aminophylline	• PVCs of most significance: may predispose to VT or VF ◦ Frequent (more than six per minute) ◦ Bigeminal ◦ Multifocal ◦ R-on-T phenomenon ◦ Couplets ◦ Runs of ventricular tachycardia (three or more PVCs in a row) • Pulse amplitude of PVC is reduced because of decreased filling time	• Treatment of cause (e.g., oxygen, electrolyte replacement, or discontinue digitalis) • No treatment required if not significant • If frequent: amiodarone, procainamide, lidocaine, or beta-blockers
Monomorphic ventricular tachycardia	• Myocardial ischemia or infarction • Reperfusion of myocardium • Ventricular aneurysm • Cardiomyopathy • Valvular heart disease • After cardiotomy • R-on-T PVC • Hypoxia • Acidosis • Electrolyte imbalance: hypokalemia • Drug toxicity: digitalis	• Ominous, for it may progress to ventricular fibrillation • Symptoms depend on underlying heart disease, rate, and duration of VT • May cause angina, HF, or shock	• Treat cause: correct electrolyte imbalance or drug toxicity • Normal left ventricular function: procainamide, amiodarone, lidocaine, sotalol • Impaired LV function: amiodarone, lidocaine, cardioversion • If having hypotension, chest pain, or pulmonary edema: immediate sedation and cardioversion • If pulseless: treat as VF (e.g., defibrillation, vasopressin or epinephrine, amiodarone)

Table 3-2 Basic Dysrhythmia and Block Management—cont'd

Rhythm	Etiology	Significance	Treatment
Polymorphic ventricular tachycardia (torsades de pointes if preceded by prolonged QT interval)	• Class IA antidysrhythmic drugs (e.g., procainamide, quinidine, or disopyramide) • Class III antidysrhythmics (e.g., sotalol or amiodarone) • Tricyclic antidepressants (e.g., amitriptyline [Elavil]) • Phenothiazines (e.g., chlorpromazine [Thorazine]) • Organic insecticides • Electrolyte imbalance (e.g., hypomagnesemia, hypocalcemia, or hypokalemia) • Congenital long QT syndrome or Brugada syndrome • Marked bradycardia • Hypothermia • Subarachnoid hemorrhage	• No effective perfusion • May go into and out of this rhythm	• Treat cause: treat ischemia and replace electrolytes • Prevent torsades de pointes: monitor QT interval closely, and discontinue any offending drug when QT interval prolongs to greater than half of the RR interval • Discontinue any offending drug if characteristic torsades pattern seen • If QRS is normal: ◦ Electrolyte replacement ◦ Amiodarone, beta-blocker, lidocaine, procainamide, sotalol • If QRS is prolonged (suggests torsades de pointes) ◦ Electrolyte replacement especially magnesium ◦ Overdrive pacing ◦ Isoproterenol ◦ Lidocaine • If impaired LV function: amiodarone, lidocaine, cardioversion
Ventricular fibrillation	• Myocardial ischemia or infarction • R-on-T PVC • Electrical shock including microshock • Brugada syndrome (familial) • Drowning • Hypothermia • Hypoxia • Drug toxicity: digitalis • Dying heart	• Lethal within 4-6 minutes • No cardiac output • Symptoms include loss of consciousness, pulse, heart sounds, ventilation; anoxic seizures	• Immediate defibrillation 360 J (or equivalent biphasic energy) • CPR • Epinephrine • Intubation • Antidysrhythmic drugs: amiodarone; lidocaine; procainamide
Idioventricular rhythm	• Vagal stimulation • Failure of higher pacemakers (e.g., ischemia or fibrosis of conduction system) • Myocardial ischemia or infarction • Third-degree AV block • Drug toxicity: digitalis	• Protects the patient from asystole but is unreliable • Do not suppress	• Accelerate higher pacemakers with atropine • Pacemaker • If pulseless: ◦ CPR ◦ Epinephrine ◦ Pacemaker
Accelerated idioventricular rhythm	• Failure of higher pacemakers (e.g., ischemia or fibrosis of conduction system) • Myocardial ischemia or infarction • Reperfusion of myocardium • Drug toxicity: digitalis	• Protects the patient from asystole, but is unreliable • Do not suppress	• Accelerate higher pacemakers with atropine • Pacemaker
Asystole	• Vagal stimulation • Myocardial ischemia or infarction • Third-degree AV block • Anaphylaxis • Drug overdosage • Hypoxia • Acidosis • Shock • Dying heart	• Lethal within 4-6 minutes • No cardiac output • Symptoms include loss of consciousness, pulse, heart sounds, ventilation; BP; anoxic seizures	• CPR • Epinephrine • Atropine • Pacemaker

AF, Atrial fibrillation; *AT,* atrial tachycardia; *AV,* atrioventricular; *BP,* blood pressure; *CHB,* complete heart block; *COPD,* chronic obstructive pulmonary disease; *CPR,* cardiopulmonary resuscitation; *ECG,* electrocardiogram; *HF,* heart failure; *INR,* international normalized ratio; *LV,* left ventricular; *MI,* myocardial infarction; *NSR,* normal sinus rhythm; *PACs,* premature atrial contractions; *PSVT,* paroxysmal supraventricular tachycardia; *RCA,* right coronary artery; *SA,* sinoatrial; *VF,* ventricular fibrillation; *VT,* ventricular tachycardia; *WPW,* Wolff-Parkinson-White.

2. Problems with impulse conduction
   a. Reentry (Figure 3-5): the most common mechanism for tachydysrhythmias
      (1) An impulse travels through an area of the myocardium and depolarizes it but then reenters the same area to depolarize it again.
      (2) Requirements
         (a) An available circuit: reentry can occur in areas of the heart where conduction velocity is abnormally slow
         (b) Unequal responsiveness of two segments of the circuit (i.e., delay in one of limb of the circuit)
         (c) An area of slowed conduction or unidirectional block
            (i) Conduction must be slow enough to allow time for the previously stimulated area to recover the ability to conduct.
            (ii) The area of unidirectional block provides a return pathway for the original stimulus to reenter a previously stimulated area to repolarize it.
      (3) Caused by any of the following:
         (a) Some ectopy
         (b) Some VTs
         (c) Most SVTs
         (d) Wolff-Parkinson-White (WPW) syndrome tachycardias

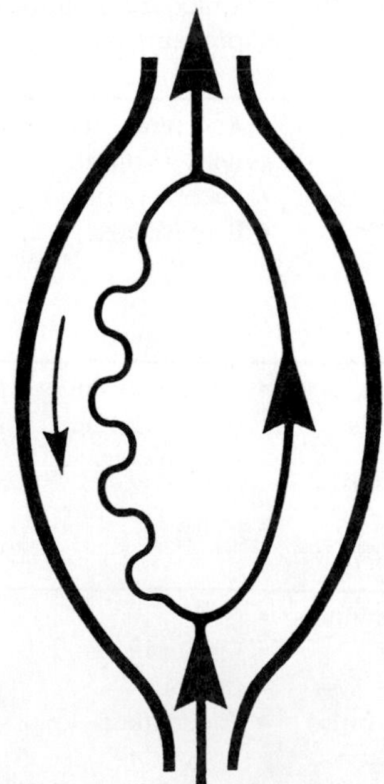

Figure 3-5 Schematic representation of a reentrant circuit depicting two limbs with varying conduction times (straight lines versus curly line). The tachycardic impulse travels around this circuit and, as it reaches the common end(s), travels to the myocardium, which then depolarizes. A similar reentrant circuit can be located around the sinus node, within the atrial or ventricular myocardium, within the AV node, or between the AV node and an accessory pathway. (From Urban, N., Greenlee, K. K, Krumberger, J. M., & Winkelman, C. [1995]. *Guidelines for critical care nursing*. St. Louis: Mosby.)

   b. Accessory pathways
      (1) Lown-Ganong-Levine syndrome
         (a) Caused by any of the following:
            (i) AV nodal bypass tract
            (ii) AV node smaller than normal
            (iii) Fibers running through AV node that do not have the built-in delay feature that nodal fibers have
         (b) Causes the following:
            (i) Short PR interval, normal QRS complex
            (ii) Tachydysrhythmias
      (2) WPW syndrome
         (a) Caused by Kent bundle, which bypasses the AV node
            (i) Type A: Kent bundle on left; R wave in V_1 with inverted T wave and depressed ST segment
            (ii) Type B: Kent bundle on right; QS interval in V_1 with upright T wave and elevated ST segment
         (b) Causes the following:
            (i) Short PR interval, wide QRS complex with slurring of first portion of QRS complex (referred to as a *delta wave*) (Figure 3-6)
            (ii) Tachydysrhythmias
               a) QRS complex morphology
                  i) Wide QRS complex: Sinus impulse may take accessory pathway around the mandatory delay in the AV node (referred to as *preexcitation*) causing

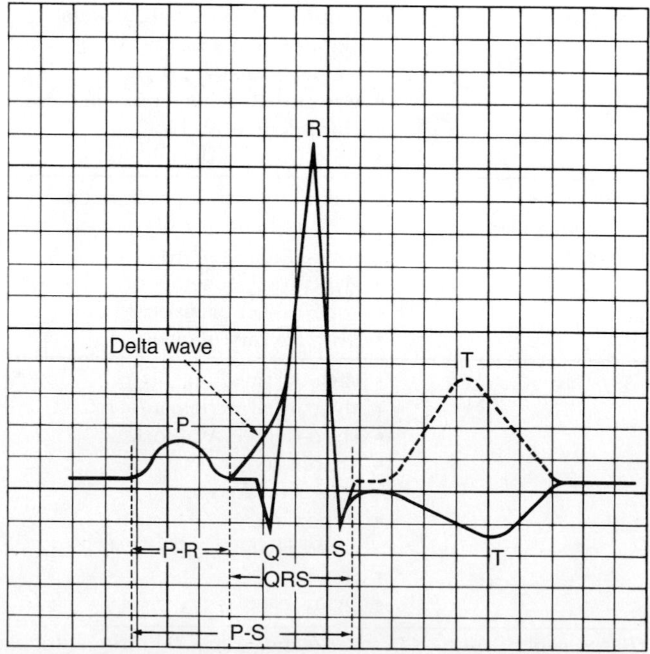

Figure 3-6 Wolff-Parkinson-White syndrome. Note the short PR interval, the delta wave, widened QRS complex, and T wave inversion characteristic of preexcitation. (From Kinney, M. R., Packa, D. R., & Dunbar, S. B. [1998]. *AACN'S clinical reference for critical-care nursing* [4th ed.]. St. Louis: Mosby.)

severe SVTs with a wide QRS complex.
- ii) Narrow QRS complex: impulse also may take atrioventricular node but reenter via accessory pathway; narrow QRS complex
- b) Treatment
  - i) Antidysrhythmic drugs: amiodarone, flecainide, procainamide, propafenone, or sotalol
  - ii) Cardioversion if drugs fail to convert
  - iii) Avoidance of adenosine, beta-blockers, calcium channel blockers, and digoxin
  - iv) Long-term treatment: ablation via catheter or surgically
- (3) Mahaim fibers
  - (a) Caused by nodoventricular or fasciculoventricular fibers
  - (b) Causes the following:
    - (i) Short PR, wide QRS
    - (ii) Tachydysrhythmias

c. Aberrant conduction
- (1) Aberrant conduction occurs most often when
  - (a) Rate is rapid.
  - (b) PACs are very premature.
  - (c) There are changes in cycle length (e.g., atrial fibrillation [AF] [QRS complex that ends a short cycle length after a long cycle length is likely to be conducted aberrantly and is referred to as *Ashman's phenomenon*]).
- (2) Because one of the bundle branches (usually the right) is still refractory when a supraventricular impulse reaches it, the impulse must travel down the nonrefractory bundle and across to the other ventricle; this causes a wide QRS complex, which frequently is mistaken for a PVC if a single complex or VT if several complexes in a row.
- (3) Unlike ectopy, aberrancy is no more serious than the supraventricular mechanism that caused it (e.g., AF with aberrancy is no more clinically significant than AF).
- (4) QRS complex morphology is the most important criterion in the differentiation between ectopy and aberrancy, but other criteria also may be helpful (Table 3-3); multiple-lead ECG is often helpful to identify P waves and to look at the morphology of the QRS complex.
- (5) Ectopy is more common than aberrancy; if in doubt, always assume ectopy and treat accordingly.

Clinical Presentation

1. Anxiety, restlessness
2. Vertigo, syncope
3. Weakness, fatigue, activity intolerance
4. Palpitations
5. Chest pain
6. Clinical indications of left ventricular failure (LVF): dyspnea; S_3; crackles
7. Clinical indications of hypoperfusion (see Table 2-2)
8. Diagnostic studies
   a. Electrocardiography: multiple-lead ECG
   b. Serum electrolyte levels
   c. Drug levels
   d. Arterial blood gases

Nursing Diagnoses (see Appendix A)

1. Decreased Cardiac Output related to changes in heart rate, rhythm, or conduction
2. Ineffective Myocardial Tissue Perfusion related to decrease in diastolic time and/or pressure
3. Ineffective Cerebral Tissue Perfusion related to change in changes in heart rate, rhythm, or conduction
4. Activity Intolerance related to changes in heart rate, rhythm, or conduction and inability to increase cardiac output in response to exercise
5. Risk for Injury related to use of an electrical device (e.g., defibrillator or pacemaker)
6. Anxiety related to acute change in health status and emergent procedures
7. Deficient Knowledge related to antidysrhythmic therapies and drugs

Collaborative Management

1. Assess for clinical manifestations of hypoperfusion (see Table 2-2): follow ACLS algorithms for lethal dysrhythmias (see Cardiopulmonary Arrest).
2. Treat etiology of dysrhythmia.
3. Correct ischemia if possible.
   a. Coronary artery vasodilators and/or antispasmodics: nitrates; calcium channel blockers
   b. Fibrinolytic drugs
   c. Percutaneous coronary intervention (PCI)
4. Correct hypoxemia/hypoxia.
   a. Improve SaO_2 (e.g., oxygen, ET intubation, mechanical ventilation, or positive end-expiratory pressure [PEEP]).
   b. Improve cardiac output (e.g., inotropes, vasodilators, or intraaortic balloon pump [IABP]).
   c. Improve hemoglobin concentration (e.g., blood).
5. Correct electrolyte imbalances.
   a. Replace deficient electrolytes.
   b. Decrease excessive electrolyte levels (e.g., electrolyte restriction, diuretics, ion exchange resins, or dialysis).
6. Correct acidosis.
   a. Improve perfusion to correct metabolic acidosis caused by lactic acid.
   b. Initiate dialysis for patients with renal failure.
   c. Provide hydration and insulin therapy for patients in diabetic ketoacidosis.
   d. Improve ventilation to correct respiratory acidosis.

Table 3-3 Differentiation between Ventricular Ectopy and Aberrancy

Features	Favoring Ventricular Ectopy	Favoring Supraventricular Origin with Abrerracy
Rate	• 130-150 beats/min	• More than 150 beats/min
Regularity	• Regular	• Irregular (since most likely to be AF)
P wave	• None or dissociated AV • Inverted P wave after QRS complex (retrograde conduction to atria)	• Premature
QRS complex width	• Greater than 0.14 second	• 0.12-0.14 second
QRS complex morphology	• Initial vector opposite normal beats • Precordial concordance (all QRS complexes V_1-V_6 positive or all QRS complexes V_1-V_6 negative) • QRS complex morphology similar to previously seen PVCs	• Initial vector same as normal beats
QRS complex morphology in V_1 NOTE: Upper case letters indicate large waves; lower case letters indicate small waves.	• Monophasic R wave • Rr′ with left peak taller • Biphasic qR interval • Biphasic Rs or rS interval	• Monophasic QS interval • Biphasic rS interval • Triphasic rSR′ or rR′ interval
QRS complex morphology in V_6 NOTE: Upper case letters indicate large waves; lower case letters indicate small waves.	• Monophasic QS interval • Biphasic qR interval • Biphasic rS interval	• Monophasic R wave • Triphasic qRs complex
Fusion beats	• Yes	• No
Compensatory pause after single beat or at end of run	• Yes	• No
Axis	• Indeterminate or LAD of −30 or greater	• Normal or RAD
Patient history	• History of PVCs, • History of heart disease	• History of premature atrial complexes, AF • History of preexisting BBB
Response to carotid massage	• No effect on ventricular rate	• Often causes at least temporary slowing of ventricular rate
BP	• Usually very low or absent (but may be normal)	• Moderately low or normal
Consciousness	• Frequently unconscious (but may be conscious)	• May complain of light-headedness
Seizures	• Frequently present (but may be absent)	• Absent

AF, Atrial fibrillation; *AV,* atrioventricular; *BBB,* bundle branch block; *BP,* blood pressure; *LAD,* left axis deviation; *PVCs,* premature ventricular complexes; *RAD,* right axis deviation.

7. Eliminate cause of catecholamine release or block effects.
   a. Treat pain.
   b. Decrease anxiety with relaxation techniques and anxiolytic drugs.
   c. Administer beta-blockers for cardioprotection as prescribed.
8. Initiate standings orders (e.g., IV, oxygen, and multiple-lead ECG).
9. Initiate antidysrhythmic therapy as indicated by standing orders or as prescribed.
   a. Vaughan-Williams classification system (Table 3-4)
   b. Drugs and treatments of choice for each dysrhythmia (Table 3-2)
      (1) Information regarding indications, actions, dosage, contraindications, and adverse effects of selected antidysrhythmic agents is in Chapter 13.
   c. Monitor closely for adverse effects of antidysrhythmic agents (see Chapter 13).
10. Use electrical therapies as indicated.
    a. Cardioversion
       (1) Uses
          (a) Urgent cardioversion is used for tachydysrhythmias (other than sinus) that is rapid enough to cause hemodynamic compromise or that has not responded to antidysrhythmic drug therapy.

Table 3-4 Vaughan-Williams Antidysrhythmic Classification System

Class	Effect	Examples
IA	• Blocks sodium influx, which depresses the rate of depolarization • Prolongs repolarization and action potential duration • Decreases contractility (negative inotrope) • Prolongs QT interval (torsades de pointes potential) and QRS complex duration	• Quinidine • Procainamide (Pronestyl) • Disopyramide (Norpace)
IB	• Blocks sodium influx during phase 0, which depresses the rate of depolarization • Shortens repolarization and action potential duration • Suppresses ventricular automaticity in ischemic tissue	• Lidocaine (Xylocaine) • Tocainide (Tonocard) • Mexiletine (Mexitil) • Phenytoin (Dilantin)
IC	• Blocks sodium influx, which depresses the rate of depolarization • Does not change repolarization and action potential duration • Has proarrhythmogenic potential	• Flecainide (Tambocor) • Propafenone (Rythmol)
II	• Depresses sinoatrial node automaticity • Increases refractory period of atrial an AV junctional tissue to slow conduction • Shortens action potential duration • Inhibits sympathetic activity	• Beta-blockers ○ Propranolol (Inderal) ○ Esmolol (Brevibloc) ○ Acebutolol (Sectral) ○ Sotalol (Betapace) (both II and III)
III	• Blocks potassium movement during phase III • Increases action potential duration • Prolongs effective refractory period	• Amiodarone (Cordarone) • Sotalol (Betapace) (both II and III) • Ibutilide (Corvert) • Dofetilide (Tikosyn)
IV	• Blocks calcium movement during phase II • Depresses automaticity in the SA and AV nodes • Prolongs the conduction time in the AV junction and increases the refractory period at the AV junction • Decreases contractility (negative inotrope)	• Calcium channel blockers ○ Verapamil (Calan) ○ Diltiazem (Cardizem)
Misc.	• Blocks reentry mechanism • Shortens action potential of atrial tissue with little or no effect on action potential of ventricle • Prolongs AV nodal refractory period • Decreases SA node automaticity and slows sinus rate	• Adenosine (Adenocard)
Misc.	• Blocks parasympathetic nervous system effects to increase • SA node firing rate and improve AV nodal conduction	• Atropine
Misc.	• Slows conduction through atrioventricular node • Prolongs AV nodal refractory period • Decreases SA node automaticity and slows sinus rate	• Digitalis

AV, Atrioventricular; *SA*, sinoatrial.

(b) Elective cardioversion is performed for tachydysrhythmias that are reasonable well tolerated hemodynamically but have not responded to antidysrhythmic drug therapy.

(2) Contraindications
  (a) Tachydysrhythmias that result from digitalis toxicity
  (b) Nonsustained tachydysrhythmias
  (c) Long-standing AF
  (d) AF with normal or slow ventricular rate in the absence of atrioventricular nodal blocking drugs
  (e) Multifocal atrial tachycardia

(3) Method—as for defibrillation except:
  (a) Conscious patients should be sedated with diazepam (Valium), lorazepam (Ativan), or midazolam (Versed).
  (b) Elective procedures should be preceded by at least a 6-hour fast.
  (c) Anterior-posterior electrode placement is preferable for cardioversion of AF.
  (d) Emergency equipment and drugs must be available.
  (e) Synchronizer switch is on so that charge is delivered only during QRS complex, avoiding the descending limb of the T wave.
  (f) Voltage is from 25 to 200 J.
  (g) Antidysrhythmic drug therapy is used after sinus rhythm is restored.

(4) Complications: as for defibrillation

b. Defibrillation: See Cardiopulmonary Arrest.

11. Use pacemaker therapies for patients who have problem with impulse formation and/or conduction.

Table 3-5 Indications for Temporary Transvenous Pacemaker in Presence of Acute Myocardial Infarction

Degree of Block	Inferior Myocardial Infarction	Anterior Myocardial Infarction
First-degree AV block	No	No
Second-degree AV block, type I	No	NA
Second-degree AV block, type II	NA	Yes
Third-degree AV block with junctional escape rhythm	No if asymptomatic Yes if symptomatic	NA
Third-degree AV block with ventricular escape rhythm	Yes	Yes

AV, Atrioventricular; *NA*, not applicable because patients with inferior myocardial infarction do not develop type II second-degree block and patients with anterior myocardial infarction do not develop type I second-degree block or have junctional escape rhythms.

a. Definition: an electronic device that delivers an electrical stimulus to the heart to cause depolarization of the myocardium and increase or decrease the heart rate
b. Indications for pacemaker
   (1) Sick sinus syndrome with syncope
      (a) Symptomatic bradydysrhythmias
      (b) Sinus block or sinus arrest with ventricular asystole
      (c) Alternating tachycardia and bradycardia (called *tachy-brady syndrome*)
   (2) Hypersensitive carotid sinus syndrome
   (3) AV blocks (Table 3-5 gives indications in acute myocardial infarction [MI])
      (a) Second-degree AV block, Mobitz type II
      (b) Third-degree AV block
   (4) Bifascicular block with acute MI
   (5) Trifascicular block (e.g., bilateral bundle branch block)
   (6) Refractory tachydysrhythmias unresponsive to drug therapy or cardioversion (referred to as *tachycardia overdrive*); an important treatment modality for torsades de pointes
c. Components (Figure 3-7)
   (1) Pulse generator
      (a) Battery
      (b) Circuitry
   (2) Lead(s)
      (a) Atrial
      (b) Ventricular
   (3) Electrode(s)
      (a) Unipolar
         (i) Negative only
         (ii) Metal of pulse generator acts as positive
      (b) Bipolar
         (i) Positive: proximal; sensing
         (ii) Negative: distal; pacing
d. Types of pacemakers
   (1) Temporary or permanent
      (a) Temporary (external pulse generator): hours to weeks
         (i) Transthoracic epicardial (Figure 3-8)

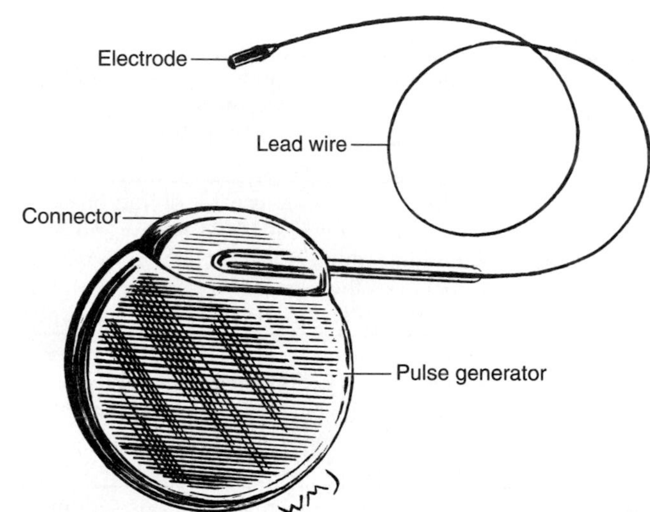

Figure 3-7 Components of a pacemaker. (Drawing by Wendy M. Johnson.)

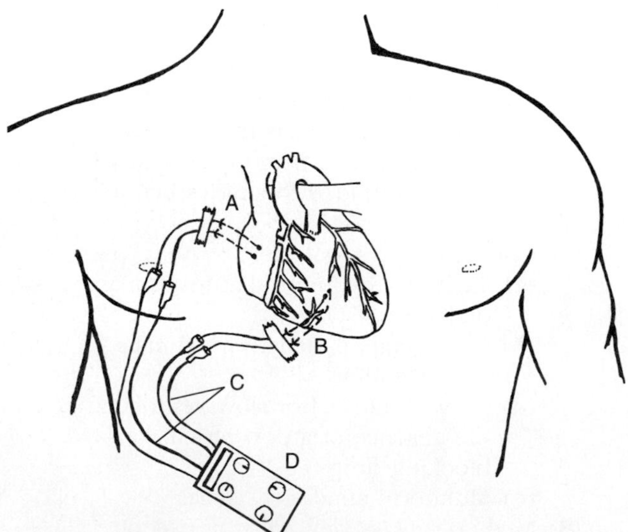

Figure 3-8 Temporary transthoracic epicardial pacing. *A*, Atrial electrodes. *B*, Ventricular electrodes. *C*, Leads. *D*, External pulse generator. (Drawing by Ann M. Walthall.)

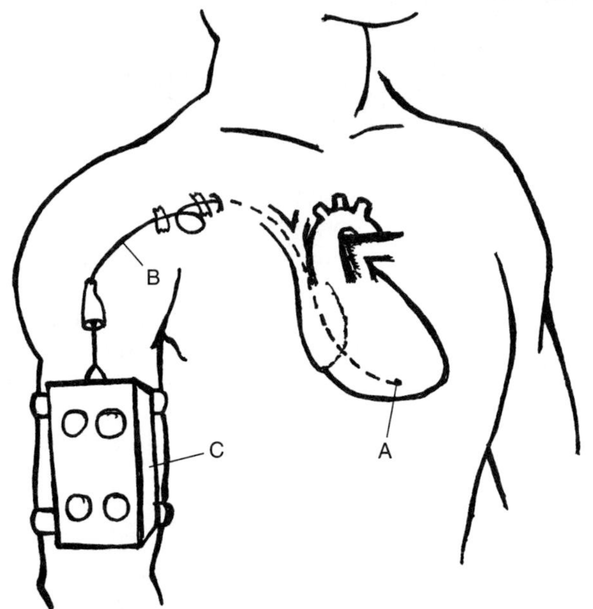

Figure 3-9 Temporary transvenous endocardial pacing. *A*, Electrode. *B*, Lead. *C*, External pulse generator. (Drawing by Ann M. Walthall.)

a) Electrodes attached to epicardium of atrium, ventricle, or both during cardiac surgery and brought through the chest wall

(ii) Transvenous endocardial (Figure 3-9)

a) Pacing lead(s) inserted percutaneously via internal jugular or subclavian vein and advanced into RA or RV or both

(iii) Transcutaneous (Figure 3-10)

a) Percutaneous leads applied to chest and back; used during cardiac arrests until transvenous pacer can be inserted

(b) Permanent (internal pulse generator): months to years

(i) Transvenous endocardial (Figure 3-11): lead inserted into cephalic vein and advanced into RA or RV; pulse generator implanted in subcutaneous fat under clavicle

(ii) Epicardial (Figure 3-12): electrodes sewn onto epicardium (thoracotomy required); pulse generator implanted in subcutaneous fat of abdomen

(2) Asynchronous versus synchronous

(a) Asynchronous

(i) Also called *fixed rate*

(ii) The pacemaker delivers a pacing stimulus at a fixed rate regardless of the intrinsic activity of the heart.

(iii) The pacemaker will cause competition with the intrinsic activity of the heart, and the pacing stimulus may land during the descending limb of the T wave.

(iv) Rarely seen today

(b) Synchronous

(i) Also called *demand*

(ii) The pacemaker delivers a pacing stimulus only when the intrinsic pacemaker of the heart fails to function at a predetermined rate.

(iii) The pacing stimulus will be inhibited or triggered when the intrinsic activity is seen.

e. North American Society of Pacing and Electrophysiology generic code (Table 3-6) and types of pacemakers (Table 3-7)

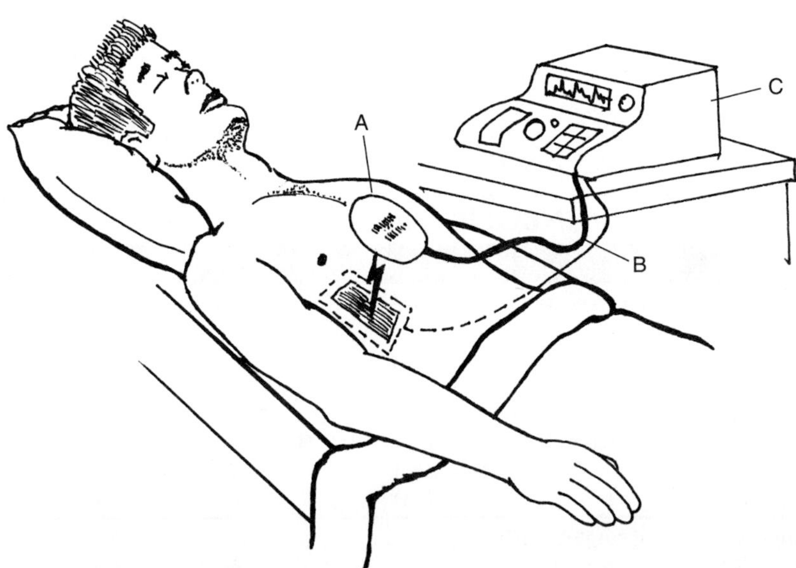

Figure 3-10 Temporary transcutaneous pacing. *A*, Electrode patches (anterior and posterior). *B*, Lead. *C*, Pulse generator. (Drawing by Ann M. Walthall.)

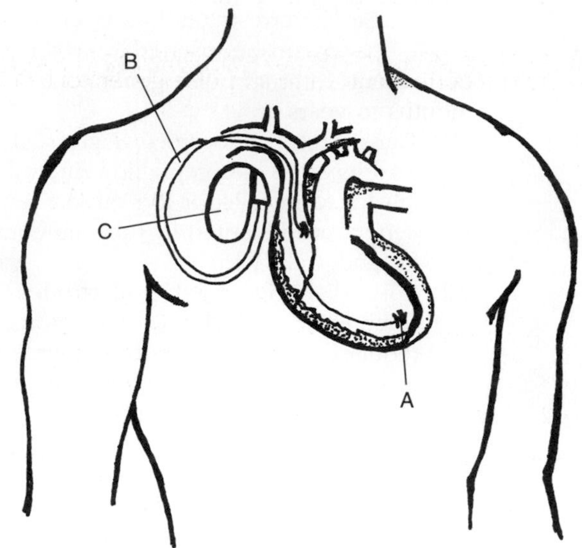

Figure 3-11 Permanent transvenous endocardial pacemaker. *A*, Electrode. *B*, Lead. *C*, Pulse generator. (Drawing by Ann M. Walthall.)

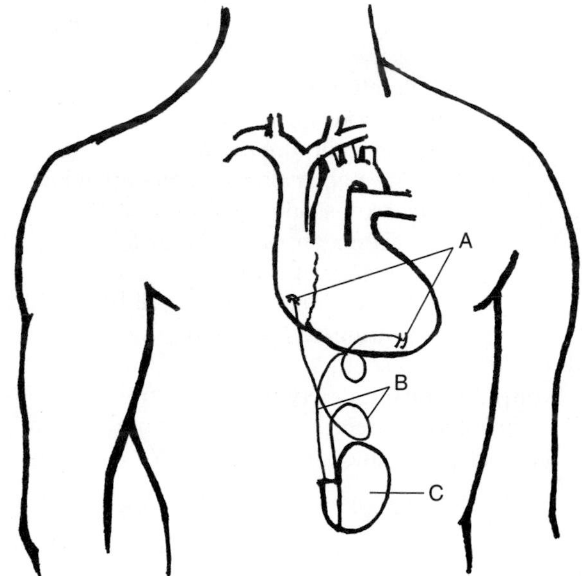

Figure 3-12 Permanent epicardial pacemaker. *A*, Electrodes. *B*, Leads. *C*, Pulse generator. (Drawing by Ann M. Walthall.)

(1) Chamber of stimulation
  (a) Atrial: AOO, AAI
    (i) Pacing stimulus occurs before the P wave
    (ii) Requires an intact AV node
  (b) Ventricular: VOO, VAT, VVI, VVT, VDD
    (i) Pacing stimulus occurs before the QRS complex
  (c) Atrioventricular sequential: DOO, DVI, DDD
    (i) Maintains AV synchrony and the hemodynamic benefit of the atrial kick
    (ii) Pacing stimulus before both or either P wave or QRS complex
    (iii) Sufficient AV delay set to allow atrial depolarization and contraction to complete ventricular filling
  (d) Atriobiventricular (also referred to as *cardiac resynchronization therapy*)
    (i) Used in severe heart failure in patients with ventricular depolarization asynchrony
    (ii) Placement of a left ventricular lead (placed directly on the left ventricle [epicardial] by thoracotomy approach or endocardially via the coronary sinus) along with right ventricular and right atrial leads
    (iii) An atrioventricular delay adequate to allow atrial contraction to contribute optimally to ventricular filling
    (iv) Optimal timing of stimulation of both ventricles; this may be with one ventricle stimulated slightly before the other rather than simultaneously
    (v) May or may not include an implantable cardioverter-defibrillator
(2) Rate-responsive: the heart rate is adjusted according to demands for cardiac output
  (a) Heart rate changes are stimulated by changes in muscle activity, minute ventilation, or blood changes in temperature or pH
  (b) Rate-responsive modes: AAIR, VVIR, DDDR

Table 3-6 The NASPE/BPEG Generic (NBG) Pacemaker Code

Position	I	II	III	IV	V
Category	Chamber(s) paced **O** = None **A** = Artium **V** = Ventricle **D** = Dual (A+V)	Chamber(s) sensed **O** = None **A** = Artium **V** = Ventricle **D** = Dual (A+V)	Response to sensing **O** = None **T** = Triggered **I** = Inhibited **D** = Dual (T+I)	Programmability, rate modulation **O** = None **P** = Simple Programmable **M** = Multiprogrammable **C** = Communicating **R** = Rate modulation	Antitachyarrhythmia function(s) **O** = None **P** = Pacing (antitachyarrhythmia) **S** = Shock **D** = Dual (P+S)
Manufacturers' designation only	**S** = single (**A** or **V**)	**S** = single (**A** or **V**)			

Note: Positions I through III are used exclusively for antibradyarrhythmia function.

Table 3-7 **Types of Pacemakers**

Code	Description	Indications	Advantages	Disadvantages
AOO	Fixed rate atrial pacer	• Consistently slow sinus rate with intact AV nodal conduction	• Single lead • Maintains AV synchrony	• Atrial competition • No protection in case of AV nodal block
AAI	Demand atrial pacer	• Sick sinus syndrome • Sinus arrest • Sinus bradycardia • Must have intact AV nodal conduction	• Single lead • Maintains AV synchrony	• No protection in case of AV nodal block
VOO	Fixed rate ventricular pacer	• Complete heart block with slow idioventricular rhythm • Rarely used today	• Single lead • Protection from ventricular asystole	• Ventricular competition with possible stimulation of ventricular dysrhythmias
VAT	Atrial triggered ventricular pacer	• Complete heart block with intact sinus node	• Synchronized AV conduction with atrial "kick" optimizes cardiac output • Ventricular rate increases with atrial rate so more exercise responsive	• Two leads • May cause pacemaker-mediated tachycardia: rapid ventricular response in sinus or atrial dysrhythmias
VVI	Demand ventricular pacer	• Sick sinus syndrome • Sinus bradycardia • Sinus arrest • Complete heart block	• Single lead • Simple and reliable • Inexpensive • Protection from ventricular asystole • Little chance of competitive rhythms	• Loss of synchronized • AV conduction and atrial "kick" may reduce cardiac output • Not rate responsive • (NOTE: VVIR is a VVI with rate-responsiveness.)
VVT	Pacing stimulus delivered if needed or not; stimulus depolarizes ventricle if no intrinsic depolarization; stimulus lands harmlessly in QRS complex if intrinsic depolarization	• Sick sinus syndrome • Sinus bradycardia • Sinus arrest • Complete heart block	• Single lead • Can evaluate pacer function even if intrinsic activity faster than pacer rate	• Loss of synchronized AV conduction and atrial "kick" may reduce cardiac output • Not rate responsive • Difficult to evaluate QRS complex morphology
VDD	Ventricular pacer that can be atrial triggered or inhibited by intrinsic ventricular depolarization	• Sick sinus syndrome • Sinus bradycardia • Sinus arrest • Complete heart block	• Maintains AV synchrony • If atrial activity is present as pacer functions in atrial triggered mode; if no atrial activity, paces the ventricle in demand mode with inhibition to intrinsic ventricular depolarization	• Two leads • May cause pacemaker-mediated tachycardia • Does not pace the atria, so loss of atrial contraction if no intrinsic atrial activity
DOO	Fixed rate AV sequential pacer	• Consistently slow atrial and ventricular rate	• Synchronized AV conduction with atrial "kick" optimizes cardiac output	• Two leads • Not rate responsive • Atrial and ventricular competition

Continued

Table 3-7 Types of Pacemakers—cont'd

Code	Description	Indications	Advantages	Disadvantages
DVI	Fixed rate atrial pacer with demand ventricular pacer	• Sick sinus syndrome • Sinus bradycardia • Sinus arrest • Complete heart block	• Synchronized AV conduction with atrial "kick" optimizes cardiac output	• Two leads • Not rate responsive • Blind to intrinsic atrial activity, so atrial competition and even AF may occur
DDD	Demand atrial and ventricular pacer; ventricular pacing may be atrial triggered or ventricular inhibited	• Sick sinus syndrome • Sinus bradycardia • Sinus arrest • Complete heart block	• Synchronized AV conduction with atrial "kick" optimizes cardiac output • Near normal physiologic function	• Two leads • Most expensive • May cause pacemaker-mediated tachycardia • Difficult troubleshooting • Is not used in AF

AF, Atrial fibrillation; *AV,* atrioventricular.

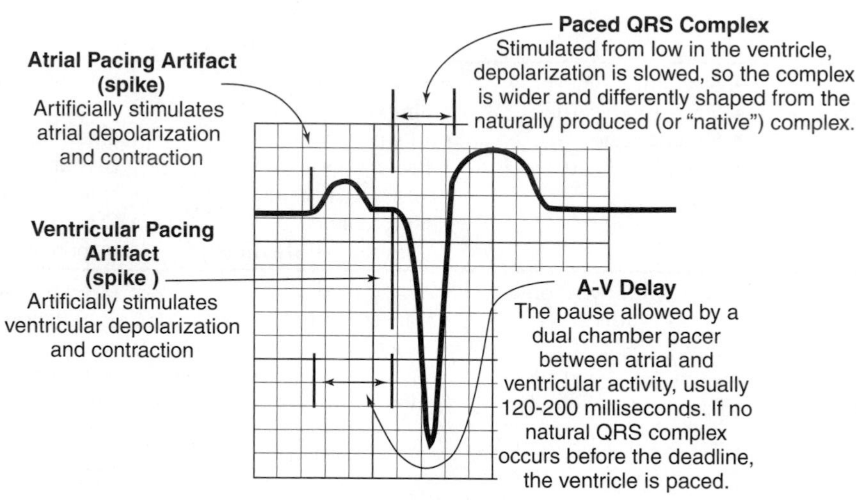

Figure 3-13 ECG evidence of pacing. (From Witherell, C. [1990]. Questions nurses ask about pacemakers. *American Journal of Nursing, 90*[12], 20.)

f. ECG evidence of pacing (Figure 3-13)
  (1) Spike before paced event
  (2) Wide QRS complex if ventricular pacer
  (3) Presence of T wave confirms ventricular depolarization
  (4) Presence of fusion beats (Figure 3-14)
g. Complications
  (1) Infection
  (2) Pneumothorax
  (3) Myocardial perforation
  (4) Hematoma
  (5) Frozen shoulder
  (6) Dysrhythmias
  (7) Electrical malfunction (Table 3-8)
h. Collaborative management
  (1) Temporary
    (a) Maintain electrical safety.
      (i) Ensure proper grounding of equipment.
      (ii) Touch side rails before touching patient to discharge static electricity.
      (iii) Wear rubber gloves when making adjustments.
      (iv) Avoid sources of electromagnetic interference (EMI) (e.g., electrocautery, defibrillation, magnetic resonance imaging (MRI), transcutaneous electrical nerve stimulation (TENS) units, radiation therapy, and lithotripsy).
    (b) Prevent complications.
      (i) Cover dial to prevent accidental changes in settings.
      (ii) Limit mobility of affected extremity to prevent accidental catheter dislodgment.
      (iii) Observe catheter site for signs of infection.
      (iv) Assist with establishment of pacing threshold and set milliamperae (mA) slightly above this; usually initially set at between 3 and 5 mA depending on pacing threshold.

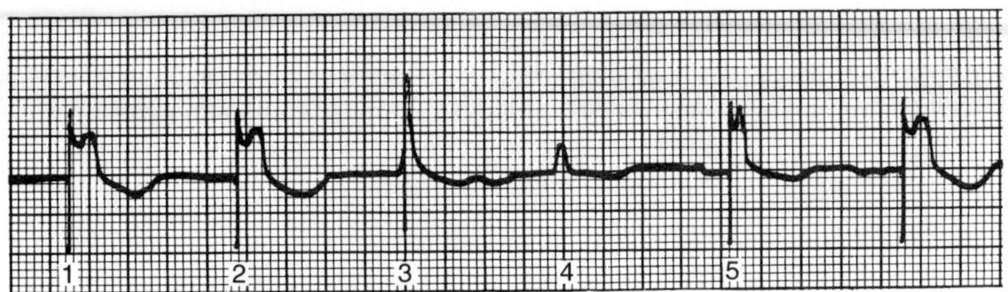

Figure 3-14 Fusion beat. Complexes 1 and 2 are paced complexes; complex 3 is a fusion beat with the paced impulse and an intrinsic impulse merging to cause this ventricular depolarization; complex 4 is an intrinsic complex; complex 5 is a paced complex. (From Guzzetta, C. E., & Dossey, B. M. [1992]. *Cardiovascular nursing: Holistic practice.* St. Louis: Mosby.)

Table 3-8 Pacemaker Electrical Malfunctions

Malfunction	Causes	Interventions
Failure to fire (pace): Pacemaker does not fire when it is physiologically indicated for it to fire • Recognized by pauses longer than the automatic interval and absence of pacer spike at end of escape interval	• Loose connections • Battery depletion • Lead displacement • Lead fracture • Sensing malfunction (e.g., EMI)	• Tighten connections if temporary. • Replace battery or pulse generator. • Lead repositioning or replacement may be needed. • Evaluate patient's own rhythm and patient's response; if inadequate, administer atropine and/or apply external transcutaneous pacemaker; CPR may be required. • Failure may be caused by sensing malfunction; to identify a sensing malfunction, convert pacemaker to asynchronous by placing a magnet over an implanted pacemaker or switching to asynchronous on an external pacemaker; if pacer spikes are visible in asynchronous mode, sensing malfunction exists. • Remove source of EMI.
Failure to capture: Pacemaker fires but depolarization does not occur • Recognized by spike not followed by depolarization (e.g., P wave if atrial pacer or QRS complex if ventricular pacer)	• Displacement of lead • Lead fracture • Increased pacing thresholds (e.g., electrolyte imbalance, drug toxicity, acid-base imbalance, or ischemia) • Fibrosis or scar tissue at the lead tip • Battery failure • Chamber perforation • Complexes not visible	• Position patient on left side or to whatever position patient was in when capture was last seen. • Increase MA. • May require lead repositioning or lead replacement. • Replace battery or pulse generator. • Check chest x-ray film for lead fracture and lead placement. • Correct metabolic or electrolyte imbalance. • Consider drugs levels and toxicity. • Check for diaphragmatic pacing and monitor or cardiac tamponade if catheter perforation is suspected. • Change monitoring lead or increase ECG size (gain). • Patient may require external transcutaneous pacing or CPR.
Failure to sense: Pacemaker fails to recognize intrinsic activity (e.g., P wave or QRS complex) • Recognized by pacer spikes falling closer to the intrinsic beats than the escape interval; spikes land indiscriminately throughout the cardiac cycle including potentially on the descending limb of the T wave	• Displacement of lead • Lead fracture • Sensitivity set too low or set on asynchronous • Disconnection of sensing circuit • Inadequate signal (e.g., low P wave or QRS complex voltage) • Battery failure	• Position patient on left side or to whatever position sensing was last seen. • Lead repositioning or replacement may be necessary. • Make sure that pacer is not set on asynchronous. • Increase sensitivity. • Check connections on temporary pacemaker. • Administer lidocaine if nonsensed QRS complexes are PVC

Continued

Table 3-8 **Pacemaker Electrical Malfunctions—cont'd**

Malfunction	Causes	Interventions
	• Increased sensing threshold (e.g., edema or fibrosis at lead tip) • Chamber perforation	• Check chest x-ray film for lead placement or lead fracture. • Replace battery or pulse generator. • If patient's own rhythm is adequate, turn pacer off or heart rate down to minimum. • If patient's own rhythm is inadequate, increase pacer rate to override patient's own rhythm.
Oversensing: Pacemaker recognizes extraneous electrical activity or the wrong intrinsic electrical activity as the inhibiting event • Recognized by absence of pacer spikes and failure to fire	• Sensitivity set too high • EMI • Oversensing of P waves or T waves • Myopotentials • Crosstalk (no ventricular pacing)	• Decrease sensitivity. • Remove from EMI; ensure that all equipment is grounded properly. • Decrease atrial output, decrease ventricular sensitivity, and increase ventricular blanking period. • Patient may require external transcutaneous pacing or CPR.

CPR, Cardiopulmonary resuscitation; *ECG,* electrocardiogram; *EMI,* electromagnetic interference; *PVC,* premature ventricular complexes.

(v) Observe cardiac monitor for pacemaker malfunction.

(2) Permanent

(a) Prevent complications.

(i) Limit mobility for affected upper extremity for 48 hours to prevent lead dislodgment.

(ii) Encourage arm exercise after 48 hours to prevent frozen shoulder (ankylosis).

(iii) Observe incision for signs of infection.

(iv) Observe cardiac monitor for pacemaker malfunction.

(b) Provide patient and family instruction.

(i) Teach patient how to take pulse and what symptoms to report.

(ii) Teach patient sources of EMI to avoid (e.g., MRI, metal detectors, radio transmitters, and electrical generating plants).

12. Prepare and care for the patient with an AICD.

a. Definition: implantable device to provide for immediate termination of VT or VF in patients in whom these dysrhythmias cannot be controlled pharmacologically or surgically.

b. Tiered therapy (also called *third-generation*) devices have all of the following:

(1) Antitachycardia pacing

(2) Low-energy cardioversion

(3) High-energy defibrillation

(4) Bradycardia backup pacing

c. Indications

(1) One or more episodes of spontaneous VT or VF in a patient in whom electrophysiology study (EPS) and/or spontaneous ventricular dysrhythmias cannot be used accurately to predict the efficacy of other treatment

(2) Recurrent episodes of sustained VF or VF in a patient in whom antidysrhythmic therapy is suboptimal because of intolerance or noncompliance

(3) Persistent inducibility of sustained VT or VF during EPS despite antidysrhythmic therapy and/or ablation

(4) VF in a patient with no evidence of structural heart disease and no detectable suppressing triggering factors

d. Contraindications

(1) Frequent episodes of VT or VF (more than two events per month)

(2) Uncontrolled heart failure (HF)

(3) Less than 6 to 12 months of productive life expectancy

(4) History of noncompliance

(5) Extreme psychological barriers to use of the device

e. Components (Figure 3-15)

(1) Generator

(a) Processes information from the lead system and delivers the electrical impulses

(b) Stores information about the patient's heart rhythm and therapy delivered

(c) Placed in the left upper quadrant of abdomen or under the clavicle

(d) Usually lasts about 3 to 5 years before replacement required

(2) Multilead system

(a) Two ventricular patches

(i) Sewn to the epicardium or placed outside the pericardial sac

(b) Some models include an additional subcutaneous patch

(c) Two leads that sense cardiac events

f. Method

(1) System evaluates heart rate and probability density function (PDF).

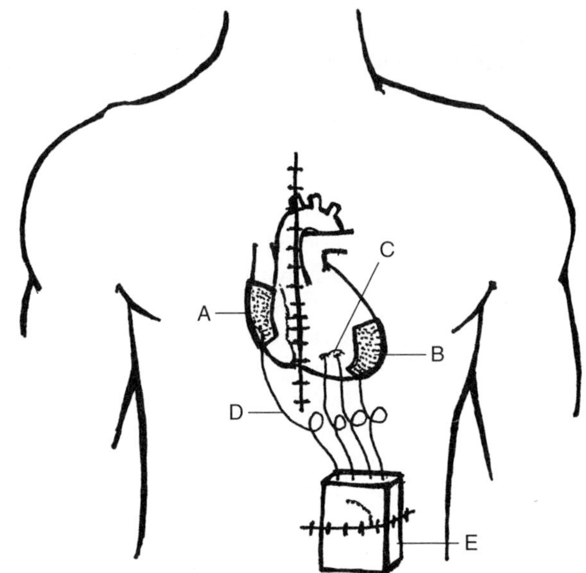

Figure 3-15 Automatic implantable cardioverter-defibrillator. *A*, Right atrial defibrillator patch. *B*, Left ventricular defibrillator patch. *C*, Two unipolar right ventricular electrodes. *D*, Leads. *E*, Pulse generator. (Drawing by Ann M. Walthall.)

(a) PDF diagnoses the amount of time the QRS complex spends away from the isoelectric baseline.
(2) System is turned on and off by using a donut-shaped magnet.
(a) Device usually is not turned on during early postoperative period because of frequent occurrence of sinus tachycardia during this period.
(3) When VT is sensed, the AICD first will initiate antitachycardia pacing.
(4) If the VT is not successfully pace-terminated, the AICD will cardiovert the rhythm with low-energy synchronized shocks.
(5) If the rhythm deteriorates to VF or if VF is the initial rhythm, the AICD will defibrillate at a higher energy level.
(6) Once a shock is delivered, the device senses the rhythm.
(7) If sinus rhythm is not restored, up to five shocks of 25 to 35 J are delivered.
(8) If the electrical rhythm deteriorates to bradycardia or asystole, the bradycardia backup pacing function is activated.

g. Complications
(1) Atelectasis
(2) Pneumonia
(3) Pneumothorax
(4) Lead migration
(5) Lead fracture

h. Collaborative management
(1) Provide postprocedure management as for pacemaker insertion.
(2) Monitor for dysrhythmias and evaluate effectiveness of AICD if firing occurs; administer antidysrhythmic agents as prescribed.
(3) If cardiopulmonary arrest occurs, do the following:
(a) Obtain emergency equipment and prepare to cardiovert or defibrillate.
(b) Treat this patient as you would any patient in cardiopulmonary arrest; do not wait for the device.
(c) Do not place defibrillator paddles within 5 to 10 cm of the generator.
(d) Anterior-posterior paddle placement may be more effective.
(4) Deactivate the AICD using a magnet as requested by the physician.
(5) Monitor for complications.
(a) Observe incision for signs of infection.
(b) Observe for clinical indications of cardiac tamponade.
(6) Encourage the patient to express fears and concerns about being shocked; consider referral to support group.

13. Prepare and care for the patient having ablation therapy.
a. Use: to eradicate dysrhythmia in patients who experience frequent, disabling, or life-threatening dysrhythmias that are not suppressed with pharmacologic therapy or in whom pharmacologic therapy is not well tolerated
b. Types
(1) Radiofrequency catheter ablation
(a) A catheter is placed in the heart via cardiac catheterization.
(b) Radiofrequency energy is applied to the area in which the dysrhythmia originates or an accessory pathway (e.g., in WPW syndrome).
(c) Controlled, localized necrosis occurs.
(d) Postprocedure care is as for cardiac catheterization or angioplasty; monitor patient closely for dysrhythmias.
(2) Surgical ablation: The area in which the dysrhythmia originates is excised or eliminated by cryosurgery or laser.

14. Prepare for and care for the patient having maze procedure for AF.
a. Procedure is performed by cardiothoracic surgery or PCI.
b. A maze of carefully planned sutures or laser-created cuts create an electrical conduction route through atrial myocardium, corralling and herding chaotic atrial impulses from the SA node to the AV node.
c. Provide postoperative management as for cardiothoracic surgery or PCI, depending on procedure performed.

Coronary Artery Disease

Definition

A progressive disease of the coronary arteries that results in their narrowing or obstruction

Etiology

Cardiac risk factors increase the incidence of premature coronary artery disease (CAD).

1. Nonmodifiable risk factors
   a. Heredity: when siblings or parents develop CAD before 55 years of age
      (1) Maternal history of CAD before 65 years conveys greater risk than paternal history in women.
      (2) Several risk factors have genetic predisposition (e.g., hypertension, hyperlipidemia, and diabetes mellitus [DM]).
   b. Advancing age: when age for males is greater than 45 years and for females greater than 55 years
   c. Gender: males have twice the risk of premenopausal females; risk increases in women after menopause
2. Modifiable risk factors
   a. Hypertension: BP greater than 140/90 mm Hg
   b. Hyperlipidemia: elevated levels of cholesterol, triglycerides, or low-density lipoproteins (LDL) and/or decreased levels of high-density lipoproteins (HDL); *desirable* levels of lipids are the following:
      (1) Cholesterol level less than 200 mg/dL
      (2) LDL level less than 100 mg/dL for patients with heart disease or DM; less than 130 for patients with two or more risk factors; less than 160 for patients with only one risk factor
      (3) HDL level greater than 40 mg/dL
      (4) Triglyceride level less than 150 mg/dL
   c. Smoking: Smoking increases platelet aggregation and fibrinogen levels and may cause vasospasm. Elevated carbon monoxide levels decrease the oxygen-carrying capacity of hemoglobin. Complete smoking cessation is desired.
   d. DM or glucose intolerance: Control of blood glucose in patients with DM is advocated to control risk of sequelae including CAD. Desirable fasting glucose level is less than 150 mg/dL.
   e. Hyperhomocysteinemia: homocysteine level greater than 14 μmol/L
      (1) Homocysteine is an essential sulfur-containing amino acid formed during the processing of dietary protein; elevated levels are toxic to the vascular endothelium and increase coagulability.
      (2) Deficiencies of folate, vitamin B_{12}, and vitamin B_6 have been implicated in elevated levels of homocysteine, and elevated levels of homocysteine may be reduced successfully by folate, vitamin B_{12}, and/or pyridoxine therapy.
   f. Sedentary lifestyle: Exercise is related inversely to cardiovascular mortality; sedentary persons also tend to be obese.
   g. Stress
      (1) Chronic stress promotes the long-term development of CAD.
      (2) Acute stress increases catecholamine levels, myocardial oxygen consumption, and dysrhythmia potential.
      (3) Personality type A with aggression also may contribute.
   h. Obesity: body weight greater than 120% of ideal body weight; ideal body weight is desirable
      (1) Obesity also contributes to hypertension, hyperlipidemia, glucose intolerance, and sedentary lifestyle.
      (2) Midline fat is of greater risk than hip and thigh fat (apple versus pear).
   i. Oral contraceptives: increase risk of MI especially in smokers; increases BP; smoking cessation is desirable for all persons but especially in women who use oral contraceptives
3. Protective factors
   a. Exercise: elevates HDL levels, decreases BP and resting heart rate, decreases body fat, and increases endogenous tissue plasminogen activator (tPA) levels
      (1) Intensity: sufficient to increase heart rate to 50% to 80% of predicted maximal heart rate
         (a) Simple formula to calculate predicted maximal heart rate is 220 minus age in years
      (2) Duration: 20 to 30 minutes
      (3) Frequency: at least 3 times per week
      (4) Type of exercise: recommendation is to vary the type of exercise to prevent boredom but walking is an excellent form of exercise for almost all patients
   b. Stress management: reduces catecholamine levels, decreases BP, reduces muscle tension
      (1) Methods include daily stretching, breathing exercises, meditation, prayer, and yoga.
   c. High-fiber, low-fat diet: reduces total cholesterol
   d. Alcohol (one to two beverages per day): increases HDL and may decrease platelet aggregation; overall health benefit diminishes after one to two alcoholic beverages per day
   e. Aspirin (81 to 325 mg daily): prevents platelet aggregation and decreases inflammation (one postulated contributor to CAD)
   f. Folic acid (0.65 mg to 1 mg daily): prevents hyperhomocysteinemia
   g. Antioxidants (vitamin C [1 g] and vitamin E [400 to 800 units] daily): prevent free radical damage
   h. International fatty acids: decrease platelet aggregation, increase HDL levels, decrease triglyceride levels
      (1) Alpha-linolenic acid found in canola oil, walnuts, and flax seeds

(2) Eicosapentaenoic acid and docosahexaenoic acid found in salmon, trout, sardines

i. Flavonoids: antioxidant effect, induce nitric oxide formation, may inhibit platelet aggregation; found in tea and cocoa

j. Loving relationships

(1) Decrease the overall incidence of CAD though mechanisms that are unclear, though loneliness and depression have been identified as contributing factors to coronary artery disease

(2) Pets also have a beneficial effect by decreasing stress and depression

Pathophysiology

1. Arteriosclerosis: a group of diseases characterized by thickening and loss of elasticity (calcification) of arterial walls
2. Atherosclerosis: the most common form of arteriosclerosis
   a. A chronic disease process characterized by the build-up of fatty plaque along the subintimal layer of arteries leading to a decrease in arterial lumen
   b. Progression (Figure 3-16)
      (1) Fatty streak: yellow, smooth lesion of lipid
         (a) Injury to the endothelial cells that line the lumen of the artery
            (i) Arteries most likely to be affected include the coronary arteries, the aorta, the cerebral arteries, and arterial bifurcations
         (b) Permeability of the endothelial cells to fatty acids and triglycerides increases
         (c) Initiation of the inflammatory/immune response
         (d) Release of vasoactive peptides, accumulation of macrophages and platelets
      (2) Fibrous plaque: raised, yellow lesion with collagen accumulation
         (a) Smooth muscle proliferation occurs
      (3) Complicated lesion: calcified lesion with ulceration, rupture, and/or hemorrhage
         (a) Platelet aggregation to the injured arterial endothelium caused by irregular surface of the intima leads to thrombosis
         (b) Decrease in arterial lumen and arterial elasticity
         (c) Decreased blood flow distal to the lesion
3. Decreased blood flow and oxygen supply to the myocardium lead to imbalance between oxygen supply and oxygen demand
   a. Gradual or partial occlusion: ischemia causing angina
      (1) Demand angina is caused by 75% occlusion of the coronary artery lumen; angina at rest caused by 99% occlusion
   b. Sudden or complete occlusion: necrosis causing MI

Nursing Diagnoses (see Appendix A)

1. Ineffective Myocardial Tissue Perfusion related to coronary artery disease and decreased cardiac output
2. Ineffective Peripheral Tissue Perfusion related to decreased cardiac output
3. Deficit Knowledge related to disease process and health maintenance
4. Anxiety related to change in health status
5. Interrupted Family Processes related to change in health status and potential life-threatening situation

Collaborative Management

1. Encourage healthful lifestyle
   a. Well-balanced diet to maintain normal weight maintenance
      (1) Low in saturated fat and transfatty acids while including monounsaturated fats (e.g., olive oil and canola oil)

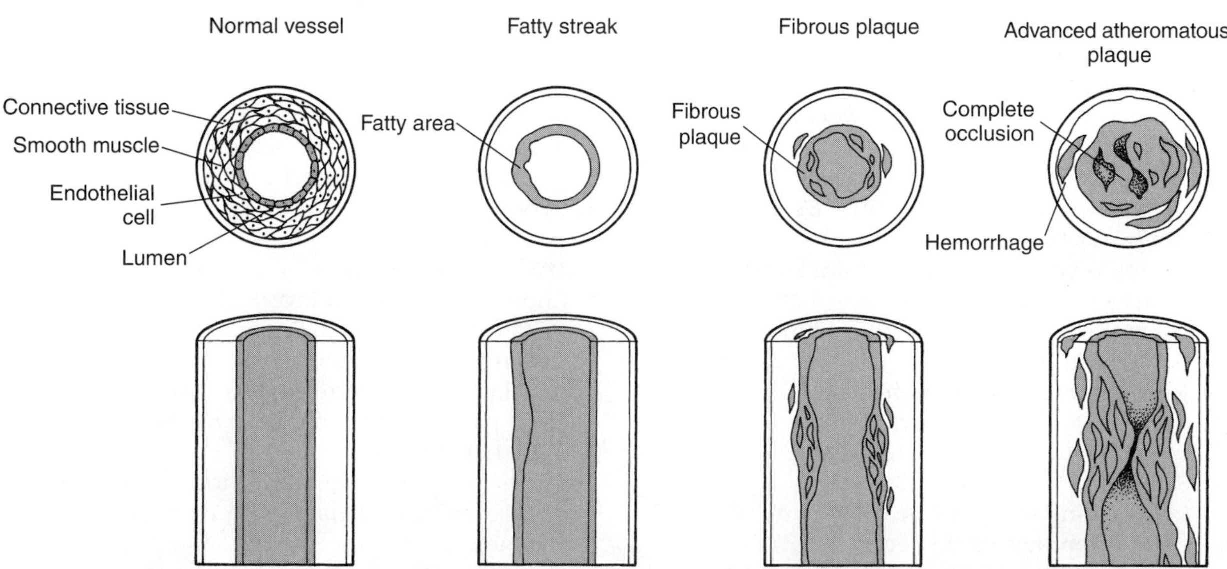

Figure 3-16 Progression of atherosclerosis. (From Thelan, L. A., Urden, L. D., Lough, M. E., & Stacy, K. M. [1998]. *Critical care nursing: Diagnosis and management* [3rd ed.]. St. Louis: Mosby.)

(2) High in fiber
(a) Fresh fruit and vegetables
(b) Whole grains
(3) Adequate low-fat proteins
b. Adequate rest and relaxation
c. Regular exercise
2. Nonpharmacologic and pharmacologic methods to reduce risk factors
3. Monitoring for progression of disease by stress tests and cardiac catheterization as indicated
4. Treatment of fixed lesions but PCI or coronary artery bypass grafting (CABG), especially if proximal or severe

Pathologic Consequences of Atherosclerosis and Arteriosclerosis

1. Angina pectoris
2. MI
3. Heart failure (HF)
4. Dysrhythmias caused by ischemia
5. Sudden death

Angina Pectoris

Definition

Transient chest pain associated with myocardial ischemia

Etiology

1. Factors that decrease supply
a. Arteriosclerosis/atherosclerosis
b. Coronary artery spasm
c. Aortitis
d. Dysrhythmias
e. Anemia
f. Shock
2. Factors that increase demand
a. Hypertension
b. Aortic valve disease
c. Tachydysrhythmias
d. HF
e. Hyperthyroidism

Pathophysiology

1. A temporary imbalance between myocardial oxygen supply and myocardial oxygen demand occurs that causes ischemia.
a. Common precipitating factors: five *E*'s and smoking
(1) Exercise: volume work (e.g., walking, running, or swimming)
(2) Exertion: pressure work (e.g., lifting, pushing, or Valsalva maneuver)
(3) Emotion: catecholamine release
(4) Eating: shunting of blood to gut
(5) Exposure to cold: vasoconstriction
(6) Smoking
(a) Nicotine increases heart rate and BP.
(b) Carbon monoxide decreases oxygen-carrying capacity of hemoglobin.
2. Ischemia leads to anaerobic metabolism and accumulation of lactic acid, causing chest pain.
3. Angina is associated with a coronary artery occlusion of 75% or more.

Clinical Presentation

1. Subjective
a. Substernal chest discomfort that usually lasts 1 to 4 minutes (but may last up to 15 minutes) and subsides with rest and/or nitroglycerin (NTG) use.
(1) Discomfort may be described as burning, squeezing, tightness, pressure, heaviness, indigestion, or aching.
(2) Pain may radiate to shoulders, back, arms, jaw, neck, and epigastrium.
(3) Precipitating factors: five *E*'s and smoking
b. Dyspnea
c. Nausea/vomiting
d. Anxiety
e. Weakness
2. Objective
a. Tachycardia
b. Hypotension or hypertension
c. Tachypnea
d. Levine's sign: clenched fist held over sternum
e. Pallor
f. Diaphoresis
g. S_4
3. Diagnostic
a. Serum
(1) Isoenzymes: negative for cardiac damage
(2) Lipid profile (fasting): to identify hyperlipidemia as a risk factor
(3) Fasting glucose: to identify DM or glucose intolerance as a risk factor
b. ECG
(1) ST segment depression in unstable angina
(2) ST segment elevation in variant angina
(3) Ventricular dysrhythmias may be present
c. Graded exercise stress test: may or may not be positive; sensitivity lower with women
d. Cardiac catheterization: coronary artery occlusion 75% or greater; may be negative in variant angina but develop occlusion from spasm
e. Echocardiography: may show segmental wall motion defects
f. Myocardial perfusion scan with thallium-201: cold areas indicating ischemia
4. Types (Table 3-9)

Nursing Diagnoses (see Appendix A)

1. Chest Pain related to myocardial ischemia
2. Ineffective Cardiopulmonary Tissue Perfusion related to coronary artery occlusion
3. Activity Intolerance related to chest pain or fear of chest pain, adverse effects of medication (e.g., beta-blockers)
4. Deficient Knowledge related to unfamiliarity with disease process, therapy, and required lifestyle changes
5. Interrupted Family Processes related to change in health status and potential life-threatening situation

Table **3-9 Types of Angina**

Type of Angina	Signs and Symptoms
STABLE	• Unchanging frequency, duration, and severity • Predictable to the patient • ST segment depression may occur during pain
UNSTABLE ANGINA • De novo angina	• Angina of new onset
• Crescendo angina: angina that has increased in frequency, intensity, or duration • Preinfarction: angina of prolonged duration that occur even at rest	• Associated with progression of CAD • Less exertion to cause pain or pain at rest • Greater severity • Longer duration • More difficult to relieve and may not be relieved with nitroglycerin • May have ST segment depression during pain
• Wellens syndrome: critical proximal stenosis of LAD coronary artery	• Associated with critical proximal stenosis of LAD coronary artery • Characteristic ECG changes that appear even in a pain-free state ○ ST segment isoelectric or elevated no more than 1 mm in V_1-V_3 ○ Symmetrical T wave inversion in V_2-V_3 ○ No loss of normal R wave progression in V_1-V_3 ○ No pathologic Q waves • Normal or slightly elevated enzymes • Emergency cardiac catheterization is indicated
• Variant (also called *Prinzmetal's* or *vasospastic*): angina related to coronary artery spasm	• Associated with coronary artery spasm ○ Pain occurs at rest ○ May be caused by tobacco, alcohol, or cocaine • Pain lasts longer than usual anginal pain: 10 minutes or more • ST segment elevation during pain

CAD, Coronary artery disease; *ECG,* electrocardiogram; *LAD,* left anterior descending.

Collaborative Management

1. Relieve chest pain.
   a. Nitroglycerin (NTG)
      (1) Usually sublingual tablets or metered-dose spray is used.
      (2) IV nitroglycerin may be used in unstable angina.
      (3) NTG is most valuable in increasing oxygen supply if good collateral circulation exists (diseased coronary arteries do not dilate well because they are relatively immobilized by calcium deposits in the media).
   b. Calcium channel blockers (e.g., nifedipine [Procardia]); especially for variant angina
   c. Morphine sulfate may be required for unstable angina
2. Increase oxygen supply.
   a. Oxygen via nasal cannula: 5 L/min during ischemic pain unless contraindicated by chronic lung disease; in patients with chronic lung disease, use pulse oximetry to guide oxygen administration: aim for an arterial oxygen saturation of 90%
   b. NTG in doses greater than 1 mcg/kg/min causes arterial and venous dilation; because diseased coronary arteries are calcified and immobilized, NTG works best to increase supply in patients who have good collateral circulation
   c. Calcium channel blockers or NTG if angina is caused by coronary artery spasm
   d. Blood transfusion if angina caused by anemia
   e. Dysrhythmias management
      (1) Tachydysrhythmias decrease the time for coronary artery filling and may decrease cardiac output
      (2) Bradydysrhythmias increase the time for coronary artery filling but may decrease cardiac output
   f. Platelet aggregation inhibitors (e.g., aspirin or ticlopidine [Ticlid]) to prevent platelet aggregation; heparin may be prescribed to prevent clotting or extension of a clot
   g. IABP may be used in unstable angina; IABP increases coronary artery perfusion pressure (CAPP)
3. Decrease oxygen demand.
   a. Removal of provoking factors
      (1) Activity cessation immediately when chest pain occurs
      (2) Bed rest during pain; semi-Fowler position usually most comfortable for the patient
   b. NTG as prescribed
      (1) NTG in doses less than 1 mcg/kg/min is a predominantly venous dilator; it decreases myocardial workload and myocardial oxygen consumption by decreasing preload.
      (2) NTG in doses greater than 1 mcg/kg/min is an arterial and venous dilator; it decreases

myocardial workload and myocardial oxygen consumption by decreasing afterload and preload.

c. Beta-blockers (e.g., metoprolol [Lopressor]) as prescribed
   (1) Beta-blockers decrease myocardial workload and myocardial oxygen demand by decreasing HR and contractility.
   (2) Beta-blockers are contraindicated in variant angina; blocking beta receptors leaves alpha receptors unopposed and perpetuates vascular spasm.
d. Calcium channel blockers as prescribed
   (1) Calcium channel blockers dilate arteries and veins, decreasing myocardial workload and myocardial oxygen consumption by decreasing preload and afterload.
   (2) Calcium channel blockers are the drugs of choice for variant angina because they are excellent antispasmodics.
e. Control dysrhythmias: tachydysrhythmias increase myocardial workload and myocardial oxygen consumption
f. Decrease catecholamine release
   (1) Establish and maintain a calm, quiet environment.
   (2) Keep the patient and the family informed.
   (3) Restrict stimulants.

4. Monitor for complications.
   a. Progression to MI
   b. Dysrhythmias
   c. Mitral regurgitation caused by ischemia and dysfunction of papillary muscles
   d. HF
5. Additional treatments
   a. Identify risk factors and encourage modification to decelerate arteriosclerotic/atherosclerotic process
   b. PCIs (Table 3-10) are used to open the lumen of diseased coronary artery (or arteries) and restore blood flow.
   c. CABG (Table 3-11) is used to provide arterial or venous conduits to redirect coronary blood flow around occluded coronary arteries.
   d. Transmyocardial revascularization
      (1) Used in patient with inoperable, Class IV angina; patient must have an ejection fraction (EF) of at least 20%
      (2) High-powered carbon dioxide laser used to create 15 to 30 transmural channels that direct nonarterial oxygenation to the ischemic myocardium
      (3) Usually done by percutaneous endocardial approach (percutaneous transluminal (PTMR) myocardial revascularization) but may be performed via left anterolateral thoracotomy
      (4) Superior to maximal medical therapy in relief of angina and improvement in exercise tolerance
   e. Enhanced external counter pulsation (EECP)
      (1) Indicated for patients with recurrent and debilitating angina despite medical therapy and revascularization, when revascularization surgery is contraindicated or would be too risky, or when the patient refuses invasive procedures
      (2) Contraindications
         (a) Dysrhythmias: AF, atrial flutter, VT
         (b) Femoral vessel cannulation within the last 7 to 14 days
         (c) Uncontrolled HF or angina
         (d) Aortic regurgitation
         (e) Severe peripheral vascular disease
         (f) BP greater than 180/110 mm Hg
         (g) Anticoagulant therapy or bleeding disorder
         (h) Pregnancy
      (3) Actions: reduces angina symptoms and increases exercise tolerance
      (4) Mechanism of action: not completely understood
         (a) May encourage development of collateral circulation
         (b) May cause release of growth factors that stimulate angiogenesis
      (5) Procedure
         (a) Pneumatic cuffs are placed on the patient's calves, thighs, and lower buttocks.
         (b) The cuffs are inflated during diastole (a plethysmograph is placed on the patient's finger).
         (c) The inflation starts at the calves, moves to the legs, and on to the lower buttocks.
         (d) The diastolic augmentation allows a backflow of aortic blood into the heart during diastole and increases CAPP.
         (e) Immediately before systole, the pressure is released, allowing a reduction in afterload and cardiac workload.
         (f) The procedure is maintained for 1 hour and is repeated 5 days per week for 7 weeks.
         (g) Course may be repeated is symptoms worsen over time.
      (6) Adverse effects: leg discomfort, skin abrasion
      (7) Nursing management
         (a) Periodically assess circulation distal to cuff when they are inflated.
         (b) Assess skin for signs of abrasion.

Acute Coronary Syndrome

Definition

Syndrome of acute myocardial ischemia caused by atherosclerotic plaque rupture and thrombus formation (Figure 3-17)

Etiology

See Coronary Artery Disease, Angina Pectoris, and Myocardial Infarction.

Table 3-10 Percutaneous Coronary Interventions

Procedures	• Percutaneous transluminal coronary angioplasty (PTCA): inflation of a balloon-tipped catheter in an area of coronary artery stenosis from plaque; plaque is pushed back against the wall of the vessel and fractured (controlled trauma) ○ Cutting balloon microsurgical dilation catheter system: microsurgical blades mounted longitudinally on an angioplasty balloon to open narrowed artery; as the balloon expands radially, the blades are exposed and incise plaque in the arteries; claimed to facilitate maximum dilation of the target lesion with more precision and less trauma than conventional angioplasty • Coronary artery stent: use of a metal that acts as a scaffolding device to support a coronary artery and maintain patency after PTCA; previously used only in case of acute closure; most PTCA procedures include planned stent placements ○ Stents are usually stainless steel but may be nitinol, tantalum, or another metal ○ Stents usually have been thought of as a coil, but they may be a mesh, slotted tube, ring, or another design ○ Stents are deployed by balloon expansion or they may be self-expanding ○ Stents may be drug-eluting to reduce the risk of neointimal hyperplasia and restenosis rates — Sirolimus, an immunosuppressive agent, to prevent proliferation of normal tissue and inflammation — Paclitaxel, an antineoplastic agent, to inhibit cell proliferation and migration • Brachytherapy: use of intracoronary irradiation to reduce risk of restenosis; combined with PTCA or stent placement • Coronary atherectomy: removal of plaque from coronary artery by a high-speed diamond-tipped (rotational) or shaving (directional) device ○ Directional coronary atherectomy: a directional device shaves pieces of the atheroma into the catheter tip ○ Coronary rotational ablation (Rotablator): a diamond-coated burr drills through the atheroma and pulverizes the plaque ○ Transluminal extraction catheter: a motorized cutting head shaves the atheroma from the arterial wall and suctions out the pieces ○ Excimer laser coronary atherectomy: use of a laser to vaporize the atheroma • AngioJet: high-speed saline jet; most effective for thrombus
Indications	• Unstable or chronic angina • Acute or postacute MI • Post–CABG with postoperative angina • Patient must be surgical candidate (in case of coronary artery dissection)
Contraindications	• Left main CAD (unless there is a patent bypass around it, referred to as *protected*) • Stenosis of coronary artery at orifice • Variant angina • Critical valvular disease
Action	The goal of PCIs is to reduce the degree of coronary artery stenosis; the intervention is considered successful is the degree of stenosis is reduced to 20% to 30% stenosis without serious complications.
Assessment	• Vital signs: BP, HR, RR, T • ECG: monitor closely for ST segment elevation • Sheath insertion site: usually femoral but may be radial • Neurovascular status of affected limb • Any complaints of chest pain • Any complaints of back pain
Nursing diagnoses	• Risk for Ineffective Cardiopulmonary Tissue Perfusion related to thrombosis, acute closure, or spasm • Risk for Chest Pain related to myocardial ischemia • Risk for Ineffective Peripheral Tissue Perfusion related to arterial trauma, mechanical occlusion by sheath, vasospasm, hematoma, swelling • Back Pain related to immobilization • Activity Intolerance related to immobilization and deconditioning • Risk for Injury (e.g., bleeding) related to arterial sheath, anticoagulation • Anxiety related to acute health alteration and recommended lifestyle changes • Deficient Knowledge related to procedure, therapy, recommended lifestyle changes

Continued

Table 3-10	Percutaneous Coronary Interventions—cont'd
Brief summary of specific nursing management	• Monitor for myocardial ischemia: note any new chest pain and ST segment elevation especially if PCI performed for acute ischemia or infarction. • Assess puncture site frequently to detect bleeding and/or hematoma formation. ◦ Control systolic BP to less than 150 mm Hg and diastolic BP to less than 90 mm Hg with antihypertensives as prescribed. ◦ Monitor platelet count and activated partial thromboplastin time (patient will receive platelet aggregation inhibitors and either unfractionated or low-molecular-weight heparin to prevent reocclusion). ◦ Immobilize groin by restraining with sheet stretched over knee on affected side and tucked on each side of bed rather than restraining ankle. ◦ Perform neurovascular checks to detect peripheral ischemia related to femoral artery thrombosis. • Monitor for clinical indications of retroperitoneal hemorrhage: postural tachycardia and/or hypotension; back and/or flank pain; Grey Turner's sign; decrease in hemoglobin and hematocrit (unfortunately, there are no early indications). • Keep affected limb straight and immobile; head of bed should be elevated no more than 30 degrees as long as the sheath is in place and for 4 to 8 hours after removal. • Assist with removal or remove sheath (depending on hospital protocol) if not completed in the cardiac catheterization laboratory; Perclose, VasoSeal, or Angio-Seal may be used when the sheath is removed in the cardiac catheterization laboratory. ◦ If heparin has been infusing intravenously, it will be discontinued and the activated clotting time needs to be less than 150 seconds; if unfractionated heparin is to be restarted, it will be restarted several hours after sheath removal; low-molecular-weight heparin subcutaneously may be used. ◦ Pain control and sedation (e.g., local infiltration with lidocaine or IV morphine and/or midazolam [Versed] or lorazepam [Ativan]). ◦ Apply pressure to where the sheath entered the artery, which is about 1 inch above the skin entry site. ◦ Manual pressure or mechanical pressure devices (e.g., C-clamp or FemoStop) may be used. ◦ Hold pressure for at least 30 minutes or until hemostasis is achieved ◦ Control of bleeding must be maintained while peripheral pulses are still palpated.
Complications: prevention and treatment	• Coronary artery dissection: caused by catheter trauma; necessitates placement of stent or, in severe cases, emergent CABG • Cardiac tamponade: caused by cardiac perforation • Dysrhythmias: caused by ischemia or reperfusion • Pseudoaneurysm: caused by catheter dissection of artery • Hemorrhage or hematoma: caused by anticoagulated state ◦ Retroperitoneal hemorrhage or hematoma ◦ Femoral artery puncture site hemorrhage or hematoma Embolic complications (e.g., MI, cerebral infarction, and peripheral emboli) • Acute reocclusion or closure: caused by the following: ◦ Trauma to intima initiating clotting cascade — Aspirin, GP IIb/IIIa platelet receptor blockers (e.g., abciximab [ReoPro], eptifibatide [Integrilin], or tirofiban [Aggrastat]), and heparin are used to prevent thrombosis; aspirin and ticlopidine (Ticlid) or clopidogrel (Plavix) are maintained after the procedure — Monitor activated partial thromboplastin time; usually maintained at 50-70 seconds ◦ Coronary artery spasm — Nitroglycerin infusion and/or calcium channel blockers are frequently used — NOTE: Report new onset chest pain or ST segment changes immediately. • Chronic restenosis: caused by intimal hyperplasia • Hypotension, bradycardia (vagal reaction): caused by increased parasympathetic nervous system during sheath removal; atropine is effective
Postprocedure education	• Information about devices placed: Give the patient a stent identification card with date, facility, type, and site of implant. • Care of site used for catheter insertion (femoral or radial) • Need for drugs to maintain stent patency: usually aspirin and clopidogrel • To avoid MRI scans within 8 weeks of stent placement • Symptoms to report: site pain, chest pain, and bleeding

BP, Blood pressure; *CABG,* coronary artery bypass graft; *CAD,* coronary artery disease; *ECG,* electrocardiogram; *HR,* heart rate; *IV,* intravenous; *MI,* myocardial infarction; *MRI,* magnetic resonance imaging; *PCI,* percutaneous coronary intervention; *PCTA,* percutaneous transluminal coronary angioplasty; *RR,* respiratory rate; *T,* temperature.

Table 3-11 Coronary Artery Bypass Grafting

Procedures	• Types of bypasses ∘ Arterial bypass (preferred because of better long-term patency rates) — Internal thoracic (also called *internal mammary*) arteries — Gastroepiploic artery — Inferior epigastric arteries — Radial arteries ∘ Vein grafts — Saphenous veins — Brachial veins • Surgical approaches ∘ Median sternotomy with cardiopulmonary bypass (CPB) — CPB provides a motionless heart and a bloodless field — Complications of CPB include systemic inflammatory response syndrome, coagulopathy, atelectasis, ARDS, cerebral microemboli, thrombotic stroke, post-CPB encephalopathy, renal insufficiency, dysrhythmias ∘ Off-pump CABG — May be performed through small median sternotomy or anterior thoracotomy — Bypass is performed on a beating heart — Avoids complications related to cardiopulmonary bypass ∘ Minimally invasive direct CABG — Performed through anterior thoracotomy — May be used for proximal LAD coronary artery and select lesions of RCA or circumflex — Bypass is performed on a beating heart — Avoids complications related to cardiopulmonary bypass — Thoracoscopy may be used
Indications	• Left main artery disease or three vessel disease • Double vessel disease if one of vessels is proximal LAD coronary artery • Single or double vessel disease with angina unresponsive to medical therapy • CAD with EF of less than 35% • Emergent conditions such as unstable angina, acute MI with persistent pain or shock, or coronary artery dissection during interventional cardiology procedures
Action	• The goal of CABG is to provide arterial or venous conduits to redirect coronary blood flow around occluded coronary arteries
Assessment	• Vital signs: HR, BP, RR, T • Hemodynamic parameters: RAP, PAP, PAOP, CO, CI, SVR, PVR, LVSWI, RVSWI • Oxygenation parameters: Sao_2, Svo_2; arterial blood gases • Serum electrolytes • Mediastinal and pleural tube drainage • Complaints of incisional pain, chest pain, and dyspnea • Incision for bleeding, separation, or redness and induration
Nursing diagnoses	• Risk for Decreased Cardiac Output related to myocardial stunning, dysrhythmias, conduction block, silent ischemia, and cardiac tamponade • Risk for Fluid Volume Deficit related to hemorrhage and third spacing • Risk for Ineffective Myocardial Tissue Perfusion related to graft occlusion, myocardial ischemia • Chest Pain related to surgical incision • Risk for Ineffective Cardiopulmonary, Cerebral, Renal, Peripheral Tissue Perfusion related to emboli, pump failure • Risk for Impaired Gas Exchange related to anesthesia, pain, immobility, atelectasis, ARDS • Impaired Skin Integrity related to chest incision, invasive procedures, and leg incisions • Risk for Injury related to epicardial pacing and intracardiac catheters • Sleep Deprivation related to noise, frequent interruptions, medications • Anxiety related to acute health alteration and recommended lifestyle changes • Deficient Knowledge related to unfamiliarity with disease process, therapy, and recommended lifestyle changes

Continued

Table 3-11 Coronary Artery Bypass Grafting—cont'd

Brief summary of specific nursing management	• Relieve pain. ◦ Administer narcotics and sedatives for relief of incisional pain. ◦ Provide instruction regarding splinting during coughing and turning. ◦ Report ischemic pain; titrate NTG for relief of ischemic pain. • Monitor patient closely for hemodynamic changes: titrate drug therapy to optimize cardiac output and minimize myocardial oxygen consumption. ◦ Pharmacologic support of this patient may include inotropes and/or vasodilators. ◦ Vasopressors may be used to increase CAPP and maintain patency of grafts; monitor for excessive afterload and myocardial oxygen consumption and for excessive vasoconstriction and peripheral hypoperfusion. • Monitor patient closely for hemorrhage: mediastinal tube, pleural tubes, incision. ◦ Administer IV fluids, blood and/or blood products, and albumin as prescribed. ◦ Maintain patency of mediastinal and pleural tubes. • Monitor patient closely for changes in perfusion. ◦ Note any complaints of chest pain, ST segment elevation, and dysrhythmias. ◦ Note any changes in appearance or volume of urine. ◦ Note any changes in level of consciousness or neurologic function. ◦ Note any changes in Sao_2, PAP, and PVR. ◦ Note any changes in bowel sounds, abdominal distention, and abdominal pain. • Monitor the ECG for dysrhythmias or blocks. ◦ Administer antidysrhythmic drugs as prescribed; antidysrhythmic drugs (e.g., amiodarone) may be given prophylactically to prevent AF. ◦ Use epicardial pacing wires for symptomatic bradycardias or blocks. • Monitor electrolytes and replace as prescribed. • Monitor for complications.
Complications: prevention and treatment	• Potential complications during surgery ◦ Cerebral or myocardial infarction ◦ Hemorrhage: greater risk with internal thoracic artery implant ◦ Inability to wean from cardiopulmonary bypass: intraaortic balloon pump and/or VAD used • Potential complications during postoperative period ◦ Immediate — Low cardiac output/hypotension — Hemorrhage — Cardiac tamponade — Dysrhythmias — MI — Hypertension — Acute respiratory failure (e.g., atelectasis or ARDS) — Renal failure — Electrolyte imbalance (e.g., hypokalemia, hypocalcemia, or hypomagnesemia) — Graft closure ◦ Intermediate — Donor site infection — Sternal wound infection: especially if patient is diabetic and/or internal thoracic (i.e., mammary) artery used for bypass

AF, Atrial fibrillation; *ARDS,* acute respiratory distress syndrome; *BP,* blood pressure; *CABG,* coronary artery bypass graft; *CAPP,* coronary artery perfusion pressure; *CI,* cardiac index; *CO,* cardiac output; *ECG,* electrocardiogram; *EF,* ejection fraction; *HR,* heart rate; *IV,* intravenous(ly); *LAD,* left anterior descending; *LVSWI,* left ventricular stroke work index; *MI,* myocardial infarction; *MRI,* magnetic resonance imaging; *NTG,* nitroglycerin; *NTP,* nitroprusside; *PAOP,* pulmonary artery occlusive pressure; *PAP,* pulmonary artery presssure; *PCI,* percutaneous coronary intervention; *PVR,* pulmonary vascular resistance; *RAP,* right atrial pressure; *RCA,* right coronary artery; *RR,* respiratory rate; *RVSWI,* right ventricular stroke work index; Sao_2, arterial oxygen saturation; Svo_2, venous oxygen saturation; *SVR,* systemic vascular resistance; *T,* temperature.

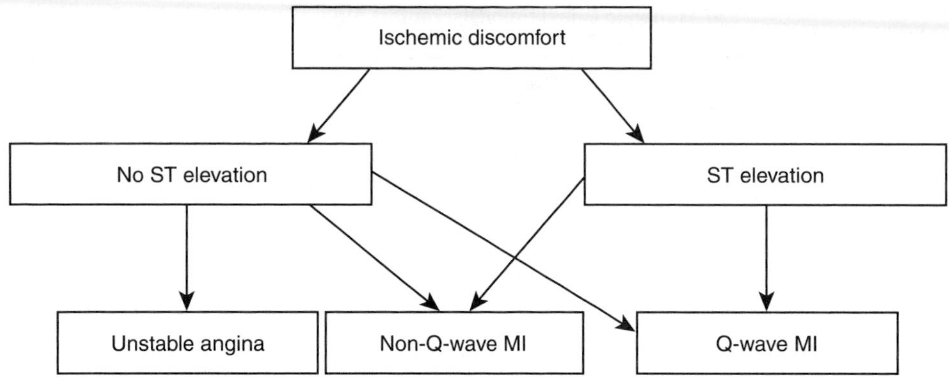

Figure 3-17 ECG decision pathway for acute coronary syndromes. *MI*, Myocardial infarction. (Ryan, T. J., Antman, E. M., Brooks, N. H., Califf, R. M., Hillis, L. D., Hiratzka, L. F., et al. [1999]. 1999 Update: ACC/AHA guidelines for the management of patients with acute myocardial infarction. *Journal of American College of Cardiology, 34*[3], 890-911.)

Non–ST Segment Elevation

1. Prolonged rest chest pain (more than 20 minutes) within the previous 24 hours without sustained ST segment elevation greater than 1 mm
   a. Unstable angina: may have ST segment depression
   b. Non–ST segment elevation MI: positive creatine kinase (myocardial bound) (CK-MB) and/or troponin
2. Pathophysiology: partial occlusion of a coronary artery with a platelet-rich thrombus
3. Goal is to prevent progression to complete occlusion of the coronary artery and resultant ST segment elevation MI
4. Collaborative management
   a. Close monitoring for progression
   b. Platelet aggregation inhibitors (e.g., aspirin and GP IIb/IIIa inhibitors) and anticoagulants (low molecular-weight heparin [e.g., enoxaparin] may be used)
   c. Beta-blocker
   d. Nitrate
   e. PCI

ST Segment Elevation

1. Prolonged rest chest pain (more than 20 minutes) within the previous 24 hours with ST segment elevation (greater than or equal to 1 mm)
   a. Non–Q wave MI: does not develop pathologic Q waves
   b. Q wave MI: does eventually (within 12 to 24 hours) develop pathologic Q waves
2. Pathophysiology: complete occlusion of a coronary artery by a thrombus
3. Goal: restore blood flow
4. Collaborative management
   a. Aspirin and beta-blocker
   b. Reperfusion therapy (e.g., acute PCI and/or fibrinolytic therapy); followed by therapies to maintain patency (e.g., aspirin, GP IIb/IIIa inhibitor, and anticoagulants)
   c. Nitrate
   d. Angiotensin-converting enzyme (ACE) inhibitor

Acute Coronary Syndromes Algorithm
(Figure 3-18)

Myocardial Infarction

Definition

Death of a portion of the myocardium

Etiology of MI

1. Arteriosclerosis/atherosclerosis
2. Coronary artery thrombosis
3. Coronary artery spasm
4. Cocaine-induced: excessive sympathetic stimulation causes tachycardia, hypertension, arterial vasoconstriction, and spasm; coronary artery spasm may cause MI, especially non–Q wave infarction
5. Combination of these factors: most MI are caused by atherosclerosis and thrombosis
6. Other less commonly seen causes
   a. Severe prolonged hypotension
   b. Chest trauma (e.g., myocardial contusion)
   c. Trauma to coronary artery or arteries
   d. Aortic stenosis or insufficiency
   e. Thyrotoxicosis
   f. Blood dyscrasias
   g. Aortic dissection
   h. Arteritis
   i. Carbon monoxide poisoning

Pathophysiology

1. Atherosclerosis with unstable plaque
2. Plaque rupture may be caused by inflammation and/or infection
   a. C-reactive protein (CRP)
      (1) Biochemical by-product that rises rapidly following an inflammatory response

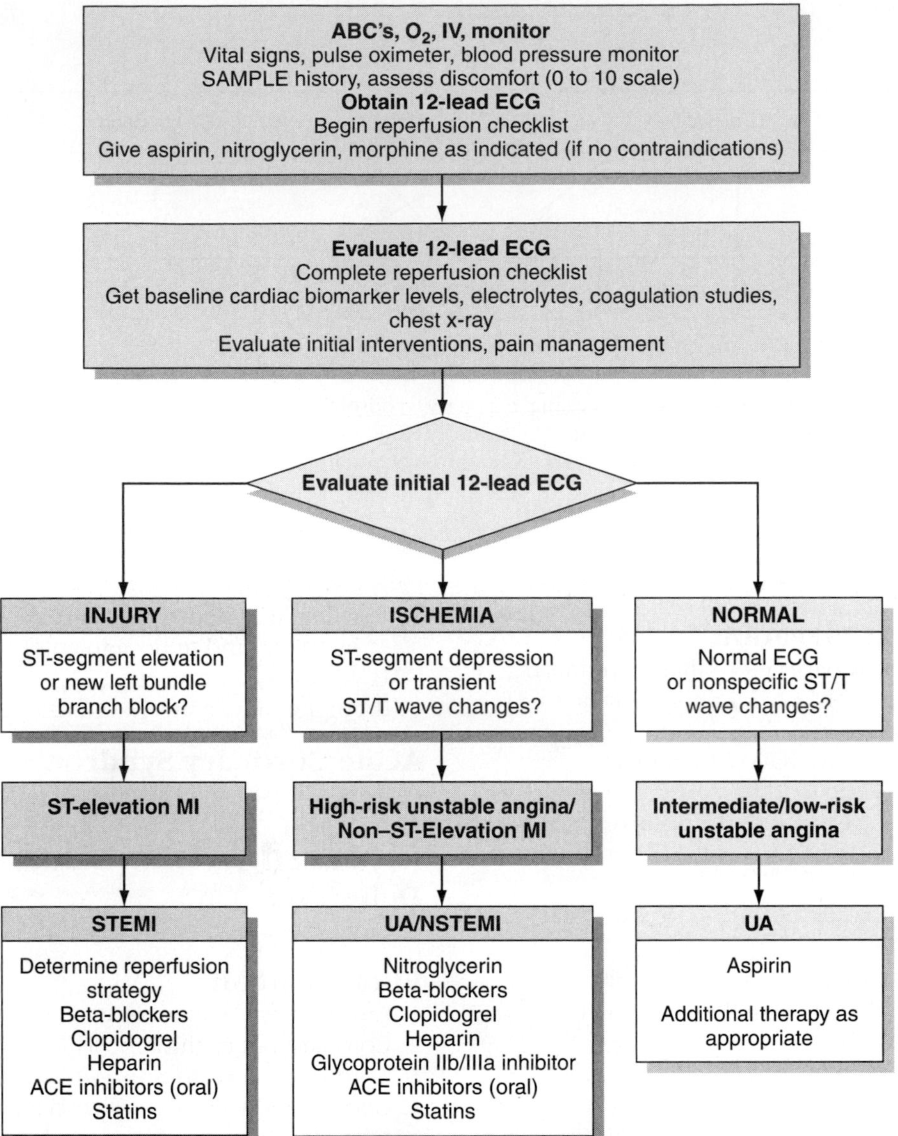

Figure 3-18 Ischemic Chest Pain/Discomfort Algorithm. (From Aehlert, B. [2007]: *ACLS Study Guide* [3rd ed.], St. Louis: Mosby.)

(2) Probably has a direct proinflammatory effect
(3) Stimulates release and expression of inflammatory mediators and has been found in atheromatous plaques

b. Interleukin-6 (IL-6)
(1) Cytokine and intercellular mediator
(2) Stimulates production of fibrinogen and CRP
(3) Stimulates the macrophages to produce platelet aggregation, tumor necrosis factor, and vascular smooth muscle proliferation

3. Platelet aggregation and blood coagulation
4. Coronary artery occlusion
5. Prolonged imbalance between myocardial oxygen supply and demand
6. Inadequate oxygenation causes anaerobic metabolism
7. Anaerobic metabolism causes lactic acidosis
8. Prolonged ischemic causes electrical and mechanical death of myocardium
   a. Electrical death causes Q waves on ECG.
   b. Mechanical death causes loss of contractility and poor wall motion on echocardiogram.
9. Contractility and compliance is decreased causing left ventricular dysfunction
   a. Decrease in contractility may cause S_3.
   b. Decrease in compliance causes S_4.
10. Ischemia, injury, and acidosis causes electrical irritability; this potentially leads to PVCs, VT, VF
11. Healing takes approximately 2 to 3 months; a firm, white scar is formed, but it does not contract or conduct electrical impulses

Classifications

1. Non–ST segment elevation MI versus ST segment elevation MI: ST segment indicates actual injury to the myocardium.
2. Q wave versus non–Q wave: Presence of Q wave correlates to mass loss of myocardium.
   a. Non–Q wave infarctions: partial occlusions or early reperfusion
      (1) Spontaneous reperfusion: cessation of spasm or endogenous tPA
      (2) Therapeutic reperfusion: fibrinolytic drugs or PCI
3. Left versus right ventricular: Table 3-12 describes wall of MI along with coronary artery affected, indicative ECG leads, and anticipated complications.
   a. Left ventricular myocardial infarction (LVMI): Most MI are LV.
      (1) Anterior LV: 42%
      (2) Septal LV: 10%
      (3) Lateral LV: 10%
      (4) Inferior LV: 33%
      (5) Posterior LV: 5%
   b. Right ventricular myocardial infarction (RVMI)
      (1) Concurrent with inferior LVMI; one third of all inferior MI have concurrent RV infarction
      (2) Rarely isolated: isolated RVMI more common in patients with right ventricular hypertrophy (e.g., COPD)
      (3) Smaller infarct caused by decreased oxygen requirements of right ventricle
      (4) Almost always transmural
4. Factors affecting mortality
   a. Age
   b. Left ventricular EF

Table 3-12 Myocardial Infarction Summary

Coronary Artery	Location of Infarct	Indicative ECG Leads	Anticipated Complications

Left main coronary artery	Extensive anterior	V_1-V_6	• Sudden cardiac death
			• Dysrhythmias, especially the following:
			  ○ Sinus tachycardia
			  ○ Atrial dysrhythmias
			  ○ Ventricular dysrhythmias
			• Blocks
			  ○ First-degree AV block
			  ○ Second-degree AV block, Mobitz type II
			  ○ Third-degree AV block with ventricular escape
			  ○ BBB
			• Ventricular rupture
			• Ventricular septal defect
			• Ventricular aneurysm
			• HF
			• Cardiogenic shock

Left anterior descending artery	Septal	V_1, V_2	• Dysrhythmias, especially:
			  ○ Sinus tachycardia
			  ○ AF
			  ○ Ventricular dysrhythmias
			• Blocks
			  ○ First-degree AV block
			  ○ Second-degree AV block, Mobitz type II
			  ○ Third-degree AV block with ventricular escape
			  ○ BBB
			• Ventricular septal rupture

	Anterior	V_3, V_4	• Dysrhythmias, especially:
			  ○ Sinus tachycardia
			  ○ AF
			  ○ Ventricular dysrhythmias
			• Blocks
			  ○ First-degree AV block
			  ○ Second-degree AV block, Mobitz type II
			  ○ Third-degree AV block with ventricular escape
			  ○ BBB
			• Ventricular aneurysm
			• HF
			• Cardiogenic shock

Left circumflex artery	Lateral	High: I, aVL Low: V_5, V_6	• Dysrhythmias • HF

Continued

Table 3-12 Myocardial Infarction Summary—cont'd

Coronary Artery	Location of Infarct	Indicative ECG Leads	Anticipated Complications
Right coronary artery	Inferior	II, III, aVF	• Dysrhythmias, especially: ◦ Sinus bradycardia ◦ Sinus arrest ◦ Junctional rhythms ◦ Ventricular dysrhythmias • Blocks ◦ Sinoatrial blocks ◦ First-degree AV block ◦ Second-degree AV block, Mobitz type I ◦ Third-degree AV block usually with AV junctional escape ◦ BBB • Papillary muscle rupture • HF
	Posterior	Reciprocal changes in V_1 and V_2 indicative of changes in V_7-V_9 (especially V_8 and V_9)	• Dysrhythmias, especially: ◦ Sinus bradycardia ◦ Sinus arrest ◦ Junctional rhythms ◦ Ventricular dysrhythmias • Blocks ◦ First-degree AV block ◦ Second-degree AV block, Mobitz type I ◦ Third-degree AV block usually with AV junctional escape • Papillary muscle rupture with acute mitral regurgitation
	Right ventricular	V_4r-V_6r (especially V_4r)	• Dysrhythmias, especially: ◦ Sinus bradycardia ◦ Sinus arrest ◦ Junctional rhythms ◦ Ventricular dysrhythmias • Blocks ◦ First-degree AV block ◦ Second-degree AV block, Mobitz type I ◦ Third-degree AV block usually with AV junctional escape ◦ BBB • Papillary muscle rupture with acute tricuspid regurgitation • RVF

AV, Atriovenous; *BBB,* bundle branch block; *ECG,* electrocardiogram; *HF,* heart failure; *RVF,* right ventricular failure.

c. Number of occluded vessels
d. Previous history of MI
e. Presence of cardiogenic shock: associated with loss of 40% of LV muscle mass; may be from one MI or several cumulative MIs
f. NOTE: Females have twice the mortality of males; this probably is related to the fact that they tend to be older and have more significant risk factors (e.g., DM or hypertension) when they develop their MI.

Clinical Presentation

1. Subjective
   a. Pain: 75% to 85% of all patients with MI have pain
      (1) Provocation: emotional or physical stress; may occur at rest
      (2) Palliation: not relieved by oxygen, rest, and/or nitrates; relieved by narcotics and/or reperfusion (e.g., fibrinolytic drugs or PCI)
      (3) Quality
         (a) Frequently prescribed as pressure on the chest
         (b) Also may be described as knifelike, stabbing, burning, or indigestion
         (c) May feel like their usual anginal pain, but more severe
         (d) Atypical pain common in women
         (e) If described as tearing or ripping, consider dissecting aortic aneurysm
      (4) Region/radiation
         (a) Primary location is usually chest but may be epigastric (especially with inferior MI).

(b) Radiation is usually to the left arm, left elbow, left shoulder, both arms, or jaw.
(c) If pain is radiating to back, consider dissecting aortic aneurysm.
(5) Severity: from vague, slight discomfort to severe pain; more intense than the patient's typical anginal pain
(6) Timing
(a) Most MIs occur within 3 hours of awakening.
(b) The pain is continuous from onset with a duration of 20 minutes or more.
(c) Pain that comes and goes for as long as several days before the actual MI is referred to as a *stuttering MI* pattern; intermittent pain before continuous pain is preinfarction angina.
b. Silent MI: as many as 25% of all patients with MI have no pain
(1) More likely in the elderly or diabetic patient
(2) Clues suggesting possible silent MI: new onset heart failure or acute change in mental status, unexplained abdominal pain, unexplained dyspnea or fatigue
c. Associated symptoms
(1) Nausea and vomiting: seen more often in inferior or posterior MI
(2) Dyspnea or orthopnea: seen more often in anterior MI
(3) Diaphoresis
(4) Palpitations
(5) Apprehension
2. Objective
a. Heart rate and rhythm
(1) Tachycardia: seen more often in anterior MI
(2) Bradycardia: seen more often in inferior MI
b. Normotension, hypotension, hypertension
(1) Hypertension: seen more often in anterior MI
(2) Hypotension: seen more often in inferior MI
(3) Equality in arms: inequality in arms indicates possible dissecting thoracic aortic aneurysm
c. Tachypnea
d. Elevated temperature: may occur 48 to 72 hours after MI
e. Levine's sign: clenched fist held over sternum
f. May have jugular venous distention (JVD): indicative of right ventricular failure (RVF); commonly seen in RV infarction
g. May have abnormal point of maximal impulse (PMI): downward and lateral displacement
h. Heart sound changes
(1) May have diminished heart sounds: related to decreased contractility
(2) May have S_4: indicative of left ventricular noncompliance; common for first 24 hours
(3) May have S_3: early sign of LVF
(4) May have pericardial friction rub: indicative of pericarditis
(5) May have systolic murmur of mitral regurgitation (high-pitched, blowing, holosystolic murmur loudest at apex that radiates to the axilla); may indicate LVF or papillary muscle dysfunction or rupture
(6) May have murmur of ventricular septal rupture (high-pitched, harsh, holosystolic murmur loudest at lower left sternal border)
i. May have carotid, aortic, or femoral bruits
j. May have clinical indications of hypoperfusion (see Table 2-2)
k. May have clinical indications of HF
(1) LVF (e.g., S_3, crackles, and dyspnea) in left ventricular infarction
(2) RVF (e.g., JVD, hepatomegaly, and peripheral edema) in right ventricular infarction
3. Serum
a. Leukocyte count: increased (usually 12,000 to 15, 000 cells/mm^3) at 48 to 72 hours
b. Erythrocyte sedimentation rate (ESR): increased at 48 to 72 hours
c. CRP: increased in acute MI
d. IL-6: increased in acute MI; marker of increased mortality in acute MI
e. Diagnostic studies for cell injury (Table 3-13)
(1) Increased serum enzymes

Table 3-13 Laboratory Diagnostic Tests for Acute Myocardial Infarction

Test	Normal Values	Time to Rise (after Injury)	Peak (after Injury)	Return to Normal (after Injury)
CK	Men: 55-170 units/L Women: 30-135 units/L	4-6 hours	24 hours	3-4 days
CK-MB	0% of total CK	6-10 hours	12-24 hours	2-3 days
LDH	90-200 units/L	24-48 hours	72 hours	8-14 days
LDH_1	17% to 25% of total LDH	8-24 hours	72 hours	8-14 days
Myoglobin	Less than 85 ng/mL	1-4 hours	6-12 hours	1-2 days
Cardiac troponin I	Less than 1.5 ng/mL	4-6 hours	18 hours	1-2 weeks
Cardiac troponin T	Less than 0.1 ng/mL	3-4 hours	24 hours	2-3 weeks

CK, Creatine kinase; *CK-MB*, creatine kinase (myocardial bound); *LDH*, L-lactate dehydrogenase.

(a) Creatine kinase (CK): elevation (usually twice normal in MI) occurs 4 to 6 hours after MI, peaks 24 hours later, and returns to normal after about 3 days; early CK peak is an indication of successful reperfusion
(b) L-Lactate dehydrogenase (LDH): elevation occurs within 24 hours after MI, peaks at 72 hours, and returns to normal within 2 weeks; may be particularly valuable for evaluation of patients who delay seeking medical attention for 2 or more days

(2) Positive serum isoenzymes
(a) CK: positive CK-MB (greater than 4%) is indicative of MI; highly specific test for MI
(i) Electrophoresis technique: traditional CK-MB; not usually diagnostic for 8 to 24 hours after onset of pain
(ii) Immunoassay technique: more sensitive earlier (within 4 hours) than electrophoresis technique; sometimes referred to as a *stat MB*
(b) LDH: normally LDH_2 is greater than LDH_1; LDH_1 greater than LDH_2 (referred to as *flipped LDH*) is indicative of MI; does not occur until 48 to 72 hours after the onset of pain

(3) Increased serum muscle proteins
(a) Myoglobin: muscle protein; high sensitivity but low specificity; excellent early negative predictive value
(b) Troponin: contractile protein
(i) Cardiac troponin I: found only in cardiac muscle; more specific but later rise and peak
(ii) Cardiac troponin T: found in cardiac muscle and in skeletal muscle; less specific than I, especially in patients with renal failure but earlier rise and peak

4. ECG
a. As a diagnostic tool for acute MI: most helpful when clearly abnormal
(1) If initial ECG nondiagnostic, repeat ECG should be done every 30 minutes until pain cessation or the ECG is clearly diagnostic and definitive therapy can be initiated.
(2) The typical criteria for prompt reperfusion therapies (e.g., PCI and fibrinolytic drugs) in acute MI include either of the following:
(a) ST segment elevation of greater than 1 mm in at least two continuous leads
(b) New left bundle branch block (LBBB)
(3) Multiple problems arise with ECG diagnosis of MI
(a) Lag time of hours (or even days) may exist before diagnostic ECG changes become evident; first ECG is diagnostic only 50% of the time.
(b) Changes may be subtle.
(c) Previous ECG may not be available for comparison.
(d) Changes may be obscured by a competitive condition.
(i) LBBB or ventricular pacemaker obscures anterior MI.
(ii) WPW syndrome obscures anterior MI.
(iii) Left anterior hemiblock obscures interior MI.
(iv) Left posterior hemiblock obscures lateral MI.
(v) Ventricular hypertrophy may obscure anterior or lateral MI.
(e) Fifteen or 18 leads are used to prevent missing an infarction in a traditionally "electrically silent" area of the heart; sensitivity and inclusion for reperfusion therapy is increased through the use of right ventricular and posterior lead.
(i) 18-lead ECG: 12 standard leads, 3 right ventricular leads, 3 posterior leads
(ii) 15-lead ECG: 12 standard leads plus V_4r, V_8, and V_9

b. ECG indicators (see Electrocardiography in Chapter 2 and Figure 2-43)
c. Locations, indicative leads, coronary artery affected (see Electrocardiography in Chapter 2 and Table 2-12)
d. Determination of the age of the MI (see Electrocardiography in Chapter 2 and Table 2-13)

5. Echocardiography
a. Normal wall motion: strong predictor of nonischemic pain
b. Reduced wall motion: strong predictor of acute occlusion
c. May show mechanical complications (e.g., ventricular septal defect and papillary muscle rupture)
6. Chest x-ray: may show cardiomegaly and indications of HF
7. Cardiac catheterization: likely will show coronary artery occlusion; PCI may be performed after diagnosis
8. Radionuclide studies
a. Technetium-99 pyrophosphate scan: infarcted areas show up as "hot spots"
b. Thallium-201 scan: ischemic or infarcted areas show up as "cold spots"

Nursing Diagnoses (see Appendix A)

1. Chest Pain related to coronary artery occlusion and resultant myocardial ischemia, infarction
2. Ineffective Cardiopulmonary Tissue Perfusion related to coronary artery occlusion
3. Risk for Decreased Cardiac Output related to alterations in contractility, dysrhythmias, rupture of cardiac structure (e.g., papillary muscle rupture and ventricular septal rupture)
4. Risk for Activity Intolerance related to decreased cardiac output and decrease in tissue oxygen delivery

5. Sleep Deprivation related to pain, dyspnea, noise, and interruptions related to care
6. Interrupted Family Processes related to change in health status and potential life-threatening situation
7. Anxiety related to acute health alteration and recommended lifestyle changes
8. Deficient Knowledge related to unfamiliarity with disease process, therapy, and recommended lifestyle changes

Collaborative Management

1. Manage cardiopulmonary arrest if needed.
   a. VF frequently occurs within 1 hour: early identification of clinical indications of MI and hospitalization is important.
   b. Manage airway, oxygenation, circulation using BCLS and ACLS.
2. Monitor ECG, vital signs, physical examination, and hemodynamic parameters for changes.
   a. Safely and accurately monitor the patient's hemodynamic parameters as indicated; indications for hemodynamic monitoring in acute MI include the following:
      (1) Persistent chest pain
      (2) Persistent tachycardia
      (3) Significant hypertension or hypotension
      (4) Significant LVF or RVF
      (5) IV inotropic or vasoactive agents
      (6) New systolic murmur
   b. Use hemodynamic parameters in evaluating clinical status for changes and responses to prescribed therapies.
3. Reduce size of MI: myocardial salvaging techniques.
   a. Treat pain promptly and adequately: decreases catecholamine release and myocardial oxygen demand.
      (1) Morphine sulfate: 2 to 4 mg IV every 5 minutes until pain relief
         (a) Actions: decreases preload; decreases catecholamine release via pain relief (which decreases heart rate and afterload); decreases anxiety and restlessness
         (b) Cautions: inferior MI; RVMI
      (2) Nitroglycerin: may be given prophylactically at 25 to 100 mcg/min IV for 24 to 48 hours
         (a) Actions
            (i) Decreases preload to decrease myocardial oxygen demand
            (ii) Dilates epicardial coronary vessels to increase myocardial oxygen supply
            (iii) Augments the analgesic effect of morphine
         (b) Caution: may cause reflex tachycardia; beta-blockers may be needed
      (3) Reperfusion therapies (e.g., fibrinolytic drugs and PCI): relieve pain by reestablishing blood flow and aerobic metabolism
      (4) IABP: may be used for intractable pain because it increases CAPP (Figures 3-19 and 3-20 and Table 3-14)
   b. Increase myocardial oxygen supply
      (1) Administer oxygen at 2 to 6 L/min per nasal cannula for 24 to 48 hours.
         (a) Oxygen probably has little effect on the myocardial arterial oxygen content of otherwise normal individuals but may improve significantly the oxygenation of an ischemic myocardium, especially in patients with hypoxemia from pulmonary edema.
         (b) Even in the absence of pulmonary edema or other complications, it seems that some patients do develop modest hypoxemia early during the course of acute MI.
      (2) Provide emergent PCI or fibrinolytic drugs to reestablish patency of the infarct-related artery (IRA) within the benchmark time frame.
         (a) PCI is preferred (especially in elderly patients) if a cardiac catheterization laboratory is available to provide opening of the IRA within 60 to 90 minutes (door, data, diagnosis, balloon); if not, fibrinolytic drugs are used and should be administered within 30 minutes (door, data, diagnosis, drug) (Table 3-15).
            (i) Assist in prompt preparation of the patient for emergent PCI if fibrinolytic drugs are contraindicated or unsuccessful.
         (b) These procedures may be preceded and/or followed by platelet aggregation inhibitor and/or anticoagulants.

Text continued on p. 160

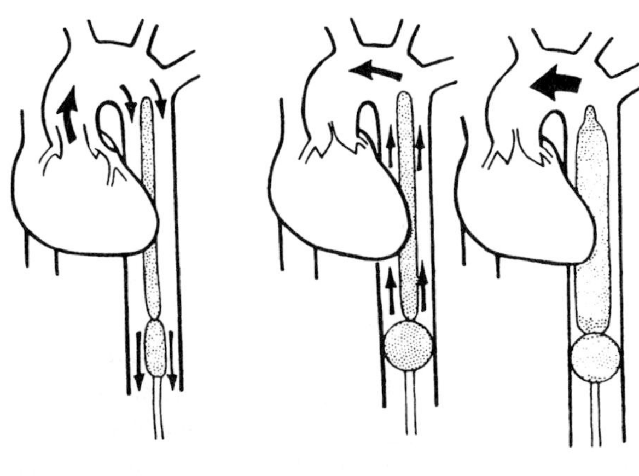

Figure 3-19 Mechanics of the intraaortic balloon pump. The balloon is deflated immediately before systole and remains deflated during systole; the balloon is inflated at the beginning of diastole and remains inflated until immediately before the next systole. (From Kinney, M. R., Packa, D. R., & Dunbar, S. B. *AACN'S clinical reference for critical-care nursing* [3rd ed.]. St. Louis: Mosby.)

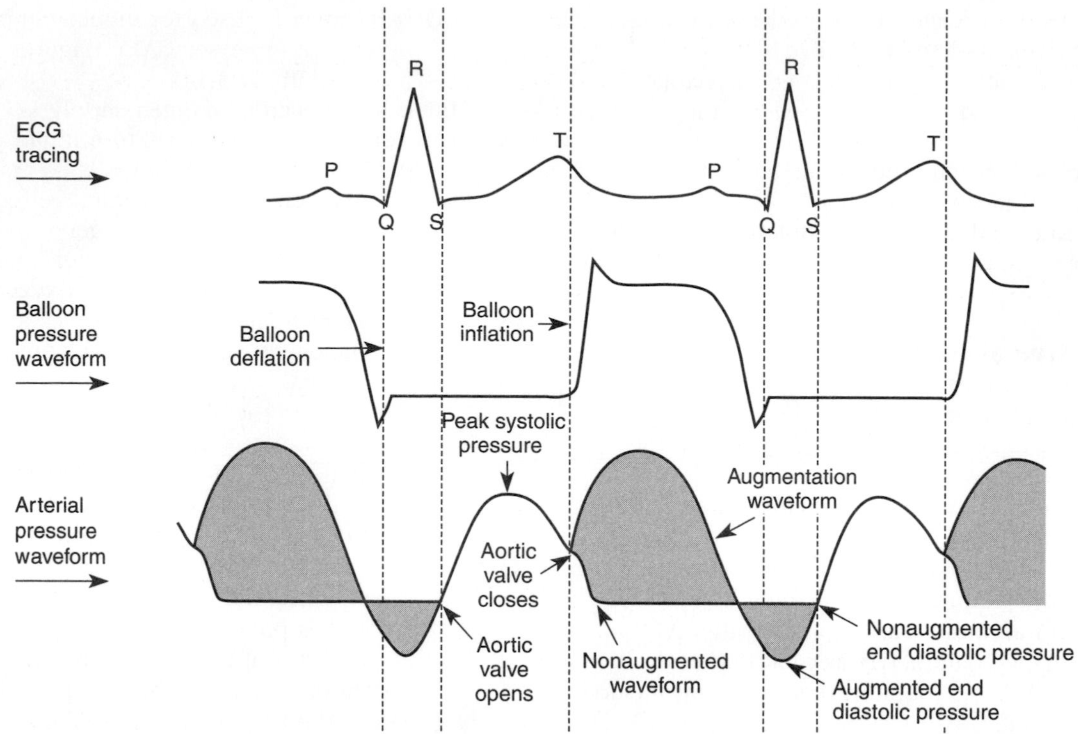

Figure 3-20 Inflation and deflation of the intraaortic balloon (*center*) timed with ECG waveform (*top*) or arterial pressure waveform (*bottom*). (From Holloway, N. M. [1988]. *Nursing care of the critically ill adult* [3rd ed.]. Boston: Addison-Wesley.)

Table 3-14 Intraaortic Balloon Pump

Indications	• Unstable angina refractory to medical therapy • Cardiogenic shock or severe LVF • HF, as a bridge to left VAD or transplant • Mechanical complications of acute MI (e.g., ruptured papillary muscle with acute mitral regurgitation or acute ventricular septal rupture) • High-risk patient undergoing CPI • Preoperative, perioperative, and/or postoperative support before CABG or other major surgery • Difficulty weaning from cardiopulmonary bypass
Contraindications	• Aortic valve regurgitation • Aortic aneurysm • Aortic dissection • Severe bilateral peripheral vascular disease (e.g., absent femoral pulse); if patient has had bilateral femoropopliteal bypass grafts, the balloon may be placed via the left axillary artery into the ascending aorta • Coagulopathy • Not recommended for patients with chronic end-stage heart disease who are not awaiting a cardiac transplant • Not recommended for patients with irreversible brain damage or terminal condition
Actions (Figure 3-19)	• Balloon is inflated during diastole to increase myocardial oxygen supply. ◦ Increases coronary artery blood flow by displacing blood retrograde toward the aortic arch and increasing diastolic BP ◦ Increases blood flow to the renal arteries and lower extremities by displaces blood antegrade toward the renal and lower extremities arteries ◦ Increases MAP to improve tissue perfusion • Balloon is deflated immediately before systole to decrease myocardial oxygen demand. ◦ Decreases left ventricular afterload by decreasing systolic BP

Table 3-14 Intraaortic Balloon Pump—cont'd

Insertion and mechanics	• Catheter with 40-mL balloon is inserted via femoral artery (NOTE: The catheter may be inserted via iliac, subclavian, or axillary artery if the femoral artery is not an option).
	• Balloon is positioned in descending thoracic aorta between left subclavian and renal arteries.
	  ○ The tip of the catheter should be at the second to third ICS just distal to the left subclavian artery by chest x-ray film.
	  ○ The balloon occludes 80% of the aortic diameter when inflated.
	• Helium to inflate the balloon is shuttled into and out of the balloon by a pump that is housed in a console at the bedside.

Timing (Figure 3-20)	• By ECG
	  ○ Inflated after the T wave
	  ○ Deflated before QRS complex
	• By arterial waveform (NOTE: New IABP catheters have fiberoptic pressure sensors in the tip that provide real-time pressure signals because the signal travels at the speed of light rather than assuming a delay with fluid-filled transducer systems.)
	  ○ Inflated at the dicrotic notch
	  ○ Deflated at the end-diastolic dip immediately before systole
	• Inflation and deflation usually are triggered by ECG, but fine timing is done by the nurse using the arterial waveform

Assessment	• HR: a normalization of heart rate is desirable. • BP: a decrease in systolic BP, an increase in diastolic BP, and an increase in MAP is desirable. • CO/CI: an increase in cardiac output/cardiac index is desirable. • PAP/PAOP: a decrease in PAP and PAOP is desirable. ○ A decrease in the amplitude of *v* wave on the PAOP waveform is desirable in patients with mitral regurgitation or ventricular septal rupture. • Sao_2: an increase in arterial Sao_2 is desirable. • Svo_2: an increase in venous Svo_2 is desirable. • Urine output: an increase in urine output is desirable. • Complaints of chest pain: an decrease in chest pain is desirable. • ECG: a decrease in the presence or frequency of dysrhythmias is desirable. • Neurovascular status of affected limb: the presence of palpable pulses and a warm limb with normal capillary refill is desirable.
Nursing diagnoses	• Decreased Cardiac Output related to balloon or pump malfunction, timing errors, catheter kink, leak, or rupture • Risk for Ineffective Peripheral Tissue Perfusion related to presence of femoral artery catheter, catheter malposition, thrombosis or embolus, or arterial spasm • Risk for Injury related to anticoagulation and invasive procedures • Impaired Physical Mobility related to bedrest, extremity restriction • Risk for Infection related to invasive catheters, devices • Anxiety related to insertion of IABP, critical illness, and critical care environment
Brief summary of nursing management	• Assess the parameters described before. • Ensure optimal timing of balloon inflation and deflation. • Titrate pharmacologic therapies to augment the mechanical therapy of the IABP. • Ensure positioning of the patient with head of bed elevation less than 30 degrees and avoidance of hip flexion. • Observe for complications, and provide appropriate management for the prevention of complications.

Complications: prevention and treatment	• Thrombosis causing lower extremity ischemia
	  ○ Insertion precautions
	  — Use the smallest sheath that will allow the catheter to be advanced through it.
	  — Select the limb with the best pulse.
	  ○ Dextran 40 as prescribed as a platelet aggregation inhibitor
	  ○ Restraint of affected leg to prevent displacement of the balloon and trauma to intima of artery
	  ○ Neurovascular assessment of the affected limb every hour
	  ○ If limb ischemia is noted, treatment may include any of the following:
	  — Removal of catheter with placement of the sheath and catheter in the other femoral artery if the IABP is still needed
	  — Catheter thrombectomy
	  — Femorofemoral graft
	  — Lidocaine or papaverine: to decrease arterial spasm

Continued

Table 3-14 Intraaortic Balloon Pump—cont'd

	• Catheter displacement causing renal or left upper extremity ischemia ◦ Elevation of head of bed no more than 20 to 30 degrees to prevent displacement of the balloon ◦ Restraint of affected limb to prevent displacement of the balloon ◦ Close monitoring of urine output ◦ Notification of physician of significant changes in urine output ◦ Neurovascular assessment of left arm every hour • Emboli ◦ Dextran 40 as prescribed as an antiplatelet aggregation agent ◦ Heparin may be prescribed ◦ Avoidance of allowing the balloon to remain static (noninflating) for more than 30 minutes; clots may form in the folds of the balloon and be embolized when the balloon then is reinflated • Infection ◦ Sterile dressing changes daily or every other day ◦ Close monitoring of the site for erythema, edema, induration, and warmth • Aortic dissection ◦ Attention to complaints of back pain and vital sign changes ◦ Removal of catheter and repair of aorta if dissection occurs • Anemia ◦ Attention to presence of petechiae or ecchymosis and platelet counts ◦ Discontinuance of heparin ◦ Blood and/or blood products may be prescribed • Balloon complications ◦ Leak — Attention to increase in volume or frequency of refilling — Replacement of catheter if leak occurs to prevent gas embolism ◦ Rupture — Attention to blood in catheter — Replacement of catheter if rupture occurs to prevent entrapment • Timing complications ◦ Inflation is too early: aortic valve closes too early, and stroke volume is decreased ◦ Inflation is too late: diastolic augmentation is decreased ◦ Deflation is too early: less increase in CAPP and less of a decrease in afterload ◦ Deflation is too late: increase in afterload • Inadequate pumping: usually caused by dysrhythmias ◦ Timing method changed from ECG to arterial line
Weaning	• Indications ◦ Cardiac index greater than 2 L/min ◦ PAOP less than 18 mm Hg ◦ MAP greater than 70 mm Hg ◦ SVR less than 1400 dynes/sec/cm^{-5} ◦ Absence of anginal pain ◦ Absence of clinical indicator of hypoperfusion • Methods ◦ May be done by decreasing the frequency (e.g., from every cardiac cycle to every other cardiac cycle to every third cardiac cycle) ◦ May be done by decreasing the volume in the balloon with each inflation (e.g., decreased by 25% with each weaning step)
Balloon removal	• Gown, mask, and eye protection must be used. • Pump is turned off, sutures are removed, and catheter is removed and inspected to ensure that the entire catheter has been removed. • Apply firm pressure to the insertion site for at least 15 minutes, but pressure may be required for more than 30 minutes if the patient has been receiving anticoagulants; a vascular hemostasis device may be used. • Monitor site frequently for the next 4 to 8 hours for bleeding or hematoma formation.

BP, Blood pressure; *CABG,* coronary artery bypass graft; *CAPP,* coronary artery perfusion pressure; *CPI,* coronary percutaneous intervention; *ECG,* electrocardiogram; *HF,* heart failure; *IABP,* intraaortic balloon pump; *ICS,* intercostal space; *MAP,* mean arterial pressure; *PAP,* pulmonary artery pressure; *PAOP,* pulmonary artery occlusive pressure; Sao_2, oxygen saturation; Svo_2, venous oxygen saturation; *VAD,* ventricular assist devices; *SVR,* systemic vascular resistance.

Table 3-15 Fibrinolytic Therapy

Actions	• Activate plasminogen to plasmin, the active agent that breaks down clots (speeds up the normal fibrinolytic process to allow early reperfusion).
	• Limit cellular necrosis and decrease infarction size.
	• Decrease mortality and morbidity.
	  ○ Short-term: reestablishing arterial patency
	  ○ Long-term: maintaining EF

Fibrinolytic agents	• Streptokinase (rarely used today)
	• rt-PA
	  ○ Alteplase (Activase): short-half life so administered as a bolus followed by infusion
	  ○ TNKase: longest half-life so administered as a one-time bolus
	• r-PA
	  ○ Reteplase (Retavase): intermediate half-life so administered as two boluses 10 minutes apart
	• Urokinase (rarely used in acute MI but frequently used in peripheral arterial occlusion)

Indications	• History strongly suggestive of MI • ST segment elevation of more than 1 mm in at least two contiguous leads or new LBBB • Pain of less than 6 hours or still having pain (NOTE: As long as the patient is having pain, salvageable myocardium is assumed because dead myocardium does not metabolize aerobically or anaerobically, producing neither lactic acid nor pain.)
Absolute contraindications	• Active internal bleeding • History of hemorrhagic stroke, intracranial neoplasm, AV malformation, or aneurysm • Intracranial or intraspinal surgery or trauma within 2 months • Known bleeding disorder (e.g., thrombocytopenia or hemophilia) • Suspected aortic aneurysm or acute pericarditis • Systolic BP greater than or equal to 200 mm Hg and/or diastolic BP greater than or equal to 120 mm Hg • Prolonged (more than 10 minutes) or traumatic CPR • Pregnancy • Streptokinase is contraindicated if the patient has received streptokinase or had a streptococcal infection within the last 6 to 9 months, but tPA still can be used
Relative contraindications	• Major surgery or trauma within 10 days • Recent gastrointestinal or genitourinary bleeding • Cerebrovascular disease • Oral anticoagulant therapy • Systolic BP greater than or equal to 180 mm Hg and/or diastolic BP greater than or equal to 110 mm Hg • Significant liver dysfunction • Septic thrombophlebitis • Subacute bacterial endocarditis • High likelihood of thrombus of left side of the heart (e.g., mitral stenosis with AF, ventricular aneurysm, or left atrial myxoma) • Diabetic hemorrhagic retinopathy • Advanced age (older than 70-75 years) with consideration of physiologic age, severity of concomitant diseases, and mental status • Any condition when bleeding would be a significant hazard or would be difficult to manage (e.g., recent femoral artery puncture or sheath)

Clinical indications of reperfusion	• Pain cessation
	• ST segment return to baseline
	• Reperfusion dysrhythmias
	  ○ Sinus bradycardia
	  ○ Idioventricular rhythm, accelerated idioventricular rhythm
	  ○ AV blocks
	  ○ Ventricular irritability: premature ventricular contractions, VT, VF
	• CK washout: early or markedly elevated creatine kinase peak

Assessment	• Heart rate • BP • ECG rhythm; note reperfusion dysrhythmias • Clinical indications of reperfusion • Bleeding (e.g., puncture points, gums, saliva, sputum, gastric secretions, stools, and urine) • Complaints of chest pain, back pain, or headache

Continued

Table 3-15 Fibrinolytic Therapy—cont'd

Nursing diagnoses	• Altered Protection related dissolution of stable protective clots by thrombolytics and delay in coagulation caused by heparin therapy • Risk for Decreased Cardiac Output related to reperfusion dysrhythmias • Risk for Alteration in Cardiac Tissue Perfusion related to reocclusion • Knowledge Deficit related to unfamiliarity with disease process, therapy, and recommended lifestyle changes

Brief summary of nursing management	• Administer adjuvant therapy: tPA is followed by aspirin, heparin (SK causes significant fibrinogen depletion, and heparin is not indicated because of increased bleeding risk).
	• Monitor for clinical indications of reperfusion; notify physician if these are not seen so that emergent PCI can be scheduled.
	• Avoid punctures: arterial; IV, intramuscular, subcutaneous.
	  ◦ Apply pressure until hemostasis achieved if punctures are required after thrombolytics initiated.
	  ◦ Insert multiple (usually two to three) IV catheters before initiation of thrombolytic therapy; one of these catheters may be used for venous sampling.
	• Monitor stools, urine, emesis, sputum, and saliva for blood.
	• Monitor for complications.

Complications	• Hemorrhage
	  ◦ At site of vascular puncture: 80% incidence
	  ◦ GI or GU bleeding: 15%-20% incidence
	  ◦ Intracranial bleed: 1% incidence
	• Reocclusion: Monitor for new pain and/or ST segment changes.
	• Allergic reactions to streptokinase
	  ◦ Monitor for urticaria, fever, bronchospasm, dyspnea, stridor, or dysrhythmias.
	  ◦ Administer diphenhydramine (Benadryl) and/or hydrocortisone (Solu-Cortef) as prescribed in attempt to prevent allergic reaction.
	• Reperfusion dysrhythmias: usually transient
	  ◦ Administer antidysrhythmic drugs or perform cardioversion or defibrillation as indicated for sustained VT or VF (prophylactic antidysrhythmic drugs are no longer recommended with fibrinolytic therapy).
	  ◦ Administer atropine or apply transcutaneous pacemaker for symptomatic bradycardia or block.

AV, Atrioventricular; *BP,* blood pressure; *CK,* Creatine kinase; *CPR,* cardiopulmonary resuscitation; *ECG,* electrocardiogram; *EF,* ejection fraction; *GI,* gastrointestinal; *GU,* genitourinary; *IV,* intravenous; *LBBB,* left bundle branch block; *MI,* myocardial infarction; *PCI,* percutaneous coronary intervention; *r-PA,* recombinant plasminogen activator; *rt-PA,* recombinant tissue plasminogen activator; *SK,* streptokinase; *TNKase,* tenecteplase; *tPA,* tissue plasminogena activator; *VF,* ventricular fibrillation; *VT,* ventricular tachycardia.

(c) Either primary PCI or fibrinolytic drugs are preceded by platelet aggregation inhibitors and/or anticoagulants.
  (i) Platelet aggregation inhibitors
    a) Aspirin (160 to 325 mg initially and daily) and/or another antiplatelet drug (e.g., clopidogrel [Plavix]) to decrease platelet aggregation and clot extension
    b) GP IIb/IIIa platelet receptor blockers (e.g., abciximab [ReoPro], eptifibatide [Integrilin], and tirofiban [Aggrastat])
  (ii) Anticoagulants
    a) Unfractionated heparin may be prescribed for 24 to 48 hours to maintain activated partial thromboplastin time (aPTT) of 45 to 60 seconds.
      i) Indirect thrombin inhibitor
      ii) Initial dosing should be weight-based; then infusion is adjusted by aPPT results.
      iii) Usual dose of unfractionated heparin: bolus of 60 units/kg and then infusion of 12 units/kg/hr
    b) Low-molecular-weight heparin, subcutaneous
      i) Indirect thrombin inhibitor
      ii) Lower incidence of heparin-associated thrombocytopenia and thrombosis (HATT) than with unfractionated heparin
    c) Bivalirudin (Angiomax)
      i) Direct thrombin inhibitor
      ii) Most frequently used after PCI
    d) Warfarin usually is prescribed for at least 3 months in patients with any of the following:
      i) Anterior Q wave MI
      ii) HF
      iii) Severe left ventricular dysfunction
      iv) AF
      v) Previous embolic event
(3) Treat anemia if present: Maintain hemoglobin concentration greater than 12 g/dL if possible.
(4) Maintain CAPP.
  (a) Use caution in administration of NTG and other vasoactive agents because they may decrease CAPP by decreasing the aortic root pressure.

(b) NTP is contraindicated during ischemic pain because it may cause coronary artery steal and decrease CAPP.

(5) Control dysrhythmias.
  (a) Tachydysrhythmias decrease the time for coronary artery filling and may decrease cardiac output.
  (b) Bradydysrhythmias increase the time for coronary artery filling but may decrease cardiac output.

(6) Administer calcium channel blockers or NTG for coronary artery spasm.
  (a) Especially important in cocaine-induced MI

(7) Use IABP as prescribed (Table 3-14)

c. Decrease myocardial oxygen consumption

(1) Administer beta-blockers as prescribed to decrease heart rate and contractility to decrease myocardial oxygen consumption.
  (a) Actions
    (i) Decrease incidence of dysrhythmias and increase VF threshold
    (ii) Block the effects of catecholamines (cardioprotection)
    (iii) Reduce infarct size and severity of HF
  (b) Agents: metoprolol (Lopressor) 5 mg IV every 2 minutes × 3 usually is given, but atenolol (Tenormin) or esmolol (Brevibloc) may be used.
  (c) Contraindications
    (i) Heart rate less than 50 beats/min
    (ii) Second or third-degree atrioventricular block
    (iii) Systolic BP less than 100 mm Hg
    (iv) HF
    (v) Bronchospasm
      a) No beta-blockers should be given to a patient with active bronchospasm.
      b) Cardioselective beta-blockers (e.g., metoprolol or esmolol) may be given to a patient with a history of bronchospastic lung disease (e.g., asthma), but noncardioselective beta-blockers (e.g., propranolol) should not be given.
    (vi) Cocaine-induced MI: Blocking beta receptors allows unopposed alpha receptors to increase vasoconstriction and vasospasm. NTG and/or calcium channel blocker (e.g., diltiazem [Cardizem]) are more likely to be prescribed along with a benzodiazepine (e.g., diazepam [Valium]) to reduce agitation and seizure potential.

(2) Administer angiotensin-converting enzyme inhibitors (e.g., captopril [Capoten] or enalapril [Vasotec]) or angiotensin-blockers (e.g., losartan [Cozaar] or valsartan [Diovan]) as prescribed to attenuate ventricular remodeling.
  (a) Action: Block the vasoconstriction and sodium and water retention associated with activation of the renin-angiotensin-aldosterone system.
  (b) Indications in acute MI: anterior or large inferior MI or evidence of HF
  (c) ACE inhibitors block the conversion of angiotensin I to angiotensin II; angiotensin-blockers block angiotensin II and do not block the breakdown of bradykinin, so are less likely to cause cough.
  (d) Caution: hypotension

(3) Administer vasodilators as prescribed.
  (a) Venous vasodilators (usually NTG) to decrease preload
  (b) Arterial vasodilators (usually NTP) to decrease afterload
  (c) Caution: hypotension; careful titration necessary to decrease myocardial oxygen consumption but to prevent hypoperfusion

(4) Provide physical and emotional rest.
  (a) Maintain bed rest for 24 hours, and then gradually increase activity as long as patient is hemodynamically stable; allow rest after meals, personal hygiene, toileting, and physical therapy.
  (b) Prevent Valsalva maneuver.
    (i) Teach patient to exhale when turning in bed.
    (ii) Administer stool softeners as prescribed.
    (iii) Provide bedside commode for elimination.
  (c) Explain procedures thoroughly: monitor alarms; equipment; visiting hours; reasons for procedures.
  (d) Keep family informed regarding patient's progress and status.
  (e) Provide for patient's comfort.
    (i) Provide prompt pain control: analgesics.
    (ii) Provide nausea control: antiemetics and mouth care.
    (iii) Provide for physical comfort: temperature control; lighting; noise control.
  (f) Instruct patient regarding relaxation techniques; encourage use of these techniques; use calming music, white noise, or nature sounds to aid in relaxation.
  (g) Provide appropriate nutrition: clear liquid to soft diet; usually low sodium.
    (i) Caffeine: Patient may have up to four to five caffeinated beverages every 24 hours as long as dysrhythmias do not occur.

(ii) Iced water: no restriction

(h) Administer anxiolytic drugs as prescribed: usually diazepam (Valium), lorazepam (Ativan), or alprazolam (Xanax).

(i) Note common emotional responses seen in acute MI, and treat appropriately (Table 3-16).

d. Use hypothermia as prescribed.

(1) Mild hypothermia (33° to 36° C) produces no serious adverse effects and has been shown to reduce infarct size in acute MI by enhancing myocardial microcirculation and protecting ischemic myocardial tissue.

(2) Use of IV meperidine (Demerol) and oral or nasogastric buspirone (BuSpar) is recommended to prevent shivering.

e. Use collaborative management specific to RV infarctions.

(1) Assess for clinical indications of RVMI, especially in the patient with acute inferior MI.

(a) ECG changes in V_4r, V_5r, and V_6r

(b) Increased right atrial pressure, decreased pulmonary artery occlusive pressure (PAOP)

(c) Decreased CO, CI, MAP and increased SVR

(d) Right-sided S_4

(e) Clinical indications of RVF: jugular venous distention (JVD), hepatojugular reflux, right-sided S_3, murmur of tricuspid insufficiency

(f) Minimal to absent pulmonary congestion

(2) Administer therapy specific to right ventricular infarction.

(a) Maintain adequate filling volumes.

(i) Measure RAP and PAOP; patients with significant right ventricular infarction usually require hemodynamic monitoring.

(ii) Administer volume: usually in the form of colloids (e.g., dextran, plasma

Table 3-16 Emotional Responses Seen in Acute Myocardial Infarction

Response	Indications	Collaborative Management
Anxiety	• Increased verbalization • Inability to concentrate • Restlessness, apprehension • Sleep disturbances • Tremors • Tachycardia, mild hypertension	• Be consistent in patient assignments. • Provide orientation to unit, procedures, and equipment. • Assess usual coping mechanisms. • Invite patient to ask questions. • Keep family informed about patient condition. • Encourage participation in rehabilitation program.
Denial	• Avoidance of discussion of heart attack • Discussions kept on a social, humorous level • Minimization of severity (e.g., "little heart attack") • Noncompliance with activity and diet restrictions; smoking • Overly cheerful demeanor • Repetition of same questions to different staff members	• Listen but do not reinforce denial. • Assess consequences of denial: denial decreases in-hospital mortality but increases incidence of sudden cardial death after discharge. • Assess the threat causing the need for denial. • Provide counseling if patient still in denial at time of discharge. • Encourage participation in rehabilitation program.
Depression	• Listlessness, disinterest • Expressions of hopelessness, pessimism • Abbreviated verbal responses (e.g., monosyllabic answers) • Slowness in movement and speech • Withdrawn behavior • Anorexia • Sad look, crying	• Voice your observations (e.g., "You look sad"). • Let the patient know that it is normal to feel this way. • Encourage verbalization of feelings. • Allow and encourage crying. • Encourage participation in rehabilitation program.
Anger	• Open opposition to treatment regimen • Expressions of disappointment or frustration • Passive-aggressive behavior • Sarcasm • Voices anger, screaming, cursing	• Acknowledge angry or hostile feelings. • Explore cause of anger. • Let patient know that these feelings are normal. • Let spouse and family know that anger is normal. • Be matter-of-fact about expressions of anger. • Encourage participation in rehabilitation program.
Aggressive sexual behavior	• Frequent seductive comments • Frequent initiation of sexually related conversion • Frequent boasts about past sexual interests and prowess • Flirtatious compliments • Attempts to hold, fondle, or kiss parts of nurse's body • Deliberate exposure of genitals	• Be honest and simply tell patient that this behavior makes you uncomfortable if it does. • Accept compliments with simple "thank you." • Arrange sexual counseling or patient and spouse. • Encourage participation in rehabilitation program.

protein fraction, or albumin). Administer fluids until PAOP is increased by more than 5 mm Hg, but PAOP and RAP should not exceed 20 mm Hg.
(iii) Avoid use of diuretics and/or venous vasodilators; if dilators are needed, use selective arterial dilators (e.g., hydralazine [Apresoline]) so that preload is not decreased.
(b) Maintain contractility: inotropes (e.g., dobutamine) are frequently needed.
f. Monitor for, prevent, and treat complications (Table 3-17).
g. Provide instruction and counseling regarding lifestyle modification and the need for pharmacologic therapy.
(1) Nonpharmacologic therapies
(a) Weight normalization
(b) Dietary modifications: low saturated fat, high fiber
(i) Low (2 to 3 g) sodium may be recommended
(ii) American Diabetic Association (ADA) diet for control of blood glucose for patient with DM
(c) Cessation of tobacco use
(d) Limitation of alcohol consumption to one to two alcoholic beverages daily
(e) Regular aerobic exercise in moderation
(f) Stress reduction: relaxation; imagery, biofeedback
(g) Differentiation between symptoms of angina and MI
(h) Changes in sexual activity that may be helpful
(2) Pharmacologic agents
(a) Prescribed medication regimen for secondary prevention of MI: aspirin, beta-blocker, ACE inhibitor (if indicated)
(b) Control of cardiac risk factors
(i) Antihypertensives for hypertension

Table 3-17 Complications of Myocardial Infarction

Complication	Clinical Indications	Prevention/Treatment
Dysrhythmias and conduction system defects	• Change in rhythm or conduction on rhythm strip or multiple lead ECG • Indications of hypoperfusion may be evident	• Close monitoring for changes in rhythm or conduction • Beta-blocker as a cardioprotective agent as prescribed • Magnesium, potassium, or calcium to correct electrolyte imbalance as prescribed ◦ Use of glucose-insulin-potassium may be prescribed; thought to deliver glucose to the ischemic myocardium • Antidysrhythmic agents as indicated and prescribed • Application of external pacemaker or insertion of transvenous pacemaker as indicated • Cardioversion or defibrillation as indicated
Heart failure	• Tachycardia, tachypnea • Clinical indications of LVF ◦ Dyspnea, orthopnea, cough ◦ S_3 ◦ Crackles in lung bases • Clinical indications of RVF ◦ Jugular venous distention ◦ Hepatomegaly, splenomegaly ◦ Peripheral edema • Chest x-ray shows pulmonary venous congestion, cardiomegaly • Increased RAP, PAP, and PAOP (PAOP usually greater than 20 mm Hg)	• Oxygen • Sodium and fluid restriction • ACE inhibitors (e.g., captopril and enalapril) • Beta-blockers (e.g., metoprolol or carvedilol) • Diuretics (e.g., furosemide or bumetanide) • Vasodilators (e.g., nitroglycerin) • Inotropic agents (e.g., dobutamine, milrinone, or digoxin)
Cardiogenic shock	• Tachycardia, tachypnea, hypotension • Clinical indications of LVF • Clinical indications of RVF • Clinical indications of hypoperfusion (see Table 2-2) • Urine output less than 0.5 mL/kg/hr • Cool to cold skin • Diminished to absent bowel sounds	• Oxygen • Sodium and fluid restrictions • ACE inhibitors (e.g., captopril and enalapril) • Inotropic agents (e.g., dobutamine) • Diuretics (e.g., furosemide or bumetanide) • Vasodilators (e.g., NTG or NGP) • IABP

Continued

Table 3-17 Complications of Myocardial Infarction—cont'd

Complication	Clinical Indications	Prevention/Treatment
	• Lethargy to confusion to coma • Chest x-ray shows pulmonary venous congestion and cardiomegaly • Decreased CO/CI (usually less than 2 L/min/m^2) • Increased PAOP (usually greater than 18 mm Hg) • Increased SVR (usually greater than 2000 dynes/sec/cm^{-5})	• Ventricular assist devices • Emergent revascularization: fibrinolytics, PCI, CABG
Papillary muscle dysfunction/rupture	• New holosystolic murmur loudest at apex • Clinical indications of LVF • Clinical indications of hypoperfusion • Increased PAP and PAOP • Large *v* waves on PAOP waveform • Echocardiography shows mitral regurgitation	• Vasodilators (e.g., NTP or NTG) • IABP • Surgical replacement of mitral valve with concurrent CABG
Ventricular septal rupture	• New holosystolic murmur loudest at lower left sternal border (LLSB) • Chest pain, dyspnea • Syncope • Increased PAP and PAOP • Increased SvO_2 • Increased CO/CI by thermodilution method of measurement (inaccurate) • Clinical evidence of hypoperfusion	• Vasodilators (e.g., NTP or NTG) • IABP • Surgical correction of ventricular septal defect with concurrent CABG
Cardiac rupture	• Clinical indications of hypoperfusion • Clinical indications of cardiac tamponade ○ Jugular venous distention ○ Muffled heart sounds ○ Hypotension ○ Increased RAP, PAP, PAOP with equalization within 5 mm Hg • Sinus tachycardia or PEA • Eventual cardiopulmonary arrest	• Pericardiocentesis. CPR; internal cardiac massage may be necessary • Surgical repair may be attempted (survival is rare)
Ventricular aneurysm	• Diffuse PMI, left ventricular heave • AF or ventricular dysrhythmias • Persistent ST segment elevation • Chest x-ray shows left ventricular dilation • Echocardiography shows dyskinesis and left ventricular dilation • Clinical indications of LVF may be present • Clinical indications of systemic emboli may be present: cerebral emboli; peripheral emboli with acute arterial occlusion	• Antidysrhythmic drugs (e.g., amiodarone) • Anticoagulants (e.g., heparin followed by warfarin) • Treatment of HF: ACE inhibitors; beta-blockers; diuretics; vasodilators; inotropes • Surgical resection may be performed • Ablative procedures may be necessary for recurrent ventricular dysrhythmias
Pericarditis	• Fever • Chest pain that worsens with deep breath and lessens sitting up and with leaning forward • Pericardial friction rub • Elevated WBC count and sedimentation rate • Diffuse ST segment elevation across the precordial leads • Chest x-ray may show pericardial effusion	• NSAIDs (e.g., ibuprofen or indomethacin) • Discontinuance of anticoagulants • Close monitoring for clinical indications of cardiac tamponade
Dressler's syndrome (also referred to as *post–myocardial infarction syndrome*): late pericarditis that is thought to be autoimmune	• Fever • Chest pain that worsens with deep breath and lessens sitting up and with leaning forward • Pericardial friction rub • Elevated WBC count and sedimentation rate • Diffuse ST segment elevation across the precordial leads • Chest x-ray may show pericardial effusion	• Corticosteroids (e.g., prednisone)

Table 3-17 Complications of Myocardial Infarction—cont'd

Complication	Clinical Indications	Prevention/Treatment
Sudden cardiac death	• Cardiopulmonary arrest	• Preventive measures include: ◦ Risk factor modification ◦ Platelet aggregation inhibitors (e.g., aspirin) ◦ Beta-blockers ◦ Encouragement of family members to learn CPR • Treatment: CPR; ACLS modalities

ACE, Angiotensin-converting enzyme; *ACLS,* advanced cardiac life support; *CABG,* coronary artery bypass graft; *CO/CI,* cardiac output/cardiac index; *ECG,* electrocardiogram; *GIK,* glucose-insulin-potassium; *HF,* heart failure; IABP, intraaortic balloon pump; *LLSB,* lower left sternal border; *NSAIDs,* nonsteroidal antiinflammatory drugs; *NTG,* nitroglycerin; NTP, nitroprusside; *PAOP,* pulmonary artery occlusive pressure; *PCI,* percutaneous coronary intervention; *PEA,* pulseless electrical activity; *RAP,* right atrial pressure; *RVF,* right ventricular failure; *SVR,* systemic vascular resistance; *SvO_2,* venous oxygen saturation; *VAD,* ventricular assist device; *WBC,* white blood cell count.

(ii) Lipid-reducing therapy (e.g., statins) for hyperlipidemia
(iii) Oral hypoglycemics and/or insulin for DM
(iv) Thyroid hormone replacement or suppressive agents for thyroid disorders

Heart Failure

Definitions

1. HF: condition in which one or both ventricles cannot pump sufficient blood to meet the metabolic needs of the body; characterized by one or both of the following:
   a. Clinical indications of intravascular and interstitial volume overload (e.g., dyspnea, crackles, and edema)
   b. Clinical indications of tissue hypoperfusion (e.g., fatigue and exercise intolerance)
2. Pulmonary edema
   a. Fluid in the alveolus
   b. Impairs gas exchange and causes hypoxemia by impairing the diffusion between alveolus and capillary
   c. May be cardiac versus noncardiac; frequently differentiated using PAOP and the difference between PA diastolic pressure and PAOP
      (1) Cardiac pulmonary edema
         (a) Caused by acute LVF
         (b) Elevated pulmonary artery pressure (PAP), elevated PAOP; difference between PA diastolic pressure and PAOP less than 5 mm Hg
         (c) Fluid is *pushed* from the pulmonary capillary into the interstitium and finally into the alveolus because of increased pulmonary capillary hydrostatic pressure
      (2) Noncardiac pulmonary edema
         (a) Most common cause is acute respiratory distress syndrome (ARDS); also may be caused by drowning
         (b) Elevated PAP, normal PAOP; difference between PA diastolic pressure and PAOP greater than 5 mm Hg
         (c) Fluid *leaks* from the pulmonary capillary into the interstitium and alveolus because of increased permeability of the damaged alveolocapillary membrane

Etiology

1. Risk factors
   a. No. 1 is CAD, especially with history of MI
   b. Congenital heart disease
   c. Valvular heart disease
   d. Hypertension
   e. Diabetes
   f. Obesity
   g. Alcoholism
   h. Smoking
   i. High or low hematocrit
   j. Sedentary lifestyle
   k. High-fat/high-salt diet
2. Etiologic factors (Table 3-18)
3. Causes of decompensation in a patient with HF
   a. Progression of left ventricular dysfunction
   b. New or worsening ischemia
   c. Hypoxemia
   d. Worsening of anemia
   e. Drugs such as nonsteroidal antiinflammatory drugs (NSAIDs), initiation of beta-blocker dosage at too high dosages
   f. Hypertension
   g. New dysrhythmia, particularly AF
   h. Missed or suboptimal medication
   i. Dietary indiscretion, such as high-salt foods
   j. Alcohol
4. Common comorbidities in a patient with HF
   a. Coronary artery disease
   b. Myocardial infarction
   c. Hypertension with systolic BP greater than 140 mm Hg
   d. Renal insufficiency

Table 3-18 Etiologic Factors of Heart Failure

Type of Heart Failure	Etiologic Factors
Left ventricular failure	• CAD/LV infarction • Cardiomyopathy • Hypertension • Dysrhythmias • Volume overload • Valvular disease: mitral or aortic • Ventricular septal defect • Coarctation of aorta • Myocarditis • Cardiac tamponade
Right ventricular failure	• LV failure • CAD/RV infarction • Pulmonary hypertension ◦ Passive: mitral valve disease ◦ Active: hypoxemia; pulmonary embolism • Dysrhythmias • Volume overload • Valvular disease: mitral or pulmonic • Ventricular septal defect • Cardiomyopathy • Myocardial contusion
Biventricular failure	**Increased demand** • Thyrotoxicosis • Anemia • Pregnancy • Systemic infection • Beriberi • Paget's disease **Electrolyte imbalance** • Hyponatremia • Hypokalemia • Hypocalcemia • Hypomagnesemia • Hypophosphatemia

CAD, Coronary artery disease; *LV,* left ventricular; *RV,* right ventricular.

e. Hyperlipidemia
f. DM
g. AF
h. COPD and/or asthma

Pathophysiology

1. Compensation → decompensation: in the short-term, these mechanisms compensate for the failing heart, but in the long-term, all of these factors trigger a process of pathologic growth and remodeling
   a. Sympathetic nervous system (SNS)
      (1) Increase in heart rate, contractility, and conductivity initially increases cardiac output.
         (a) Eventually, coronary artery blood flow is reduced by diastolic shortening caused by tachycardia.
         (b) Dysrhythmias may occur.
      (2) Vasoconstriction increases preload and afterload and therefore BP.
         (a) Increase in myocardial oxygen consumption results.
   b. Renin-angiotensin-aldosterone system: Sodium and water retention and peripheral vasoconstriction increases blood volume and preload.
      (1) Myocardial oxygen consumption is increased.
      (2) Eventually, pulmonary and peripheral edema may occur.
      (3) Ventricular dilation and hypertrophy may occur.
   c. Hypertrophy: More myofibrils increase cross-bridge cycling, and more mitochondria increase supply of adenosine triphosphate (ATP).
      (1) Eventually, a disproportionate number of ATP–consuming myofibrils to ATP–producing mitochondria.
      (2) Eventually, decreased endocardial perfusion and increased wall stress may occur.
   d. Interstitial remodeling
      (1) Initially collagen formation may reduce ventricular dilation.
      (2) Eventually, compliance is decreased and diastolic dysfunction results.
      (3) Eventually, force transmission through ventricular wall is decreased.
      (4) Ventricular remodeling causes the normal oval shape of the ventricular chamber to become more spherical.
         (a) This abnormal ventricular contour causes a decrease in contractility, stretching of the mitral valve ring leading to mitral regurgitation, and prolongation of the QRS complex with ventricular depolarization asynchrony.
         (b) Ventricular asynchrony causes the interventricular septum to move paradoxically so that the septum is displaced into the noncontracting ventricle, which decreases cardiac output and cardiac index and increases PAOP.
         (c) With more time required for ventricular systole, diastolic filling time is reduced, accentuating the backward failure.
      (5) Electrical remodeling predisposes the myocardium to malignant ventricular dysrhythmias.
2. Signal-modulating inhibitors: Primary therapies are directed toward blocking dysfunctional compensatory mechanisms.
   a. SNS: beta-blockers, alpha- and beta-blockers
   b. Renin-angiotensin-aldosterone system: ACE inhibitors and angiotensin II receptor blockers (ARBs)
   c. Aldosterone: spirnolactone (Aldactone)

Classifications

1. Location: left or right
2. Onset: acute or chronic
3. Output state: low-output (e.g., MI or cardiomyopathy) or high-output (e.g., thyrotoxicosis or anemia)

4. Type of pumping defect: backward (i.e., high volume and engorgement behind the failing ventricle) versus forward (i.e., low filling volume for the ventricle in front of the failing ventricle)
5. Relationship to the cardiac cycle: systolic (60% to 70%) or diastolic (30% to 40%)
   a. Systolic dysfunction (pump problem): inability of the ventricle to shorten against a load; the left ventricle loses its ability to contract normally against progressive increases in afterload
      (1) Possible causes: MI; myocardial contusion; myocarditis; dilated cardiomyopathy; hypertension; valvular heart disease; electrolyte imbalance; dysrhythmias
      (2) Hemodynamics: decreased contractility; EF less than 40%; increased cardiac volumes and pressures
      (3) Clinical indications: displaced PMI; JVD; S_3; crackles; dyspnea; peripheral edema; cardiomegaly
      (4) Drug therapy: diuretics if congestive symptoms; ACE inhibitor or ARB; beta-blocker or alpha- and beta-blocker but not pure alpha-blocker; inotropes may be required for diuretic-resistant congestion; antidysrhythmic drugs and anticoagulants may be indicated
   b. Diastolic dysfunction (filling problem): an impairment in left ventricular filling at near normal or mildly elevated left atrial and ventricular pressures; caused by decrease in ventricular compliance; small changes in volume are associated with a disproportionate increase in pressure
      (1) Possible causes: myocardial ischemia; hypertrophic cardiomyopathy; ventricular hypertrophy; constrictive pericarditis or cardiac tamponade; valvular heart disease; aging
      (2) Hemodynamics: increased contractility; normal EF; increased cardiac pressures with normal or slightly increased cardiac volumes
      (3) Clinical indications: S_4; crackles; dyspnea; peripheral edema; precordial heave; normal heart sound
      (4) Drug therapy: diuretics if congestive symptoms; ACE inhibitor or ARB; beta-blocker or alpha- and beta-blocker

Clinical Presentation (Box 3-1)

1. First symptoms frequently are cough, exertional dyspnea, edema, or fatigue
2. Serum
   a. Serum electrolyte levels: may reveal and/or confirm imbalances especially hypokalemia, hypocalcemia, and hypomagnesemia
   b. Serum albumin levels: may show hypoproteinemia, which can contribute to edema
   c. Arterial blood gases: may show hypoxemia (especially if pulmonary edema present) and acid-base imbalances (including lactic acidosis in severe hypoperfusion states)

BOX 3-1 Clinical Indications of Left Ventricular and Right Ventricular Failure

Left Ventricular Failure

- Tachypnea, dyspnea, orthopnea,
- PND
- Tachycardia
- Left-sided S_3
- Displaced PMI, heave at apex
- Crackles, wheezes
- Cough, frothy sputum, hemoptysis
- Diaphoresis
- Pulsus alternans
- Oliguria
- Weakness, fatigue
- Mental confusion
- Murmur of MR
- ABGs: decreased Pao_2, Sao_2
- Hemodynamics
  - Elevated PA, PAOP
  - Decreased CO/CI
- Abnormal chest X-ray
  - Cardiomegaly
  - Engorged pulmonary vasculature
  - Kerley B lines
  - Pleural effusion
- ECG
  - Left atrial enlargement
  - Left ventricular hypertrophy
  - Atrial dysrhythmias

Right Ventricular Failure

- Jugular venous distention
- Hepatojugular reflux
- Dependent pitting edema
- Heave at sternum
- Hepatomegaly/splenomegaly
- Anorexia, nausea, vomiting
- Abdominal pain and bloating
- Ascites
- Nocturia
- Weakness, fatigue
- Weight gain
- Murmur of TR
- Right-sided S_3
- Hemodynamics
  - Elevated CVP, RAP
- Abnormal liver function studies
  - ALT
  - AST
  - LDH
- ECG
  - Right atrial enlargement
  - Right ventricular hypertrophy
  - Atrial dysrhythmias

d. Drug levels: may reveal abnormal levels of digoxin and antidysrhythmic agents
e. Thyroid profile: may reveal abnormal thyroid function
f. CBC: may show anemia or leukocytosis
g. Blood urea nitrogen (BUN), creatinine: may be elevated to detect renal impairment
h. Brain-type natriuretic peptide (BNP)
   (1) Normal: less than 100 pg/mL; levels greater than 100 pg/mL indicate HF
   (2) Elevated BNP peptide level correlates with an increased left ventricular end-diastolic pressure and volume and PAOP
      (a) Other conditions associated with increased BNP levels
         (i) LVF
         (ii) Cardiac inflammation
         (iii) Primary pulmonary hypertension (PH)
         (iv) Renal failure
         (v) Cirrhosis
         (vi) Endocrine disorders (e.g., primary hyperaldosteronism and Cushing's syndrome)
         (vii) May be elevated in elderly patients
      (b) May replace chest x-ray as the test of choice in differential diagnosis of dyspnea in acute care setting
i. Urine: may show proteinuria and/or presence of red blood cells (RBCs) or casts

3. Diagnostic studies
   a. Chest x-ray shows cardiac enlargement and dilation; may show pulmonary congestion
   b. Cardiac catheterization and coronary angiography
      (1) May show coronary artery disease or valve abnormalities
      (2) Cardiac pressures increased and EF decreased in systolic dysfunction
      (3) Cardiac pressures increased and EF normal in diastolic dysfunction
   c. Computed tomography (CT): may be used to evaluate left ventricular wall motion and detect cardiac tumors, MI, and aortic aneurysm
   d. Echocardiography: shows changes in chamber size, wall thickness, and valve motion
   e. Electrocardiography
      (1) May show myocardial ischemia/infarction
      (2) May show atrial enlargement and/or ventricular hypertrophy
   f. Multiple gated acquisition (MUGA) scan: may be used to evaluate cardiac function, determine EF, and detect wall motion abnormalities
4. Hemodynamic parameters
   a. Increase in volume indicators: RAP, PAP, PAOP
   b. Decrease in cardiac output/index
   c. Increase in systemic vascular resistance (SVR)
   d. Increase in pulmonary vascular resistance (PVR)
5. New York Heart Association (NYHA) Functional Classification
   a. Class I: patients with cardiac disease but without resulting limitation of physical activity; ordinary physical activity does not cause undue fatigue, palpitation, dyspnea, or angina
   b. Class II: patients with cardiac disease resulting in slight limitation of physical activity; they are comfortable at rest; ordinary physical activity results in fatigue, palpitation, dyspnea, or angina
   c. Class III: patients with cardiac disease resulting in marked limitation of physical activity; they are comfortable at rest; less than ordinary activity causes fatigue, palpitation, dyspnea, or angina
   d. Class IV: patients with cardiac disease resulting in inability to carry on any physical activity without discomfort; symptoms of cardiac insufficiency or angina may be present even at rest; if any physical activity is attempted, discomfort is increased
6. AHA Prognostic Classification
   a. A: Risk factors for the development of structure heart disease or overt HF
   b. B: Presence of structural heart disease (e.g., MI or valvular heart disease) without symptoms of HF
   c. C: Presence of structural heart disease and current or prior symptoms of HF that is responsive to therapy
   d. D: Presence of HF refractory to conventional treatment requiring ventricular assist device (VAD), cardiac transplantation, or palliative care

Nursing Diagnoses (see Appendix A)

1. Decreased Cardiac Output related to alterations in preload, afterload, contractility, or heart rate
2. Impaired Gas Exchange related to intraalveolar fluid
3. Fluid Volume Excess related to maladaptive compensatory mechanism resulting from decreased cardiac output
4. Ineffective Peripheral Tissue Perfusion related to impaired cardiac contractility
5. Risk for Fluid/Electrolyte Imbalance related to increased body fluid, decrease in renal perfusion, diuretic therapy, and sodium restriction
6. Activity Intolerance related to decreased cardiac output, decrease in tissue oxygen delivery, and deconditioning
7. Sleep Deprivation related to dyspnea, anxiety, and nocturia
8. Anxiety related to acute health alteration and recommended lifestyle changes
9. Deficient Knowledge related to unfamiliarity with disease process, therapy, and recommended lifestyle changes
10. Interrupted Family Processes related to change in health status and potential life-threatening situation

Collaborative Management

1. Treat the cause and/or contributing factors if possible.
   a. Reperfusion in acute MI along neurohormonal antagonism with beta-blocker (or alpha/beta-blocker [e.g., carvedilol]) and ACE inhibitor

b. Revascularization of patients with coronary artery disease
c. Valve replacement if required, especially for acute valvular disorder such as ruptured papillary muscle with acute mitral regurgitation
d. Treatment of symptomatic or life-threatening dysrhythmias with antidysrhythmic agents, electrical therapies (e.g., cardioversion, defibrillation, pacemaker, or AICD), or surgical procedures (e.g., ablation)
e. Continuous positive airway pressure (CPAP) for obstructive sleep apnea, which is common in patients with HF
f. Avoidance of certain pharmacologic agents
  (1) Antidysrhythmic drugs being used to suppress asymptomatic dysrhythmias
  (2) Most calcium channel blockers
  (3) NSAIDs (increase resistance to diuretics)

2. Improve oxygenation.
  a. Oxygen by nasal cannula at 2 to 6 L/min to maintain SaO_2 saturation of 95% unless contraindicated
  b. Intubation and mechanical ventilation may be required
    (1) Noninvasive positive-pressure ventilation (biphasic positive airway pressure [BiPAP]) may be used to avert intubation.
      (a) Positive pressure ventilation during inspiration (pressure support ventilation) during inspiration decreases the work of breathing.
      (b) Continuous positive airway pressure (CPAP) during expiration increases the driving pressure of oxygen to improve oxygenation, decreases intrapulmonary shunt by opening collapsed alveoli, and decreases surface tension and work of breathing.
    (2) PEEP may be required if patient is receiving mechanical ventilation.
      (a) Increases the driving pressure of oxygen
      (b) Decreases shunt by opening alveoli that are collapsed (i.e., alveolar recruitment) and keeps alveoli open at low distending pressure if they are still open
      (c) Decreases surface tension and work of breathing
      (d) Positive alveolar pressure prevents the transudation of fluid into the alveoli
  c. Elimination of accumulated fluid: diuretics
  d. Treatment of anemia: More than half of patients with HF are anemic with hemoglobin less than 12 g/dL, and treatment of anemia improves cardiac function.
    (1) Packed RBCs may be required acutely if anemia is significant
    (2) Erythropoietin (epoetin alfa [Epogen])
    (3) Iron

3. Decrease myocardial oxygen consumption.
  a. Physical and emotional rest
    (1) Allow rest after meals, personal hygiene, toileting, and physical therapy.
    (2) Prevent Valsalva maneuver.
      (a) Teach patient to exhale when turning in bed.
      (b) Administer stool softeners as prescribed.
      (c) Provide bedside commode for elimination.
    (3) Explain procedures thoroughly: monitor alarms; equipment; visiting hours; reasons for procedures.
    (4) Keep family informed regarding patient's progress and status.
    (5) Provide for physical comfort: temperature control; lighting; noise control.
    (6) Instruct patient regarding relaxation techniques; encourage use of these techniques.
    (7) Provide appropriate nutrition: soft low-sodium (2 to 3 g/day) diet.
    (8) Administer anxiolytic drugs as prescribed: usually diazepam (Valium), lorazepam (Ativan), or alprazolam (Xanax).
  b. Beta-blocker (or alpha- and beta-blocker) as prescribed
    (1) Indications: HF as the result of systolic and diastolic dysfunction; usually used for Class II or III HF
    (2) Actions
      (a) Acts as a cardioprotective agents to protect the heart from excessive catecholamines
      (b) Decreases left ventricular mass and volume
      (c) Changes the shape of the ventricle from spherical to elliptical
      (d) Increase exercise capacity
    (3) Agents
      (a) Carvedilol (Coreg): alpha-blocker and noncardioselective beta-blocker
      (b) Metoprolol (Lopressor): cardioselective beta-blocker
      (c) Esmolol (Brevibloc): short-acting cardioselective beta-blocker administered by IV infusion
      (d) Dosages are started low and gradually increased while one monitors closely for decompensation because beta-blockers decrease contractility.
    (4) Contraindications for the use of beta-blockers in HF
      (a) Decompensated HF
      (b) Cardiogenic shock
      (c) Acute pulmonary edema
      (d) Hemodynamic instability (requiring IV inotropic support)
      (e) Bronchial asthma (cardioselective beta-blockers may be used cautiously)
      (f) Second- or third-degree AV block
      (g) Sick sinus syndrome
      (h) Severe hepatic impairment

4. Decrease preload
  a. Positioning: low Fowler's position with legs dependent
  b. Sodium and fluid restrictions acutely

(1) Fluid restriction to less than 2000 mL per 24 hours
(2) Sodium restriction to less than 2 to 3 grams per 24 hours
(3) Daily measurement of weight to detect early fluid retention

c. Diuretics
(1) Indication: HF with evidence of or a predisposition to fluid retention
(2) Action: eliminate symptoms and physical signs of fluid retention, such as JVD and/or edema
(3) Agents
(a) Usually loop diuretics are used (e.g., furosemide [Lasix] or bumetanide [Bumex]).
(i) Continuous infusion may be superior to intermittent boluses.
(b) Aldosterone antagonists (e.g., spironolactone [Aldactone] or eplerenone [Inspra]) may be used with loop diuretics or alone.
(i) These are relatively weak diuretics in patients with normal renin; however, they are much more effective in patients who have edema associated with increased production or decreased elimination of renin.
(ii) Benefits are additive to the benefits of ACE inhibitors.
(iii) Close monitoring of potassium levels is necessary, especially when patient also is taking an ACE inhibitor or ARB.
(iv) These are contraindicated in patients with renal insufficiency.
(c) Two or more diuretics may be prescribed together.
(d) Short-term use of a drug that increases renal blood flow, such as fenoldopam (Corlopam), may be prescribed.
(4) Cautions
(a) Overuse will decrease blood volume, decrease CO, and lead to organ hypoperfusion and prerenal azotemia.
(b) Diuretics may alter the efficacy and toxicity of other drugs used to treat HF (e.g., ACE inhibitors and beta-blockers).

d. ACE inhibitors and ARBs
(1) Indications: HF as the result of systolic and diastolic dysfunction
(2) Action
(a) ACE inhibitors block conversion of angiotensin I to angiotensin II and the resultant vasoconstriction and aldosterone release.
(b) ARBs block angiotensin II and the resultant vasoconstriction and aldosterone release.
(i) ARBs frequently are used if a patient has angioedema or cough as a result of angiotensin-converting enzyme inhibitors; they also are preferred with African-Americans.
(3) Agents
(a) ACE inhibitors: captopril (Capoten), enalapril (Vasotec), lisinopril (Zestril, Prinivil), ramipril (Altace), benazepril (Lotensin), quinapril (Accupril), fosinopril (Monopril), moexipril (Univasc), trandolapril (Mavik)
(b) ARBs: losartan (Cozaar), valsartan (Diovan), telmisartan (Micardis), irbesartan (Avapro)
(c) If neither ACE inhibitors or ARBs are tolerated, the combination of nitrates and hydralazine (Apresoline) may be prescribed.
(4) Cautions
(a) Hypotension
(b) Angioedema, especially ACE inhibitors
(c) Hyperkalemia especially when in combination with an aldosterone antagonist such as spironolactone (Aldactone)
(d) Proteinuria and renal failure

e. Nesiritide (Natrecor): recombinant form of B-type natriuretic peptide (BNP)
(1) Indication: decompensated HF in patients who have dyspnea at rest or with minimal activities and clinical evidence of fluid overload
(a) Systolic and diastolic dysfunction
(b) Decompensation is defined as sustained deterioration in function of at least one NYHA class, usually associated with evidence of total body salt and water overload.
(2) Action: binds to the alpha-type natriuretic peptide receptor on the surface of vascular smooth muscle and endothelial cells
(a) Dilates arteries and reduces SVR
(b) Dilates veins and reduces PAOP
(c) Decreases aldosterone and norepinephrine levels
(d) Inhibits renin-angiotensin-aldosterone system and endothelin pathways, prompting the release of fluid and sodium from the body
(e) Improves symptoms of decompensated HF more than NTG with less proarrhythmogenesis and tachycardia than dobutamine
(3) Contraindications
(a) Hypovolemia
(b) Profound hypotension (e.g., cardiogenic shock)
(c) Aortic stenosis
(d) Hypertrophic or restrictive cardiomyopathy
(e) Constrictive pericarditis or cardiac tamponade

f. Endothelin receptor antagonist: tezosentan (Veletri)

(1) Action: vasodilation
(2) Does not increase heart rate, but higher doses were associated with hypotension
g. Venous vasodilators (e.g., NTG [Tridil] and morphine)
(1) Not recommended in diastolic dysfunction
h. Dialysis: if the patient is in renal failure
i. Continuous renal replacement therapy: under investigation to manage the overhydration in HF refractory to traditional therapies such as fluid restriction and diuretics
5. Decrease afterload.
a. NTP: particularly helpful for hypertensive patients
b. Calcium channel blockers
(1) Most calcium channel blockers should be avoided in the treatment of HF; amlodipine (Norvasc) and felodipine (Plendil) may be used in diastolic dysfunction.
c. ACE inhibitors or ARBs: prevent activation of angiotensin II with the resultant vasoconstriction and increase in afterload
d. Renal artery angioplasty, stents: indicated for patient with renal artery stenosis
e. Pulmonary vasodilators may be used to reduce PH
f. IABP: especially helpful in patients who have very high afterload that is refractory to arterial vasodilators or who are too hypotension to use arterial dilators to reduce afterload
6. Increase contractility.
a. Inotropic agents (e.g., dobutamine [Dobutrex])
(1) Indications: temporary treatment of diuretic-refractory decompensation
(2) Agents
(a) Cardiac glycosides (e.g., digoxin)
(i) Recommended to improve symptoms in patients with HF caused by left ventricular systolic dysfunction with dilated ventricle and should be used together with diuretics, angiotensin-converting enzyme inhibitors, and beta-blockers
(ii) Actions
a) Improve cardiac contractility by inhibiting Na^+,K^+-ATPase; increases EF and exercise tolerance
b) Inhibit SNS and reduce norepinephrine and renin activity
c) Slow the heart rate in AF
(iii) Major drawback: the narrow therapeutic/toxic ratio
(b) Sympathetic stimulants (e.g., dobutamine)
(i) Used primarily with HF in presence of acute MI
(ii) Actions
a) Increases contractility by stimulating beta receptors and so may increase ectopy potential
b) Dobutamine is preferred (unless patient is hypotensive) because it causes less tachycardia than dopamine does and decreases afterload rather than increases afterload such as dopamine does
(iii) Parenteral only
(c) Phosphodiesterase inhibitors (e.g., milrinone [Primacor])
(i) Used only if no response to digitalis, diuretics, or vasodilators
(ii) Actions
a) Increases contractility by inhibiting phosphodiesterase
b) Causes vasodilation to decrease preload and afterload
(iii) Parenteral only
b. Mechanical cardiac support devices
(1) The supply of acceptable donor hearts remains insufficient for the number of patients who require them; mechanical devices offer an at least temporary alternative, and devices continue to be developed and tested as a permanent alternative to cardiac transplantation.
(2) Goal: to stabilize and improve the hemodynamic condition of the patient with loss of ventricular function
(3) Complications: infection and thromboembolism are most significant; bleeding; hypertension
(4) VAD: used in severe cases especially if patient is a candidate for cardiac transplantation (Table 3-19)
c. Surgical approaches
(1) Dynamic cardiomyoplasty
(a) Latissimus dorsi muscle wrapped around the heart and stimulated by electrical impulses to contract with each heartbeat
(b) High perioperative mortality in NYHA Class IV patients along with overall high long-term mortality and lack of demonstrated survival advantage over medical therapy; not recommended at this time
(2) Partial left ventriculectomy (also referred to as the *Batista HF procedure*): most suited for dilated cardiomyopathy
(a) Resection of a wedge of left ventricular wall to restore the volume-mass-diameter relationship of the left ventricle; mitral and/or tricuspid valve may be replaced concurrently
(b) American College of Cardiology/American Heart Association (ACC/AHA) guidelines conclude that procedure currently is considered not useful/effective and in some cases can be harmful
(3) Dor procedure (also referred to as *endoventricular circular patch plasty*)

Table 3-19 Ventricular Assist Device

Indications	• Bridge to recovery: persistent HF despite aggressive therapy but with potential for recovery if the heart is given time to rest • Inability to wean patient from cardiopulmonary bypass • Cardiogenic shock refractory to pharmacologic or IABP therapy • Bridge to transplant: end-stage heart disease awaiting suitable donor for cardiac transplant • Permanent long-term: use of implantable device for patients with Class IV HF with EF less than 25%, on continuous inotropic therapy, but not a candidate for cardiac transplantation; may be referred to as "destination therapy" • Physiologic indications despite pharmacologic support or IABP therapy ○ MAP less than 60 mm Hg ○ Systolic BP less than 90 mm Hg ○ PAOP or RAP greater than 20-25 mm Hg ○ Urine output less than 20 mL/hr ○ Cardiac index less than 2 L/min/m^2 ○ EF less than 25% ○ May be used with IABP
Contraindications	• Irreversible, extensive heart disease; no possibility of being weaned from VAD, and patient not a candidate for cardiac transplant • Prolonged cardiac arrest with resultant neurologic damage • Multiple organ failure • Significant complications or disease (e.g., chronic renal failure, cancer with metastasis, severe hepatic disease, significant blood dyscrasias, or severe COPD)
Actions	• Maintains systemic circulation and tissue perfusion with flow assistance • Decreases myocardial workload to promote ventricular recovery • Reversal of ventricular dilation, regression of left ventricular hypertrophy, reversal of ventricular remodeling
Devices	Categorized by purpose • Bridge to recovery: Abiomed BV, BioMedicus • Bridge to transplant: Novacor 100, HeartMate (implanted pneumatic), Thoratec (pneumatic) • Long-term: HeartMate (vented electric) Categorized by device type • Implantable: Novocor; HeartMate • External: Thoratec; Abiomed • Fully implantable (no drive or venting lines through the skin): Arrow LionHeart and AbioMed AbioCor in clinical trials All devices have cannula, pump, and external power source
Insertion and mechanics	Requires an extended median sternotomy Left ventricular assist device (LVAD) • Outflow circuit anastomosed to patient aorta or femoral artery. • Inflow circuit anastomosed to left atrium or ventricle. • Left atrium usually is used in the pending recovery patient. • Left ventricle usually is used in the bridge to transplant patient. Right ventricular assist device (RVAD) • Outflow circuit anastomosed to patient's pulmonary artery. • Inflow circuit anastomosed to right atrium. Biventricular assist device • Both ventricles are supported; the main advantage here is that with LVAD or RVAD the unassisted ventricle may fail. Implanted device • The pump unit may be implanted into the abdominal wall. • Controller unit and power source are attached to the pump unit by a percutaneous lead.
Assessment	• HR: a normalization of heart rate is desirable. • BP: an increase in MAP is desirable. • CO/CI: an increase in cardiac output/cardiac index is desirable. ○ Thermodilution CO will not be accurate in patients with RVAD; use Fick formula (calculation of CO using mixed venous oxygen saturation and arterial oxygen saturation). • PAP/PAOP: a decrease in PAP and PAOP is desirable. • SaO_2: an increase in Sao_2 is desirable. • SvO_2: an increase in Svo_2 is desirable.

Table 3-19 Ventricular Assist Device—cont'd

	• Urine Output: an increase in urine output is desirable. • Complaints of chest pain: a decrease in chest pain is desirable. • ECG: a decrease in the presence or frequency of dysrhythmias is desirable. • Neurovascular status of affected limb: the presence of palpable pulses and a warm limb with normal capillary refill is desirable.
Nursing diagnoses	• Decreased Cardiac Output related to pump failure, dysrhythmias, and mechanical problems with the VAD • Risk for Impaired Gas Exchange related to pulmonary vascular congestion, pulmonary infection, or air embolism • Risk for Fluid Volume Deficit related to third spacing and coagulopathies • Risk for Injury related to mechanical malfunction of the VAD • Risk for Infection related to invasive catheters, devices, and sternotomy • Anxiety related to insertion of VAD, noise from device, critical illness, and critical care environment
Brief summary of nursing management	• Assess the parameters described previously. • Titrate pharmacologic therapies to augment the mechanical therapy of the VAD. • Adjust fluid balance by administering colloids, crystalloids, or diuretics as prescribed. • Prevent hazards of immobility: turn patient side to side when hemodynamics are stabilized; use passive range of motion; use special mattresses and beds as indicated. • Observe for complications and provide appropriate management for the prevention of complications. • Provide emotional support to the patient and family; use social services, pastoral care, and support groups as indicated.

Complications: prevention and treatment	• Thromboembolism: heparin may be prescribed
	• Hemolysis
	• Bleeding
	  ○ Monitor ACT while patient is receiving heparin.
	  ○ Monitor for bleeding, including cardiac tamponade.
	  ○ Administer blood and blood products as indicated.
	  ○ Prevent tubing disconnection; all connections should be clearly visible and securely connected.
	• Infection: risk increased by CD4 reduction that accompanies VAD implantation
	  ○ Monitor CBC, body temperature, and heart rate.
	  ○ Monitor for pain, tenderness, heat, and redness at exit site and abdominal pump pocket.
	  ○ Assess breath sounds and chest x-ray film; pneumonia is common because of immobilization; ventilatory assistance is required with some VADs.
	• Dysrhythmias
	• Cerebral emboli
	• Respiratory failure
	• Renal failure
	• Air embolism
	• Mechanical failure
	• Psychological complications (e.g., depression and anxiety)
	• Anxiety concerning device failure and infection

Weaning	• The following parameters with VAD off are required before weaning the patient from the VAD:
	  ○ MAP greater than 60 mm Hg
	  ○ RAP (RVAD) or PAOP (LVAD) less than 25 mm Hg
	  ○ CI greater than 2 L/min/m^2
	• The VAD flow is decreased.
	• Anticoagulation is recommended during weaning.
	• VAD removal is done in the OR.

ACT; Activated clotting time; *BP,* blood pressure; *CBC,* complete blood count; *CI,* cardiac index; *CO,* cardiac output; *COPD;* chronic obstructive pulmonary disease; *ECG,* electrocardiogram; *EF,* ejection fraction; *HF,* heart failure; *IABP,* intraaortic balloon pump; *MAP,* mean arterial pressure; *OR,* operating room; *PAOP,* pulmonary artery occlusive pressure; *PAP,* pulmonary artery pressure; *rt-PA,* recombinant tissue plasminogen activator; *SaO_2,* arterial oxygen saturation; *SvO_2,* venous oxygen pressure; *VAD,* ventricular assist device.

(a) Areas of hypofunctioning myocardium are cut out and the opening in the wall is repaired with a synthetic or autologous tissue circular patch.
(b) Evidence is unclear, and the current ACC/AHA guidelines do not address this procedure.
(4) Left-ventricular splints and wraps: in clinical trials
(a) Goal: arrest and reverse remodeling of the failing heart
(b) Devices
(i) Myocor Myosplint: two epicardial pads and a transventricular tension member; the two pads are placed on the surface of the heart with the load-bearing tension member passing through the ventricle, connecting the pads and drawing the ventricular walls toward one another
(ii) Acorn Cardiac Support Device: wraps the heart in a mesh bag to prevent further dilation and failure; the Dacron wrap is pulled over the base of the heart and is attached with sutures
(iii) Evidence is unclear, and the current ACC/AHA guidelines do not address these procedures.
(5) Cardiac transplantation
(a) Indications for cardiac transplantation in HF patient
(i) Class III or IV and a life expectancy of less than 24 hours
(ii) Under 65 years of age at the time of listing; if retransplantation or heart-kidney or heart-liver, the age of 55 years generally is used
(iii) Acute HF or cardiogenic shock as a result of acute MI that is refractory to medical therapy and requires mechanical support or patients who cannot be weaned from cardiopulmonary bypass are candidates unless they has contraindications.

7. Manage dysrhythmias.
a. Atrial
(1) Atrial dysrhythmias frequently resolve with treatment of HF because atrial stretch, and therefore atrial irritability, is decreased.
(2) Digoxin decreases ventricular response rate by increasing refractoriness of AV node.
(3) Anticoagulants are used to prevent mural thrombi and embolic events.
b. Ventricular
(1) Antidysrhythmic drugs as prescribed
(a) Class I antidysrhythmic drugs (e.g., procainamide or lidocaine) should not be used except for immediately life-threatening ventricular dysrhythmia.
(b) Some Class III antidysrhythmic drugs, such as amiodarone, do not appear to increase the risk of death and are preferred over Class I agents.
(2) Correction of electrolyte deficiencies that may cause dysrhythmias and alter the efficacy and safety of antidysrhythmic agents
c. Dual-chamber pacemaker with rate modulation
(1) Beneficial for patients with severe HF with poor activity tolerance
(2) Increases heart rate in response to physical activity
d. Cardiac resynchronization therapy (CRT) atriobiventricular pacing
(1) Indications in HF patients: 30% to 50% of patients with HF have ventricular asynchrony, and the 80% of patients with advanced HF have LBBB with resultant ventricular asynchrony
(a) EF of 35% or less
(b) QRS complex of at least 130 milliseconds (0.13 second)
(c) NYHA Class III to IV
(2) Actions
(a) Restores synchronous ventricular contraction to optimize left ventricular filling and improve cardiac output
(b) Improved exercise tolerance
(c) Improved quality of life
(d) Reduction in mortality
(3) Collaborative management: as for newly implanted pacemakers and for HF
(a) Monitor for 100% ventricular capture and for any lengthening of the QRS complex that might indicate loss of capture of one of the ventricles (usually the left ventricle).
(b) Restrict movement of the arm to prevent lead dislodgment or bleeding in the pacemaker pocket; give instructions regarding avoidance of pushing, pulling, or lifting anything heavier than 5 lb for 1 to 2 weeks after surgery or what symptoms to report and other instruction as for implanted pacemaker.
(c) Monitor for complications: infection.

8. Monitor for complications.
a. Deep vein thrombosis/pulmonary embolism
b. Progressive deterioration
c. Dysrhythmias: common cause of sudden death
d. Complications of therapy
(1) Fluid and electrolyte imbalance: hypokalemia; hypocalcemia; hypomagnesemia resulting from diuretic therapy
(2) Digitalis toxicity
e. Depression
f. Anxiety
g. Sleep disturbances

9. Provide instruction and counseling regarding lifestyle modification and need for pharmacologic therapy.

a. Nonpharmacologic therapies
   (1) Weight normalization
   (2) Dietary modifications
      (a) Low saturated fat
      (b) Low (2 to 3 g) sodium
      (c) ADA diet for control of blood glucose for patient with DM
   (3) Cessation of tobacco use
   (4) Limitation of alcohol consumption to one to two alcoholic beverages daily
   (5) Regular aerobic exercise in moderation
   (6) Complementary therapies: relaxation; imagery, biofeedback
   (7) Stress reduction
   (8) Yearly flu and pneumococcal vaccines
   (9) Recognition of symptoms of HF and when to call the physician
   (10) Measurement of body weight is the best way to monitor when to initiate and titrate diuretic therapy
      (a) Teach the patient to notify the physician if the patient gains 2 lb/day for more than 2 days or a total of 5 lb in 1 week.
b. Pharmacologic agents
   (1) Prescribed medication regimen for HF
   (2) Control of hypertension, hyperlipidemia, DM, and thyroid disorders
   (3) Avoidance of drugs that may worsen HF: NSAIDs

10. Provide collaborative management specific to RVF (cor pulmonale)
   a. Treat the cause.
      (1) Hypoxemia: oxygen to maintain SaO_2 of at least 90%
      (2) Pulmonary embolism
         (a) Anticoagulants
         (b) Fibrinolytic drugs RVF and/or refractory hypoxemia
   b. Pulmonary vasodilators (e.g., nitric oxide or epoprostenol [Flolan]) may be indicated depending on etiology.

Cardiomyopathy

Definition

Disorder involving the structure and function of the myocardium (Figure 3-21)

Dilated (previously called *congestive*)

1. Etiology
   a. Idiopathic
   b. Infection, especially viral (e.g., coxsackievirus B and arbovirus)
   c. Toxins (e.g., doxorubicin [Adriamycin], daunorubicin [Cerubidine], alcohol, lead, arsenic, and cobalt)
   d. Electrolyte, vitamin, or nutrient deficiency
      (1) Hypokalemia
      (2) Hypocalcemia
      (3) Hypophosphatemia
      (4) Thiamine deficiency
   e. Pregnancy
   f. Neuromuscular disorders (e.g., myasthenia gravis or muscular dystrophy)
   g. Connective tissue disorders (e.g., lupus or scleroderma)
   h. Infiltrative disorders (e.g., sarcoidosis or amyloidosis)
   i. Hyperthyroidism
2. Pathophysiology
   a. Damage to myofibrils causing a decrease in contractility and systolic dysfunction
   b. Preload and afterload increased by stimulation of the renin-angiotensin-aldosterone system
   c. Gross dilation of heart, often affecting all four chambers
   d. Refractory HF
3. Clinical presentation
   a. Subjective
      (1) Fatigue, weakness
      (2) Chest pain
      (3) Palpitations
      (4) Syncope
      (5) Symptoms of HF: dyspnea; edema

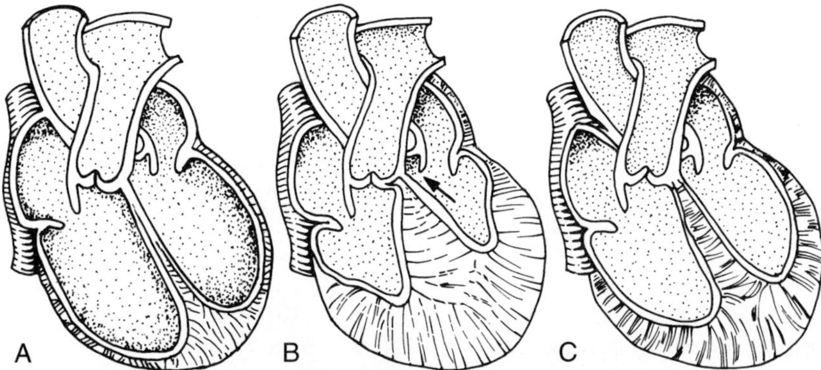

Figure 3-21 Cardiomyopathies. **A**, Dilated. **B**, Hypertrophic. **C**, Restrictive. (From Kinney, M. R., Packa, D. R., & Dunbar, S. B. [1993]. *AACN'S clinical reference for critical-care nursing* [3rd ed.]. St. Louis: Mosby.)

b. Objective
  (1) Orthostatic BP changes
  (2) May have murmurs of tricuspid and/or mitral regurgitation
  (3) Signs of biventricular failure
    (a) LVF: S_3; crackles; PMI displaced laterally
    (b) RVF: JVD; peripheral edema; hepatomegaly
c. Diagnostic
  (1) Chest x-ray
    (a) Cardiomegaly
    (b) Pulmonary congestion
    (c) Possibly pleural effusion
  (2) Electrocardiography
    (a) Biventricular hypertrophy, biatrial enlargement
    (b) Dysrhythmias: AF common
    (c) Blocks: BBB may be seen
  (3) Echocardiography
    (a) Decreased ventricular wall motion
    (b) Decreased EF
    (c) Enlarged chamber size
    (d) Abnormal wall motion
  (4) Cardiac catheterization
    (a) Elevated PAP, left atrial pressure (LAP), left ventricular end-diastolic pressure (LVEDP)
    (b) Decreased cardiac output
    (c) Decreased EF
    (d) Mitral and/or tricuspid regurgitation
    (e) RAP, RVEDP may be elevated if RVF present

4. Nursing Diagnoses (see Appendix A)
  a. Decreased Cardiac Output related to decreased contractility
  b. Impaired Gas Exchange related to intraalveolar fluid
  c. Fluid Volume Excess related to maladaptive compensatory mechanism resulting from decreased cardiac output
  d. Activity Intolerance related to decreased tissue oxygenation
  e. Anxiety related to health alteration and recommended lifestyle changes
  f. Interrupted Family Processes related to change in health status and potential life-threatening situation
  g. Deficient Knowledge related to disease process, therapy, and recommended lifestyle changes
5. Collaborative management
  a. Provide care as for HF.
    (1) Oxygen by nasal cannula at 2 to 6 L/min to maintain SaO_2 of 95% unless contraindicated
    (2) ACE inhibitor (e.g., captopril)
    (3) Beta-blocker (e.g., metoprolol) or alpha- and beta-blocker (e.g., carvedilol) may be prescribed
    (4) Vasodilators (e.g., nitrates)
    (5) Diuretics (e.g., furosemide)
    (6) Inotropes (e.g., digoxin) may be required
    (7) CRT: atriobiventricular pacing
  b. Decrease myocardial oxygen consumption.
    (1) Activity restrictions
    (2) Sodium restrictions
    (3) Physical comfort: temperature; lighting; noise control
    (4) Anxiolytic drugs as prescribed and indicated: usually diazepam (Valium); lorazepam (Ativan); or alprazolam (Xanax)
  c. Monitor for complications.
    (1) Dysrhythmias
      (a) AF: digoxin
      (b) Ventricular dysrhythmias: antidysrhythmic agents (e.g., amiodarone), AICD
    (2) Systemic emboli: anticoagulation frequently prescribed especially for patients with EFs less than 30%
  d. Assist in preparation of the patient for mitral valve replacement or cardiac transplantation as requested

Hypertrophic (previously called *idiopathic hypertrophic subaortic stenosis [IHSS]*)

1. Etiology
  a. Idiopathic
  b. Heredity: genetically transmitted autosomal dominant trait
  c. Neuromuscular disorders
  d. Hypoparathyroidism
2. Pathophysiology
  a. Hypertrophy of heart muscle, including ventricular septum and ventricular free wall
  b. Rigid, noncompliant ventricles will not stretch to fill, causing diastolic dysfunction with a decrease in preload and cardiac output
  c. Mitral regurgitation caused by papillary muscles and mitral valve pulled out of alignment
  d. With severe hypertrophy, left ventricular outflow tract obstruction, especially when contractility is increased by increase in circulating catecholamines
  e. Decrease in blood flow to coronary arteries (angina) and brain (syncope)
  f. Sudden cardiac death may result
3. Clinical presentation
  a. Subjective
    (1) Dyspnea, orthopnea, paroxysmal nocturnal dyspnea (PND)
    (2) Chest pain
    (3) Palpitations
    (4) Syncope
  b. Objective
    (1) PMI displaced laterally
    (2) Crackles
    (3) S_4
    (4) Murmurs
      (a) Subaortic stenosis: systolic ejection murmur loudest along left sternal border;

increases with Valsalva maneuver, decreases with squatting position
(b) Mitral regurgitation: holosystolic blowing murmur loudest at apex radiates to axilla
c. Diagnostic
(1) Chest x-ray
(a) Left atrial dilation
(b) Cardiomegaly
(c) Pulmonary congestion
(2) Electrocardiography
(a) Left atrial enlargement and left ventricular hypertrophy
(b) ST and T wave abnormalities
(c) Dysrhythmias
(i) AF frequently seen
(ii) Ventricular dysrhythmias may be seen
(d) Blocks: left anterior hemiblock frequently seen
(3) Echocardiography
(a) Left atrial enlargement
(b) Increased thickness of the left ventricular free wall and interventricular septum causing narrowing of the left ventricular outflow tract
(c) Abnormal wall motion especially of septum
(d) Mitral regurgitation possible
(4) Cardiac catheterization
(a) Elevated LVEDP
(b) Mitral regurgitation may be evident
(c) Left ventricular outflow pressure gradient
4. Nursing Diagnoses (see Appendix A)
a. Ineffective Cardiopulmonary and Cerebral Tissue Perfusion related to ventricular outflow obstruction
b. Decreased Cardiac Output related to pump failure
c. Anxiety related to health alteration and recommended lifestyle changes
d. Interrupted Family Processes related to change in health status and potential life-threatening situation
e. Deficient Knowledge related to disease process, therapy, and recommended lifestyle changes
5. Collaborative management
a. Prevent obstruction of the left ventricular outflow tract.
(1) Administer beta-blockers and/or calcium channel blockers as prescribed to decrease contractility and myocardial oxygen consumption; these agents also decrease the heart rate to improve ventricular filling.
(2) Avoid inotropic agents, which would increase the outflow tract obstruction.
(3) Prepare patient for percutaneous or surgical procedures as requested.
(a) Percutaneous transluminal septal myocardial ablation (PTSMA)
(i) Perform PCI to isolate the septal perforator branch of the left anterior descending coronary artery, and inject 98% ethanol to cause selective infarction of a portion of the septum to prevent movement of the septum toward the left ventricular free walls to keep the outflow tract open.
a) Contraindications include inadequate septal thickness, RBBB, mitral valve disease, greater than 50% occlusion of the RCA.
(ii) Temporary pacemaker is usually in place for 24 to 48 hours.
(iii) CK-MB and troponin should peak 7 hours after ablation.
(iv) IV or oral analgesics may be required.
(v) Care is as for any other PCI along with monitoring for dysrhythmias, heart blocks, stroke, cardiac tamponade, and hypotension.
(b) Ventricular septal myectomy
(i) Surgical removal of a portion of the hypertrophied septum
(ii) Requires thoracotomy and cardiopulmonary bypass
(iii) Mitral valve usually replaced concurrently
(iv) Complications include septal perforation, blocks, and dysrhythmias along with the complications of cardiac surgery with cardiopulmonary bypass
(c) Dual-chamber pacing
(i) Shortening of the AV interval minimizes contraction of the septum and decreases the outflow tract obstruction
(ii) Usually used along with pharmacologic agents
b. Maintain adequate filling volumes.
(1) Administer IV fluids as prescribed.
(2) Administer beta-blockers and calcium channel blockers to decrease the heart rate, allowing more time for filling.
(3) Use caution or avoid drugs that decrease preload, such as venous vasodilators and diuretics.
c. Monitor for complications.
(1) Dysrhythmias
(a) Atrial: digoxin is not used because it may increase outflow tract obstruction; diltiazem or verapamil may be used
(b) Ventricular: antidysrhythmic drugs (e.g., amiodarone)
(2) Systemic emboli: anticoagulants frequently prescribed, especially for patients with EFs less than 30%
d. Assist in preparation of the patient for cardiac transplantation as requested

Restrictive

1. Etiology
a. Idiopathic

   b. Infiltrative disorders (e.g., sarcoidosis or amyloidosis)
   c. Endomyocardial fibrosis
   d. Glycogen deposition
   e. Radiation
   f. Lymphoma
   g. Connective tissue disorders (e.g., scleroderma)
2. Pathophysiology
   a. Fibrous tissue infiltrates myocardium, endocardium, and subendocardium
   b. Heart becomes noncompliant and cannot stretch, fill, or contract well
   c. Decreased preload and contractility
   d. Decreased CO
   e. HF
3. Clinical presentation
   a. Subjective
      (1) Chest pain
      (2) Fatigue, weakness
      (3) Dyspnea, orthopnea, PND
   b. Objective
      (1) Signs of RVF: JVD, hepatomegaly, peripheral edema, right-sided S_3
      (2) Also may have signs of LVF: left-sided S_3, crackles
   c. Diagnostic
      (1) Chest x-ray
         (a) Cardiomegaly
         (b) Pulmonary congestion
         (c) Possibly pleural effusion
      (2) Electrocardiography
         (a) Low QRS complex voltage
         (b) AV blocks are common
      (3) Echocardiography
         (a) Atrial enlargement
         (b) Enlarged ventricular outside dimension but small ventricular chamber
         (c) Pericardial effusion may be evident
      (4) Cardiac catheterization: elevated RAP, RVEDP, PAP, LAP, LVEDP
4. Nursing Diagnoses (see Appendix A)
   a. Decreased Cardiac Output related to inability of the heart to stretch and fill
   b. Fluid Volume Excess related to maladaptive compensatory mechanism resulting decreased cardiac output
   c. Activity Intolerance related to pump failure
   d. Anxiety related to health alteration and recommended lifestyle changes
   e. Interrupted Family Processes related to change in health status and potential life-threatening situation
   f. Deficient Knowledge related to disease process, therapy, and recommended lifestyle changes
5. Collaborative management
   a. Treat the cause, which may include use of steroids.
   b. Provide care as for HF.
      (1) Oxygen by nasal cannula at 2 to 6 L/min to maintain Sao_2 of 95% unless contraindicated
      (2) ACE inhibitors (e.g., captopril)
      (3) Beta-blockers (e.g., metoprolol)
      (4) Vasodilators (e.g., nitrates)
      (5) Diuretics (e.g., furosemide)
      (6) Inotropes (e.g. digoxin)
   c. Monitor for complications.
      (1) Dysrhythmias
         (a) AF: digoxin
         (b) Ventricular dysrhythmias: antidysrhythmic agents (e.g., amiodarone)
      (2) AV blocks: pacemaker may be needed
      (3) Systemic emboli: anticoagulants frequently prescribed, especially for patients with EFs less than 30%
   d. Assist in preparation of the patient for cardiac transplantation as requested

Indications for Cardiac Transplantation

For more information about organ transplantation, see Chapter 8.

1. Heart disease
   a. Severe functional limitations
   b. Poor prognosis
   c. Not surgically correctable
   d. Unresponsive to medical therapy
   e. Pulmonary vascular resistance (PVR) normal or reversible with therapy (if PH is severe and irreversible, the patient may be a candidate for a heart-lung transplant)
2. Age of 70 years of less
3. Lack of intrinsic disease in other organ systems that would limit long-term survival or would be worsened by immunosuppressive therapy
4. Favorable psychosocial profile
5. Blood negative for HIV and HBV

Pulmonary Hypertension

Definition

Abnormal elevation of the pressure in the blood vessels of the lungs

Etiology

1. Primary PH
   a. Idiopathic; risk factors include the following:
      (1) Usually seen in women between the age of 20 and 40 years
      (2) Oral contraceptives, elevated catecholamines, and hepatic dysfunction are contributing factors
   b. May be sporadic or familial
2. Secondary
   a. Passive: pulmonary venous congestion caused by LVF liver disease
   b. Obstructive: pulmonary embolism
   c. Vasoconstrictive: hypoxemic pulmonary vasoconstriction; sleep apnea
   d. Obliterative: interstitial lung disease; connective tissue disease; HIV
   e. Hyperkinetic: congenital heart disease with left-to-right shunt
   f. Drug-related: fen-phen (phentermine with fenfluramine or dexfenfluramine)

Pathophysiology

1. Primary
   a. Vasoconstriction, hypertrophy of the vascular smooth muscle along with formation of fibrous constriction around the vessels, and thrombosis
   b. Small pulmonary arteries become narrowed or obliterated
   c. Increase in pulmonary vascular resistance
   d. Increase in the workload on the right ventricle
   e. Right ventricular hypertrophy and, eventually, failure
2. Secondary
   a. Active: Hypoxemia causes constriction of the pulmonary vasculature (referred to as *hypoxemic pulmonary vasoconstriction*), which increases the workload on the right ventricle and eventually right ventricular hypertrophy and failure.
   b. Passive: Back pressure from a failing left ventricle or mitral valve disease causes pulmonary vascular engorgement, increase in pulmonary pressures, increase in the workload on the right ventricle and eventually right ventricular hypertrophy and failure.

Clinical Presentation

1. Subjective
   a. Dyspnea; initially exertional progressing to dyspnea with mild exertion to dyspnea at rest
   b. Fatigue, lethargy
   c. Chest discomfort
   d. Palpitations
   e. Syncope
   f. Cyanosis may be present
2. Objective
   a. Tachypnea
   b. Use of accessory muscles
   c. Cough; may exhibit hemoptysis
   d. Accentuated P_2: the second component of S_2
   e. May have clinical indications of right ventricular hypertrophy (RVH): right ventricular heave; right-sided S_4
   f. May have clinical indications of RVF: JVD, peripheral edema, hepatomegaly, murmur of tricuspid regurgitation
3. Diagnostic
   a. Hemodynamic monitoring
      (1) Diastolic PAP more than 5 mm Hg greater than PAOP
      (2) PAP greater than 30/15 mm Hg
      (3) PAP mean greater than 25 mm Hg at rest or greater than 30 mm Hg with activity
      (4) Pulmonary vascular resistance more than 250 dynes/sec/cm^{-5}
   b. Serum
      (1) Hemoglobin and hematocrit may be elevated; polycythemia is caused by erythropoietin release triggered by hypoxemia.
      (2) Liver function studies may be elevated.
      (3) Arterial blood gases may be normal at rest, but hypoxemia occurs with exertion; eventually hypoxemia occurs at rest.
   c. Chest x-ray: may show cardiomegaly, dilated central pulmonary vessels
   d. Electrocardiography: right atrial enlargement, right ventricular strain and hypertrophy
   e. Echocardiograms: used to evaluate heart size, function, and blood flow
   f. Ventilation-perfusion scan: used to evaluate for presence of pulmonary embolism
   g. Cardiac catheterization: elevated right heart and pulmonary pressures

Nursing Diagnoses (see Appendix A)

1. Decreased Cardiac Output related to increased workload on the right ventricle and RVF leading to low left ventricular preload
2. Impaired Gas Exchange related to PH
3. Fluid Volume Excess related to RVF
4. Risk for Fluid/Electrolyte Imbalance related to increased body fluid, decrease in renal perfusion, diuretic therapy, and sodium restriction
5. Activity Intolerance related to decreased cardiac output, decrease in tissue oxygen delivery, and deconditioning
6. Sleep Deprivation related to dyspnea and anxiety
7. Anxiety related to acute health alteration and recommended lifestyle changes
8. Interrupted Family Processes related to change in health status and potential life-threatening situation
9. Knowledge Deficit related to unfamiliarity with disease process, therapy, and recommended lifestyle changes

Collaborative Management

1. Treat cause if possible.
   a. Oxygen for hypoxemia; maintain $Sa{O_2}$ greater than 90%
   b. Fibrinolytic drugs or pulmonary embolectomy if caused by pulmonary emboli
   c. Phlebotomy may be performed for patients with significant polycythemia
   d. Discontinue any causative drug.
2. Decrease pulmonary vascular pressures.
   a. Anticoagulants: warfarin (Coumadin) to maintain INR between 2 to 3
   b. Pulmonary vasodilators may be prescribed
      (1) Calcium channel blockers (e.g., nifedipine [Procardia] or diltiazem [Cardizem]) may be prescribed
      (2) Prostacyclin
         (a) A prostaglandin with potent vasodilatory effects along with platelet aggregation inhibition
         (b) Monitor for chest pain, bradycardia, syncope, and severe headache
         (c) Do not discontinue abruptly
         (d) Agents
            (i) Epoprostenol [Flolan]
               a) Administered intravenously; being investigated for inhalation use

b) Requires refrigeration; infusion requires the use of gel ice packs to keep the solution between 36° and 45° F
(ii) Treprostinil sodium (Remodulin)
a) Administered subcutaneously via a microinfusion pump; monitor for pain, local reaction at injection site
b) Stable at room temperature
c) Longer half-life than epoprostenol
(3) Bosentan (Tracleer) may be prescribed
(a) May be administered intravenously or orally
(b) Endothelin receptor antagonist
(c) Monitor liver function studies
(4) Nitric oxide by inhalation
(a) Local vasodilator
(b) Monitor closely for methemoglobinemia
(5) Sildenafil (Viagra): being investigated for use in PH
3. Provide treatment for HF if present.
a. Diuretics may be required for congestive symptoms
b. Digoxin if concurrent LVF is present
c. Sodium restriction to 2 to 3 g/day
4. Prepare patient for surgery as requested.
a. Surgery for treatment of cause (e.g., valve repair or replacement)
b. Balloon dilation atrial septostomy
(1) Palliative treatment for patients with primary PH refractory to vasodilator therapy
(2) Atrial septal defect is created; right-to-left shunting that occurs improves left ventricular filling and cardiac output offsetting the desaturation of the blood that bypassed the lung
c. Lung transplant or heart-lung transplant
(1) Single or double lung transplant is indicated for patients with primary PH who fail to respond to therapy.
(2) Heart-lung transplantation is indicated for patients with left ventricular disease or congenital structural abnormalities.
5. Provide instruction and counseling regarding lifestyle modification and need for pharmacologic therapy.
a. Oxygen therapy
(1) Usually recommended for continuous use
(2) Avoidance of high altitude, which would decrease the driving pressure of oxygen and worsen hypoxemia; oxygen should be used when flying
b. Low (2 to 3 g) sodium diet
c. Cessation of nicotine use
d. Moderate exercise avoiding overexertion
e. Energy conservation methods
f. Avoidance of drugs that may accentuate PH, cause thrombogenesis, or interfere with anticoagulant therapy: oral anticoagulants (pregnancy should be avoided, so another method of birth control is recommended); decongestants; aspirin and NSAIDs, herbal medications

Acute Inflammatory Heart Disease

Pericarditis

1. Definition: inflammatory process involving the visceral or parietal pericardium
2. Etiology
a. Idiopathic: most common cause
b. MI
(1) Acute: usually occurs within 7 days; related to inflammation and the healing process
(2) Subacute (referred to as *Dressler's syndrome*): occurs later (usually 2 weeks or more); thought to be an autoimmune response
c. Trauma
d. After cardiotomy or thoracotomy
e. Connective tissue diseases (e.g., systemic lupus erythematosus, scleroderma, or rheumatoid arthritis)
f. Infection: viral or bacterial (e.g., tuberculosis)
g. Malignancy
h. Dissecting thoracic aortic aneurysms
i. Radiation therapy
j. Uremia
k. Myxedema
l. Drugs: procainamide (Pronestyl); hydralazine (Apresoline); minoxidil (Loniten); phenytoin (Dilantin); daunorubicin (Cerubidine); isoniazid (INH); penicillin
3. Pathophysiology
a. Inflammation of the layers of the pericardium occurs.
b. Increased capillary permeability caused by inflammation may cause fluid leak into the pericardial space; cardiac tamponade is possible.
(1) As little as 50 to 100 mL may cause cardiac tamponade if the fluid accumulation is acute and rapid (e.g., trauma or after cardiotomy).
(2) As much as 2 L may not cause cardiac tamponade if the fluid accumulation is chronic and slow (e.g., uremia with pleural effusion).
c. If scarring, thickening, and fibrosis of the pericardium occurs, constrictive pericarditis develops.
d. Either constrictive pericarditis or cardiac tamponade decreases diastolic filling of the heart, causing systemic and/or pulmonary venous congestion and decreased cardiac output and cardiac index, leading to shock.
4. Clinical presentation
a. Subjective
(1) Precordial or left pleuritic chest pain
(a) Persistent sharp or stabbing pain
(b) Radiates to the left shoulder, neck, or abdomen

(c) Aggravated by inspiration, cough, and supine position
(d) Relieved by sitting up and/or leaning forward: referred to as *Mohammed's sign*
(2) Hoarseness, dysphagia, and dyspnea if pericardial effusion compresses adjacent structures
(3) Cough
(4) Hemoptysis
b. Objective
(1) Tachypnea
(2) Tachycardia
(3) Fever, malaise
(4) Heart sound changes
(a) Pericardial friction rub
(b) Muffled heart sounds if pericardial effusion or cardiac tamponade occur
(c) Pericardial knock (loud, early-diastolic sound heard best at lower LSB) may be heard if constrictive pericarditis occurs
c. Diagnostic
(1) Serum
(a) White blood cell (WBC) count: increased
(b) Sedimentation rate: increased
(c) C-reactive protein: increased
(d) CK-MB and troponin: negative
(e) ANA: positive if due to connective tissue disease
(f) Blood cultures: positive if due to infection
(2) Chest x-ray
(a) Pericardial effusion causes water bottle silhouette
(b) Pleural effusion and pulmonary infiltrates may be seen
(3) Electrocardiography
(a) Diffuse concave ST segment elevation in all leads except aVL, aVR, and V_1; upright T waves; no Q waves
(b) PR segment depression
(c) Low voltage if pericardial effusion
(d) Dysrhythmias: AF, atrial flutter, premature atrial contractions, paroxysmal atrial tachycardia
(4) Echocardiography
(a) Pericardial effusion may be seen
(b) If constrictive pericarditis: pericardial thickening or calcification
(5) CT or MRI: pericardial effusion; thickened or calcified pericardium in constrictive pericarditis
(6) Pericardial fluid analysis
5. Nursing Diagnoses (see Appendix A)
a. Pain related to pericardial inflammation
b. Ineffective Breathing Patterns related to guarding because of chest pain
c. Risk for Decreased Cardiac Output related to decreased preload and contractility with cardiac tamponade
d. Interrupted Family Processes related to change in health status
6. Collaborative management
a. Relieve pain and discomfort.
(1) Semi-Fowler or high Fowler's positions
(2) NSAIDs
(a) Aspirin
(b) Indomethacin (Indocin)
(3) Steroids if no response to NSAIDs or if effusion present
(4) Narcotic analgesics if necessary
b. Administer drugs and therapies for treatment of cause.
(1) Antibiotics if bacterial
(2) Steroids if connective tissue disorders
(3) Dialysis for uremia
(4) Thyroid hormone replacement for myxedema
(5) Withdrawal of suspect drugs
c. Discontinue anticoagulants as ordered.
(1) If anticoagulants must be continued, heparin will be used because it is much easier to reverse than dicumarol.
(2) If anticoagulants are not discontinued, monitor the patient closely for clinical indications of cardiac tamponade.
d. Monitor for complications.
(1) Dysrhythmias
(2) Constrictive pericarditis
(3) Cardiac tamponade: see Cardiac Tamponade.
(4) HF
e. Assist in preparation of patient for surgical procedures
(1) Pericardiocentesis and biopsy if etiology unclear, if purulent pericarditis suspected, or if cardiac tamponade occurs
(2) Pericardial resection
(a) Pericardial window: for recurrent effusion
(b) Pericardiectomy: if constrictive pericarditis

Myocarditis

1. Definition: inflammation of the myocardium
2. Etiology
a. Viral infections (e.g., coxsackievirus A and B [most common cause], poliomyelitis, influenza, rubella, rubeola, adenoviruses, or echoviruses)
b. Bacterial infections (e.g., diphtheria, tuberculosis, typhoid fever, tetanus, staphylococcus, pneumococcal, or gonococcal infections)
c. Parasitic infections (e.g., trypanosomiasis or toxoplasmosis)
d. Helminthic infections (e.g., trichinosis)
e. Fungal infections (e.g., candidiasis or aspergillosis); usually seen in patients with immunosuppression
f. Hypersensitivity reactions (e.g., rheumatic fever, postcardiotomy syndrome)
g. Radiation therapy to the chest
h. Chronic alcoholism
3. Pathophysiology
a. Three stages
(1) I: viral infection triggers the immune response, which should attenuate viral proliferation

(2) II: autoimmunity
(a) If the immune system does not down-regulate after viral proliferation is controlled, autoimmune disease occurs.
(b) T cells target the patient's own tissue.
(c) Cytokine activation and cross-reacting antibodies may accelerate the process further.
(3) III: dilated cardiomyopathy may occur
(a) Caused by the direct effect of coxsackie viral protease, cytokines such as tumor necrosis factor activating proteinases, and the effect of viruses on the myocyte
(b) Ventricular dilation and remodeling occurs
(c) Progressive HF develops, which may cause death or necessitate cardiac transplantation
b. Damage to myocardium may be diffuse to focal
(1) Diffuse injury frequently causes HF
(2) Focal injury may cause necrosis of portions of the conduction system and blocks
4. Clinical presentation
a. Subjective
(1) Chest soreness, burning, or pressure: increased by inspiration and supine position
(2) Easy fatigability
(3) Syncope
(4) Clinical indications of upper respiratory or gastrointestinal viral infection
(5) Sudden, unexplained dyspnea, orthopnea, PND
b. Objective
(1) Fever
(2) Crackles
(3) Heart sound changes
(a) Distant heart sounds
(b) S_3, S_4
(c) Murmur of mitral regurgitation may be heard
(d) Pericardial friction rub may be heard
c. Diagnostic
(1) Serum
(a) WBC count: increased
(b) CK-MB and troponin: may be increased
(c) Sedimentation rate: increased
(2) Chest x-ray
(a) Cardiomegaly
(b) Pleural or pericardial effusion
(c) Pulmonary congestion
(3) Electrocardiography
(a) Diffuse ST segment and T wave abnormalities
(b) Low voltage
(c) Left axis deviation
(d) Dysrhythmias: supraventricular or ventricular
(e) Blocks: AV or BBBs
(4) Endomyocardial biopsy: done for definitive diagnosis
(a) Virologic diagnosis
(b) Lymphocyte infiltration
(c) Myocyte necrosis
5. Nursing Diagnoses (see Appendix A)
a. Decreased Cardiac Output related to pump failure
b. Activity Intolerance related to pump failure
c. Anxiety related to health alteration and recommended lifestyle changes
d. Interrupted Family Processes related to change in health status and potential life-threatening situation
e. Deficient Knowledge related to disease process, therapy, and recommended lifestyle changes
6. Collaborative management
a. Administer drugs therapies for treatment of cause.
(1) Antibiotics for bacterial infections
(2) Amphotericin B for fungal infections
(3) Corticosteroids for connective tissue diseases (contraindicated in early infectious viral myocarditis because they may enhance myocardial damage by increasing tissue necrosis and viral replication, and so should not be used)
(4) Withdrawal of offending agent
b. Diminish viral activity during phase I.
(1) Antivirals may be prescribed
(2) Support of the patient's immune system and avoidance of potentially harmful immunosuppression.
(3) Immune globulin and interferon may be prescribed.
c. Modulate the immune response during phase II.
(1) Corticosteroids, azathioprine, cyclosporine, and OKT3 monoclonal antibody may be prescribed.
d. Provide treatment as for dilated cardiomyopathy in phase III.
(1) Decrease myocardial oxygen consumption.
(a) Bed rest and activity restrictions until fever and cardiac symptoms subside
(b) Oxygen by nasal cannula at 2 to 6 L/min to maintain SaO_2 of 95% unless contraindicated
(c) Antipyretics for fever
(d) Sodium restrictions
(e) Physical comfort: temperature control; lighting; noise control
(f) Anxiolytic drugs as prescribed: usually diazepam (Valium); lorazepam (Ativan); or alprazolam (Xanax)
(2) Prevent further ventricular remodeling and clinical deterioration.
(a) ACE inhibitors (e.g., captopril)
(b) Aldosterone antagonists (e.g., spirolactone [Aldactone])
(c) Alpha- and beta-blockers (e.g., carvedilol [Coreg])
(d) Vasodilators (e.g., nitrates)
(e) Diuretics (e.g., furosemide)
(f) IABP may be required
(3) Improve contractility: inotropes.
(a) Dobutamine usually is used initially.

(b) Digitalis may be used especially if supraventricular tachydysrhythmias are present.
(c) Milrinone (Primacor) may be used.
e. Monitor for complications.
(1) Dilated cardiomyopathy
(2) Dysrhythmias
(a) Atrial: may be treated with digoxin, amiodarone, or cardioversion
(b) Ventricular
(i) Usually treated with amiodarone, cardioversion, or defibrillation
(ii) Implantable defibrillator may be used for those with documented life-threatening ventricular dysrhythmias
(3) Blocks: temporary or permanent pacemaker frequently required
(4) Pericarditis: monitor closely for clinical indications of cardiac tamponade
(5) Systemic emboli: anticoagulants may be prescribed; if so, monitor closely for clinical indications of cardiac tamponade

Infective Endocarditis

1. Definition: inflammation of the endocardium, usually occurring in the membranous lining of the heart valves but also may involve cardiac prosthesis
2. Etiology
a. Predisposing factors include the following:
(1) Congenital or acquired valvular heart disease
(a) Septal defects
(b) Bicuspid aortic valve
(c) Mitral valve prolapse (with murmur)
(d) Rheumatic heart disease
(e) Degenerative heart disease
(f) History of endocarditis
(2) Cardiac surgery: especially valve repairs or replacements
(3) Invasive tests or monitoring
(a) Intracardiac catheters (e.g., cardiac catheterization, pulmonary artery catheter, or transvenous pacing catheters)
(b) IV catheters (e.g., central vein catheters or dialysis catheter)
(c) Gastrointestinal or genitourinary procedures (e.g., bladder catheterization)
(d) Gynecologic or obstetric surgeries
(4) Skin, bone, or pulmonary infections
(5) Poor oral hygiene
(6) Dental procedures
(7) IV drug use
(8) Body piercing
(9) Immunosuppressed state (e.g., AIDS, cancer, DM, burns, hepatitis, or immunosuppressive drugs or steroids)
b. Causative agents
(1) Bacteria
(a) *Staphylococcus aureus*
(b) *Streptococcus viridans*
(c) Group A nonhemolytic *Streptococcus*
(d) *Streptococcus pneumoniae* (pneumococcus)
(e) *Staphylococcus epidermidis*
(f) *Streptococcus faecalis* (enterococci)
(g) *Pseudomonas aeruginosa*
(h) *Enterococcus*
(i) *Haemophilus*
(j) *Serratia marcescens*
(2) Fungi
(a) *Aspergillus fumigatus*
(b) *Candida albicans*
(3) Viruses such as coxsackievirus or adenovirus
3. Pathophysiology
a. Infective endocarditis may be described as acute or subacute.
(1) Acute infective endocarditis
(a) Typically a fulminant systemic illness of brief duration
(b) Most frequently occurs with normal valves and causes severe damage to the valves
(c) Organism is usually *Staphylococcus aureus*
(2) Subacute endocarditis
(a) Manifests initially as a flulike illness and progresses slowly
(b) Most frequently associated with already damaged valves (e.g., rheumatic heart disease and mitral valve prolapse)
(c) Outcome is usually good with adequate treatment
(d) Organism is usually *Streptococcus viridans*
b. Infection may affect right-sided or left-sided valves.
(1) Left-sided valves are affected most often, with the aortic valve affected twice as often as the mitral valve.
(2) Right-sided valves are affected more often in IV drug abusers.
c. Bacteria and/or blood products adhere to structural irregularities in the cardiac valves.
d. Lesions form as a result of colonization of bacteria.
(1) These lesions, called *vegetations*, contain bacteria, RBCs, platelets, fibrin, collagen, and necrotic tissue.
e. Valvular tissue is damaged by the vegetations.
f. Valve becomes incompetent and may later scar to become stenotic.
g. Other problems include allergic vasculitis and embolization of vegetations and bacteria.
4. Clinical presentation
a. Subjective
(1) Infectious symptoms (e.g., fever, chills, diaphoresis, malaise, weakness, anorexia, myalgias, arthralgias, and headache)
(2) Chest pain
(3) Abdominal pain
(4) May have symptoms of HF: dyspnea, orthopnea, PND
b. Objective
(1) Fever

(2) Heart sound changes
(a) New or changed murmur
(b) Pericardial friction rub
(3) Confusion or delirium
(4) Embolic or allergic vasculitis signs
(a) Splinter hemorrhages
(b) Petechiae: conjunctiva, chest, abdomen, oral mucosa
(c) Roth's spots: round white lesions on retina
(d) Janeway lesions: flat, painless erythematous lesion on palms, soles of feet, or extremities
(e) Osler's nodes: painful nodules on fingers and toes
(f) Clinical indications of embolic stroke (e.g., hemiparesis or hemiplegia, aphasia, or ataxia)
(5) May have signs of HF: S_3, crackles, JVD; hepatomegaly, splenomegaly, peripheral edema

c. Diagnostic
(1) Serum
(a) WBC count: increased
(b) RBC count: decreased
(c) Hemoglobin: decreased
(d) Sedimentation rate: elevated
(e) Blood cultures: persistently positive
(2) Urine: microscopic hematuria, proteinuria
(3) Chest x-ray
(a) If tricuspid or pulmonic valve
(i) Multiple, bilateral infiltrates primarily in lower lobes
(ii) Infiltrates
(b) If mitral or aortic valve
(i) Cardiomegaly
(ii) Pulmonary congestion
(4) Electrocardiography
(a) Dysrhythmias
(i) Atrial: supraventricular tachydysrhythmias including PAT, AF, and atrial flutter
(ii) Ventricular: PVCs
(b) Blocks: AV blocks or BBBs
(5) Echocardiography: transesophageal is more sensitive and specific than transthoracic
(a) Oscillating intracardiac vegetations
(b) Valve dysfunction

5. Nursing Diagnoses (see Appendix A)
a. Infection related to causative organism
b. Risk for Decreased Cardiac Output related to valvular damage and resultant valve regurgitation
c. Risk for Ineffective Tissue Perfusion related to emboli
d. Interrupted Family Processes related to change in health status and potential life-threatening situation
e. Deficient Knowledge related to unfamiliarity with disease process, therapy, and recommended lifestyle changes

6. Collaborative management
a. Prevent endocarditis.
(1) Persons with valvular heart disease should receive antibiotics prophylactically before intrusive procedures (e.g., dental procedures or cardiac catheterization).
(2) Good hygiene, especially oral, also may help to prevent endocarditis, especially in susceptible persons.
(3) Intrusive procedures should be avoided if possible.
(4) Injection of contaminated substances (e.g., street drugs) should be avoided.
b. Decrease myocardial oxygen consumption
(1) Bed rest and activity restrictions until fever and cardiac symptoms subside
(2) Oxygen by nasal cannula at 2 to 6 L/min to maintain SaO_2 of 95% unless contraindicated
(3) Sodium restrictions
c. Control and treat infection.
(1) Blood cultures
(2) Antibiotics as prescribed
(a) Antibiotic therapy for endocarditis is usually for 4 to 8 weeks' duration.
(b) Long-term antibiotic therapy generally requires central venous catheter placement.
d. Control hyperthermia.
(1) Antipyretics
(2) Cooling measures
e. Maintain hydration: oral or IV fluid as indicated.
f. Monitor for complications.
(1) Extension of the infection with abscess or fistula formation; purulent pericardial effusion
(2) HF, cardiogenic shock, or pulmonary edema may occur as a result of valve perforation or dehiscence, ruptured chordae tendineae, or valvular obstruction by vegetation
(3) Systemic emboli
(a) Monitor for clinical manifestations.
(i) Neurologic: visual field defects; hemiplegia; aphasia; change in level of consciousness; seizures
(ii) Cardiac: chest pain; ECG indicators of ischemia, injury, or infarction
(iii) Pulmonary: tachypnea; dyspnea; hemoptysis; pleuritic chest pain
(iv) Renal: hematuria; flank pain; oliguria
(v) Splenic: pain in upper left quadrant; abdominal rigidity
(vi) Peripheral vascular: pain; pallor; pulselessness; paresthesia; paralysis; polar (coldness)
(b) Maintain hydration.
(c) Administer anticoagulants as prescribed.
(4) Bacterial or mycotic aneurysm (localized abnormal expansion of a vessel resulting from destruction of a part or all of the vessel wall by growth of bacteria or fungus): intracranial, intrathoracic, abdominal, or peripheral
(5) Pericarditis or myocarditis

(6) Dysrhythmias or blocks
(7) Septic shock
g. Assist in preparation of patient for surgery for valve repair or replacement if indicated

Valvular Heart Disease

Definition

An acquired or congenital disorder of a cardiac valve; characterized by stenosis (obstruction) or regurgitation (backward flow) of blood

Mitral Insufficiency (Regurgitation, Incompetence)

1. Etiology
   a. Trauma
   b. Rheumatic heart disease (RHD) or other form of endocarditis
   c. Papillary muscle dysfunction or rupture, rupture of chordae tendineae
   d. Congenital malformation of mitral valve
   e. Mitral valve prolapse (MVP) (also referred to as *Barlow's syndrome* or *floppy mitral valve syndrome*)
   f. LV dilation from LVF
   g. Hypertrophic cardiomyopathy
   h. Marfan syndrome
   i. Calcification of mitral valve leaflets
   j. Scleroderma
   k. Prosthetic valve dysfunction
2. Pathophysiology
   a. Portion of LV volume is ejected back into the LA during ventricular systole because of incompetent mitral valve
      (1) Increased LAP
      (2) Increased PAP
      (3) PH
      (4) RVF (and eventually hypertrophy)
   b. Because the mitral valve does not close, blood enters the left ventricle during the entire phase of diastole (including isovolumetric relaxation); this leads to LVF (and eventually hypertrophy)
3. Clinical presentation
   a. Subjective
      (1) Dyspnea, orthopnea, PND; patient may have cough
      (2) Chest pain may occur but is not common
      (3) Palpitations may occur
      (4) Weakness, fatigue
      (5) Anxiety
   b. Objective
      (1) Tachycardia
      (2) Diaphoresis
      (3) Confusion
      (4) PMI displaced laterally; may be more diffuse
      (5) Crackles may be present
      (6) Heart sound changes
         (a) S_2 may be widely split
         (b) Right-sided S_3 and S_4 may be heard
         (c) Holosystolic murmur: high-pitched, blowing, loudest at apex, and radiates to axilla
      (7) Signs of RVF: JVD; hepatomegaly; peripheral edema
   c. Diagnostic
      (1) Hemodynamic monitoring: PAOP waveform shows large *v* waves
      (2) Chest x-ray
         (a) Cardiomegaly
         (b) Left atrial enlargement
         (c) Left ventricular hypertrophy
         (d) Pulmonary congestion may be present
      (3) Electrocardiography
         (a) Left atrial enlargement
         (b) Left and/or right ventricular hypertrophy
         (c) Dysrhythmias: most frequently AF
      (4) Echocardiography
         (a) Thickening, prolapse, and calcification of mitral valve
         (b) Right ventricular, left atrial, and left ventricular enlargement
      (5) Cardiac catheterization
         (a) Increased left atrial and ventricular pressures
         (b) Regurgitation of blood from the left ventricle to the left atrium

Mitral Stenosis

1. Etiology
   a. RHD
   b. Endocarditis
   c. Congenital
   d. Tumors of left atrium (e.g., atrial myxoma)
   e. Calcification of mitral annulus
2. Pathophysiology
   a. Mitral valve will not open well because of progressive fibrosis, scarring, calcification, or fusion of commissures
   b. LAP increases
   c. Dilation of LA (may cause AF)
   d. PH; pulmonary edema may occur
   e. Right ventricular hypertrophy
   f. RVF
3. Clinical presentation
   a. Subjective
      (1) Dyspnea, orthopnea, PND, crackles
      (2) Cough, hemoptysis
      (3) Fatigue, weakness
      (4) Palpitations
      (5) Dysphagia
      (6) Hoarseness
      (7) Syncope may occur
      (8) Chest pain may occur but is rare
   b. Objective
      (1) Ruddy face (mitral facies)
      (2) Right ventricular heave palpable at sternum
      (3) Heart sound changes
         (a) Loud S_1: referred to as *closing snap*
         (b) Loud P_2
         (c) Right-sided S_3 and S_4

(d) Opening snap
(e) Middiastolic murmur: harsh, rumbling, loudest at apex; may have associated thrill
(4) Signs of RVF: JVD; hepatomegaly; peripheral edema
c. Hemodynamic parameters: PAOP waveform shows large *a* waves
d. Diagnostic
(1) Chest x-ray may show the following:
(a) Left atrial enlargement
(b) Pulmonary congestion
(c) Right ventricular hypertrophy
(d) Mitral valve calcification
(2) Electrocardiography
(a) Left atrial enlargement (frequently referred to as *P-mitrale*)
(b) Right ventricular hypertrophy
(c) Dysrhythmias: most frequently AF
(3) Echocardiography
(a) Abnormal movement and thickening of valve leaflets and narrowing of mitral valve orifice
(b) Left atrial enlargement
(c) Right ventricular hypertrophy
(4) Cardiac catheterization
(a) Elevated pressure gradient across mitral valve
(b) Elevated RAP, PAP, LAP

Aortic Insufficiency (Regurgitation, Incompetence)

1. Etiology
a. RHD
b. Calcification
c. Congenital malformation (e.g., bicuspid aortic valve)
d. Endocarditis
e. Syphilis
f. Marfan syndrome
g. Hypertension
h. Connective tissue disease (e.g., lupus erythematosus)
i. Aortic dissection
j. Trauma
2. Pathophysiology
a. Incompetent aortic valve allows blood from the aorta to reenter left ventricle during diastole.
b. LVEDV and LVEDP increase.
c. Left ventricle dilates and fails.
d. Left atrium dilates.
e. PH; pulmonary edema may occur.
f. Low aortic root pressure decreases coronary artery filling pressure, causing myocardial ischemia.
3. Clinical presentation
a. Subjective
(1) Fatigue
(2) Cough
(3) Symptoms of HF: dyspnea; orthopnea; PND
(4) Exertional chest pain
(5) Syncope
(6) Palpitations
b. Objective
(1) Musset's sign: nodding of the head with each systole
(2) Widened pulse pressure
(3) Water-hammer (also called *Corrigan's*) pulse: rapid rise that collapses suddenly
(4) PMI displaced laterally and downward
(5) Hill's sign: popliteal BP is greater than brachial BP by 40 mm Hg or more
(6) Quincke's sign: visible capillary pulsation of nail beds when fingertip is pressed
(7) Signs of HF: S_3, crackles, JVD, hepatomegaly, peripheral edema
(8) Heart sound changes
(a) Diastolic murmur: high-pitched, blowing, decrescendo, loudest at base, may radiate to the apex; may have associated thrill
(b) May have aortic ejection click
(c) Systolic murmur: may have systolic ejection murmur
c. Diagnostic
(1) Chest x-ray
(a) Left atrial enlargement
(b) Left ventricular hypertrophy
(c) Pulmonary congestion
(2) Electrocardiography
(a) Sinus tachycardia
(b) Left ventricular hypertrophy
(c) Left atrial enlargement
(3) Echocardiography
(a) Poor aortic valve motion
(b) Thickening of aortic valve
(c) Left ventricular hypertrophy
(d) Left atrial enlargement
(4) Cardiac catheterization
(a) Elevated LAP, LVEDP
(b) Regurgitation from aorta to left ventricle

Aortic Stenosis

1. Etiology
a. RHD
b. Calcification
c. Congenital bicuspid valve
d. Aortic coarctation
2. Pathophysiology
a. Incomplete aortic valve opening
b. Increased afterload
c. Increased left ventricular workload
d. Left ventricle hypertrophy
e. LVF
f. Left atrial enlargement
g. PH; pulmonary edema may occur
h. RVF
i. Low aortic root pressure decreases coronary artery filling pressure causing myocardial ischemia
3. Clinical presentation
a. Subjective
(1) Chest pain, especially on exertion

(2) Syncope, especially on exertion
(3) Symptoms of LVF: dyspnea; orthopnea; PND
(4) Fatigue, weakness
(5) Palpitations

b. Objective
(1) Narrow pulse pressure
(2) PMI displaced laterally and/or downward
(3) Signs of LVF: S_3; crackles
(4) Heart sound changes
(a) May have split S_1
(b) Paradoxical split of S_2
(c) Systolic ejection murmur: harsh, crescendo/decrescendo, loudest at aortic area radiating to the neck
(d) May have aortic ejection click

c. Diagnostic
(1) Chest x-ray
(a) Calcification of aortic valve may be seen
(b) Cardiomegaly
(c) Left atrial enlargement
(d) Left ventricular hypertrophy
(e) Pulmonary congestion
(f) Right ventricular hypertrophy
(2) Electrocardiography
(a) Left atrial enlargement (P-mitrale)
(b) Left ventricular hypertrophy
(c) Dysrhythmias: most frequently AF
(d) Blocks: AV blocks; LBBB
(3) Echocardiography
(a) Aortic valve leaflet thickening and decreased movement of the leaflets
(b) Calcification of aortic valve
(c) High-pressure gradient between left ventricle and aorta
(d) Left ventricular hypertrophy
(e) Possibly right ventricular hypertrophy
(4) Cardiac catheterization
(a) Significant pressure gradient
(b) Elevated LAP, LVEDP

Nursing Diagnoses (see Appendix A)

1. Decreased Cardiac Output related to pump failure
2. Risk for Injury related to anticoagulant therapy
3. Activity Intolerance related to pump failure
4. Anxiety related to health alteration and recommended lifestyle changes
5. Interrupted Family Processes related to change in health status and potential life-threatening situation
6. Deficient Knowledge to disease process, therapy, and recommended lifestyle changes

Collaborative Management for Valvular Heart Disease

1. Decrease myocardial oxygen consumption.
a. Oxygen by nasal cannula at 2 to 6 L/min to maintain arterial oxygen saturation of 95% unless contraindicated
b. Sodium restrictions
c. Physical comfort: temperature, lighting, noise control
d. Anxiolytic drugs as prescribed: usually diazepam (Valium); lorazepam (Ativan); or alprazolam (Xanax)
2. Provide care for HF.
a. Oxygen at 2 to 6 L/min via nasal cannula as indicated by pulse oximetry and/or arterial blood gases
b. ACE inhibitors (e.g., captopril)
c. Beta-blockers (e.g., metoprolol) may be prescribed
d. Vasodilators (e.g., nitrates) but avoid in severe AS
e. Diuretics (e.g., furosemide) but use with caution in severe AS
f. Inotropic agents
(1) Digitalis may be used especially if supraventricular tachydysrhythmias are present.
(2) Dobutamine or milrinone may be used.
3. Monitor for complications.
a. Dysrhythmias: usually AF
b. Blocks: permanent pacemaker may be necessary
c. Emboli (mural thrombi): potential for pulmonary, cerebral, renal, splenic, mesenteric embolus; antiembolic measures including anticoagulation
d. Endocarditis: prophylactic antibiotics before any invasive procedures, dental procedures for prevention
4. Prepare patient for surgical repair or replacement of the affected valve as requested
a. Valvuloplasty: PCI to repair a valve using a balloon-tipped intracardiac catheter; considered palliative because restenosis rate is high
b. Commissurotomy: surgical separation of the thickened adherent leaves of a stenotic valve (usually mitral)
c. Valve repair: repair of a valve; fibrous pericardium frequently is used
d. Valve replacement
(1) Types of valve replacement
(a) Bioprosthetic valves: last 5 to 10 years
(i) Types
a) Homografts: human cadaver valves that have been specially treated for surgical use
b) Heterograft: valve from an animal, usually a pig or cow, that has been prepared for surgical use
(ii) Anticoagulation
a) Short-term (~3 months after valve replacement) anticoagulation (INR of 2 to 3) is recommended.
b) Long-term anticoagulation is recommended if AF or left atrial thrombus.
(b) Mechanical valves: last 10 to 15 years
(i) Stainless steel, carbon, or other durable material
(ii) Long-term anticoagulation is recommended (INR of 2 to 3.5 depending on type of valve).

(c) Pulmonary autograft (also referred to as *Ross procedure*)
(i) The patient's own pulmonic valve is used to replace the diseased aortic valve with a homograft or heterograft implanted into the pulmonic position.
(2) Postoperative management as for CABG with close monitoring for atrioventricular nodal blocks

Hypertensive Crises

Definitions

1. Hypertension: increase in BP greater than 140/90 mm Hg on at least three separate occasions
2. Hypertensive crisis: rapid rise in BP and occurs when BP elevation is severe enough to cause the threat of immediate vascular necrosis and end organ damage; BP usually greater than 180/120 mm Hg or MAP greater than 150 mm Hg
   a. Hypertensive urgencies: an acute or chronic BP elevation not associated with any observable acute organ damage
      (1) Do not usually require critical care unit admission
      (2) Usually safely treated with oral antihypertensive agents
      (3) May be associated with the following:
         (a) Uncontrolled hypertension in the patient who requires emergency surgery
         (b) Postoperative hypertension
         (c) Severe hypertension following kidney transplant
         (d) Monoamine oxidase (MAO) inhibitor and tyramine interaction
   b. Hypertensive emergencies: an acute elevation of BP that is associated with acute and ongoing organ damage to the kidneys, brain, heart, eyes, or vascular system
      (1) No absolute BP level, but BP is usually greater than 240/140 mm Hg
      (2) BP must be lowered within minutes to a few hours to reduce potential complications of new or progressive end organ damage
      (3) Requires immediate hospitalization in a critical care unit and IV antihypertensive agents
      (4) May be associated with the following:
         (a) Acute aortic dissection
         (b) Acute MI
         (c) Acute LVF with pulmonary edema
         (d) Pheochromocytoma crisis
         (e) Intracranial hemorrhage
         (f) Eclampsia, preeclampsia
         (g) Hypertension associated with severe burns
         (h) Acute glomerulonephritis
         (i) Postoperative CABG
         (j) Withdrawal of antihypertensive drugs
         (k) Substance abuse (e.g., cocaine or methamphetamine)
         (l) Hypertensive encephalopathy: usually associated with BP greater than 250/150 mm Hg

Etiology

1. Primary
   a. Untreated or inadequately treated essential (idiopathic) hypertension
      (1) Risk factors: family history; black race; obesity; hyperlipidemia; diabetes or glucose intolerance; tobacco use; excessive alcohol intake; high-fat and/or high-sodium diet; stress; sedentary lifestyle; aging; oral contraceptives
      (2) Poor compliance frequently a factor in hypertensive crisis; factors closely related to poor compliance include lack of symptoms (i.e., the silent killer), side effects of pharmacologic agents, and costs of pharmacologic agents
      (3) Mechanisms
         (a) Hyperactivity of the SNS: epinephrine and norepinephrine cause increased cardiac contractility and vasoconstriction
         (b) Hyperactivity of the renin-angiotensin-aldosterone system
            (i) Angiotensin causes vasoconstriction and release of aldosterone.
            (ii) Aldosterone causes sodium and water retention.
         (c) Endothelial dysfunction: Endothelin causes vasoconstriction and, along with other persistent vasoconstrictors, leads to hypertrophy of vascular smooth muscle and vascular remodeling.
2. Secondary
   a. Renal disease
      (1) Increased renin-angiotensin levels
         (a) Renin-secreting tumor
         (b) Renovascular disease
      (2) Acute glomerulonephritis
      (3) Chronic pyelonephritis
   b. Eclampsia or preeclampsia of pregnancy
   c. CNS injuries
      (1) Head injury
      (2) Spinal cord injury: Autonomic dysreflexia is hypertension with bradycardia that occurs in patients with spinal cord injury at T6 or above in response to noxious stimuli.
   d. Burns
   e. Drug side effects: oral contraceptives; steroids; cocaine; amphetamines; methamphetamine; decongestants
   f. Drug interactions: MAO inhibitors and tyramine; disulfiram (Antabuse) and alcohol
   g. Drug withdrawal: clonidine; beta-blockers; alcohol
   h. Pheochromocytoma
   i. Polycythemia
   j. Coarctation of the aorta
   k. Pituitary or adrenocortical hyperfunction (e.g., Cushing's syndrome and primary hyperaldosteronism)
   l. Vasculitis
   m. Scleroderma or other connective tissue disease

Pathophysiology

1. Hypertension produces changes in the arterioles and decrease in blood flow to vital organs
   a. Severe hypertension causes necrosis of the intima and media of the arteries
   b. Systolic hypertension now considered to more contributory to left ventricular hypertrophy/failure and stroke than diastolic hypertension
2. Organ ischemia occurs from platelet aggregation, intravascular coagulation, arteriolar spasm, and edema
3. Target organs most likely to be damaged by hypertensive crises
   a. Heart: increased afterload; hypertensive cardiovascular disease; left ventricular hypertrophy and failure; angina; MI
   b. Kidney: decreased renal perfusion; proteinuria; renal failure
   c. Retina: hemorrhages, blindness
   d. Brain: hypertensive encephalopathy
      (1) Excessive cerebral hydrostatic pressure
      (2) When cerebral perfusion pressure exceeds 150 mm Hg, cerebral autoregulation fails
      (3) Increased capillary pressure and permeability
      (4) Vasospasm, ischemia, cerebral edema and hemorrhage

Clinical Presentation

1. General
   a. Significant elevation in BP above normal (Table 3-20)
   b. Epistaxis may occur
2. Cardiovascular involvement may be present.
   a. Chest pain
   b. Signs of left ventricular hypertrophy: PMI displaced to left, S_4, ECG indicators of left ventricular hypertrophy (i.e., deep S in V_1 and V_2 and tall R in V_5 and V_6)
   c. Signs of LVF/pulmonary edema: dyspnea; orthopnea; left ventricular heave; S_3; crackles
3. Renal involvement may be present.
   a. Nocturia
   b. Pressure-related diuresis
   c. Hematuria
   d. Elevated BUN and creatinine
4. Retinal involvement may be present.
   a. Visual disturbances (e.g., blurred vision, reduced visual acuity, photophobia, and temporary loss of vision)
   b. Funduscopic changes (Keith-Wagener-Barker classification)
      (1) Grade I: arteriolar narrowing
      (2) Grade II: focal arteriolar spasm
      (3) Grade III: hemorrhages and exudates
      (4) Grade IV: papilledema
5. Neurologic involvement may be present especially in hypertensive encephalopathy.
   a. Occipital or anterior headache especially in the morning; may be severe
   b. Nausea, vomiting
   c. Seizures
   d. Altered mental status: irritability, confusion, agitation progressing to lethargy and coma
   e. Focal neurologic signs (e.g., cranial nerve palsy, sensory or motor deficits, aphasia; positive Babinski's reflex)
6. Diagnostic
   a. Serum
      (1) Potassium: hypokalemia occurs in primary hyperaldosteronism
      (2) BUN and creatinine may be elevated
      (3) Lipid profile to evaluate additional cardiac risk
      (4) Aldosterone may be elevated
   b. Captopril challenge test: plasma renin level is measured before and 1 hour after 25 mg of captopril (Capoten) to confirm or rule out renovascular hypertension
   c. Urine: hematuria or proteinuria may be present
   d. Chest x-ray
      (1) Cardiomegaly may be present.
      (2) Widening of mediastinum suggests dissecting thoracic aortic aneurysm.
   e. Electrocardiography: may show left atrial enlargement, left ventricular hypertrophy
   f. CT of brain: may show cerebral edema and/or hemorrhage

Table 3-20 New Classification of Blood Pressure Levels according to the Seventh Report of the Joint National Committee on Prevention, Detection, Evaluation, and Treatment of High Blood Pressure (JNC7)

Blood Pressure Category	Systolic (mm Hg)	and/or	Diastolic (mm Hg)
Optimal	Less than 120	and	Less than 80
Normal	Less than 130	and	Less than 85
Hypertensive			
Stage 1	140 to 159	or	90 to 99
Stage 2	160 or greater	or	100 or greater

Modified from Chobanian, A. V., Bakris, G. L., Black, H. R., Cushman, W. C., Green, L. A., Izzo, J. L., Jr., et al. (2003). The Seventh Report of the Joint National Committee on Prevention, Detection, Evaluation, and Treatment of High Blood Pressure: the JNC 7 report. *JAMA, 289*(19), 2560-2572.

Nursing Diagnoses (see Appendix A)

1. Impaired Cardiopulmonary, Cerebral, and Renal Tissue Perfusion related to uncontrolled hypertension and adverse effects of antihypertensive therapy (hypotension)
2. Anxiety related to threat to or change in health status

3. Risk for Ineffective Therapeutic Regimen Management related to complexity of regimen, cost of medication, and side effects of therapy
4. Interrupted Family Processes related to change in health status and potential life-threatening situation
5. Deficient Knowledge related to unfamiliarity with disease process, therapy, and recommended lifestyle changes

Collaborative Management

1. Maintain airway, ventilation, and oxygenation.
   a. Oxygen: 2 to 6 L/minute via nasal cannula
   b. Airway maintenance
      (1) Oropharyngeal or nasopharyngeal airway or ET intubation may be required especially if altered level of consciousness or pulmonary edema
   c. Ventilation: mechanical ventilation may be required especially if neurologic impairment or pulmonary edema
2. Decrease myocardial oxygen consumption.
   a. Activity restriction initially
   b. Sodium restriction to less than 2 g per 24 hours
   c. Smoking cessation
   d. Physical comfort: temperature control; lighting; noise control
   e. Anxiolytic drugs as prescribed: usually diazepam (Valium); lorazepam (Ativan); or alprazolam (Xanax)
3. Decrease BP gradually.
   a. Reduction of MAP by no more than 20% to 25% during the first 2 hours because BP decreased too aggressively may cause neurologic damage by significantly decreasing cerebral perfusion pressure (NOTE: If aortic dissection has occurred, BP is reduced more aggressively but within 5 to 10 minutes.)
      (1) Monitor BP closely.
         (a) An invasive arterial catheter is indicated in hypertensive emergency.
         (b) If neurologic changes occur, BP reduction should be slowed or temporarily stopped.
   b. Antihypertensive agents
      (1) Vasodilators
         (a) NTP (Nipride)
            (i) Mixed arterial and venous vasodilator
            (ii) Usually first-line agent for hypertensive emergency
         (b) Fenoldopam mesylate (Corlopam)
            (i) Arterial vasodilator with dopaminergic stimulation
            (ii) Particularly helpful in patients with postoperative hypertension or renal insufficiency
         (c) NTG
            (i) Effects are dose-dependent
               a) Venous vasodilator at doses of less than 1 mcg/kg/min
               b) Mixed arterial and venous vasodilator when dose greater than 1 mcg/kg/min
            (ii) Particularly helpful in patients with acute coronary syndrome or HF
         (d) Hydralazine (Apresoline)
            (i) Arterial vasodilator
            (ii) Use with caution because this drug may cause severe, prolonged, and uncontrolled hypotension
            (iii) Frequently used for eclampsia
         (e) Nicardipine (Cardene)
            (i) Mixed arterial and venous vasodilator
            (ii) Only calcium channel blocker available for IV use
            (iii) Particularly helpful in postoperative hypertension
            (iv) Contraindicated in HF
         (f) Nifedipine (Procardia)
            (i) Mixed arterial and venous vasodilator
            (ii) Oral agent only; sublingual use concluded by U.S. Food and Drug Administration (FDA) to be neither safe nor efficacious
      (2) Sympathetic blockers
         (a) Alpha-blockers block vasoconstriction
            (i) Phentolamine (Regitine): especially helpful if hypertension is caused by autonomic dysreflexia, because bradycardia contraindicates beta-blocker; also particularly helpful in pheochromocytoma
         (b) Beta-blockers block the reflex tachycardia associated with vasodilators
            (i) Esmolol (Brevibloc): rapid acting, cardioselective beta-blocker
            (ii) Contraindicated in HF and heart block
         (c) Alpha- and beta-blockers: block vasoconstriction and tachycardia
            (i) Labetalol (Normodyne): alpha-blocker and noncardioselective beta-blocker
               a) Particularly helpful in patients with intracranial hypertension because direct vasodilators would increase intracranial volume and pressure
               b) Also used in intraoperative hypertension and aortic dissection
               c) Contraindicated in HF, asthma, and heart block
      (3) ACE inhibitor
         (a) Enalapril (Vasotec) (only IV ACE inhibitor)
         (b) Particularly helpful with HF
      (4) Diuretics: usually loop diuretics (e.g., furosemide [Lasix] or bumetanide [Bumex])
         (a) Use of diuretics is controversial because these patients may have had significant diuresis related to excessive glomerular filtration rate

4. Assist in preparation of patient for surgical procedures to treat cause of hypertension if appropriate.
   a. Angioplasty may be done for renovascular disease.
   b. Adrenalectomy is done for pheochromocytoma after tachycardia and hypertension have been controlled adequately.
5. Monitor for complications.
   a. Cerebral infarction
   b. MI
   c. HF/pulmonary edema
   d. Dissection of aorta
   e. Renal failure
6. Provide instruction and counseling regarding lifestyle modification and need for pharmacologic therapy.
   a. Nonpharmacologic management
      (1) Weight normalization
      (2) Dietary modifications
         (a) Low-fat, no added salt (2 to 3 g/day) diet
         (b) Fresh fruits and vegetables
         (c) Fish, especially fatty fish such as salmon and trout
         (d) Nuts
         (e) Low-fat dairy
         (f) Monounsaturated fatty acids (from extra virgin olive oil)
         (g) Increase potassium, magnesium, and calcium
      (3) Aerobic exercise
      (4) Alcohol moderation (e.g., one glass of wine or equivalent per day)
      (5) Complementary therapies: relaxation, biofeedback, acupuncture, pets
   b. Pharmacologic management
      (1) Indications for pharmacologic management
         (a) Mild hypertension with end organ damage or DM
         (b) Moderate hypertension that has not responded to conservative treatment
         (c) Severe hypertension
      (2) Choice of drug and/or combinations
         (a) Diuretics and beta-blockers are first-line usually
         (b) If HF or DM: ACE inhibitor
         (c) If history of MI: beta-blocker and ACE inhibitor
         (d) If elderly with isolated systolic hypertension: diuretic or calcium channel blocker
         (e) If hypertensive and hypercholesteremic: statin (e.g., pravastatin)

Vascular Disease

Peripheral Arterial Disease

1. Definition: partial or total occlusion of an artery by atherosclerosis/arteriosclerosis obliterans
2. Etiology
   a. Arteriosclerosis/atherosclerosis (same risk factors as in discussion of coronary artery disease)
      (1) Atherosclerosis: most common cause
      (2) Arteriosclerosis: significant cause in older patients
   b. Hypertension
   c. Arteritis
3. Pathophysiology
   a. Most significant occlusion usually occurs at bifurcations (Figure 3-22)
   b. Damage to intima with progressive deterioration and thrombus formation
   c. Partial or complete occlusion
   d. Fontaine classification correlates progression of obstruction and symptomatology
      (1) Stage 1: pathologic changes within the artery but no clinical symptoms
      (2) Stage 2: intermittent claudication; 75% occlusion
      (3) Stage 3: pain at rest; ~90% to 95% occlusion
      (4) Stage 4: necrosis: ~99% to 100% occlusion
4. Clinical presentation
   a. Occlusive disease of terminal aorta and iliac
      (1) Subjective

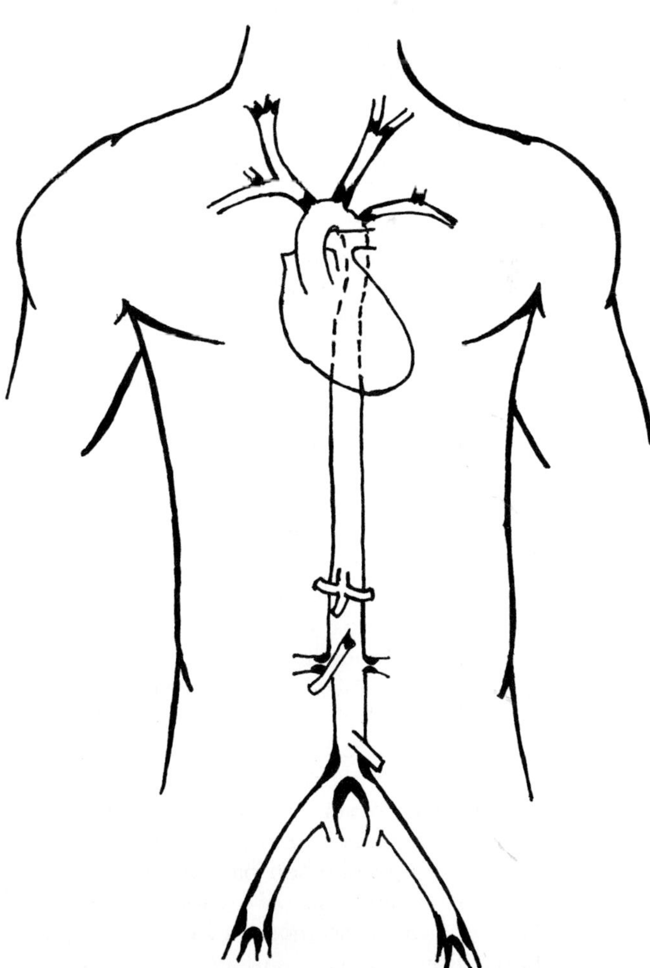

Figure 3-22 Common sites for atherosclerotic plaque deposition. (Drawing by Ann M. Walthall.)

(a) Intermittent claudication in thigh and hip: pain increases with exercise and decreases with rest
(b) Impotence
(2) Objective
(a) Cool lower extremities
(b) Hair loss over lower extremities
(c) Decreased or absent iliac or femoral pulses
(d) Bruit or thrill over iliac area

b. Occlusive disease of femoral and popliteal arteries
(1) Subjective
(a) Intermittent claudication in lower leg progressing to pain at rest
(b) Decreased sensation or paresthesia of lower extremities
(2) Objective
(a) Coolness of lower extremities
(b) Hair loss over lower extremities
(c) Pallor, mottling of lower extremities
(d) Nonhealing ulcers on toes or points of trauma
(e) Decrease motor strength in lower extremities
(f) Decreased or absent femoral and popliteal pulses
(g) Bruit or thrill over femoral or popliteal area
(3) Diagnostic
(a) Arteriography: shows partial or complete arterial occlusion
(b) Doppler and duplex ultrasonography show partial to complete vascular occlusion

5. Nursing Diagnoses (see Appendix A)
a. Risk for Ineffective Breathing Patterns related to incisional pain and retained secretions
b. Risk for Ineffective Peripheral Perfusion related to graft occlusion, hematoma, or bleeding
c. Risk for Infection related to surgery and invasive procedures
d. Pain related to surgery and ischemia
e. Activity Intolerance related to intermittent claudication
f. Risk for Impaired Skin Integrity related to decreased tissue perfusion
g. Anxiety related to health alteration and recommended lifestyle changes
h. Interrupted Family Processes related to change in health status and potential limb-threatening situation
i. Deficient Knowledge related to disease process, therapy, and recommended lifestyle changes

6. Collaborative management
a. Decrease peripheral oxygen requirements
(1) Activity cessation when pain occurs
(2) Bed rest during acute occlusion
(3) Maintenance of normothermia
(4) Prevention of trauma
b. Administer appropriate pharmacologic agents to reestablish blood flow: fibrinolytic drugs (e.g., urokinase; streptokinase; rt-PA)
(1) These agents may be administered locally by an intraarterial infusion or systemically intravenously
(2) Followed by an anticoagulant such as heparin
c. Assist in preparation of the patients for percutaneous procedures aimed at decreasing occlusion (e.g., percutaneous balloon angioplasty, laser angioplasty, or atherectomy); may be accompanied by insertion of flexible coil stent
(1) Postprocedure care is as for PCI.
(2) Monitor catheter insertion site closely for bleeding and/or hematoma formation.
(3) Monitor peripheral perfusion closely; report any indications of arterial occlusion (i.e., six P's) immediately.
(4) Administer anticoagulants and/or platelet aggregation inhibitors as prescribed.
d. Assist in preparation of the patient for surgery aimed at improving flow (Figure 3-23), and provide postoperative management.
(1) Surgical procedures
(a) Arterial embolectomy: removal of an occlusive clot from an artery; frequently accomplished with a balloon-tipped catheter
(b) Thromboendarterectomy: excision of thickened layer of artery; aortofemoral, aortoiliac, or femoropopliteal thromboendarterectomy
(c) Bypass: Graft is anastomosed proximal and distal to the occlusion.
(i) Graft may be autologous vein (usually saphenous), human umbilical vein, or an artificial graft (Dacron or polytetrafluoroethylene).
(ii) Commonly performed bypasses include aortobifemoral, femoral to femoral, femoropopliteal, and femorotibial
(d) Extraanatomical bypass (EAB): prosthetic material is tunneled subcutaneously
(i) May be used femoral to femoral or axillary to femoral
(ii) Used for patients who are high risk for an open abdominal procedure or who have numerous previous surgical procedures or peritonitis (sometimes referred to as a *hostile abdomen*)
(e) Sympathectomy: interruption of sympathetic tract to decrease local vascular resistance to improve local blood flow
(f) Amputation: removal of limb performed only when attempts to revascularize the limb have failed
(2) Postoperative management
(a) Maintain airway, oxygenation, and ventilation.
(i) Assess ventilatory status frequently: rate; rhythm; excursion; effort; use of accessory muscles; presence of stridor

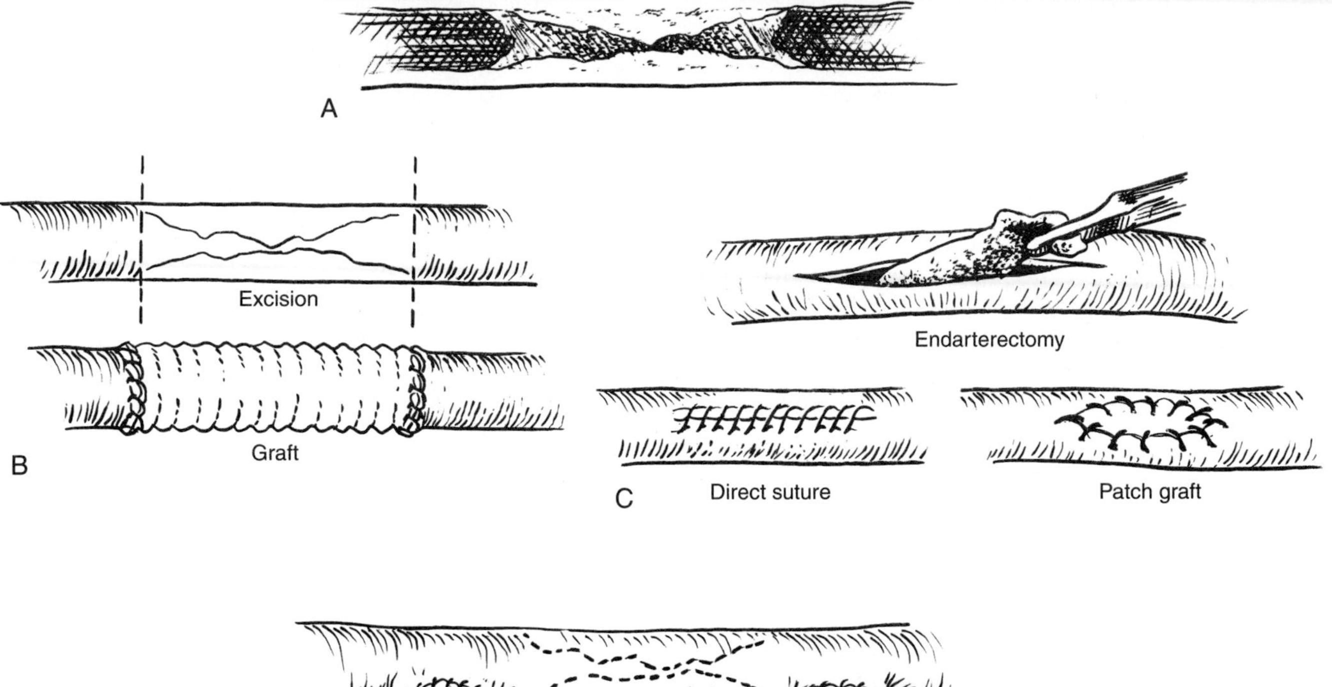

Figure 3-23 Surgical procedures for peripheral vascular disease. **A,** Occluded vessel. **B,** Excision and circumferential graft. **C,** Endarterectomy with direct suture or patch graft. **D,** Bypass graft. (Drawing by Wendy M. Johnson.)

or other adventitious sounds; pulse oximetry.

(ii) Encourage deep breathing and incentive spirometry.

(iii) Assess frequently for edema, hematoma, tracheal deviation, and dysphagia.

(iv) Elevate head of the bed (HOB) 30 degrees.

(v) Have equipment for cricothyroidotomy, tracheostomy, and suction.

(vi) Prevent aspiration: high Fowler's position while eating; NPO until gag reflex returns; suction fluids as necessary.

(vii) Administer oxygen at 2 to 5 L/min as prescribed.

(b) Maintain adequate flow and pressure at graft site.

(i) Maintain and control systolic BP under 120 mm Hg.

a) NTP

b) Nicardipine (Cardene)

c) Analgesics as indicated

(ii) Prevent emboli by using antiembolic techniques.

a) Dextran 40 often is used as platelet aggregation inhibitor.

b) Heparin also may be used.

(iii) Avoid pressure on incision sites.

a) Elevate HOB no greater than 45 degrees for first 72 hours.

b) Elevate legs 20 to 30 degrees.

c) Encourage foot and leg exercises.

d) Mobilize from lying to standing; avoid sitting position and flexing or crossing of legs after femoral artery revascularization.

(iv) EAB specifically

a) Position patient on nonoperative side.

b) Prevent external pressure on graft and avoid flexion of graft.

c) Feel for thrill over graft.

d) Assess for vascular steal: clinical indications of hypoperfusion of limb from which blood was diverted.

e) Monitor for brachial plexus injury if axillofemoral bypass.

(c) Assess for clinical indications of hypoperfusion.

(i) Perform neurovascular assessment of extremities hourly; monitor for pain, pallor, pulselessness, paresthesia, paralysis, polar (cold).

(ii) Measure pressures by Doppler ultrasonography, and calculate ankle-brachial index (ABI).
a) Report any decrease in ABI of 0.15 or more.
b) Do not measure pressure by Doppler ultrasonography if the bypass is performed to the most distal arteries of the leg (painful for the patient and may cause graft compression).
(iii) Maintain normal body temperature: heated blankets or automatic warming blanket, warming lights.
(d) Treat pain.
(i) Administer analgesics as indicated.
(ii) Position patient for comfort.
(e) Prevent skin breakdown related to ischemia and immobility.
(i) Inspect skin, bony prominences, and affected extremities frequently.
(ii) Reposition patient often.
(iii) Use egg crate, alternating air mattress, or special bed depending on other risk factors.
(iv) Keep heels elevated off bed.
(f) Maintain adequate hydration.
(i) Administer IV fluids as indicated.
(ii) Monitor urine output closely, and report urine output of less than 0.5 mL/kg/hr.
(g) Monitor for postoperative complications.
(i) Hemorrhage
(ii) Infection
a) Assess incision and wounds for indications of infection.
b) Monitor WBC count and body temperature.
c) Provide aseptic wound care.
d) Administer antibiotics as prescribed.
(iii) Arterial thrombosis
(iv) Cerebral embolus (blood or plaque)
(v) Peripheral ischemia, infarction, loss of limb
(vi) Graft infection
a) Monitor for fever, malaise, back pain, anorexia, paralytic ileus, and leukocytosis.
b) Administer antibiotics as prescribed.
c) Prepare patient for removal and replacement of graft as requested.
e. Provide instruction and counseling regarding lifestyle modification and need for pharmacologic therapy.
(1) Nonpharmacologic therapies
(a) Weight normalization
(b) Dietary modifications
(i) Low saturated fat
(ii) ADA diet for control of blood glucose for patient with DM
(c) Cessation of tobacco use
(d) Regular aerobic exercise in moderation; should not exercise to the point of pain
(e) Foot care: special attention to any lesions because healing may be impaired by decreased circulation
(f) Avoidance of constrictive clothing
(g) Complementary therapies: relaxation; imagery, biofeedback
(2) Pharmacologic agents
(a) Platelet aggregation inhibitors (e.g., aspirin, clopidogrel [Plavix])
(b) Agents that increase the flexibility of the RBCs: pentoxifylline (Trental)
(c) Peripheral vasodilators
(i) Papaverine: rarely used today
(ii) Cilostazol (Pletal): phosphodiesterase III inhibitor; inhibits platelet aggregation and causes vasodilation
(d) Anticoagulants: warfarin (Coumadin)
(e) Antihypertensives if indicated

Acute Arterial Occlusion

1. Definition: acute complete occlusion of an artery by thrombosis in an already narrowed artery, embolism, or trauma
2. Etiology
a. Arterial embolization
(1) AF
(2) Ventricular aneurysm
(3) Bacterial endocarditis
b. Injury to arterial intima causing arterial thrombosis
(1) Postcardiac catheterization or angioplasty
(2) IABP
(3) Postarterial bypass or aneurysm
c. Compression of artery with swelling
(1) Fracture (compartment syndrome)
(2) Circumferential burn
3. Pathophysiology
a. Occlusion of an artery occurs.
b. Ischemia occurs.
c. Vasoactive factors, such as serotonin, may be released that cause vasospasm and worsen the ischemia.
d. Ischemia progresses to necrosis if not promptly resolved.
4. Clinical presentation
a. Six *P*'s
(1) Pain: severe and sudden
(2) Pallor, cyanosis
(3) Pulselessness
(4) Paresis or paralysis
(5) Paresthesia or anesthesia
(6) Polar
b. Doppler stethoscope indicates diminished or absent blood flow.
c. Diagnostic study: Angiography indicates arterial occlusion.

5. Nursing Diagnoses (see Appendix A)
   a. Risk for Ineffective Peripheral Perfusion related to graft occlusion, hematoma, or bleeding
   b. Risk for Infection related to surgery and invasive procedures
   c. Pain related to surgery and ischemia
   d. Risk for Impaired Skin Integrity related to decreased tissue perfusion
   e. Anxiety related to health alteration and recommended lifestyle changes
   f. Interrupted Family Processes related to change in health status and potential life-threatening surgery
   g. Deficient knowledge related to disease process, therapy, and recommended lifestyle changes
6. Collaborative management
   a. Initiate emergencies measures immediately.
      (1) Oxygen at 2 to 5 L/min to maintain Sao_2 at 95% unless contraindicated
      (2) Proper positioning of limb: Keep extremity straight, warm, and dependent.
      (3) Notification of physician immediately of perfusion defect
      (4) IV infusion of normal saline at keep-vein-open rate in unaffected limb
      (5) Narcotics (e.g., morphine) for pain
   b. Assist in preparation of diagnostic studies: angiogram.
   c. Reestablish patency of artery.
      (1) Intraarterial fibrinolytic (e.g., urokinase or rt-PA) followed by anticoagulant
      (2) Preparation for surgical procedures if indicated
         (a) Procedures
            (i) Surgical embolectomy especially for large arteries
            (ii) Balloon embolectomy
            (iii) Thromboendarterectomy
            (iv) Bypass grafting
      (3) Postoperative care as described in Peripheral Arterial Disease
   d. Explain procedures thoroughly to patient to minimize stress.
   e. Monitor closely for complications.
      (1) Reocclusion
      (2) Loss of limb
      (3) Infection
   f. Provide patient teaching as for peripheral arterial disease.

Aortic Aneurysm

1. Definition: a permanent localized dilation of the aorta with an increase of at least 1.5 times its normal diameter
2. Etiology
   a. Degenerative changes caused by aging or familial predisposition
   b. Congenital weakness of the aorta
   c. Hypertension
   d. Pregnancy: especially third trimester
   e. Coarctation of the aorta
   f. Syphilis
   g. Severe systemic infection (e.g., bacterial aneurysm or mycotic aneurysm)
   h. Marfan syndrome
   i. Trauma: especially blunt trauma with acceleration-deceleration injury
   j. Arterial cannulation (e.g., PCI or IABP)
3. Pathophysiology
   a. Elastin provides elasticity of the vessel wall, and collagen is responsible for mechanical strength; abnormal proteolytic enzyme activity (elastase and collagenase) causes increased synthesis and degradation of elastin and collagen.
   b. Elastin destruction may be the triggering event of aneurysm formation followed by weakening of the collagen, which allows the dilation of the aorta to occur.
   c. An expanding hematoma compresses or occludes the arteries that branch off the aorta and may compress structures.
   d. Hematoma formation in the medial layer causes longitudinal separation of the layers of the aorta (dissection).
      (1) Hypertension is a factor in most dissections.
      (2) As the heart contracts, more blood enters the false lumen and the dissection expands.
      (3) Blood leaking into the pericardial sac may cause cardiac tamponade.
   e. The resultant thin-walled channel can rupture easily and hemorrhage into mediastinal, pleural, or abdominal cavities.
   f. Types (Figure 3-24)
      (1) False: does not involve all layers of the artery; pulsating hematoma that results from arterial trauma such as arterial cannulation
      (2) True: involves all layers of the arterial wall; usually saccular arising from a distinct portion of the wall
      (3) Saccular: outpouching from an artery that results from localized thinning and stretching of the media
      (4) Fusiform: involves the total circumference of the artery with diffuse dilation
      (5) Dissecting: a cavity is formed by dissection by blood between the layers of the arterial wall
      (6) Rupture: artery wall ruptures and leaks arterial blood into the mediastinum if thoracic or into abdominal cavity if abdominal
4. Clinical presentation
   a. Subjective: usually asymptomatic until dissection or rupture occur
   b. Objective
      (1) Normal to high BP; hypotension suggests cardiac tamponade or aortic rupture
      (2) Pulsatile mass
      (3) Increased aortic diameter on palpation
      (4) Bruit over aorta
   c. Specifically ascending thoracic aorta
      (1) May be asymptomatic
      (2) Dyspnea
      (3) Chest pain

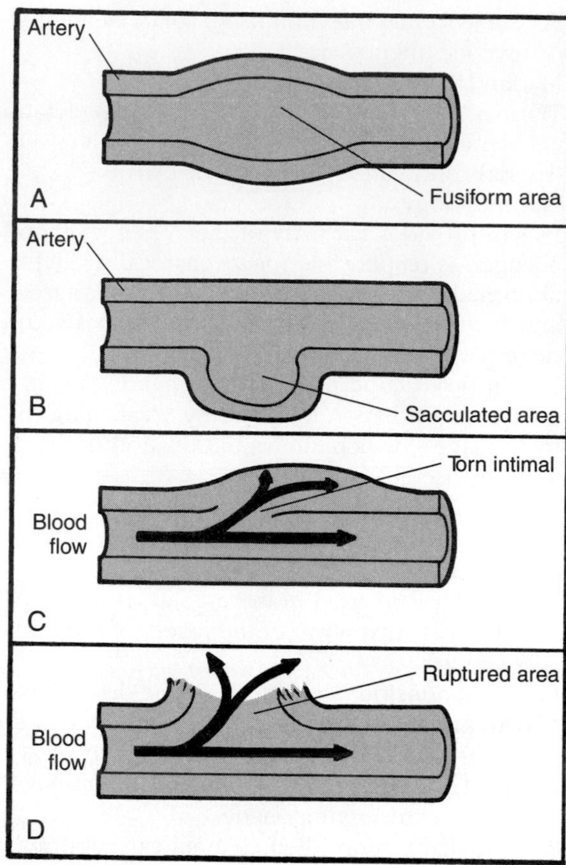

Figure 3-24 Types of aneurysms. **A,** Fusiform. **B,** Saccular. **C,** Dissecting. **D,** Ruptured. (From Urden, L.D., et al. [2005]. *Thelan's critical care nursing: Diagnosis and management* [5th ed.], St. Louis: Mosby.)

(4) Clinical indications of aortic regurgitation: diastolic murmur; LVF; widened pulse pressure

d. Specifically aortic arch
(1) Dyspnea
(2) Stridor
(3) Cough
(4) JVD
(5) Hoarseness
(6) Weak voice

e. Specifically descending thoracic arch
(1) Dull chest pain and upper back pain
(2) Hoarseness

f. Dissecting TAA
(1) Sudden, sharp, tearing, or ripping pain in chest radiating to shoulders, neck, or back
(2) Hypotension
(3) Dyspnea
(4) Syncope
(5) Leg weakness, transient paralysis
(6) May have BP and pulse difference between arms or between arms and legs
(7) May have clinical indications of thrombotic stroke
(8) May have clinical indications of cardiac tamponade (see Cardiac Tamponade)

g. Specifically abdominal aorta
(1) Dull abdominal and back pain
(2) Nausea and vomiting
(3) Abdominal bloating
(4) Pulsation in abdomen

h. Specifically ruptured (AAA)
(1) Severe, sudden, dull, continuous abdominal pain radiating to low back, hips, and scrotum; pain unaffected by movement
(2) Feeling of abdominal fullness
(3) Nausea and vomiting
(4) Syncope and shock
(5) Pulsation in abdomen: periumbilical area

i. Diagnostic
(1) Serum: hemoglobin and hematocrit may be decreased
(2) Chest x-ray
(a) Mediastinal widening in thoracic aneurysm
(b) Aortic calcification
(3) Electrocardiography
(a) May show left ventricular hypertrophy
(b) May show nonspecific ST-T wave changes
(c) Absence of ECG indicators of MI
(4) Transesophageal echocardiography: may show aortic root dilation, intimal flap dividing true and false lumen in dissection
(5) Aortography: lumen of aneurysm; size and location of aneurysm
(6) CT scan, MRI: presence and location of aneurysm
(7) Ultrasound: presence, size, shape, location of aneurysm
(8) Flat plate of abdomen (kidney, ureter, and bladder): outline of aneurysm

5. Nursing Diagnoses (see Appendix A)
a. Risk for Ineffective Breathing Patterns related to incisional pain, retained secretions
b. Risk for Ineffective Tissue Perfusion related to aneurysm dissection and decreased peripheral blood flow
c. Risk for Decreased Cardiac Output related to aneurysm dissection or rupture
d. Fluid Volume Deficit related to vascular disruption
e. Risk for Impaired Skin Integrity related to decreased peripheral blood flow
f. Anxiety related to health alteration and recommended lifestyle changes
g. Interrupted Family Processes related to change in health status and potential life-threatening situation
h. Deficient Knowledge related to disease process, therapy, and recommended lifestyle changes

6. Collaborative management
a. Control pain.
(1) Narcotics are required in rupture or dissection.
(2) Use extreme caution if patient is hypotensive.
b. Maintain and control mean arterial pressure at 60 to 75 mm Hg if dissection occurs.

(1) If patient is hypertensive, administer the following:
   (a) NTP; may be used with propranolol (Inderal)
   (b) Labetalol (Normodyne)
(2) If patient is hypotensive, provide the following:
   (a) IV access: two large-bore, short IV catheters; blood for type and crossmatch
   (b) Normal saline or lactated Ringer's solution by rapid infusion until blood is available; colloids (e.g., albumin, hetastarch, or dextran) also may be used
   (c) Blood and blood products

c. Decrease tissue oxygenation requirements.
   (1) Activity restriction
   (2) Oxygen by nasal cannula at 2 to 6 L/min to maintain Sao_2 of 95% unless contraindicated
   (3) Intubation and mechanical ventilation may be necessary
   (4) Physical comfort: temperature control; lighting; noise control
   (5) Anxiolytic drugs as prescribed: usually diazepam (Valium); lorazepam (Ativan); or alprazolam (Xanax)

d. Assist in preparation of patient for surgical repair.
   (1) Indication for surgical repair: aneurysmal dilation of 5 to 6 cm in diameter; indications for immediate surgical repair include the following:
      (a) Involvement of ascending aorta; aortic insufficiency
      (b) Failure of drug therapy to control progression of dissection as evidenced by continued pain and progressive symptoms
      (c) Cardiac tamponade
      (d) Compromise of a major branch of aorta
      (e) Indications of cerebral or cardiac ischemia
   (2) Procedures
      (a) Surgical procedure: resection of aneurysm and circumferential (fusiform aneurysm) or patch graft (saccular aneurysm)
         (i) Repair of thoracic aortic aneurysm involving the ascending aorta and/or aortic arch requires cardiopulmonary bypass; concurrent aortic valve repair or replacement may be needed for ascending thoracic aneurysms.
         (ii) Descending thoracic aortic aneurysms usually are repaired by thoracotomy and do not require cardiopulmonary bypass.
         (iii) AAA repairs are done through abdominal incisions; a bowel preparation is performed unless surgery is emergent.
      (b) Endovascular grafts for aneurysm repair
         (i) Modular device that expands to fit and seal the aorta, lines the inside of the aneurysm like a sleeve providing a new path for blood flow and reducing the pressure on the aneurysm; uses a stent or hooks to secure the sleeve
         (ii) Implanted through a delivery catheter into the femoral artery
         (iii) Advantages over traditional surgical aneurysm repair
            a) May be used in patients at high risk for traditional aneurysm repair
            b) Intubation not required; may not require critical care unit stay
            c) Fewer complications
               i) Less blood loss than open repair
               ii) Less hypothermia than with laparotomy
            d) Shorter hospital stay
            e) Lower early mortality; long-term mortality is comparable between the two options
         (iv) Disadvantages compared with traditional surgical repair
            a) Conventional surgery still is required in one half of all patients with AAA; not all patients are candidates because the location of the aneurysm and the size of the patient's arteries above and below the aneurysm may preclude the implant; AAA must be infrarenal
            b) More costly in the short-term and in the long-term (life-long surveillance required)
   (3) Postoperative management
      (a) Maintain airway, oxygenation, and ventilation.
         (i) Assess ventilatory status frequently: rate; rhythm; excursion; effort; use of accessory muscles; presence of stridor or other adventitious sounds; pulse oximetry.
         (ii) Encourage deep breathing and incentive spirometry.
         (iii) Assess frequently for edema, hematoma, tracheal deviation, and dysphagia.
         (iv) Elevate HOB 30 degrees.
         (v) Have equipment for cricothyroidotomy, tracheostomy, and suction.
         (vi) Prevent aspiration: high Fowler's position while eating; NPO until gag reflex returns; suction as necessary.
         (vii) Administer oxygen at 2 to 5 L/min as prescribed.
      (b) Maintain adequate flow and pressure at graft site.
         (i) Maintain and control systolic BP under 120 mm Hg.
            a) NTP

b) Nicardipine (Cardene)
c) Analgesics as indicated
(ii) Prevent emboli by using antiembolic techniques.
a) Dextran 40 often is used as platelet aggregation inhibitor.
b) Heparin also may be used.
(iii) Avoid pressure on incision sites.
a) Elevate HOB no greater than 45 degrees for first 72 hours.
b) Elevate legs 20 to 30 degrees.
c) Encourage foot and leg exercises.
d) Mobilize patient from lying to standing; instruct patient to avoid sitting position, flexing, or crossing of legs after femoral artery revascularization.
(c) Assess patient for clinical indications of hypoperfusion.
(i) Perform neurovascular assessment of extremities hourly; monitor for pain; pallor; pulselessness; paresthesia; paralysis; polar (cold).
(ii) Maintain normal body temperature: heated blankets or automatic warming blanket, warming lights.
(d) Treat pain.
(i) Administer analgesics as indicated.
(ii) Position patient for comfort.
(e) Prevent skin breakdown related to ischemia and immobility.
(i) Inspect skin, bony prominences, and affected extremities frequently.
(ii) Reposition patient often.
(iii) Use an egg crate, alternating air mattress, or special bed depending on other risk factors.
(iv) Keep heels elevated off bed.
(f) Maintain adequate hydration.
(i) Administer IV fluids as indicated.
(ii) Monitor urine output closely, and report urine output of less than 0.5 mL/kg/hr.
(g) Monitor patient for postoperative complications.
(i) For acute respiratory failure, monitor for all of the following:
a) Dyspnea
b) Hypoxemia
c) Tachypnea
d) Tachycardia
e) Fever
(ii) For hemorrhage, hypovolemia, and hematoma, monitor for all of the following:
a) Hypotension
b) Tachycardia
c) Clinical manifestations of hypoperfusion
d) Decreased RAP, PAP, and PAOP
(iii) For myocardial ischemia and infarction, monitor for all of the following:
a) Chest pain
b) Dyspnea
c) Decreased cardiac output
d) Dysrhythmias
e) ECG: ST segment changes
(iv) For cerebral ischemia and infarction, monitor for all of the following:
a) Change in LOC
b) Pupillary change
c) Aphasia
d) Motor or sensory changes
(v) For pulmonary ischemia and infarction, monitor for all of the following:
a) Dyspnea
b) Chest pain
c) Pleural friction rub
d) Hypoxemia
(vi) For renal ischemia and infarction, monitor for all of the following:
a) Flank pain
b) Decreased urine output
c) Changes in BUN or creatinine
d) Hematuria
(vii) For mesenteric ischemia and infarction, monitor for all of the following:
a) Watery, bloody diarrhea
b) Abdominal pain
c) Change in bowel sounds
(viii) For splenic ischemia and infarction, monitor for all of the following:
a) Pain in left upper quadrant radiating to left shoulder
b) Abdominal rigidity
(ix) Spinal cord ischemia, infarction
a) Monitor for all of the following:
i) Paralysis of lower extremities
ii) Bowel/bladder paralysis
b) Drainage of cerebrospinal fluid, naloxone, osmotic diuretics, steroids, and/or calcium channel blockers may be prescribed to prevent/treat spinal cord hyperemia/edema.
(x) Arterial thrombosis
a) Sudden, painful ischemia of feet (sometimes referred to as *trash foot*) and or lower leg
b) Diminished or absent peripheral pulses; decreased ABI
(xi) Complications specific to endovascular aneurysm repair
a) Endoleak: persistence of blood flow outside the lumen of the endoluminal graft but within the aneurysmal sac
i) May be managed by observation, further endovascular procedures, or open repair

ii) Risk for continued aneurysm expansion and risk of rupture
b) Postimplant-syndrome
i) Back pain and fever without a leukocytosis or other signs of infection
ii) May last up to 7 days
iii) Cause unknown
c) Graft limb thrombosis
i) Thrombectomy or embolectomy may be required.
e. Provide instruction and counseling regarding lifestyle modification and need for pharmacologic therapy as for Peripheral Arterial Disease.

Carotid Arterial Stenosis (may be referred to as *extracranial cerebrovascular disease*)

1. Etiology
a. Atherosclerosis/arteriosclerosis: risk factors as for coronary artery disease and peripheral vascular disease
b. Trauma
c. Fibromuscular dysplasia
d. Cervical irradiation
e. Arteritis
2. Pathophysiology
a. Atherosclerotic plaque accumulates at the bifurcation of the internal and external carotid arteries.
b. Fragments of this plaque or associated thrombi may break away from the plaque, causing cerebral emboli.
c. Eventually, ischemia or infarction of the brain may occur.
(1) Ischemia
(a) Transient ischemic attack (TIA): focal neurologic deficit lasting less than 24 hours
(2) Infarction: a completed ischemic stroke
(a) Permanent neurologic deficit though some improvement may occur over time
(b) Carotid artery stenosis is the cause of 15% to 25% of strokes
3. Clinical presentation
a. Subjective: usually asymptomatic unless TIA or completed stroke is experienced; symptoms may include the following:
(1) Visual changes: diplopia; ipsilateral monocular blindness (referred to as *amaurosis fugax*)
(2) Memory loss
(3) Vertigo
(4) Syncope
b. Objective
(1) Bruit or thrill over one or both carotid arteries
(2) Signs of transient ischemic attacks (TIA) or stroke may include the following:
(a) Slurred speech/aphasia
(b) Ataxia
(c) Paresis or paralysis
(d) Temporary loss of consciousness
c. Diagnostic
(1) Doppler ultrasonography of the carotid arteries
(2) Digital subtraction angiography
(3) Computerized tomography: used to rule out other etiologic factors
(4) Magnetic resonance angiography
(5) Cerebral arteriography
4. Nursing Diagnoses (see Appendix A)
a. Risk for Ineffective Breathing Patterns related to incisional pain, retained secretions, and airway compromise
b. Risk for Ineffective Cerebral Tissue Perfusion related to carotid artery stenosis, thrombosis, and embolization
c. Risk for Decreased Cardiac Output related to hypotension, hypertension, and hypovolemia
d. Risk for Fluid Volume Deficit related to hemorrhage
e. Risk for Injury to the cranial nerves during surgery
f. Anxiety related to health alteration and recommended lifestyle changes
g. Interrupted Family Processes related to change in health status and potential life-threatening surgery
h. Deficient Knowledge related to disease process, therapy, and recommended lifestyle changes
5. Collaborative management
a. Administer pharmacologic agents as prescribed
(1) Platelet aggregation inhibitors (e.g., aspirin, clopidogrel [Plavix], aspirin plus dipyridamole [Aggrenox])
(2) Agents that increase the flexibility of the RBCs: pentoxifylline (Trental)
(3) Anticoagulants: warfarin (Coumadin)
(4) Antihypertensives if indicated
b. Prepare patient for percutaneous or surgical procedure as requested.
(1) Indications
(a) Occlusion of 70% or greater occlusion of the internal carotid artery or mild stroke within the previous 6 months
(b) No contraindications for surgery
(2) Procedures
(a) Carotid angioplasty and stenting
(i) Balloon dilation of the stenotic area and placement of a crush-resistant stent
(ii) Especially useful in patients with recurrent carotid stenosis, lesions distal in the internal carotid artery or high in the neck, or patients with history of cervical irradiation
(b) Carotid endarterectomy: removal of an atheroma at the carotic artery bifurcation
(3) Postoperative management
(a) Maintain airway, oxygenation, and ventilation.
(i) Assess ventilatory status frequently: rate; rhythm; excursion; effort; use of

accessory muscles; presence of stridor or other adventitious sounds; pulse oximetry.
(ii) Encourage deep breathing and incentive spirometry.
(iii) Assess frequently for edema, hematoma, tracheal deviation, and dysphagia.
(iv) Elevate HOB 30 degrees.
(v) Have equipment for cricothyroidotomy, tracheostomy, and suction.
(vi) Prevent aspiration: high Fowler's position while eating; nothing by mouth until gag reflex returns; suction fluids as necessary.
(vii) Administer oxygen at 2 to 5 L/min as prescribed.

(b) Monitor for/prevent alteration in cerebral perfusion related to cerebral embolism, ischemia, and infarction.
(i) Assess BP and heart rate frequently: BP usually is maintained within ±20 mm Hg of preoperative values.
(ii) Report immediately clinical indications of cerebral hypoperfusion: change in level of consciousness, pupil changes, paresis or plegia, visual changes, dysphasia or aphasia, seizures, and headache.
(iii) Check neurologic and cranial nerve function. (NOTE: There is no risk of injury to the cranial nerves with carotid angioplasty.)
a) Level of consciousness
b) Pupils
c) Motor function
d) Sensory function
e) Cranial nerves
i) VII: Ask patient to smile.
ii) IX, X: Check swallowing, speech, and gag reflex.
iii) XI: Ask patient to shrug against your hands.
iv) XII: Ask patient to stick tongue out; check for midline position.
v) Recurrent laryngeal nerve: check speech.
vi) Great auricular nerve: Note perception of sensation on face and ear.
(iv) Administer antiplatelet aggregation drugs (e.g., aspirin, clopidogrel [Plavix], or dextran 40) as prescribed.

(c) Monitor for hemorrhage or hematoma.
(i) Assess BP and heart rate frequently.
(ii) Assess neck dressing for hematoma, hemorrhage; check back of neck and assess drainage from drain if present.
(iii) Check for tracheal deviation.
(iv) Monitor hemoglobin and hematocrit.
(v) Administer antihypertensives (e.g., nitroprusside (Nipride) and labetalol (Normodyne) as prescribed to maintain BP: systolic, 100 to 160 mm Hg; diastolic, less than 100 mm Hg.

(d) Monitor for complications.
(i) MI
(ii) Cerebral hemorrhage/embolism/infarction
(iii) Carotid hemorrhage
(iv) Hematoma
(v) Cranial nerve injury
(vi) Seizures

c. Provide instruction and counseling regarding lifestyle modification and need for pharmacologic therapy as for Peripheral Arterial Disease.

Cardiovascular Trauma

Myocardial Contusion

1. Definition: transient or permanent myocardial dysfunction caused by blunt trauma to the heart and may include myocardial necrosis without coronary artery disease
2. Etiology
   a. Usually acceleration/deceleration injury sustained in motor vehicle collision; sternum may hit steering wheel or dashboard; injury also may be caused by shoulder strap of seat belt
   b. Other vehicular accidents: motorcycle collisions, auto-pedestrian collisions
   c. Kicking of chest by large animal
   d. Assault with blunt instrument
   e. Industrial crush injury
   f. Explosion
   g. Vigorous CPR
   h. Projectile objects (e.g., baseball or hockey puck)
3. Pathophysiology
   a. The heart is compressed between the sternum and spine.
   b. RBCs extravasate around myocardial fibers (i.e., bruising of the myocardium).
   c. Subpericardial and subendocardial myocardial fibers become edematous and may fragment; necrosis may even occur in severe cases.
   d. The atria and the right ventricle are the primary sites of injury because of their anterior position.
   e. Decreased right ventricular contractility causes an increase in right ventricular end-diastolic volume and a decrease in right ventricular EF (i.e., backward failure of the right ventricle).
   f. This decrease in right ventricle EF decreases preload to the left ventricle (i.e., forward failure of the left ventricle).
   g. Dilation of RV shifts interventricular septum to the left, compromising left ventricular compliance.
   h. An increase in PVR frequently is seen, increasing RV afterload and further decreasing RV EF.

i. Damage to cardiac valves may occur, especially mitral and aortic, because LV pressures are higher.
j. In addition to the effect of blunt trauma on myocardial contractility, sudden cardiac death may occur as a result of a blunt, nonpenetrating blow to the precordium or left lateral chest during the electrically vulnerable period of the cardiac cycle, causing fatal ventricular dysrhythmias; this sudden cardiac death is referred to as *commotio cordis*.

4. Clinical presentation
   a. Subjective
      (1) Precordial angina-like chest pain
         (a) Frequently increases with inspiration, cough, and movement
         (b) Unresponsive to nitroglycerin but frequently responsive to oxygen, antiinflammatory agents, or narcotics
      (2) Dyspnea
      (3) Palpitations
   b. Objective
      (1) Tachycardia
      (2) Ecchymosis may be present on anterior chest
      (3) Clinical indications of RVF: JVD; peripheral edema; hepatomegaly
      (4) Cardiac arrest as a result of fatal ventricular dysrhythmias may occur
   c. Diagnostic
      (1) Serum: CK-MB and cardiac troponin may be positive depending on the severity of the injury
      (2) Electrocardiography with right ventricular leads
         (a) ST segment changes, T wave inversion; Q waves may be seen if injury is severe or if a coronary artery is lacerated or thromboses
         (b) QT interval may be prolonged
         (c) Dysrhythmias
            (i) Atrial dysrhythmias: PACs, AF, atrial flutter
            (ii) Ventricular dysrhythmias: PACs, VT, VF
            (iii) Blocks: AV blocks; RBBB
      (3) Echocardiography
         (a) Decreased regional wall motion (especially right ventricular)
         (b) Increased end-diastolic wall thickness
         (c) Decreased RV EF
         (d) May show complications (e.g., apical thrombi; pericardial effusion; cardiac tamponade)
      (4) Radionuclide studies may be done: decreased RV EF
5. Nursing Diagnoses (see Appendix A)
   a. Decreased Cardiac Output related to pump failure, tamponade, and hemorrhage
   b. Risk for Impaired Peripheral Tissue Perfusion related to emboli
   c. Impaired Gas Exchange related to pulmonary edema
   d. Activity Intolerance related to pump failure
   e. Anxiety related to health alteration and recommended lifestyle changes
   f. Interrupted Family Processes related to change in health status and potential life-threatening situation
   g. Deficient Knowledge related to disease process, therapy, and recommended lifestyle changes
6. Collaborative management
   a. Treat pain.
      (1) Morphine sulfate usually is used.
      (2) Antiinflammatory agents also may be helpful.
   b. Ensure adequate right ventricular contractility, left ventricular filling, and cardiac output.
      (1) Isotonic fluids as prescribed to ensure adequate left ventricular filling; avoid venous vasodilators and diuretics
      (2) Inotropes (e.g., dobutamine) as prescribed to improve right ventricular contractility
   c. Decrease myocardial oxygen demand.
      (1) Bed rest
      (2) Oxygen by nasal cannula at 2 to 6 L/min to maintain Sao_2 of 95% unless contraindicated
      (3) Anxiolytic drugs as prescribed and indicated
   d. Treat dysrhythmias.
      (1) Atrial: digitalis; cardioversion
      (2) Ventricular: usually amiodarone
      (3) Blocks: temporary pacemaker; permanent pacemaker may be necessary
   e. Assist in assessment for other thoracic injuries (e.g., fractured ribs, sternum, clavicle, or pulmonary contusion)
   f. Monitor for complications.
      (1) Ventricular rupture
      (2) Cardiac tamponade
      (3) Coronary artery thrombosis
      (4) Valve rupture
      (5) Conduction defects
      (6) HF
      (7) Ventricular aneurysm
      (8) Cardiogenic shock: monitor for clinical manifestations of hypoperfusion
      (9) Systemic emboli
         (a) Sequential compression devices may be used on the legs
         (b) Anticoagulation avoided unless there are intramural thrombi

Penetrating Cardiac Trauma

1. Definition: puncture of the heart with a sharp object or rib
2. Etiology
   a. Violence (e.g., knife wound, gunshot wound, or ice pick)
   b. Industrial accident (e.g., scaffolding)
   c. Motorcycle collision (e.g., handlebar impalement)
   d. Sports injury
   e. Explosion
   f. Crush injury

3. Pathophysiology
   a. Puncture of the heart (usually RV) with sharp object or rib
   b. Loss of blood into the pericardial space or into the mediastinum
   c. Cardiac tamponade or shock may occur
4. Clinical presentation
   a. Subjective: chest pain
   b. Objective
      (1) Visible wound; object causing penetration may be seen
      (2) Bleeding from chest
      (3) Hypotension
      (4) Clinical indications of hypoperfusion (see Table 2-2)
      (5) Clinical indications of cardiac tamponade (see Cardiac Tamponade)
   c. Hemodynamic parameters
      (1) Decrease in RAP, PAP, PAOP if hemorrhage; increase in RAP, PAP, PAOP if cardiac tamponade
      (2) Decrease in CO and CI
      (3) Decrease in Svo_2
   d. Diagnostic: hemoglobin and hematocrit decreased
5. Nursing Diagnoses (see Appendix A)
   a. Decreased Cardiac Output related to pump failure
   b. Impaired Gas Exchange related to pulmonary edema
   c. Activity Intolerance related to pump failure
   d. Anxiety related to health alteration and recommended lifestyle changes
   e. Interrupted Family Processes related to change in health status and potential life-threatening situation
   f. Deficient Knowledge related to unfamiliarity with disease process and therapy
6. Collaborative management
   a. Manage cardiopulmonary arrest if indicated: manage airway, oxygenation, and circulation using BCLS and ACLS if needed.
   b. Control hemorrhage.
      (1) Do not remove an impaled object; objects may be stabilized with IV bags and dressings
      (2) Apply pressure to site if the object has been removed and there is a bleeding wound.
      (3) Apply pressure around site if the object has not been removed already and there is bleeding around the wound.
      (4) Assist in insertion of chest tube for hemothorax or pneumothorax.
      (5) Assist with pericardiocentesis for cardiac tamponade.
   c. Improve oxygen delivery.
      (1) Oxygen by nasal cannula at 2 to 6 L/min to maintain Sao_2 of 95% unless contraindicated
      (2) Intubation and mechanical ventilation may be necessary
      (3) IV access: two large-bore, short IV catheters; blood for type and crossmatch
      (4) Normal saline or lactated Ringer's solution by rapid infusion until blood is available; colloids (e.g., albumin, hetastarch, or dextran) also may be used
      (5) Blood and blood products
   d. Assist in preparation of the patient for exploratory thoracotomy.
   e. Monitor for complications.
      (1) Hemorrhagic shock
      (2) Cardiac tamponade
      (3) Hemothorax
      (4) Pneumothorax

Great Vessel Injury

1. Definition: injury or tear to great vessel or vessels, usually the aorta but possibly the pulmonary artery
2. Etiology
   a. Acceleration-deceleration injury (e.g., motor vehicle collision)
   b. Compression injury
   c. Penetrating trauma
3. Pathophysiology: disruption of major vessel integrity causes loss of effective circulating blood volume leading to shock
4. Clinical presentation
   a. Subjective
      (1) Chest pain frequently radiating to back or back pain
      (2) Dyspnea
      (3) Dysphagia or hoarseness
      (4) Sensory or motor changes in lower extremities
   b. Objective
      (1) Tachycardia
      (2) BP changes
         (a) Hypertension or hypotension
         (b) Difference between left and right arms
         (c) Difference (greater than normal) between upper and lower extremities
      (3) Tracheal shift
      (4) Clinical indications of hypoperfusion
      (5) Harsh systolic murmur may be audible along the precordium
   c. Hemodynamic parameters
      (1) Decrease in RAP, PAP, and PAOP
      (2) Decrease in CO and CI
      (3) Decrease in Svo_2
   d. Diagnostic
      (1) Serum: hemoglobin and hematocrit decreased
      (2) ECG: may show dysrhythmias or ST-T wave changes indicative of ischemia
      (3) Chest x-ray
         (a) Mediastinal widening
         (b) Loss of aortic knob shadow
      (4) Transesophageal echocardiography or spiral CT
      (5) Aortogram: will show extravasation of dye
5. Nursing Diagnoses (see Appendix A)
   a. Fluid Volume Deficit related to hemorrhage
   b. Risk for Decreased Cardiac Output related to cardiac tamponade

c. Anxiety related to health alteration and recommended lifestyle changes
d. Interrupted Family Processes related to change in health status and potential life-threatening situation
e. Deficient Knowledge related to disease process and therapy

6. Collaborative management
   a. Manage cardiopulmonary arrest if needed: manage airway, oxygenation, and circulation using BCLS and ACLS if needed.
   b. Improve oxygen delivery.
      (1) Oxygen by nasal cannula at 2 to 6 L/min to maintain Sao_2 of 95% unless contraindicated
      (2) Intubation and mechanical ventilation may be necessary
      (3) IV access: two large-bore, short IV catheters; blood for type and crossmatch
      (4) Normal saline or lactated Ringer's solution by rapid infusion until blood is available; colloids (e.g., albumin, hetastarch, or dextran) also may be used
      (5) Blood and blood products
   c. Control bleeding: antihypertensive drugs may be needed to keep MAP less than 90 mm Hg.
   d. Assist in preparation of the patient for exploratory thoracotomy as soon as possible; it is not possible truly to stabilize this patient except in the operating room with vascular repair.
   e. Monitor for complications.
      (1) Hemorrhagic shock
      (2) Cardiac tamponade
      (3) Hemothorax
      (4) False aneurysm

Cardiac Tamponade

Definition

1. When fluid (blood, effusion fluid, pus) in the pericardial space compromises cardiac filling and cardiac output
2. Tamponade does not depend on the amount of fluid in the pericardial space but on the presence of hemodynamic consequences of pericardial fluid

Etiology

1. Blunt or penetrating injury to heart
2. After cardiotomy
   a. If mediastinal tube is occluded or after removal of mediastinal tube
   b. After removal of epicardial pacing wires
3. After MI
   a. Pericarditis especially in the anticoagulated patient
   b. Cardiac rupture
4. Iatrogenic causes: perforation of the myocardium by transvenous pacemaker wires, invasive catheters, intracardiac injection, cardiac needle biopsy
5. Transmyocardial revascularization
6. After CPR or electrical cardioversion
7. Fibrinolytic or anticoagulant therapy
8. Rupture of great vessels
9. Dissecting aortic aneurysms
10. Malignancy and/or radiation therapy
11. Connective tissue disease: rheumatoid arthritis; systemic lupus erythematosus; scleroderma
12. Metabolic disease: renal failure; hepatic failure; myxedema
13. Inflammation: pericarditis
14. Infection: viral; bacterial; fungal
    a. Tuberculosis
15. Drugs: procainamide (Pronestyl); hydralazine (Apresoline); minoxidil (Loniten); phenytoin (Dilantin); daunorubicin (Cerubidine); methyldopa (Aldomet); sulfasalazine (Azulfidine); isoniazid (INH); methysergide (Sansert); sargramostim (Leukine); tetracycline derivatives

Pathophysiology

1. Fluid or blood accumulate in the pericardial space.
   a. The pericardial space normally contains less than 50 mL.
   b. If the fluid accumulates rapidly (e.g., cardiac trauma or surgery), a relatively small volume (~100 to 200 mL) may cause cardiac tamponade.
   c. If the fluid accumulates slowly (e.g., uremia or myxedema), a large volume may be accommodated before hemodynamic consequences related to poor cardiac filling occurs.
2. When intrapericardial pressure is very high and approaches atrial pressures and ventricular diastolic pressure, the transmural cardiac pressure falls, leading to inability of the heart to fill.
3. End-diastolic volume (preload) decreases.
4. Contractility decreases.
5. Stroke volume decreases.
6. Cardiac output decreases.
7. LVF, RVF, and shock may occur.

Clinical Presentation

1. Subjective
   a. Precordial fullness or pain
   b. Dyspnea with improved when sitting upright
   c. Anxiety or feeling of impending doom
2. Objective
   a. Early sign is usually tachycardia, but as the impairment in ventricular filling progresses, the patient may be pulseless (PEA)
   b. Hypotension, narrowed pulse pressure
   c. Increased JVD: may not be seen if patient is hypotensive
   d. Absent PMI
   e. Dullness to percussion below the left scapula (Ewart's sign)
   f. Heart sound changes
      (1) Pericardial friction rub may be heard, especially if tamponade is associated with pericarditis.
      (2) Heart sounds may be distant, muffled, or absent.
   g. Beck's triad: hypotension; distended neck veins; muffled heart sounds

h. Excessive mediastinal tube drainage that suddenly stops in a cardiac surgery or trauma patient
3. Hemodynamic parameters
a. Increased RAP (central venous pressure)
b. Pulsus paradoxus on arterial waveform or by auscultation
c. Equalization of left and right filling pressures of the heart with hemodynamic monitoring: RAP, PAd pressure, PAOP within 5 mm Hg of each other
d. Change in PAOP waveform: large *a* wave, large *v* wave (M sign)
e. Decrease in CO/CI
f. Decrease in Svo_2
4. Diagnostic
a. Chest x-ray
(1) Widened mediastinum
(2) Dilated superior vena cava
(3) Enlarged heart (i.e., water-bottle silhouette)
b. Electrocardiography
(1) Diffuse ST segment elevation across the precordial leads
(2) Decrease in the amplitude of the QRS complex or electrical alternans (i.e., alternating tall and small QRS complexes) across the precordial leads
(3) Bradycardia may indicate impending PEA
(4) Ventricular dysrhythmias
c. Echocardiogram: 2D or transesophageal
(1) Echo-free space evident between the pericardium and epicardium
(2) Right atrial and ventricular collapse
(3) Respiratory variation in cardiac chamber dimension and transvalvular flow velocities
(4) Transesophageal echocardiogram or CT imaging may be required
d. CT of chest
e. Fluoroscopy of chest: may be used during pericardiocentesis

Nursing Diagnoses (see Appendix A)

1. Decreased Cardiac Output related to decreased preload and decreased contractility
2. Fluid Volume Deficit related to hemorrhage into pericardial space
3. Anxiety related to health alteration
4. Interrupted Family Processes related to change in health status and potential life-threatening situation
5. Deficient Knowledge related to disease process and therapy

Collaborative Management

1. Maintain airway, ventilation, oxygenation, and perfusion.
a. Airway, oxygenation, circulation support using BCLS and ACLS if needed
b. 100% oxygen by face mask; intubation and mechanical ventilation as indicated
c. Circulating volume replacement
(1) Initiate two large-bore IVs: replace vascular volume as necessary
(a) Normal saline: 200 to 500 mL over 10 to 15 minutes
(b) Fresh frozen plasma, dextran, or albumin also may be used
(c) Blood replacement also may be necessary
d. Inotropes (e.g., dobutamine) as prescribed
e. Atropine or transcutaneous pacing may be necessary for bradydysrhythmias
2. Administer drugs or therapies related to cause.
a. Discontinuance of drug that contributed to the tamponade
b. Protamine or vitamin K if patient is taking anticoagulants
c. Dialysis for patients with renal failure
d. Antibiotics if purulent effusion
e. Thyroid hormone replacement for myxedema
f. Corticosteroids may be prescribed in drug-related pericardial effusions, uremia, and pericarditis
3. Prepare to assist with pericardiocentesis (Figure 3-25) for emergency cardiac tamponade.
a. Place patient in semi-Fowler position; subxiphoid or left parasternal approach is most commonly used.
b. Apply ECG machine and electrodes.
(1) Apply limb leads.
(2) Attach chest lead wire to the exploring needle with an alligator clamp if requested; this technique is used to assess needle position because when needle touches epicardium, ST segment elevation is seen and PVCs may occur.
c. Have echocardiography technician available to assist with 2D echo guidance if requested; fluoroscopy also may be used.
d. Have emergency equipment available, including transcutaneous pacemaker.
e. Assist with administration of local anesthetic.
f. Administer sedation if the patient is anxious.

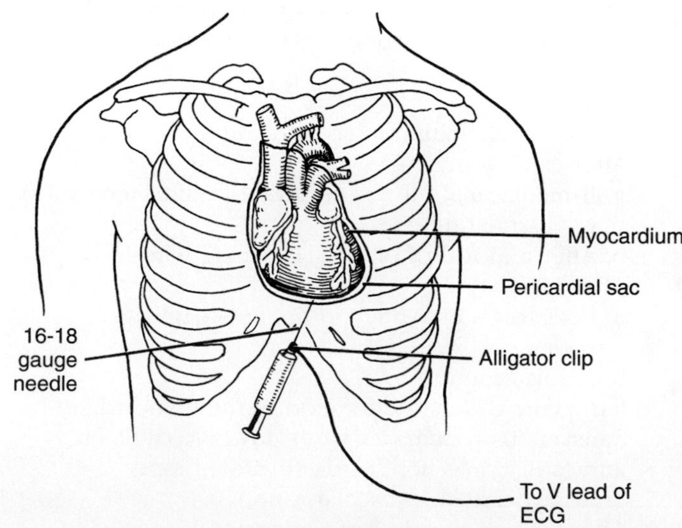

Figure 3-25 Pericardiocentesis. *ECG*, Electrocardiogram.

g. Assist with slow aspiration of the fluid and sending it to the laboratory department for analysis.
h. Assist with placement of pericardial catheter if indicated; may be used for injection of sclerosing agents, corticosteroids, fibrinolytic drugs, or chemotherapeutic agents.
i. Monitor for complications.
   (1) Laceration of coronary artery or conduction system
   (2) Myocardial perforation
   (3) Pneumothorax
   (4) Dysrhythmias
   (5) Hypotension (usually reflexogenic)

4. Assist in preparation of patient for surgical intervention.
   a. Pericardiocentesis may not resolve the tamponade if effusion is posterior; surgical drainage is indicated if purulent or hemorrhagic effusion.
   b. Subxiphoid pericardiotomy or thoracoscopic procedures may be necessary.
5. Monitor/assist with treatment of recurrent pericardial effusion or tamponade occurs.
   a. Monitor for recurrence of clinical indications of tamponade.
   b. Prepare the patient for the selected procedure.
      (1) Percutaneous balloon pericardiotomy
      (2) Intrapericardial instillation of sclerosing agent
      (3) Pleuropericardial or peritoneal-pericardial window

LEARNING ACTIVITIES

1. DIRECTIONS: Match the dysrhythmia with the most appropriate treatment summary.

________	1. VF	a. CPR intubate, transcutaneous pacing, epinephrine, atropine
________	2. Stable monomorphic VT	b. Treatment of cause, beta-blockers or sedatives
________	3. Asystole	c. Calcium channel blocker, beta-blocker, amiodarone, ibutilide, cardioversion
________	4. Symptomatic bradycardia	d. Amiodarone, beta-blocker, or calcium channel blocker; do not cardiovert
________	5. PEA	e. Magnesium, overdrive pacing, isoproterenol
________	6. Stable SVT	f. Defibrillation, CPR vasopressin or epinephrine, intubate, amiodarone
________	7. Acute onset AF	g. Amiodarone, synchronized cardioversion
________	8. Pulseless VT	h. Atropine and/or transcutaneous pacing
________	9. Junctional tachycardia	i. CPR intubate, assess for possible causes, epinephrine, atropine
________	10. Sinus tachycardia	j. Vagal maneuvers and adenosine, calcium channel blocker, beta-blocker, digoxin
________	11. Torsades de pointes	

2. DIRECTIONS: Complete the following table by identifying the Vaughn-Williams antidysrhythmic classification of the following drugs. Some drugs are of more than one class.

Adenosine (Adenocard)	
Amiodarone (Cordarone)	
Atropine	
Digoxin	
Diltiazem (Cardizem)	
Dofetilide (Tikosyn)	
Esmolol (Brevibloc)	
Flecainide (Tambocor)	
Ibutilide (Corvert)	
Lidocaine (Xylocaine)	
Metoprolol (Lopressor)	
Procainamide (Pronestyl)	
Propranolol (Inderal)	
Quinidine	
Sotalol (Betapace)	
Verapamil (Calan)	

3. DIRECTIONS: Complete the following table to identify the North American Society of Pacing and Electrophysiology code for the pacemaker that would have the capabilities of the others together.

AOO		VVI	a.
VVI		VAT	b.
AAI	VAT	VVI	c.

4. DIRECTIONS: Analyze the following ECG rhythm strips. Identify the type of pacemaker and whether there is a pacemaker malfunction.

a.

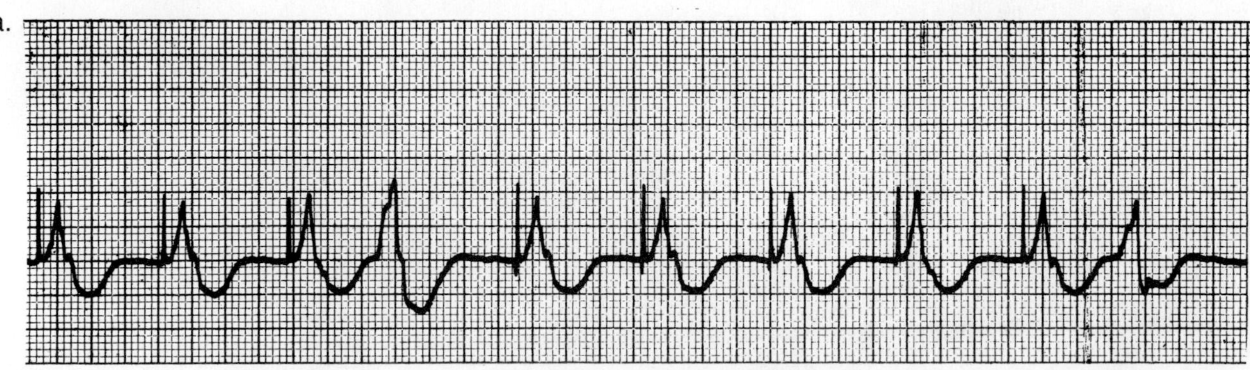

Interpretation ____

b.

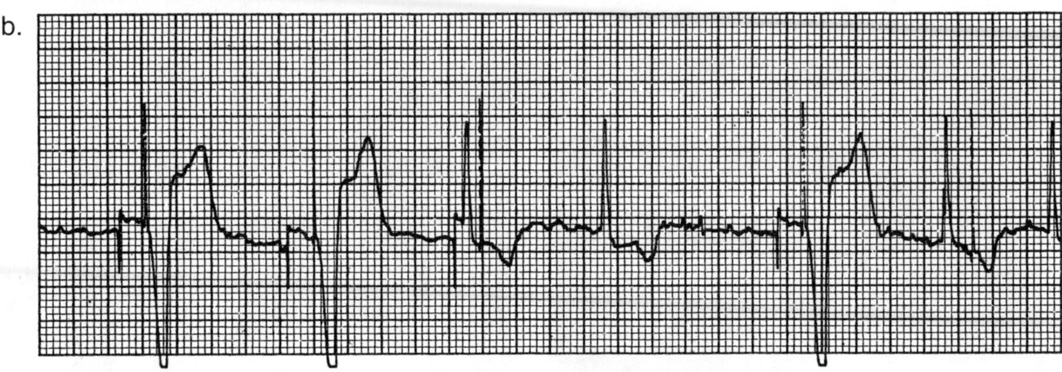

Interpretation ____

c.

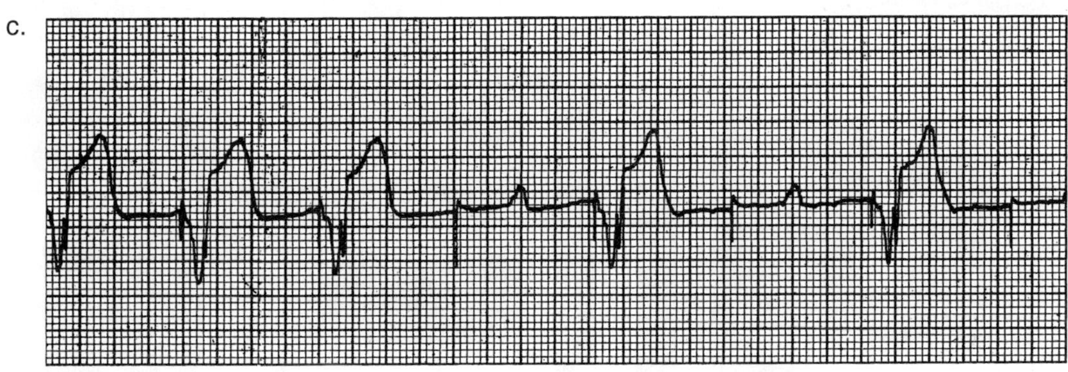

Interpretation ____

5. **Directions:** Complete the following table, differentiating cardiac risk factors as nonmodifiable or modifiable.

Nonmodifiable	Modifiable

6. **Directions:** Match the following treatments for acute MI with rationales for use. More than one may apply.

____ 1. Fibrinolytic drugs
____ 2. PCI procedures such as angioplasty and atherectomy
____ 3. ACE inhibitors
____ 4. Nitroglycerin
____ 5. Calcium channel blockers
____ 6. Beta-blockers
____ 7. Aspirin
____ 8. Heparin
____ 9. Glycoprotein IIb/IIIa inhibitors
____ 10. IABP

a. Increases myocardial oxygen supply by reestablishing patency of the infarct-related artery
b. Decreases myocardial oxygen demand by blocking the effects of catecholamines
c. Increases myocardial oxygen supply by reducing spasm
d. Decreases myocardial oxygen demand by reducing preload
e. Prevents extension of a clot by decreasing platelet aggregation
f. Prevents extension of a clot by preventing the conversion of prothrombin to thrombin
g. Prevents ventricular dilation and adverse remodeling of the myocardium
h. Used for secondary prevention after MI
i. Decreases myocardial oxygen consumption by decreasing afterload
j. Increases myocardial oxygen supply by increasing coronary artery perfusion pressure

7. **Directions:** Complete the following crossword puzzle dealing with CAD and acute MI.

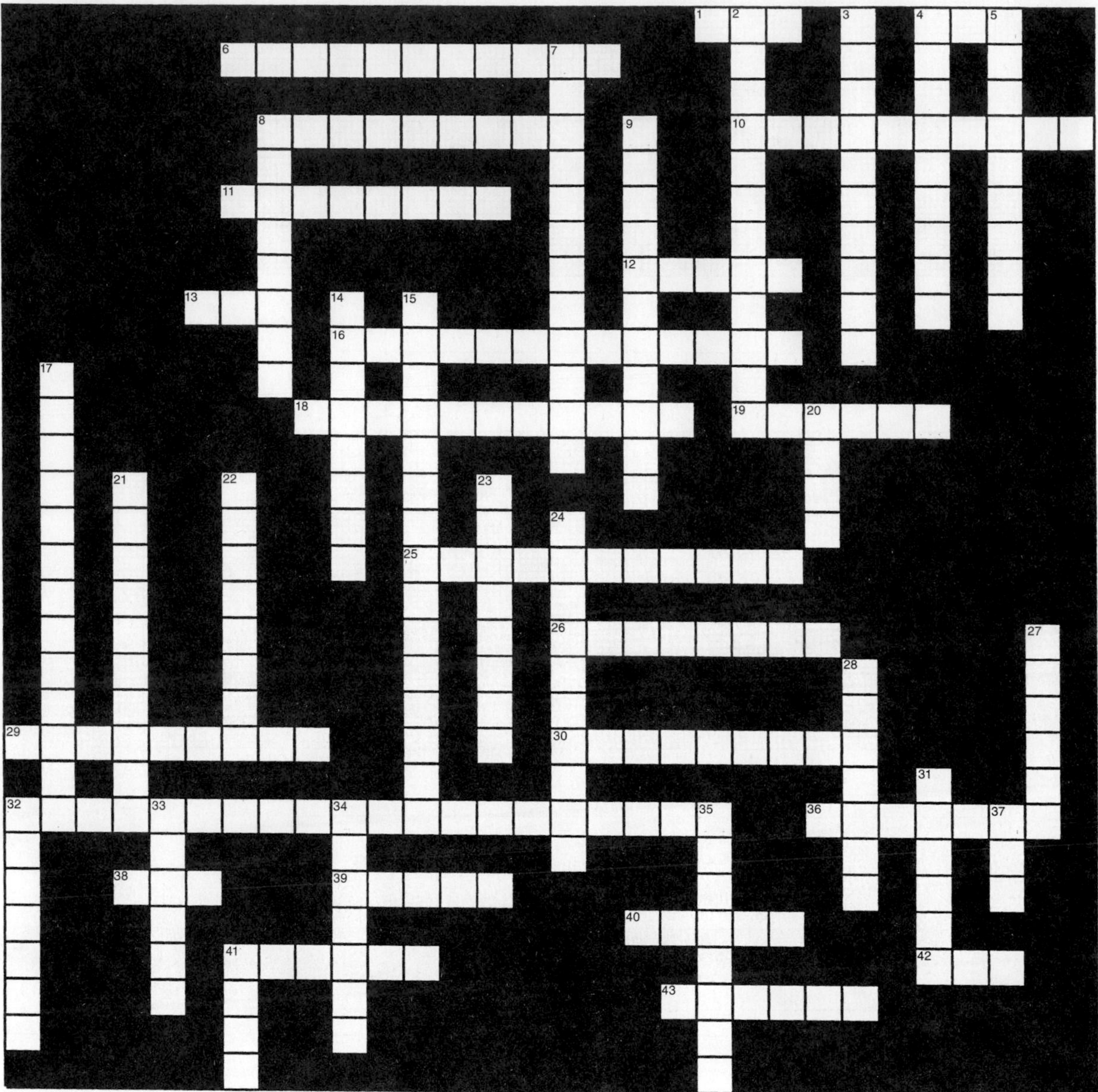

ACROSS

1. Good cholesterol (abbreviation)
4. Platelet aggregation inhibitor (abbreviation)
6. PCI procedure that opens an occluded artery using balloon dilation
8. Muscle protein sensitive but not specific for MI
10. ACE inhibitors are used after MI to prevent this
11. Cardiac muscle protein measured in diagnosing MI
12. This coronary artery supplies RA, RV, and the inferior wall of LV
13. Preferred method of reperfusion for acute MI (abbreviation)
16. Nitrate used for acute chest pain
18. Evidenced by cessation of pain, ST segment return to baseline, dysrhythmias
19. New holosystolic murmur at lower sternum, increase SVo_2 and shock indicates rupture of the ___.
25. Oral platelet aggregation inhibitor frequently used for after PCI
26. An activity that is likely to decrease body weight, BP, lipids, and stress
29. Rupture of the ___ muscle causes acute mitral regurgitation.
30. Indicative leads for this cardiac wall are V_8 and V_9.
32. Risk factor for CAD treated with folic acid
36. Indicative leads for this cardiac wall are I and aVL and/or V_5 and V_6.
38. Bad cholesterol (abbreviation)
39. CABG performed on a beating heart through a small sternotomy
40. Device used during PCI to prevent closure
41. Evidenced on ECG by ST segment elevation
42. S_3, dyspnea, crackles indicate what complication of acute MI (abbreviation)

43. CABG done through small thoracotomy incision used for left anterior mammary artery–left anterior descending coronary artery anastomosis (abbreviation)

DOWN

2. The most common complication of MI
3. Cardioselective beta-blocker used more often for acute MI
4. tPA with short half-life and so must be given as bolus followed by infusion
5. GP IIb/IIIa inhibitor frequently used after PCI (generic)
7. tPA that has a longer half-life and is administered as a single bolus
8. Analgesic of choice for acute MI
9. PCI procedure that opens an occluded artery using a shaving device
14. Indicative leads for this cardiac wall are II, III, and aVF.
15. The most likely cause of acute MI
17. Irradiation method used during PCI procedure
20. Percutaneous procedure for patients with inoperative, Class IV angina that involves laser-created channels (abbreviation)
21. The inotropic agent most likely to be used for cardiogenic shock with MI
22. Evidenced on ECG by T wave inversion
23. The internal mammary now is referred to as the internal ___.
24. Calcium channel blocker used for coronary artery spasm
27. Indicative leads for this cardiac wall are V_1 and V_2.
28. Type of angina caused by spasm
31. A major cause for delay in seeking assistance for chest pain
32. Anticoagulant used to prevent extension of a clot or reocclusion
33. Artery sometimes used for CABG that has a high spasm potential
34. Acute chest pain and/or ST segment elevation after PCI may indicate acute ___.
35. Indicative leads for this cardiac wall are V_3 and V_4.
37. General term used for undifferentiated chest pain (abbreviation)
41. Device used to decrease afterload and increase myocardial perfusion in cardiogenic shock (abbreviation)

8. DIRECTIONS: Identify the physical findings from the following list that are seen in these pathologic conditions. More than one physical finding may be listed for each pathologic condition.

_________ 1. RVF
_________ 2. LVF
_________ 3. Left ventricular MI
_________ 4. Pulmonary embolism
_________ 5. Tension pneumothorax
_________ 6. Cardiac tamponade
_________ 7. Valvular dysfunction
_________ 8. Pericarditis
_________ 9. Endocarditis
_________ 10. Hyperlipidemia
_________ 11. Chronic arterial insufficiency
_________ 12. Chronic venous insufficiency

a. Jugular venous distention
b. Displaced PMI
c. S_3 at apex
d. S_3 at sternum
e. S_4 at apex
f. S_4 at sternum
g. Murmur
h. Pericardial friction rub
i. Muffled heart sounds
j. Splinter hemorrhages
k. Intermittent claudication
l. Xanthelasma
m. Peripheral edema
n. Peripheral pallor
o. Peripheral rubor
p. Fever
q. Crackles in lung bases
r. Corneal arcus
s. Hepatomegaly
t. Pulsus paradoxus

9. **DIRECTIONS:** Identify whether the following causes or clinical findings are associated with LVF or RVF. Some may be associated with biventricular failure.

Causes	Left	Right
Aortic stenosis		
Cardiac tamponade		
Cardiomyopathy		
Mitral stenosis		
MI (left)		
MI (right)		
Pulmonary embolism		
Pulmonary hypertension		
Systemic hypertension		
Sign/Symptom	**Left**	**Right**
Abnormal liver function studies		
Ascites		
Atrial dysrhythmias		
Crackles audible over lungs		
Dyspnea		
Elevated PAOP		
Elevated RAP		
Hepatomegaly		
JVD		
Mental confusion		
Murmur of mitral regurgitation		
Murmur of tricuspid regurgitation		
Orthopnea		
Peripheral edema		
S_3, S_4 at apex		
S_3, S_4 at sternum		
Weight gain		

10. a. List two primary effects of IABP.
   (1) ______________________________
   (2) ______________________________

   b. List two major contraindications of IABP.
   (1) ______________________________
   (2) ______________________________

   c. In IABP the balloon is inflated during which phase of the cardiac cycle?
   ____

   d. In IABP the balloon is deflated immediately before which phase of the cardiac cycle?
   ____

   e. List two complications caused by displacement of the balloon in the aorta.
   (1) ______________________________
   (2) ______________________________

11. DIRECTIONS: Identify the labeled portions of the IABP waveform.

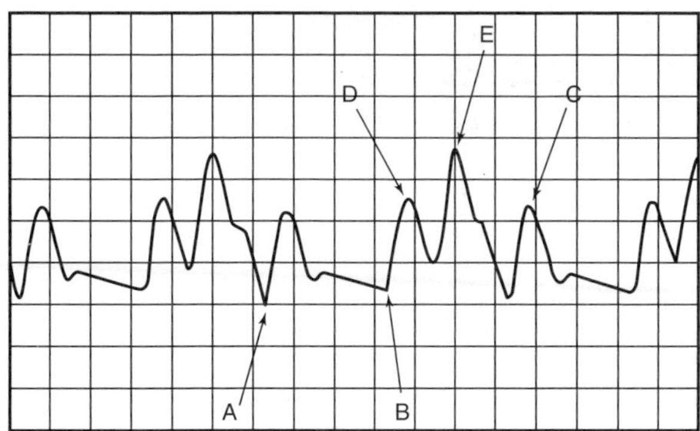

A ______________________

B ______________________

C ______________________

D ______________________

E ______________________

12. DIRECTIONS: Identify the following signs, symptoms, causes, or treatments as associated with dilated, hypertrophic, or restrictive cardiomyopathy. You may identify more than one type of cardiomyopathy for each feature.

Feature	Dilated	Hypertrophic	Restrictive
Associated with alcoholism or infection			
Do not give inotropes			
Clinical presentation: syncope, chest pain, sudden death			
Clinical presentation similar to HF			
May be candidate for cardiac transplantation			
AF common			
Treatment includes beta-blockers and calcium channel blockers			
Do not give diuretics or nitrates			
Associated with infiltrative and connective tissue disorders			
Treated with diuretics, ACE inhibitors, digoxin			
Associated with genetically transmitted autosomal dominant trait			
Atrioventricular blocks are common			
Hemiblock is common			
Treatment may include steroids			
May be treated with therapeutic septal infarction			

13. DIRECTIONS: Identify the following signs, symptoms, causes, or treatments as associated with pericarditis, myocarditis, or endocarditis. You may identify more than one type of cardiomyopathy for each feature.

Feature	Pericarditis	Myocarditis	Endocarditis
Associated with MI			
May cause cardiomyopathy			
Causes splinter hemorrhages, petechiae			
Treated with antiinflammatory drugs			
Sudden onset of HF			
Causes pericardial friction rub			
Valve replacement may be necessary			
Usually associated with viral infection			
Associated with cardiac surgery			
Definitive diagnosis requires biopsy			
May cause systemic emboli			
Monitor closely for cardiac tamponade			
Causes murmur			
Associated with uremia			
Associated with ST segment elevation			
Treated with antimicrobials			
Increased incidence in patients with rheumatic heart disease			

14. Directions: Complete the following table regarding antihypertensive agents.

Description	Drug
IV calcium channel blocker used for hypertension	
IV beta-blocker that also blocks alpha receptors	
IV vasodilator that may cause coronary artery steal and intrapulmonary shunt	
IV vasodilator that is particularly helpful in patients with chest pain	
IV ACE inhibitor	
Oral ACE inhibitor that was the first ACE inhibitor	
Two oral calcium channel blockers used for hypertension	
IV vasodilator frequently used in pregnancy-related hypertension	
IV vasodilator with dopaminergic stimulation effects	

15. Directions: Complete the following crossword puzzle dealing with cardiovascular pharmacology. Use only generic names.

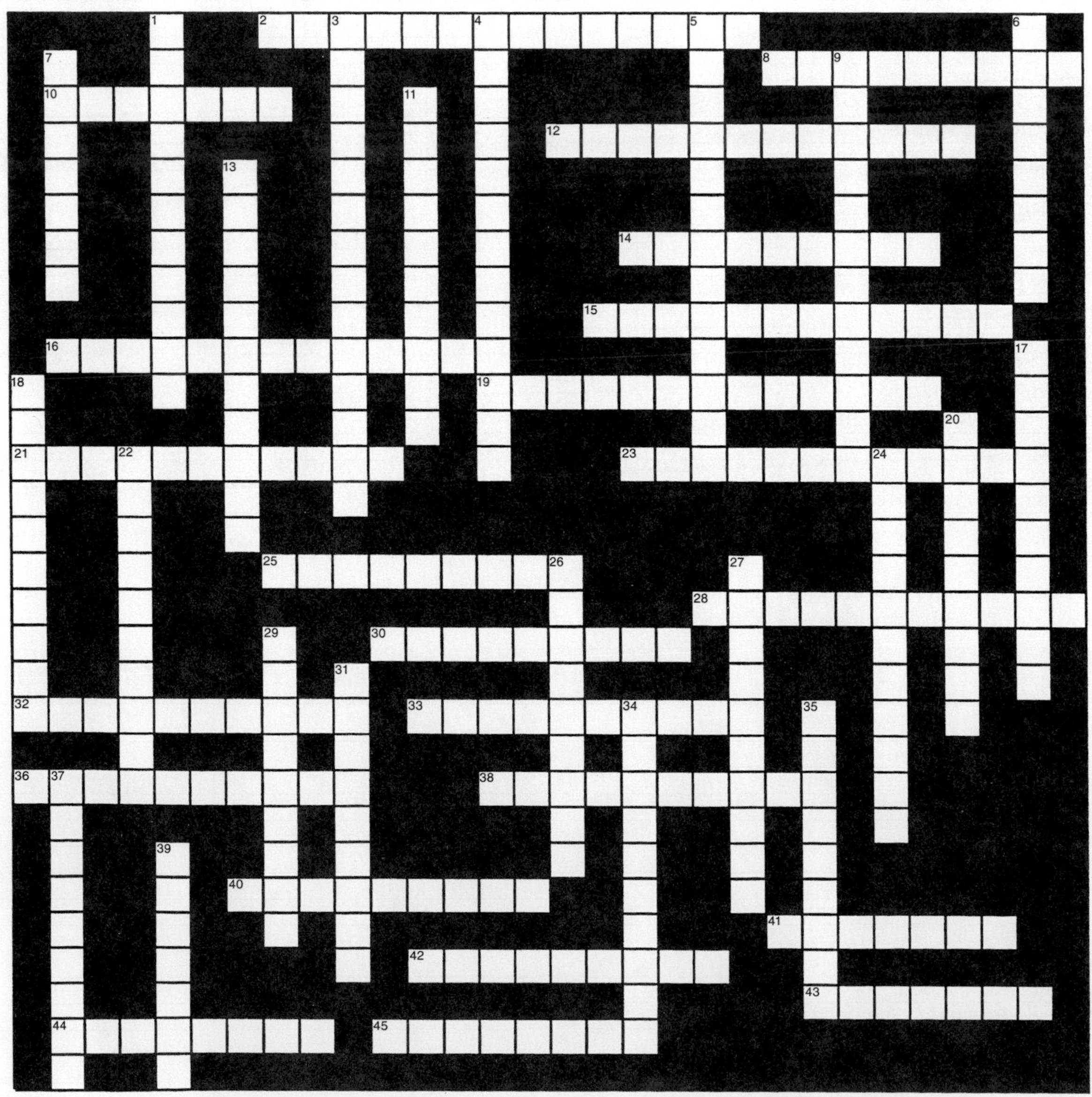

ACROSS

2. Drug used in peripheral arterial disease to increase the flexibility of the RBCs
8. ACE inhibitor; may cause rash or cough
10. Platelet aggregation inhibitor used for primary and secondary prevention of MI
12. IV pulmonary vasodilator used in PH
14. Phosphodiesterase inhibitor; more potent and with fewer side effects than amrinone
15. Class IA antidysrhythmic; may cause prolongation of the QT interval and torsades de pointes
16. Alpha-selective sympathomimetic
19. Predominantly arterial nitrate-type vasodilator
21. Calcium channel blocker used for hypertension; available for IV use
23. Tissue plasminogen activator with a longer half-life; given as a single bolus
25. Class IB antidysrhythmic; monitor for indications of toxicity such as paresthesia, confusion, and seizures
28. Hormone used in pulseless VT or VF as an alternative to epinephrine; longer half-life than epinephrine
30. Alpha- and beta-blocker; used for hypertension
32. Cardioselective beta-blocker; used for secondary prevention of acute MI
33. Class IC antidysrhythmic; used for refractory ventricular dysrhythmias
36. Calcium channel blocker frequently used in variant angina
38. Loop diuretic; rapid administration may cause temporary deafness
40. Class IV antidysrhythmic; frequently used in SVT
41. Cardiac glycoside; decreases ventricular response rate in AF and atrial flutter
42. Electrolyte; usually included in postoperative fluid replacement
43. Cardioselective beta-blocker with short half-life
44. Sympathomimetic with dose-dependent effects
45. Analgesic of choice in acute MI venous vasodilator

DOWN

1. Sympathomimetic used in pulseless VT, VF, asystole, and PEA
3. Alpha-dominant sympathomimetic
4. Pure beta-stimulant; may be used in torsades de pointes
5. Predominantly venous nitrate-type vasodilator
6. Benzodiazepine anxiolytic
7. Electrolyte used in hyperkalemia, hypermagnesemia, hypocalcemia, and calcium channel blocker toxicity
9. Alpha-blocker; frequently used for sympathomimetic drug infiltration to prevent tissue necrosis
11. Sympathomimetic inotopic agent most frequently used in cardiogenic shock
13. Arterial dilator administered by IV injection; used in hypertension especially if pregancy related
17. Oral Class III antidysrhythmic agent used for new onset AF requires hospitalization and ECG monitoring during initiation of therapy
18. Arterial dilator with dopaminergic stimulation used in hypertension and to improve renal flow
20. Electrolyte; indicates in torsades de pointes
22. Class III antidysrhythmic; first-line antidysrhythmic agent for pulseless VT or VF
24. Noncardioselective beta-blocker
26. ACE inhibitor not available in IV form
27. Alpha- and beta-blocker used in HF
29. Class IV antidysrhythmic agent that decreases contractility less than verapamil
31. Tissue plasminogen activator with short half-life; given as a bolus followed by an infusion
34. Beta-type natriuretic hormone used in HF
35. Nucleoside used to break reentrant mechanism in paroxysmal SVT
37. IV Class III antidysrhythmic used for acute onset AF
39. Low-molecular-weight form used as a platelet aggregation inhibitor especially after vascular surgery

Learning Activities Answers

1.

1. f
2. g
3. a
4. h
5. i
6. j
7. c
8. f
9. d
10. b
11. e

2.

Adenosine (Adenocard)	Unclassified
Amiodarone (Cordarone)	III
Atropine	Unclassified
Digoxin	Unclassified
Diltiazem (Cardizem)	IV
Dofetilide (Tikosyn)	III
Esmolol (Brevibloc)	II
Flecainide (Tambocor)	IC
Ibutilide (Corvert)	III
Lidocaine (Xylocaine)	IB
Metoprolol (Lopressor)	II
Procainamide (Pronestyl)	IA
Propranolol (Inderal)	II
Quinidine	IA
Sotalol (Betapace)	II & III
Verapamil (Calan)	IV

3.

<table>
<tr><td colspan="2">AOO</td><td colspan="2">VVI</td><td>a. DVI</td></tr>
<tr><td colspan="2">VVI</td><td colspan="2">VAT</td><td>b. VDD</td></tr>
<tr><td>AAI</td><td colspan="2">VAT</td><td>VVI</td><td>c. DDD</td></tr>
</table>

4. a. Interpretation: VVI with normal function; complex No. 4 is a PVC and it is sensed appropriately.
b. Interpretation: DVI function with failure to sense; complex No. 5 shows atrial pacing with an intrinsic ventricular complex that is not sensed.
c. Interpretation: VVI with intermittent failure to capture; after the third paced complex, there is a nonconducted pacing spike; after the fourth paced complex, there is a nonconducted pacing spike.

5.

Nonmodifiable	Modifiable
Heredity	Hypertension
Advancing age	Diabetes mellitus or glucose intolerance
Male sex	Hyperlipidemia
	Hyperhomocysteinemia
	Sedentary lifestyle
	Stress
	Obesity
	Cigarette smoking
	Oral contraceptives (especially in smokers)

6. 1. a
2. a
3. g
4. d, c
5. c
6. b
7. e
8. e, f
9. e
10. i, j

7.

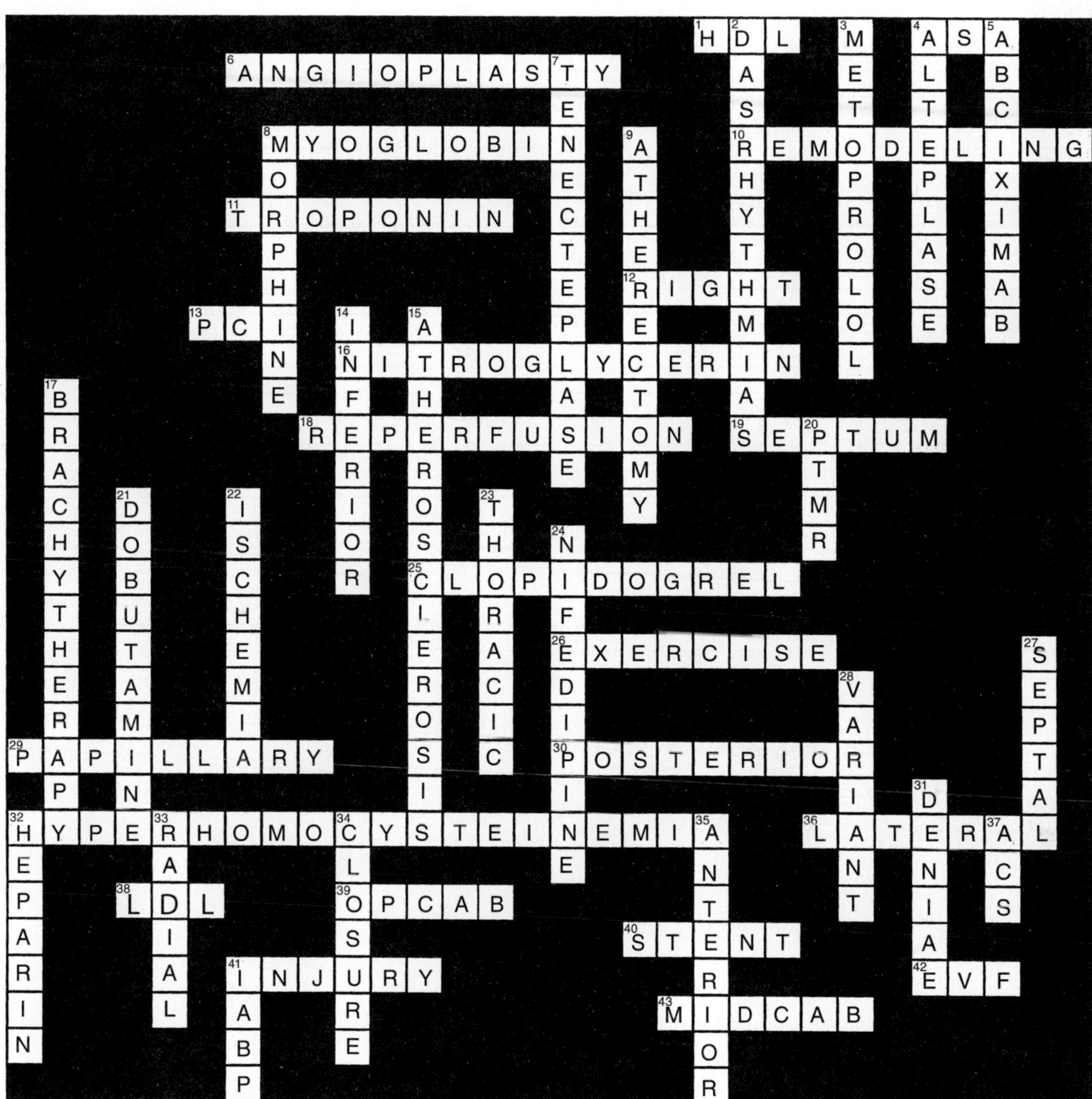

8.

a, b, d, g, m, s	1. RVF
b, c, g, q	2. LVF
e	3. Myocardial infarction
f	4. Pulmonary embolism
a, b	5. Tension pneumothorax
a, i, t	6. Cardiac tamponade
g	7. Valvular dysfunction
h, p	8. Pericarditis
g, j, p	9. Endocarditis
l, r	10. Hyperlipidemia
k, n	11. Chronic arterial insufficiency
m, o	12. Chronic venous insufficiency

9.

Causes	Left	Right
Aortic stenosis	✔	
Cardiac tamponade	✔	✔
Cardiomyopathy	✔	
Mitral stenosis	✔ (forward failure)	✔(backward failure)
Myocardial infarction (left)	✔	
Myocardial infarction (right)		✔
Pulmonary embolism	✔ (forward failure)	✔(backward failure)
PH		✔
Systemic hypertension	✔	
Sign/Symptom	**Left**	**Right**
Abnormal liver function studies		✔
Ascites		✔
Atrial dysrhythmias	✔	✔
Crackles audible over lungs	✔	
Dyspnea	✔	
Elevated PAOP	✔	
Elevated RAP		✔
Hepatomegaly		✔
Jugular venous distention		✔
Mental confusion	✔	
Murmur of mitral regurgitation	✔	
Murmur of tricuspid regurgitation		✔
Orthopnea	✔	
Peripheral edema		✔
S_3, S_4 at apex	✔	
S_3, S_4 at sternum		✔
Weight gain	✔	✔

10. a. (1) Increases coronary artery perfusion pressure
(2) Decreases afterload
b. (1) Aortic regurgitation
(2) Aortic aneurysm
c. Diastole
d. Systole
e. (1) Ischemia of left arm
(2) Renal ischemia

11. A. Assisted aortic end-diastolic pressure
B. Unassisted aortic end-diastolic pressure
C. Assisted systole
D. Unassisted systole
E. Diastolic augmentation

12.

Feature	Dilated	Hypertrophic	Restrictive
Associated with alcoholism or infection	✔		
Do not give inotropes		✔	
Clinical presentation: syncope, chest pain, sudden death		✔	
Clinical presentation similar to CHF	✔		✔
May be candidate for cardiac transplantation	✔	✔	✔
AF common	✔	✔	
Treatment includes beta-blockers and calcium channel blockers		✔	
Do not give diuretics or nitrates		✔	
Associated with infiltrative and connective tissue disorders	✔		✔
Treated with diuretics, ACE inhibitors, digoxin	✔		✔
Associated with genetically transmitted autosomal dominant trait		✔	
AV blocks are common			✔
Hemiblock is common		✔	
Treatment may include steroids			✔
May be treated with therapeutic septal infarction		✔	

13.

Feature	Pericarditis	Myocarditis	Endocarditis
Associated with MI	✔		
May cause cardiomyopathy		✔	
Causes splinter hemorrhages, petechiae			✔
Treated with antiinflammatory drugs	✔		
Sudden onset of CHF		✔	
Causes pericardial friction rub	✔		
Valve replacement may be necessary			✔
Usually associated with viral infection		✔	
Associated with cardiac surgery	✔		✔
Definitive diagnosis requires biopsy		✔	
May cause systemic emboli		✔	✔
Monitor closely for cardiac tamponade	✔		
Causes murmur			✔
Associated with uremia	✔		
Associated with ST segment elevation	✔		
Treated with antimicrobials		✔	✔
Increased incidence in patients with rheumatic heart disease		✔	✔

14.

Description	Drug
IV calcium channel blocker used for hypertension	Nicardipine (Cardene)
IV beta-blocker that also blocks alpha receptors	Labetalol (Normodyne)
IV vasodilator that may cause coronary artery steal and intrapulmonary shunt	Nitroprusside (Nipride)
IV vasodilator that is particularly helpful in patients with chest pain	Nitroglycerin (Tridil)
IV ACE inhibitor	Enalapril (Vasotec IV)
Oral ACE inhibitor that was first ACE inhibitor	Captopril (Capoten)
Two oral calcium channel blockers used for hypertension	Nifedipine (Procardia); diltiazem (Cardizem)
IV vasodilator frequently used in pregnancy-related hypertension	Hydralazine (Apresoline)
IV vasodilator with dopaminergic stimulation effects	Fenoldopam (Corlopam)

15.

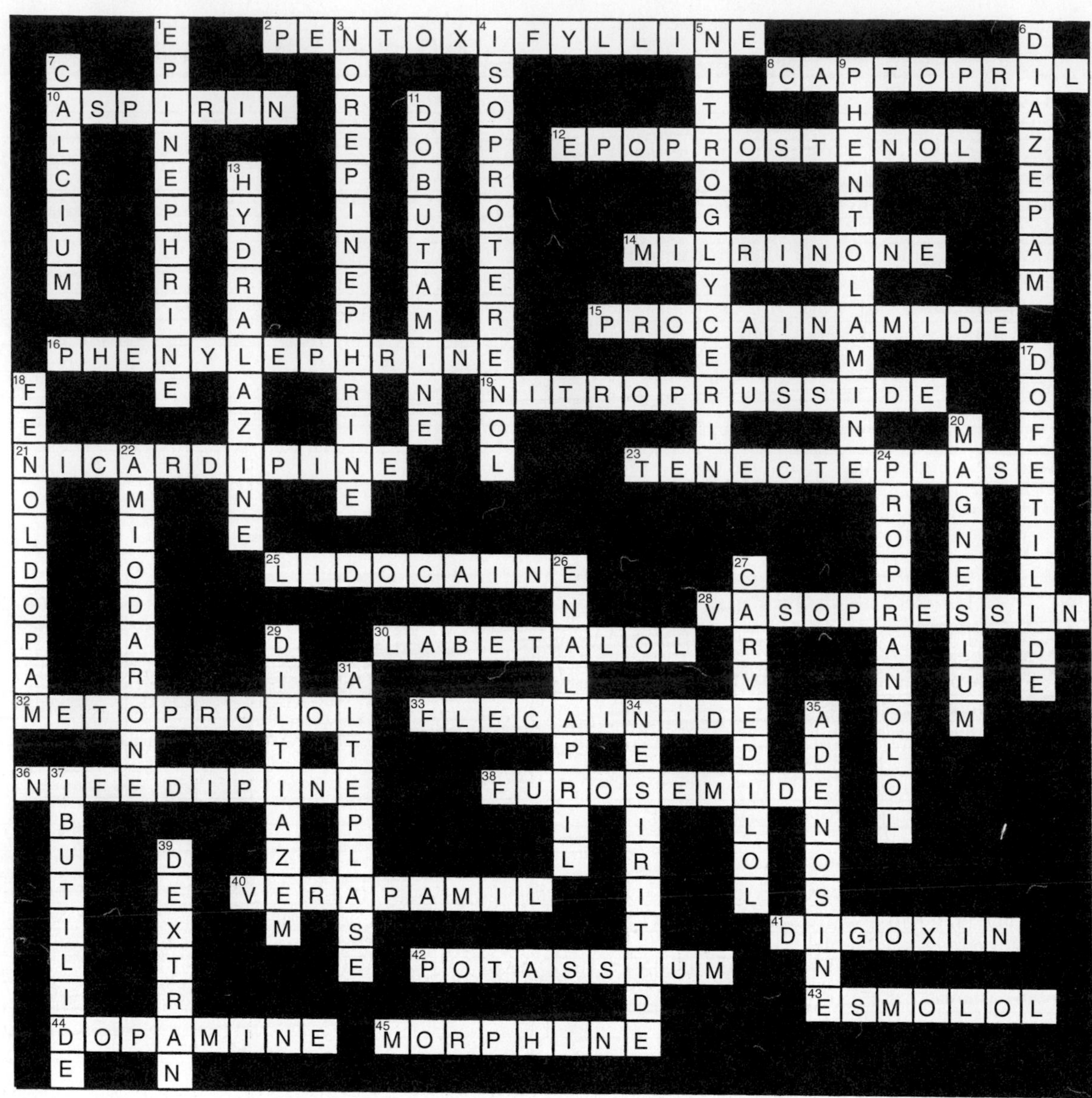

Bibliography

Accorda, R. (2000). Advances in the surgical treatment of coronary artery disease. *Nursing Clinics of North America, 35*(4), 913.

Adams-Hamoda, M. G., Caldwell, M. A., Stoots, N. A., & Drew, B. J. (2003). Factors to consider when analyzing 12-lead electrocardiograms for evidence of acute myocardial ischemia. *American Journal of Critical Care, 12*(1), 9-18.

Aehlert, B. (2002a). *ACLS: Quick review study guide* (2nd ed.). St. Louis, MO: MosbyJEMS.

Aehlert, B. (2002b). *ECGs made easy* (2nd ed.). St. Louis, MO: Mosby.

Ahrens, T. A., Schallom, L., Bettorf, K., Ellner, S., Hurt, G., Val, O. M., et al. (2001). End-tidal carbon dioxide measurements as a prognostic indicator of outcome in cardiac arrest. *American Journal of Critical Care, 10*(6), 391-389.

Albert, N. M., Eastwood, C. A., & Edwards, M. L. (2004). Evidence-based practice for acute decompensated heart failure. *Critical Care Nurse, 24*(6), 14-31.

American Association for Critical-Care Nurses. (2004). Practice Alert: Family presence during CPR and invasive procedures. Retrieved December 29, 2006, from http://www.aacn.org//AACN/practiceAlert.nsf/Files/Family%20Presence%20During%20CPR%20and%20Invasive%20Procedures/$file/AACN.PracticeAlert.Family%20Presence.10-4-04.pdf

American Heart Association. (2005a). Part 3: Overview of CPR. *Circulation, 112*(24 suppl), IV12-IV18.

American Heart Association. (2005b). Part 4: Adult basic life support. *Circulation, 112*(24 suppl), IV19-IV34.

American Heart Association. (2005c). Part 5: Electrical therapies: Automated external defibrillators, defibrillation, cardioversion, and pacing. *Circulation, 112*(24 suppl), IV35-IV46.

American Heart Association. (2005d). Part 6: CPR techniques and devices. *Circulation, 112*(24 suppl), IV47-IV50.

American Heart Association. (2005e). Part 7.1: Adjuncts for airway control and ventilation. *Circulation, 112*(24 suppl), IV51-IV57.

American Heart Association. (2005f). Part 7.2: Management of cardiac arrest. *Circulation, 112*(24 suppl), IV58-IV66.

American Heart Association. (2005g). Part 7.3: Management of symptomatic bradycardia and tachycardia. *Circulation, 112*(24 suppl), IV67-IV77.

American Heart Association. (2005h). Part 7.4: Monitoring and medications. *Circulation, 112*(24 suppl), IV78-IV83.

American Heart Association. (2005i). Part 7.5: Postresuscitation support. *Circulation, 112*(24 suppl), IV84-IV88.

American Heart Association. (2005j). Part 8: Stabilization of the patient with acute coronary syndromes. *Circulation, 112*(24 suppl), IV89-IV110.

Aminoff, U. B., & Kjellgren, K. I. (2001). The nurse: A resource in hypertension care. *Journal of Advanced Nursing, 35*(4), 582-589.

Anderson, L. A. (2001). Abdominal aortic aneurysm. *Journal of Cardiovascular Nursing, 15*(4), 1-14.

Artinian, N. T. (2003). The psychosocial aspects of heart failure. *American Journal of Nursing, 103*(12), 32-44.

Berke, W. J., & Ecklund, M. M. (2003). Keep pace with step-down care. *Critical Care Nurse, 23*(1), 56-58.

Bestul, M. B., McCollum, M., Stringer, K. A., & Burchenal, J. (2004). Impact of a critical pathway on acute myocardial infarction quality indicators. *Pharmacotherapy, 24*(2), 173-178.

Bither, C., & Apple, S. (2001). Home management of the failing heart. *American Journal of Nursing, 101*(12), 41.

Bond, A. E., Nelson, K., Germany, C. L., & Smart, A. N. (2003). The left ventricular assist device. *American Journal of Nursing, 103*(1), 32-41.

Branum, K. (2003). Management of decompensated heart failure. *AACN Clinical Issues, 14*(4), 498-511.

Broyles, L. M., & Korniewicz, D. M. (2002). The opiate-dependent patient with endocarditis: Addressing pain and substance abuse withdrawal. *AACN Clinical Issues, 13*(3), 431-451.

Bruni, K. R. (2001). Renovascular hypertension. *Journal of Cardiovascular Nursing, 15*(4), 78-90.

Bubien, R. S., & Sanchez, J. E. (2001). Atrial fibrillation: Treatment rational and clinical utility of nonpharmacologic therapies. *AACN Clinical Issues, 12*(1), 140-155.

Caldwell, D. A., & Lovasik, D. (2002). Endocarditis in the immunocompromised. *American Journal of Nursing, 102*(5), S32-S36.

Callahan, H. E. (2003). Families dealing with advanced heart failure: A challenge and an opportunity. *Critical Care Nursing Quarterly, 26*(3), 230-243.

Callans, D. J. (2002). Management of the patient who has been resuscitated from sudden cardiac death. *Circulation, 105*, 2704-2707.

Candela, L. (2002). Caring for a patient with *Listeria* endocarditis: Use of antibiotic desensitization. *Critical Care Nurse, 22*(5), 38-43.

Carelock, J., & Clark, A. (2001). Heart failure: pathophysiologic mechanisms. *American Journal of Nursing, 101*(12), 26.

Carlsson, E., Olsson, B., & Herterveg, E. (2002). The role of the nurse in enhancing quality of life in patients with an implantable cardioverter-defibrillator: The Swedish experience. *Progress in Cardiovascular Nursing, 17*(1), 18-25.

Carter, T., & Ellis, K. (2005). Right ventricular infarction. *Critical Care Nurse, 25*(2), 52-62.

Chen-Scarabelli, C. (2002). Beating-heart coronary artery bypass graft surgery: Indications, advantages, and limitations. *Critical Care Nurse, 22*(5), 44-58.

Chernecky, C., Alichnie, M. C., Garrett, K., George-Gay, B., Hodges, R. K., & Terry, C. (2002). *ECGs and the heart*. Philadelphia: W. B. Saunders.

Cherrington, C. C., Moser, D. K., Lennie, T. A., & Kennedy, C. W. (2004). Illness representation after acute myocardial infarction: Impact on in-hospital recovery. *American Journal of Critical Care, 13*(2), 136-145.

Chittock, D. R., Dhingra, V. K., Ronco, J. J., Russell, J. A., Forrest, D. M., Tweeddale, M., et al. (2004). Severity of illness and risk of death associated with pulmonary artery catheter use. *Critical Care Medicine, 32*(4), 911-915.

Cianci, P., Lonergan-Thomas, H., Slaughter, M., & Silver, M. A. (2003). Current and potential applications of left ventricular assist devices. *Journal of Cardiovascular Nursing, 18*(1), 17-22.

Collins, E., Langbeing, W. E., Dilan-Koetje, J., Bammert, C., Hanson, K., Reda, D., et al. (2004). Effects of exercise training on aerobic capacity and quality of life in individuals with heart failure. *Heart and Lung, 33*(3), 154-161.

Connaughton, M. (2001). *Evidence-based coronary care*. London: Churchill Livinstone.

Cooke, H. (2000). *When someone dies*. Oxford: Butterworth Heinemann.

Costello, F. (2002). Guidelines 2000: Changes in ACLS. *American Journal of Nursing, 102*(7), 24AA-24HH.

Crouch, M. A., Limon, L., & Cassano, A. T. (2003). Clinical relevance and management of drug-related QT interval prolongation. *Pharmacotherapy, 23*(7), 881-908.

Davis, S. (2002). How the heart failure picture has changed. *Nursing 2002, 32*(11), 36-46.

DeVon, H. A., & Zerwic, J. J. (2004). Differences in the symptoms associated with unstable angina and myocardial infarction. *Progress in Cardiovascular Nursing, 19*(1), 6-11.

Donohue, M. A. T. (2005). Best practice protocols: Evidence-based care for acute myocardial infarction. *Nursing Management, 36*(8), 23-27.

Doss, M., Martens, S., & Hemmer, W. (2002). Emergency endovascular interventions for ruptured thoracic and abdominal aortic aneurysms. *American Heart Journal, 144*(3), 544-548.

Dougherty, C. M., Pyper, G. P., & Frasz, H. A. (2004). Description of a nursing intervention program after an implantable cardioverter defibrillator. *Heart and Lung, 33*(3), 183-197.

Eells, P. L. (2004). Advances in prostacyclin therapy for pulmonary arterial hypertension. *Critical Care Nurse, 24*(2), 42-54.

Fenton, J. (2001). The clinician's approach to evaluating patients with dysrhythmias. *AACN Clinical Issues, 12*(1), 72-86.

Finkelmeier, B. A., & Marolda, D. (2001). Aortic dissection. *Journal of Cardiovascular Nursing, 15*(4), 15-24.

Fowler, R. A., & Pearl, R. G. (2002). The airway: Emergent management for nonanesthesiologists. *Western Journal of Medicine, 176*(1), 45-50.

Freeman, J. J., & Hedges, C. (2003). Cardiac arrest: The effect on the brain. *American Journal of Nursing, 103*(6), 50-55.

Futterman, L. G., & Lemberg, L. (2001b). Brugada. *American Journal of Critical Care, 10*(5), 360-364.

Futterman, L., & Lemberg, L. (2001a). Heart failure: update on treatment and prognosis. *American Journal of Critical Care, 10*(4), 285.

Futterman, L., & Lemberg, L. (2002). Novel markers in the acute coronary syndrome: BNP, IL-6, PAPP-A. *American Journal of Critical Care, 11*(2), 168-172.

Futterman, L. G., & Lemberg, L. (2004). The significance of hypothermia in preserving ischemic myocardium. *American Journal of Critical Care, 13*(1), 79-84.

Geiter, H. B., Jr. (2003a). Treating preexcitation tachycardias. *Nursing 2003, 33*(12), 32cc31-32cc32.

Geiter, H. B., Jr. (2003b). Understanding Wolff-Parkinson-White and preexcitation syndromes. *Nursing 2003, 33*(11), 32cc31-32cc34.

Geiter, H. B., Jr. (2004). Wellens syndrome: Subtle clues to big trouble. *Nursing 2004, 34*(6), 32cc31-32cc34.

Gilbert, C. J. (2001). Common supraventricular tachycardias: mechanisms and management. *AACN Clinical Issues, 12*(1), 100-113.

Gilski, D. J., & Borkenhagen, B. (2005). Risk evaluation in action for cardiovascular health. *Critical Care Nurse, 25*(1), 26-37.

Goldrick, B. A. (2003). Endocarditis associated with body piercing. *American Journal of Nursing, 103*(1), 26-27.

Gordon, P. A. (2004). Effects of diabetes on the vascular system: Current research evidence and best practice recommendations. *Journal of Vascular Nursing, 22*(1), 2-12.

Granger, B., & Miller, C. (2001). Acute coronary syndrome. *Nursing 2001, 31*(11), 36.

Greenberg, B. H. (2002). Endothelin and endothelin receptor antagonists in heart failure. *CHF, 8*(5), 257-261.

Gregoratos, G., Abrams, J., Epstein, A. E., Freedman, R. A., Hayes, D. L., Hlatky, M. A., et al. (2002). ACC/AHA/NASPE 2002 guideline update for implantation of cardiac pacemakers and antiarrhythmia devices: Summary article. A report of the American College of Cardiology/American Heart Association Task Force on Practice Guidelines. *Circulation, 106*, 2145-2161.

Hamlin, S. K., Villars, P. S., Kanusky, J. T., & Shaw, A. D. (2004). Role of diastole in left ventricular function, II: Diagnosis and treatment. *American Journal of Critical Care, 13*(6), 453-468.

Hamner, J. B., Dubois, E. J., & Rice, T. P. (2005). Predictors of complications associated with closure devices after transfemoral percutaneous coronary procedures. *Critical Care Nurse, 25*(3), 30-37.

Hardin, S., & Hussey, L. C. (2003). AACN synergy model for patient care: Case study of a CHF patient. *Critical Care Nurse, 23*(1), 73-76.

Hatchett, R., & Thompson, D. (Eds.). (2002). *Cardiac nursing: A comprehensive guide*. Edinburgh: Churchill Livingstone.

Hawley, J., & Dreher, H. M. (2002). Cardiac tamponade: The pressure's on. *Nursing 2002, 32*(4), 32cc31-32cc34.

Helms, S. V., & Lingle, C. (2004). Tap into safer telemetry. *Nursing Management, 35*(12), 54-59.

Hobbs, R. (2001). Should patients with severe heart failure be treated with beta-blockers? *Cleveland Clinic Journal of Medicine, 68*(5), 469.

Hoit, B. D. (2002). Management of effusive and constrictive pericardial heart disease. *Circulation, 105*, 2939-2942.

Hravnak, M., Hoffman, L. A., Saul, M., Zullo, T. G., Cuneo, J. F., & Pellegrini, R. V. (2004). Short-term complications and resource utilization in matched subjects after on-pump or off-pump primary isolated coronary artery bypass. *American Journal of Critical Care, 14*(6), 499-508.

Humphreys, D. (2001). Enhanced external counter pulsation: Beating angina. *Nursing 2001, 31*(10), 54.

Hussey, L. C., & Hardin, S. (2003). Sex-related differences in heart failure. *Heart and Lung, 32*(4), 215-223.

Iqbal, M. B., Taneja, A. K., Lip, G. Y. H., & Flather, M. (2005). Recent developments in atrial fibrillation. *British Medical Journal, 5*, 127-137.

Jowett, N. I., & Thompson, D. R. (2003). *Comprehensive cardiac care*. London: Bailliere Tindall.

Kantachuvessiri, A. (2002). Pulmonary veins: Preferred site for catheter ablation of atrial fibrillation. *Heart and Lung, 31*(4), 271-278.

Keller, K. B., & Lemberg, L. (2003). The cocaine-abused heart. *American Journal of Critical Care, 12*(6), 562-566.

Keller, K. B., & Lemberg, L. (2004). Prinzmetal's angina. *American Journal of Critical Care, 13*(4), 350-354.

Kurowski, V., Hartmann, F., Killermann, D. P., Giannitsis, E., Wiegand, U. K. H., Frey, N., et al. (2002). Prognostic significance of admission cardiac troponin T in patients treated successfully with direct percutaneous interventions for acute ST-segment elevation myocardial infarction. *Critical Care Medicine, 30*(10), 2229-2234.

Lanza, M. (2001). Right ventricular myocardial infarction: When the power fails. *Nursing 2001, 31*(9), 32cc31.

LeRoy, S. S. (2001). Clinical dysrhythmias after surgical repair of congenital heart disease. *AACN Clinical Issues, 12*(1), 87-99.

Lewis, C. D. (2001). Peripheral arterial disease of the lower extremity. *Journal of Cardiovascular Nursing, 15*(4), 45-63.

Lewis, P. S., Boyd, C. M., Hubert, N. E., & Steele, M. (2001). Ethanol-induced therapeutic infarction to treat hypertrophic obstructive cardiomyopathy. *Critical Care Nurse, 21*(2), 20-34.

Little, C. (2004). Your guide to the intra-aortic balloon pump. *Nursing 2004, 34*(12), 32cc31-32cc32.

Liu, P. P., & Mason, J. W. (2001). Advances in the understanding of myocarditis. *Circulation, 104*, 1076-1082.

Lorenz, B. T., & Coyte, K. (2002). Coronary artery bypass graft surgery without cardiopulmonary bypass: A review and nursing implications. *Critical Care Nurse, 22*(1), 51-60.

Lusardi, P., & Brown, V. (2003). Inhaled epoprostenol. *American Journal of Nursing, 103*(7), 64AA-64HH.

MacKlin, M. (2001). Managing heart failure: a case study approach. *Critical Care Nurse, 21*(2), 36.

Mair, M. (2003). Monophasic and biphasic defibrillators. *American Journal of Nursing, 103*(8), 58-60.

Malacaria, B., & Feloney, C. D. H. (2003). Going with the flow of anticoagulant therapy. *Nursing 2003, 33*(3), 36-44.

Marrone, L., & Fogg, C. (2003). Should the family be present during resuscitation? *Nursing 2003, 33*(10), 32cc31-32cc32.

McAvoy, J. (2004). Case studies of ST-segment elevation before and after percutaneous coronary intervention. *Critical Care Nurse, 24*(6), 32-39.

McBride, B. F., & White, C. M. (2003). Acute decompensated heart failure: A contemporary approach to pharmacotherapeutic management. *Pharmacotherapy, 23*(8), 997-1020.

McCabe, P. J. (2005). Spheres of clinical nurse specialist influence: Evidence-based care for patients with atrial fibrillation. *Clinical Nurse Specialist, 19*(6), 308-319.

McIntyre, K. M. (2004). Vasopressin in asystolic cardiac arrest. *New England Journal of Medicine, 350*(2), 179-181.

McLaughlin, V. V., Presberg, K. W., Doyle, R. L., Abman, S. H., McCrory, D. C., Fortin, T., et al. (2004). Prognosis of pulmonary artery hypertension. *Chest, 126*(1 suppl), 78S-92S.

Milgrom, L. B., Brooks, J. A., Qi, R., Bunnell, K., Wuestefeld, S., & Beckman, D. (2004). Pain levels experienced with activities after cardiac surgery. *American Journal of Critical Care, 13*(2), 116-125.

Miller, J. M., & Zipes, D. P. (2002). Catheter ablation of arrhythmias. *Circulation, 106*, e203-e205.

Neutel, J. (2002). The use of combination drug therapy in the treatment of hypertension. *Progress in Cardiovascular Nursing, 17*(2), 81-88.

Nickolaus, M. (2000). Advances in interventional cardiology: beyond the balloon. *Nursing Clinics of North America, 35*(4), 897.

Nienaber, C. A., & Eagle, K. A. (2003a). Aortic dissection: New frontiers in diagnosis and management. Part I: From etiology to diagnostic strategies. *Circulation, 108*, 628-635.

Nienaber, C. A., & Eagle, K. A. (2003b). Aortic dissection: New frontiers in diagnosis and management. Part II: Therapeutic management and follow-up. *Circulation, 108*, 772-778.

Nunnelee, J. D., & Spaner, S. D. (2004). The quality of research on physical examination for abdominal aortic aneurysm. *Journal of Vascular Nursing, 22*(1), 14-18.

Oliver, B., & Ayello, E. (2005). How drug-eluting stents keep coronary blood flowing. *Nursing 2005, 35*(2), 36-42.

Oliver-McNeil, S. (2001). Treating hypertrophic cardiomyopathy without surgery. *Nursing 2001, 31*(2), 32cc31-32cc34.

Olson, K. K., & Autio, L. A. (2001). Measuring quality of care for essential hypertension. *Holistic Nursing Practice, 15*(4), 22-34.

Palatnik, A. (2000). Acute coronary syndrome: new advances and nursing strategies. *Dimensions of Critical Care Nursing, 19*(5), 22.

Palek, D. (2001). Endovascular repair of abdominal aortic aneurysm. *American Journal of Nursing, 101*(4), 24AA.

Parsons, C., Sole, M., & Byers, J. (2000). Noninvasive positive-pressure ventilation: averting intubation of the heart failure patient. *Dimensions of Critical Care Nursing, 19*(6), 18.

Patronis Jones, R. A., & Stephens, R. (2001). Issues and trends in care of the hypertensive client. *Holistic Nursing Practice, 15*(4), vi-xi.

Paul, S. (2001). Understanding advanced concepts in atrioventricular block. *Critical Care Nurse, 21*(1), 56.

Peacock, W. F., IV. (2002). The B-type natriuretic peptide assay: A rapid test for heart failure. *Cleveland Clinic Journal of Medicine, 69*(3), 243-256.

Pooler, C., & Barkman, A. (2002). Myocardial injury: Contrasting infarction and contusion. *Critical Care Nurse, 22*(1), 15-26.

Porter, B. (2002). The role of the advanced practice nurse in anticoagulation. *AACN Clinical Issues, 13*(2), 221-233.

Powers, C. C., & Martin, N. K. (2002). When seconds count, use an AED. *American Journal of Nursing, 102*(9), 8-10.

Prahash, A., & Lynch, T. (2004). B-type natriuretic peptide: A diagnostic, prognostic, and therapeutic tool in heart failure. *American Journal of Critical Care, 13*(1), 46-55.

Pyne, C. C. (2004). Classification of acute coronary syndromes using the 12-lead electrocardiogram as a guide. *AACN Clinical Issues, 15*(4), 558-567.

Reid, M. B., & Cottrell, D. (2005). Nursing care of patients receiving intra-aortic balloon counterpulsation. *Critical Care Nurse, 25*(5), 40-49.

Reimer-Kent, J. (2003). From theory to practice: Preventing pain after cardiac surgery. *American Journal of Critical Care, 12*(2), 136-143.

Rempher, K. J. (2003). Continuous renal replacement therapy for management of overhydration in heart failure. *AACN Clinical Issues, 14*(4), 512-519.

Reynolds, J., & Apple, S. (2001). A systematic approach to pacemaker assessment. *AACN Clinical Issues, 12*(1), 114-126.

Rodgers, J., & Reeder, S. (2001a). Current therapies in the management of systolic and diastolic dysfunction. *Dimensions of Critical Care Nursing, 20*(6), 2.

Rodgers, J., & Reeder, S. (2001b). Managing heart failure, part 1. *Nursing 2001, 31*(11), 32cc31.

Rodgers, J., & Reeder, S. (2001c). Managing heart failure, part 2. *Nursing 2001, 31*(12), 32cc31.

Roosens, C., Heerman, J., De Somer, F., Caes, F., Van Belleghem, Y., & Poelaert, J. I. (2002). Effects of off-pump coronary surgery on the mechanics of the respiratory system, lung, and chest wall: Comparison with extracorporeal circulation. *Critical Care Medicine, 30*(11), 2430-2437.

Rosenow, D. J., & Russell, E. (2001). Current concepts in the management of hypertensive crisis: Emergencies and urgencies. *Holistic Nursing Practice, 15*(4), 12-21.

Rosenthal, K. (2004). Case study: Using ultrafiltration to manage CHF. *Nursing Management, 35*(3), 41-46.

Rosenthal, K. (2005). Is electromagnetic interference still a risk? *Nursing Management, 36*(4), 68-71.

Ryan, C. J., DeVon, H. A., & Zerwic, J. J. (2005). Typical and atypical symptoms. *American Journal of Nursing, 105*(2), 34-36.

Saksena, S., & Madan, N. (2002). Management of the patient with an implantable cardioverter-defibrillator in the third millennium. *Circulation, 106*, 2642-2646.

Saul, L., & Shatzer, M. (2003). B-type natriuretic peptide testing for detection of heart failure. *Critical Care Nursing Quarterly, 26*(1), 35-39.

Savage, L. (2003). Quality of life among patients with a left ventricular assist device: What is new? *AACN Clinical Issues, 14*(1), 64-72.

Schnautz, L., Glines, E., Rowley, D., Harris, D., & Petty, M. (2005). To freeze or not to freeze. *American Journal of Nursing, 105*(2), 72AA-72DD.

Shaffer, R. (2002). ICD therapy: the patient's perspective. *American Journal of Nursing, 102*(2), 46-49.

Shubrooks, S. J., Nesto, R. W., Leeman, D., Waxman, S., Lewis, S. M., Fitzpatrick, P., et al. (2001). Urgent coronary bypass surgery for failed percutaneous coronary intervention in the stent era: Is backup still necessary? *American Heart Journal, 142*(1), 190-196.

Steinbis, S. (2003). Hypertrophic obstructive cardiomyopathy and septal ablation. *Critical Care Nurse, 23*(3), 47-50.

Sutherland, J. (2001). Selected complementary methods and nursing care of the hypertensive client. *Holistic Nursing Practice, 15*(4), 4-11.

Thomas, S. A., Friedmann, E., Khatta, M., Cook, L. K., & Lann, A. L. (2003). Depression in patients with heart failure. *AACN Clinical Issues, 14*(1), 3-12.

Thompson, C., & Tsiperfal, A. (2002). When do we monitor the effects of a "therapeutic" myocardial infarction? *Progress in Cardiovascular Nursing, 17*(3), 152-154.

Tokarczyk, T. R. (2003). Cardiac transplantation as a treatment option for the heart failure patient. *Critical Care Nursing Quarterly, 26*(1), 61-68.

Urden, L., Stacy, K., & Lough, M. (2006). *Thelan's critical care nursing: Diagnosis and management* (5th ed.). St. Louis, MO: Mosby.

Vaught, K., & Ostrow, L. (2001). Bed rest after percutaneous transluminal coronary angioplasty: How much is enough? *Dimensions of Critical Care Nursing, 20*(4), 46.

Villars, P. S., Hamlin, S. K., Shaw, A. D., & Kanusky, J. T. (2004). Role of diastole in left ventricular function, I: Biochemical and biomechanical events. *American Journal of Critical Care, 13*(5), 394-405.

Wagner, J. M. (2004). Lived experience of critically ill patients' family members during cardiopulmonary resuscitation. *American Journal of Critical Care, 13*(5), 416-420.

Wennberg, D. E., Lucas, F. L., Siewers, A. E., Kellett, M. A., & Malenka, D. J. (2004). Outcomes of percutaneous coronary interventions performed at centers without and with onsite coronary artery bypass graft surgery. *Journal of the American Medical Association, 292*(16), 1961-1968.

Wenzel, V., Krismer, A. C., Arntz, H. R., Sitter, H., Stadlbauer, K. H., & Lindner, K. H. (2004). A comparison of vasopressin and epinephrine for out-of-hospital cardiopulmonary resuscitation. *New England Journal of Medicine, 350*(2), 105-113.

White, M. (2002). Psychosocial impact of the implantable cardioverter defibrillator: Nursing implications. *Journal of Cardiovascular Nursing, 16*(6), 53-61.

Wiegand, D. L.-M. (2003). Advanced in cardiac surgery: Valve repair. *Critical Care Nurse, 23*(2), 72-91.

Woods, A. (2001). Improving the odds against hypertension. *Nursing 2001, 31*(8), 36.

Woods, S., Froelicher, E. S. S., & Motzer, S. U. (2004). *Cardiac nursing* (5th ed.). Philadelphia: Lippincott.

Zevola, D. R., Raffa, M., & Brown, K. (2002). Using clinical pathways in patients undergoing cardiac valve surgery. *Critical Care Nurse, 22*(1), 31-50.

Zhang, J. (2002). Sudden cardiac death: Implantable cardioverter defibrillators and pharmacological treatments. *Critical Care Nursing Quarterly, 26*(1), 45-49.

The Pulmonary System: Physiology, Assessment, and Ventilatory Support

CHAPTER 4

Selected Concepts in Anatomy and Physiology

General Information

1. The pulmonary system consists of lungs, conducting air passages, muscles of ventilation, central nervous system control, thoracic cage, and alveoli (Figure 4-1).
2. Functions of the pulmonary system include the following:
   a. Allows interchange of gases between the atmosphere and the bloodstream
   b. Assists in maintenance of acid-base balance
   c. Contributes to phonation
   d. Acts as a reservoir for blood for the left atrium and ventricle
   e. Assists in metabolism

Functional Anatomy

1. Conducting airways: nose to terminal bronchioles
   a. Conduct airflow toward gas exchange units; no gas exchange occurs in these airways
      (1) Consists of branching tubes with diminishing diameter
      (2) Accounts for approximately 2 mL/kg of inspired tidal volume (this volume is referred to as *anatomic dead space*)
   b. Upper airway (Figure 4-2): nose or mouth to external opening of vocal cords; serves as a passageway for food and inspired gas
      (1) Mouth: not as effective as the nose in conditioning the inspired air
         (a) Smaller surface area
         (b) No ciliated epithelium to trap dust or bacteria from inspired air
      (2) Nose
         (a) Structure
            (i) Mucous membrane lining contains cilia and mucus-producing cells.
            (ii) Rich supply of blood vessels lies under the mucous membranes to provide warmth.
            (iii) Skeletal rigidity maintains patency during inspiration.
            (iv) Turbinates increase surface area.
            (v) Four sinuses surround and drain into the nasal cavity: frontal, maxillary, ethmoid, sphenoid.
            (vi) Septum divides the nose into two fossae.
            (vii) Small inlet with larger outlet allows air to have maximal contact with the nasal mucosa.
         (b) Functions
            (i) Warms inspired gas to body temperature
            (ii) Humidifies inspired gas to relative humidity of approximately 80% to 100% at body temperature; accounts for insensible water loss of 400 mL/24 hours
            (iii) Protects the lower airway from foreign material; filters inspired air of particles 5 micrometers or larger
            (iv) Prevents inspiration of potentially dangerous environmental gases
            (v) Assists in production of sound in phonation
            (vi) Provides sense of olfaction: olfactory area located in the superior turbinate (sniffing directs air toward this area)
         (c) More resistance (2 to 3 times) than the mouth; this is rationale for why dyspneic patients are more likely to breathe through their mouth
      (3) Pharynx: posterior nasal cavity to esophagus
         (a) Structure

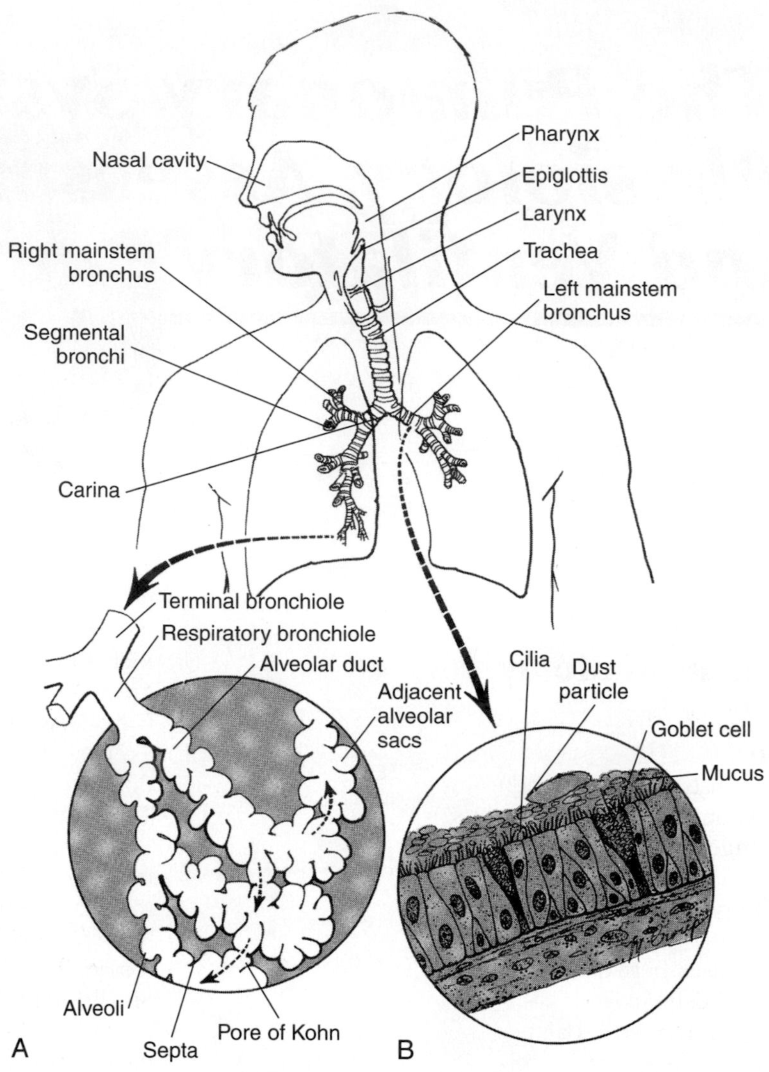

Figure 4-1 The respiratory system. **A,** Acinus. **B,** Mucociliary escalator. (From Price, S. A., & Wilson, L. M. [1997]. *Pathophysiology: Clinical concepts of disease processes* [5th ed.]. St. Louis: Mosby.)

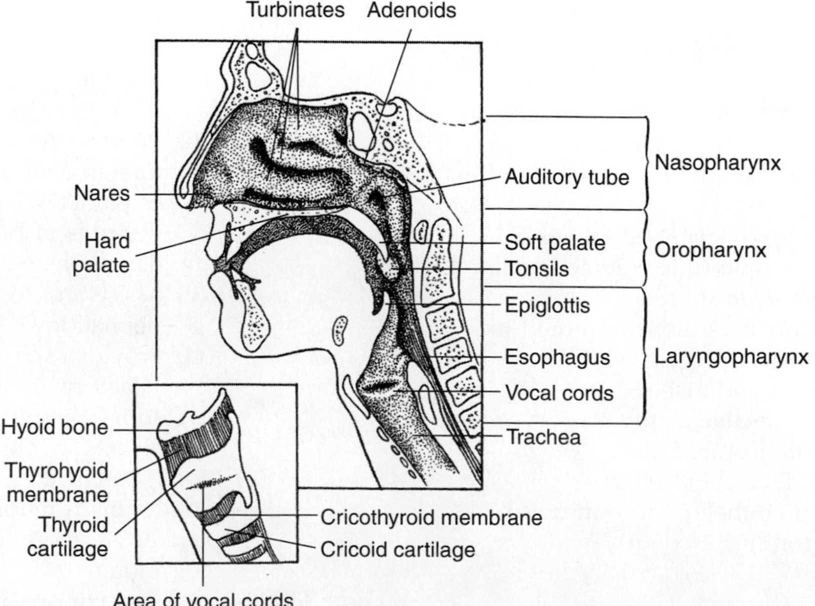

Figure 4-2 The upper airway (lateral view). (From Luce, J. M., & Pierson, D. J. [1998]. *Critical care medicine*. Philadelphia: W. B. Saunders.)

(i) Nasopharynx: between posterior nasal cavity and soft palate; contains the pharyngeal tonsils and eustachian tubes
a) Pharyngeal tonsils (also called *adenoids*): dense concentration of lymphatic tissue; guards entryway into respiratory and gastrointestinal (GI) tracts
b) Eustachian tubes: connection between nasopharynx and middle ear; opens during swallowing to equalize pressure in the middle ear
i) Middle ear pain or infection may develop during upper respiratory infection if eustachian tube closes.
ii) Nasal intubation may block eustachian tubes and cause otitis media.
(ii) Oropharynx: between the soft palate and base of tongue
a) Location of the palatine and lingual tonsils
b) Center of the gag reflex that defends the lower airway against aspiration; gag reflex controlled by cranial nerves IX (glossopharyngeal) and X (vagus)
(iii) Laryngopharynx (also called the *hypopharynx*): from base of tongue to the epiglottis
(b) Functions
(i) Swallowing: uvula and soft palate move posteriorly and superiorly to keep food and liquid from entering the nasopharynx
(ii) Protection: area is rich in lymphatic tissue
(4) Larynx: upper portion of the trachea; connects the laryngopharynx with the trachea
(a) Structure: consists of thyroid cartilage, vocal cords, cricoid cartilage
(i) Epiglottis: flexible cartilage attached to the thyroid cartilage that overhangs the larynx like a lid; prevents food from entering the larynx and trachea during swallowing
(ii) Thyroid cartilage: largest laryngeal cartilage
a) Contains the vocal cords
b) Also referred to as the *Adam's apple*
(iii) Vocal folds: two pairs of membranes that protrude into the lumen of the larynx; controlled by recurrent laryngeal nerve, a branch of the vagus nerve
a) False vocal cords: upper pair; play no part in vocalization
b) True vocal cords: lower pair
i) Form a triangular opening between them that leads to the trachea
ii) Change shape and vibrate in response to contraction of muscles in the larynx to result in phonation
c) Glottis: passage through the vocal cords
(iv) Cricothyroid membrane: avascular structure that connects the thyroid and cricoid cartilage; cricothyrotomy, an emergency opening of the airway, is performed at this membrane
(v) Cricoid cartilage: complete ring located below the thyroid cartilage
(b) Functions
(i) Allows speech
(ii) Prevents aspiration through the valve action of epiglottis
(iii) Allows for cough reflex and Valsalva maneuver
c. Lower airway (Figure 4-3): below larynx; conducts air to the gas exchange surface
(1) Structure
(a) Trachea: first portion of tracheobronchial tree
(i) Consists of 16 to 20 C-shaped rings; 10 to 12 cm long
(ii) The esophagus and trachea share a common wall; erosion through this wall (tracheoesophageal fistula) may be caused by an overinflated endotracheal (ET) tube or tracheostomy tube cuff

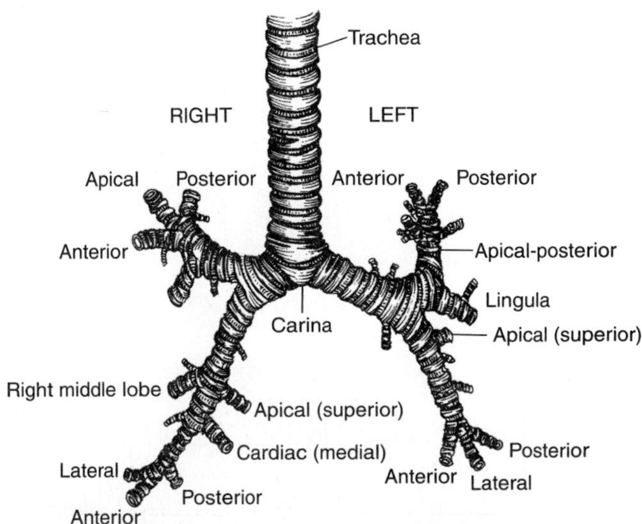

Figure 4-3 The lower airway. (Modified from Frownfelter, D. L. [Ed.]. [1978]. *Chest physical therapy and pulmonary rehabilitation.* Chicago: Mosby.)

(b) Carina: bifurcation of trachea into left and right mainstem bronchi
   (i) The carina is rich in parasympathetic nervous system fibers and cough receptors.
   (ii) Suctioning may cause bradycardia and hypotension because of stimulation of the carina with the suction catheter.

(c) Bronchi
   (i) Right mainstem bronchus is almost straight (25 degrees) off trachea and larger in diameter than the left (40 to 60 degrees); aspiration of liquid or food, foreign bodies, suction catheter, and ET tube goes to the right preferentially.
   (ii) Conducting airways branch from mainstem bronchi branch to lobar bronchi, from lobar bronchi branch to segmental bronchi, from segmental bronchi branch to subsegmental bronchi, and so on.
      a) These branches are called *generations* or *levels* (Figure 4-4): mainstem (first level), lobar (second), segmental (third), subsegmental (fourth through ninth), bronchioles (tenth through fifteenth branches).
   (iii) Bronchi are supported by cartilage and smooth muscle.

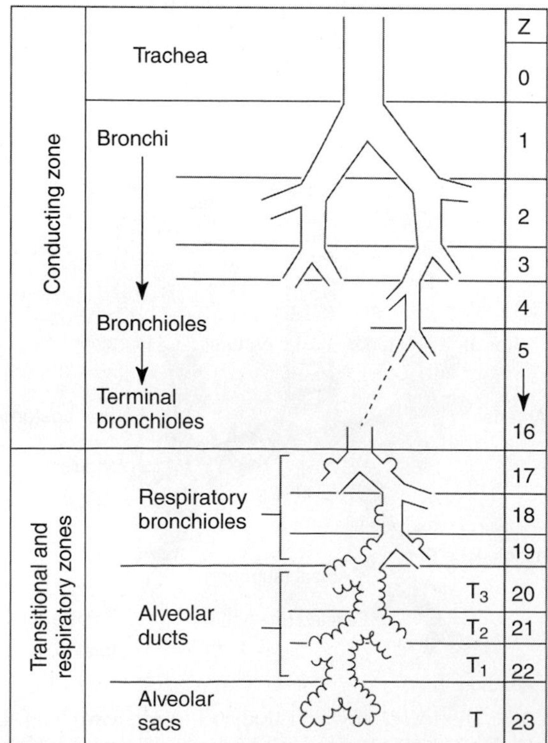

Figure 4-4 Airway generations.

   (iv) Mast cells lie just beneath the bronchial epithelium near the smooth muscle and blood vessels.

(d) Function
   (i) The lower airway conducts, warms, cleanses, and humidifies air.
   (ii) The bronchi are responsible for most of total airway resistance in a healthy person.
   (iii) Mast cells secrete histamine and other mediators of the inflammatory process when stimulated by antigen-antibody response.

(2) Terminal bronchioles
   (a) Structure
      (i) Sixteenth branch
      (ii) One millimeter in diameter; fibrous, elastic smooth muscle with no cartilage; no mucus glands or cilia
   (b) Function
      (i) Terminal bronchioles are particularly sensitive to carbon dioxide (CO_2) and dilate in response to increased CO_2 levels.
      (ii) Bronchospasm may significantly narrow the lumen and increase airway resistance.

2. Lung
   a. Lobes separated by fissures
      (1) Right: three lobes
      (2) Left: two lobes
         (a) The upper left lobe is divided by a fissure.
         (b) The lower portion of the left upper lobe is referred to as the *lingula;* it is approximately the same size as the right middle lobe.
   b. Segments
      (1) Right: 10 segments
      (2) Left: eight segments
   c. Subsegments
   d. Lobules
      (1) Primary functional units of lung
      (2) Consists of terminal bronchiole, alveolar ducts, alveolar sacs, alveoli, pulmonary circulation
   e. Gas exchange units (Figure 4-5): respiratory bronchioles to alveoli
      (1) Acinus: a term used to refer to the terminal respiratory unit distal to the terminal bronchioles; has an alveolar-capillary membrane for gas exchange
      (2) Respiratory bronchioles
         (a) Structure
            (i) Composed of the seventeenth though twentieth branches
            (ii) Less than 1 mm in diameter; bronchioles less than 1 mm are subject to collapse when compressed

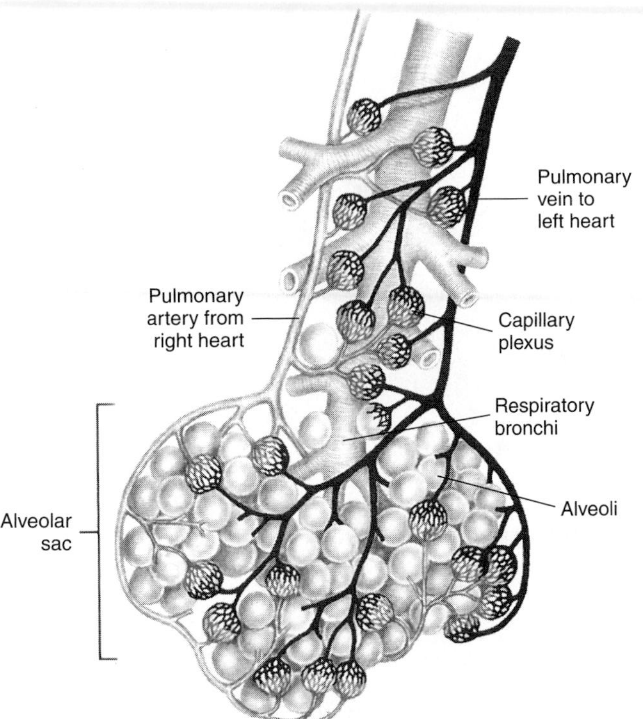

Figure 4-5 The acinus. (From Wilson, S. F., & Thompson, V. M. [1990]. *Mosby's clinical nursing series: Respiratory disorders.* St. Louis: Mosby.)

(b) Function
  (i) Increasing number of alveoli are attached.
  (ii) Gas exchange takes place here.

(3) Alveolar ducts, alveolar sacs, and alveoli
  (a) Structure
    (i) Alveolar ducts: twentieth to twenty-second levels
    (ii) Alveolar sacs: level 23
    (iii) Alveoli: 300 million alveoli
      a) 200-300 micrometers in diameter
      b) One half of alveoli in ducts and one half in alveolar sacs in grapelike clusters of 15 to 20 alveoli
      c) Surface area approximately 80 m^2
      d) Contain pores of Kohn: openings between alveoli in intraalveolar septa
        i) Thought to allow collateral ventilation
        ii) Also may contribute to movement of microorganisms between alveoli and rapid transmission of infection
    (iv) Lined with alveolar epithelium: site of diffusion of oxygen (O_2) and CO_2 between inspired air and blood
    (v) Type I pneumocytes
      a) Cover 90% of total alveolar surface
      b) Flat, large, squamous cells; susceptible to injury
      c) Responsible for integumentary air-blood barrier; cytoplasmic junctions tight and impermeable to water under normal circumstances
    (vi) Type II pneumocytes
      a) These small, cuboidal, granular cells cover only 5% total alveolar surface.
      b) They produce, store, and secrete surfactant, a lipoprotein that lines the inner aspect of the alveolus.
        i) Surfactant decreases surface tension of the fluid lining the alveoli and prevents alveolar collapse at the end of expiration, especially at low volumes.
        ii) Surfactant is especially important in inferior portions of lung where alveoli are small and distending pressures are low.
        iii) A deficiency of surfactant causes alveolar collapse, poorly compliant lungs, and alveolar edema.
        iv) The half-life of surfactant is only 14 hours; injury to these cells quickly results in massive atelectasis.
      c) If type I pneumocytes are injured, type II pneumocytes increase mitosis to replicate and form a cuboidal cell line and may differentiate to type I.

f. Alveolar-capillary membrane
  (1) Structure
    (a) Lines respiratory bronchioles to alveoli
    (b) Surface area of 1 m^2/kg body mass and 0.2 micrometers in thickness
    (c) Diffusion pathway (Figure 4-6): gases travel through the pathway from alveolus to blood (O_2) or blood to alveolus (CO_2)
      (i) Alveolar epithelium
      (ii) Epithelial basement membrane
      (iii) Interstitial space
      (iv) Capillary basement membrane
      (v) Capillary endothelium
  (2) Function
    (a) Immense surface area and thinness of membrane allow for rapid gas exchange by diffusion.
    (b) Pulmonary capillary endothelial cells produce and degrade prostaglandins, metabolize vasoactive amines, convert angiotensin I to angiotensin II, and at least partly produce coagulation factor VIII.

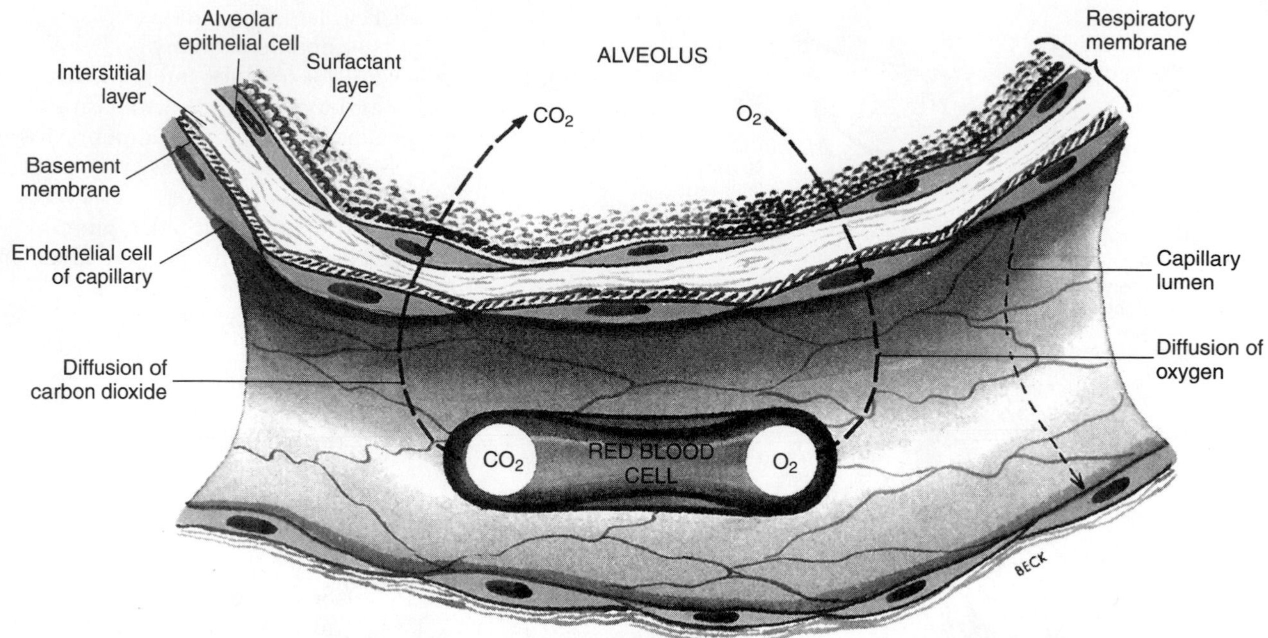

Figure 4-6 The diffusion pathway. (From Lewis, S. M., & Collier, I. C. [1992]. *Medical-surgical nursing* [3rd ed.]. St. Louis: Mosby.)

g. Defense mechanisms
   (1) Upper airway
      (a) Nasal cilia
      (b) Sneeze: reaction to irritation in the nose
      (c) Cough: reaction to irritation in the upper airway distal to the nose
         (i) Vocal cords close and intrathoracic pressure increases.
         (ii) Sudden opening of glottis allows propulsion of mucus.
      (d) Mucociliary escalator
         (i) Combination of mucus and cilia
         (ii) Particles not filtered by nasal cilia (smaller than 5 micrometers) are trapped in mucus and then are propelled upward by the pulsatile motion of the cilia; this mucus then is coughed and expectorated or swallowed
      (e) Lymphatics
   (2) Lower airway
      (a) Cough: especially at level of carina
      (b) Mucociliary escalator
      (c) Lymphatics
   (3) Alveoli
      (a) Immune system
      (b) Lymphatics
      (c) Alveolar macrophages: mononuclear phagocytes
         (i) Engulf and remove bacteria and other foreign substances
         (ii) Move from alveolus to alveolus through the pores of Kohn
   (4) Loss of normal defense mechanisms
      (a) Disease
      (b) Injury
      (c) Anesthesia
      (d) Corticosteroids
      (e) Smoking
      (f) Malnutrition
      (g) Ethanol
      (h) Uremia
      (i) Hypoxia or hyperoxia
      (j) Artificial airways

3. Lymphatics
   a. Structure: surround lobule
   b. Functions
      (1) Remove interstitial fluid to keep lung free of excess fluid
         (a) Normal lymph drainage is approximately 20 mL/hr; it may be 200 mL/hr in pulmonary edema.
         (b) When interstitial lymphatic vessels become enlarged through increased fluid filtration such as pulmonary edema, horizontal linear opacities referred to as *Kerley's B lines* are seen on chest x-ray.
      (2) Remove inhaled particles from distal areas of lung
4. Circulation (Figure 4-7)
   a. Pulmonary circulation: low-pressure, low-resistance system
      (1) Lungs receive the full cardiac output (approximately 5 L/min)
      (2) Right ventricle → main pulmonary artery → left and right pulmonary arteries → arterioles → capillaries that spread over the surface of the alveoli → red blood cells (RBCs) move through in single file to allow the diffusion of gases and the attachment of O_2 to hemoglobin

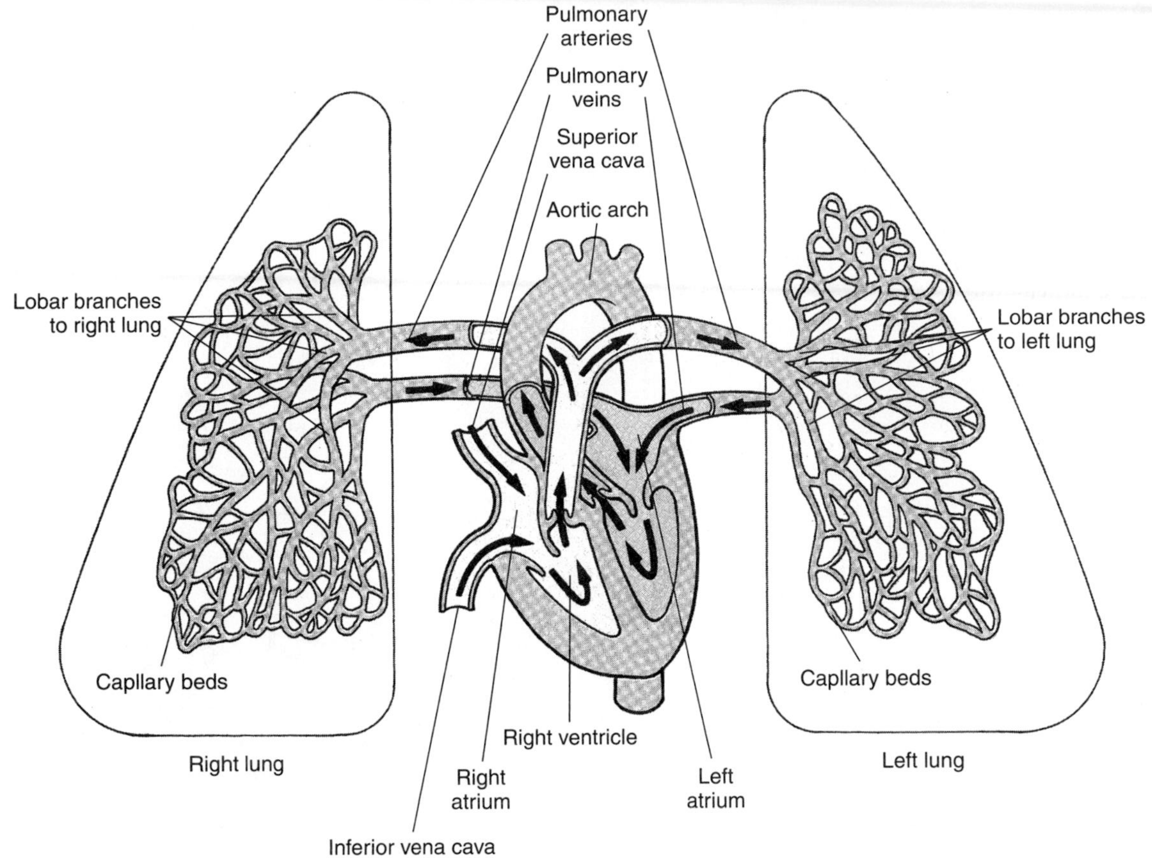

Figure 4-7 The pulmonary circulation. (From Wilson, S. F., & Thompson, V. M. [1990]. *Mosby's clinical nursing series: Respiratory disorders*. St. Louis: Mosby.)

(a) A corresponding arteriole and venule exists for every bronchiole.
(b) The network of capillaries is dense and frequently is described as a sheet of blood
(c) The pulmonary capillaries are small and barely accommodate erythrocyte passage.

(3) Veins move out of lung toward pleura
(a) Numerous veins gradually form four pulmonary veins that empty into the left atrium.
(b) The venous system serves as an immense reservoir of blood for the left atrium and left ventricle.

(4) Mean pressure in pulmonary artery: 10 to 20 mm Hg
(a) Pulmonary hypertension (median pulmonary artery pressure greater than 20 mm Hg)
(i) Primary pulmonary hypertension: idiopathic
(ii) Secondary pulmonary hypertension
a) Passive pulmonary hypertension: result of back pressure
i) Mitral stenosis
ii) Left ventricular failure
b) Active pulmonary hypertension
i) Constriction of the pulmonary circulation is caused by decreased alveolar O_2 concentration (called *hypoxemic pulmonary hypertension*), acidosis, or endogenous agents such as epinephrine, norepinephrine, and angiotensin II
ii) Obstruction in pulmonary circuit: pulmonary embolus
(b) Dilation of the pulmonary circulation caused by
(i) O_2
(ii) Pulmonary vasodilators (e.g., isoproterenol, aminophylline, epoprostenol [Flolan], bosentan [Tracleer], nitric oxide)

b. Bronchial circulation
(1) This system consists of the nutrient and O_2 circulation for the tracheobronchial tree down to terminal bronchioles, visceral pleura, interstitial and connective tissue, some arteries and veins, lymph nodes, and nerves within the thoracic cavity.
(a) Two bronchial arteries to the left lung: directly off the aorta
(b) One bronchial artery to the right lung: from the intercostal artery that originates from the right subclavian or internal mammary artery

(2) Gas exchange units are supplied with nutrients and O_2 by the pulmonary circulation.
(3) Bronchial venous blood enters the pulmonary veins and causes some desaturation of the oxygenated blood in the pulmonary vein; this venous blood and the blood from the thebesian veins account for the normal physiologic shunt of 3% to 5%.

5. Thoracic cage (Figure 4-8)
   a. Muscular walls reinforced by bones
      (1) Sternum anterior: three connected flat bones
         (a) Manubrium
         (b) Body
         (c) Xiphoid
      (2) Spine posterior: twelve pairs of ribs are attached to the vertebrae
      (3) Ribs anterior, lateral, and posterior
         (a) Seven pairs of ribs, called *true ribs*, are attached to sternum
         (b) Five pairs of ribs are attached to the rib above it
      (4) Clavicles superior
      (5) Diaphragm: inferior border of the thoracic cage
   b. Properties
      (1) Rigid to protect the lungs
      (2) Resilient to allow expansion and reduction of lung volume that occurs during ventilation
   c. Contents
      (1) Heart
      (2) Lungs
      (3) Esophagus
      (4) Great vessels
      (5) Liver
      (6) Spleen
6. Pleural cavities (Figure 4-9)
   a. Each lung hangs in its own pleural cavity attached only at the hilum; the hilum is where

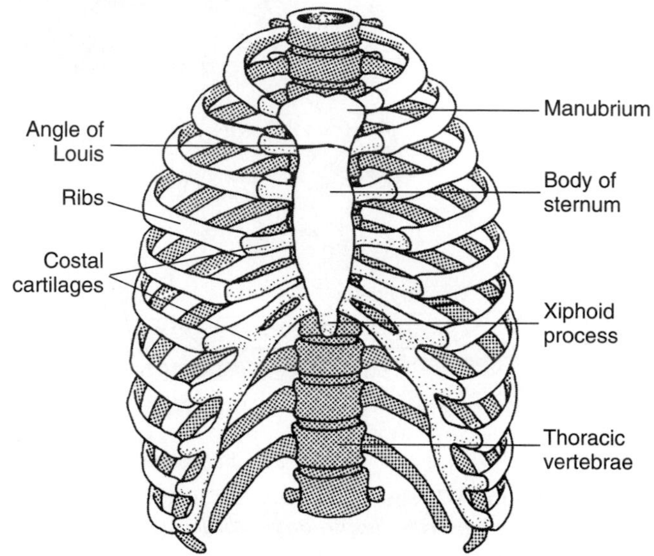

Figure 4-8 The thoracic cage. (From Scanlan, C. L., Spearman, C. B., & Sheldon, R. L. (Eds.). [1990]. *Egan's fundamentals of respiratory care* [6th ed.]. St. Louis, MO: Mosby.)

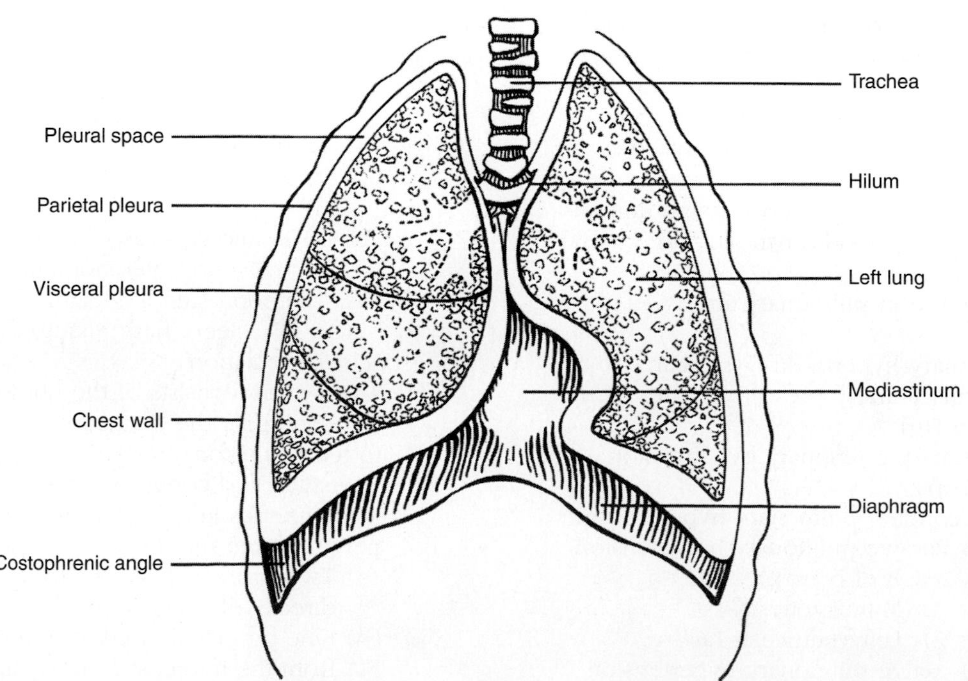

Figure 4-9 Internal structures of the thorax, including pleural cavities. (From Dettenmeier, P. A. [1992]. *Pulmonary nursing care*. St. Louis: Mosby.)

the two mainstem bronchi branch and where the pulmonary vessels enter and leave the thoracic space.

b. Pleural cavities are independent of one another.
c. The borders of pleural cavities are as follows:
   (1) Chest wall lateral
   (2) Mediastinum medial
   (3) Diaphragm inferior
d. Pleural linings consist of two layers:
   (1) Visceral: contiguous with lung
   (2) Parietal: contiguous with chest wall
   (3) Pleural space
      (a) Contains a few milliliters of serous fluid, which acts as a lubricant and adhesive between the visceral and parietal pleurae as they slide along each other with each ventilatory cycle
      (b) Maintains a negative intrapleural pressure of approximately −5 mm Hg below atmospheric pressure; this pressure becomes more negative (−10 mm Hg) during inspiration; loss of this negative intrapleural pressure causes the lung to collapse (e.g., pneumothorax)

7. Mediastinum: center of thoracic cavity; contains the following:
   a. Heart and great vessels
   b. Trachea and mainstem bronchi
   c. Esophagus
   d. Phrenic, vagus, and other nerves
   e. Lymph nodes and ducts
   f. Thymus gland
8. Muscles of ventilation (Figure 4-10)
   a. Inspiratory
      (1) Diaphragm
         (a) Innervation occurs via phrenic nerves (C3 to C5).
         (b) The diaphragm consists of two hemidiaphragms connected by a central membranous tendon; this tendon is contiguous with the fibrous pericardium.
         (c) Contraction flattens the diaphragm.
            (i) Increases size of thorax superior to inferior
            (ii) Normally accounts for 70% of tidal volume (V_T) during quiet breathing
         (d) Relaxation makes the diaphragm dome shaped and decreases the volume of the thoracic cavity.
      (2) External intercostal muscles
         (a) Innervation occurs from T1 to T12.
         (b) Contraction raises the ribs, increasing the size of the thorax anteroposteriorly.
      (3) Accessory muscles of inspiration
         (a) Scalene
            (i) Located in the neck; stretch from the first cervical vertebrae to the first and second ribs
            (ii) Enlarge the upper rib cage
         (b) Sternocleidomastoid
            (i) Located in the neck; stretch from the manubrium and clavicle to the mastoid process and occipital bone
            (ii) Elevate the sternum to increase the anteroposterior and transverse diameter of the chest
         (c) Not used in normal resting ventilation but used during exercise and in respiratory distress; also used in the inspiratory phase of sneeze or cough
   b. Expiratory
      (1) Expiration is normally passive

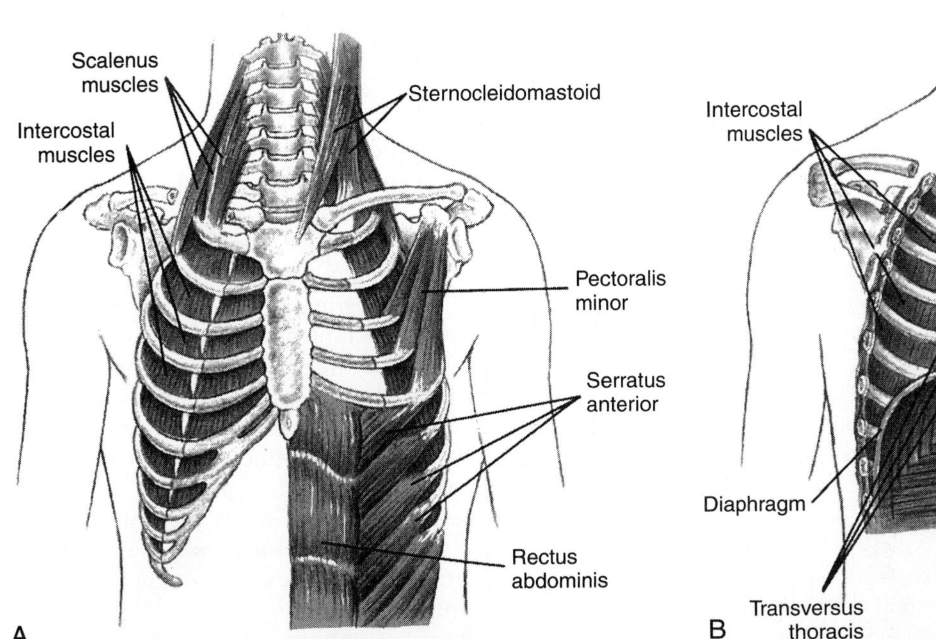

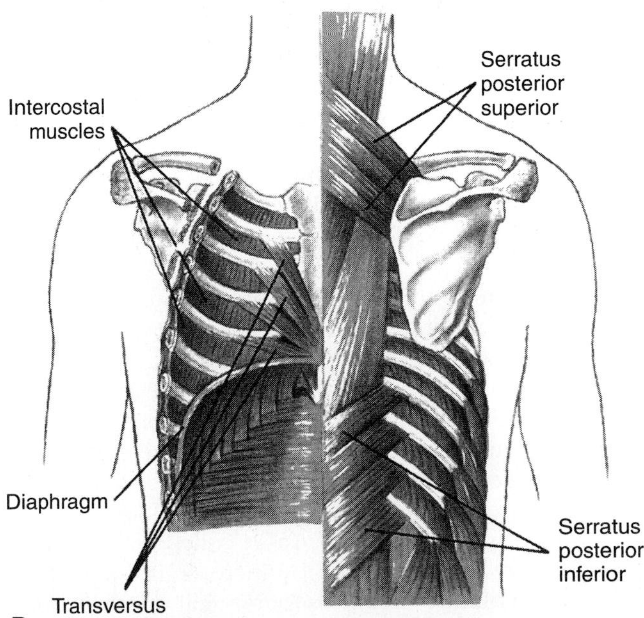

Figure 4-10 Muscles of ventilation. **A,** Anterior. **B,** Posterior. (From Thelan, L. A., Urden, L. D., Lough, M. E., & Stacy, K. M. [1998]. *Critical care nursing: Diagnosis and management* [3rd ed.]. St. Louis: Mosby.)

(a) Expiration occurs when diaphragm and external intercostal muscles relax and return to resting position.
(b) The natural tendency of the lungs is to collapse because they are made of elastic tissue; elastance is the quality of the lungs to recoil after inspiration.
(2) Accessory muscles of expiration: internal oblique, external oblique, rectus abdominis, internal intercostal, and transversus abdominis
(a) Depress the lower ribs and pull down the anterior portion of the lower chest
(b) Increase pressure in abdominal cavity and compress the abdominal viscera up against the diaphragm
(c) Used when increased levels of ventilation are needed
(d) Important in forceful expiration, coughing, and sneezing

9. Neuroanatomy
a. Medulla: central chemoreceptors sensitive to cerebrospinal fluid pH (↑ $Paco_2$ → acidosis)
(1) Primary control of ventilation is by these central chemoreceptors and $Paco_2$ and pH levels.
(2) They respond to minimal changes in $Paco_2$ quickly.
(3) Adjustment of alveolar ventilation occurs.
(a) Increase in $Paco_2$ causes an increase in the rate and depth of ventilation.
(b) Decrease in $Paco_2$ causes a decrease in the rate and depth of ventilation.
b. Arterial chemoreceptors in aortic arch and carotid bodies: sensitive to pH and Pao_2
(1) These peripheral chemoreceptors and Pao_2 levels provide secondary control of ventilation.
(2) They will not respond to $Paco_2$ levels until a 10 mm Hg change is seen.
(3) They respond when Pao_2 falls below approximately 60 mm Hg; particularly important in patients with chronically elevated levels of $Paco_2$.
c. Pontine: control rhythmic ventilation
(1) Apneustic center stimulates inspiratory center.
(2) Pneumotaxic center inhibits inspiratory activity.
d. Stretch receptors in alveoli (Hering-Breuer reflex): inhibit further inspiration to prevent overdistention of alveoli; may cause bronchodilation, tachycardia, vasodilation
e. Proprioceptors in muscles and tendons: increase ventilation in response to body movements
f. Baroreceptors in aortic arch and carotid bodies: increase in blood pressure (BP) inhibits ventilation
g. Juxtacapillary receptors (also called *pulmonary J-receptors*): stimulated by increase in interstitial fluid volume; may cause laryngeal constriction, hypotension, bradycardia, mucus production, dyspnea
h. Chest wall pain receptors
(1) Lung parenchyma does not have pain receptors
(2) Parietal pleura does have pain receptors; transmit impulses via intercostal nerves and thoracic ganglia
i. Irritant receptors: stimulated by pulmonary edema, chemical or mechanical irritation; may cause bronchospasm, cough, mucus production
j. Modifying influences: drugs; brain trauma, edema, or increased intracranial pressure; chronic hypercapnia

Physiology (Figure 4-11)

1. Ventilation: movement of air between atmosphere and alveoli and distribution of air within the lungs to maintain appropriate concentrations of O_2 and CO_2 in the alveoli
a. Process (Figure 4-12)
(1) Inspiration (inhalation): the movement of atmospheric air into the alveoli
(a) Message from medulla travels down phrenic nerve to diaphragm.
(b) Diaphragm and external intercostal muscles contract.
(c) Size of thorax increases.
(d) Lungs are stretched and intrapulmonary pressure is decreased to less than atmospheric pressure (−1 cm H_2O).
(e) Air moves into lungs to equalize the difference between atmospheric and alveolar pressure.
(2) Expiration (exhalation): movement of air from alveoli to the atmosphere
(a) Relaxation of diaphragm and external intercostal muscles
(b) Recoil of lungs to their resting size and a concomitant increase in alveolar pressure above atmospheric pressure (+1 cm H_2O)
(c) Air movement out of lungs to equalize the pressure difference
b. Efficiency of ventilation: evaluated by $Paco_2$
(1) $Paco_2$ greater than 45 mm Hg indicates hypoventilation.
(2) $Paco_2$ less than 35 mm Hg indicates hyperventilation.
c. Lung volumes (Figure 4-13 and Table 4-1)
(1) Alveolar ventilation is the volume of air per minute participating in gas exchange; it is the most important portion of minute ventilation; minute ventilation minus dead space ventilation.
(2) Dead space ventilation (Figure 4-14) is the volume of air per minute that does not participate in gas exchange.
(a) Anatomic dead space is the volume of air in conducting airways and does not participate in gas exchange; approximately 2 mL/kg of V_T.
(b) Alveolar (pathologic) dead space is the volume of air in contact with nonperfused alveoli.

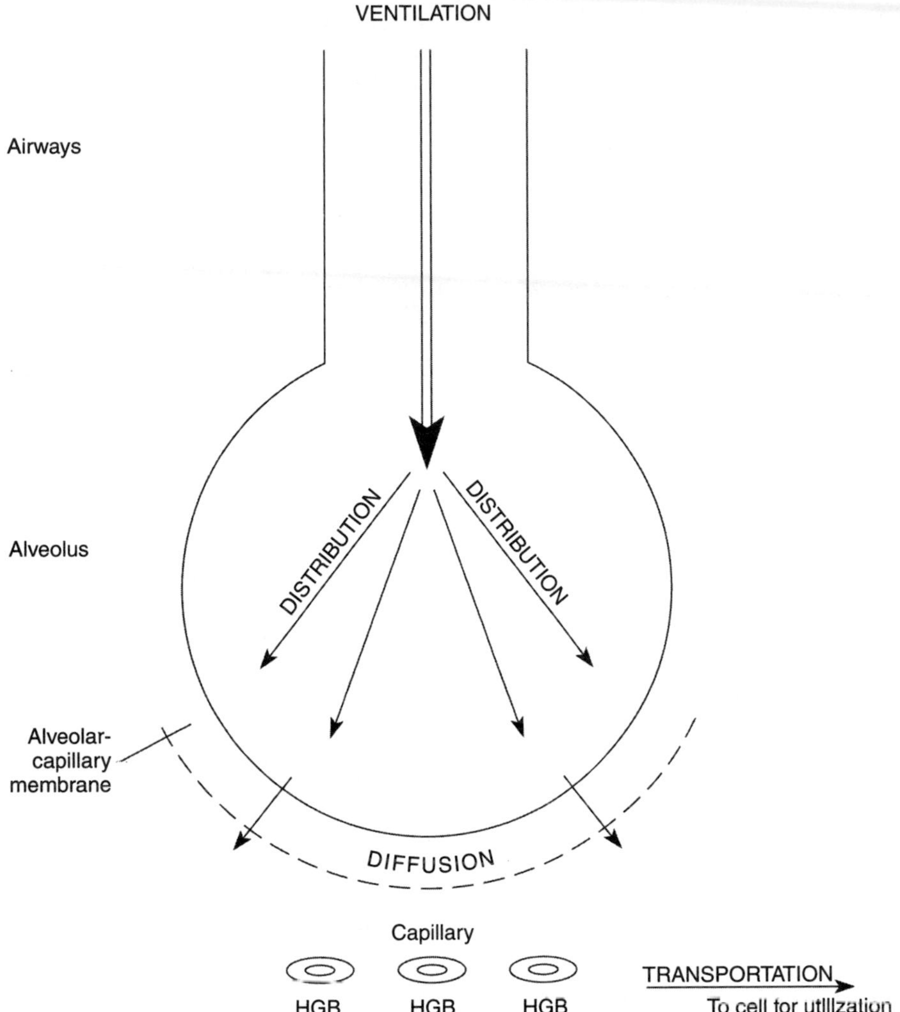

Figure 4-11 Respiratory process: ventilation, distribution, diffusion, transportation, cellular utilization. *HGB*, Hemoglobin. (Drawing by Ann M. Walthall.)

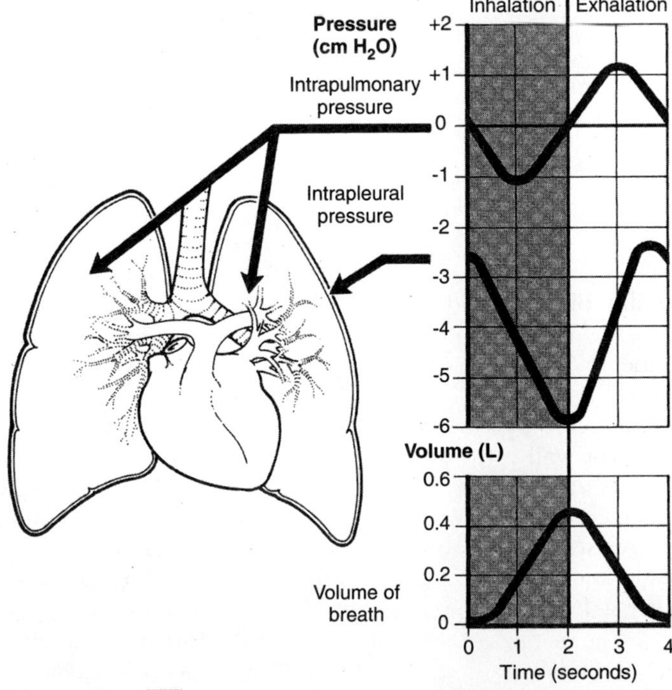

Figure 4-12 Pressure changes during ventilation. (From Thelan, L. A. Urden, L. D., Lough, M. E., & Stacy, K. M. [1998]. *Critical care nursing: Diagnosis and management* [3rd ed.]. St. Louis: Mosby.)

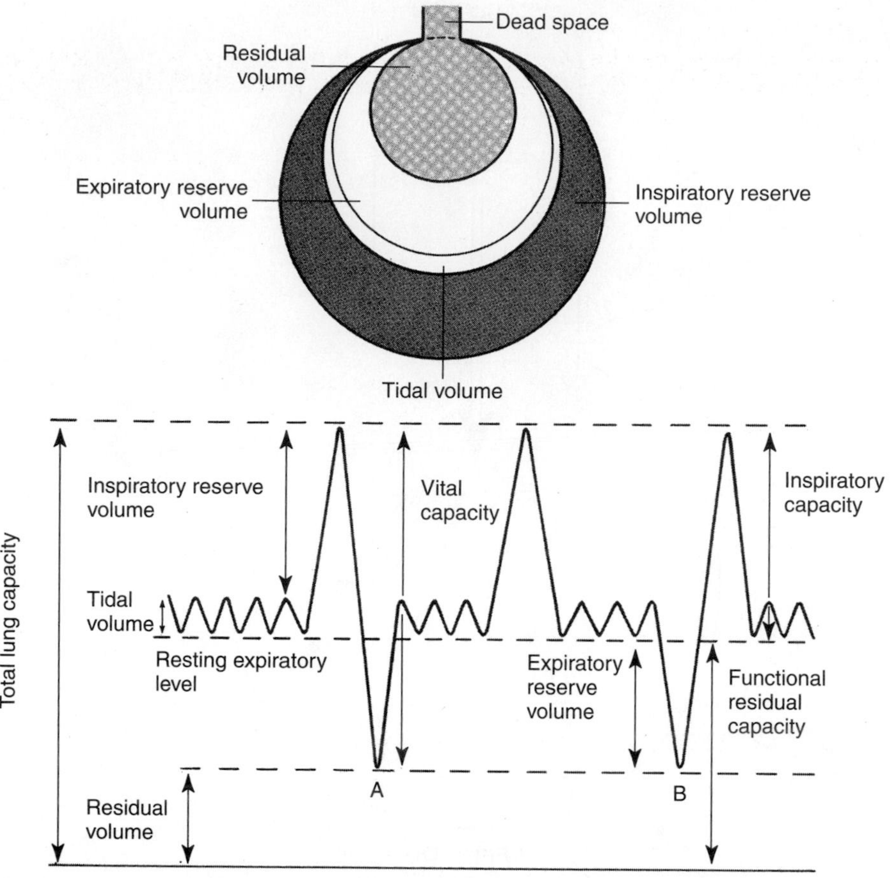

Figure 4-13 Lung volumes and capacities: upward deflection reflects inspiration, and downward deflection reflects expiration. (From Dettenmeier, P. A. [1992]. *Pulmonary nursing care*. St. Louis: Mosby.)

(c) Physiologic dead space is anatomic plus alveolar dead space.

(i) Calculated by: $V_D = \dfrac{Paco_2 - P_Eco_2}{V_T \; Paco_2}$

where P_Eco_2 is partial pressure of CO_2 on expiration

Normal: 0.2 to 0.4

d. Work of breathing = Work of deforming the elastic system + Work of producing airflow through the airways (Figure 4-15)

(1) Usually the work of breathing is negligible: 2% to 3% of total energy expenditure by the body

(2) Compliance

(a) Measure of expandability of lungs and/or thorax

(b) $C = \dfrac{\text{Change in volume}}{\text{Change in pressure}}$

(i) Static compliance: affected by changes in compliance of chest wall or lung

(ii) Dynamic compliance: affected by changes in compliance of chest wall or lung or airway resistance

(iii) Calculation of static and dynamic compliance (Figure 4-16 and Table 4-2)

(c) Factors affecting static compliance

(i) Chest wall changes

a) Kyphoscoliosis

b) Flail chest

c) Thoracic pain with splinting

d) Obesity

(ii) Lung changes

a) Atelectasis

b) Pneumonia

c) Pulmonary edema

d) Pulmonary fibrosis

e) Pleural effusion

f) Pneumothorax

(d) Additional factors affecting dynamic compliance

(i) As for factors affecting static compliance and airway resistance changes; the difference between static and dynamic compliance represents airway resistance

(3) Airway resistance

(a) Pressure differential required to produce a unit flow change; affected by airway caliber and length

(b) Factors affecting airway resistance (and dynamic compliance)

(i) Bronchospasm

(ii) Mucus

(iii) Artificial airways

(iv) Water condensation in ventilator tubing

(v) Mucosal edema

(vi) Bronchial tumor

Table 4-1 **Lung Volumes, Capacities, and Mechanics**

Volume	Definition	Normal
Tidal volume (V_T)	The volume of air moved in and out of the lungs with each normal breath	7 mL/kg or approximately 500 mL
Inspiratory reserve volume (IRV)	The volume of air that can be maximally inspired above the normal inspiratory level	3000 mL
Expiratory reserve volume (ERV)	The volume of air that can be maximally exhaled beyond the normal expiratory level	1000 mL
Residual volume (RV)	The volume of air remaining in the lungs at the end of a maximal expiration	1000 mL
Inspiratory capacity (IC)	V_T + IRV; the volume of air that can be maximally inspired from a normal expiratory level	3500 mL
Functional residual capacity (FRC)	RV + ERV; the volume of air remaining in the lungs at the end of normal expiration	2000 mL
Vital capacity (VC)	V_T + IRV + ERV; the volume of air that can be maximally expired after a maximal inspiration	4500 mL
Total lung capacity (TLC)	V_T + IRV + ERV + RV; the volume of air that the lungs can hold with maximal inspiration	5500-6000 mL
Respiratory rate or frequency (f)	The number of breaths per minute	12-20 breaths per minute
Minute ventilation (M_E)	$V_T \times f$; the volume of air expired per minute	5-10 L
Dead space (V_D)	$V_D/V_T = Paco_2 - P_Eco_2/Paco_2$ $Paco_2$ (arterial); P_Eco_2 (exhaled) The volume or percentage of the V_T that does not participate in gas exchange; includes the volume of air in the conducting pathways (anatomic dead space) plus the volume of alveolar air that is not involved in gas exchange because of a pathologic condition (alveolar dead space)	V_D/V_T ratio is normally less than 0.4; V_D/V_T greater than 0.6 usually an indication for mechanical ventilation
Alveolar ventilation (V_A)	$V_T - V_D$; the volume of tidal air that is involved in alveolar gas exchange	350 mL
Forced vital capacity (FVC)	The volume of air in a forceful maximal expiration	Normally same as VC: 4500 mL
Forced expiratory volume (FEV)	The volume of air exhaled in a given time period; FEV_1: the volume of air exhaled in 1 second; FEV_3: the volume of air exhaled in 3 seconds	FEV_1: greater than 75% of VC FEV_3: greater than 95% of VC

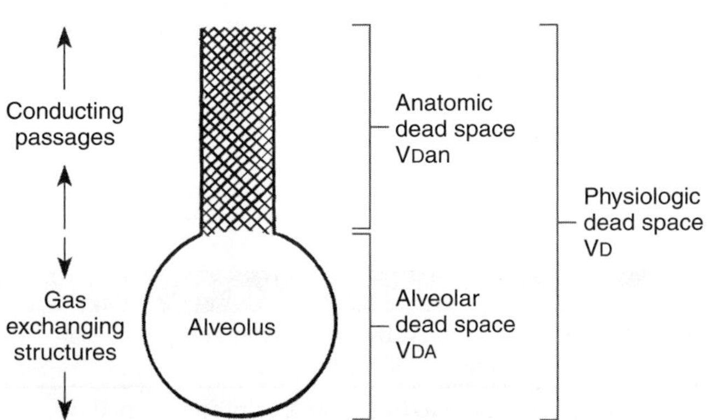

Figure 4-14 Physiologic dead space: anatomic dead space and alveolar dead space. (Drawing by Wendy W. Johnson.)

2. Perfusion: movement of blood through the pulmonary capillaries
   a. Pulmonary vasculature: resistance varies to accommodate the blood flow that it receives
   b. Distribution of perfusion
      (1) Related to gravity and intraalveolar pressures
         (a) Gravity causes the pressure in the capillaries in the bases to be higher than the pressure in the capillaries in the apices; preferential blood flow is to the gravity-dependent areas of the lungs.
         (b) The intraalveolar pressures are generally equal throughout the lungs.
         (c) This creates the potential for intraalveolar pressure to exceed capillary hydrostatic pressure in some areas of the lung, causing absence of blood flow to these areas.

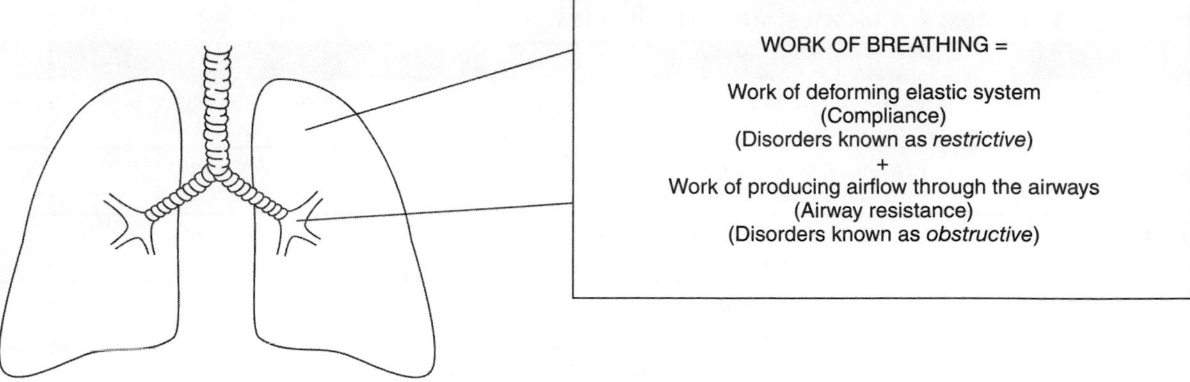

WORK OF BREATHING =
Work of deforming elastic system
(Compliance)
(Disorders known as *restrictive*)
+
Work of producing airflow through the airways
(Airway resistance)
(Disorders known as *obstructive*)

Figure 4-15 The work of breathing.

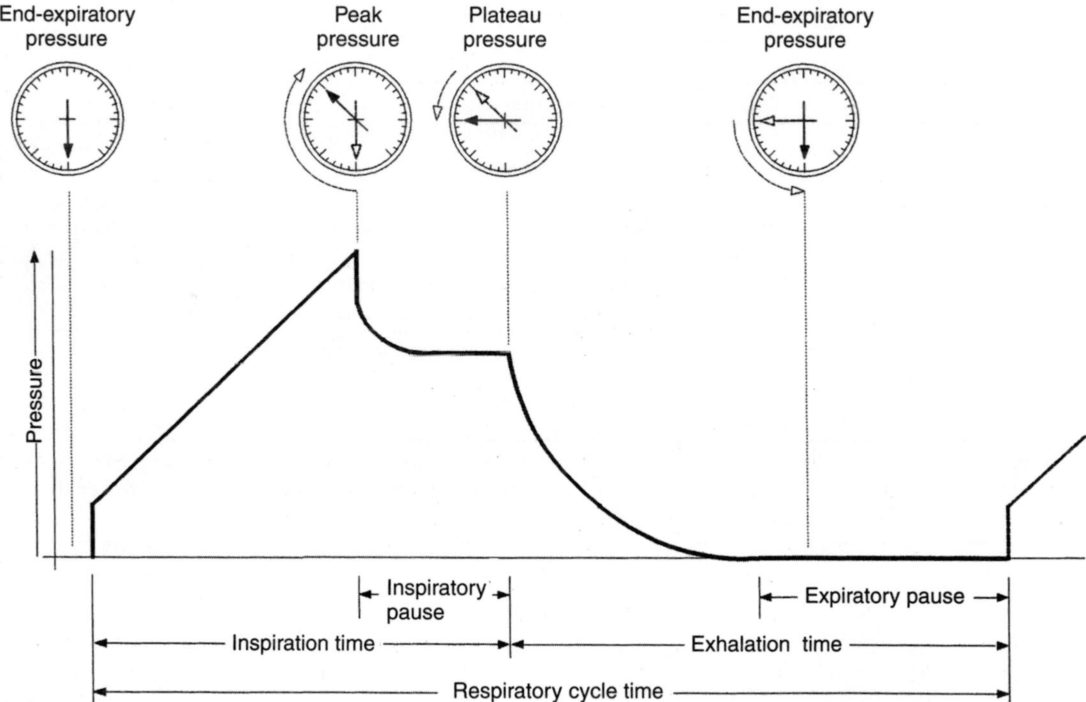

Figure 4-16 Airway pressure in a patient on positive pressure ventilation. Plateau pressure is used to calculate static compliance. Peak pressure is used to calculate dynamic compliance. The difference between static and dynamic compliance represents airway resistance. Remember that PEEP levels are subtracted from the plateau or peak pressures before calculation of compliance. (From Dupuis, Y. G. *Ventilators: Theory and clinical application* [2nd ed.]. St. Louis: Mosby-Year Book.)

Table 4-2 Types of Compliance

Type	Formula	Normal	Significance
Static compliance	$\frac{\text{Tidal volume}}{\text{Plateau pressure} - \text{PEEP}}$	50-100 mL/cm H_2O	Affected by changes in compliance of chest wall or lung
Dynamic compliance	$\frac{\text{Tidal volume}}{\text{Peak pressure} - \text{PEEP}}$	35-55 mL/cm H_2O	Affected by changes in compliance of chest wall or lung or airway resistance

PEEP, Positive end-expiratory pressure.

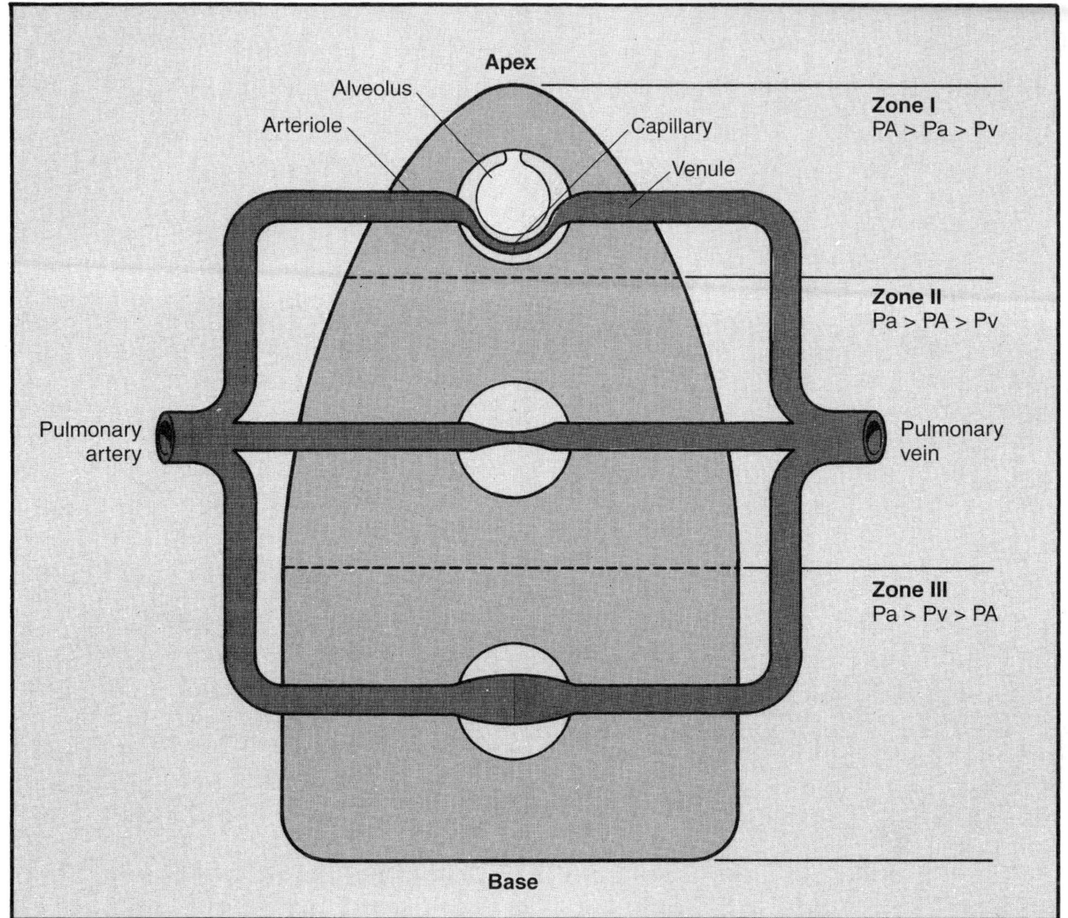

Figure 4-17 Zones of distribution of perfusion: relationship of alveolar pressure *(PA)* and gravitational forces to pulmonary vascular pressures and blood flow. The upright lung can be divided into three zones. In zone I, the upper third of the lung, alveolar pressure exceeds pulmonary venous *(Pv)* and pulmonary arterial *(Pa)* pressures. In zone II, the middle third of the lung, the pulmonary artery pressure is greater than alveolar pressure, which is greater than pulmonary venous pressure. In zone III, the lower third of the lung, pulmonary artery pressure is greater than pulmonary venous pressure, which is greater than alveolar pressure. NOTE: Pulmonary artery catheters are positioned in zone III for accurate measurement of PAOP as a reflection of left atrial pressure. (From McCance, K. L., & Huether, S. E. [1990]. *Pathophysiology: The biologic basis for disease in adults and children*. St. Louis: Mosby.)

(2) Zones (Figure 4-17)
  (a) Zone 1: nondependent portion of the lung; potential for no perfusion
  (b) Zone 2: middle portion of the lung; varying blood flow
  (c) Zone 3: gravity-dependent area of the lung; receives constant blood flow; pulmonary artery catheters ideally are placed in zone 3 for accurate reflection of left atrial pressure by the pulmonary artery occlusive pressure (PAOP)
(3) Hypoxemic pulmonary vasoconstriction
  (a) Localized
    (i) Protective mechanism that decreases blood flow to an area of poor ventilation so that blood can be shunted to areas of better ventilation
    (ii) Stimulated by decreased alveolar O_2 levels
  (b) Generalized
    (i) If all alveoli have low O_2 levels as occurs with alveolar hypoventilation, hypoxemic pulmonary vasoconstriction may be distributed over the lungs
    (ii) Increases pulmonary vascular resistance (PVR) and pulmonary artery pressure (PAP)
    (iii) Right ventricular hypertrophy and failure (cor pulmonale) may result
      a) Chronic cor pulmonale: chronic conditions such as chronic obstructive pulmonary disease (COPD)
      b) Acute cor pulmonale: acute conditions such as pulmonary embolism

c. Ventilation/perfusion (V/Q) ratio
  (1) Normal (Figure 4-18): alveolar minute ventilation equals ~4 L; normal cardiac output (100% goes to lungs) equals ~5 L; normal V/Q ratio equals 0.8

(2) Pathologic mismatch (Figure 4-19)
  (a) Dead space: V greater than Q
    (i) V/Q ratio greater than 0.8 (i.e., high V/Q ratio)
    (ii) Examples include pulmonary embolism, shock, and decrease in perfusion to the lung caused by excessive V_T or positive end-expiratory pressure (PEEP)
  (b) Shunt: Q greater than V
    (i) V/Q ratio less than 0.8 (i.e., low V/Q ratio)
    (ii) Examples include atelectasis, acute respiratory distress syndrome (ARDS), and pneumonia
    (iii) PaO_2 less than 60 mm Hg with a fraction of inspired oxygen (FiO_2) of 0.5 or greater suggests clinically significant shunt
    (iv) There are several methods of estimating shunt (Table 4-3)
  (c) Silent: no V or Q

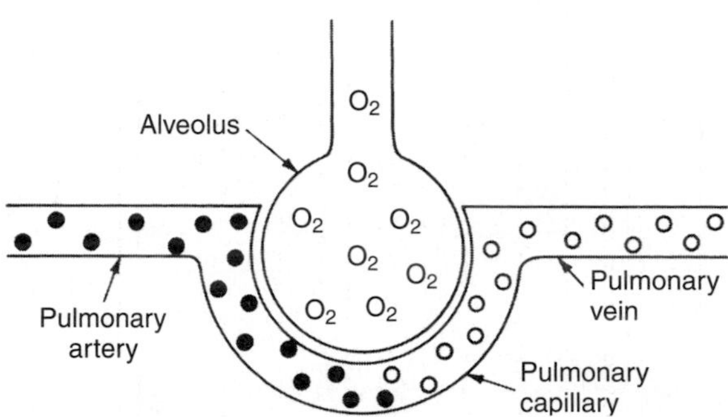

Figure 4-18 Normal V/Q ratio: normal alveolar ventilation per minute is approximately 4 L, and normal perfusion (cardiac output) is approximately 5 L/min; normal V/Q ratio is 0.8. (From Kinney, M. R., Packa, D. R., & Dunbar, S. B. [1998]. *AACN's clinical reference for critical-care nursing*. [4th ed.]. St. Louis: Mosby.)

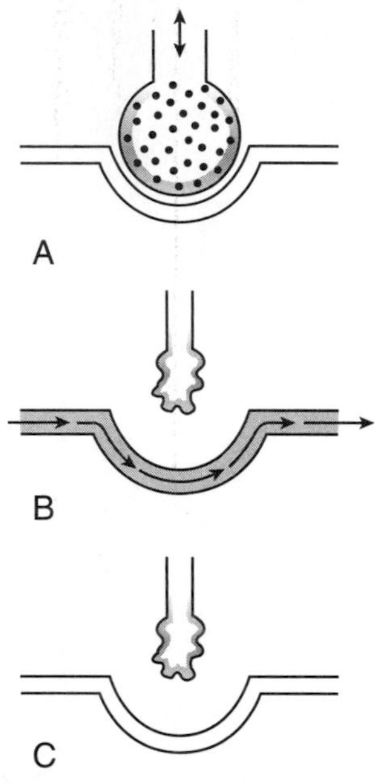

Figure 4-19 Abnormal V/Q ratio. **A,** High V/Q ratio with ventilation exceeding perfusion; also called a *dead space unit.* **B,** Low V/Q ratio with perfusion exceeding ventilation; also called a *shunt unit.* **C,** Absent ventilation and perfusion, referred to as a *silent unit.* (From Kinney, M. R., Packa, D. R., & Dunbar, S. B. [1998]. *AACN's clinical reference for critical-care nursing* [4th ed.]. St. Louis: Mosby.)

Table 4-3 Methods of Estimating Intrapulmonary Shunt

Parameter	Formula	Normal
a/A ratio	(PaO_2/PAO_2)	• Normal, greater than 0.8 • Moderate, 0.5-0.8 • Significant, 0.25-0.5 • Critical, less than 0.25
A:a gradient	$PAO_2 - PaO_2$	• Less than 10 mm Hg • A:a gradient × 0.05 = approximate percentage of shunt
PaO_2/FiO_2 (or P/F) ratio	$\frac{PaO_2}{FiO_2}$	• Greater than 300 • 300 = ~15% shunt • 200 = ~20% shunt
Respiratory index	$\frac{PAO_2 - PaO_2}{PaO_2}$	• Less than 1
Clinical shunt (Cs/Ct)	$\frac{(PAO_2 - PaO_2) \times 0.003}{[(CaO_2 - CvO_2) + (PaO_2 - PaO_2)] \times 0.003}$	3%-5%
Alternate clinical shunt equation	$\frac{(Hgb \times 1.34)(1 - SaO_2) + (0.003)\ PaO_2 - PaO_2}{(Hgb \times 1.34)(1 - SvO_2) + (0.003)\ PaO_2 - PvO_2}$	3%-5%

CaO_2, Arterial oxygen content; CvO_2, venous oxygen content; FiO_2, fraction of inspired oxygen (written as a decimal); *Hgb*, hemoglobin concentration; PAO_2, alveolar oxygen tension; PaO_2, arterial oxygen tension; *Pb*, barometric pressure (760 mm Hg at sea level, adjust for higher altitudes); PvO_2, partial oxygen pressure in mixed venous blood; SaO_2, arterial oxygen saturation; SvO_2, venous oxygen saturation.
NOTE: PaO_2 is obtained by arterial blood gas measurement. PAO_2 is calculated as FiO_2 (Pb − 47) − ($PaCO_2$/0.8). The pressure of water vapor at sea level is 47, and this number is subtracted from barometric pressure. The usual respiratory quotient is 0.8.

(3) Positional mismatch (Figure 4-20)
  (a) Greatest ventilation in superior areas
  (b) Greatest perfusion in inferior areas
  (c) This is rationale for "good lung down" in unilateral lung conditions
    (i) Improves ventilation to the "bad lung" (e.g., atelectasis, pneumonia, or pneumothorax) and optimizes perfusion to the "good lung"
    (ii) Exception is pneumonectomy: patient is positioned on the operative side or back

3. Distribution: movement of inspired air into lobes, segments, and lobules
  a. Transpulmonary pressure or distending pressure is equal to alveolar pressure minus pleural pressure
    (1) Alveolar pressure is the pressure that reaches the alveoli after resistance has been overcome
    (2) Pleural pressure is determined by gravity
  b. Closing volume is lung volume present when a significant number of small alveoli close
4. Diffusion: movement of gases between the alveoli, plasma, and RBCs
  a. Gases diffuse from areas of higher concentration to areas of lower concentration regardless of medium until concentration is the same throughout the chamber.

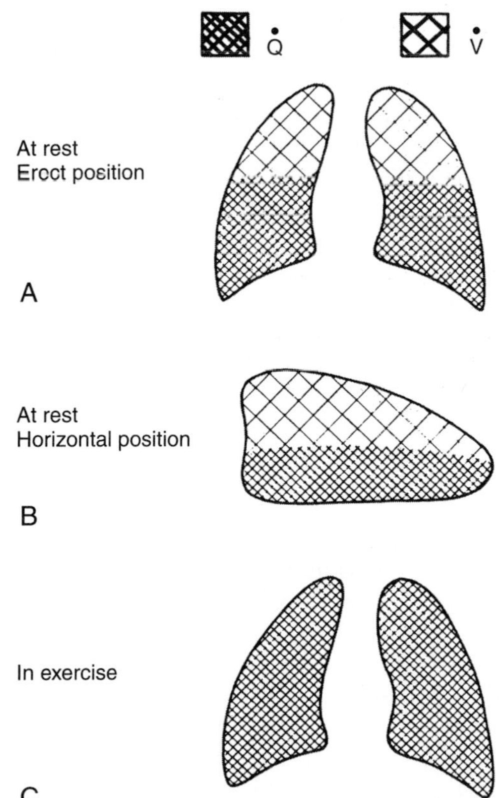

Figure 4-20 Positional changes in ventilation and perfusion. **A,** While one is sitting or standing, the upper lobes are ventilated best and the lower lobes are perfused best. **B,** While one is lying on one side, the superior lung is ventilated best and the inferior lung is perfused best. **C,** In exercise, ventilation and perfusion are increased and optimally matched throughout. (From Wade, J. F. [1982]. *Comprehensive respiratory care.* St. Louis: Mosby.)

  b. Dalton's law of partial pressure (Figure 4-21): In a mixture of gases, the pressure exerted by each gas is independent of the other gases and directly corresponds to the percentage of the total mixture that it represents.
    (1) Atmospheric (or barometric) pressure, the pressure exerted by the weight of the atmosphere, is 760 mm Hg at sea level; adjustments should be made when at high altitudes.
      (a) Components and pressures in the atmosphere
        (i) O_2 represents 20.9% of 760 mm Hg and exerts 159 mm Hg.
        (ii) Nitrogen represents 79% of 760 mm Hg and exerts 0.2 mm Hg.
        (iii) CO_2 represents 0.03% of 760 mm Hg and exerts 0.2 mm Hg.
        (iv) Water vapor represents 0.5% of 760 mm Hg and exerts 3.8 mm Hg.
    (2) During inspiration, the upper airway warms and humidifies atmospheric air, which increases the pressure of the vapor to 47 mm Hg; the partial pressures of the other gases must decrease because the total cannot exceed barometric pressure of 760 mm Hg; for example: (760 [barometric pressure at sea level] − 47 [pressure of water vapor at body temperature]) × 0.21 (FiO_2 of room air) = 150 mm Hg.
    (3) As the inspired gas mixes with gas that was not expired, the concentrations of CO_2 and O_2 change again.
    (4) Alveolar air is high in O_2 pressure and low in CO_2 pressure, and the pulmonary capillary blood is high in CO_2 pressure and low in O_2 pressure.
    (5) This differential in partial pressure of oxygen (PO_2) and CO_2 causes the gases to move across the alveolar-capillary membrane toward the lower side of the respective pressure gradients (e.g., O_2 moves from the alveolus to the capillary and CO_2 moves from the capillary to the alveolus).
  c. Determinants of diffusion
    (1) Surface area available for gas transfer
      (a) Fick's law of diffusion: the rate of transfer of a gas through a sheet of tissue is proportional to the tissue area; alveolar surface area is normally immense
      (b) Negatively affected by pulmonary resection (e.g., lobectomy or pneumonectomy) or emphysema
    (2) Thickness of the alveolar-capillary membrane: negatively affected by pulmonary edema or fibrosis
    (3) Diffusion coefficient of gas
      (a) CO_2 is 20 times more diffusible than O_2

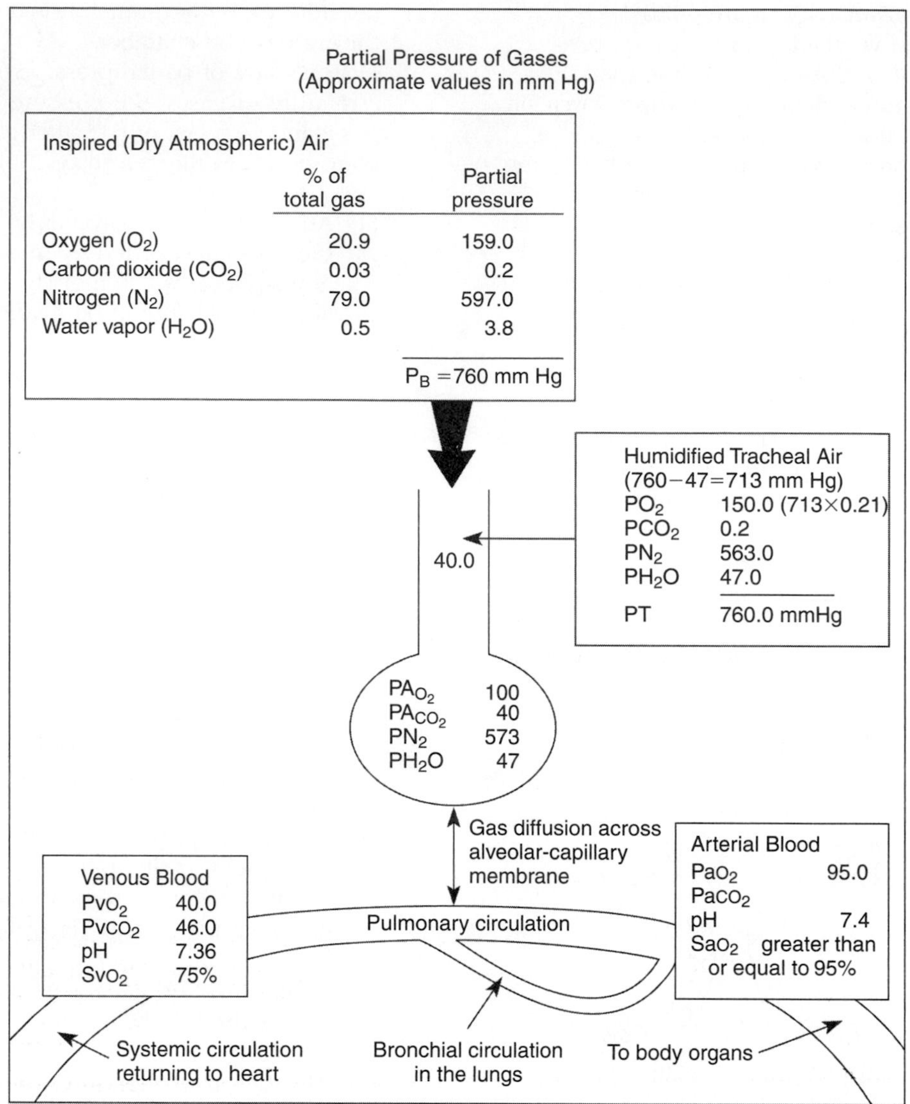

Figure 4-21 Dalton's law of partial pressure. P_T, Pressure of tracheal air; PAO_2, alveolar pressure of oxygen; $PACO_2$, alveolar pressure of carbon dioxide; PvO_2, partial oxygen pressure in mixed venous blood; $PvCO_2$, partial carbon dioxide pressure in mixed venous blood; PH_2O, partial pressure of water vapor; PN_2, partial pressure of nitrogen; SvO_2, venous oxygen saturation; SaO_2, arterial oxygen saturation.

(i) Diffusion problems cause hypoxemia, but they do not cause hypercapnia.
(ii) Hypercapnia indicates hypoventilation (e.g., respiratory muscle fatigue).

(4) Driving pressure
(a) Fraction of the gas multiplied by barometric pressure
(b) Negatively affected by low inspired fraction of oxygen (FIO_2) (e.g., smoke inhalation) or low barometric pressure (e.g., high altitudes)
(c) Positively affected by higher than normal FIO_2 (e.g., supplemental O_2) or higher than normal barometric pressure (e.g., hyperbaric O_2 chamber)
(i) Continuous positive airway pressure (CPAP) and PEEP increase the driving pressure of O_2 by keeping the pressure above zero throughout the entire ventilatory cycle.

5. Transport of gases in blood: movement of O_2 and CO_2 through the circulatory system; O_2 being moved from the alveolus to the tissues to be used and CO_2 being moved from the tissues to the alveolus for exhalation
a. O_2
(1) Mode of transport
(a) Hemoglobin (Hgb): 97% of O_2 is combined with Hgb; represented by the arterial oxygen saturation (SaO_2)
(i) One molecule of Hgb can carry four molecules of O_2
(ii) The amount of O_2 that the Hgb actually carries depends on the affinity

of the Hgb for O_2; there is normally more affinity at the lung level and less affinity at the tissue level because of the Bohr effect, which controls the reaction between Hgb and O_2 and CO_2

a) Oxygenated Hgb is a stronger acid than deoxygenated Hgb.
   i) This change in pH facilitates the release of O_2 from the Hgb at the tissue level.
   ii) As the Hgb gives up the O_2, it becomes a weaker acid and picks up CO_2 for transport back to the lung.

b) Deoxygenated Hgb is a weaker acid than oxygenated Hgb.
   i) This change in pH facilitates the attraction of O_2 to the Hgb at the lung level.
   ii) As the Hgb picks up O_2, it becomes a stronger acid and releases CO_2 at the lung level.

(iii) Ability of Hgb to deliver O_2 to the tissues is affected negatively by the following:
   a) Anemia
   b) Abnormal Hgb (e.g., methemoglobinemia, carboxyhemoglobin, or hemoglobin S [sickle cell])

(b) Plasma: 3% of O_2 is dissolved in the plasma; represented by the PaO_2

(2) Oxyhemoglobin dissociation curve: shows the relationship between PaO_2 and Hgb saturation (Figure 4-22)
   (a) Critical point: PaO_2 60 mm Hg
      (i) PaO_2 above 60 mm Hg: horizontal limb of curve; increase in PaO_2 above 60 mm Hg results in minimal increases in SO_2
      (ii) PaO_2 below 60 mm Hg: vertical limb of curve; decrease in PaO_2 below 60 mm Hg results in dramatic decreases in SO_2
   (b) Correlation between PaO_2 and SaO_2 with a normal curve (Table 4-4)
      (i) P_{50}: the PO_2 at which hemoglobin is 50% saturated with a pH of 7.40; usually PaO_2 of 27 mm Hg
   (c) Shifting of the oxyhemoglobin dissociation curve

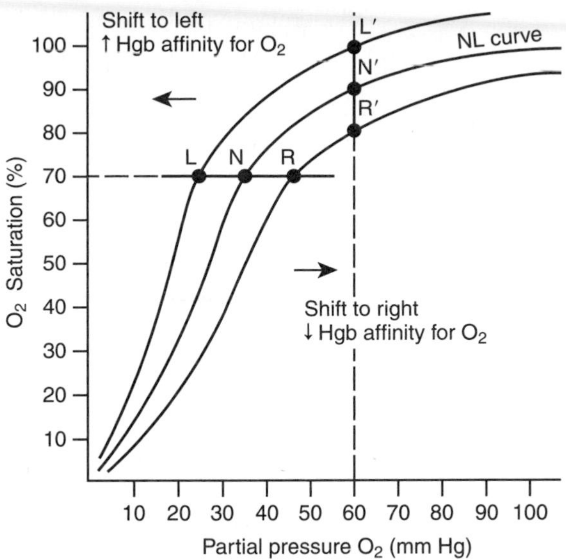

Figure 4-22 Oxyhemoglobin dissociation curve. Normal curve *(N)* optimizes pickup of O_2 at the lung and drop-off of O_2 at the tissue level; left shift *(L)* increases the affinity between O_2 and Hgb, which optimizes pickup of O_2 at the lung level but impairs drop-off of O_2 at the tissue level; right shift *(R)* decreases affinity between O_2 and Hgb, which impairs pickup of O_2 at the lung level but optimizes drop-off of O_2 at the tissue level. (From Dettenmeier, P. A. [1992]. *Pulmonary nursing care*. St. Louis: Mosby.)

Table 4-4 Correlation between PaO_2 and SaO_2

PaO_2 (in mm Hg)	SaO_2 (in %)
100	98
90	97
80	95
70	93
60	90
50	85
40	75
30	57
27	50

(i) Decreased P_{50} and shifting of the oxyhemoglobin dissociation curve to the left
   a) Affinity of Hgb for O_2 is increased; therefore Hgb is more saturated for a given PaO_2 and less O_2 is unloaded for a given PaO_2.
   b) This means that it is easier to pick up O_2 at the lung level but more difficult to drop off O_2 at the tissue level.
   c) Factors that shift the oxyhemoglobin dissociation curve to the left:

alkalemia, hypothermia, hypocapnia, decreased 2,3-diphosphoglycerate (DPG).

(ii) Increased P_{50} and shifting of the oxyhemoglobin dissociation curve to the right

a) Affinity of Hgb for O_2 is decreased; therefore Hgb is less saturated for a given PaO_2 and more oxygen is unloaded for a given PaO_2.

b) This means that it is more difficult to pick up O_2 at the lung level but easier to drop off O_2 at the tissue level.

c) Factors that shift the oxyhemoglobin dissociation curve to the right: acidemia, hyperthermia, hypercapnia, increased 2,3-DPG.

(iii) Discussion of 2,3-DPG (Box 4-1)

(3) O_2 capacity

(a) Maximal amount of O_2 the blood can carry

(b) Formula: Hgb × 1.34, where *Hgb* is hemoglobin concentration

(i) Hgb in grams per deciliter

(ii) 1.34 represents the amount of O_2 1 g of Hgb can carry; it is a constant

(4) O_2 content in arterial blood (CaO_2)

(a) Actual amount of O_2 that arterial blood is carrying

(b) O_2 capacity multiplied by SO_2; amount of O_2 dissolved in the plasma (0.0031 × PaO_2) may be added but is such a minute factor in most situations that it is inconsequential unless the patient is hyperoxemic (e.g., hyperbaric O_2 therapy)

(c) Formula: Hgb × 1.34 × SaO_2

(i) Hgb in grams per deciliter

(ii) 1.34 represents the amount of O_2 1 g of Hgb can carry; it is a constant

(iii) Saturation as a decimal (e.g., 95% is 0.95)

(d) Normal: 18 to 20 mL/dL (~20 mL/dL)

(5) O_2 content in venous blood (CvO_2)

(a) Actual amount of O_2 in venous blood

(b) Formula: 1.34 × Hgb × SvO_2, where SvO_2 is the venous O_2 saturation

(i) Hgb in grams per deciliter

(ii) 1.34 represents the amount of O_2 1 g of Hgb can carry; it is a constant

(iii) Saturation as a decimal (e.g., 95% is 0.95)

(c) Normal: 12 to 16 mL/dL (~15 mL/dL)

b. CO_2 most transported as bicarbonate

(1) Carbonic acid and water in the presence of carbonic anhydrase form bicarbonate in the erythrocyte

(2) Five percent is dissolved in plasma ($PaCO_2$)

(3) Five percent is combined with Hgb as carbaminohemoglobin; CO_2 attaches to Hgb at a different bonding site from O_2

c. Diffusion between systemic capillary bed and body tissues: pressure gradients allow diffusion

(1) Haldane effect: in the tissue, as O_2 leaves Hgb, increased CO_2 can be picked up by Hgb; in the lungs, the binding of O_2 with Hgb tends to displace CO_2

(2) O_2 diffusion to peripheral tissues is affected by

(a) Quantity and rate of blood flow

(b) Difference in capillary and tissue O_2 pressures

(c) Capillary surface area

(d) Capillary permeability

(e) Intracapillary distance

6. O_2 delivery (DO_2) to the tissue

a. DO_2: volume of O_2 delivered to the tissues by thc left ventricle each minute

BOX 4-1 Important Information about 2,3-Diphosphoglycerate (2,3-DPG)

What Is 2,3-DPG?

- A substance in the erythrocyte that affects the affinity of Hgb for O_2
- A chief end product of glucose metabolism and a link in the biochemical feedback control system that regulates the release of O_2 to the tissues

What Does 2,3-DPG Do to the Oxyhemoglobin Dissociation Curve?

- Increased amounts of 2,3-DPG shift the curve to the right, decreasing the affinity between Hgb and O_2.
- Decreased amounts of 2,3-DPG shift the curve to the left, increasing the affinity between Hgb and O_2.

What Causes Amounts of 2,3-DPG to Increase or Decrease?

- Increased
  - Chronic hypoxemia, such as high altitude or congenital heart disease
  - Anemia
  - Hyperthyroidism
  - Pyruvate kinase deficiency
- Decreased
  - Multiple blood transfusions of banked blood (i.e., total body exchange [~10 units] over minutes to hours)
  - Hypophosphatemia (e.g., malnutrition, refeeding syndrome, or treatment of diabetic ketoacidosis)
  - Hypothyroidism
  - Hexokinase deficiency

(1) Product of cardiac output and arterial O_2 content
(a) Cardiac output is a product of heart rate and stroke volume; stroke volume is affected by preload, afterload, and contractility.
(b) Arterial O_2 content is a product of Hgb and arterial saturation.
(2) Formula: CO × Hgb × Sao_2 × 13.4, where *CO* is cardiac output
(a) CO in liters per minute
(b) Hgb in grams per deciliter
(c) Saturation as a decimal (e.g., 95% is 0.95)
(3) Normal Do_2: 900 to 1100 mL/min (~1000 mL/min)
(4) O_2 delivery index (Do_2I): Do_2 divided by body surface area; considers body size
(a) Formula for Do_2I: CI × Hgb × Sao_2 × 13.4, where *CI* is cardiac index
(i) CI in liters/minute/m^2
(ii) Hgb in grams per deciliter
(iii) Saturation as a decimal (e.g., 95% is 0.95)
(b) Normal: 550 to 650 mL/min/m^2 (~600 mL/min/m^2)

b. O_2 consumption (Vo_2): volume of O_2 consumed by the tissues each minute
(1) Determined by comparing the O_2 content in the arterial blood to the O_2 content in the mixed venous blood (e.g., drawn from the distal tip of pulmonary artery catheter)
(2) Formula: CO × Hgb × 13.4 × (Sao_2 − Svo_2)
(3) Normal Vo_2: 200 to 300 mL/min (~250 mL/min)
(4) O_2 consumption index (Vo_2I): Vo_2 divided by body surface area; considers body size
(a) Formula for Vo_2I: CI × Hgb × 13.4 × (Sao_2 − Svo_2)
(b) Normal: 110 to 160 mL/min/m^2 (~150 mL/min/m^2)

c. O_2 extraction ratio (O_2ER)
(1) Evaluation of the amount of O_2 that is extracted from the arterial blood as it passes through the capillaries; ratio of the difference between the content of O_2 in the arterial blood and the content of O_2 in venous blood to the content of O_2 in the arterial blood
(2) Formula: Cao_2 − Cvo_2/Cao_2
(3) Normal: 22% to 30% (~25%)

d. O_2 extraction index
(1) Estimation of O_2ER calculated using only saturations
(2) Formula: (Sao_2 − Svo_2)/Sao_2
(3) Normal: 20% to 27% (~25%)

e. O_2 reserve in venous blood
(1) Determined by mixed Svo_2
(2) Normal: 60% to 80% (~75%)
(3) Note that normal Sao_2 is 99% and Svo_2 is 75% (the tissues used 25%); note that normal Cao_2 is 20 mL/dL and Cvo_2 is 15 mL/dL (the tissues used 25%; note that normal Do_2 is 1000 mL/min and Vo_2 is 250 mL/min (the tissues used 25%); there is normally a 75% O_2 reserve

7. Cellular respiration: use of O_2 by the cell
a. Estimated by the amount of CO_2 produced and the O_2 consumed
(1) Respiratory quotient: ratio of these two values
(a) Normally 0.8, but changes occur according to the nutritional substrate being used; primary carbohydrate metabolism changes the ratio to 1 because carbohydrate metabolism produces more CO_2 than does the metabolism of protein or fat
(b) Simplified Krebs cycle: food is converted by the body to H_2O and CO_2 and cellular energy (adenosine triphosphate [ATP])
(2) Variables affecting O_2 consumption
(a) Increased O_2 consumption
(i) Increased work of breathing
(ii) Hyperthermia
(iii) Trauma
(iv) Sepsis
(v) Anxiety
(vi) Hyperthyroidism
(vii) Muscle tremors or seizures
(b) Decreased O_2 consumption
(i) Hypothermia
(ii) Sedation
(iii) Neuromuscular blockade
(iv) Anesthesia
(v) Hypothyroidism
(vi) Inactivity
b. O_2 is used by the mitochondria in the production of cellular energy; O_2 deficit may result in lethal cell injury if prolonged

8. Metabolic functions of the lung
a. Synthesis of interferon and tumor-inhibiting factor
b. Production, conversion, or removal of many vasoactive substances in the pulmonary circulation; bradykinin, serotonin, heparin, histamine, prostaglandins E and F, and certain polypeptides such as angiotensin I

Pulmonary Assessment

Interview

1. Chief complaint: why the patient is seeking help and duration of the problem; possible symptoms related to pulmonary disorders that may be identified as chief complaint may include any of the following:
a. Dyspnea or shortness of breath
(1) Onset
(2) Duration
(3) Frequency
(4) Timing: time of day; weather or season; activity; eating; talking; deep breathing

(5) Position (e.g., orthopnea)
(6) Severity
(a) Subjective scale
(i) Grade 1: shortness of breath with mild exertion, such as running a short distance or climbing a flight of stairs
(ii) Grade 2: shortness of breath while walking a short distance at a normal pace on level grade
(iii) Grade 3: shortness of breath with mild daily activity such as shaving or bathing
(iv) Grade 4: shortness of breath while sitting at rest
(v) Grade 5: shortness of breath while lying down
(b) Effect on ability to do activities of daily living
(c) Frequently accentuated by anxiety
(7) Palliation: What is effective in relieving dyspnea?
(8) Accompanying symptoms
(a) Cough
(b) Chest pain
(c) Wheezing

b. Cough
(1) Onset
(2) Duration
(3) Frequency
(4) Timing: time of day, weather or season, activity, eating, talking, deep breathing
(5) Position
(6) Pattern: regular or occasional
(7) Dry or productive
(8) Accompanying symptoms
(a) Sputum production
(b) Hemoptysis
(c) Chest pain
(d) Wheezing
(e) Dyspnea
(9) Medication history: may be side effect of angiotensin-converting enzyme inhibitors (e.g., captopril [Capoten] and enalapril [Vasotec])

c. Sputum production
(1) Duration
(2) Frequency
(3) Amount: use household measurements (e.g., teaspoons, tablespoons, shot glass, Dixie cup, iced tea glass)
(4) Color: may assist with identification of most likely microorganism
(a) Pinkish-orange: *Staphylococcus*
(b) Rusty: *Streptococcus*
(c) Greenish: *Pseudomonas*
(d) Currant-colored: *Klebsiella*
(5) Consistency
(6) Odor
(7) Hemoptysis
(8) Usual treatment (e.g., expectorants, cough drops, or a cigarette)

d. Hemoptysis
(1) May be related to tuberculosis, lung cancer, bronchiectasis, pneumonia, or pulmonary embolism
(2) Character
(a) Grossly bloody
(b) Blood-tinged
(c) Blood-streaked
(d) Hematest positive
(3) Differentiation from hematemesis
(a) Hemoptysis: frothy, alkaline, accompanied by sputum
(b) Hematemesis: nonfrothy, acidic, dark red or brown, accompanied by food particles

e. Chest pain: See Table 2-5.
(1) P
(a) Provocation: Pulmonary pain frequently is provoked by trauma, coughing, deep breathing, or movement.
(b) Palliation: Pulmonary pain may be relieved by sitting upright or by narcotics.
(2) Q
(a) Quality: Pulmonary pain is most frequently sharp and is increased by coughing, inspiration, and movement.
(3) R
(a) Region: Pulmonary pain usually is located at the lateral chest.
(b) Radiation: Pulmonary pain may radiate to the shoulder and neck.
(4) S
(a) Severity: Pulmonary pain is usually moderate but may be severe.
(5) T
(a) Timing
(i) Onset: Pulmonary pain onset is usually gradual.
(ii) Duration: Pulmonary pain duration is usually days to weeks.

f. Wheezing
(1) Onset
(2) Duration
(3) Timing: time of day, weather or season, activity, eating, talking, deep breathing; position
(4) Identified triggers (e.g., dust, pollen, or propellants)
(5) Usual treatment

g. Nasal or sinus problems
(1) Epistaxis
(2) Nasal stuffiness
(3) Postnasal drip
(4) Sinus pain

h. Hoarseness: chronic hoarseness may be related to cancer of larynx

i. Ascites: may be related to cor pulmonale

j. Abdominal pain: may be related to cor pulmonale

k. Edema or weight gain: may be related to cor pulmonale

l. Fatigue or weakness: may be related to cor pulmonale

m. Fever: may be related to pulmonary infections
n. Night sweats: may be related to tuberculosis
o. Anorexia: may be related cor pulmonale, dyspnea, or drug side effects (e.g., xanthine bronchodilators)
p. Weight loss: may be related to dyspnea, fatigue (preventing food preparation), or hypermetabolism
q. Sleep disturbances: may be related to dyspnea or coughing

2. History of present illness
   a. PQRST
   b. Associated symptoms
3. Medical history
   a. Childhood diseases
      (1) Frequent respiratory infections
      (2) Allergies
      (3) Asthma
      (4) Scarlet fever
   b. Past illnesses
      (1) Recurrent respiratory infections
      (2) Pneumonia
      (3) Cystic fibrosis
      (4) Asthma
      (5) COPD
         (a) Possible components
            (i) Chronic bronchitis: dominant reported symptom is coughing with sputum production
            (ii) Emphysema: dominant reported symptom is dyspnea
            (iii) Patients with COPD often also have asthma: dominant reported symptom is wheezing
         (b) Most patients have two, if not all three, of these components
      (6) Tuberculosis
      (7) Lung cancer
      (8) Pulmonary fibrosis: frequently related to occupational lung disease
         (a) Pneumoconiosis (coal worker's lung disease)
         (b) Asbestosis
         (c) Silicosis
      (9) Fungal disease (e.g., histoplasmosis)
      (10) Pulmonary embolism
      (11) Pneumothorax
      (12) Granulomatous diseases (e.g., sarcoidosis)
      (13) Connective tissue disorders (e.g., lupus or scleroderma)
      (14) Immunosuppression
      (15) Cor pulmonale: right ventricular hypertrophy and/or failure as a result of pulmonary disease
   c. Past injury: chest trauma
   d. Past surgical procedures: thoracotomy
   e. Allergies and type of reaction
   f. Past diagnostic studies
      (1) Allergy testing
      (2) Tuberculin and/or fungal skin tests
      (3) Chest x-ray
      (4) Pulmonary function studies
      (5) Bronchoscopy
      (6) Laryngoscopy
4. Family history of genetically predisposed disease
   a. Asthma
   b. Emphysema: particularly emphysema related to $alpha_1$-antitrypsin deficiency
   c. Tuberculosis
   d. Cystic fibrosis
   e. Cancer
5. Social history
   a. Work environment
      (1) Occupation
      (2) Environmental hazards: chemicals, vapors, dust, pulmonary irritants, allergens
      (3) Use of protective devices
   b. Home environment
      (1) Allergens: pets, plants, trees, molds, dust mites
      (2) Type of heating
      (3) Use of air conditioner and/or humidifier
   c. Recreational habits: exposure to inhalants and allergens
   d. Exercise habits
   e. Tobacco use: present and past
      (1) Type of tobacco
      (2) Duration and amount
         (a) Cigarettes: record as pack-years (number of packs per day times the number of years person has been smoking)
         (b) Chewing or rubbing tobacco: type and amount per day
         (c) Marijuana: joints per day
      (3) Efforts to quit: previous and current desire to quit
      (4) Second-hand smoke exposure
   f. Fluid consumption
      (1) Volume of water per day
      (2) Caffeine-containing beverages
      (3) Alcohol-containing beverages: alcoholic beverages per day or week
   g. Eating habits
      (1) Quality and quantity of meals
      (2) Number of meals per day
      (3) Pulmonary symptoms during meals: dyspnea, cough, wheezing
6. Medication history
   a. Prescribed drug, dose, frequency, and time of last dose
   b. Nonprescribed drugs
      (1) Over-the-counter drugs, including herbs
      (2) Substance abuse
   c. Patient understanding of drug actions, side effects; knowledge of how to use and clean inhaler if prescribed

Landmarks (See Figure 2-28)

1. Anatomic
   a. Clavicle
   b. Sternum

c. Ribs
d. Intercostal spaces
e. Angle of Louis: sternal angle between manubrium and body of sternum
f. Xiphoid process
g. Costal margin
h. Costal angle
2. Imaginary
a. Midsternal line
b. Midclavicular line (MCL)
c. Anterior axillary line
d. Midaxillary line (MAL)
e. Posterior axillary line
f. Scapular line
g. Midspinal line
3. Location of lungs (Figure 4-23)
a. The apex of the lungs extends 2 to 4 cm above the inner third of the clavicle.
b. The inferior border anteriorly is at the sixth rib at the MCL and at the eighth rib at the MAL, posteriorly at T10 on expiration and at T12 with deep inspiration.
c. Fissure dividing upper and lower lobes is at T3 posteriorly.
d. Upper lobes are primarily anterior; lower lobes are primarily posterior.
e. Trachea bifurcates at the angle of Louis anteriorly or T4 posteriorly.

Inspection and Palpation

1. Vital signs
a. BP
b. Heart rate
c. Respiratory (ventilatory) rate
d. Temperature
e. Height
f. Weight
2. General survey
a. Apparent health status: Compare apparent age relative to chronologic age.
b. Level of consciousness: Note restlessness and/or confusion (frequently the first sign of hypoxia).
c. Increased work of breathing: Note use of accessory muscles.
d. Speech pattern: Note pausing midsentence to take a breath.
e. Presence of injury, abrasion, deformity
f. Nutritional status
g. Stature/posture
3. Mouth or nose
a. Pursed lip breathing: may be instinctive or the patient may have been taught to use this technique during times of dyspnea
b. Artificial airway
(1) Type
(2) Size
(3) Placement (e.g., centimeter mark at teeth for oral ET tube)
(4) Cuff pressure (measured with a cuff pressure gauge or sphygmomanometer with three-way stopcock)
c. O_2 therapy
(1) Administration device and flow rate
(2) FiO_2
d. Nasogastric tube, nasointestinal tube, orogastric tube, or orointestinal tube
(1) Size
(2) Placement confirmation
(a) Aspiration of gastric (acidic) or intestinal (alkaline) contents
(b) Radiologic confirmation
e. Condition of nasal or oral mucosa
f. Presence of halitosis: suggests poor oral hygiene, poor dental health, or sinus infection

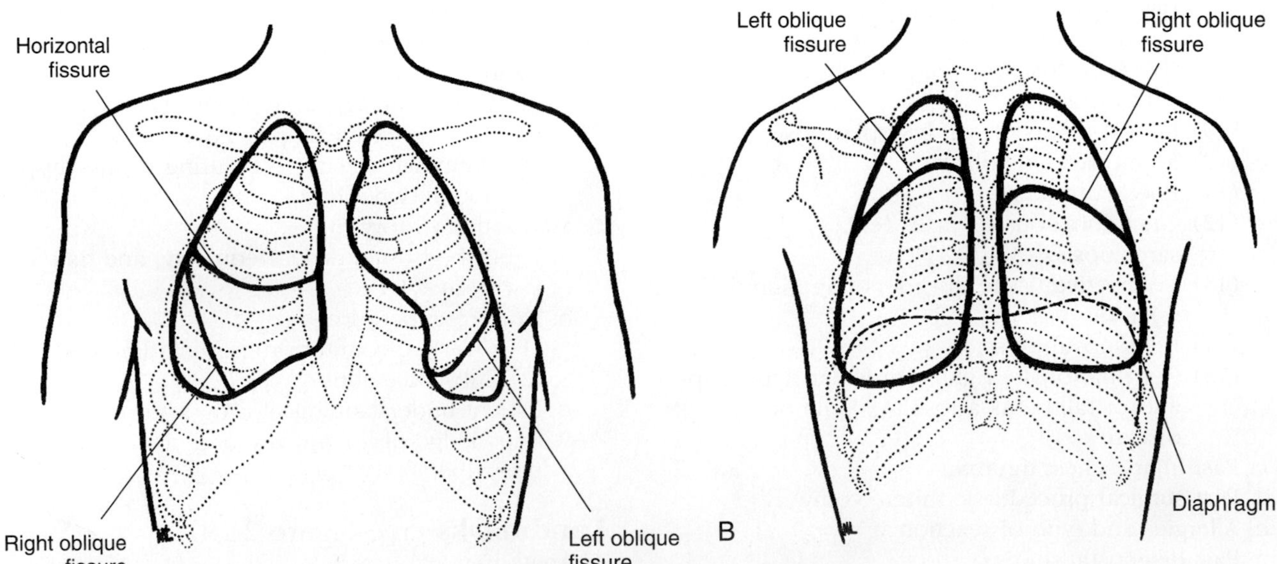

Figure 4-23 Location of the lungs. **A,** Anterior. **B,** Posterior. (From Wilkins, R. L., Sheldon, R. L., & Krider, S. J. [1994]. *Clinical assessment in respiratory care.* St. Louis: Mosby.)

4. Skin, mucous membranes, and appendages
   a. Color
      (1) Pallor: may indicate anemia
      (2) Rubor: may indicate hypercapnia or polycythemia
      (3) Cyanosis
         (a) Peripheral (or cold) cyanosis
            (i) Seen on fingertips and toes
            (ii) Associated with peripheral hypoperfusion or vasoconstriction
         (b) Central (or warm) cyanosis
            (i) Seen on lips and mucous membranes
            (ii) Associated with 5 g/dL of deoxygenated Hgb
               a) Will be a late sign of hypoxemia in anemic patients; patients with Hgb levels of less than 5 g/dL will not be cyanotic, regardless of degree of hypoxemia
               b) May be a relatively early sign of hypoxemia in polycythemic patients because they will be cyanotic when they have 5 g/dL of Hgb desaturated even though they may have a normal (~15 g/dL) still saturated; this is why patients with chronic bronchitis are nicknamed "blue bloaters"
                  i) Blue because of chronic cyanosis
                  ii) Bloaters because of chronic RVF
         (c) In dark-skinned patients, cyanosis appears as an ashen color
      (4) Cherry-red: may indicate carbon monoxide intoxication
      (5) Tobacco stains on fingertips
   b. Scars: especially thoracic
   c. Petechiae: may indicate any of the following:
      (1) Blood dyscrasias affecting platelets
         (a) Disseminated intravascular coagulation
         (b) Platelet aggregation inhibitors (e.g., aspirin, nonsteroidal antiinflammatory agents, or clopidogrel [Plavix])
      (2) Liver disease
      (3) Fat embolism
   d. Edema: may be associated with cor pulmonale
   e. Nailbeds
      (1) Color: note cyanosis
      (2) Clubbing
         (a) Indicates chronic decrease in O_2 supply to body tissues
            (i) Especially indicative of restrictive lung diseases (e.g., pulmonary fibrosis or lung cancer)
            (ii) Also indicative of right-to-left cardiac shunting (e.g., cyanotic heart disease)
            (iii) May be seen in late obstructive lung disease
         (b) Normal angle between nailbed and nail less than 180 degrees
         (c) Early clubbing angle equal to 180 degrees
         (d) Late clubbing greater than 180 degrees
5. Neck
   a. Tracheal deviation
      (1) Local causes: hematoma; goiter
      (2) Mediastinal causes
         (a) Shifts toward affected side
            (i) Spontaneous pneumothorax
            (ii) Atelectasis
            (iii) Pneumonectomy
         (b) Shifts away from affected side
            (i) Tension pneumothorax
            (ii) Large pleural effusion
            (iii) Hemothorax
   b. Lymph nodes (infraclavicular, supraclavicular, and/or axillary nodes): may be enlarged in lung cancer
   c. Jugular neck vein distention: may indicate any of the following:
      (1) RVF (e.g., cor pulmonale)
      (2) Tension pneumothorax
      (3) Cardiac tamponade
      (4) Superior vena cava syndrome
         (a) Edema of neck, eyelids, and hands also seen
         (b) May occur in lung cancer
   d. Accessory muscle use: indicates respiratory distress
6. Thorax
   a. Posture: tripod position
      (1) Sitting up and leaning forward (e.g., over bedside table)
      (2) Position for optimal ventilation
      (3) Indicates respiratory distress
   b. Contour
      (1) Normal
         (a) Slope of ribs: ribs are normally at 45-degree angle to vertebrae
         (b) Costal angle: normally less than 90 degrees
         (c) Anterior-posterior (AP) diameter: normally one half of lateral diameter so that normal ratio of AP to lateral diameter is 1:2
         (d) Symmetric
      (2) Abnormalities
         (a) Pectus excavatum (funnel chest)
            (i) Sternum pushed inward
            (ii) May cause hypoventilation or restrictive lung disease
         (b) Pectus carinatum (pigeon chest)
            (i) Sternum pushed outward
            (ii) May cause hypoventilation or restrictive lung disease
         (c) Scoliosis
            (i) S curvature to spine
            (ii) May cause hypoventilation or restrictive lung disease

(d) Kyphosis (hunchback)
(i) Frequently occurs with aging because of osteoporosis
(ii) May cause hypoventilation or restrictive lung disease
(e) Increased AP diameter: indicates obstructive lung disease

c. Intercostal spaces
(1) Retraction of interspaces during inspiration
(a) Tracheal obstruction
(b) Asthma
(2) Bulging of interspaces during expiration
(a) Asthma
(b) Tension pneumothorax
(c) Pleural effusion

d. Chest movement
(1) Impaired movement
(a) Thoracic pain with splinting
(b) Restrictive lung disease
(2) Unequal expansion
(a) Massive unilateral atelectasis
(b) Massive pleural effusion
(c) Pneumonia
(d) Pneumothorax
(e) Pulmonary resection: lobectomy, pneumonectomy
(f) Right main stem intubation (no movement on left)
(g) Flail chest
(3) Respiratory excursion: normally 3 to 6 cm during normal breathing

e. Respiratory rate, rhythm, and quality
(1) Rate and rhythm (Table 4-5)
(2) Type
(a) Abdominal: males or supine females
(b) Thoracic or costal: upright females
(3) Inspiration-to-expiration (I:E) ratio
(a) Normally 1:2 with expiration lasting twice as long as inspiration
(b) Obstructive lung diseases causes prolonged expiratory time with ratios 1:3 or greater

f. Chest wall
(1) Point of maximal impulse
(a) Normally palpated at fifth left intercostal space at the MCL
(b) Frequently shifted medially in patients with chronic lung disease and pulmonary hypertension caused by right ventricular hypertrophy
(c) May be shifted in either direction with mediastinal shift depending on side and type of condition creating mediastinal shift
(2) Heave: right ventricular heave may be felt at the sternum or in epigastric area because of right ventricular hypertrophy and/or failure
(3) Tenderness: may be caused by any of the following:
(a) Fracture
(b) Tumor
(c) Costochondritis
(4) Fremitus
(a) Vocal fremitus
(i) Evaluated by asking the patient to say "99" while palpating the patient's thorax with the ball of the examiner's hand
(ii) Decreased vocal fremitus
a) Thick chest wall
b) Bronchial obstruction
c) Pleural effusion
d) Pleural thickening
e) Pneumothorax
f) Emphysema
(iii) Increased vocal fremitus
a) Over large airways
b) Pneumonia
c) Tumor
d) Pulmonary fibrosis
e) Pulmonary infarction
(b) Pleural friction fremitus: grating sensation that occurs with pleural inflammation
(c) Rhonchal fremitus: vibration felt with movement of secretions through the tracheobronchial tree
(5) Subcutaneous emphysema (air in subcutaneous tissue)
(a) Assess for subcutaneous emphysema around tracheostomy, chest tube, or stab wound
(b) Assess for subcutaneous emphysema after bronchoscopy; indicates perforation of tracheobronchial tree
(6) Chest tubes (see Table 5-1)
(7) Central venous catheters
(a) Location
(b) Patency
(c) Rate and type of solutions
(8) Wounds

7. Abdomen
a. Liver
(1) May be palpable in patients with normal liver but not with hyperinflated lungs because liver is pushed downward
(2) May be enlarged and tender because of cor pulmonale
b. Abdominal muscles (accessory muscles of expiration): frequently used by patients with obstructive lung disease to help push the air out of the lungs

8. Ventilatory support
a. Mode
(1) Inspiratory (e.g., control, assist-control, intermittent mandatory ventilation, or pressure-support)
(2) Expiratory (e.g., PEEP or CPAP)
b. V_T
c. Rate
d. FiO_2
e. PEEP
f. Peak inspiratory pressure and calculated dynamic compliance
g. Plateau pressure and calculated static compliance

Table 4-5 Respiratory Rhythms

Rhythm	Description	Possible Causes
Eupnea	Rate 12-20 breaths/min and normal depth of ventilation; regular with occasional sigh	• Normal
Bradypnea	Slow (less than 10 breaths/min), regular ventilation	• Depression of respiratory center with opium, alcohol, or tumor • Sleep • Increased intracranial pressure • Carbon dioxide narcosis • Metabolic alkalosis
Tachypnea	Rapid (greater than 30 breaths/min) ventilation; depth may be normal or decreased	• Restrictive lung disease • Pneumonia • Pleurisy • Chest pain • Fear • Anxiety • Respiratory insufficiency
Hypopnea	Shallow ventilation; normal rate	• Deep sleep • Heart failure • Shock • Meningitis • Central nervous system depression • Coma
Hyperpnea	Deep ventilation; rate may be normal or increased	• Exercise • Hypoxia • Fever • Hepatic coma • Midbrain or pons lesions • Acid-base imbalance • Salicylate overdosage
Cheyne-Stokes	Increasing and decreasing rate and depth of ventilation followed by apnea lasting 20 to 60 seconds	• Increased intracranial pressure • Heart failure • Renal failure • Meningitis • Cerebral hemisphere damage • Drug overdosage
Kussmaul's	Deep, gasping, rapid (usually greater than 35 breaths/min) ventilation	• Metabolic acidosis (e.g., diabetic ketoacidosis; renal failure) • Peritonitis
Apneustic	Prolonged gasping inspiration followed by short, inefficient expiration	• Lesion of pons
Biot's	Periods of apnea alternating with a series of breaths of equal depth; breathing may be slow and deep or rapid and shallow	• Meningitis • Encephalitis • Head trauma • Increased intracranial pressure
Ataxic	Lack of any pattern to ventilation	• Brainstem lesion
Obstructive	Inspiration/expiration ratio of 1:4 or greater	• Asthma • Emphysema • Chronic bronchitis
Apnea	Cessation of ventilation for longer than 15 seconds	• Central nervous system damage • Sleep apnea

9. Clinical indications of respiratory distress (Box 4-2)
10. Clinical indications of hypoxemia/hypoxia
    a. Hypoxemia (decreased O_2 in the blood): noted by Pao_2 less than 80 mm Hg and Sao_2 less than 95% on arterial blood gas (ABG) samples or Sao_2 less than 95% by pulse oximetry
    b. Hypoxia (decreased O_2 in the tissues): noted by clinical indications of hypoxia (Box 4-3) and increased serum lactate level

11. Clinical indications of hypercapnia (increased CO_2 in the blood): noted by increased $PaCO_2$ on ABG samples and clinical indications of hypercapnia (Box 4-4)

Percussion

1. Description of percussion tones (Table 4-6)
2. Thorax
   a. Percussion tones normally heard
      (1) Lung: resonance
      (2) Diaphragm: flat
      (3) Heart: dull
   b. Abnormal percussion tones over thorax
      (1) Hyperresonant: asthma, emphysema, pneumothorax
      (2) Dull: atelectasis, pneumonia, tumor
      (3) Flat: pleural effusion
   c. Diaphragmatic excursion
      (1) Evaluated by percussing the position of the diaphragm at expiration and then during full inspiration
      (2) Normal diaphragmatic excursion is 3 to 5 cm
      (3) May be decreased by the following:
         (a) Increased intrathoracic volume: emphysema
         (b) Increased intraabdominal volume and pressure:
            (i) Ascites
            (ii) Hepatomegaly
            (iii) Pregnancy
            (iv) Gaseous abdominal distention
         (c) Decreased chest excursion and V_T: thoracic or abdominal pain
         (d) Phrenic nerve injury
3. Abdomen
   a. Liver
      (1) Normal liver span in the right MCL is 6 to 12 cm.
      (2) Hepatomegaly (liver span greater than 12 cm in left MCL) may be seen in cor pulmonale.
         (a) Assessment by percussion is necessary before specifying hepatomegaly because patients with hyperinflated lungs may have a palpable normal liver because it is pushed downward.

Auscultation

1. Method of lung auscultation
   a. Use diaphragm
   b. Ask patient to take deep breaths through the mouth
   c. Listen at least one full breath at each location
   d. Compare symmetric areas
2. Breath sounds
   a. Intensity
      (1) Increased
         (a) Hyperventilation
         (b) Anything that decreases the distance between the lung and your stethoscope (e.g., thin chest wall)
      (2) Decreased
         (a) Hypoventilation
            (i) Emphysema

BOX 4-2 Clinical Indications of Respiratory Distress

Pursed lip breathing
Tripod positioning
Speaking only one or two words between breaths
Cough
Use of accessory muscles
Intercostal retractions

BOX 4-3 Clinical Indications of Hypoxia

Restlessness → confusion → lethargy → coma
Tachycardia → dysrhythmias
Tachypnea
Dyspnea
Use of accessory muscles
Mild hypertension (early) → hypotension (late)
Cyanosis may be present (depending on hemoglobin level)

BOX 4-4 Clinical Indications of Hypercapnia

Headache
Irritability
Confusion
Inability to concentrate → somnolence → coma
Bradypnea
Tachycardia → dysrhythmias
Hypotension
Facial rubor (plethora)

Table 4-6 Percussion Tones

Tone	Intensity	Pitch	Duration	Quality	Normal Location
Tympanic	Loud	High	Medium	Drumlike	Stomach, bowel
Hyperresonant	Loud	Low	Long	Booming	Hyperinflated lungs
Resonant	Medium	Low	Long	Hollow	Normal lung
Dull	Soft	High	Medium	Thudlike	Liver, spleen, heart
Flat	Soft	High	Short	Extreme dullness	Muscle, bone

(ii) Thoracic pain
(iii) Restrictive lungs (e.g., atelectasis or pulmonary fibrosis)
(b) Anything that increases the distance between the lung and your stethoscope
(i) Muscular or obese chest
(ii) Pneumothorax (may be diminished or absent)
(iii) Hemothorax (may be diminished or absent)
(iv) Pleural effusion
(3) Absent
(a) Severe bronchospasm
(b) Massive atelectasis
(c) Pneumonectomy
(d) Pneumothorax
(e) Hemothorax
(f) Malpositioned ET tube (absent breath sounds over left lung)

b. Quality
(1) Descriptions and normal locations (Figure 4-24 and Table 4-7)
(2) Implications
(a) Bronchial in areas other than normal location: consolidation (e.g., atelectasis, pneumonia, or tumor)
(b) Bronchovesicular in areas other than normal location: partial consolidation, partial aeration

c. Adventitious sounds (Table 4-8): pathologic extra sounds that may be heard at points in the ventilatory cycle or throughout the ventilatory cycle

d. Voice sounds: abnormal and indicative of consolidation
(1) Bronchophony: increase in clarity of voice sounds
(a) Ask patient to say "99."
(b) Voice sounds are normally muffled.
(c) If voice sounds are clear over a particular area, bronchophony is present.
(2) Egophony: "e" to "a" conversion of voice sounds
(a) Ask patient to say "e."
(b) Muffled "e" should be heard over normal lung.
(c) If "a" is heard over a particular area, egophony is present.
(3) Whispered pectoriloquy: increase in clarity of whispered sounds
(a) Ask the patient to whisper "99."
(b) Whispered sounds are normally muffled.

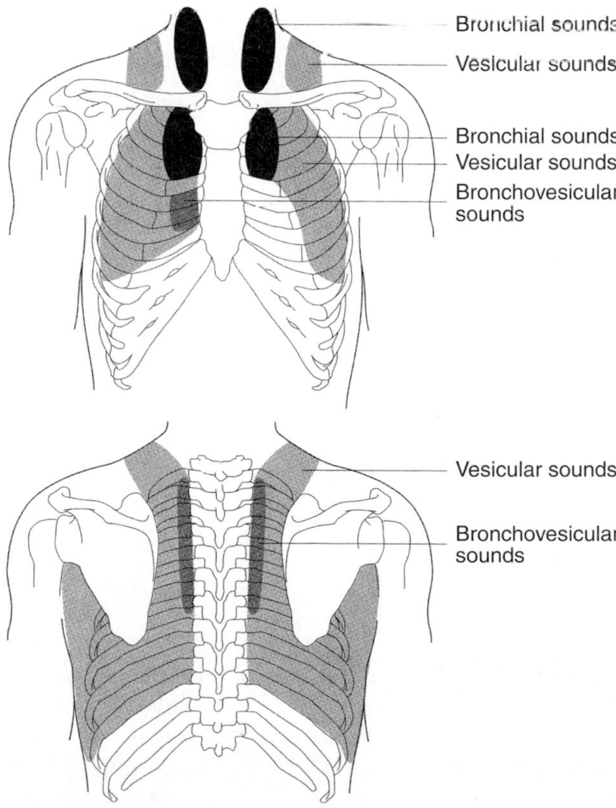

Figure 4-24 Quality of breath sounds: normal locations. (From Barkauskas, V. H., et al. [1994]. *Health and physical assessment*. St. Louis: Mosby.)

Table 4-7 **Breath Sounds: Quality**

Quality	I:E Ratio	Intensity	Pitch	Quality	Normal Location
Bronchial	I less than E	Loud	High	Hollow	Trachea
Bronchovesicular	I = E	Medium	Medium	Breezy	Mainstem bronchi
Vesicular	I greater than E	Soft	Low	Swishy	Peripheral lung

E, Expiration; *I*, inspiration.

Table 4-8 **Adventitious Breath Sounds**

Sound	Alternative Terms	Phase	Description	Cause
Stridor	Croupy	Inspiratory	High-pitched whistle audible without a stethoscope	• Upper airway obstruction • Epiglottis • Foreign body • Laryngospasm • Laryngeal edema
Crackles	Rales	Inspiratory	Discontinuous crackling sound; similar to rubbing hair between fingers	• Pulmonary edema • Atelectasis • Pulmonary fibrosis
Rhonchi	Gurgles, sonorous rhonchi	Expiratory	Continuous gurgling sound	• Fluid or mucus in airways
Wheezes	Whistles; sibilant rhonchi	Inspiratory or expiratory	High-pitched whistling sound	• Decrease in airway lumen ○ Bronchospasm ○ Mucous plug ○ Tumor
Pleural friction rub		Inspiratory and expiratory	Grating or scratching sound	• Pulmonary infarction • Pleurisy • Tuberculosis • Lung cancer

(c) If whispered sounds are clear over a particular area, whispered pectoriloquy is present.

Bedside Assessment of Pulmonary Function

1. Bedside parameters (also referred to as *ventilatory mechanics*)
   a. Spirometry: measured with Wright respirometer
      (1) V_T
         (a) Amount of air moved in and out each breath
         (b) Normal: 7 mL/kg
            (i) V_T less than 5 mL/kg indicates need for artificial airway and/or mechanical ventilation.
            (ii) V_T greater than 5 mL/kg indicates that the patient can be weaned and/or extubated.
      (2) Vital capacity (VC)
         (a) Maximal amount of air that can be exhaled after a maximal inspiration
         (b) Normal: 15 mL/kg
            (i) VC less than 10 mL/kg indicates need for artificial airway and/or mechanical ventilation.
            (ii) VC greater than 10 mL/kg indicates that the patient can be weaned and/or extubated.
      (3) Minute ventilation
         (a) $f \times V_T$, where *f* is respiratory frequency
         (b) Normal: 5 to 10 L/min
      (4) Maximal voluntary ventilation
         (a) Volume of air moved into and out of the lungs with maximal effort over a short period of time (usually 10 to 15 seconds)
         (b) Normal is 170 L/min (NOTE: One quarter this total actually is measured in the 15-second period; patients are not asked to ventilate at this intensity for an entire minute.)
         (c) Reflects the status of the ventilatory muscles, compliance of the lung and thorax, and airway resistance; may provide a quick assessment of the patient's ventilatory reserve before surgery
   b. Maximal inspiratory pressure (MIP): measured with negative inspiratory pressure meter
      (1) Also referred to as *negative inspiratory force*
      (2) Normal is greater than (more negative than) −60 to −80 cm H_2O
         (a) MIP of less than −25 cm H_2O indicates need for artificial airway and/or mechanical ventilation.

(b) MIP of greater than −25 cm H_2O indicates that the patient can be weaned and/or extubated.

c. Rapid shallow breathing index (RSBI)
(1) Calculated as f/V_T using frequency in 1 minute and average V_T over 1 minute
(2) Provides an indication of the perception in the brain of how well the respiratory muscles tolerate the work of breathing; if the brain senses that the workload is too high for the respiratory muscles to tolerate, the reflex ventilatory pattern is rapid, shallow breathing
(3) RSBI of 105 breaths/min/L indicates readiness for weaning

2. Capnography (may also be referred to as *end-tidal CO_2 monitoring*)
a. Continuous noninvasive method for evaluating the adequacy of CO_2 exchange in the lungs; assesses $Paco_2$ indirectly by detecting the level of CO_2 in the exhaled air
(1) Measurement of expired CO_2 tension
(2) Display of the CO_2 waveform from breath to breath (Figure 4-25)
b. Indications
(1) Verification of tracheal intubation
(a) Esophageal intubation is reflected by decreased $P_{ET}CO_2$ (end-tidal pressure of carbon dioxide) or an abnormal waveform.
(b) Inexpensive, disposable, colorimetric CO_2 indicators frequently are used for this purpose; they do not display waveform.
(2) Verification of adequacy of chest compression during cardiopulmonary resuscitation
(a) In the absence of pulmonary blood flow, $P_{ET}CO_2$ decreases rapidly because no CO_2 is being returned to the lungs.
(b) $P_{ET}CO_2$ is decreased when chest compressions are inadequate, and $P_{ET}CO_2$ increases when effectiveness of compression is increased.
(3) Evaluation of ventilation and $Paco_2$
(a) This use is limited in critically ill patients because the relationship between $Paco_2$ and $P_{ET}CO_2$ is affected by changes in pulmonary dead space and perfusion.
(b) Gradient of $Paco_2$ minus $P_{ET}CO_2$ may be used as an indication of changes in pulmonary dead space or a drop in cardiac output.
(c) This gradient may be used during procedural sedation to monitor for changes in ventilation.
c. Description
(1) The CO_2 in the expired air is measured; the end-tidal CO_2 is assumed to represent alveolar gas and may be used to estimate the $Paco_2$; because this relationship depends on the ventilation-perfusion (V/Q) ratios throughout the lung, this assumption may be particularly erroneous in critically ill patients.
d. Normal value: the $P_{ET}CO_2$ is usually 1 to 5 mm Hg below the $Paco_2$
(1) Increased $P_{ET}CO_2$ assumes hypoventilation.
(2) Decreased $P_{ET}CO_2$ assumes hyperventilation.
e. Implication: changes in $P_{ET}CO_2$ indicate that the patient requires prompt assessment and ABG samples for analysis

3. Pulse oximetry (Spo_2, or functional oxygen saturation)
a. Continuous noninvasive method of monitoring arterial oxygen saturation
b. Indications
(1) Recovery from anesthesia
(2) Assessment of adequacy of oxygenation (does not adequately evaluate ventilation because $Paco_2$ increases with hypoventilation, but Pao_2 and O_2 saturation do not decrease until much later)
c. Description
(1) Sensor with light source is placed on the fingertip, toe, bridge of nose, forehead, or ear lobe; one must take care to use the appropriate sensor for the location (i.e., a finger sensor should not be attached to the ear lobe)
(2) The amount of arterial Hgb that is saturated with O_2 is determined by beams of light passed through the tissue
d. Normal value: greater than 95%; moderate to severe hypoxemia should be suspected if less than 90%; causes of decreased Spo_2
(1) Decrease in Sao_2 and Pao_2
(2) Decrease in CO
e. Limitations
(1) Inadequate pulsations may result from the following:
(a) Significant hypotension
(b) Vasopressor use

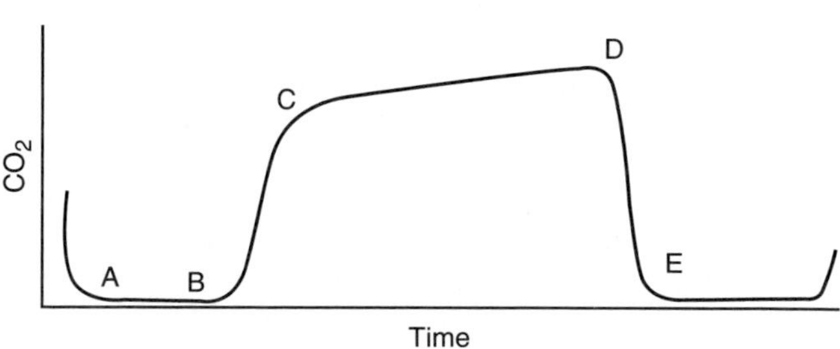

Figure 4-25 Typical normal CO_2 waveform. *A* to *B*, Exhalation of CO_2-free gas from dead space. *B* to *C*, Combination of dead space and alveolar gases. *C* to *D*, Exhalation of mostly alveolar gas. *D*, Exhalation of CO_2 at maximal point (end-tidal point). *D* to *E*, Inspiration begins and CO_2 concentration rapidly falls to baseline or zero. (From St. John, R. E. [2004]. Airway management. *Critical Care Nurse, 24*[2], 93-96.)

(c) Severe hypothermia
(d) Arterial compression
(2) Tends to overestimate Sao_2 by 2% to 5%; accuracy of Spo_2 below 70% is questionable; the lower the Sao_2, the larger the difference between it and the Spo_2
(3) Does not accurately reflect O_2 tissue delivery in patients with anemia or abnormal Hgb
(a) Carboxyhemoglobin
(i) Results in overestimation of O_2 saturation reading because Hgb is saturated but with carbon monoxide
(ii) Smokers may have elevated carboxyhemoglobin levels
(b) Methemoglobin
(i) Results in overestimation of Sao_2
(ii) Methemoglobin is a form of Hgb that cannot carry O_2
(iii) May be related to the administration of nitroglycerin, nitroprusside, sulfonamides, or local anesthetics
(c) Hgb S: sickle cell anemia
(4) Other variables may impair accuracy
(a) Intravenous dyes (e.g., methylene blue or indocyanine green): result in inaccurate readings
(b) Increased bilirubin (greater than 20 mg%): results in inaccurately low readings
(c) Ambient light: may affect accuracy
(d) Motion artifact: may affect accuracy
(e) Edema: may result in inaccurately low readings
(f) Nail polish: blue, green, gold, black, or brown nail polish needs to be removed
(g) Pierced ear lobe: results in inaccurate reading

f. Implication: changes in Spo_2 indicate that the patient requires prompt assessment and ABGs for analysis

4. Transcutaneous Pao_2 ($P_{tc}O_2$) monitoring
a. Continuous noninvasive method of monitoring Pao_2
b. Indications: as for pulse oximetry
c. Description
(1) Sensor is placed on the skin; electrode has a heating element to warm skin and cause capillaries to dilate and increase blood flow
d. Normal value: greater than 80 mm Hg; moderate to severe hypoxemia should be suspected if less than 60 mm Hg
e. Limitations
(1) Affected by skin blood flow, thickness, temperature, skin O_2 consumption, subcutaneous emphysema, and edema
(2) Tends to underestimate Pao_2
(3) Less reliable in adults than in infants
f. Implications
(1) Pao_2 will always be equal to or greater than $P_{tc}O_2$.
(2) Changes in $P_{tc}O_2$ indicates that the patient requires prompt assessment and ABGs for analysis.

5. Mixed Svo_2
a. Oxygen saturation of the blood as it returns to the lung for reoxygenation; reflects how well the demand of the body for O_2 is met by the amount of O_2 supplied
b. Normal Svo_2: 60% to 80%
c. Complete discussion of Svo_2 monitoring is in the Hemodynamic Monitoring section of Chapter 2

6. Continuous airway pressure monitoring
a. Noninvasive technique for displaying the patient's airway pressure waveforms on a bedside monitoring system; provides a visual representation of the patient's own spontaneous effort and the function of the ventilator
b. Description
(1) Air-filled (i.e., not primed with fluid) pressure tubing is connected to the ventilator tubing at the Y connector.
(2) Tubing is connected to a transducer, and the transducer is attached to a channel of the bedside monitor.
(3) Zeroing is at any level.
(4) Positive waveform deflections indicate positive pressure ventilation, and negative deflections indicate spontaneous inspiratory effort.
c. Implications
(1) Assessment of asynchrony between patient and ventilator
(2) Identification of ventilator mode
(3) Detection of PEEP, including auto–PEEP
(4) Improvement of accuracy of hemodynamic waveforms
(5) Identification of respiratory efforts when muscle paralysis and/or sedation is inadequate

Diagnostic Studies

1. Serum chemistries
a. Sodium: normal 136 to 145 mEq/L
b. Potassium: normal 3.5 to 5.5 mEq/L
c. Chloride: normal 96 to 106 mEq/L
d. Calcium: normal 8.5 to 10.5 mg/dL
e. Phosphorus: normal 3 to 4.5 mg/dL
f. Magnesium: normal 1.5 to 2.2 mEq/L or 1.8 to 2.4 mg/dL
g. Glucose: normal 70 to 110 mEq/L
h. Blood urea nitrogen: normal 5 to 20 mg/dL
i. Creatinine: normal 0.7 to 1.5 mg/dL
j. Lactate: 1 to 2 mmol/L
2. ABGs

a. pH: normal 7.35 to 7.45
b. $Paco_2$: normal 35 to 45 mm Hg
c. HCO_3^-: normal 22 to 26 mM
d. Pao_2: normal 80 to 100 mm Hg
e. Sao_2: greater than 95%

3. Hematology
   a. Hematocrit: normal 40% to 52% for males; 35% to 47% for females
   b. Hgb: normal 13 to 18 g/dL for males; 12 to 16 g/dL for females
   c. White blood cells (WBCs): normal 3500 to 11,000 cells/mm^3
   d. D dimer: normally negative
4. Sputum analysis: specimen may be obtained in morning by cough, induced tracheobronchial aspiration, transtracheal aspiration, or bronchoscopy
   a. Characteristics: color; odor; viscosity; presence of blood
   b. Culture and sensitivity tests: identifies infecting organism and effective antibiotic agent
   c. Gram's stain: differentiates between gram-negative and gram-positive bacteria
   d. Acid-fast stain: determines presence of acid-fast bacilli (tuberculosis)
   e. Cytologic studies: determines presence of malignant cells
5. Pleural fluid analysis
   a. Total protein: differentiates between exudative pleural effusion and transudative pleural effusion
   b. Gram's stain: differentiates between gram-negative and gram-positive bacteria
   c. Acid-fast stain: determines presence of acid-fast bacilli (tuberculosis)
   d. Cytologic studies: determines presence of malignant cells
6. Skin tests
   a. Type I hypersensitivity tests (allergy tests)
   b. Type II hypersensitivity tests: purified protein derivative for tuberculosis
   c. Fungal diseases (e.g., *Candida*)
7. Other diagnostic studies (Table 4-9)

Acid-Base Balance and Arterial Blood Gas Interpretation

Physiology Review

1. Acid: a substance that can give up a H^+; acids are produced by the body as a result of cellular metabolism
   a. Volatile (e.g., carbonic acid)
      (1) Exhalable
      (2) Results from aerobic metabolism of glucose
      (3) Eliminated by the lungs
   b. Nonvolatile (also called *fixed;* e.g., sulfuric, phosphoric, and uric)
      (1) Nonexhalable and cannot be converted into a gas
      (2) Results from aerobic metabolism of protein and fat and the anaerobic metabolism of glucose
      (3) Eliminated by the kidney
   c. Elimination or neutralization necessary
2. Acidemia: the condition of the blood with a pH of below 7.35
3. Acidosis: the process that causes the acidemia
4. Base: a substance that can accept a H^+ (the primary base in the body is bicarbonate [HCO_3^-])
5. Alkalemia: the condition of the blood with a pH of above 7.45
6. Alkalosis: the process that causes the alkalemia
7. pH
   a. Indirect measurement of H^+ concentration
   b. Reflection of the balance between carbonic acid (acid regulated by the lungs) and HCO_3^- (base regulated by the kidneys)
   c. Inversely proportional to H^+ concentration
      (1) Increase in H^+ concentration: lower pH, more acid

Table 4-9 Pulmonary Diagnostic Studies

Study	Evaluation	Comments
Bronchography	• Detects obstruction or malformation of the tracheobronchial tree	• Patient inspires radiopaque substance and then x-rays are taken • Inquire about possibility of pregnancy
Chest x-ray	• Detects pathologic lung condition (e.g., pneumonia, pulmonary edema, atelectasis, or tuberculosis) • Determines size and location of lung lesions and tumors • Verifies placement of endotracheal tube, central venous catheters, and chest tubes	• Noninvasive test with minimal radiation exposure • Inquire about possibility of pregnancy • Posteroanterior and lateral films are done most commonly, but in critical care areas, anteroposterior portable films are frequently necessary because of inability to transport patient • Lateral decubitus films aid in identification of pleural effusion
Exercise testing	• Identify early disability • Differentiate between cardiac and pulmonary disease	• Monitor for changes in functional oxygen saturation during exercise • Monitor closely for exercise-induced hypotension or ventricular dysrhythmias

Continued

Table 4-9 **Pulmonary Diagnostic Studies—cont'd**

Study	Evaluation	Comments
Laryngoscopy, bronchoscopy, mediastinoscopy	• Obtain cytologic specimen or biopsy • Identify tumors, obstructions, secretions, or foreign bodies in tracheobronchial tree • Locate a bleeding site • May be used therapeutically to remove secretions, foreign bodies, and other contaminants	• Patient is sedated before the procedure, usually with a benzodiazepine (e.g., diazepam or midazolam) • Monitor the patient for subcutaneous emphysema after study; indicates tracheal or bronchial tear • Monitor for hemoptysis; some blood in sputum is normal after biopsy but frank hemoptysis requires immediate attention
Lung biopsy Transthoracic needle lung biopsy Open lung biopsy	• Obtain specimen for cytologic evaluation	• Transthoracic needle biopsy performed under fluoroscopy; inquire about possibility of pregnancy • Open lung biopsy requires thoracotomy
Magnetic resonance imaging	• Distinguishes tumors from other structures (e.g., tumor, pleural thickening, or fibrosis)	• Noninvasive test • Contraindicated for patients with pacemakers or implanted metallic devices
Pulmonary angiography	• Detects changes in lung tissue (e.g., masses) • Diagnoses abnormalities in pulmonary vasculature, including thrombi and emboli • Identifies congenital abnormalities of the circulation	• Invasive test • Inquire about possibility of pregnancy • Contrast media injected into pulmonary artery: ensure adequate hydration after study • Monitor arterial puncture point for hematoma or hemorrhage
Pulmonary function studies (See Table 4-1 for lung volumes and parameters with normal values.) Spirometry: volumes and capacities Residual volume, functional residual capacity, and total lung capacity require nitrogen washout technique Ventilatory mechanics Flow-volume loop studies Diffusing capacity	• Measures lung volumes, capacities, and flow rates • Identifies features of restrictive or obstructive lung disease • Evaluates responsiveness to bronchodilator therapy • Aids in evaluation of surgical risk • Documents a disability or cause of dyspnea	• Noninvasive study • Frequently repeated after bronchodilator therapy
Sleep studies	• Diagnose and differentiate between obstructive sleep apnea, central sleep apnea, and cardiac sleep apnea	• Restrict caffeine before testing • Usually done during normal sleep hours
Thoracentesis (may include pleural biopsy)	• Obtain pleural fluid and/or tissue specimen • May be used therapeutically to remove pleural fluid	• Monitor patient for indications of pneumothorax • Monitor for leakage from puncture point
Thoracic computerized tomography	• Defines lesions, masses, cavities, or shadows seen on normal chest x-rays • Evaluates tracheal or bronchial narrowing • Aids in planning radiation therapy	• X-rays are taken at different angles
Ultrasonography	• Evaluates pleural disease • Visualizes diaphragm and detects disease around diaphragm (e.g., subphrenic hematoma or abscess)	• Noninvasive test
Ventilation scan Lung perfusion scan Ventilation/perfusion scan	• Diagnoses ventilation and/or perfusion abnormalities including emphysema and pulmonary emboli	• Invasive test: radioisotope inspired and injected intravascularly • Inquire about possibility of pregnancy • Nuclear scan study: assure patient that amount of radioactive material is minimal

(2) Decrease in H^+ concentration: higher pH, more base

d. Must be maintained within a narrow range to allow functioning of enzymatic systems in the body

(1) pH below 6.8 or above 7.8 is incompatible with life

(2) Note that this is a 0.6 change toward acidosis but only a 0.4 change toward alkalosis (from midline normal of 7.4); this is because the shift of the oxyhemoglobin dissociation curve caused by alkalosis affects tissue oxygenation more adversely than does the shift caused by acidosis

8. Henderson-Hasselbalch equation

a. pH is determined by the logarithm of the ratio of HCO_3^- concentration to arterial $Paco_2$.

(1) $$pH = \frac{pK \text{ (constant of 6.1)} + \log HCO_3^-}{Paco_2}$$

b. Ratio of 20 HCO_3^- to 1 carbonic acid maintains normal pH (Figure 4-26).

Acid-Base Regulation

1. Chemical buffers

a. Weak acid and strong base

b. Immediate response when a change in acid-base status occurs by combining with excess acid or base

c. Buffer systems

(1) Bicarbonate-carbonic acid buffer system

(a) The most important buffer system

(b) HCO_3^- is generated by the kidney and aids in the elimination of H^+

(c) $CO_2 + H_2O \leftrightharpoons H_2CO_3^- \leftrightharpoons H^+ + HCO_3^-$
LUNGS KIDNEYS

(2) Phosphate system: aids in excretion of H^+ by the kidney

(3) Ammonium: H^+ is added to ammonia in the renal tubule to form ammonium; allows greater excretion of H^+ by the kidney

(4) Hgb and other proteins: aids in buffering extracellular fluid

2. Respiratory system

a. Regulates the excretion or retention of carbonic acid

(1) If pH decreases, the rate and depth of ventilation increase.

(2) If pH increases, the rate and depth of ventilation decrease.

b. Responds within minutes: fast but weak

3. Renal system

a. Regulates the excretion or retention of HCO_3^- and the excretion of hydrogen and nonvolatile acids

(1) If pH decreases, the kidney retains HCO_3^-.

(2) If pH increases, the kidney excretes HCO_3^-.

b. Responds within 48 hours: slow but powerful

Acid-Base Imbalances (Table 4-10)

1. Acidemia: pH below 7.35

a. Acidosis: the process causing acidemia

(1) Caused by acid gain

(a) If acid is volatile (reflected by increase in $Paco_2$): respiratory acidosis

(b) If acid is nonvolatile (reflected by decrease in HCO_3^-): metabolic acidosis

(2) Caused by base loss or metabolic acid gain (reflected by decrease in HCO_3^-): metabolic acidosis

(3) Anion gap is used to differentiate between metabolic acid gain or base loss as cause of metabolic acidosis

(a) Calculated: $(Na^+ + K^+) - (Cl^- + CO_2^-)$

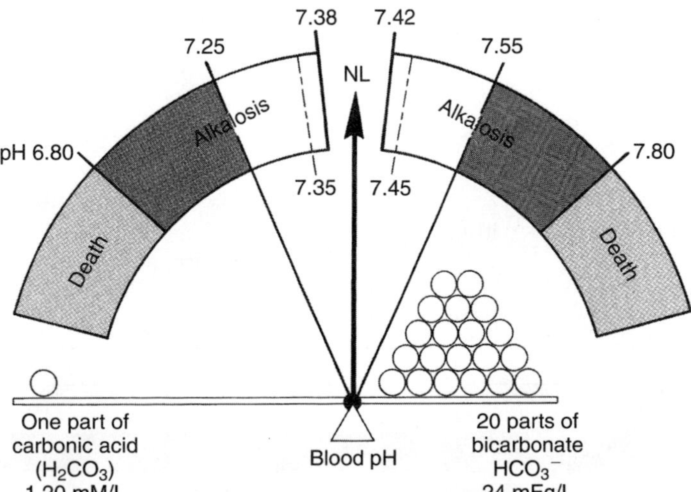

Figure 4-26 Acid-base balance. Twenty parts of HCO_3^- are required to buffer one part carbonic acid; pH normally is maintained within the narrow range *(NL)* of 7.35 to 7.45; pH below 6.8 or above 7.8 is incompatible with life. (From Price, S. A., & Wilson, L. M. [1994]. *Pathophysiology: Clinical concepts of disease processes.* [4th ed.]. St. Louis: Mosby.)

(b) Normal: 5 to 15
(c) If anion gap is normal (between 5 and 15), metabolic acidosis is due to a base loss
(d) If anion gap is increased (greater than 15), metabolic acidosis is due to acid gain
(e) More information on anion gap is in Chapter 6

2. Alkalemia: pH above 7.45
   a. Alkalosis: the process causing alkalosis
      (1) Caused by acid loss
         (a) If acid is volatile (reflected by decrease in $Paco_2$): respiratory alkalosis
         (b) If acid is nonvolatile (reflected by increase in HCO_3^-): metabolic alkalosis
      (2) Caused by base gain or metabolic acid loss (reflected by increase in HCO_3^-): metabolic alkalosis
3. Compensation
   a. Respiratory acidosis
      (1) The kidneys reabsorb more HCO_3^- or excrete more H^+
      (2) The HCO_3^- and base excess levels increase
      (3) This change will be slow and may take as long as 2 to 3 days
   b. Respiratory alkalosis
      (1) The kidneys excrete more HCO_3^-
      (2) The HCO_3^- and base excess levels decrease
      (3) This change will be slow and may take as long as 2 to 3 days
         (a) Because respiratory alkalosis is almost always a short-term process (e.g., hyperventilation anxiety syndrome), compensation for respiratory alkalosis rarely is seen because it takes too long and the problem would be resolved
   c. Metabolic acidosis
      (1) The lungs increase the rate and depth of ventilation.
      (2) The $Paco_2$ level decreases.
      (3) This change will be rapid, usually within minutes to hours.
   d. Metabolic alkalosis
      (1) The lungs decrease the rate and depth of ventilation.
      (2) The $Paco_2$ level increases.
      (3) This change will be rapid, usually within minutes to hours.
   e. Correction versus compensation
      (1) Correction may be a physiologic process or the result of appropriate therapeutic measures; correction is achieved when the pH is normal and both indicators ($Paco_2$, HCO_3^-) are normal.
      (2) Compensation is a physiologic process; the pH is normal and both indicators are abnormal.
         (a) Partial compensation: pH is still abnormal but the secondary parameter is outside normal range in the direction to move the pH toward normal
         (b) Full compensation: pH is normal and the secondary parameter is outside normal range in the direction to move the pH toward normal
4. Mixed disorders (Table 4-11)
   a. More than one disorder may coexist.
   b. The degree of respiratory component versus metabolic component can be calculated using these formulae.
      (1) As the $Paco_2$ changes by 10 torr (from normal of 40 torr), it is associated with a change in pH of 0.08 in the opposite direction.
      (2) As the pH changes by 0.15 (from normal of 7.4), it is associated with a change in base of 10 mEq.
   c. Compensation cannot exist in mixed disorders because each system is independently abnormal and cannot help the other.

Analysis of Arterial Blood Gases

1. Purposes of ABGs.
   a. Evaluate ventilation: $Paco_2$
   b. Evaluate acid-base status: pH; to determine the cause of the acid-base imbalance, determine which parameter is abnormal
      (1) Respiratory: $Paco_2$
      (2) Metabolic: HCO_3^-
   c. Evaluate oxygenation: Pao_2
2. Parameters and normals (Box 4-5)
   a. pH: negative logarithm of H^+ concentration in arterial blood
      (1) Normal pH is 7.35 to 7.45.
      (2) Levels below 7.35 indicate an acidosis.
      (3) Levels above 7.45 indicate an alkalosis.
   b. $Paco_2$
      (1) Normal $Paco_2$ is 35 to 45 mm Hg

Table 4-10 Acid-Base Imbalances

Imbalance	pH	Primary Change	Compensatory Change
Respiratory acidosis	Less than 7.35	↑ $Paco_2$	↑ HCO_3^-
Metabolic acidosis	Less than 7.35	↓ HCO_3^-	↓ $Paco_2$
Respiratory alkalosis	Greater than 7.45	↓ $Paco_2$	↓ HCO_3^-
Metabolic alkalosis	Greater than 7.45	↑ HCO_3^-	↑ $Paco_2$

(2) Levels below 35 mm Hg indicate a respiratory alkalosis or respiratory compensation for a metabolic acidosis
(3) Levels above 45 mm Hg indicate a respiratory acidosis or respiratory compensation for a metabolic alkalosis

c. HCO_3^- level in arterial blood
(1) Normal HCO_3^- is 22 to 26 mEq/L.
(2) Levels below 22 mEq/L indicate a metabolic acidosis or metabolic compensation for respiratory alkalosis.
(3) Levels above 26 mEq/L indicate a metabolic alkalosis or metabolic compensation for respiratory acidosis.

d. Base excess: difference between acid and base levels in arterial blood
(1) Normal base excess is +2 to −2.
(2) Levels below −2 (actually a base deficit) indicate a metabolic acidosis or metabolic compensation for respiratory alkalosis.
(3) Levels above +2 indicate a metabolic alkalosis or metabolic compensation for respiratory acidosis.

e. Pao_2
(1) Normal Pao_2 is 80 to 100 mm Hg.
(2) Levels above 100 mm Hg indicate hyperoxemia.
(3) Levels below 80 mm Hg indicate mild hypoxemia.
(4) Levels below 60 mm Hg indicate moderate hypoxemia.
(5) Levels below 40 mm Hg indicate severe hypoxemia.

f. Sao_2 saturation of Hgb by O_2
(1) Normal Sao_2 is 95% or greater.
(2) Levels below 95% indicate mild desaturation of Hgb.
(3) Levels below 90% indicate moderate desaturation of Hgb.
(4) Levels below 75% indicate severe desaturation of Hgb.

3. Steps in analysis
a. Is pH acidotic, alkalotic, or normal?
b. Which parameter is abnormal?
(1) $Paco_2$: respiratory
(2) HCO_3^- metabolic
c. If the pH is normal, is it leaning? If so, consider compensation.
(1) Compensation causes a leaning pH: the pH leans toward the *initial* disorder.
(a) The body never overcompensates; a normal nonleaning pH with two abnormal indicators ($Paco_2$ and HCO_3^-) suggests a mixed disorder (e.g., one alkalotic process and one acidotic process).
(2) For compensation to be occurring, one parameter change must help the other.
(a) Full compensation: normal pH with both indicators abnormal
(b) Partial compensation
(i) pH is still abnormal
(ii) Both indicators ($Paco_2$ and HCO_3^-) are abnormal with the secondary indicator moving in the direction to help normalize the pH
d. Assess oxygenation.
(1) Pao_2 less than 80 mm Hg is hypoxemia.
(2) Pao_2 less than 60 mm Hg on room air is usually an indication for O_2 administration.
(3) Acceptable Pao_2 should be adjusted for age; one method is to subtract 1 mm Hg for each year greater than 60 years from 80 mm Hg; this gives acceptable Pao_2 on room air for a patient of that age.

4. Technical problems that may affect accuracy of ABG values
a. Too much heparin: decrease in $Paco_2$, decrease in HCO_3^-, increase in base excess
b. Air bubble: increase in pH, decrease in $Paco_2$, increase in Pao_2
c. Not chilled immediately: decrease in pH, decrease in Pao_2, increase in $Paco_2$
d. Inadequate discard volume when drawing from catheter with flush solution: decreased $Paco_2$
e. Discussion of acid-base imbalances (Table 4-12)

Table 4-11 Mixed Acid-Base Disorders

Mixed Disorder	Clinical Example
Mixed acidosis	Cardiac and respiratory arrest
Mixed alkalosis	Compensated respiratory acidosis (e.g., COPD) being excessively mechanically ventilated
Respiratory acidosis and metabolic alkalosis	Patient with COPD who are taking diuretics
Respiratory alkalosis and metabolic acidosis	Hepatic and renal failure

COPD, Chronic obstructive pulmonary disease.

Box 4-5 Arterial Blood Gas Normal Values

pH	7.35-7.45
$Paco_2$	35-45 mm Hg
Bicarbonate	22-26 mEq/L
Pao_2	80-100 mm Hg

Airway Management

Etiology of Airway Obstruction

1. Upper airway
a. Relaxation of tongue against hypopharynx: primary cause of obstruction in unconscious patient

Table 4-12 Discussion of Acid-Base Imbalances

Imbalance	Etiology	Clinical Presentation	Collaborative Management
Respiratory acidosis: pH low; $Paco_2$ high	Hypoventilation • Airway obstruction • CNS depression from drugs, injury, or disease • Chest wall injury (e.g., flail chest) • Obstructive lung disease (e.g., chronic bronchitis, emphysema, or late asthma) • Restrictive lung disease (e.g., kyphoscoliosis or obesity hypoventilation syndrome) • Oxygen-induced hypoventilation in patients with chronic hypercapnia • Neuromuscular abnormality (e.g., Guillain-Barré syndrome, myasthenia gravis, or multiple sclerosis) • Atelectasis, pneumonia • Pulmonary edema • Respiratory arrest	*Initially* • Sympathetic nervous system stimulation symptoms (e.g., tachycardia, tachypnea, or diaphoresis) *Later* • Bradypnea • Hypotension • Dysrhythmias • Confusion • Headache • Blurred vision • Flushed face (plethora) • Somnolence leading to coma (these late symptoms also are referred to as *carbon dioxide narcosis*)	Increase ventilation and treat cause. • Maintain patent airway. • Position patient for optimal ventilation. • Implement bronchial hygiene measures. • Administer drug therapy (e.g., bronchodilators, mucolytics, or antibiotics). • Mechanical ventilation may be necessary. • If patient is on mechanical ventilation: ◦ Increase rate ◦ Increase V_T
Respiratory alkalosis: pH high; $Paco_2$ low	Hyperventilation • Anxiety or hysteria • Thoracic pain • Early asthma • Pneumothorax • Pulmonary embolus • Early salicylate intoxication • Hyperthyroidism • Hepatic failure • Fever • Gram-negative septicemia • CNS infection or injury • Excessive mechanical ventilation	• Tachycardia • Palpitations • Dry mouth • Anxiety • Profuse perspiration • Paresthesia around mouth and extremities • Dizziness, vertigo, syncope • Increased muscle irritability, twitching • Tetany • Inability to concentrate • Seizures • Coma	Decrease ventilation and treat cause. • Provide reassurance and maintain a calm attitude. • Administer sedatives (frequently given IV). • Ask patient to breathe into and out of a paper bag or use a rebreathing mask. • If patient is on mechanical ventilation: ◦ Decrease rate ◦ Decrease V_T ◦ Change from assist-control to intermittent mandatory ventilation ◦ Consider sedation ◦ Consider addition of dead space tubing
Metabolic acidosis: pH low; HCO_3^- low	*Acid gain (increased anion gap)* • Tissue hypoxia (e.g., shock [lactic acidosis]) • Ketoacidosis (DKA or starvation) • Renal failure • Drugs and toxins (e.g., salicylates; methanol, ethylene glycol) *HCO_3^- loss (normal anion gap)* • Bile drainage • Pancreatic fistula • Diarrhea • Acetazolamide (Diamox) therapy	• Nausea, vomiting, abdominal discomfort • Weakness • Tremors • Malaise • Headache • Tachypnea progressing to Kussmaul's respirations • Hypotension • Dysrhythmias • Confusion • Lethargy → coma	• Treat cause as appropriate: ◦ Improve oxygenation and/or perfusion (lactic acidosis) ◦ Give insulin (DKA) ◦ Dialysis (renal failure) ◦ Antidiarrheals (diarrhea) • Administer buffer: ◦ Bicarbonate IV or orally for pH 7.0 or less
Metabolic alkalosis: pH high; HCO_3^- high	*Acid loss* • Nasogastric suction or severe vomiting • Potassium-wasting diuretic therapy • Steroid therapy • Cushing's disease • Hyperaldosteronism • Hepatic disease • Hypokalemia, hypochloremia *HCO_3^- gain* • Dosing with HCO_3^- • Excess infusion of lactated Ringer's solution	• Bradypnea • Nausea, vomiting, diarrhea • Paresthesia around mouth and extremities • Confusion • Dizziness • Increased muscle irritability • Tetany • Seizures • Coma	• Treat cause: ◦ Antiemetic ◦ Electrolyte replacement: potassium and/or chloride ◦ Discontinuance of sodium bicarbonate or lactated Ringer's solution • Administer carbonic anhydrase inhibitor: ◦ Acetazolamide (Diamox) Administer buffer: ◦ Arginine monohydrochloride ◦ Ammonium chloride ◦ Weak hydrochloric acid solution

CNS, Central nervous system; *DKA*, diabetic ketoacidosis; *HCO_3^-*, bicarbonate; *IV*, intravenous; V_T, tidal volume.

b. Foreign body aspiration
(1) Aspiration of food: primary cause of obstruction in conscious patient
(2) Vomitus
(3) Dentures
c. Tumor
d. Hematoma
e. Laryngeal spasm, edema
f. Vocal cord paralysis
g. Infection (e.g., epiglottis)
h. Trauma (e.g., fractured trachea)
2. Lower airway
a. Foreign bodies
b. Secretions
c. Hemorrhage
d. Pneumonia
e. Space-occupying lesions, tumors
f. Bronchospasm

Clinical Presentation of Airway Obstruction

1. Partial obstruction
a. Presence of air movement
b. Restlessness, agitation, anxiety
c. Respiratory distress: tracheal tug; intercostal retractions; use of accessory muscles
d. Cyanosis
e. Coughing
f. Altered speech
g. Inspiratory sounds: snoring; stridor
h. Breath sound changes: wheezes; rhonchi
2. Complete obstruction
a. Lack of air movement
b. Extreme anxiety in conscious patient
c. Respiratory distress: tracheal tug; intercostal retractions; use of accessory muscles
d. Cyanosis
e. Inability to speak, cough, or produce any sound
f. Universal sign of choking: patient clutches throat with hand
g. Unconsciousness within seconds

Collaborative Management of Airway Obstruction and/or Respiratory Distress

1. Evaluate the patency of the airway: look, listen, and feel for airflow.
2. Maintain optimal airway and thoracic position.
a. Used head tilt–chin lift (also called *sniffing*) position for optimal airway position.
(1) True hyperextension should be avoided
(2) Contraindicated if cervical spine fracture possible (instead use jaw thrust)
b. Position head of bed for optimal chest excursion: semi-Fowler to high Fowler's position.
3. Remove any obstruction.
a. Inspect the mouth for blood, teeth, loose dentures, food, or anything else that may cause obstruction.
b. Remove any visible obstruction.
(1) Use fingers to remove visible foreign bodies; blind sweeps are not recommended because of concern that the obstruction may be pushed deeper into the airway.
(2) Magill forceps may be used, but one must take care to prevent pushing the obstruction deeper into the airway.
c. Use abdominal thrusts (also referred to as *Heimlich maneuver*): subxiphoid thrusts to relieve upper airway obstruction.
(1) Alternate five abdominal thrusts with attempts to ventilate in unconscious patient.
(2) Avoid abdominal thrusts (use chest thrusts) in any of the following situations:
(a) Patient is too obese for you to get your arms around him or her.
(b) Patient has had recent abdominal surgery.
(c) Patient is pregnant.
d. Place patient in recovery position: side-lying on left side.
4. Encourage deep breathing: sustained inspiratory effort.
a. Purposes of deep breathing include the following:
(1) Increases air in the alveoli, preventing atelectasis
(2) Makes coughing more effective
b. Incentive spirometry also may be used to provide graded incentives for sustained inspiration.
5. Remove secretions as required.
a. Cough: forceful expiration to dislodge and remove secretions from the tracheobronchial tree
(1) Indications
(a) Breath sound changes: especially rhonchi; wheezes caused by mucous plugs also may clear with coughing
(b) With postural drainage: between position changes but never in a head-down position
(c) NOTE: While coughing should be encouraged in the foregoing identified situations, routine coughing may increase the incidence of atelectasis; preventive measures (e.g., in postoperative patients) should focus on deep breathing with sustained inspiration rather than forced expiration (e.g., coughing).
(2) Technique for effective coughing
(a) Assist patient to comfortable position.
(b) Instruct patient to do the following:
(i) Inhale deeply.
(ii) Cough 2 to 3 times with mouth open.
(iii) Expectorate any sputum.
(iv) Inhale slowly and deeply.
(3) Special techniques
(a) Huff coughing
(i) Forced expiration with glottis open
(ii) May be helpful for patients with COPD to keep airways open
(b) Augmented coughing
(i) Requires an assistant to deliver a subxiphoid thrust during expiration

(ii) May be necessary for patients with abdominal muscle weakness or paralysis

b. Suctioning of oropharynx: removal of secretions from the oropharynx through the use of a suction catheter and negative pressure

(1) Indications

(a) Before deflation of ET tube cuff to prevent oropharyngeal secretions from draining into tracheobronchial tree

(b) After suctioning of tracheobronchial tree to prevent accumulation of oropharyngeal secretions that can be aspirated silently around ET tube cuff

(c) With mouth care of patients with artificial airways in place

(2) Equipment

(a) Yankauer suction device usually is used.

(b) If the suction catheter that was used to suction the tracheobronchial tree is used, suction oropharynx only *after* suctioning the tracheobronchial tree and rinsing the catheter.

c. Suctioning of tracheobronchial tree: removal of secretions from the tracheobronchial tree through the use of a suction catheter and negative pressure

(1) Clinical indications for the need to suction; suctioning of the airway should not be routine but should be performed when indicated

(a) Sympathetic nervous system stimulation (tachycardia, tachypnea)

(b) Change in BP: increased or decreased

(c) Dyspnea

(d) Noisy or shallow ventilation

(e) Rhonchi

(f) Obvious visible secretions

(g) Excessive coughing during inspiratory cycle of ventilator

(h) High-pressure alarm on ventilator

(i) Clinical indications of hypoxia (Box 4-3) or hypercapnia (Box 4-4)

(2) Technique for suctioning the tracheobronchial tree using principles to prevent complications

(a) Suction only if indicated, and limit number of passes to minimum required.

(b) Use an appropriate size of suction catheter: the outer diameter of the catheter should be no more than one half the inner diameter of the ET tube or tracheostomy.

(c) Use a closed suction system or a special adaptor for open suction system that allows suctioning without discontinuing mechanical ventilation for patients on therapeutic levels of PEEP (more than 5 cm H_2O) because these patients frequently have significant oxygen desaturation during suctioning.

(d) Use a special curved-tip catheter (Coudé catheter) if it is required to enter the left mainstem bronchus; it is usually adequate to use a regular suction catheter to suction the trachea because the coughing stimulated effectively clears both mainstem bronchi into the trachea.

(e) Use sterile technique if suctioning is performed through ET tube or tracheostomy; aseptic technique is used if suctioning nasotracheally.

(i) Use two gloves.

(ii) Wear goggles to protect your eyes if open suction system is used.

(f) Explain procedure to the patient; protect the patient's eyes if open suction system is used.

(g) Provide hyperoxygenation (100% oxygen) before, during, and after suctioning; monitor functional oxygen saturation (Spo_2) during suctioning for indications of oxygen desaturation.

(h) Monitor electrocardiogram (ECG) during and after suctioning for vagal stimulation (bradycardia) and for dysrhythmias related to hypoxemia (premature ventricular contractions)

(i) Advance the catheter only 1 cm past the length of the ET tube or tracheostomy tube (i.e., shallow suctioning) to avoid mucosal trauma.

(i) Though traditionally it has been recommended to advance the catheter to the point of obstruction and then to pull back slightly before applying suction, evidence now indicates that it is the catheter contact rather than the suction that traumatizes the mucosa.

(ii) If resistance is met, withdraw the suction catheter slightly before applying suction.

(j) Apply suction while withdrawing the catheter; though traditionally it has been advised to apply suction intermittently during withdrawal of catheter, tracheal mucosal damage is similar with intermittent and continuous suction application.

(k) Limit suctioning to 10 seconds; hyperoxygenate the patient for 30 seconds between passes.

(l) Avoid excessive negative pressure.

(i) Keep pressure 100 mm Hg or less if open suction system.

(ii) Keep pressure 120 mm Hg if closed suction system.

(m) Liquefy secretions through humidification and hydration.

(i) Instillation of saline (also referred to as *saline lavage*) has been proved ineffective and potentially harmful.

a) Ineffective: successful humidification requires small particle size, not bolus administration
b) Causes hypoxemia
c) Contributes to nosocomial pneumonia

(ii) If increased oral or parenteral fluids cannot be given (e.g., renal failure), either of the following may be indicated:
a) Saline by inhalation (small particle size allows deeper penetration into tracheobronchial tree and liquefies mucus)
b) Acetylcysteine (Mucomyst) given by inhalation: breaks down disulfide bonds to liquefy mucus; may cause bronchospasm, so a bronchodilator frequently is required

(n) Rinse the catheter.
(i) In an open suction system: suction sterile water through the catheter and appropriately discard the disposable catheter; most suction catheter kits have a disposable cup to put water in for rinsing the catheter.
(ii) If using a closed suction system, rinse the catheter by pulling it out of the airway (to indicator on device) and then injecting saline into the irrigation port while continuously applying suction (this is irrigation, not lavage) and then closing the irrigation port and the suction valve.

(o) Monitor of complications.
(i) Hypoxemia
(ii) Dysrhythmias
(iii) Hypertension
(iv) Intracranial hypertension
(v) Tracheal trauma

(p) Stop suctioning if the following occur: change in heart rate, ECG rhythm, or skin color; significant change in Spo_2 or Svo_2.

(q) Assess breath sounds after suctioning to evaluate effectiveness.

(3) If doing nasotracheal suctioning in a patient who does not have an ET or tracheostomy tube:
(a) Provide O_2 with a non-rebreathing mask before suctioning.
(b) Place patient in "sniffing" position while sitting up, or place towel roll between shoulders if patient is supine.
(c) Lubricate catheter with water-soluble lubricant before insertion.
(d) Prevent injury to the nasal mucosa.
(i) Placement of a nasopharyngeal airway may be done to prevent injury to the nasal mucosa if frequent suctioning is required.
(ii) ET intubation or tracheostomy also may be required if frequent suctioning is required.
(e) Ask the patient to cough and advance the catheter during that time because the glottis is open; if the patient cannot follow commands, advance the catheter during inspiration.
(f) Note indications that the catheter is in the trachea.
(i) Patient becomes anxious.
(ii) Patient cannot speak.
(g) Complete suctioning as for a patient with an ET or tracheostomy tube.

(4) Advantages of closed suction system
(a) Continued oxygenation and reduction in loss of PEEP so decreased incidence of hypoxemia
(b) Decreased cost and nursing time
(c) Decreased chance of aerosolization of secretions, which protects patient's and nurse's eyes
(d) Decreased risk of introducing bacteria into airway

(5) Specialized ET tube to allow for continuous aspiration of subglottic secretions has been shown to reduce the incidence or delay the onset of nosocomial pneumonia (see Pneumonia in Chapter 5)

6. Provide chest physiotherapy as indicated.
a. Purposes
(1) To promote bronchial hygiene
(2) To improve breathing efficiency
(3) To promote physical reconditioning
b. Postural drainage (PD): sequential positioning of the patient
(1) Purpose: use gravity to drain secretions from peripheral areas into the major bronchi or trachea so that they can be coughed and expectorated or suctioned
(2) Indication: prevention and treatment of respiratory complications
(a) Lobar atelectasis
(b) Disorders with significant mucus production (e.g., cystic fibrosis, bronchiectasis, or COPD)
(3) Technique
(a) Administer bronchodilator before PD if prescribed.
(b) Turn off enteral feedings for 30 minutes before PD; ensure that cuff of ET or tracheostomy tube is inflated.
(c) Place patient in position to drain selected segment of lung or alternate through the following positions.

(i) Left side with hips higher than head
(ii) Right side with hips higher than head
(iii) Supine with hips higher than head
(iv) Prone with hips higher than head
(d) Maintain each position for 10 to 30 minutes.
(e) Cough between position changes but never in a head-down position.
(f) Avoid PD for at least 1½ hours after meals.
(4) Contraindications
(a) Obesity
(b) Spinal fracture, rib fracture, flail chest
(c) Pulmonary hemorrhage, embolism, malignancy
(d) Pneumothorax, empyema, large pleural effusion
(e) Tuberculosis
(f) Asthma, acute bronchospasm
(g) Bleeding disorder
(h) Seizures, intracranial hypertension
(i) Acute myocardial infarction, heart failure, hemodynamic instability
(j) Recent pacemaker insertion
(k) Increased risk of aspiration

c. Percussion: clapping the chest with cupped hands
(1) Purpose: mechanically dislodge secretions from the bronchial walls into the major bronchi or trachea so that they can be coughed and expectorated or suctioned
(2) Technique
(a) May be done with hands or mechanical device; if using hands:
(i) Cup hands as if holding water.
(ii) Tap chest with cupped hands, listening for a cupping, not slapping, sound.
(b) Avoid: spine; liver; kidneys; spleen; female patient's breasts
(3) Contraindications
(a) Known bleeding disorder
(b) Lung cancer
(c) Pneumothorax
(d) Extreme caution in elderly patients with osteoporosis, after thoracotomy

d. Vibration: vibration during expiration of areas of the chest with an open hand or a vibrating device
(1) Purpose: loosen secretions from the bronchial walls into the major bronchi or trachea so that they can be coughed and expectorated or suctioned
(2) Technique
(a) Hold hand flat against chest and vibrate hand during expiration
(b) Hand vibrator also may be used
(3) Contraindications: as for percussion

7. Turn patient at least every 2 hours; use a special bed as appropriate

a. Consider "good lung down" principle for patients with unilateral lung conditions (exception: pneumonectomy).

b. Consider kinetic therapy through the use of continuous lateral rotational therapy bed if appropriate.
(1) Effect: promotes redistribution of ventilation, promotes redistribution of perfusion, and optimizes V/Q matching
(2) Indications
(a) Acute lung injury (ALI)/acute respiratory distress syndrome (ARDS) or high risk for these
(b) Pneumonia
(c) Prevention of ventilator-associated pneumonia and lobar atelectasis
(3) Guidelines
(a) Start as early as possible.
(b) Explain the process to the patient before turning.
(c) Monitor BP and Spo_2 frequently, especially initially until acclimation.
(4) Contraindications
(a) Table rotational beds
(i) Severe claustrophobia, though most of these patients will be sedated
(ii) Uncontrolled diarrhea
(iii) Weight greater than 500 lb
(b) Cushion-based beds and mattress replacement beds
(i) Severe claustrophobia, though most of these patients will be sedated
(ii) Uncontrolled diarrhea
(iii) Weight greater than 300 lb
(iv) Unstable spinal cord injury
(v) Skeletal traction

c. Consider placing the patient in prone position periodically if appropriate; frequently used in ALI and ARDS.
(1) Effects
(a) Improved compliance of the dorsal chest wall, which increases reexpansion of dependent lung regions and thus optimizes V/Q matching
(b) Reduction in the amount of lung volume compressed by the heart
(c) Lessening of the compression on the lower lobes by the pressure of the abdominal contents against the diaphragm, which improves ventilation of the lower lobes
(d) Reduction of the gradients of pleural and transpulmonary pressures, causing more even distribution of ventilation
(e) PEEP is more likely to result in more homogeneous perfusion in the lung in prone position, whereas PEEP tends to redistribute blood flow away from well-ventilated ventral areas of the lung in supine position

(2) Contraindications
(a) Intracranial hypertension
(b) Unstable fractures, especially cervical, thoracic, or lumbar fractures
(c) Cervical or skeletal traction
(d) Left ventricular failure
(e) Hemodynamic instability
(f) Active intraabdominal process
(g) Pregnancy
(h) Weight greater than 300 lb may be a contraindication depending on method of turning and/or special bed
(3) Complications
(a) Skin breakdown, particularly the face, ears, nose, eyes, mouth, shoulders, elbows, hips, knees, genitalia, and breasts
(i) Take extra care with breast and penile implants
(b) Dependent edema
(c) Corneal abrasions
(d) Inadvertent extubation or removal of catheters
(e) Obstructed chest tube
(f) Nerve injury
(g) Transient supraventricular tachycardia
(h) Aspiration
(4) Methods
(a) Requires three to four persons depending on patient size; one person should be at the head to stabilize items such as the ET tube and central venous catheters.
(b) Explain the procedure to the patient and administer sedation and/or analgesia
(c) Withhold enteral feedings for the hour before turning to prone but continue feedings once in prone position
(d) Equipment
(i) Use of pillows to position patient in swimming position and elevate abdomen off the bed to prevent impairment in diaphragmatic excursion
(ii) KCI RotoProne bed
(iii) Use of special bed with pronating capability (e.g., KCI TriaDyne II with proning accessory)
(iv) Use of Hillrom Vollman Prone Positioner
(e) Monitor BP and Spo_2
(f) Frequent repositioning still is required to prevent pressure ulcers
(5) Though dramatic improvement in oxygenation frequently occurs, improved survival has not be demonstrated

8. Use artificial airways safely and appropriately.
a. Indications for emergency airway management
(1) Apnea
(2) Upper airway obstruction
(3) Need for airway protection (e.g., vomiting, bleeding, or altered mental status)
(4) Intracranial hypertension
(5) Acute respiratory failure or impending respiratory failure
b. General principles
(1) Provide humidification because natural humidification mechanisms are bypassed.
(2) Use aseptic technique with upper airway artificial airways; use sterile technique with lower airway artificial airways.
(3) Suction as indicated; because ET tubes splint the epiglottis open, effective coughing is impaired.
(4) Provide method of communication; this is the most significant stressor experienced by intubated patients.
(a) Picture communication board, alphabet board, or magic slate, or felt-tip pen or marker and paper may be used; avoid pencils and ball-point pens, which require more pressure
(b) Fenestrated or Passy-Muir tracheostomy tubes may be used in some patients; these allow air to leak over the vocal cords
(c) Lip reading is usually *not* an acceptable method, especially if oral tube is in place
c. Summary of artificial airways (Table 4-13)
(1) Upper airway artificial airways (Figure 4-27)
(a) Oropharyngeal airway
(b) Nasopharyngeal airway
(c) Cricothyrotomy
(2) Lower airway artificial airways
(a) Esophageal-tracheal Combitube (Figure 4-28)
(b) Laryngeal mask airway (LMA) (Figure 4-29)
(c) ET tube (Figure 4-30)
(i) Nasotracheal tube
(ii) Orotracheal tube
(d) Tracheostomy (Figure 4-30)
d. ET intubation
(1) Indications
(a) Ventilatory parameters
(i) V_T less than 5 mL/kg
(ii) VC less than 10 mL/kg
(iii) MIP less than −25 cm H_2O
(b) Need for sealed airway (e.g., mechanical ventilation or risk for aspiration)
(c) Loss of protective reflexes
(d) Inability to cough adequately and clear airways
(2) Insertion of ET tube
(a) Prepare the oxygen delivery system to be used after intubation: usually T piece with nebulizer or mechanical ventilator; manual resuscitation bag with reservoir bag with 100% may be used during cardiac arrest or until mechanical ventilator is ready.
(b) Collect supplies and select tube size.
(i) Tube: females usually 7.5 to 8; males usually 8 to 8.5

Table 4-13 **Summary of Artificial Airways**

Type of Airway	Advantages	Disadvantages	Miscellaneous
Oropharyngeal airway	• Easy to insert • Inexpensive • Effectively holds tongue away from pharynx	• Improper insertion technique can push tongue back and occlude airway • Easily dislodged • Poorly tolerated by conscious patients because it may stimulate gag reflex • Causes increased oral secretions • Contraindicated in patients with trauma to lower face, recent oral surgery, or loose or avulsed teeth	• Determine appropriate size: with flange at teeth, end of airway should not extend beyond the angle of the jaw ◦ Large adult: usually 100 mm (size 5) ◦ Medium adult: usually 90 mm (size 4) ◦ Small adult: usually 80 mm (size 3) • Insert by holding tongue down with tongue blade and sliding into place; alternative method: insert upside down and turn over when into pharynx; take care not to traumatize palate • Do not use as a bite block; likely to cause vomiting and potential aspiration in conscious patients • Remove, wash, and give mouth care every 4 hours; check mucous membranes for ulcerations
Nasopharyngeal airway (also called a *trumpet airway*)	• Easy to insert • Inexpensive • Effectively holds tongue away from pharynx • May be used in conscious or unconscious patients • Prevents trauma to nasal mucosa during nasotracheal suctioning • May be inserted when mouth cannot be opened (e.g., during seizures or jaw fractures)	• May cause nosebleeds, pressure necrosis, or sinus infection • Kinks and clogs easily • Contraindicated in patients predisposed to nosebleeds, nasal obstruction, bleeding disorder, and sepsis and in patients with basal skull fracture	• Determine appropriate size: 1 inch longer than nose to ear lobe; lumen smaller than naris ◦ Large adult: usually 8-9 internal diameter ◦ Medium adult: usually 7-8 internal diameter ◦ Small adult: usually 6-7 internal diameter • Insert with bevel against septum • Use viscous lidocaine (Xylocaine) as a lubricant for insertion to decrease discomfort • Do not use in patients receiving anticoagulants • Provide humidification of inspired air • Confirm placement by visualizing the tip of the airway next to the uvula • Rotate naris to naris every 8 hours • Limit the duration of use to reduce risk of sinus infection
Esophageal-tracheal Combitube	• Allows ventilation whether the tube is inserted into the trachea or the esophagus • Reduces risk of aspiration over mask ventilation • Permits easier placement over ET tube because visualization of the vocal cords is not necessary • Provides ventilation and oxygenation comparable to that achieved with an ET tube	• Incorrect identification of the position of the distal lumen may result in absence of ventilation • May cause esophageal trauma • Cannot mechanically ventilate the patient with a Combitube	• Use of an end-tidal carbon dioxide or esophageal detector device is recommended to confirm placement as being in the trachea or esophagus

Table 4-13 Summary of Artificial Airways—cont'd

Type of Airway	Advantages	Disadvantages	Miscellaneous
LMA	• Permits easier placement than ET tube because visualization of the vocal cords is not necessary • Provides ventilation and oxygenation comparable to that achieved with an ET tube • Allows placement when there is a possibility of unstable neck injury or when appropriate positioning of the patient for tracheal intubation is impossible • Reduces risk of aspiration over mask ventilation Permits coughing and speech	• Small proportion of patients cannot be ventilated with an LMA so an alternative strategy is needed • Cannot prevent aspiration because it does not separate the gastrointestinal tract from the respiratory tract • May cause laryngospasm and bronchospasm • May be difficult to ventilate patients who require high airway pressures to attain adequate tidal volumes	• If lubrication is required, lubricate only the posterior aspect of the airway • If used for mechanical ventilation, an audible air leak may occur
ET tube (general)	• Provides relatively sealed airway for mechanical ventilation and prevention of aspiration • Permits easy suctioning • Prevents gastric distention with air during cardiopulmonary resuscitation	• Requires skilled personnel for insertion • Splints epiglottis open and prevents effective cough • Causes loss of physiologic PEEP because epiglottis is splinted open; patient should receive 3-5 cm H_2O PEEP to reestablish physiologic PEEP • May kink and clog Causes aphonia • May cause laryngeal or tracheal damage • Contraindicated in patients with laryngeal obstruction caused by tumor, infection, or vocal cord paralysis	• Determine appropriate size: ◦ Females: usually 7.5-8 internal diameter ◦ Males: usually 8-8.5 internal diameter ◦ Tube may need to be 0.5-1 smaller if to be inserted nasally • Provide humidification of inspired air • Mark tube at corner of mouth or at naris to assess any movement • Use minimal occlusive volume or minimal leak volume for cuff inflation; ensure that cuff pressure does not exceed 18 mm Hg (if pressure greater than 18 mm Hg required to achieve seal and that tube is too small and needs to be replaced with larger tube) • Confirm placement by chest x-ray: tip of tube should be 3-5 cm above carina • Provide mouth care every 4 hours; observe oral or nasal mucosa for signs of ulcerations or necrosis • Position to prevent kinking; use mechanical ventilator support arms to support ventilator tubing
Oral (specific) ET tube	• Easier insertion than nasal intubation • Permits larger tube than nasal intubation	• Less stable and comfortable than nasal tube • May stimulate gag reflex • May be bitten or chewed • May cause necrosis at corner of mouth • Increases oral secretions; makes mouth care more difficult • Contraindicated in patients with acute unstable cervical spine injury because of need for neck extension (blind nasotracheal intubation may be attempted in these patients)	• Reposition tube from one side of the mouth to the other and retape when indicated; avoid unnecessary manipulation of tube

Continued

Table 4-13 Summary of Artificial Airways—cont'd

Type of Airway	Advantages	Disadvantages	Miscellaneous
Nasal (specific) ET tube	• More comfortable for patient than oral • ET tube • Permits good oral hygiene • Cannot be bitten or chewed	• More difficult insertion than oral intubation • May cause pressure necrosis or sinus infection • Requires smaller size • Contraindicated in patients with nasal obstruction, fractured nose, sinusitis, bleeding disorder, or basal skull fracture	• Monitor for clinical indications of sinus infection: fever; increased pharyngeal drainage; halitosis; leukocytosis; sinus pain or headache
Cricothyrotomy	• Provides immediate airway access, especially helpful if complete upper airway obstruction	• May cause bleeding • Only temporary; very small opening if established with large needle; larger opening if airway opened with scalpel and small tracheostomy tube is used	• Provide humidification of inspired air • Use large bore over-the-needle catheter; adaptor required to attach to manual resuscitation bag • Physician may use scalpel and insert small tracheostomy tube • Monitor for bleeding and subcutaneous emphysema
Tracheostomy	• Provides long-term airway access • Minimizes risk of vocal cord damage from an • ET tube during long-term airway maintenance • Decreases dead space and decreases work of breathing • Provides a relative seal to prevent aspiration • Allows the patient to eat and swallow • Allows easier suctioning • Permits Valsalva maneuver and effective cough • Is more comfortable for patient • Is less likely to be dislodged than ET tube • Bypasses upper airway obstruction	• May require surgery but may be performed percutaneously • Causes aphonia • May cause false passage anterior to trachea in patients with thick necks • May cause erosion of innominate artery with tip of tube or low stoma • Causes scar • May cause tracheocutaneous or tracheoesophageal fistula	• Usually considered if artificial airway is required longer than 2 to 3 weeks • Determine appropriate size: usually 5-6 • Requires humidification of inspired air • Preferred if airway obstruction (e.g., tumor or laryngeal edema or spasm) • Provide tracheostomy care that includes cleaning stoma and tube every 8 hours with saline; keep stoma dry (if 4 × 4 used, change often if secretions present) • Keep obturator, extra tracheostomy tube, and tracheal spreader at bedside

ET, Endotracheal, *LMA*, laryngeal mask airway, *PEEP*, positive end-expiratory pressure.

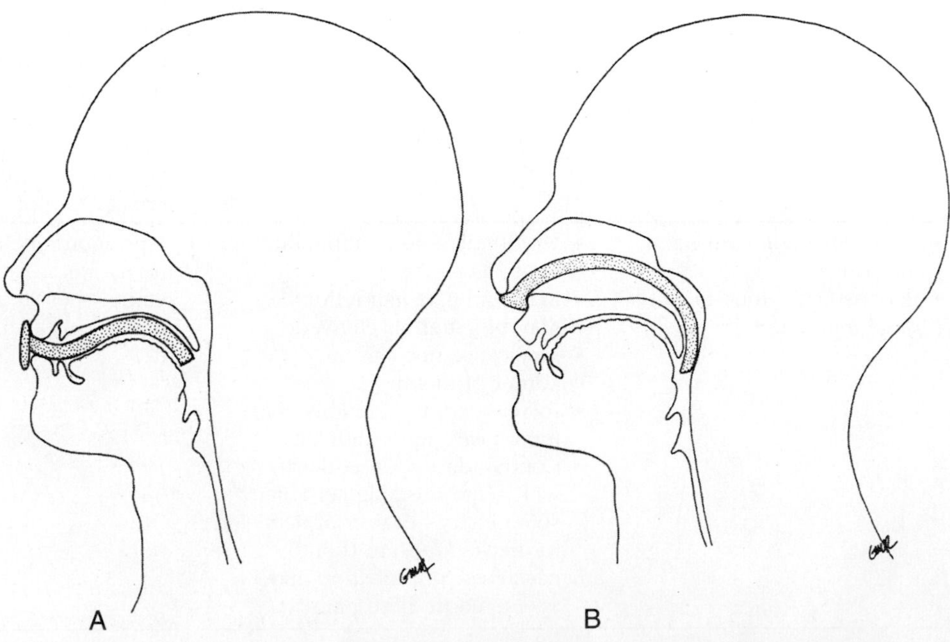

Figure 4-27 Upper airway artificial airways. **A,** Oropharyngeal airway. **B,** Nasopharyngeal airway. (From Sheehy, S. B. [1992]. *Emergency nursing: Principles and practice* [3rd ed.]. St. Louis: Mosby.)

(ii) Equipment to insert and secure tube: laryngoscope with straight (Miller) and curved (MacIntosh) blades with working lights, stylet, Magill forceps, lubricant, syringe, tape or device for stabilization of tube
(iii) Suction equipment including suction catheter and Yankauer suction device
(c) Monitor ECG and Spo_2 during intubation.
(d) Hyperoxygenate patient with 100% O_2 for at least 2 minutes.
(e) Place patient in head tilt–chin lift position.
(f) The most qualified person available who has been trained in ET intubation and frequently performs the procedure (usually physician or nurse anesthetist) should perform intubation.
(g) Complete intubation within 30 seconds; if not, cease attempts and hyperoxygenate the patient again.
(h) Confirm placement of ET tube.
(i) Feel air movement through tube.
(ii) Assess bilateral chest excursion.
(iii) Auscultate bilateral breath sounds; if breath sounds are audible on the right but not on the left, right mainstem intubation has occurred; pull the tube back slightly and then recheck breath sounds.
(iv) Use a capnometer to confirm consistent exhalation of CO_2.
(v) Auscultate over epigastrium: air movement should not be audible.

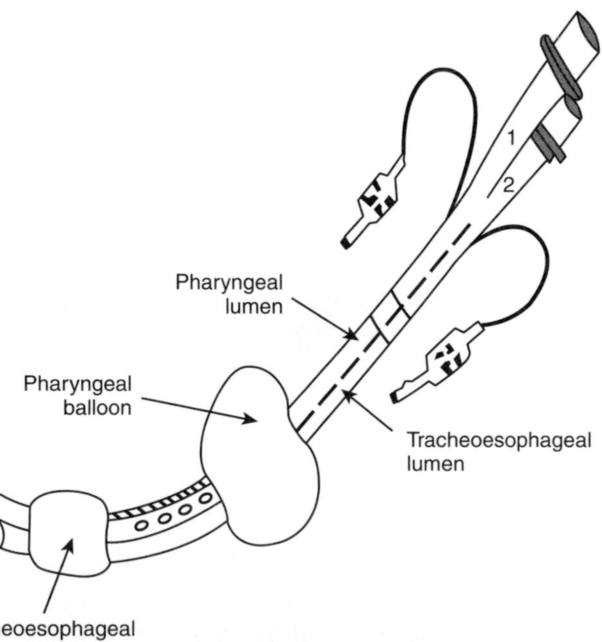

Figure 4-28 Esophageal tracheal Combitube. (From Urtubia, R. M., Aguila, C. M., & Cumsille, M. A. [2000]. Combitube: A study for proper use. *Anesthesia and Analgesia, 90*[4], 958-962.)

(vi) Confirm tube positioning by chest x-ray film; distal tip of tube should be 2 cm above the carina.
(i) Inflate the cuff using the minimal occlusive volume or minimal leak volume (see section on cuffs).
(j) Tape tube in place.
(i) Secure tape to minimize pressure areas on the face; tape with tension to both sides to avoid excessive pressure on corner of mouth if oral tube.
(ii) If a commercial stabilization device is used, assess lips and oral mucosa frequently for evidence of excessive pressure.
(k) Note the depth marking on the side of the tube.
(i) Usually at 19 to 23 cm for an average adult.
(ii) Cut tube so that only 2 to 3 inches of tube extends beyond mouth or nose to decrease airway resistance and potential for kinking.
(l) Attach O_2 delivery system or mechanical ventilator.
(3) Rapid sequence intubation: use of pharmacologic agents for sedation and paralysis to secure an airway in the most rapid way possible
(a) Monitor Spo_2, ECG rhythm, and BP throughout procedure.
(b) Administer high concentration of O_2 by non-rebreathing mask.
(c) Administer (or prepare for administration) of pharmacologic agents (as allowed by state Nurse Practice Act and hospital policy).
(i) Sedation
a) Any of the following may be used:
i) Etomidate (Amidate)
ii) Thiopental sodium (Pentothal): avoid if head injury, eye injury, or hypotension
iii) Propofol (Diprivan)
iv) Fentanyl (Sublimaze) and midazolam (Versed)
v) Ketamine and atropine and midazolam (Versed)
b) NOTE: Sedative may need to be repeated so that sedation lasts as long as neuromuscular blockade (depends on duration of neuromuscular blockade agent).
(ii) Neuromuscular blockade: any of the following may be used:
a) Succinylcholine (Anectine)
b) Rocuronium (Zemuron)
c) Vecuronium (Norcuron)
(d) Apply cricoid pressure until intubated
(e) Assist with preparation and insertion of the ET tube

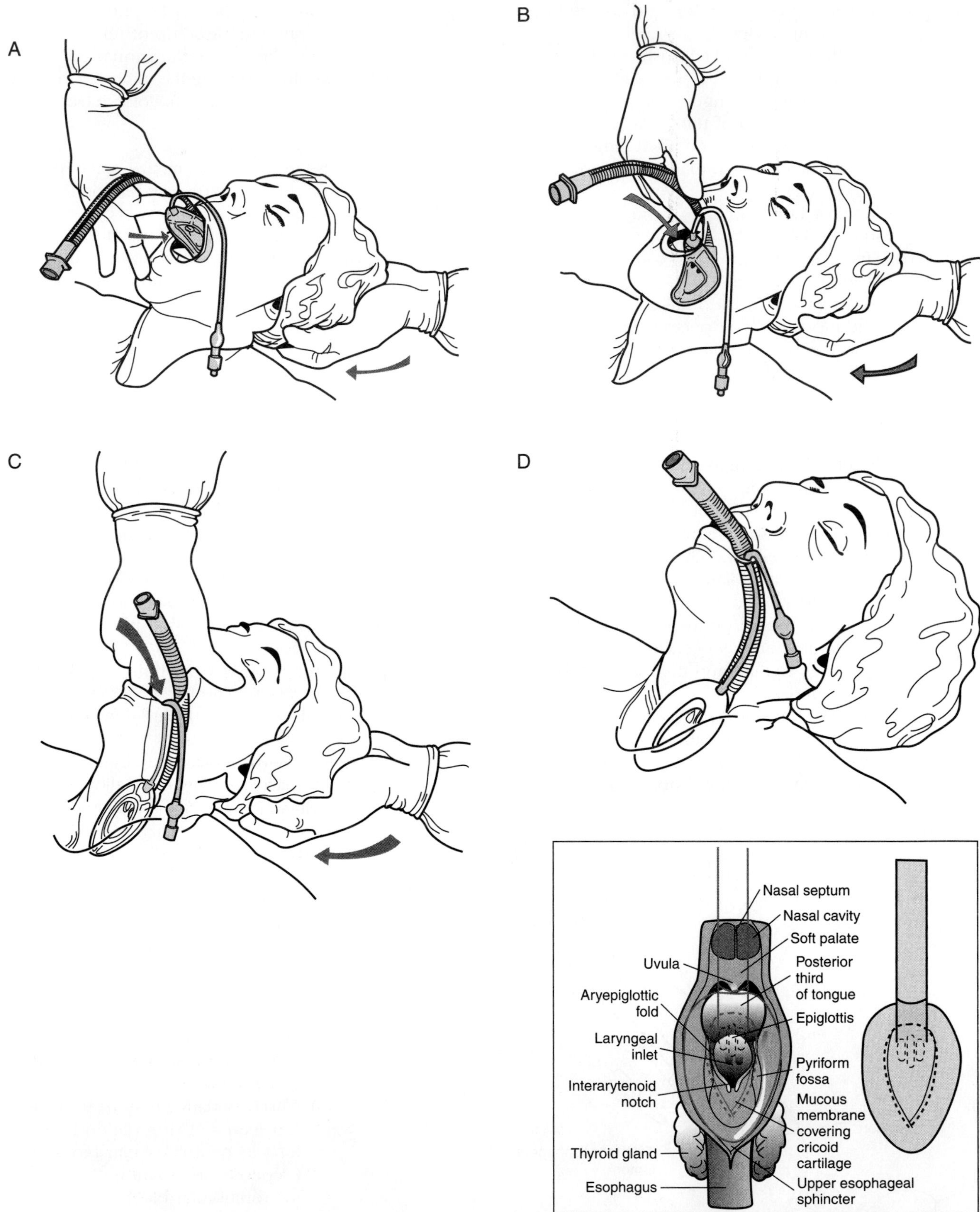

Figure 4-29 Laryngeal mask airway (LMA). **A,** LMA is an adjunctive airway that consists of a tube with a cuffed masklike projection at distal end. **B,** LMA is introduced through mouth into pharynx. **C,** Once LMA is in position, a clear, secure airway is present. **D** (anatomic detail), During insertion, LMA is advanced until resistance is felt as distal portion of tube locates in hypopharynx. Cuff then is inflated. This seals larynx and leaves distal opening of tube just above glottis, providing a clear, secure airway. (From Part 6: Advanced cardiovascular life support. Section 3: Adjuncts for oxygenation, ventilation, and airway control. European Resuscitation Council. [2000]. *Resuscitation, 46*[1-3], 115-125.)

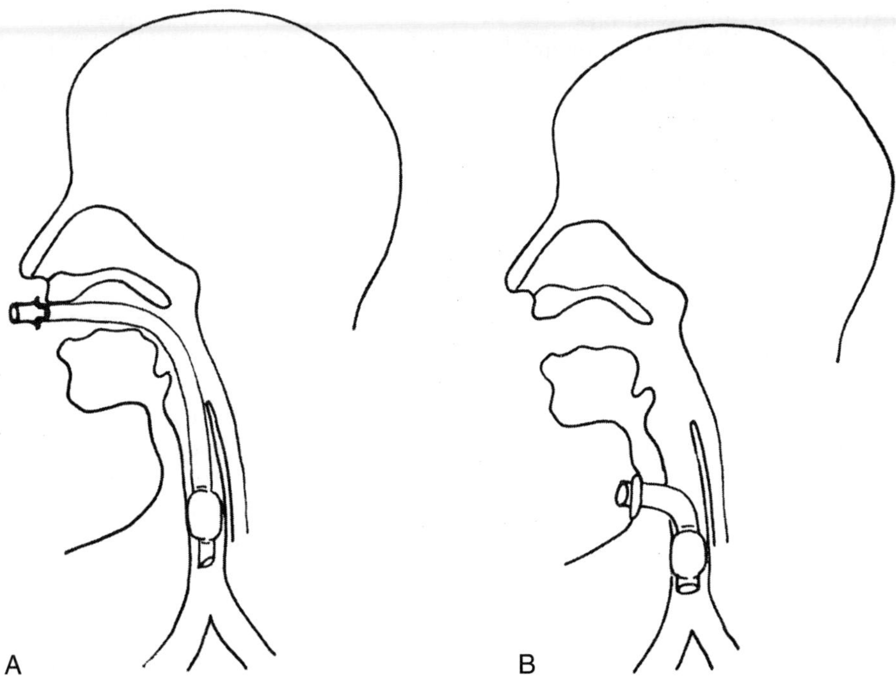

Figure 4-30 Lower airway artificial airways. **A,** ET tube. **B,** Tracheostomy tube. (From Phipps, W. J. et al. [1995]. *Medical-surgical nursing: Concepts and clinical practice* [5th ed.]. St. Louis: Mosby.)

(f) Confirm placement of ET tube
(g) Provide ventilation with bag-valve-mask or mechanical ventilator

(4) Extubation of intubated patients
- (a) Criteria
  - (i) Patient awake and oriented or able to keep airway open
    - a) Protective reflexes must be intact (e.g., gag).
    - b) Patient should not be paralyzed or excessively narcotized or sedated.
  - (ii) Vital signs stable; acceptable Hgb and hemodynamics
  - (iii) ABGs within acceptable limits after a trial of 30 minutes on nebulizer (T piece) trial at 40% O_2: Pao_2 60 mm Hg or greater, Sao_2 90% or greater, and $Paco_2$ 35 to 45 mm Hg or consistent with patient's normal values
  - (iv) Acceptable bedside ventilatory parameters:
    - a) V_T 5 mL/kg or greater
    - b) VC 10 mL/kg or greater
    - c) MIP of −25 cm H_2O or greater (more negative)
- (b) Technique
  - (i) Have postextubation O_2 delivery system ready; intubation kit also should be available.
  - (ii) Suction fluids from trachea and then pharynx.
  - (iii) Deflate cuff.
  - (iv) Remove tube during expiration.
  - (v) Apply O_2 delivery system.
  - (vi) Encourage patient to cough; apply suction if needed.
  - (vii) Repeat ABGs 20 to 30 minutes after extubation and as indicated thereafter.
  - (viii) Observe for laryngospasm: stridor, dyspnea, tachypnea; treatment may include high humidity, steroids, racemic epinephrine, or reintubation.
  - (ix) Monitor patient's tolerance to extubation by clinical observation, ventilatory measurements, and blood gas studies.
- (c) Prevention of unplanned extubation
  - (i) Identify patients at high risk for unplanned extubation: restless, confused, anxious, recovering from anesthesia, history of psychiatric disorders, or on rotating bed.
  - (ii) Explain to the patient the purpose of the ET tube and that it temporarily prevents the patient from speaking; explain the hazards of self-extubation.

(iii) Secure the ET tube with tape around head or with a commercially available stabilization device.
(iv) Note the size of the ET tube and the position of the tube at the teeth.
(v) Provide sedation as indicated.
(vi) Restrain the patient's hands as necessary; indications of the need to restrain include reaching for the tube, moving head side to side, and agitation.
(vii) Ensure support of ventilator tubing to decrease tension on the ET tube.
(viii) Assess the need for continued intubation frequently; self-extubation is frequently an indication that intubation is no longer required.
(ix) Place call bell within reach and explain to the patient how to use it.
(x) Ensure that appropriate equipment is available at the bedside: bag-valve-mask, replacement ET tube, and suction equipment.

(d) Treatment of unplanned extubation
(i) Assess patency of airway, respiratory rate, Spo_2, breath sounds, and neurologic status.
(ii) Administer O_2 with bag-valve-mask if the patient requires ventilatory assistance or by mask or cannula if the patient is breathing spontaneously.
(iii) Notify the physician and emergency personnel (e.g., code team), and assemble equipment for emergency reintubation.
(iv) Reassure the patient and the family.

e. Weaning patients from tracheostomy tube
(1) Indications same as for ET extubation
(2) Techniques
(a) Progression to a smaller size uncuffed (or cuff not inflated) tracheostomy tube
(i) Allows the patient to use his or her upper airway and the opening of the tracheostomy tube
(ii) Increases airway resistance and work of breathing
(b) Change to fenestrated tube: opening at the top of tube allows air to leak upward so that the patient can use the upper airway (and can speak)
(c) Deflate cuff
(i) Allows the patient to use his upper airway and the opening of the tracheostomy tube
(ii) Increases airway resistance and work of breathing
(d) Tracheostomy button
(i) Closes the opening in the trachea so that the patient uses his upper airway
(ii) Increases airway resistance and work of breathing

f. Cuffs
(1) Cuffs in current use are high-volume, low-pressure cuffs; these cuffs distribute the pressure over a larger areas of the trachea and decrease the incidence of tracheal ischemia and stenosis; laryngectomy patients may have uncuffed laryngectomy tube.
(2) Cuffed tubes provide *relative* seal for patients receiving mechanical ventilation and aid in prevention of aspiration; note that cuffs do not establish an absolute seal and that silent aspiration of oropharyngeal or gastric secretions is common in critically ill patients.
(3) Inflate cuff using minimal occlusive volume or minimal leak volume.
(a) Minimal occlusive volume
(i) Listen over trachea with stethoscope.
(ii) Inflate cuff until no air leak is audible during the inspiratory cycle of the ventilator.
(b) Minimal leak volume
(i) Listen over trachea with stethoscope.
(ii) Inflate cuff until no air leak is audible during the inspiratory cycle of the ventilator.
(iii) Remove 0.1 cm of air or until a minimal leak is audible during the inspiratory cycle of the ventilator.
(4) Intracuff pressure should not exceed capillary filling pressure but should be adequate to prevent the drainage of excessive subglottic secretions.
(a) Measure and record cuff pressure every 4 to 8 hours with a cuff pressure gauge or a mercury manometer and three-way stopcock.
(b) Recommended pressure is between 20 and 25 mm Hg (20 and 30 cm H_2O).
(5) Routine deflation is not necessary with high-volume, low-pressure cuffs and may contribute to nosocomial pneumonia by allowing oropharyngeal secretions to drain into the tracheobronchial tree

g. Complications of airway intubation
(1) Physiologic alterations created by airway diversion
(a) Inadequate humidification of inspired air
(b) Increased risk of nosocomial pneumonia caused by accumulation of secretions
(i) Increased mucus caused by tube because it is a foreign body
(ii) Impaired ciliary movement
(c) Aphonia: most significant stressor identified by patients

(d) Ineffective cough: ET tubes splint the epiglottis open, preventing effective intrathoracic pressure to achieve an effective cough; patients can cough with a tracheostomy because the epiglottis is not splinted open
(e) Loss of physiologic PEEP
(i) ET tubes splint the epiglottis open and remove physiologic PEEP.
(ii) Physiologic PEEP is reestablished with 3 to 5 cm H_2O of PEEP for intubated patients. (NOTE: This may be contraindicated in patients with a thoracotomy.)
(2) During placement
(a) ET intubation
(i) Trauma: damage to teeth or mucous membranes; perforation or laceration of pharynx, larynx, or trachea
(ii) Aspiration
(iii) Laryngospasm, bronchospasm
(iv) Tube malposition: esophageal or endobronchial intubation
(v) Hypoxia or anoxia if attempts are prolonged
(b) Tracheostomy
(i) Barotrauma: pneumothorax; pneumomediastinum
(ii) Hemorrhage
(iii) Tracheoesophageal fistula
(iv) Laryngeal nerve injury
(v) Cardiopulmonary arrest
(3) While tube is in place
(a) Tube obstruction or displacement
(b) Cuff rupture
(c) Disconnection between tracheal tube and ventilator including self-extubation
(d) Pressure necrosis
(i) At corners of mouth if oral ET tube
(ii) At superior nasal concha if nasal ET tube
(e) Local infection; otitis media; sinus infection with nasotracheal tubes
(f) Bronchospasm
(g) Leaks because of broken cuff balloon
(h) Trauma: laryngeal injury; tracheal ischemia, necrosis, dilation
(i) Transition from ET to tracheostomy usually occurs approximately 2 weeks after intubation but several studies have shown benefit (e.g., decreased length of mechanical ventilation and shorter critical care and hospital stay) in earlier tracheostomy (within 3 days when it is anticipated that the patient will require prolonged mechanical ventilation)
(4) Postextubation
(a) ET tube
(i) Acute laryngeal edema
(ii) Hoarseness (common)
(iii) Aspiration if swallowing is impaired
(iv) Stenosis of larynx or trachea (late complication)
(b) Tracheostomy
(i) Difficulties with decannulation of a tracheostomy
(ii) Tracheoesophageal fistula
(iii) Tracheoinnominate artery fistula
(iv) Tracheocutaneous fistula
(v) Tracheal stenosis

9. Provide oral care for patient comfort and to aid in prevention of nosocomial pneumonia.
a. Recognize factors contributing to poor oral hygiene.
(1) Artificial airways
(2) Poor nutrition
(3) Nothing by mouth status
(4) Mouth breathing, tachypnea
(5) O_2 administration
(6) Anxiety
(7) Drugs such as antihistamines, antiemetics, and antibiotics
b. Assess the lips, oral mucosa, tongue, gums, teeth, and soft and hard palate at least twice daily.
c. Provide oral care periodically.
(1) Every 2 to 4 hours
(a) Use suction foam swabs over teeth, tongue, and oral mucosa followed by moisturizing swabs and water-soluble lip balm
(i) Foam swabs stimulate the oral mucosa.
(ii) Avoid lemon glycerin swabs, which are drying to the oral mucosa.
(b) Suction fluids from oropharynx.
(i) Rinse catheter (e.g., Yankauer) with sterile water or saline after each use.
(ii) Store oropharyngeal suction catheter in a nonsealed bag when not in use.
(iii) Replace oropharyngeal suction device, tubing, and suction canister every 24 hours.
(2) Twice daily
(a) Brush teeth to prevent dental plaque colonization.
(i) Brushing the teeth with a toothbrush removes dental plaque and reduces the number of oral microorganisms.
(ii) A soft-bristle pediatric toothbrush should be used along with toothpaste, preferably with an alkaline pH.
(iii) Removable partial dentures should be removed and thoroughly cleaned.
(b) Administer chlorhexidine gluconate (Peridex) by spray or rinse as prescribed.
(i) Chlorhexidine: broad-spectrum antibacterial agent that is not

absorbed through the skin or mucous membranes
a) Concentration recommendations vary from 0.12% to 0.2%
(ii) Effectiveness in prevention of ventilator-associated pneumonia inconclusive
(iii) Initiated preoperatively if surgical patient

Oxygen Therapy

Definitions

1. Hypoxemia
   a. Decrease in arterial blood O_2 tension
   b. Diagnosis by ABGs
   c. Decrease in Pao_2 and Sao_2
      (1) Mild hypoxemia: Pao_2 less than 80 mm Hg (~Sao_2 95%)
      (2) Moderate (significant) hypoxemia: Pao_2 less than 60 mm Hg (~Sao_2 90%)
      (3) Severe hypoxemia: Pao_2 less than 40 mm Hg (~Sao_2 75%)
2. Hypoxia
   a. Decrease in tissue oxygenation
   b. Diagnosis by clinical indications (Box 4-3)
   c. Affected by Pao_2 and Sao_2, hemoglobin, CO, patent vessels, cellular demand

Etiology

1. Hypoxemia
   a. Low inspired O_2 concentration (e.g., high altitudes)
   b. Hypoventilation (e.g., asthma)
   c. V/Q mismatching (e.g., pulmonary embolism)
   d. Shunt (e.g., ARDS)
   e. Diffusion abnormalities (e.g., pulmonary fibrosis)
2. Hypoxia
   a. Hypoxemic hypoxia: resulting from a gas exchange problem (e.g., V/Q mismatch, shunt, or diffusion abnormalities)
   b. Anemic hypoxia: resulting from reduced O_2-carrying capacity of the blood (e.g., anemia, carbon monoxide poisoning, or methemoglobinemia)
   c. Circulatory hypoxia: resulting from a reduced blood flow in the body or a reduction in CO (e.g., shock)
   d. Histotoxic hypoxia: resulting from the inability of the cells to use O_2 (e.g., cyanide poisoning)

Pathophysiology

1. Decrease in Pao_2 initially stimulates the sympathetic nervous system.
2. O_2 extraction at tissue level increases.
3. As Pao_2 becomes critically low, tissue oxygenation becomes inadequate and hypoxia occurs.
4. Nutrient metabolism changes from aerobic to anaerobic, which results in 20 times less ATP than aerobic metabolism and lactic acid as a waste product.
5. Acidosis and decreased cellular energy results.

Assessment

1. Evidence of altered perfusion
   a. Tachycardia
   b. Hypotension
   c. Changes in skin color and temperature
2. Evidence of anaerobic metabolism: lactic acidosis (serum arterial lactate level greater than 2 mM/L)
3. Evidence of organ dysfunction
   a. Cerebral: altered sensorium
   b. Myocardial: decreased CO; dysrhythmias
   c. Renal: decreased urine output
4. Parameters of O_2 delivery
   a. Pao_2, Sao_2, Spo_2
   b. Hgb, hematocrit
   c. CO, CI
5. Hemodynamic monitoring parameters
   a. CO
   b. Svo_2
      (1) Measured by Svo_2 port of a fiberoptic oximetric pulmonary artery catheter or by mixed venous blood gas analysis
      (2) Normal: 60% to 80%

Indications for Oxygen Therapy

1. Significant hypoxemia: Pao_2 less than 60 mm Hg; Sao_2 or Spo_2 less than 90%
2. Suspected hypoxemia (e.g., asthma, pulmonary embolism, aspiration, drug overdose, seizure or postictal state, pneumothorax, or trauma)
3. Increased myocardial workload (e.g., heart failure, hypertensive crisis, or myocardial infarction)
4. Decreased CO (e.g., shock, hypotension, or cardiopulmonary arrest)
5. Increased O_2 demand (e.g., sepsis or increased ventilatory work)
6. Decreased O_2 carrying capacity (e.g., carbon monoxide or cyanide poisoning, methemoglobinemia, sickle cell disease, or anemia)
7. Before procedures that may cause hypoxemia (e.g., suctioning, during and after anesthesia, transport of unstable patient, or bronchoscopy)

Principles of Oxygen Therapy

1. Airway is always the first priority; O_2 is useless without an adequate airway.
2. O_2 is a potent drug that is administered as prescribed; it may be prescribed as flow rate, O_2 concentration (expressed as a percent), or Fio_2 (expressed as a decimal)
3. The objective is to improve tissue oxygenation.
   a. Maintain Pao_2 at least 60 mm Hg and Sao_2 at 90%; serial serum lactate levels are also helpful in monitoring progression

or improvement of hypoxia and degree of anaerobic metabolism.
b. Determine the effectiveness of O_2 therapy: determined by pathology.
   (1) O_2 therapy is ineffective for shunt; alveoli must be opened (also referred to as *alveolar recruitment*) to get the O_2 to the alveolar-capillary membrane; PEEP is required in these cases.

4. If high concentrations are necessary, limit duration to prevent O_2 toxicity.
   a. Frequent ABG samples are mandatory if Fio_2 is above 0.4.
   b. Exact concentration of inspired O_2 should be measured with O_2 analyzer.
5. Fio_2 can be estimated by counting number of reservoirs.
   a. Nose and pharynx only (1) less than 40%: example, nasal cannula
   b. Nose and pharynx + mask (2) 40% to 60%: example, simple face mask
   c. Nose and pharynx + mask + reservoir bag (3) 60% to 80%: example, partial rebreathing mask
   d. Nose and pharynx + mask + reservoir bag + one-way valves (three + decrease in dilution) 80% to 100%: example, non-rebreathing mask
6. Safety guidelines
   a. Keep O_2 source at least 10 feet from open flame.
   b. Do not allow smoking in a room with supplemental O_2.
   c. Do not use electrical appliances within 5 feet of O_2 source.
   d. Do not use petroleum-based products around O_2 source; use only water-soluble lubricants and creams.
   e. Turn the O_2 off when not in use.
   f. Secure the O_2 tanks to prevent accidental dropping; keep O_2 source away from heat or direct sunlight.

High-Flow versus Low-Flow Oxygen Delivery Systems

1. Low-flow O_2 delivery systems
   a. Do not provide total inspired gas; remainder of patient's inspiratory volume is met by patient breathing varying amounts of room air
   b. Fio_2 depends on rate and depth of ventilation and fit of device
      (1) If minute ventilation increases, O_2 concentration decreases because the amount of room air (diluent) increases in relation to the amount of O_2 via the O_2 delivery system.
      (2) If minute ventilation decreases, O_2 concentration increases.
   c. Does not necessarily mean low Fio_2
   d. Criteria indicating that low-flow O_2 delivery system is acceptable
      (1) Normal or near-normal V_T (~7 mL/kg of ideal body weight [IBW])
      (2) Respiratory rate normal or near normal (~15 to 25 breaths/min)
      (3) Regular respiratory rate
      (4) Specific O_2 concentration not critical to patient's care
   e. Devices
      (1) Nasal cannula
      (2) Reservoir systems
         (a) Simple face mask
         (b) Partial rebreathing mask
         (c) Non-rebreathing mask
2. High-flow O_2 delivery systems
   a. Provide the entire inspired gas by high flow of gas or entrainment of room air
   b. Provide a predictable Fio_2
   c. Does not necessarily mean high Fio_2
   d. Criteria indicating that high-flow O_2 delivery system is needed
      (1) Tidal volume is significantly less than or more than normal (~7 mL/kg of IBW)
      (2) Respiratory rate less than 15 breaths/min or more than 25 breaths/min
      (3) Irregular respiratory rate
      (4) Specific O_2 concentration is critical to patient's care
      (5) Evidence of alveolar hypoventilation with hypercapnia
   e. Devices
      (1) Venturi mask
      (2) T piece: may be high or low flow depending on flow rate
      (3) Tracheostomy collar: may be high or low flow depending on flow rate
      (4) Mechanical ventilator

Oxygen Delivery Systems (Table 4-14)

Hazards of Oxygen Therapy

1. O_2-induced hypoventilation
   a. Greatest risk if $Paco_2$ greater than 50 mm Hg because low Pao_2 becomes primary stimulus to breathe
      (1) Airway obstruction
      (2) COPD
      (3) Respiratory center depression
   b. Use O_2 with caution but remember low Pao_2, not Fio_2, is stimulus to breathe; use only enough O_2 to bring Pao_2 up to approximately 60 mm Hg or Sao_2 up to approximately 90%
2. Absorptive atelectasis
   a. Causes: High concentrations of O_2 (an absorbable gas) wash out the nitrogen (a nonabsorbable gas) that normally holds the alveoli open at the end of expiration and the effects of O_2 on pulmonary surfactant.
   b. Prevention: Do not administer O_2 that is not indicated.

Table 4-14 Summary of Oxygen Delivery Systems

System	Advantages	Disadvantages	Miscellaneous
Nasal cannula 1-6 L/min delivers 24%-44% O_2 (3% increase with each liter)	• Safe and simple • Comfortable • Effective for low O_2 concentration • Allows eating and talking • Inexpensive	• Contraindicated in nasal obstruction • May cause drying and irritation of nasal mucosa • May cause necrosis at ears • Cannot be used when patient has nasal obstruction • Variable concentrations of O_2 depending on tidal volume, ventilatory rate, flow rate, and nasal patency	• Ensure that flow rates do not exceed 6 L/min • Provide humidification if flow rates exceed 4 L/min • Use gauze pads under cannula at tops of ears to prevent pressure ulceration • Give oral and nasal care every 8 hours; moisten lips and nose with water-soluble lubricant
Simple face mask 6-10 L/min delivers 40%-60% O_2	• Delivers high O_2 concentration • Does not dry mucous membranes of nose and mouth • Can be used in patients with nasal obstruction	• Hot, confining, uncomfortable • Tight seal necessary • Frequently poorly tolerated in dyspneic patient • Interferes with eating and talking • May cause CO_2 retention if flow rate is less than 6 L/min • Variable concentrations of O_2 depending on tidal volume, ventilatory rate, and flow rate • Cannot deliver less than 40% • Potential for O_2 toxicity • Impractical for long-term therapy	• Place pads between mask and bony facial parts • Wash and dry face every 4 hours • Clean mask every 8 hours • Ensure flow rate of at least 6 L/min • Check ABGs frequently • Watch for signs of O_2 toxicity
Partial rebreathing mask 6-10 L/min delivers 35%-60%	• Delivers high O_2 concentrations • Does not dry mucous membranes	• As for face mask • May cause CO_2 retention if reservoir bag is allowed to collapse	• Ensure that bag is not totally deflated during inhalation (increase flow rate) • Keep mask snug • Check ABGs frequently • Watch for signs of O_2 toxicity
Non-rebreathing mask 6-12 L/min delivers 60%-90%	• As for other masks • One-way valves prevent rebreathing of CO_2 and increase O_2 concentrations	• As for other masks except does not cause CO_2 retention	• As for partial rebreathing mask • Check ABGs frequently • Watch for signs of O_2 toxicity
Venturi mask 4 L/min delivers 24%-28% 8 L/min delivers 35%-40%	• Delivers accurate O_2 concentration depending on flow rate and diluter jet inserted despite changes in patient's respiratory pattern • O_2 concentration can be changed • Does not dry mucous membranes	• Fraction of inspired O_2 can be lowered if mask does not fit snugly, if tubing is kinked, if O_2 intake ports are blocked, or if less than recommended liter flow is used • Hot, confining, uncomfortable • Tight seal necessary • Frequently poorly tolerated in dyspneic patient • Interferes with eating and talking	• Check ABGs frequently • Watch for signs of O_2 toxicity • As for other masks
Tracheostomy collar 21%-70% 10 L or to provide visible mist	• Does not pull on tracheostomy • Elastic ties allow movement of mask away from tracheostomy without removing it	• O_2 diluted by room air • Increased likelihood of infection and skin irritation around stoma because of high humidity • Condensation can collect in the tubing and drain into patient's airway, especially during turning	• Ensure that O_2 is warmed and humidified • Empty condensation from tubing frequently; empty into water trap or container for appropriate discard; do not empty water back into humidifier

Table 4-14 Summary of Oxygen Delivery Systems—cont'd

System	Advantages	Disadvantages	Miscellaneous
T piece or tube flow rate set at 2.5 times patient's minute ventilation to deliver 21%-100%	• Delivers variable concentrations • Less moisture around tracheostomy than with tracheostomy collar	• May cause CO_2 retention at low flow rates • Weight of T piece can pull on tracheostomy tube • Condensation can collect in the tubing and drain into patient's airway, especially during turning	• Requires heated nebulizer • Use extension on open side to act as a reservoir and increase O_2 concentration as prescribed • Empty condensation from tubing frequently • Check ABGs frequently • Watch for signs of O_2 toxicity
Mechanical ventilation 21%-100%	• Delivers predictable, constant concentrations of O_2 • Supports ventilation and oxygenation • Addition of positive end-expiratory pressure augments the driving pressure of O_2; this aids in the achievement of acceptable Pao_2 levels at lower O_2 concentrations	• Requires skilled personnel • Requires electricity and backup power generator (plug into red outlet) • Condensation can collect in the tubing and drain into patient's airway, especially during turning	• Requires heated humidifier • Empty condensation from tubing frequently • Check ABGs frequently • Watch for signs of O_2 toxicity

ABGs, Arterial blood gases; *Co_2,* carbon dioxide; *O_2,* oxygen.

3. O_2 toxicity
   a. Cause: too high a concentration over too long a time (hours to days)
   b. Pathophysiology
      (1) Overproduction of O_2 free radicals
      (2) Large numbers of O_2 free radicals overwhelms the supply of neutralizing enzymes
      (3) Injury to capillary endothelium and increase in interstitial edema
      (4) Injury to type I pneumocytes and intraalveolar edema
      (5) Proliferation of type II pneumocytes
      (6) Thickening of alveolar-capillary membrane
      (7) Scarring and pulmonary fibrosis
   c. Clinical indications
      (1) Early
         (a) Substernal chest pain that increases with deep breathing
         (b) Dry cough and tracheal irritation
         (c) Dyspnea
         (d) Upper airway changes (e.g., nasal stuffiness, sore throat, and eye and ear discomfort)
         (e) Anorexia, nausea, vomiting
         (f) Fatigue, lethargy, malaise
         (g) Restlessness
      (2) Late
         (a) Chest x-ray changes: atelectasis, patches of pneumonia
         (b) Progressive ventilatory difficulty: decreased VC; decreased compliance; hypercapnia
         (c) Increased intrapulmonary shunt: increasing A:a gradient and decreased Pao_2/Fio_2 ratio; hypoxemia
   d. Prevention
      (1) Use the lowest Fio_2 possible to maintain a Pao_2 of at least 60 mm Hg (Sao_2 90%)
         (a) Limit duration of 1 Fio_2 to 24 hours if at all possible.
         (b) Limit the use of Fio_2 above 0.6 to 2 to 3 days if at all possible.
         (c) Assess ABGs frequently if Fio_2 is above 0.4 to ensure that high concentration is still required.
         (d) Fio_2 of 0.4 is considered relatively safe.
      (2) Use PEEP to increase the driving pressure of O_2; use of PEEP achieves the following:
         (a) The same Pao_2 at a lower Fio_2
         (b) A better Pao_2 at the same Fio_2
      (3) Remember that hypoxia is far more common than O_2 toxicity and must be corrected; *actual* hypoxemia should never be allowed to persist because of concern regarding *potential* O_2 toxicity

Hyperbaric Oxygenation

1. Definition: administration of high concentration (usually 100%) O_2 under greatly increased pressure (usually 2 to 3 atm)
2. Indications: carbon monoxide or cyanide poisoning; air embolism; radiation therapy; gas gangrene; burns; nonhealing wounds, necrotizing fasciitis, decompression illness, osteomyelitis, intracranial abscess

3. Actions: can cause a twenty-twofold increase in Pao_2, which increases the amount of O_2 dissolved in the blood to enhance tissue oxygenation
4. Complications: O_2 toxicity; absorptive atelectasis; ARDS, bleeding and edema of eustachian tubes, rupture of tympanic membrane

Mechanical Ventilation

Indications for Mechanical Ventilation

1. Acute ventilatory failure with respiratory acidosis not relieved by ordinary methods
2. Hypoxemia despite maximum O_2 therapy
3. Relief of hypoxemia causes increased CO_2 retention
4. Apnea: consideration needs to be given to the reversibility of the situation (i.e., mechanical ventilation is not indicated to prolong a terminal condition)
5. Physiologic indications
   a. VC less than 10 mL/kg or twice predicted V_T
   b. Unable to achieve maximal inspiratory force of −25 cm H_2O
   c. Pao_2 less than 60 mm Hg with Fio_2 greater than 0.6
   d. Arterial $Paco_2$ below 30 or above 50 mm Hg
      (1) Hypercapnia alone is not an indication for mechanical ventilation and must be accompanied by acidosis to be an indication for mechanical ventilation: for example, a patient with COPD has chronic hypercapnia (not an indication for mechanical ventilation) but develops an even greater $Paco_2$ level and decompensated respiratory acidosis with acute respiratory infection (a potential indication for mechanical ventilation).
   e. Dead space/tidal volume ratio (V_D/V_T) greater than 0.6
   f. Respiratory rate greater than 30 to 35 breaths/min
6. Also may be used for the following purposes:
   a. Reduce oxygen consumption by reducing the work of breathing (e.g., shock).
   b. Stabilize the chest wall (e.g., flail chest).
   c. Allow sedation and neuromuscular paralysis.

Types of Ventilators

1. Negative pressure ventilators
   a. Types: iron lung; chest cuirass; poncho style; body wrap
   b. Ventilatory process
      (1) Negative pressure is generated outside of body, excluding the upper airway.
      (2) Negativity is transmitted to intrapleural and intraalveolar spaces.
      (3) Pressure gradient occurs, and air moves into lungs.
      (4) Expiration passively occurs by removing negative pressure around the chest wall.
   c. Uses
      (1) Restricted to nonpulmonary (e.g., neuromuscular) problems
      (2) Long-term ventilator support without an artificial airway
      (3) Primarily in-home or rehabilitation settings
   d. Advantages
      (1) Artificial airway not required
      (2) Normal breathing mechanics maintained, so it avoids harmful changes in intrathoracic pressure caused by positive pressure ventilators
   e. Disadvantages
      (1) Not helpful for patients with lung disease
      (2) Not possible to regulate V_T and alveolar ventilation precisely
      (3) Large size required (e.g., iron lung)
      (4) Restriction of patient movement
      (5) Patient care difficult because the body is enclosed in ventilator
      (6) Difficulty obtaining a seal around chest
      (7) May cause venous pooling in the abdomen leading to decreased CO particularly in hypovolemic patients
2. Positive pressure ventilators
   a. Ventilatory process
      (1) Inspiration is created by positive pressure being pushed into the airway.
      (2) Expiration occurs passively when the positive pressure stops.
   b. Cycling classifications
      (1) Time-cycled: deliver inspiratory flow until preset time interval has ended; used in neonates and children
      (2) Pressure-cycled: deliver inspiratory flow until preset pressure is met
         (a) Advantages
            (i) Relatively inexpensive
            (ii) Mobile
            (iii) Run on compressed air or O_2
         (b) Disadvantages
            (i) V_T varies depending on compliance of the lung and the integrity of the ventilatory circuit
            (ii) Sealed airway (e.g., cuffed ET tube or tracheostomy tube) required
            (iii) Positive intrathoracic pressure decreases venous return to the right heart and may decrease CO especially in hypovolemic patients
            (iv) Risk of ventilator-induced lung injury (VILI)
      (3) Volume-cycled: deliver inspiratory flow until preset volume is met
         (a) Advantages: delivers the set V_T regardless of changes in lung compliance

(b) Disadvantages
(i) Sealed airway required
(ii) Positive intrathoracic pressure decreases venous return to the right heart and may decrease CO especially in hypovolemic patients
(iii) Risk of VILI

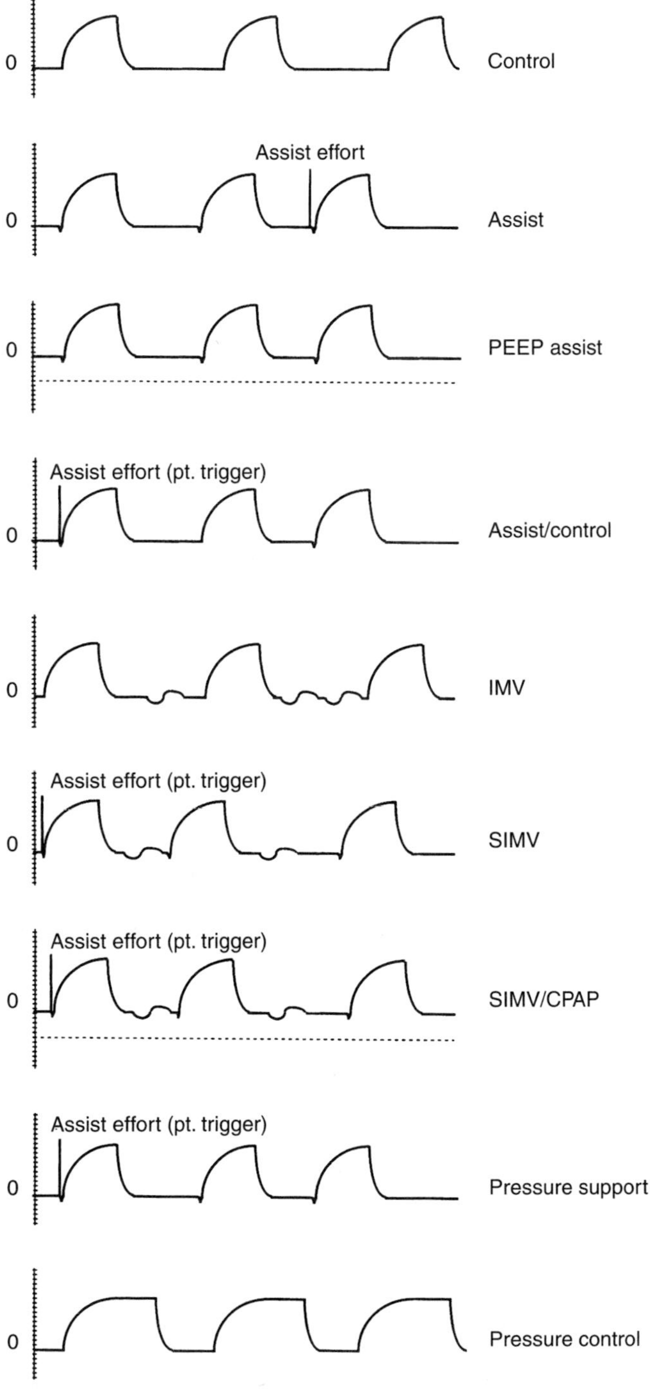

Figure 4-31 Common modes of mechanical ventilation. *PEEP*, Positive end-expiratory pressure; *IMV*, intermittent mandatory ventilation; *SIMV*, synchronized intermittent mandatory ventilation; *CPAP*, continuous positive airway pressure. (From McPherson, S. P., & Spearman, C. B. [1990]. *Respiratory therapy equipment*. St. Louis: Mosby.)

Inspiratory Modes

Refers to how the machine senses or signals the initiation of inspiration (Figure 4-31 and Table 4-15)

Expiratory Maneuvers

1. PEEP
   a. Definition: maintenance of pressure above atmospheric at airway opening at end-expiration
      (1) Physiologic: 3 to 5 cm H_2O
      (2) Therapeutic: greater than 5 cm H_2O
         (a) Adjustment of PEEP
            (i) Begin with 3 to 5 cm H_2O of PEEP
            (ii) Increase in increments of 3 to 5 cm H_2O until an O_2 saturation of 90% until SaO_2 (or SpO_2) is achieved
         (b) There is no true upper limit, but the higher the level, the greater the chance of barotrauma
         (c) Levels greater than 20 cm H_2O may be referred to as *super PEEP*
      (3) Best (or optimal) PEEP: PEEP that provides SaO_2 of at least 90% without compromising cardiac output (remember that tissue O_2 delivery is affected by SaO_2, Hgb, and CO; if SaO_2 is increased but CO is decreased, no true gains in tissue O_2 delivery are achieved, and tissue O_2 delivery may even by decreased)
      (4) Auto–PEEP (also called *occult PEEP* or *intrinsic PEEP*): adds to therapeutic PEEP (Figure 4-32)
         (a) Cause: inadequate emptying of the lungs
            (i) May be caused by airway obstruction or decreased compliance
            (ii) May be inherent in modes with very rapid rates and/or short expiratory time
         (b) Adverse effects
            (i) Increased risk of barotrauma and volutrauma
            (ii) Accentuation of hemodynamic compromise
            (iii) Increased work of breathing
            (iv) Patient anxiety
         (c) Measurement: difference between the mean alveolar pressure and external airway pressure at end-expiration
            (i) Newer ventilators may provide automated assessment
            (ii) May be determined manually
               a) Place patient on assist-control
               b) Occlude airway at end-expiration
               c) Observe increase in airway pressure

Table 4-15 Modes of Mechanical Ventilation

Mode	Description	Comments
Control	• Preset tidal volume and rate; the ventilator delivers the tidal volume at the rate, and the circuit is closed in between these mandatory breaths	• Patient must be apneic or paralyzed or they "fight" the ventilator • Guarantees ventilation with a specific minute ventilation • Allows ventilatory muscle rest
Assist-control (AC) (also called *assisted mandatory ventilation*)	• Preset tidal volume, minimum rate (control rate), and inspiratory effort required to "trigger" the ventilator to cycle to assist breaths (sensitivity); the ventilator delivers the control breaths of the specified tidal volume and responds by cycling additionally if the patient's inspiratory effort (negative pressure) is adequate	• More comfortable than control mode • Less work of breathing for patient than spontaneous breathing or IMV • Allows ventilatory muscle rest • Risk for hyperventilation because each assisted breath is delivered at the same tidal volume as mandatory breaths; sedation may be necessary to decrease the number of spontaneously triggered breaths
Synchronized intermittent mandatory ventilation	• Preset tidal volume and minimum rate; the ventilatory circuit is open between the mandatory breaths so that the patient may take additional breaths; because the ventilator does not cycle to assist these breaths, the tidal volume of these breaths varies • Mandatory breaths are synchronized so that they do not occur during the patient's ventilatory efforts	• Allows muscle reconditioning better than control or assist-control • Less potential for hyperventilation because patient-initiated breaths are at the tidal volume determined by the patient • More work of breathing for patient than assist-control because patient-initiated breaths are not assisted • Less need for sedation than assist-control or control modes • Does not decrease cardiac output as much as Assist-Control or Control modes • Frequently used for weaning
Pressure support ventilation (PSV)	• Preset inspiratory support pressure level; when the patient initiates a breath, this positive pressure flows to assist the patient's spontaneous breaths; tidal volume and rate are patient controlled	• Low level (5-10 cm H_2O) helps to eliminate the increased work of breathing associated with an ET tube; higher levels help to augment the patient's own intrinsic tidal volume • Lessens work of breathing but also allows use of respiratory muscles to lessen muscular atrophy • Lower mean airway pressures than volume ventilation • May be used with IMV or alone; if used alone, patient must be spontaneously breathing • There is no preset ventilatory rate, and apnea occurs if the patient does not initiate a breath; newer models provide a volume ventilation backup (called VAPSV)
Biphasic positive airway pressure (Bi-PAP)	• Preset pressure to be delivered during inspiration and preset pressure to be maintained during expiration • Combination of PSV (inspiratory positive airway pressure) and CPAP (Expiratory positive airway pressure)	• Frequently used as an interim method to avoid intubation and mechanical ventilation; may be delivered by mask • May be delivered by a mechanical ventilator or specialized noninvasive positive pressure ventilation machine
Pressure-controlled ventilation (PCV)	• Preset inspiratory pressure limit, rate, and I:E ratio; the ventilator delivers air until the pressure limit is reached and maintains this pressure throughout inspiration • Tidal volumes vary because of changes in the patient's lung compliance, inspiratory time, and airway resistance	• Lower mean airway pressures than volume ventilation • Allows more even distribution of air and improves arterial oxygenation at lower FiO_2 levels • Does not provide a guaranteed tidal volume • Requires sedation

Table 4-15 Modes of Mechanical Ventilation—cont'd

Mode	Description	Comments
Volume-assured pressure support ventilation (VAPSV)	• Preset inspiratory pressure limit, target tidal volume, and terminal flow rate • When the preset tidal volume has been achieved, inspiratory flow ends; if the preset tidal volume has not been achieved, inspiratory time is extended at the terminal flow rate until the set tidal volume is achieved • Starts as a pressure breath but ends as a volume breath if the preset tidal volume is not achieved	• Provides guarantee of adequate tidal volume lacking from PSV
Inverse ratio ventilation (IRV)	• Preset I:E ratio with inspiratory time to be greater than expiratory time; I:E ratio of 2:1 or greater; may be volume controlled or pressure controlled	• Improves distribution of ventilation • Prevents collapse of alveoli • Increases Pao_2 and arterial oxygen saturation • Increases mean airway pressure without further increases in peak inspiratory pressures • May decrease cardiac output • Makes the patient uncomfortable; patients require sedation to decrease discomfort and anxiety; muscle paralysis may be required along with sedation • May cause auto-PEEP, which, when added to therapeutic PEEP, increases risk of barotrauma • Do not use in patients with chronic obstructive pulmonary disease
Pressure-controlled/inverse ratio ventilation (PC/IRV)	• Combination of pressure support ventilation and inverse ratio ventilation	• Improves oxygenation and allows reduction of Fio_2 • May be used in ARDS with refractory hypoxemia • As for PSV and IRV
Airway pressure release ventilation (APRV)	• CPAP with short (1 to 1½ seconds) releases to allow further expiration and carbon dioxide elimination	• Prevents lung overdistention while maintaining inflation of newly recruited alveoli • Maintains lower mean and peak airway pressures • Less hemodynamic compromise than traditional modes
Bi-level	• CPAP with two different levels; CPAP-high and CPAP-low	• Contraindicated in patients with obstructive lung disease
Pressure-regulated volume-controlled (PRVC) (may also be referred to as *adaptive pressure ventilation* or *autoflow*)	• Preset target tidal volume and pressure limit; the ventilator automatically sets the initial flow rate and flow waveform to deliver the desired volume at the desired pressure • Inspiratory pressure changes breath to breath to augment the tidal volume delivery of subsequent breaths accounting for changes in compliance, resistance, and patient effort • Measurement of compliance at predetermined intervals and adjusts the flow rate and pressure support to deliver the set tidal volume at or below the maximal pressure	• Preferred mode for patients with high airway pressures • Produces a guaranteed tidal volume but minimizes the risk of barotrauma and volutrauma • Requires special ventilator
High-frequency ventilation	• Preset (very low) tidal volumes delivered at preset (very high) rates; ventilation and oxygenation are achieved by gas diffusion and convection • High-frequency positive pressure ventilation: 60-120 breaths/min • High-frequency jet ventilation: 120-600 breaths/min • High-frequency oscillation ventilation: 500-1200 oscillations per minute	• May be used in some cases of chest trauma, bronchopleural fistula, or ARDS • Causes lower airway and intrathoracic pressures than traditional mechanical ventilation; may reduce the incidence of barotrauma and decreased cardiac output • Muscle paralysis along with sedation required • May cause increased oral secretions • Auscultation of heart and lung sounds is difficult • Requires special ventilator

Continued

Table 4-15 Modes of Mechanical Ventilation—cont'd

Mode	Description	Comments
Independent lung ventilation (ILV) (also called *differential lung ventilation* or *split-lung ventilation*)	• Ventilation technique that ventilates each lung separately • Separate modes, flow rates, and PEEP may be used for each lung • May be synchronized	• Used for unilateral pathologic conditions or thoracic trauma • Requires double-lumen tube and separate ventilators to each lumen, (and a synchronizer if synchronized independent lung ventilation) • Asynchronous lung ventilation is better tolerated hemodynamically in most patients • Patient requires sedation and/or paralysis
Liquid ventilation	• Conventional ventilation along with the substitution of nitrogen with inert perfluorochemical fluids	• Perfluorochemical fluids serve as a liquid PEEP recruiting alveoli and as a local antiinflammatory • Fluids are replaced as evaporation occurs • Chest x-ray interpretation is complicated by the fluid
Extracorporeal membrane oxygenation	• Transfer of blood from the patient through an artificial lung to oxygenate the blood that then is returned to the body	• Provides blood oxygenation while allowing the lung to rest and heal • Not available in all medical centers and no survival benefit shown thus far

ARDS, Acute respiratory distress syndrome; *CPAP*, continuous positive airway pressure; *ET*, endotracheal; *Fio*$_2$, fraction of inspired oxygen; *I:E*, inspiration: expiration; *IMV*, intermittent mandatory ventilation; *IRV*, inverse ratio ventilation; *PEEP*, positive end-expiratory pressure; *PSV*, pressure support ventilation; *VAPSV*, volume-assured pressure support ventilation.

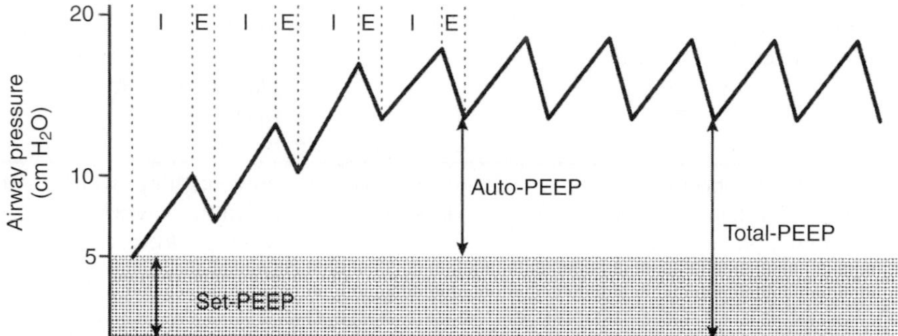

Figure 4-32 Auto-PEEP (positive end-expiratory pressure) as frequently is seen in inverse ratio ventilation. Insufficient expiratory time permits the trapping of gases in the lung. This trapped gas creates pressure, which is known as *auto-PEEP*. This PEEP is added to therapeutic PEEP for total PEEP. *I*, Inspiration; *E*, expiration. (From Pierce, L. [1995]. *Guide to mechanical ventilation and intensive respiratory care.* Philadelphia: Saunders.)

(d) Goal: reduce auto–PEEP to the lowest practical level
(i) Reduce bronchospasm
(ii) Adjust flow rates and I:E ratio

b. Actions of PEEP
(1) Increases driving pressure of O_2
(a) Improves the Pao$_2$ without increasing the Fio$_2$
(b) Allows the use of lower Fio$_2$ to achieve the same Pao$_2$, thereby decreasing risk of O_2 toxicity
(2) Decreases surface tension to prevent alveolar collapse at end-expiration
(3) Decreases intrapulmonary shunt by opening alveoli that are collapsed (referred to as *alveolar recruitment*); increases functional residual capacity
(4) Minimizes the risk of VILI by stabilizing the lung units and reducing the repeated opening and collapsing of alveoli

c. Uses of PEEP
(1) ARDS (also referred to as *noncardiac pulmonary edema*)
(2) Cardiac pulmonary edema
(3) Acute respiratory failure with persistent hypoxemia
(4) Occasionally used to increase intrapulmonic pressure in patients with intrathoracic bleeding
(5) Physiologic PEEP is used to mimic the PEEP exerted by the closed glottis in intubated patients

d. Adverse effects of PEEP
(1) Hemodynamic consequences of positive pressure ventilation are accentuated
(a) Decreased venous return
(b) Increased right ventricular afterload
(c) Decreased left ventricular distensibility
(d) Decreased CO

(2) Barotrauma
(3) Increased intracranial pressure (ICP)

e. Contraindications to PEEP
(1) Untreated hypovolemia
(2) Extreme caution in hypotensive states
(3) Increased risk of barotrauma in patients with COPD

f. Nursing management to maintain PEEP
(1) Monitor vital signs and hemodynamic parameters closely.
(2) Maintain prescribed levels of PEEP; patients with an inspiratory effort pull a negative pressure and negate the level of PEEP; these patients require sedation and/or muscle paralysis to maintain the therapeutic effects of PEEP.
(a) Sedation: benzodiazepines such as lorazepam (Ativan) or diazepam (Valium) are recommended for long-term use; propofol (Diprivan) frequently is used for short-term mechanical ventilation when rapid reversibility is desired (e.g., cardiac surgery patient) (for more on sedatives, see Chapter 14)
(b) Analgesics: morphine intermittently or infusion may be needed especially in patients who have chest trauma or surgery
(c) Muscle paralysis (e.g., pancuronium [Pavulon], vecuronium [Norcuron], or rocuronium [Zemuron]) (for more on neuromuscular blocking agents, see Chapter 14)
(i) Sedatives and/or analgesics must always be given with these agents.
(ii) Inform the patient that the effect is temporary.
(iii) Patient does not have blink reflex; protect the cornea by instilling saline or artificial tears into each eye at least every 4 hours.
(iv) May cause residual muscle weakness; use peripheral nerve stimulation unit to evaluate appropriateness of dose.
(v) Discontinue muscle paralytics at least 24 hours before weaning.

2. CPAP: nonventilator technique for maintaining positive pressure during spontaneous ventilation
a. Uses: may be used by mask or in the intubated patient
(1) As an interim treatment to prevent the need for intubation
(2) May be used to wean a patient from PEEP
(3) Sleep apnea
b. Actions, adverse effects, contraindications as for PEEP

Mechanical Ventilator Parameters

1. Mode
2. V_T: 5 to 10 mL/kg of IBW; 4 to 8 mL/kg of IBW in patients with ALI/ARDS
3. Respiratory rate: varies according to ventilator flow rate, I:E ratio, and whether ventilator is on control or assist mode; usually 8 to 16 breaths/min
4. FiO_2
a. Initially 1 (i.e., 100%) for 20 minutes especially if cardiac arrest
b. Adjusted so that PaO_2 is 60 mm Hg
c. Use lowest FiO_2 that achieves desired PaO_2
d. PEEP may be added to maintain acceptable PaO_2 with lower FiO_2 to reduce the risk of O_2 toxicity
5. PEEP or CPAP
6. Sensitivity: if assist mode is used
a. Amount of inspired effort required to initiate an assisted breath
b. Usually set at −1 to −2 cm H_2O
7. Sigh
a. Volume: 1.5 to 2 times the inspired V_T
b. Frequency: 10 to 15 times/hour
c. Though sighing was done infrequently when large V_Ts were used, they may be helpful in preventing atelectasis now that more physiologic V_Ts are being used
8. Humidification
a. Continuous humidification is required with inspired air warmed to body temperature; temperature is maintained at 32° to 37° C and humidity at 100%
b. Methods of adding moisture
(1) Humidifiers: inspiratory gas passes over or bubbles through heated water to produce water vapor
(a) Water condensation (may be referred to as *rainout*) must be emptied frequently into a water trap or container for discard
(2) Nebulizers: high-frequency sound waves (ultrasonic) or a gas-powered airstream (pneumatic) focused on a water source produces an aerosol
(3) Heat-and-moisture exchange devices (also referred to as an *artificial nose*)
(a) Contain materials that absorb exhaled moisture and heat with each breath so it "recycles" heat and moisture from the patient's exhaled air
(b) Cannot provide as much humidity as a heated humidifier
(c) A new version incorporates electric heating and a gravity-drive saline drip
c. Methods of adding warmth

(1) Heated wire circuit
(a) An electrically heated wire runs through the ventilator circuit to warm the inspired gas to the desired temperature
(b) Eliminates water condensation in ventilator tubing because the wire heats the tubing so that it is the same temperature as gas leaving the ventilator
(2) Servomechanism: a thermal sensor at the patient Y sends information to the ventilator humidity system so that the humidifier is adjusted to match the desired temperature
9. Flow rate
a. Usually 40 to 80 L/min but adjusted so that inspiratory volume can be completed in time allowed, based on desired ventilatory rate and I:E ratio
(1) Slower the flow rate, better distribution in normal lung
(2) Faster the flow rate, better for patients with COPD so that more time is allowed for expiration
b. Patient comfort is also a consideration: does the patient feel like he or she is getter enough air?
10. I:E ratio
a. Usually 1:1.5 or 1:2
b. Inverse ratio ventilation: more time for inspiration than expiration; thought to improve distribution of inspired air, especially in ARDS
11. Alarm settings: all alarms should be ON
a. High-pressure alarm: set alarm 10 to 20 cm H_2O above the patient's peak inspiratory pressure
(1) Causes for high pressure alarm
(a) Increased airway resistance: secretions; bronchospasm; kink in tubing; displacement of artificial airway; patient coughing during inspiration; patient biting on ET tube; water condensation in tubing
(b) Decreased compliance: pneumothorax (sudden increase); development of pulmonary edema, atelectasis, pneumonia, ARDS (gradual increase)
b. Low exhaled volume alarm: set alarm at 50 to 100 mL below inspired V_T; causes for low exhaled volume alarm
(1) Disconnection
(2) Cuff leak
(3) Leak in circuitry
(4) Overbreathing: occurs when the patient deeply inspires as the ventilator is delivering inspiration; the ventilator senses low pressure; this patient may require sedation to prevent recurrent ventilator alarms
c. Apnea setting: ON
(1) Patient fatigue
(2) Overmedication
(3) Decrease in level of consciousness
d. Low FiO_2: ON
(1) O_2 disconnect
(2) Break in inspiratory circuit
12. Power: the mechanical ventilator must be pulled into a grounded electrical outlet that is backed up by the emergency generator; this is usually red

Assessment of the Mechanically Ventilated Patient

1. Pulmonary
a. Airway: type; size; position; cuff pressure
b. Chest excursion, use of accessory muscles
c. Breath sounds
d. Secretions: amount; color; consistency; odor
e. Spontaneous ventilatory mechanics: at least every 24 hours without sedation (i.e., sedation vacation) though sedation withdrawal is contraindicated for some patients (e.g., neurologically injured patients)
(1) Respiratory rate
(2) Patient's own V_T
(3) VC
(4) Minute ventilation
(5) MIP
(6) Rapid shallow breathing index: best single index for assessing readiness for weaning
(a) Calculated: f/V_T
(b) RSBI of 105 indicates readiness to wean
f. Ventilator parameters
(1) Mode: as set
(2) V_T as set and exhaled
(3) Respiratory rate: ventilator and patient initiated
(4) FiO_2: confirmed with O_2 analyzer
(5) PEEP: airway pressure at the end of expiration (on pressure gauge not just what it is set to be)
(6) Peak inspiratory pressure: airway pressure at the peak of inspiration; calculate dynamic compliance
(7) Plateau pressure: airway pressure with an inflation hold; calculate static compliance
(8) Alarms: check that all are ON
g. Ventilator circuitry: leaks; condensation; temperature of inspired air
h. Pulse oximetry: SpO_2
i. Chest x-ray: usually done daily unless chronic situation
j. ABGs: usually done daily and 20 to 30 minutes after any ventilator changes and as indicated by change in patient status
(1) Table 4-16 describes mechanical ventilator parameter changes to make in response to ABG results; note that only one change should be made at a time
2. Cardiovascular
a. Heart rate
b. ECG rhythm
c. Heart sounds

Table 4-16 Mechanical Ventilator Parameter Changes to Make According to Arterial Blood Gases

Parameter	Change
If $Paco_2$ is greater than 45 mm Hg (or above the patient's normal if patient has chronic obstructive pulmonary disease)	• Increase ventilation ○ Increase rate ○ Increase tidal volume (if it does not currently exceed 10 mL/kg)
If $Paco_2$ is less than 35 mm Hg (unless therapeutic hypocapnia is being maintained, such as increased intracranial pressure)	• Decrease ventilation ○ Decrease rate ○ Decrease tidal volume ○ If patient on assist-control mode: change mode from assist-control to intermittent mechanical ventilation ○ Consider sedation and/or analgesia ○ Mechanical dead space may be considered (tubing that acts as a rebreathing device)
If Pao_2 is less than 60 mm Hg	• Increase Fio_2 • Add or increase PEEP (especially if Fio_2 already greater than 0.6 [60%])
If Pao_2 is >100 mm Hg	• Decrease Fio_2 • Decrease PEEP (especially if Fio_2 is less than 0.4 [40%])

Fio_2, Fraction of inspired oxygen; *PEEP*, positive end-expiratory pressure.

   d. BP: direct (arterial catheter) or indirect (auscultated)
   e. Hemodynamic parameters: right atrial pressure; PAP; PAOP; CO/CI; systemic vascular resistance/systemic vascular resistance index; PVR/PVR index; Svo_2
3. Neurologic
   a. Level of consciousness
   b. Airway reflexes: gag; swallowing; corneal
   c. Sedation level (see Chapter 14 for sedation scales)
4. Renal/metabolic
   a. Urine output
   b. Urine specific gravity
   c. Serum electrolytes
5. GI
   a. Abdominal distention
   b. Bowel sounds
   c. Guaiac testing: NG aspirate; vomitus; stools
6. Nutritional status
   a. Daily weight
   b. Total protein, albumin, and serum transferrin levels
   c. Calorie counts and nutrient balance
7. Immunologic
   a. Temperature
   b. Sputum cultures
   c. WBC count
8. Psychologic
   a. Complaints of pain or anxiety
   b. Clinical indicators of pain or anxiety

Potential Complications of Positive Pressure Ventilation (Table 4-17)

1. Use of bundles to prevent serious complications
   a. Bundle concept: evidence-based interventions "bundled" together to improve patient outcomes; a small number (three to five) interventions is recommended (Institute for Healthcare Improvement, 2005)
   b. Interventions typically included in a "vent" bundle (Institute for Healthcare Improvement, 2005)
      (1) Elevation of the head of the bed
      (2) Daily "sedation vacations" and assessment of readiness to extubate
      (3) Peptic ulcer disease prophylaxis
      (4) Deep venous thrombosis prophylaxis
      (5) Regularly scheduled oral care has been added by many institutions

Weaning (also referred to as *Liberation*)

1. Definition: the gradual withdrawal of ventilatory support for patients who have been mechanically ventilated more than 24 hours
2. Phases of weaning
   a. Preweaning phase: assessment to determine whether the patient is capable of attempting spontaneous ventilation
      (1) Respiratory factors
         (a) Resolution or improvement of disease process that necessitated mechanical ventilation
         (b) Oxygenation
            (i) Patient does not require more than 5 cm H_2O of PEEP or Fio_2 greater than 0.5 to maintain acceptable Pao_2 (60 mm Hg) and Sao_2 (90%)
            (ii) Pao_2/Fio_2 ratio greater than or equal to 150 mm Hg
         (c) Ventilation
            (i) Respiratory rate less than 30 breaths/min
            (ii) $Paco_2$ less than 45 mm Hg or equal to the patient's baseline $Paco_2$
            (iii) V_T greater than 5 mL/kg

Table 4-17 Complications of Mechanical Ventilation

Complication	Causes	Prevention	Clinical Presentation	Treatment
Decreased cardiac output	• Increased intrathoracic pressures that decrease venous return to the right heart, • Increase right ventricular afterload • Decrease left ventricular distensibility	• Ensure adequate preload before mechanical ventilation. • Avoid excessive tidal volumes. • Adjust PEEP carefully.	• Tachycardia, hypotension • Cool, clammy skin • Decrease in urine output • Change in level of consciousness	• Administer fluids to increase preload. • Administer inotropes as prescribed.
Ventilator-induced lung injury	• Barotrauma: high inflation pressures may cause pneumothorax, pneumomediastinum, or subcutaneous emphysema • Volutrauma: high inflation volumes and repeated end-expiratory collapse followed by repeated reopening during inspiration may cause release of inflammatory mediators, injury to the lung ultrastructure, and ALI/ARDS • Oxygen toxicity • High end-inspiratory lung volume, such as occurs with high levels of PEEP, auto-PEEP (e.g., inverse ratio ventilation), and high functional residual capacity, such as elderly patients (i.e., senile emphysema) or patients with COPD	• Avoid excessive tidal volumes; now recommended to be within 5-10 mL/kg of IBW with even lower tidal volumes for patients with ALI/ARDS (~6 mL/kg of IBW). • Keep plateau pressure less than 30 cm H_2O. • Keep Fio_2 less than 0.6 (60%). • Adjust PEEP carefully.	• Pneumothorax: chest pain, dyspnea, sudden increase in peak inspiratory pressure, decreased breath sounds and chest movement on affected side, tracheal shift, hypotension, jugular venous distention if tension pneumothorax, clinical indications of hypoxia, decreased Spo_2, changes on chest x-ray • ALI/ARDS: high peak and plateau pressures, refractory hypoxemia (Pao_2/Fio_2 ratio less than 300 mm Hg), noncardiac (pulmonary artery occlusive pressure less than 18 mm Hg), pulmonary edema, patchy atelectasis on chest x-ray	• If pneumothorax suspected, take patient off ventilator and manually ventilate with a manual resuscitation bag; assist with insertion of chest tube for pneumothorax. • Decrease tidal volume or PEEP if possible to decrease mean airway pressure and prevent alveolar overdistention.
Fluid retention	• Decrease in insensible loss via respiratory system • Overhydration by humidification • Decreased urine output because of antidiuretic hormone and aldosterone secretion	• Avoid decrease in cardiac output, which stimulates renin-angiotensin-aldosterone system.	• Weight gain • Intake greater than output • Crackles • Decreased compliance	• Use therapies to prevent decrease in cardiac output.
Atelectasis	• Airway obstruction • Small tidal volumes or lack of sighing • Infrequent turning of patient	• Use periodic sighing. • Turn patient frequently. • Provide adequate humidification. • Perform tracheal suctioning as indicated. • Provide chest PT as indicated. • Reposition patient frequently	• Diminished breath sounds • Crackles • Abnormal chest x-ray • Increased A:a gradient ($PAo_2 - Pao_2$) • Decreased compliance	• Provide periodic sighing. • Provide chest PT

Table 4-17 Complications of Mechanical Ventilation

Complication	Causes	Prevention	Clinical Presentation	Treatment
Hypercapnia; hypocapnia	• Inadequate or excessive ventilation • Hypermetabolism may contribute to hypercapnia	• Initiate ventilation with tidal volume at 10-15 mL/kg and rate of 8-12 breaths/min. • Make ventilator changes after initial ABGs.	• Increased (greater than 45 mm Hg) or decreased (less than 35 mm Hg) $Paco_2$	• Hypercapnia: increase tidal volume (or rate). • Hypocapnia: decrease rate (or tidal volume); change to intermittent mechanical ventilation or pressure support ventilation.
Oxygen toxicity	• Too high a concentration of O_2 over too long a time	• Maintain Fio_2 as low as possible to maintain an Sao_2 (or Spo_2) of 90% and limit duration of Fio_2 of greater than 0.4 if possible; addition of PEEP allows reduction of Fio_2 while maintaining the same Sao_2. • REMEMBER: Hypoxemia is far more common than O_2 toxicity and must be corrected.	• Substernal distress • Paresthesias in extremities • Anorexia, nausea, vomiting • Fatigue, lethargy, malaise • Restlessness • Dyspnea, progressive respiratory difficulty • Decreased compliance • Increased A:a gradient	• Decrease O_2 concentration as soon as possible. • Provide supportive management.
Aspiration	• Stomach contents • Tube feedings • Oral secretions • Gastric distention • Impaired gastric emptying • Esophageal reflux	• Maintain cuff inflation using minimal occlusive volume. • Keep head of bed elevated 30 to 45 degrees. • Check for gastric retention at least every 4 hours. • Check NG tube placement at least every 4 hours.	• Increased tracheal secretions • Fever • Rhonchi, wheezes • Signs/symptoms of hypoxemia/hypoxia • Infiltrate shown on chest x-ray	• Provide supportive management. • Administer antibiotics as prescribed. • Administer steroids as prescribed.
GI effects: stress ulcer, ileus, gastric dilation	• Hyperacidity • Endogenous or exogenous steroids • Gastric or mesenteric ischemia • Inadequate nutrition	• Use enteral feedings. • Administer antacids; H_2 receptor antagonists (e.g., cimetidine [Tagamet]); barrier agents (e.g., sucralfate [Carafate]) as prescribed.	• NG aspirate, vomitus, or stools positive for blood • Decreased bowel sounds • Gastric distention • Increased gastric retention	• Note effect of hemoglobin loss of tissue oxygenation; blood administration may be necessary. • Administer PPI, antacids, H_2 receptor antagonists, sucralfate as prescribed.
Infection	• Immunosuppression • Artificial airways bypass normal upper airway defense mechanisms • Ventilatory equipment: warm, moist environment is good for bacterial growth • Suctioning procedure • Silent aspiration of GI bacteria when PPIs, H_2 antagonists, or antacids used for ulcer prophylaxis; controversial issue	• Use good hand-washing techniques. • Use sterile technique for suctioning. • Provide aseptic airway management and tubing changes. • Avoid change in usual acidic gastric pH; use enteral feedings for ulcer prophylaxis if gastric mobility adequate. • Keep head of bed elevated during tube feedings.	• Tachycardia, tachypnea • Fever • Crackles, rhonchi, or wheezes • Hypoxemia • Change in color or character of sputum • Positive cultures • Infiltrate shown on chest x-ray	• Administer antibiotic specific to culture.

Continued

Table 4-17 Complications of Mechanical Ventilation—cont'd

Complication	Causes	Prevention	Clinical Presentation	Treatment
	• Cross-contamination may be cause	• Keep ET tube or tracheostomy cuff inflated to 18 mm Hg. • Drain humidifier condensation into water trap or container and not back into humidifier. • Routine change of ventilator circuit is no longer indicated, but the circuit should be changed if visibly soiled or malfunctioning. • Additional information is in Pneumonia section of Chapter 5.		
Patient-ventilator asynchrony (patient "fighting" ventilator)	• Incorrect ventilator setup for the patient's needs • Acute change in patient's status • Obstructed airway • Ventilator malfunction • Anxiety	• Ensure proper setup of ventilator equipment; monitor settings every hour. • Monitor peak inspiratory pressure. • Suction fluids as indicated. • Talk to patient, keep him or her informed. • Administer anxiolytics as indicated.	• Anxiety, agitation • Increase in peak inspiratory pressure • Ventilator alarm sounding • Change in pulse oximetry or ABGs	• Perform rapid check of patient and ventilator. • Disconnect patient from ventilator and provide manual ventilation via manual resuscitation bag. • Check vital signs, breath sounds, and pulse oximetry. • Assess ABGs. • Suction fluids from airway. • Check patency of ET or tracheostomy tube.
Anxiety	• Loss of autonomy over vital body function (breathing) • Inability to communicate • Sensory overload (e.g., alarms, repeated interruptions for vital signs, and noise of ventilator) • Sensory deprivation (e.g., separation from family, work, and meaningful activities) • Discomfort (e.g., arterial punctures, ET tube, NG tube, and Foley catheter)	• Explain to patient why he or she cannot speak; provide method of communication. • Explain all procedures thoroughly; keep patient informed regarding progress and plans. • Add familiar objects to patient's environment (e.g., family photos and cards). • Have calendar, clock in room; have window shades or curtains open to orient patient to light and dark. • Allow uninterrupted time for rest and sleep. • Put eyeglasses and hearing aid on patient if appropriate. • Encourage expression of fears. • Be available; answer call bell promptly. • Promote as much independence as possible.	• High-pressure alarm because the patient is breathing out of synchrony with ventilator • Tachycardia • Tachypnea, excessive triggering of ventilator is on assist-control, potentially causing hypocapnia and respiratory alkalosis • Complaints of being "nervous"	• Stay with patient during times of extreme anxiety. • Use therapeutic touch (e.g., hold hand). • Use soft restraints only as necessary to prevent self-extubation. • Encourage family visitation and participation if appropriate.

Table 4-17 Complications of Mechanical Ventilation—cont'd

Complication	Causes	Prevention	Clinical Presentation	Treatment
		• Provide emotional support to the family. • Avoid uncomfortable or painful procedures if possible (e.g., arterial catheter instead of arterial punctures). • Use complementary therapies such as music and aromatherapy.		
Inability to wean	• COPD: occurs when $Paco_2$ is corrected instead of pH • Malnutrition: catabolism and muscle breakdown • Neuromuscular blocking agents: disuse syndrome	• Correct pH instead of $Paco_2$ in patients with COPD. • Provide adequate calories to prevent catabolism; adequate protein and high calories are given; adequate calories must be given to prevent the protein from being used for energy; calories given are predominantly fat since carbohydrate metabolism produces more carbon dioxide. • Avoid neuromuscular blocking agents if possible; limit duration of use.	• Increased $Paco_2$, increased ventilatory rate, tachycardia with weaning efforts	• COPD: Allow $Paco_2$ to increase so that the kidney will hold on to bicarbonate to compensate; keep Pao_2 close to patient's normal (e.g., 60-65 mm Hg). • Provide adequate protein and calories; avoid high-carbohydrate weaning. feedings during • Discontinue several days before to weaning.

ABG, Arterial blood gas; *ALI/ARDS*, acute lung injury/acute respiratory distress syndrome; *COPD*, chronic obstructive pulmonary disease; *ET*, endotracheal, *Fio₂*, fraction of inspired oxygen; *GI*, gastrointestinal; *IBW*, ideal body weight, *NG*, nasogastric; *O₂*, oxygen; *PEEP*, positive end-expiratory pressure; *PPI*, proton pump inhibitor; *PT*, physical therapy; *Sao₂*, arterial oxygen saturation; *Spo₂*, functional oxygen saturation.

(iv) VC greater than 10 mL/kg
(v) Minute ventilation less than 10 L/min
(d) Lung mechanics
(i) MIP greater that −25 cm H_2O
(ii) Rapid shallow breathing index of 105 breaths/min/L
(2) Nonrespiratory factors
(a) Neurologic status: conscious
(b) Hemodynamics: stable
(c) Hgb: adequate
(d) Fluid and electrolytes: corrected and normal
(e) Nutrition: adequate nutritional status
(f) Psychological factors: psychologically prepared and cooperative
(g) Medications: cessation of deep sedation and muscle paralytics

b. Weaning phase
(1) Methods of weaning
(a) Spontaneous breathing trial with T piece (Figure 4-33) for short-term mechanical ventilation (i.e., less than 72 hours)
(i) Spontaneous breathing for 120 minutes through ventilator with pressure support ventilation of 0; CPAP of up to 5 cm H_2O allowed
a) If successful, extubation or tracheostomy
b) If unsuccessful, allow patient to rest and try again the next day
(ii) Advantage: may be able to wean patient more quickly than intermittent mechanical ventilation or pressure support ventilation methods
(iii) Disadvantage: recurrent ventilatory failures discourage and frighten the patient
(b) Intermittent mechanical ventilation
(i) Gradually reduce intermittent mechanical ventilation rate
(ii) Advantages
a) Provides exercise for ventilatory musculature

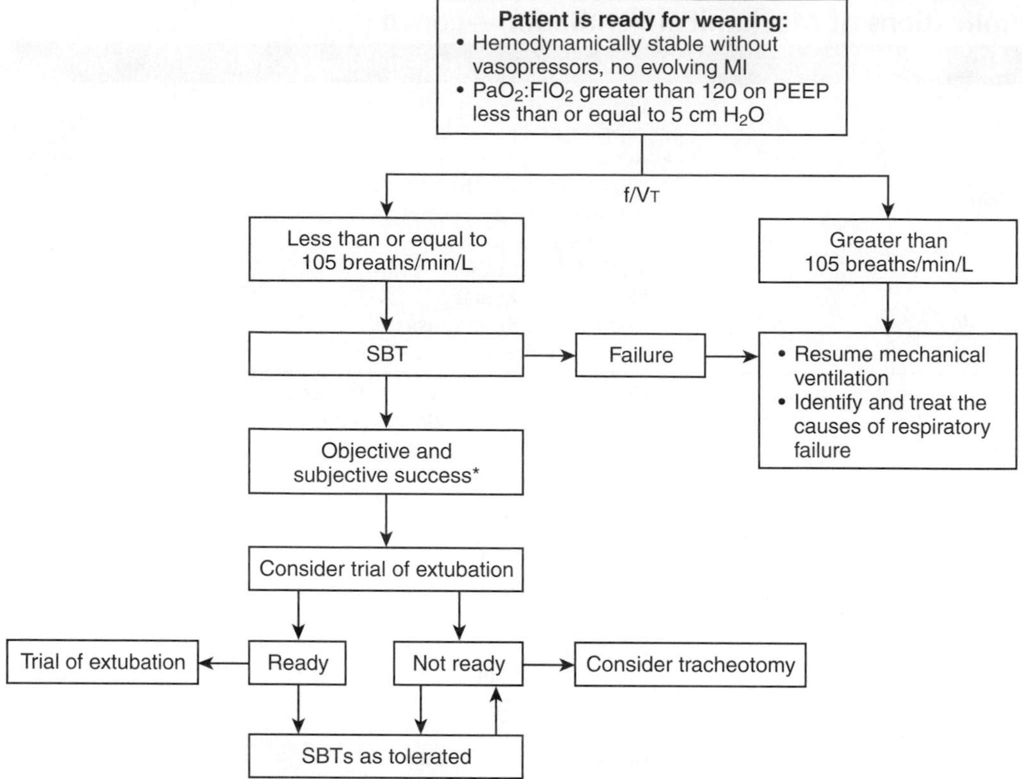

Figure 4-33 Algorithm for ventilator weaning using daily RSBI (f/V_T) measurements and SBTs. *f*, Respiratory frequency; *Fio*$_2$, fraction of inspired oxygen; *MI*, myocardial infarction; *Pao*$_2$, arterial oxygen tension; *PEEP*, positive end-expiratory pressure; *RSBI*, rapid shallow breathing index; *SBT*, spontaneous breathing trial; V_T, tidal volume. *Objective criteria for success or failure of SBTs include heart and respiratory rate, blood pressure, and arterial blood gases. Subjective criteria include diaphoresis and anxiety. (Adapted from Manthous, C. A. [2000]. Liberation from mechanical ventilation: Translating science to clinical practice. *Journal of Critical Illness, 15*[4], 208-210.)

b) More physiologic $Paco_2$ may be achieved
c) Large ventilator-provided breaths help to prevent atelectasis
d) Safer than trail-and-error method
e) Good acceptance by patients

(iii) Disadvantages: may take longer than T piece method

(c) Pressure support ventilation method

(i) Gradually decrease the amount of pressure support assisting the patient
a) Usually started at 15 to 25 cm H_2O
b) Gradually decreased by 3 to 6 cm H_2O every 1 to 3 days as long as maintaining a satisfactory minute ventilation
c) When the patient can maintain adequate ventilation with the pressure support ventilation at 5 cm H_2O, conduct a T piece trial

(ii) Advantages
a) Patient comfort frequently greater with pressure support ventilation
b) Less work of breathing than with intermittent mechanical ventilation or T piece method

(d) CPAP

(i) May be used for patients whose Pao_2 is PEEP– dependent; the patient is weaned from the ventilator by one of the foregoing methods but is left on CPAP to provide the improved driving pressure needed to maintained an adequate Pao_2

(2) Criteria used to stop a weaning trial

(a) Neurologic

(i) Change in level of consciousness
(ii) Extreme anxiety

(b) Pulmonary
(i) Respiratory rate greater than 35 breaths/min or less than 10 breaths/min
(ii) Use of accessory muscle of ventilation
(iii) Paradoxical chest wall motion
(iv) Complaints of dyspnea, fatigue, or pain
(v) Sao_2 less than 90%
(vi) Increase in $Paco_2$ of 5 to 8 mm Hg and/or pH less than 7.3
(c) Cardiovascular
(i) Systolic BP greater than 180 mm Hg or less than 90 mm Hg
(ii) Heart rate greater than 140 beats/min or sustained increase 20% above baseline
(iii) Premature ventricular contractions greater than six per minute, couplets, or runs of ventricular tachycardia
(iv) ST segment changes
(3) Therapies to facilitate weaning
(a) Coordination and communication among disciplines: flow sheets, communication boards
(b) Multidisciplinary weaning protocol
(c) Multidisciplinary rounds
(d) Recognition of likely reasons for failure to wean
(i) Underlying illness has not resolved sufficiently
(ii) Malnutrition
(iii) Excessive secretions
(iv) Presence of auto–PEEP
(v) Impaired muscle function resulting from electrolyte imbalance (e.g., hypokalemia, hypophosphatemia, or hypomagnesemia)
(vi) Respiratory muscle fatigue
c. Weaning outcomes phase
(1) Complete weaning: the patient is able to maintain a normal respiratory rate and V_T while breathing spontaneously
(2) Partial weaning: the patient is able to maintain spontaneous ventilation for short periods
(3) Terminal weaning followed by death
3. General guidelines
a. Position patient for optimal ventilation: usually semi-Fowler to high Fowler's.
b. Avoid depressing the patient's ventilatory drive and muscle strength by avoiding sedatives and muscle paralyzants; treat pain but do not overnarcotize.
c. Reduce carbohydrates if indicated; equivalent calories can be provided in the form of fats.
(1) Use Pulmocare if patient is being fed enterally: high fat and protein but low carbohydrates.
(2) Decrease glucose and increase fat (Intralipids) if patient is being fed parenterally.
d. Begin weaning attempts in the early morning; do not attempt to wean the patient at night.
e. Complementary therapies such as biofeedback and music may be helpful.
f. Because the mechanical ventilator may provide security for the patient, it may be helpful to leave ventilator in room with patient for 24 hours after weaning.
g. Monitor patient closely for clinical indicators of fatigue and ventilatory failure and abort weaning if necessary.

Noninvasive Positive Pressure Ventilation

Description

Positive pressure ventilation (usually CPAP or biphasic positive airway pressure [Bi-PAP]) of a nonintubated spontaneously breathing patient, primarily with a face or nasal mask attached to a standard ventilator or a machine specifically for noninvasive ventilation with the purpose of augmenting alveolar ventilation

Indications

1. Acute respiratory failure
2. Pulmonary edema
3. Weaning of a patient from traditional mechanical ventilation and/or PEEP
4. Sleep apnea

Advantages over Traditional Mechanical Ventilation

1. Avoidance of intubation and complications of intubation
2. Improved patient comfort
3. Lower incidence of nosocomial pneumonia
4. Lower sedation requirements
5. No loss of speech
6. Shorter critical care unit stays

Contraindications

1. Absolute
   a. Hemodynamic instability
   b. Problems with airway patency (e.g., copious secretions)
   c. Risk for aspiration
   d. Altered level of consciousness (i.e., patients without airway protective reflexes)
2. Relative
   a. Uncooperative patient
   b. Morbid obesity
   c. Unstable angina or acute myocardial infarction
   d. Inability to fit mask

Complications

1. Facial skin breakdown
2. Nasal congestion
3. Conjunctivitis
4. Gastric distention
5. Aspiration
6. Pneumothorax

LEARNING ACTIVITIES

1. **DIRECTIONS:** Complete the following crossword puzzle to review pulmonary anatomy and physiology.

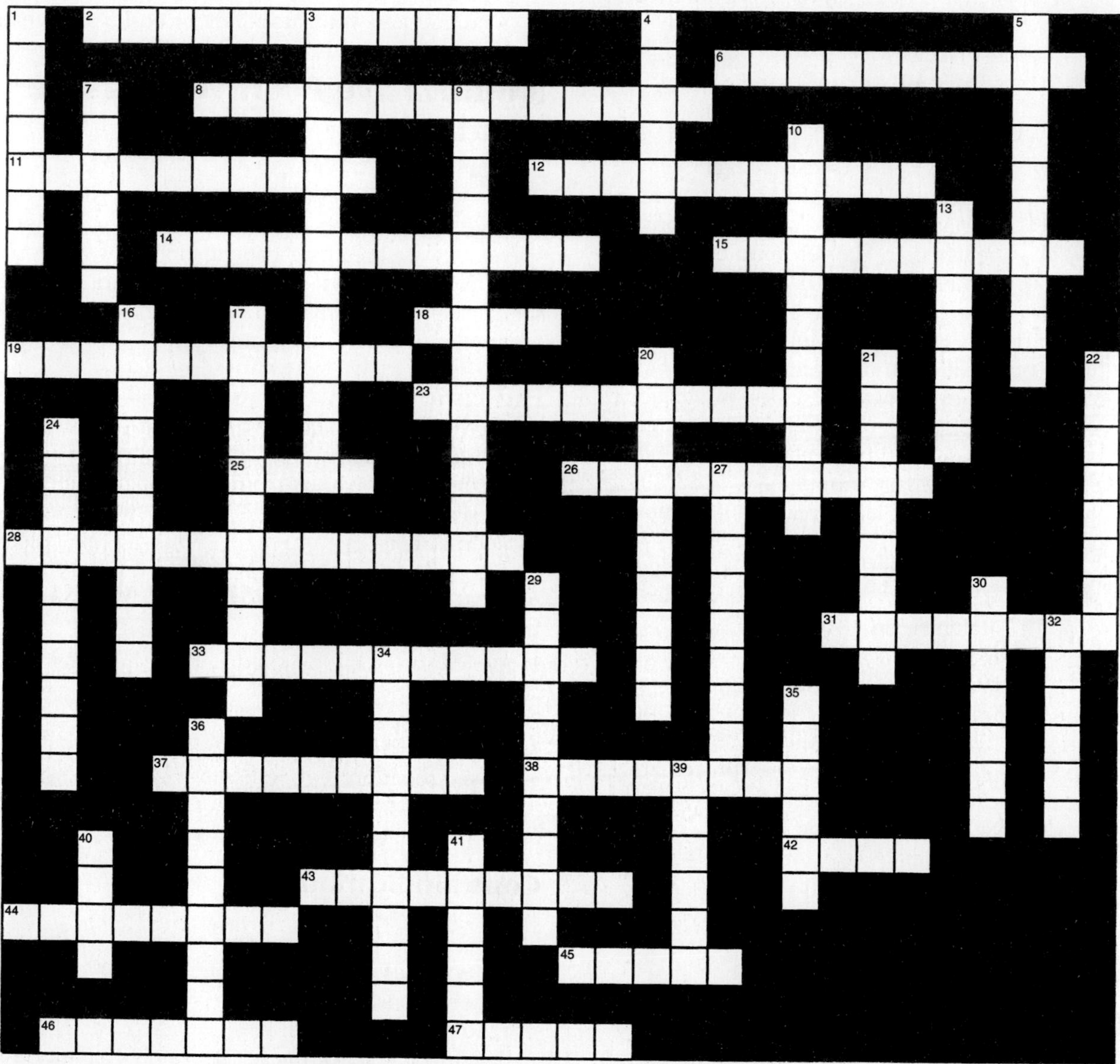

ACROSS

2. These cellular organelles use oxygen and nutrients to make ATP
6. The passive phase of ventilation
8. The lowest portion of the pharynx
11. These structures increase the surface area in the nose
12. The center of the thoracic cavity
14. The avascular membrane that can be punctured or opened with a scalpel to provide an emergency airway
15. The type of dead space that describes the air in conducting pathways
18. These openings between the alveoli are called pores of _____
19. The first bronchial branch that is part of the gas exchange unit is the _____ bronchiole
23. The movement of air into and out of the lungs
25. The area of the brain that controls rhythmic ventilation; contains both the apneustic and pneumotaxic centers
26. A lipoprotein that decreases surface tension and keeps the alveoli open at low distending pressure
28. These receptors are stimulated by an increase in interstitial fluid volume
31. The pleural layer that is contiguous with the chest wall
33. The active phase of ventilation
37. The process by which oxygen and carbon dioxide move across the alveolar-capillary membrane
38. The type of dead space that describes the air in the alveoli that are not perfused; V greater than Q
42. This structure is primarily responsible for warming, humidifying, and filtering inspired air

43. The ability of the lung to return to its original size after inspiration
44. The pleural layer that is contiguous with the lung
45. When deoxygenated blood comes in contact with nonventilated alveoli; V less than Q
46. The type of compliance that reflects both compliance of the lung and airway resistance
47. Hairlike projections that move mucus with entrapped particles upward to be coughed out

DOWN

1. The passage through the vocal cords
3. The _____ dissociation curve shows the relationship between PaO_2 and SaO_2
4. A dense concentration of lymphatic tissue that guards entryways into the GI or respiratory tracts
5. The change in pressure for a given change in volume
7. The area at the bifurcation of the trachea; rich in parasympathetic fibers
9. These receptors cause an increase in ventilation rate in response to body movement
10. Most carbon dioxide is transported in the blood as _____
13. The area of the left lung that corresponds to the right middle lobe
16. The flexible cartilage attached to the thyroid cartilage; closes to protect the larynx
17. The eustachian tubes open into the ____
20. A phagocyte in the alveoli
21. The nutrient circulation of the lung is supplied by this artery
22. The last branch of the conducting airways is the _____ bronchiole
24. Surfactant is produced by the type II _____
27. The main accessory muscles of expiration are the internal intercostal and _____ muscles
29. The area between the soft palate and the base of the tongue; the center for the gag reflex is located here
30. Central chemoreceptors are located in this area of the brain
32. The terminal respiratory unit that has an alveolar-capillary membrane for the exchange of oxygen and carbon dioxide
34. Airway _____ affects the work of breathing
35. The first portion of the trachea
36. The primary muscle of inspiration
39. The primary responsibility of the pulmonary system is to ensure the delivery of _____ to the tissues
40. The type of cell that secretes histamine
41. The type of compliance that reflects the compliance of the lung and the chest wall

2. **DIRECTIONS:** Fill in the primary and accessory muscles of inspiration and expiration.

	Primary	Accessory
Inspiration		
Expiration		

3. **DIRECTIONS:** Identify whether the following factors cause a shift of the oxyhemoglobin curve to the left or right.

	Left	Right
Increased 2,3-DPG		
Hypothermia		
Hypercapnia		
Hyperthermia		
Acidosis		
Decreased 2,3-DPG		
Hypocapnia		
Alkalosis		
Hypophosphatemia		
Massive blood transfusion		

4. **DIRECTIONS:** Identify the following conditions as restrictive or obstructive. Remember: if compliance of the lung or chest wall is affected, the condition is restrictive; if airway resistance is affected, the condition is obstructive.

	Restrictive	Obstructive
Obesity hypoventilation syndrome		
Asthma		
Pneumothorax		
Atelectasis		
Pneumonia		
Kyphoscoliosis		
Pulmonary edema		
Mucous plugs		
Lung cancer (bronchial)		
Lung cancer (parenchymal)		
Tuberculosis		
Chronic bronchitis		
Artificial airway		
Bronchospasm		

5. **DIRECTIONS:** Identify the primary breath sound change that occurs in the following conditions.

Condition	Breath Sound Change or Changes
Emphysema	
Atelectasis	
Pneumonia	
Chronic bronchitis	
Pneumothorax	
Pulmonary fibrosis	
Asthma	
Pulmonary edema	
Pleurisy	
Hemothorax	
Pleural effusion	
Pulmonary embolism	

6. **DIRECTIONS:** Identify normal values for the following parameters.

Tidal volume	
Vital capacity	
Maximal inspiratory pressure	
PaO_2	
SaO_2	
SvO_2	
DO_2	
VO_2	
O_2ER	

DO_2, Oxygen delivery; *O_2ER*, oxygen extraction ratio; *PaO_2*, partial pressure of oxygen; *SaO_2*, arterial oxygen saturation; *SvO_2*, venous oxygen saturation; *VO_2*, oxygen consumption.

7. **DIRECTIONS:** Identify the acid-base imbalance likely to occur in each of these situations.

a.	A patient is admitted to your unit with epidural analgesia being delivered. Her ventilatory rate is 8 breaths/min.	
b.	A patient has had large volumes of NG drainage for the last several shifts.	
c.	A postoperative patient has a history of COPD. He is now having problems with retained secretions.	
d.	A postoperative patient has a history of heart failure. She has been taking diuretics before and after surgery.	
e.	A postoperative thoracotomy patient is complaining of chest pain and has a respiratory rate of 32 breaths/min. She is complaining of tingling around her mouth and fingertips.	
f.	A postoperative patient has large volumes of ileal drainage from the new ileostomy.	

8. DIRECTIONS: Analyze the following ABGs. Identify any acid-base imbalance, any partial or total compensation, and the presence of hypoxemia. Assume all patients to be under 60 years of age.

	pH	$Paco_2$	HCO_3^-	Pao_2	Answer
1.	7.30	54	26	64	
2.	7.48	30	24	96	
3.	7.30	40	18	85	
4.	7.50	40	33	92	
5.	7.35	54	30	55	
6.	7.21	60	20	48	
7.	7.54	25	30	95	
8.	7.40	58	33	72	
9.	7.40	30	18	89	

9. DIRECTIONS: Match the O_2 delivery system with the O_2 concentration range that it can deliver. Choices may be used more than once.

a. Nasal cannula
b. Simple face mask
c. Partial rebreathing mask
d. Non-rebreathing mask
e. Venturi mask
f. T piece
g. Mechanical ventilator

___ 1. 21% to 100%
___ 2. 24% to 40%
___ 3. 24% to 44%
___ 4. 35% to 60%
___ 5. 40% to 60%
___ 6. 60% to 80%

10. DIRECTIONS: Identify the type of artificial airway in each of the following situations. More than one may be listed.

Problem	Preferred Artificial Airway
Tongue against hypopharynx	
Need for frequent nasotracheal suctioning	
Inability to open mouth, such as seizure	
Facial or jaw fracture	
Complete upper airway obstruction when ET intubation is impossible (e.g., laryngeal edema or spasm, or tracheal fracture)	
Need for sealed airway (e.g., mechanical ventilation or potential for aspiration)	
Need for long-term lower airway access and sealed airway	

11. DIRECTIONS: Match the following modes to the description of the mode.

a. Control
b. Assist-control
c. Synchronized intermittent mandatory ventilation
d. Pressure support ventilation
e. Pressure-controlled ventilation
f. Independent lung ventilation
g. High-frequency ventilation
h. Pressure-regulated volume-controlled
i. Bi-PAP
j. Airway pressure release ventilation

___ 1. Provides positive pressure when the patient initiates a breath to reduce the work of breathing
___ 2. Allows the patient to trigger additional assisted breaths between control breaths
___ 3. Combines pressure support ventilation and CPAP
___ 4. Useful for patients with unilateral lung disease, such as a pulmonary contusion
___ 5. Provides an open circuit to allow the patient to take breaths between control breaths
___ 6. Varies the flow rate and flow waveform to deliver the desired volume at the desired pressure
___ 7. Provides short periods of lower pressure during CPAP to allow further expiration
___ 8. Uses small V_Ts and rapid rates to keep airway pressures lower
___ 9. Maintains a closed circuit between control breaths so the patient cannot take additional breaths
___ 10. Ends inspiration when a preset pressure is reached; V_T is variable

12. **DIRECTIONS:** Identify four physiologic effects of PEEP and CPAP.
   a. ____________________
   b. ____________________
   c. ____________________
   d. ____________________

13. **DIRECTIONS:** Identify whether the following factors will cause a high pressure or low exhaled volume alarm.

	High Pressure	Low Exhaled Volume
Cuff leak		
Bronchospasm		
Need for suctioning		
Disconnect		
Water condensation in tubing		
Pneumothorax		
ARDS		

14. **DIRECTIONS:** Identify the values for the following parameters that indicate that the patient may be weaned successfully from mechanical ventilation.
   a. Spontaneous V_T __________
   b. Spontaneous VC __________
   c. MIP __________
   d. PaO_2 of at least __________ on an FIO_2 of no greater than __________ with no more than __________ cm H_2O PEEP
   e. RSBI __________

LEARNING ACTIVITIES ANSWERS

1.

1 GLOTTIS
2 MITOCHONDRIA
3 OXYHEMOGLOBIN
4 TONSIL
5 COMPLIANCE
6 EXPIRATION
7 CARINA
8 LARYNGOPHARYNX
9 PROPRIOCEPTORS
10 BICARBONATE
11 TURBINATES
12 MEDIASTINUM
13 LINGULA
14 CRICOTHYROID
15 ANATOMICAL
16 EPIGLOTTIS
17 NASOPHARYNX
18 KOHN
19 RESPIRATORY
20 MACROPHAGE
21 BRONCHIAL
22 TERMINAL
23 VENTILATION
24 PNEUMOCYTE
25 PONS
26 SURFACTANT
27 ABDOMINAL
28 JUXTACAPILLARY
29 OROPHARYNX
30 MEDULLA
31 PARIETAL
32 ACINUS
33 INSPIRATION
34 RESISTANCE
35 LARYNX
36 DIAPHRAGM
37 DIFFUSION
38 ALVEOLAR
39 OXYGEN
40 MAST
41 STATIC
42 NOSE
43 ELASTANCE
44 VISCERAL
45 SHUNT
46 DYNAMIC
47 CILIA

2.

	Primary	Accessory
Inspiration	Diaphragm External intercostal muscles	Scalene Sternocleidomastoid
Expiration	None; expiration is normally passive	Internal oblique External oblique Rectus abdominis Internal intercostal muscles Transversus abdominis

3.

	Left	Right
Increased 2,3-DPG		x
Hypothermia	x	
Hypercapnia		x
Hyperthermia		x
Acidosis		x
Decreased 2,3-DPG	x	
Hypocapnia	x	
Alkalosis	x	
Hypophosphatemia	x	
Massive blood transfusion	x	

4.

	Restrictive	Obstructive
Obesity hypoventilation syndrome	x	
Asthma		x
Pneumothorax	x	
Atelectasis	x	
Pneumonia	x	
Kyphoscoliosis	x	
Pulmonary edema	x	
Mucous plugs		x
Lung cancer (bronchial)		x
Lung cancer (parenchymal)	x	
Tuberculosis	x	
Chronic bronchitis		x
Artificial airway		x
Bronchospasm		x

5.

Condition	Breath Sound Change or Changes
Emphysema	Diminished breath sounds
Atelectasis	Diminished breath sounds Bronchial or bronchovesicular breath sounds Crackles
Pneumonia	Diminished breath sounds Bronchial or bronchovesicular breath sounds
Chronic bronchitis	Rhonchi Wheezes also may be present
Pneumothorax	Diminished or absent breath sounds
Pulmonary fibrosis	Diminished breath sounds Crackles
Asthma	Wheezes Rhonchi
Pulmonary edema	Crackles Wheezes (referred to as *cardiac asthma*) may be present
Pleurisy	Pleural friction rub
Hemothorax	Diminished or absent breath sounds
Pleural effusion	Diminished breath sounds
Pulmonary embolism	Crackles Pleural friction rub if pulmonary infarction develops

6.

Tidal volume	7 ml/kg
Vital capacity	Greater than 15 mL/kg
Maximal inspiratory pressure	Greater than (more negative than) –60 cm H_2O
Pao_2	80-100 mm Hg
Sao_2	Greater than 95%
Svo_2	60%-80%
Do_2	~1000 mL/min
Vo_2	~250 mL/min
O_2ER	~25%

7.

a.	Respiratory acidosis
b.	Metabolic alkalosis
c.	Respiratory acidosis (but with elevated bicarbonate; chronic compensated respiratory acidosis with decompensation)
d.	Metabolic alkalosis
e.	Respiratory alkalosis
f.	Metabolic acidosis

8.

	pH	$Paco_2$	HCO_3^-	Pao_2	ANSWER
1.	7.30	54	26	64	Respiratory acidosis with mild hypoxemia
2.	7.48	30	24	96	Respiratory alkalosis
3.	7.30	40	18	85	Metabolic acidosis
4.	7.50	40	33	92	Metabolic alkalosis
5.	7.35	54	30	55	Compensated respiratory acidosis with moderate hypoxemia
6.	7.21	60	20	48	Mixed disorder: respiratory and metabolic acidosis with moderate hypoxemia
7.	7.54	25	30	95	Mixed disorder: respiratory alkalosis and metabolic alkalosis
8.	7.40	58	33	72	Mixed disorder: respiratory acidosis and metabolic alkalosis NOTE: Compensation causes the pH to lean toward either end of the normal pH range; the nonleaning pH indicates that this is a mixed disorder rather than compensation.
9.	7.40	30	18	89	Mixed disorder: Respiratory alkalosis and metabolic acidosis NOTE: Compensation causes the pH to lean toward either end of the normal pH range; the nonleaning pH indicates that this is a mixed disorder rather than compensation.

9.

f, g	1. 21%-100%
e	2. 24%-40%
a	3. 24%-44%
c	4. 35%-60%
b	5. 40%-60%
d	6. 60%-90%

10.

Problem	Preferred Artificial Airway
Tongue against hypopharynx	Oropharyngeal or nasopharyngeal
Need for frequent nasotracheal suctioning	Nasopharyngeal
Inability to open mouth (e.g., seizure)	Nasopharyngeal
Facial or jaw fracture	Nasopharyngeal or nasotracheal tube
Complete upper airway obstruction when ET intubation is impossible (e.g., laryngeal edema or spasm, or tracheal fracture)	Cricothyrotomy or tracheostomy
Need for sealed airway (e.g., mechanical ventilation or potential for aspiration)	ET tube or tracheostomy LMA, but less protection from aspiration
Need for long-term lower airway access and sealed airway	Tracheostomy

11.

d 1. Provides positive pressure when the patient initiates a breath to reduce the work of breathing
b 2. Allows the patient to trigger additional assisted breaths between control breaths
i 3. Combines pressure support ventilation and CPAP
f 4. Useful for patients with unilateral lung disease, such as a pulmonary contusion
c 5. Provides an open circuit to allow the patient to take breaths between control breaths
h 6. Varies the flow rate and flow waveform to deliver the desired volume at the desired pressure
j 7. Provides short periods of lower pressure during CPAP to allow further expiration
g 8. Uses small V_Ts and rapid rates to keep airway pressures lower
a 9. Maintains a closed circuit between control breaths so the patient cannot take additional breaths
e 10. Ends inspiration when a preset pressure is reached; V_T is variable

12. a. Increases the driving pressure of O_2
b. Decreases surface tension
c. Decreases intrapulmonary shunt (alveolar recruitment)
d. Aids in prevention of VILI

13.

	High Pressure	Low Exhaled Volume
Cuff leak		x
Bronchospasm	x	
Need for suctioning	x	
Disconnect		x
Water condensation in tubing	x	
Pneumothorax	x	
ARDS	x	

14. a. Spontaneous V_T: at least 5 mL/kg
b. Spontaneous VC: at least 10 mL/kg
c. MIP greater than (more negative than) −25 cm H_2O
d. PaO_2 of at least *60 mm Hg* on an FiO_2 of no greater than *0.5* with no more than *5* cm H_2O PEEP.
e. RSBI: Less than or equal to 105 breaths/min/L

Reference

Institute for Healthcare Improvement. (2005). *Bundle up for safety.* Retrieved January 1, 2006, from http://www.ihi.org/IHI/Topics/CriticalCare/IntensiveCare/ImprovementStories/BundleUpforSafety.htm

Bibliography

Ackerman, M. H. (1998). Instillation of normal saline before suctioning in patients with pulmonary infections: A prospective randomized controlled trial. *American Journal of Critical Care, 7*(4), 261-266.

Acton, R. D., Hotchkiss, J. R., Jr., & Dries, D. J. (2002). Noninvasive ventilation. *Journal of Trauma, 53*(3), 593-601.

Ahrens, T. A., Kollef, M. H., Stewart, J., & Shannon, W. (2004). Effect of kinetic therapy on pulmonary complications. *American Journal of Critical Care, 13*(5), 376-382.

American Heart Association. (2005). Part 7.1: Adjuncts for airway control and ventilation. *Circulation, 112*(24 suppl), IV51-IV57.

Bateman, S., & Grap, M. J. (2003). Sedation and analgesia in the mechanically ventilated patient. *American Journal of Nursing, 103*(5), 64AA-64HH.

Berry, B. E., & Pinard, A. E. (2002). Assessing tissue oxygenation. *Critical Care Nurse, 22*(3), 22-42.

Brook, A. D., Sherman, G., Malen, J., & Kollef, M. H. (2000). Early versus late tracheostomy in patients who require prolonged mechanical ventilation. *American Journal of Critical Care, 9*(5), 352-359.

Brooks, D., Anderson, C. M., Carter, M. A., Downes, L. A., Keenan, S. P., Kelsey, C. J., et al. (2001). Clinical practice guidelines for suctioning the airway of the intubated and nonintubated patient. *Canadian Respiratory Journal, 8*(3), 163-181.

Burns, S. M. (2001). Safely caring for patients with a laryngeal mask airway. *Critical Care Nurse, 21*(4), 72-77.

Burns, S. M. (2004). Continuous airway pressure monitoring. *Critical Care Nurse, 24*(6), 70-74.

Burns, S. M. (2005). Mechanical ventilation of patients with acute respiratory distress syndrome and patients requiring weaning. *Critical Care Nurse, 25*(4), 14-24.

Burns, S. M., Earven, S., Fisher, C. J., Lewis, R., Merrell, P., Schubart, J. R., et al. (2003). Implementation of an institutional program to improve clinical and financial outcomes of mechanically ventilated patients: One-year outcomes and lessons learned. *Critical Care Medicine, 31*(12), 2752-2763.

Capovilla, J., VanCouwenberghe, C., & Miller, W. (2000). Noninvasive blood gas monitoring. *Critical Care Nursing Quarterly, 23*(2), 79-86.

Cereda, M., Villa, F., Colombo, E., Greco, G., Nacoti, M., & Pesenti, A. (2001). Closed system endotracheal suctioning maintains lung volume during volume-controlled mechanical ventilation. *Intensive Care Medicine, 27*(4), 648-654.

Chulay, M. (2001). Endotracheal or tracheostomy tube suctioning. In D. Lynn-McHale & K. Carlson (Eds.), *AACN procedure manual for critical care* (5th ed., pp. 41-48). Philadelphia: W. B. Saunders.

Danks, R. R., & Danks, B. (2004). Laryngeal mask airway: Review of indications and use. *Journal of Emergency Nursing, 30*(1), 30-35.

Dries, D. J., McGonigal, M. D., Malian, M. S., Bor, B. J., & Sullivan, C. (2004). Protocol-driven ventilator weaning reduces use of mechanical ventilation, rate of early reintubation, and ventilator-associated pneumonia. *Journal of Trauma, 56*(5), 943-952.

Dumont, C. P., & Tiep, B. L. (2002). Using a reservoir nasal cannula in acute care. *Critical Care Nurse, 22*(4), 41-46.

Epstein, C. D., El-Mokadem, N., & Peerless, J. R. (2002). Weaning older patients from long-term mechanical ventilation: A pilot study. *American Journal of Critical Care, 11*(4), 369-377.

Esmond, G. (Ed.). (2001). *Respiratory nursing*. Edinburgh: Bailliere Tindall.

Evans, B. (2005). Best-practice protocols: VAP prevention. *Nursing Management, 36*(12), 10-16.

Fernstermacher, D., & Hong, D. (2004). Mechanical ventilation. What have we learned? *Critical Care Nursing Quarterly, 27*(3), 258-294.

Fowler, R. A., & Pearl, R. G. (2002). The airway: Emergent management for nonanesthesiologists. *Western Journal of Medicine, 176*(1), 45-50.

Frakes, M. A. (2001). Measuring end-tidal carbon dioxide: Clinical applications and usefulness. *Critical Care Nurse, 21*(5), 23-37.

Frawley, P. M., & Habashi, N. M. (2001). Airway pressure release ventilation: Theory and practice. *AACN Clinical Issues, 12*(2), 234-246.

Gay, S. E., Ankney, N., Cochran, J. B., & Highland, K. B. (2005). Critical care challenges in the adult ECMO patient. *Dimensions of Critical Care Nursing, 24*(4), 157-162.

Goodfellow, L. T., & Jones, M. (2002). Bronchial hygiene therapy. *American Journal of Nursing, 102*(1), 37-44.

Grap, M. J. (2002). Pulse oximetry. *Critical Care Nurse, 22*(3), 69-74.

Grap, M. J., Strickland, D., Tormey, L., Keane, K., Lubin, S., Emerson, J., et al. (2003). Collaborative practice: Development, implementation, and evaluation of a weaning protocol for patients receiving mechanical ventilation. *American Journal of Critical Care, 12*(5), 454-460.

Happ, M. B. (2001). Communicating with mechanically ventilated patients: State of the science. *AACN Clinical Issues, 12*(2), 247-258.

Henneman, E. A. (2001). Liberating patients from mechanical ventilation. A team approach. *Critical Care Nurse, 21*(3), 25-33.

Henneman, E., Dracup, K., Ganz, T., Molayeme, O., & Cooper, C. (2002). Using a collaborative weaning plan to decrease duration of mechanical ventilation and length of stay in the intensive care unit for patients receiving long-term ventilation. *American Journal of Critical Care, 11*(2), 132-149.

Hynes-Gay, P., & MacDonald, R. (2001). Using high-frequency oscillatory ventilation to treat adults with acute respiratory distress syndrome. *Critical Care Nurse, 21*(5), 38-47.

Ibrahim, E. H., & Kollef, M. H. (2001). Using protocols to improve the outcomes of mechanically ventilated patients: Focus on weaning and sedation. *Critical Care Clinics, 17*(4), 989-1001.

Jagim, M. (2003). Airway management: Rapid sequence intubation in trauma patients. *American Journal of Nursing, 103*(10), 32-35.

Kinloch, D. (1999). Instillation of normal saline during endotracheal suctioning: Effects on mixed venous oxygen saturation. *American Journal of Critical Care, 8*(4), 231-240; quiz, 241-232.

Kollef, M. H. (2004). Prevention of hospital-associated pneumonia and ventilator-associated pneumonia. *Critical Care Medicine, 32*(6), 1396-1405.

Kollef, M. H., Skubas, N. J., & Sundt, T. M. (1999). A randomized clinical trial of continuous aspiration of subglottic secretions in cardiac surgery patients. *Chest, 116*(5), 1339-1346.

Kruse, J. A., Fink, M. P., & Carlson, R. W. (2003). *Saunders manual of critical care*. Philadelphia: Saunders.

Leifer, G. (2001). Hyperbaric oxygen therapy. *American Journal of Nursing, 101*(8), 26-35.

Lindgren, V. A., & Ames, N. J. (2005). Caring for patients on mechanical ventilation. *American Journal of Nursing, 105*(5), 50-61.

Manthous, C. A. (2000). Liberation from mechanical ventilation: Translating science to clinical practice. *Journal of Critical Illness, 15*(4), 208-210.

Munro, C. L., & Grap, M. J. (2004). Oral health and care in the intensive care unit: State of the science. *American Journal of Critical Care, 13*(1), 25-33.

Nakagawa, N. K., Macchione, M., Petrolino, H. M., Guimaraes, E. T., King, M., Saldiva, P. H., et al. (2000). Effects of a heat and moisture exchanger and a heated humidifier on respiratory mucus in patients undergoing mechanical ventilation. *Critical Care Medicine, 28*(2), 312-317.

O'Brynan, L., Von Rueden, K., & Malila, F. (2002). Evaluating ventilator weaning best practice: A long-term acute care hospital system-wide quality initiative. *AACN Clinical Issues, 13*(4), 567-576.

Olson, D. M., Chioffi, S. M., Macy, G. E., Meek, L. G., & Cook, H. A. (2003). Potential benefits of bispectral index monitoring in critical care: A case study. *Critical Care Nurse, 23*(4), 45-52.

O'Neal, P. V., Grap, M. J., Thompson, C., & Dudley, W. (2001). Level of dyspnoea experienced in mechanically ventilated adults with and without saline installation prior to endotracheal suctioning. *Intensive and Critical Care Nursing, 17*, 356-363.

Parrish, C. R., & McCray, S. F. (2003). Nutritional support of the mechanically ventilated patient. *Critical Care Nurse, 23*(1), 77-80.

Parthasarathy, S. (2004). Sleep during mechanical ventilation. *Current Opinion in Pulmonary Medicine, 10*(6), 489-494.

Pierce, L. N. (2002). Traditional and nontraditional modes of mechanical ventilation. *Critical Care Nurse, 22*(4), 56-59.

Pyne, C. C. (2004). Classification of acute coronary syndromes using the 12-lead electrocardiogram as a guide. *AACN Clinical Issues, 15*(4), 558-567.

Raymond, S. J. (1995). Normal saline instillation before suctioning: helpful or harmful? A review of the literature. *American Journal of Critical Care, 4*(4), 267-271.

Resar, R., Pronovost, P., Haraden, C., Simmonds, T., Rainey, T., & Nolan, T. (2005). Using a bundle approach to improve ventilator care processes and reduce ventilator-associated pneumonia. *Joint Commision Journal on Quality and Patient Safety, 31*(5), 243-248.

Richmond, A. L., Jarog, D. L., & Hanson, V. M. (2004). Unplanned extubation in adult critical care: Quality improvement and education payoff. *Critical Care Nurse, 24*(1), 32-37.

Salipante, D. M. (2002). Developing a multidisciplinary weaning unit through collaboration. *Critical Care Nurse, 22*(4), 30-39.

Schwenker, D., Ferrin, M., & Gift, A. G. (1998). A survey of endotracheal suctioning with instillation of normal saline. *American Journal of Critical Care, 7*(4), 255-260.

Siela, D. (2002). Using chest radiography in the intensive care unit. *Critical Care Nurse, 22*(4), 18-29.

Simmons, C. L. (1997). How frequently should endotracheal suctioning be undertaken? *American Journal of Critical Care, 6*(1), 4-6.

Smith, C., & Fultz, J. (2000). Airway management in a patient with penetrating chest trauma: A postflight case review. *Journal of Emergency Nursing, 26*(4), 352-354.

Smulders, K., van Der Hoeven, H., Weers-Pothoff, I., & Vandenbroucke-Grauls, C. (2002). A randomized clinical trial of intermittent subglottic secretion drainage in patients receiving mechanical ventilation. *Chest, 121*(3), 858-862.

Smyrnios, N. A., Connolly, A., Wilson, M. M., Curley, F. J., French, C. T., Heard, S. O., et al. (2002). Effects of a multifaceted, multidisciplinary, hospital-wide quality improvement program on weaning from mechanical ventilation. *Critical Care Medicine, 30*(6), 1224-1230.

Sole, M. L., Byers, J. F., Ludy, J. E., & Ostrow, C. L. (2002a). Suctioning techniques and airway management practices: Pilot study and instrument evaluation. *American Journal of Critical Care, 11*(4), 363-368.

Sole, M. L., Byers, J. F., Ludy, J. E., Zhang, Y., Banta, C. M., & Brummel, K. (2003). A multisite survey of suctioning techniques and airway management practices. *American Journal of Critical Care, 12*(3), 220-232.

Sole, M. L., Poalillo, F. E., Byers, J. F., & Ludy, J. E. (2002b). Bacterial growth in secretions and on suctioning equipment of orally intubated patients: a pilot study. *American Journal of Critical Care, 11*(2), 141-149.

St. John, R. E. (2003). End-tidal carbon dioxide monitoring. *Critical Care Nurse, 23*(4), 83-88.

St. John, R. E. (2004). Airway management. *Critical Care Nurse, 24*(2), 93-96.

Tamul, P. C., & Peruzzi, W. T. (2004). Assessment and management of patients with pulmonary disease. *Critical Care Medicine, 32*(4 Suppl.), S137-S145.

Thomas, L. A. (2003). Clinical management of stressors perceived by patients on mechanical ventilation. *AACN Clinical Issues, 14*(1), 73-81.

Twibell, R., Siela, D., & Mahmoodi, M. (2003). Subjective perceptions and physiological variables during weaning from mechanical ventilation. *American Journal of Critical Care, 12*(2), 101-112.

Urden, L., Stacy, K., & Lough, M. (2006). *Thelan's critical care nursing: Diagnosis and management* (5th ed.). St. Louis: Mosby.

Urtubia, R. M., Aguila, C. M., & Cumsille, M. A. (2000). Combitube: A study for proper use. *Anesthesia and Analgesia, 90*(4), 958-962.

Wiegand, D. L.-M. J., & Carlson, K. K. (2005). *AACN procedure manual for critical care* (5th ed.). Philadelphia: W. B. Saunders.

Wilkins, R. L., Stoller, J. K., & Scanlan, C. L. (2003). *Egan's fundamentals of respiratory care* (Vol. 8). St. Louis: Mosby.

Winters, A. C., & Munro, N. (2004). Assessment of the mechanically ventilated patient: An advanced practice approach. *AACN Clinical Issues, 15*(4), 525-533.

The Pulmonary System: Pathologic Conditions

CHAPTER 5

Chest Surgery and Chest Tubes

Surgical Procedures

1. Thoracotomy: opening into the thorax or pleural cavity
2. Exploratory thoracotomy: opening of the thorax in order to perform a biopsy or locate bleeding
3. Lobectomy: removal of one or more lobes of the lung
4. Segmental resection: removal of segment(s) of a lobe
5. Wedge resection: removal of a small peripheral section of the lung without regard to segments
6. Pneumonectomy: removal of an entire lung; indicated when tumor is centrally located at hilus or bronchus
7. Thoracoplasty: surgical collapse of a portion of chest wall by multiple rib resections to decrease volume in the hemithorax; may be used after pulmonary resection if lung cannot reexpand to fill thoracic space or after pneumonectomy: reduces the size of the thoracic cavity on the operative side and decreases the chance of mediastinal shift toward that side
8. Decortication of lung: removal of fibrinous membrane covering visceral and parietal pleura; used for recurrent spontaneous pneumothorax
9. Pleurodesis: process of fusing the two layers of the pleura through the use of agents (e.g., doxycycline, monocycline, or sterile talc) that cause a fibrotic reaction to prevent pleural fluid formation; used for recurrent malignant pleural effusion
10. Bullectomy: removal of cysts or bullae in lung
11. Reduction pneumoplasty (lung volume reduction surgery): resection of hyperinflated areas of lung to allow more normal function of diaphragm and expansion of more normal areas of the lung
12. Closed thoracostomy: insertion of chest tube through intercostal space (ICS) into pleural space; tube is connected to chest drainage system
13. Open thoracostomy: insertion of chest tube during rib resection; usually used in empyema when pleural space is fixed
14. Thymectomy: removal of the thymus; frequently performed for myasthenia gravis
15. Chest trauma surgery: repair of penetrating or nonpenetrating trauma; drainage of pleural cavity and control of hemorrhage
16. Removal of mediastinal masses: removal of cysts, tumors, abscesses from mediastinum
17. Tracheal resection: resection of a portion of the trachea with end-to-end anastomosis; removal of stenotic area of trachea or tumor
18. Esophagogastrectomy: resection of a part of the esophagus and upper portion of the stomach with end-to-end anastomosis; colon interposition using a portion of the large intestine may performed as an alternative to end-to-end anastomosis; for cancer of esophagus or corrosive esophagitis

Chest Tubes (Also Called *Thoracostomy Tube* or *Thoracic Catheter*)

1. Indications for chest tube drainage
   a. Pneumothorax: greater than 15% or on mechanical ventilator
   b. Hemothorax: greater than 500 mL
   c. Pneumohemothorax
      (1) Surgically induced during thoracotomy
      (2) Traumatic
   d. Pleural effusion
2. Purposes of chest tubes
   a. Pleural tubes
      (1) To remove free air: tube placed anterior and superior (usually at second ICS at midclavicular line [MCL]); pneumothorax: air in the pleural space
      (2) To drain the intrapleural space: tube placed lateral and inferior (usually at fifth or sixth ICS at midaxillary line)
         (a) Hemothorax: blood in the pleural space
         (b) Pleural effusion: liquid in the pleural space; may be transudate or exudate
            (i) Transudate: occurs if there is a rise in pulmonary venous pressure

(e.g., heart failure [HF]) or hypoproteinemia (e.g., malnutrition or cirrhosis); tends to accumulate at the base of the lungs

(ii) Exudate: occurs as a result of increased capillary permeability or impaired lymphatic absorption (e.g., involvement of the pleura by inflammation or malignancy); the fluid has a higher specific gravity and protein content than a transudate

(c) Empyema (also called *pyothorax*): pus in the pleural space

(d) Chylothorax: chyle (lymph fluid and triglyceride fat) in the pleural space

(e) Hydrothorax: water (e.g., IV fluid) in the pleural space

(3) To reestablish negative pressure in pleural space

b. Mediastinal tubes: to drain air and blood from the mediastinum after cardiac or other mediastinal surgery

3. Chest drainage system

a. Components

(1) Drainage collection bottle or chamber collects liquid drainage.

(2) Water-seal bottle or chamber provides a one-way valve to allow air to escape but does not allow atmospheric air to go into the pleural space.

(3) Suction control bottle or chamber controls the amount of suction.

b. Systems (Figure 5-1)

(1) Three-bottle system

(a) The drainage collection bottle is the bottle closest to the patient; this bottle is connected to the water-seal bottle.

(b) The water-seal bottle is filled so that the tube from the chest tube is submerged 2 cm under the water.

(c) The water-seal bottle must have a vent open at the top of the bottle to allow air to escape.

(d) The third bottle is the suction control bottle.

(i) It has one tube to connect it to the water-seal bottle.

(ii) Another tube connects it to the suction device (usually wall suction, but it may be a free-standing Emerson-type suction device).

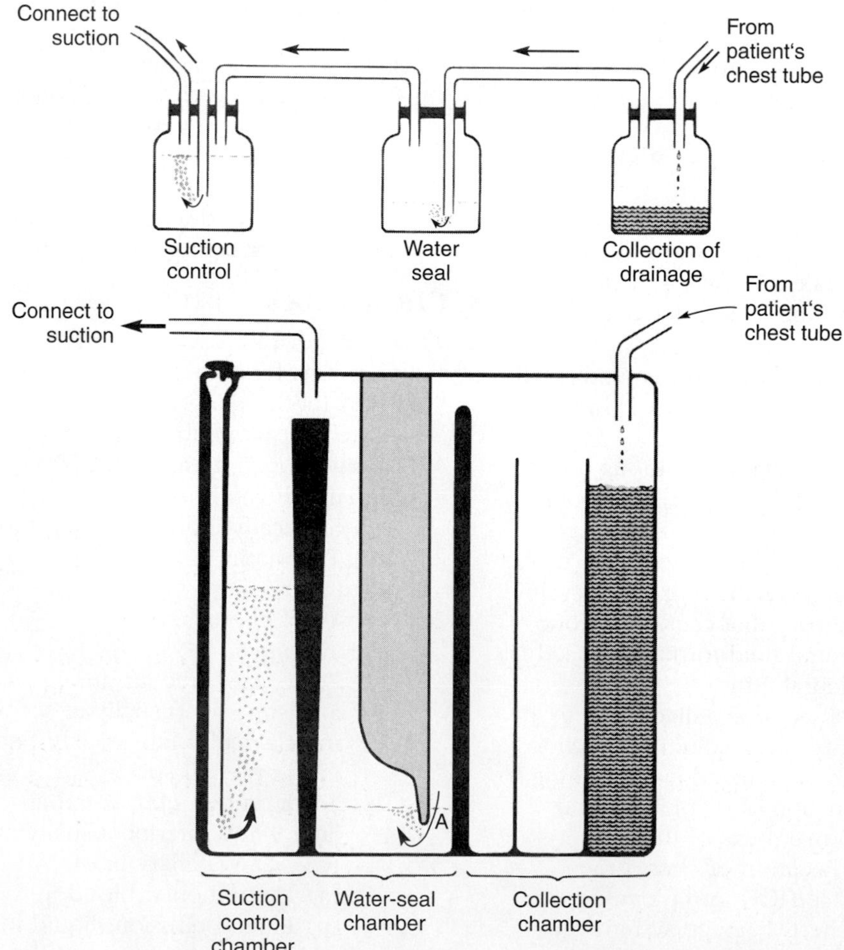

Figure 5-1 Comparison of a commercially available chest tube drainage system with a three-bottle system. (From Urden, L. D., Stacy, K. M., & Lough, M. E. [2006]. *Thelan's critical care nursing: Diagnosis and management* [5th ed.]. St. Louis, MO: Mosby.)

(iii) The third tube is submerged under water to the prescribed suction amount in centimeters of water (usually 20 cm H_2O); the other end of this tube is open to air.

(iv) Suction is adjusted so that a gentle bubbling occurs in this bottle.

a) Remember that vigorous bubbling just makes the water evaporate more quickly so that you must keep refilling it.

b) The actual amount of suction is determined by the depth that the tube is submersed minus the water-seal depth.

c) Suction is not necessary to remove air and free-flowing fluid; if the pleural air or liquid not does respond to gravity water-seal drainage, suction may be applied.

(2) All-in-one system

(a) More convenient

(b) Only the water-seal and drainage collection chambers may be used, or all three will be used if suction is desired.

(c) In a wet system (e.g., Atrium, Pleur-evac, Thora Seal, Aqua Seal, or Medi-Vac), adjust the amount of suction by filling the water level in the suction control chamber; adjust wall suction so that gentle bubbling occurs in the suction control chamber.

(i) Again, remember that the actual amount of suction is the height of the suction control chamber minus the height of the water-seal chamber.

(d) In a dry system (e.g., Sentinel Seal, Thora-Klex, Argyle Altitude, Pleur-evac Sahara, Atrium Oasis), adjust the amount of suction until the indicator appears.

(3) Portable chest drainage system (e.g., Atrium Express)

(a) Only one chamber to collect chest drainage

(b) Has a dry seal

(c) Usually used as a gravity drain only but may be used with suction; automatically regulated to −20 cm H_2O when connected to wall suction

(4) Heimlich valve (Figure 5-2)

(a) One-way valve that is used for uncomplicated pneumothorax with little or no liquid drainage

(i) May be connected to a small drainage bag to the valve but usually is not used if more than 50 mL of fluid

(ii) May be connected to wall suction (but is not usually)

(iii) Note fluttering of the valve as air escapes from the pleural space

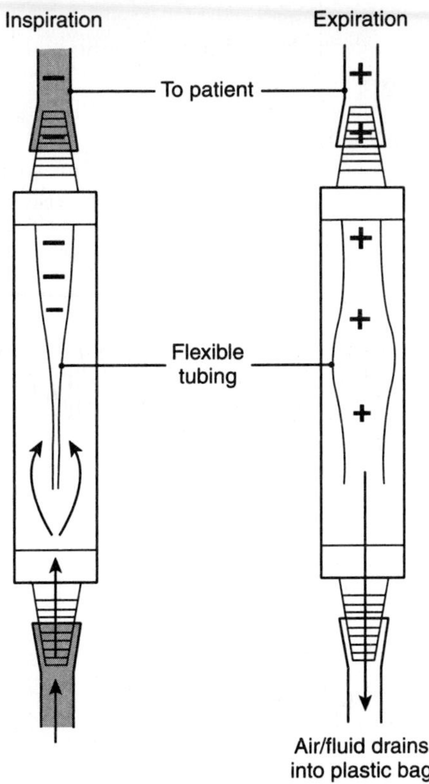

Figure 5-2 Heimlich one-way valve. **A,** During inspiration, negative pressure collapses the flexible tubing and prevents outside air from entering the pleural space. **B,** During expiration, positive pressure opens the flexible tubing and allows air and fluid to drain into an attached plastic bag. (From Kersten, L. D. [1989]. *Comprehensive respiratory nursing: A decision-making approach*. Philadelphia: W. B. Saunders.)

(b) Advantages: small, lightweight, and allows the patient to move around more easily; patient may be discharged with a chest tube attached to a Heimlich valve

4. Autotransfusion

a. Definition: the reinfusion of the patient's own blood; consists of collecting, filtering, and reinfusing the patient's own blood

b. Indications for autotransfusion of blood from a chest drainage system

(1) Chest trauma

(2) Chest surgery

(3) Consider autotransfusion if volume in chamber is 400 mL within 4 hours and hematocrit is less than 30%

c. Advantage: eliminates risk of potentially fatal transfusion reactions and transmission of blood-borne diseases

d. Contraindications

(1) Malignancy

(2) Sepsis

(3) Coagulopathies

(4) Contamination of blood with urine or feces

(5) Traumatic wounds more than 4 hours after injury

e. Method
   (1) Large-bore chest tube is connected to a closed drainage system.
   (2) The blood passes through a filter into a collection bag.
   (3) Collection bag may contain a preservative (usually citrate phosphate dextrose).
   (4) When filled, this bag is removed, inverted, and infused into the patient IV.
f. Complications
   (1) Disturbances in coagulation: thrombocytopenia; disseminated intravascular coagulopathy (DIC)
   (2) Acute renal failure caused by hemolysis and hemoglobinuria
   (3) Emboli
   (4) Sepsis
   (5) Spread of malignancy
   (6) Citrate toxicity: hypocalcemia

Assessment (Table 5-1)

Table 5-1 Assessment Parameters for the Patient with a Chest Tube

Parameter	Note
Patient	• Ventilatory effort • Chest discomfort or pain • Anxiety • Level of understanding • Cough • Sputum production
Breathing	• Rate • Regularity • Depth • Breath sounds (disconnection of suction from suction control chamber is required for accurate assessment of breath sounds)
Entry site	• Intactness of dressing • Drainage on dressing • Subcutaneous emphysema around insertion site
Tubing	• Tight, taped connections • Absence of kinks, compressions, or dependent loops
Drainage collection chamber	• Volume (normal 50-100 mL/hr for first few hours after thoracotomy and then 10-20 mL/hr) • Type: color; consistency; odor • Bottle below chest level
Water-seal chamber	• Filled to 2 cm or prescribed amount • Fluctuations with respirations (also referred to as *tidaling*) • Any bubbling • If not on suction, air vent open
Suction control chamber	• Filled to prescribed amount (usually −20 cm H_2O) • Gentle, continuous bubbling
Suction source	• If no control bottle, suction set at ordered level • If control bottle, suction set so that gentle, continuous bubbling occurs

Nursing Diagnoses

1. Ineffective Breathing Pattern related to incisional pain and inadequate lung expansion
2. Impaired Gas Exchange related to alveolar hypoventilation
3. Ineffective Airway Clearance related to retained secretion
4. Risk for Injury related to malfunctioning chest tube or chest drainage system
5. Risk for Infection related to surgical incision, trauma, invasive procedures, and poor airway clearance
6. Pain related to thoracic incision
7. Imbalanced Nutrition, Less than Body Requirements related to lack of exogenous nutrients and increased nutrient requirements
8. Activity Intolerance related to imbalance between oxygen supply and oxygen demand and pain
9. Anxiety related to acute change in health status
10. Anticipatory Grieving related to diagnosis of malignancy (if thoracotomy performed for lung cancer)

Collaborative Management

1. Control pain.
   a. Administer analgesics and/or local anesthetics as prescribed to relieve pain and encourage deep breathing.
      (1) IV analgesia: by regularly scheduled IV injection or by patient-controlled analgesia
      (2) Interpleural analgesia: local anesthetic (e.g., bupivacaine [Marcaine]) injected into pleural space during surgery; a new type of chest tube now available with injection port for periodic administration of lidocaine
      (3) Epidural analgesia: opiate and/or local anesthetic injected into epidural space
      (4) Nonsteroidal antiinflammatory agent (e.g., ketorolac [Toradol]) to augment the pain relief of narcotics
   b. Instruct the patient how to splint the chest when coughing; instruct the family how to assist.
2. Maintain airway patency and adequate oxygenation and ventilation.
   a. Position the patient for optimal ventilation/perfusion (V/Q) matching.
      (1) Elevate head of the bed (HOB) to 30 to 45 degrees.
      (2) "Good lung down" optimizes ventilation to encourage the reexpansion of the surgical lung and optimizes perfusion to the nonaffected "good" lung.
         (a) Exception: Pneumonectomy patients are positioned on their operative side or back.

b. Assess the position of the trachea; report immediately any shift from the normal midline.
c. Encourage deep breathing and use of the incentive spirometer.
   (1) Note that air is removed from the pleural space by the positive pressure of expiration and the negative pressure of suction on the chest tube; deep breathing is *important* in reexpansion of the lung.
d. Maintain airway clearance.
   (1) Encourage the patient to cough if indicated (e.g., rhonchi audible).
      (a) Routine coughing is not indicated because of the following:
         (i) Coughing is forceful expiration that actually may increase the risk of atelectasis.
         (ii) Coughing causes pain and may cause splinting and decrease in chest excursion and increase the risk of atelectasis.
      (b) Focus on sustained inspiration maneuver; this frequently stimulates the patient to cough if coughing is needed.
   (2) Suction only if the patient is unable to clear secretions.
      (a) Use caution when suctioning the patient because leakage from the bronchial stump may occur (especially with pneumonectomy patients).
e. Administer bronchodilators as prescribed.
f. Prevent gastric distention; gastric suction may be required.
g. Administer oxygen as indicated by arterial blood gases and functional oxygen saturation (SpO_2).
h. Assist with weaning from mechanical ventilation and extubation as soon as possible because positive pressure ventilation increases risk of air leak.

3. Maintain water-seal drainage system and patency of chest tubes.
   a. Assess chest drainage system hourly.
      (1) Ensure that connections are spiral taped.
      (2) Position tubing to prevent kinks and dependent loops.
      (3) Maintain suction level at prescribed level; water may need to be added to the suction control chamber because water evaporates in wet chest drainage systems.
      (4) Assess the water-seal chamber for fluctuation with ventilation (also referred to as *tidaling*); lack of fluctuation may be caused by any of the following:
         (a) The lung is reexpanded; confirm by assessment of chest x-ray.
         (b) The tube is kinked; follow the tube from chest to chest drainage system and position tube to prevent kinking.
         (c) The tube is occluded.
            (i) The risk of an occluded tube, especially in a patient on mechanical ventilation, is tension pneumothorax, mediastinal shift, and potential tearing of great vessels.
            (ii) Though routine milking or stripping is not recommended, make efforts to reestablish patency of an occluded tube (and prevent tension pneumothorax).
               a) Milk the tube first; if unsuccessful in reestablishing fluctuation in the water-seal chamber, strip short sections.
                  i) Milking is hand-over-hand squeezing of the chest tube; stripping is to clamp with the thumb and forefinger of the nondominant hand while pulling the tube between the thumb and forefinger of the dominant hand followed by release of the thumb and forefinger of the nondominant hand.
                  ii) Milking and stripping of chest tubes create negative pressure within the pleural space; although these may help to move a clot along, they may create trauma to the pleura.
               b) If milking or stripping of short sections is unsuccessful in reestablishing fluctuation in the water-seal chamber, notify the physician; a new tube may be required.
      (5) Assess for air leak and differentiate between expected removal of air from pleural space (occasional bubble) and a break in the chest tube system.
         (a) An occasional bubble indicates that the tube is still needed because air is still escaping from the pleural space.
         (b) Excessive bubbling indicates the need to search for a leak in the system.
            (i) Brief clamping with hemostats moving from the chest drainage system to the insertion site can be helpful in identifying the location of the leak.
            (ii) Ensure that all connections are connected and spiral taped.
            (iii) Assess the insertion site for displacement of the tube so that the proximal eyelet is outside the skin; notify the physician so that the tube can be repositioned.
            (iv) Suspect bronchopleural fistula if no external air leak can be identified.
   b. Keep the chest drainage system lower than the patient's chest.

c. Avoid intentionally occluding (e.g., clamping) the tube.
   (1) Clamp the tube only if one of the following occurs:
      (a) The chest drainage system must be lifted above the level of the chest (e.g., putting patient in helicopter for transport) so that chest drainage does not drain back into the pleural space; clamp as briefly as possible
         (i) NOTE: Heimlich valves or portable chest drainage systems (gravity drainage) frequently are used for transports.
      (b) If the drainage collection is full (e.g., large pleural effusions), have the new chest drainage system ready and clamp as briefly as possible while connecting the chest tube to the new chest drainage system
      (c) If specifically instructed to do so by the physician before chest tube removal
         (i) This is done to see whether the patient is likely to tolerate not having the chest tube.
         (ii) Monitor patient closely for clinical indications of tension pneumothorax.
   (2) If there has been a significant air leak and the chest drainage system breaks, submerse the tube about 2 cm into a bottle of sterile water or sterile saline; if a bottle of sterile water or saline is not available, put tap water into a clean Styrofoam cup and submerse the tube about 2 cm into the cup
      (a) NOTE: The patient is better off with an open pneumothorax than a tension pneumothorax.
   (3) If there has been a significant air leak and the tube accidentally comes out of the chest, apply a dressing to the chest with your hand or tape it on three sides (i.e., as you would for a sucking chest wound) and notify the physician immediately.

4. Monitor for common complications.
   a. Hemorrhage/shock
      (1) Replace blood and fluid volume as prescribed; thoracic surgery patients generally receive less fluid than nonthoracic surgery patients in the early postoperative period to prevent acute respiratory distress syndrome (ARDS) and pulmonary edema.
      (2) Monitor patient for clinical indications of hypoperfusion (Table 2-2).
   b. Infection
      (1) Use sterile technique while dressing the insertion site, setting up the chest drainage system, and replacing the system.
      (2) Monitor patient for fever and other clinical indications of infection.
      (3) Assess the incision and the chest tube insertion site for redness, induration, and drainage; culture drainage if purulent.
      (4) Monitor sputum and chest drainage for signs of infection; culture as necessary.
      (5) Administer antibiotics as prescribed.
   c. Tension pneumothorax
      (1) Maintain patency of the chest tube and functioning of chest drainage system.
      (2) Avoid clamping chest tube except for reasons identified previously.
      (3) Monitor for clinical indications of tension pneumothorax: dyspnea; chest pain; tracheal shift away from affected side; hyperresonance to percussion; decreased breath sounds on affected side.
   d. Dysrhythmias: especially atrial dysrhythmias
      (1) Most likely in patients having pneumonectomy; prophylactic antidysrhythmics may be initiated preoperatively
   e. Pulmonary edema: related to capillary leak and pulmonary hypertension
      (1) Use caution with fluid administration.
      (2) Hemodynamic monitoring may be necessary.
   f. ARDS: devastating after pneumonectomy
      (1) Monitor for changes in ventilatory effort and Spo_2.
   g. Pulmonary embolism (PE)
      (1) Have patient sit on edge of bed the evening of surgery, get out of bed into a chair within 24 to 36 hours, and ambulate as soon as possible until contraindicated by hemodynamic instability.
   h. Bronchopleural fistula: usually related to empyema
      (1) Very small tidal volumes used with mechanical ventilation (e.g., high-frequency jet ventilation)
   i. Empyema
      (1) Treat infection.
   j. Frozen shoulder: impairment in shoulder mobility
      (1) Encourage range of motion to shoulder on operative side.
      (2) Administer analgesics to allow movement.
      (3) Encourage use of arm for self-care activities.

5. Assist with removal of chest tube: usually removed when there has been no air leak from anterior tube or less than 100 mL per 24 hours for posterior tube.
   a. Clamp tube for up to 24 hours before removal as requested.
   b. Administer analgesics before chest tube removal; music also may be helpful.
      (1) Recommended analgesics include the following:
         (a) Ketorolac (Toradol) 30 mg IV 60 minutes before
         (b) Morphine 4 mg IV 20 minutes before
   c. Instruct the patient to hold his or her breath when requested.
      (1) There is no difference in the rate of post–chest tube removal pneumothoraces using either end-inspiration or end-expiration (Bell, Ovadia, Abdullah, Spector, & Rabinovici, 2001)

d. Apply occlusive dressing after the physician removes the tube at the end of expiration.
e. Monitor the patient for clinical indications of recurrent pneumothorax: dyspnea, chest pain, asymmetric chest excursion, and diminished breath sounds.

Acute Respiratory Failure

Definitions

1. Acute respiratory failure: failure of the respiratory system to provide for the exchange of oxygen and carbon dioxide between the environment and tissues in quantities sufficient to sustain life
   a. Hypoxemic normocapnic respiratory failure (type I): low Pao_2 with normal $Paco_2$
   b. Hypoxemic hypercapnic respiratory failure (type II): low Pao_2 with high $Paco_2$
2. Chronic obstructive pulmonary disease (COPD) with acute exacerbation: acute process in a patient with a chronic condition; usually caused by respiratory infection
   a. COPD: a disease state characterized by the presence of airflow obstruction caused by chronic bronchitis or emphysema; the airflow obstruction is progressive, may be accompanied by airway hyperactivity, and may be partially reversible (American Thoracic Society)
      (1) Chronic bronchitis: defined clinically by excessive mucus secretion in the bronchi
      (2) Emphysema: defined pathophysiologically by enlargement of the air spaces distal to the terminal bronchioles with destruction of alveolar walls
   b. Acute exacerbation of COPD: worsening dyspnea, increase in sputum volume, and increase in sputum purulence

Etiology

1. Type I respiratory failure
   a. Pneumonia
   b. Pulmonary edema
   c. Pulmonary fibrosis
   d. Pleural effusion
   e. Pneumothorax
   f. Asthma
   g. Atelectasis
   h. Aspiration pneumonitis
   i. ARDS (early)
   j. Smoke inhalation
   k. PE
   l. Kyphoscoliosis
   m. Fat embolism
2. Type II respiratory failure (may also be called *acute ventilatory failure*)
   a. COPD with acute exacerbation
   b. Status asthmaticus
   c. Central nervous system (CNS) depressant drugs
   d. Anesthesia
   e. Neuromuscular blocking drugs
      (1) Muscle paralytics
      (2) Aminoglycosides
      (3) Organophosphate poisoning
   f. Head trauma
   g. Poliomyelitis
   h. Amyotrophic lateral sclerosis
   i. Spinal cord injury
   j. Guillain-Barré syndrome
   k. Myasthenia gravis
   l. Multiple sclerosis
   m. Muscular dystrophy
   n. Morbid obesity
   o. Chest trauma
   p. Surgery: especially thoracic, abdominal, flank incision
   q. Sleep apnea
   r. Tracheal obstruction
   s. Epiglottis
   t. Cystic fibrosis
   u. Near drowning

Pathophysiology (Table 5-2)

1. Hypoventilation
2. V/Q mismatching
3. Shunting
4. Diffusion defects

Clinical Presentation

1. Subjective
   a. History of precipitating factor
   b. Clinical indications of respiratory distress (Box 4-2)
   c. Clinical indications of hypoxia (Box 4-3)
   d. Clinical indications of hypercapnia (Box 4-4)
2. Objective
   a. Clinical indications of respiratory distress (Box 4-2)
   b. Hypoxemia: decrease in Spo_2, arterial oxygen saturation (Sao_2), Pao_2
   c. Clinical indications of hypoxia (Box 4-3)
   d. Clinical indications of hypercapnia (Box 4-4)
3. Diagnostic
   a. Arterial blood gas (ABG) changes
      (1) Pao_2 less than 50 to 60 mm Hg
      (2) $Paco_2$ greater than 50 mm Hg with a pH of less than 7.3
   b. Chest x-ray: may identify cause

Nursing Diagnoses

1. Impaired Gas Exchange related to V/Q mismatching and intrapulmonary shunt
2. Ineffective Breathing Pattern related to increased work of breathing and fatigue
3. Ineffective Airway Clearance related to retained secretion
4. Risk for Infection related to invasive procedures and poor airway clearance

Table 5-2 Mechanisms of Hypoxemia

Mechanism	Pathophysiology	Etiology	Diagnosis	Treatment
Hypoventilation	Hypoventilation causes carbon dioxide retention and hypoxemia	Damage to/depression of the neurologic control of ventilation: • Head injury • Cerebral thrombosis or hemorrhage • CNS system depressant drugs • Oxygen-induced hypoventilation Neuromuscular defects in the ventilatory mechanism: • Myasthenia gravis • Multiple sclerosis • Muscular dystrophy • Guillain-Barré syndrome • Poliomyelitis • Spinal cord injuries • Botulism • Tetanus • Neuromuscular blocking drugs Obstructive lung conditions • Asthma • Chronic bronchitis • Emphysema • Airway obstruction • Cystic fibrosis Restrictive lung conditions • Kyphoscoliosis • Obesity hypoventilation syndrome • Recent thoracic, abdominal, or flank incision • Lung cancer • Flail chest • Pleural effusion • Pneumothorax	• Physical examination ◦ Neurologic status may be altered ◦ Abnormal chest wall motion ◦ Abnormal breath sounds ◦ Clinical indications of hypoxemia or hypercapnia • ABGs: hypoxemia with increased $Pa{CO_2}$ and normal A:a gradient • May have abnormal chest x-ray and PFTs	• Improve oxygenation by increasing alveolar ventilation (e.g., positioning, bronchial hygiene, and drug therapy) • Specific therapy depends on the specific etiology
V/Q mismatching	• Low V/Q units, with perfusion in excess of ventilation, result in hypoxemia because the blood traversing these alveolar units is not fully oxygenated • High V/Q units, with ventilation in excess of perfusion, result in oxygenated alveolar units that are not perfused	Regional ventilation abnormalities • Asthma • Chronic bronchitis • Emphysema • Atelectasis • Pneumonia • Bronchospasm • Mucous plugs • Foreign bodies • Tumor Regional perfusion abnormalities • PE	• Physical examination ◦ Abnormal chest wall motion ◦ Abnormal breath sounds ◦ Clinical indications of hypoxemia • ABGs: hypoxemia with a widened A:a gradient; $Pa{CO_2}$ dependent on ventilation status • Abnormal chest x-ray PFTs, and/or V/Q scan	• Oxygen ◦ Specific therapy depends on the specific etiology

Table 5-2 Mechanisms of Hypoxemia—cont'd

Mechanism	Pathophysiology	Etiology	Diagnosis	Treatment
		• Decreased cardiac output/index • Excessive (PEEP)		
Shunt	Blood transverses from the right side of the heart to the left side of the heart without being oxygenated: anatomic shunt is when the blood bypasses the alveolar-capillary unit, and physiologic shunt is when the blood goes through the alveolar-capillary unit but it is nonfunctional	Anatomic shunts • Normal anatomic shunts: bronchial, pleural, thebesian veins • Intrapulmonary shunts: pulmonary (AV) fistula • Intracardiac shunts: tetralogy of Fallot • Other pathologic shunts (e.g., shunts associated with neoplasms) Physiologic shunts • Alveolar collapse ◦ Atelectasis ◦ Pneumothorax ◦ Hemothorax ◦ Pleural effusion • Alveoli filled with a fluid or foreign material ◦ Cardiac pulmonary edema ◦ Noncardiac pulmonary edema (e.g., near drowning and ARDS) ◦ Pneumonias	• Physical examination ◦ Abnormal breath sounds ◦ Clinical indications of hypoxemia • ABGs: hypoxemia with a normal or decreased $Paco_2$ ◦ Widened A:a gradient ◦ Shunt greater than 6% • May have abnormal chest x-ray and PFTs	• Oxygen administration has little or no effect • Specific therapy depends on the specific etiology • PEEP frequently is used for physiologic shunt
Diffusion abnormalities	• Increased diffusion pathway: diffusion between alveolar oxygen and pulmonary capillary blood is impaired; blood exiting the gas exchange unit is hypoxemic • Decreased diffusion area: decrease in alveolar-capillary membrane surface area available for diffusion and/or loss of pulmonary capillary bed	Increased diffusion pathway • Accumulation of fluid • Pulmonary edema: cardiac or noncardiac • Accumulation of collagen in the pulmonary interstitium • Pulmonary fibrosis • Sarcoidosis • Collagen-vascular Decreased diffusion area • Pulmonary resection such as lobectomy or pneumonectomy • Destructive lung diseases ◦ Emphysema ◦ Tumor ◦ Obliterative pulmonary vascular diseases	• History and physical exam findings are compatible with the diagnosis • ABGs: hypoxemia with normal or low $Paco_2$ ◦ Widened A:a gradient ◦ Further decrease in Pao_2 with exercise • PFTs: decreased diffusing capacity for cardiac output • Chest x-ray may show cause	• Oxygen • Home oxygen therapy frequently is indicated

5. Imbalanced Nutrition, Less than Body Requirements related to lack of exogenous nutrients and increased nutrient requirements
6. Activity Intolerance related to imbalance between oxygen supply and oxygen demand
7. Anxiety related to change in health status

Collaborative Management

1. Treat the cause.
2. Maintain patent airway and optimal ventilation.
   a. Position the patient for optimal ventilation.
      (1) HOB to 30 to 45 degrees
      (2) Overbed table for patient to lean on
      (3) "Good lung down" if unilateral lung condition exists
      (4) Prone position especially in ARDS
   b. Maintain adequate hydration: usually 2 to 3 L per 24 hours unless contraindicated by cardiac or renal disease.
      (1) Oral fluids: noncaffeinated
      (2) IV fluids: usually 5% dextrose in normal saline (D_5NS)
   c. Provide bronchial hygiene and chest physiotherapy as indicated.
      (1) Inspiratory maneuvers: deep breathing; incentive spirometry
      (2) Analgesics in doses adequate to allow patient to deep breathe and cough as indicated
      (3) Encouragement of the patient to cough if rhonchi are audible; suction secretions if the patient is unable to clear airways
      (4) Postural drainage, percussion, and vibration may be necessary
      (5) Bronchoscopy may be necessary if airway clearance techniques are inadequate
      (6) Intubation and mechanical ventilation may be necessary if $Paco_2$ continues to rise and acidosis develops
         (a) The goal of mechanical ventilation is to normalize the pH, not necessarily the $Paco_2$.
         (b) Normalization of the $Paco_2$ is not appropriate in patients with COPD and chronic hypercapnia (this causes metabolic alkalosis, eventual excretion of sodium bicarbonate, and weaning difficulties).
   d. Administer appropriate drug therapy.
      (1) Bronchodilators may be indicated
         (a) $Beta_2$-adrenergic agonists (these agents are preferred over nonrespiratory-selective beta stimulants such as epinephrine and isoproterenol because they cause fewer cardiovascular side effects)
            (i) Terbutaline (Brethine)
            (ii) Albuterol (Proventil)
            (iii) Isoetharine HCl (Bronkosol)
            (iv) Metaproterenol (Alupent)
         (b) Parasympatholytics (e.g., ipratropium [Atrovent])
         (c) Xanthines (e.g., aminophylline or theophylline)
         (d) Magnesium
      (2) Expectorants (e.g., guaifenesin [Robitussin] or potassium iodide [SSKI]) may be used, but hydration is most important)
      (3) Mucolytics (e.g., acetylcysteine [Mucomyst]) may be used to decrease the tenacity of the mucus; frequently causes bronchospasm and so is given with a bronchodilator
      (4) Sedatives: generally avoided unless patient is very agitated
      (5) Antitussives: avoid use of antitussives unless nonproductive cough is causing patient fatigue
3. Optimize oxygen delivery and decrease oxygen consumption.
   a. Administer oxygen as indicated for hypoxemia.
      (1) Nasal cannula or mask; masks are contraindicated in hypercapnic patients because the high concentration of oxygen provided by these delivery systems likely would eliminate the hypoxic drive
      (2) Flow rate or oxygen concentration to keep Spo_2 approximately 95% unless contraindicated; in patients with chronic hypercapnia, adjust flow rate or oxygen concentration to keep Spo_2 approximately 90%
   b. Use PEEP as necessary to maintain adequate Sao_2 and Pao_2.
   c. Ensure rest periods especially after meals or activities.
   d. Provide a quiet, restful environment.
   e. Treat fever (controversial because pyrogens are helpful in mobilizing the immune system).
      (1) Antipyretics (e.g., acetaminophen [Tylenol])
      (2) Cooling blankets may be used, but shivering should be avoided because of the effect on oxygen consumption
   f. Improve delivery of oxygen to the tissues.
      (1) Improve Sao_2: oxygen or PEEP as required.
      (2) Improve cardiac index (CI): for example, fluid administration, inotropes, intraaortic balloon pump, or vasoactive agents as required.
      (3) Increase hemoglobin: packed red blood cells as required.
      (4) Use extracorporeal membrane oxygenator as indicated and available: viewed primarily as a rescue therapy when other therapies have failed.
4. Treat infection if present.
   a. Administer antimicrobials as indicated: empirically or specific to cultured microorganism.
   b. Use bronchial hygiene techniques.
5. Monitor for and prevent complications.
   a. Dysrhythmias
   b. Pulmonary infections: pneumonia
   c. Pulmonary edema

d. PE
e. Barotrauma (e.g., pneumothorax)
f. Pulmonary fibrosis
g. Oxygen toxicity
h. Renal failure
i. Acid-base imbalance
   (1) Respiratory acidosis
   (2) Respiratory alkalosis occurs in patients with chronic hypercapnia when $PaCO_2$ is normalized rather than the pH because of long-term renal retention of bicarbonate
j. Electrolyte imbalance
k. Gastrointestinal (GI) complications: abdominal distention; ileus; ulcer; hemorrhage
l. Thromboembolism
m. DIC
n. Sepsis; septic shock
o. Psychological responses: psychosis; depression

Acute Respiratory Distress Syndrome

Definitions

1. Acute lung injury
   a. A syndrome of lung inflammation and increased alveolar-capillary permeability characterized by hypoxemia resistant to oxygen therapy
   b. The less severe end of the spectrum of the pulmonary component of systemic inflammatory response syndrome (SIRS)
   c. PaO_2/fraction of inspired oxygen (FIO_2) ratio less than 300 mm Hg
2. ARDS
   a. A syndrome of acute respiratory failure characterized by noncardiac pulmonary edema and manifested by refractory hypoxemia caused by intrapulmonary shunt
   b. May be considered the severe end of the spectrum of the pulmonary component of SIRS
   c. PaO_2/FIO_2 ratio less than or equal to 200 mm Hg
   d. Synonyms: shock lung, pump lung (postperfusion lung), Da Nang lung, wet lung, posttraumatic lung, respirator lung, congestive atelectasis, pulmonary fat embolism syndrome, alveolar-capillary leak syndrome, noncardiac pulmonary edema

Etiology

Risk increases if more than one of the following occurs simultaneously.

1. Direct injury
   a. Chest trauma: pulmonary contusion
   b. Near drowning
   c. Hypervolemia, pulmonary edema
   d. Inhalation of toxic gases and vapors
      (1) Smoke
      (2) Chemicals
      (3) Oxygen toxicity
   e. Pneumonia: viral, bacterial, or fungal
   f. Aspiration pneumonitis
   g. Radiation pneumonitis
   h. PE: particularly fat or amniotic fluid
   i. Radiation
   j. Drugs: bleomycin
2. Indirect injury
   a. Sepsis: most likely cause
   b. Shock or prolonged hypotension
      (1) Septic shock
      (2) Hypovolemic shock
      (3) Cardiogenic shock
      (4) Anaphylactic shock
      (5) Neurogenic shock
   c. Multisystem trauma, especially multiple fractures
   d. Burns
   e. Cardiopulmonary bypass
   f. DIC
   g. Toxemia of pregnancy
   h. Acute pancreatitis
   i. Diabetic coma
   j. CNS injury
   k. Drug overdosage: heroin; methadone; barbiturates; aspirin; thiazide diuretics
   l. Blood transfusion
   m. Abdominal trauma

Pathophysiology

1. Initial injury
   a. Direct or indirect injury to the lung
   b. Acute lung injury reduces normal perfusion to the lungs, causing platelet aggregation and stimulation of the inflammatory-immune system
      (1) Activation of the classical cascade systems: complement, kallikrein-kinin, coagulation, fibrinolysis
      (2) Activation of the cellular systems: neutrophils, macrophages, monocytes, mast cells, endothelial cells, fibroblasts
      (3) Activation of the final mediator systems: proteases, oxygen radicals, eicosanoids
   c. These mediators activate or stimulate neutrophils, macrophages, and other cells to release toxic substances that cause microvascular injury
2. Early exudative phase: days 1 to 3
   a. Acute and diffuse injury to endothelium and epithelium surface of lung
   b. Damage to alveolar-capillary membrane and increase in capillary permeability
   c. Capillary leak allows proteins and fluids to spill into the interstitium and alveolar spaces; pulmonary lymphatic drainage capacity is overwhelmed and alveolar flooding occurs
   d. Pulmonary edema results and causes interference with oxygen diffusion and inactivation of surfactant; damage to type II pneumocytes results in decreased production of surfactant
      (1) Hyaline membranes are formed (probably from transudated plasma proteins) that increase the thickness of the alveolar-capillary

membrane and therefore the diffusion pathway
   (2) Alveolar collapse and massive atelectasis occur that decrease functional residual capacity and lung compliance
  e. Profound hypoxemia occurs related to extensive intrapulmonary shunting
  f. Vasoconstrictive mediators cause increased pulmonary vasoconstriction and pulmonary hypertension
3. Intermediate proliferative phase: days 3 to 10
  a. Type I pneumocytes are destroyed and replaced by type II pneumocytes, which proliferate
  b. Interstitial space expands by edema fluid, fibers, and proliferating fibroblasts
  c. Continuing decrease in lung compliance and increasing alveolar dead space
4. Late fibrotic phase: beyond day 10
  a. Cellular alveolar infiltrates resolve
  b. Interstitial collagen deposition
  c. Pulmonary fibrosis may occur
  d. Hypertrophy of the right ventricle may occur

Clinical Presentation

1. Phases of ARDS (Table 5-3)
2. Criteria used in ARDS diagnosis
  a. Presence of a predisposing condition
  b. Severe oxygenation defect: hypoxemia is the hallmark of ARDS
   (1) Pao_2 less than 60 mm Hg on Fio_2 greater than 0.5
   (2) Pao_2/Fio_2 ratio less than or equal to 200 mm Hg
  c. Chest x-ray: diffuse bilateral parenchymal infiltrates
  d. Static compliance: significantly less than the normal of 50 to 100 mL/cm H_2O (usually 15 to 25 mL/cm H_2O)
  e. Pulmonary artery occlusive pressure (PAOP): less than 18 mm Hg
  f. No other explanation for the foregoing findings
3. Recommended criteria for acute lung injury and ARDS: American-European Consensus Conference on ARDS (1992) (Table 5-4)
4. Hemodynamic parameters
  a. PAOP differentiates cardiac from noncardiac pulmonary edema
   (1) ARDS (noncardiac pulmonary edema) causes elevated pulmonary artery pressure (PAP) with normal PAOP
   (2) Cardiac pulmonary edema causes elevated PAP and PAOP
  b. Pulmonary vascular resistance (PVR) is increased

Table 5-3 Phases of Acute Respiratory Distress Syndrome

Parameter	Phase I	Phase II	Phase III	Phase IV
Heart rate	Tachycardia	Tachycardia	Tachycardia	Bradycardia
Cardiac index	Normal	Increased	Increased	Decreased
Tidal volume/minute ventilation	Increased	Increased	Normal or decreased	Decreased
$Paco_2$	Decreased	Decreased	Normal or increased	Increased
Acid-base	Respiratory alkalosis	Respiratory alkalosis	Metabolic (and possibly respiratory) acidosis	Respiratory and metabolic acidosis
Pao_2 on room air	Normal	Normal or slightly decreased (~60 mm Hg)	Significantly decreased (~40 mm Hg)	Severely decreased (~25 mm Hg)
Shunt	Less than 6%	10%	20%	Greater than 30%
Compliance	Normal	Slightly decreased	Moderately decreased	Severely decreased
Pulmonary clinical manifestations	Dyspnea	Dyspnea; fatigue; retractions	Dyspnea; fatigue; retractions; cyanosis	Dyspnea; fatigue (may have had respiratory arrest); cyanosis; rusty sputum
Breath sounds	Clear	Fine crackles	Coarse crackles and/or wheezes	Crackles, rhonchi, and/or wheezes
Chest x-ray	Normal	Patchy infiltrates usually in dependent areas	Diffuse infiltrates	Consolidation
Other signs/ symptoms	Tachycardia	Tachycardia	Tachycardia; dysrhythmias; decreasing sensorium	Bradycardia; dysrhythmias; hypotension; decreasing sensorium

Table 5-4 Hemodynamic Parameters

	Onset	Oxygenation: Pao_2/Fio_2 Ratio	Frontal Chest X-Ray	PAOP
Acute lung injury	Acute	Less than 300 mm Hg (regardless of PEEP)	Bilateral infiltrates	Less than 18 mm Hg or no clinical evidence of left atrial enlargement
ARDS	Acute	Less than or equal to 200 mm Hg (regardless of PEEP)	Bilateral infiltrates	Less than 18 mm Hg or no clinical evidence of left atrial enlargement

Fio_2, Fraction of inspired oxygen; *PEEP*, positive end-expiratory pressure; *PAOP*, pulmonary artery occlusive pressure; *ARDS*, acute respiratory distress syndrome.

5. Diagnostic
   a. May give clues to cause
   b. ABGs (see Table 5-3): refractory hypoxemia (hypoxemia despite high concentration of oxygen); Pao_2 of less than 60 mm Hg despite Fio_2 0.5 or greater for 24 hours
   c. Sputum analysis: tracheal protein/plasma protein ratio greater than 0.7 (cardiac pulmonary edema less than 0.5)
   d. Pulmonary function studies
      (1) Lung volumes decreased: tidal volume; vital capacity
      (2) Functional residual capacity decreased
      (3) Static and dynamic compliance decreased
   e. Chest x-ray
      (1) May be normal initially
      (2) Bilateral diffuse interstitial and alveolar infiltrates
      (3) Ground glass appearance
      (4) "Whiteout" caused by massive atelectasis
      (5) Heart size is normal (one factor that differentiates ARDS from cardiac pulmonary edema)
   f. Computed tomography (CT) of thorax
      (1) Gravity-dependent infiltrates
      (2) Lack of homogeneity of infiltrates
   g. Bronchoalveolar lavage: prevalent polymorphonuclear leukocytes

Nursing Diagnoses

1. Impaired Gas Exchange related to V/Q mismatching and intrapulmonary shunt
2. Ineffective Breathing Pattern related to reduced lung compliance, increased work of breathing and fatigue, and anxiety
3. Ineffective Airway Clearance related to fatigue, altered consciousness, and increased pulmonary secretions
4. Decreased Cardiac Output related to decreased preload caused by positive pressure mechanical ventilation and PEEP
5. Risk for Infection related to invasive procedures and poor airway clearance
6. Imbalanced Nutrition: Less than Body Requirements related to lack of exogenous nutrients, increased nutrient requirements
7. Activity Intolerance related to imbalance between oxygen supply and oxygen demand
8. Anxiety related to change in health status

Collaborative Patient Management

1. Prevent acute lung injury (ALI)/ARDS or detect ALI/ARDS as early as possible.
   a. Use standard infection control measures (sepsis is the most common etiology).
   b. Treat precipitating factors (e.g., antimicrobials if infection is present).
   c. Provide nutritional support.
      (1) Enteral feeding preferred
         (a) Effects of enteral nutritional support significant to ARDS, SIRS, and multiple organ dysfunction syndrome (MODS)
            (i) Prevents villous atrophy and increases blood flow to the GI tract
            (ii) Retards transmigration (translocation) of bacteria or lipopolysaccharides that play a significant role in sepsis and MODS
         (b) Orogastric feeding tube or percutaneous endoscopic gastroscopy tube is preferred in order to avoid the complications of nasogastric tube, such as sinusitis and epistaxis
      (2) Parenteral nutrition if enteral feeding is contraindicated
         (a) Selective decontamination of digestive tract may be used in patients who cannot be fed enterally to prevent bacterial translocation from the GI tract
   d. Monitor patients at high risk for ALI/ARDS closely.
      (1) Assess patient for indications of respiratory distress (e.g., tachypnea or use of accessory muscles).
      (2) Monitor pulse oximetry for drop in Spo_2.
      (3) Monitor static and dynamic compliance in patients on a mechanical ventilator.
2. Maintain airway, oxygenation, and ventilation; the goal is to maintain acceptable oxygenation (arterial oxygen saturation [Sao_2] of at least 90%) with nontoxic

FiO_2 levels (less than 60%) and acceptable plateau pressures (30 cm H_2O).

a. Position the patient for optimal ventilation.
   (1) Elevate HOB to 30 to 45 degrees.
   (2) Turn the patient every 2 hours; kinetic therapy with 60 degrees of lateral rotation may be used.
   (3) Position the patient in prone or semiprone position periodically (NOTE: Recommended frequency has not been established, but the patient is likely to be kept prone for 4 to 8 hours with frequent repositioning to reduce pressure injury).
b. Provide bronchial hygiene and chest physiotherapy as indicated.
   (1) Encourage the patient to cough and/or use suction as indicated.
   (2) Chest physiotherapy may be indicated.
c. Administer oxygen as indicated.
   (1) May require high concentrations (up to 100%) with non-rebreathing mask before intubation and mechanical ventilation
   (2) FiO_2 should be maintained as low as possible to prevent oxygen toxicity; positive pressure (continuous positive airway pressure [CPAP] or PEEP) will increase driving pressure, allowing the use of a lower FiO_2 to maintain an acceptable oxygenation (e.g., PaO_2 60 mm Hg; SaO_2 of 90%)
      (a) CPAP may be administered via mask before intubation
      (b) Mechanical ventilation with PEEP sedation and/or muscle paralysis may be necessary to maintain PEEP
      (c) NOTE: These patients are usually dependent on PEEP and will quickly desaturate when PEEP is discontinued temporarily; use a closed suction system or PEEP valve on a manual resuscitation bag before and after suctioning.
d. Ensure adequate ventilation.
   (1) Noninvasive positive pressure ventilation (e.g., pressure support ventilation [PSV] or biphasic positive airway pressure [bi-PAP]) with face mask before need for intubation as prescribed
   (2) Endotracheal intubation: indicated to deliver mechanical ventilation and PEEP when FiO_2 greater than 0.5 is required to maintain acceptable oxygenation or as patient fatigues
   (3) Mechanical ventilation to maintain adequate ventilation and oxygenation while preventing ventilation-induced lung injury (VILI)
      (a) Modes: pressure controlled/inverse ratio ventilation, pressure-regulated volume-controlled ventilation, airway pressure release ventilation, or high-frequency ventilation may be used
      (b) Tidal volume: limitation of peak inspiratory pressure and reduction of regional lung overdistention by the use of low tidal volumes with permissive hypercapnia may reduce VILI and improve outcome in severe ARDS
         (i) Tidal volume at 4 to 8 mL/kg (~6 mL/kg) of ideal body weight (IBW)
            a) Large tidal volumes are avoided because the ARDS lung is like a "baby lung" and large tidal volumes have been shown to cause increased alveolar edema and worsening of lung injury; large tidal volumes cause more injury than high pressure
            b) Lung injury occurs as the result of the following:
               i) Overdistention and shearing of open alveoli
               ii) Repeated reopening of collapsed alveoli
      (c) Rate: usually less than 30 respirations per minute to reduce the risk of dynamic hyperinflation and auto–PEEP
      (d) Flow rates and tidal volume are adjusted to keep plateau pressure at less than 35 cm H_2O
         (i) Peak inspiratory flow rate usually 70 to 80 L/min
      (e) Permissive hypercapnia
         (i) Limitation of the tidal volume and minute ventilation may permit the accumulation of carbon dioxide.
         (ii) Permissive hypercapnia stems from the hypothesis that the adverse effects of alveolar overdistention are more detrimental to patient outcome than the adverse effects of respiratory acidosis.
            a) Overdistention of the alveoli causes the following:
               i) Barotrauma and volutrauma (VILI)
               ii) Release of inflammatory cytokines
               iii) Decrease in surfactant production
         (iii) Contraindication: intracranial hypertension
         (iv) Treatment of resultant respiratory acidosis
            a) Bicarbonate may be used if pH is less than 7.2
            b) Extracorporeal carbon dioxide removal ($ECCO_2R$): similar to ECMO used to remove carbon dioxide
            c) Tracheal gas insufflation: gas flow near the carina to wash carbon dioxide out of the large airways during expiration
   (4) CPAP or PEEP
      (a) Effects of CPAP or PEEP in the ARDS patient

(i) Decreases surface tension to keep alveoli open at low distending pressures at the end of expiration
(ii) Aids in reopening collapsed alveoli to reduce intrapulmonary shunt
(iii) Increases the driving pressure of oxygen to allow achievement of same PaO_2 on a lower FiO_2 or a higher PaO_2 on the same FiO_2 this effect therefore decreases risk of oxygen toxicity

(b) Usual level is 5 to 15 cm H_2O, but higher levels may be needed to maintain SaO_2 and PaO_2; titrated upward in increments of 2 cm H_2O until oxygenation ceases to improve and/or CI is decreased despite adequate circulating blood volume
(c) Adverse effects in the ARDS patient, particularly with high levels of CPAP or PEEP
(i) VILI
(ii) Decreased cardiac output related to decrease in venous return
a) Ensure adequate preload
b) Remember that a decrease in cardiac output is more detrimental to tissue oxygenation than is borderline hypoxemia

e. Administer aerosolized surfactant (e.g., colfosceril [Exosurf] or beractant [Survanta]) as prescribed.
(1) Effects
(a) Recognition that surfactant is deficient and dysfunctional in ARDS; so surfactant replacement is intended to decrease surface tension, allow more equitable distribution of tidal volume among the alveoli to decrease VILI, and aid in the prevention of alveolar collapse along with reinflation of already collapsed alveoli
(2) Administration by aerosolization; direct instillation into the endotracheal tube is being studied
(3) Though an oxygenation benefit has been demonstrated, no survival benefit has been shown in adults

f. Use partial liquid ventilation with perfluorocarbon (PFC) (e.g., perflubron) as prescribed.
(1) Effects: PFC is a noncompressible liquid with a low surface tension and high solubility for oxygen and carbon dioxide
(a) Allows for effective gas transfer
(b) Reduces surface tension of surfactant-deficient lung tissue, which increases pulmonary end-expiratory volume and improves lung compliance; acts as a liquid PEEP
(c) Accumulates in dependent regions of the lung (because it is heavier than water), which concentrates its action in areas of the lung most susceptible to VILI
(d) Redistributes pulmonary blood flow to nondependent lung issues, which allows more effective gas exchange through fully aerated alveoli
(e) Reduces lung inflammation by reduction of proinflammatory cytokines
(f) Mobilizes mucus and purulent secretions from the alveoli; they float to the top of the PFC layer and can be removed easily
(2) Method
(a) PFC is instilled via endotracheal tube to replace all or some of the functional residual capacity, and conventional mechanical ventilation is maintained.
(b) Sedation and neuromuscular blockade is required.
(3) Complication: mucous plugging of the airways and endotracheal tube
(4) Though an oxygenation benefit has been demonstrated, no survival benefit has been shown

g. Decrease intraalveolar fluid.
(1) Avoid overhydration as may occur in fluid resuscitation of trauma patients.
(2) Administer diuretics as prescribed.
(a) May be given to prevent further fluid sequestration into the alveoli
(b) Guided by PAOP: maintain PAOP at ~12 mm Hg
(c) May be given along with albumin in patients with hypoproteinemia with fluid retention
(3) Use CPAP or PEEP to increase intraalveolar pressure and aid in prevention of further fluid sequestration into the alveoli.

h. Maintain cardiac output and tissue oxygenation.
(1) Administer volume as indicated by PAOP readings: maintain PAOP ~12 mm Hg.
(a) Crystalloids versus colloids debate
(i) Colloids leak across the alveolar-capillary membrane as readily as crystalloids in this patient because of damage to the alveolar-capillary membrane.
(ii) No advantage accrues for one over the other in these patients; balanced amounts may be used, or crystalloids may be used because they have a cost benefit.
(2) Administer inotropes as indicated by left ventricular stroke work index and CI.
(a) Dobutamine is usually the first choice.
(b) CI greater than 4.5 L/min/m^2 has been recommended as goal (supranormal oxygen delivery goal of greater than 600 mL/min/m^2).
(3) Use hemodynamic monitoring, including venous oxygen saturation (SvO_2), to guide therapy.
(a) Volume or diuretics
(b) Inotropic therapy

(c) Best PEEP: level of PEEP to achieve Sao_2 of ~90% but without decreasing the CI

(4) Administer blood as indicated: hemoglobin less than 10 to 12 g/dL especially in the presence of hypoxemia.

(5) Use ECMO when available and indicated.

(a) Form of cardiopulmonary bypass in which the blood is removed from the patient, passed through large membrane lungs, and then placed back into circulation; mechanical ventilation can be maintained without the high levels of Fio_2 and PEEP that may cause VILI

(b) Effects

(i) Provides oxygenation of blood along with removal of carbon dioxide

(ii) Allows time for the lungs to heal

(iii) Prevents possible VILI and oxygen toxicity

(c) May be used as a salvage therapy in patients with life-threatening respiratory failure without multiple organ dysfunction in tertiary centers with capability and experience

(d) No survival benefit has been demonstrated

(6) Use $ECCO_2R$ when available and indicated.

(a) Similar to ECMO and may be used to correct pH especially in patients with significant hypercapnia

(b) No survival benefit has been demonstrated

i. Decrease oxygen consumption.

(1) Eliminate unnecessary activity.

(2) Provide rest periods after meals and other activities that increase oxygen consumption.

(3) Decrease anxiety: anxiolytics; sedatives.

(a) Neuromuscular blockers reduce oxygen requirements and may be necessary to maintain adequate ventilation especially in a restless patient.

(4) Treat fever using antipyretics (acetaminophen [Tylenol]) and cooling blanket.

(a) Debate continues regarding the benefits of fever reduction because the pyrogens are thought to be essential in mobilizing the immune system.

(b) Reduction of fever does reduce oxygen requirements and may be necessary to reduce the tissue oxygen deficit.

(c) Take care while using cooling blanket to prevent shivering.

3. Treat pulmonary hypertension.

a. Use oxygen and CPAP or PEEP to reduce the hypoxemia that causes hypoxemic pulmonary vasoconstriction.

b. Administer vasodilators as prescribed.

(1) Nitric oxide

(a) Endogenously synthesized by vascular endothelium and acts as a natural local vasodilator; exogenously administered by inhalation

(i) Nitroglycerin and nitroprusside work by a nitric oxide–activated pathway; however, these drugs given IV would dilate all vessels (including vessels to nonventilated alveoli), interfere with hypoxic vasoconstriction, and lead to increased intrapulmonary shunting; systemic hypotension also likely would occur

(ii) Effects of nitric oxide by inhalation

a) Dilates vessels only to ventilated alveoli

b) Reduces pulmonary hypertension

c) Acts as a potent bronchodilator

(iii) Nitric oxide is likely to have best results when used at an earlier, less severe stage of acute lung injury; effect also augmented by prone position

(iv) Though dramatic improvement in oxygenation frequently occurs, no survival benefit has been demonstrated

(b) Dosage of nitric oxide: 2 to 80 ppm; usual dose range is 5 to 40 ppm; low dosages seem to have best effects

(c) Adverse effects

(i) Methemoglobinemia

a) Hemoglobin-bound nitric oxide is transformed to methemoglobin, the oxidized form of hemoglobin that cannot carry oxygen; results in severe hypoxia.

b) Methemoglobin levels should be measured every 8 to 24 hours or as indicated during nitric oxide administration.

i) Normal methemoglobin level is 0% to 2%.

c) Treatment of methemoglobin is discontinuance of causative agent (nitric oxide in this case) if possible and administration of the antidote, which is methylene blue.

(ii) Lung injury as a result of nitrogen dioxide

a) Nitric oxide and oxygen can combine to form nitrogen dioxide, which is injurious to the lung.

b) Risk is greatest with high levels of nitric oxide and high Fio_2.

c) Prevention: Keep levels as low as possible and monitor nitrogen dioxide levels.

(iii) Weaning difficulties

a) Monitor closely for tachycardia, pulmonary hypertension, and hypoxemia with dosage reduction; weaning usually occurs over a 24-hour period

(2) Prostacyclin (epoprostenol [Flolan])

(a) Effect: decreases vascular resistance

(i) Intravenously administered prostaglandin I_2 (PGI_2) decreases pulmonary and systemic arterial pressures but may increase intrapulmonary shunt.
(ii) Inhaled PGI_2 decreases PVR without increase in intrapulmonary shunt and without causing adverse systemic hemodynamic effects.
(b) Usual dose is 10 to 25 ng/kg/min
(3) Prostaglandin E_1
(a) Effect: decrease in PVR, but some studies have shown a decrease in PaO_2/FiO_2 ratios
(b) Usual dose is 30 ng/kg/min
4. Modify mediator release and effect (under continuing investigation).
a. Administer corticosteroids as prescribed.
(1) While not effective in preventing the onset of ARDS, may be helpful during the fibroproliferative phase
(2) Reduces some proinflammatory cytokines
(3) Methylprednisolone usually used
b. Administer antioxidants as prescribed.
(1) Toxic oxygen radicals produced by activated neutrophils, macrophages, and endothelial cells play a key role in lung injury
(2) Action: may shorten the duration of lung injury
(3) Examples: N-acetylcysteine or procysteine (OTZ)
c. Administer antiinflammatory agents: anticytokines; antiprostaglandins (e.g., ketorolac [Toradol], ibuprofen [Motrin], or indomethacin [Indocin]) as prescribed.
d. Administer ketoconazole (Nizoral) as prescribed.
(1) Actions
(a) Inhibits the production of leukotrienes and thromboxane by the alveolar macrophages
(b) May prevent ARDS in patients with sepsis
(2) Administered through enteral tube
5. Provide nutritional support to prevent respiratory muscle atrophy.
a. Use enteral route if possible.
b. Administer high-protein and high-calorie diet rich in omega-3 and omega-6 fatty acids.
(1) 1 to 2 g/kg of IBW of protein
(a) Conditionally essential amino acids glutamine and arginine may be particularly helpful in reducing endotoxemia and should be included
(2) 20 to 25 kcal/kg of IBW of nonprotein calories to prevent exogenous protein and muscle tissue from being catabolized to meet nutritional requirements
(3) Nonprotein calories in the form of carbohydrates increase carbon dioxide production; reduced carbohydrate formulas, such as Pulmocare, may be preferable, especially in patients with hypercapnia
c. Replace multivitamins and minerals: vitamins A, C, and E; zinc; and selenium.
6. Monitor for complications.
a. Secondary infections: nosocomial pneumonia
b. Sepsis
c. Shock
d. MODS
e. Airway trauma
f. Dysrhythmias
g. PE
h. Pulmonary fibrosis
i. Pneumothorax
j. GI hemorrhage
k. DIC
l. HF
m. Renal failure

Pneumonia

Definitions

1. Pneumonia: inflammatory process of the lung parenchyma, including alveolar spaces and interstitial tissue, produced by an infectious agent
2. Community-acquired pneumonia (CAP): pneumonia
3. Hospital-acquired pneumonia (HAP): acute pneumonia that develops after 48 hours of hospitalization; also referred to as *nosocomial pneumonia*
a. Assumption of a more virulent organism; these organisms are often resistant to multiple antibiotics
b. Ventilator-associated pneumonia (VAP): subtype of HAP associated with intubation and mechanical ventilation

Etiology

1. Causative agents
a. Bacteria
(1) CAP
(a) *Streptococcus pneumoniae:* most common
(b) *Staphylococcus aureus*
(c) *Haemophilus influenzae*
(d) *Klebsiella pneumoniae*
(e) *Legionella pneumophila*
(f) *Bacteroides fragilis*
(g) *Mycobacterium tuberculosis*
(2) HAP
(a) *Pseudomonas* species
(b) *Staphylococcus aureus*
(c) *Enterobacter* species
(d) *Klebsiella pneumoniae*
(e) *Escherichia coli*
(f) *Haemophilus influenzae*
(g) *Serratia marcescens*
(h) *Streptococcus* species
(i) *Proteus mirabilis*
(j) *Acinetobacter* species
(k) *Legionella pneumophila*
(3) VAP
(a) *Pseudomonas aeruginosa*
(b) *Staphylococcus aureus*

(c) *Klebsiella pneumoniae*
(d) *Acinetobacter* species
(e) *Enterobacter* species
(f) *Serratia marcescens*

b. Viruses
(1) Adenovirus
(2) Hantavirus
(3) Influenza types A and B
(4) Respiratory syncytial virus

c. Fungi
(1) *Histoplasma capsulatum*
(2) *Coccidioides immitis*
(3) *Candida* species
(4) *Aspergillus* species

d. Parasites (e.g., *Pneumocystis carinii*)
e. Mycoplasma: *Mycoplasma pneumoniae*

2. Predisposing factors
a. Patient-related
(1) Advanced age
(2) History of smoking
(3) Periodontal disease
(4) Altered level of consciousness
(5) Chronic illness
(a) COPD
(b) Diabetes mellitus
(c) Cardiovascular disease
(d) Malignancy
(6) Severe acute illness
(a) Shock
(b) Head injury
(c) Chest trauma
(7) Malnutrition: alcoholism, malignancy, eating disorder, poverty
(8) Immunocompromise
(a) Patients with neutropenia resulting from acute leukemia or cytotoxic agents usually have gram-negative bacilli as a source
(b) Severely immunocompromised patient also may develop pneumonia caused by the following:
(i) Gram-negative aerobic bacteria
a) *Haemophilus influenzae*
b) *Klebsiella pneumoniae*
c) *Legionella pneumophila*
d) *Escherichia coli*
e) *Pseudomonas aeruginosa*
f) *Proteus mirabilis*
g) *Klebsiella pneumoniae*
h) *Enterobacter* species
(ii) Viruses
a) Cytomegalovirus
b) Varicella-zoster
c) Herpes simplex
(iii) Fungi
a) *Candida albicans*
b) *Aspergillus fumigatus*
c) *Cryptococcus neoformans*
(iv) Protozoa: *Pneumocystis carinii*
(9) Chronic immobility

b. Treatment-related
(1) Surgery, especially if the following:
(a) Thoracic, abdominal, or flank incisions
(b) Craniotomy
(c) Long anesthesia time
(d) Prolonged hospitalization
(2) Artificial airway, especially self-extubation and reintubation
(3) Saline lavage during suctioning of endotracheal tube or tracheostomy
(a) Ineffective in liquifying secretions
(b) Dislodges 5 times the number of bacterial colonies than suction catheter alone (Hagler & Traver, 1994)
(c) Not completely removed with suctioning, allowing colonized saline to lie in lungs
(4) Bronchoscopy
(5) Mechanical ventilation
(6) Nasogastric tube
(7) Aspiration of colonized material related to therapies
(a) Oropharyngeal colonization
(i) Previous or concurrent antibiotic therapy: predisposes the patient to colonization of the oropharynx
(ii) Leakage of pharyngeal flora around the endotracheal tube (ET) cuff
(b) Gastric colonization
(i) Gastric colonization likely with a gastric pH of greater than 4; bacteria in the stomach then migrate upward to be aspirated silently into the lungs;
a) Effects of drugs on gastric pH
i) H_2 receptor antagonist, proton pump inhibitors (PPIs), and antacids alter the pH of the stomach (normally between 1 and 3).
ii) Sucralfate (Carafate) does not significantly alter the pH and is associated with a lower incidence of pneumonia than PPIs, H_2 receptor antagonists, or antacids.
b) Continuous enteral feedings also may alter gastric pH
(ii) Pneumonia rates of patients receiving mechanical ventilation correlate directly with increased gastric pH levels (Daschner et al., 1988)
(8) Supine position
(9) Broad-spectrum antibiotic therapy, especially cephalosporins

c. Infection control–related
(1) Poor hand washing
(2) Inadequate disinfection/sterilization of devices
(3) Contaminated water for humidification
(4) Contaminated respiratory therapy or anesthesia equipment

(5) Changing of ventilator tubing more often than every 48 hours

Pathophysiology

1. Causative agent is inhaled or enters the pharynx through direct contact.
   a. Nosocomial pneumonia specifically
      (1) Cross-colonization
      (2) Altered defenses of intubated and mechanically ventilated patient
         (a) Normal anatomic barriers are bypassed
         (b) Impairment of cough reflex
         (c) Increase in mucus production
         (d) Stagnation of mucus
         (e) Impairment of mucociliary apparatus
      (3) Contaminated aerosol generation
         (a) Inadequate disinfection/sterilization of devices
         (b) Contaminated water for humidification
         (c) Contaminated respiratory therapy or anesthesia equipment
         (d) Saline lavage during suctioning of endotracheal tube or tracheostomy
      (4) Aspiration of colonized material
         (a) Oropharyngeal colonization
            (i) Concurrent antibiotic therapy: predisposes the patient to colonization of the oropharynx
            (ii) Leakage of pharyngeal flora around the ET cuff
         (b) Gastric colonization
            (i) Gastric colonization is likely with a gastric pH of greater than 4.
            (ii) H_2 receptor antagonists, PPIs, and antacids contribute to alter the normal acidic pH of the stomach, allowing proliferation of bacteria in the stomach that then migrate upward to be aspirated silently into the lungs; sucralfate (Carafate) is associated with a lower incidence of pneumonia than PPIs, H_2 receptor antagonists, or antacids.
            (iii) Pneumonia rates of patients receiving mechanical ventilation correlate directly with increased gastric pH levels (Daschner et al., 1988).
      (5) Hematogenous spread from another site
2. Alveoli become inflamed and edematous.
3. Alveolar spaces fill with exudate and consolidate.
4. Alveoli are not ventilated but they are perfused: V/Q mismatch; shunt.
5. Diffusion of oxygen is obstructed, causing hypoxemia and hypercapnia.
6. Stimulation of goblet cells increases mucus, which causes increased airway resistance and increased work of breathing.
7. Acute respiratory failure occurs.
8. Abscesses may form and rupture into the pleural space to form pneumothorax and/or empyema.

Clinical Presentation

1. Subjective
   a. Frequently begins with cold or flulike symptoms; infectious symptoms: chills, fever, malaise, tachycardia, headache, myalgia
   b. Chest pain (frequently pleuritic-type pain)
   c. Confusion: especially in elderly patients
2. Objective
   a. Tachycardia
   b. Tachypnea
   c. Fever though elderly patients may be hypothermic
   d. Productive cough; sputum mucoid, rusty, bloody, or purulent; may have foul odor
   e. Diaphoresis
   f. Cyanosis may be seen (dependent on hemoglobin and Sao_2 levels)
   g. Splinting of chest; decreased chest excursion
   h. Use of accessory muscles
   i. Increased tactile fremitus
   j. Clinical indications of dehydration
   k. Dullness to percussion over areas of consolidation
   l. Breath sound changes: diminished; bronchial breath sounds; crackles and/or rhonchi; rub may be audible
   m. Voice sounds: egophony; bronchophony; whispered pectoriloquy
3. Diagnostic
   a. Serum
      (1) White blood cells (WBCs)
         (a) Elevated with shift to left if bacterial but may be normal in elderly patient, immunocompromised patient, or in overwhelming infection
         (b) Normal or decreased if viral
      (2) ABGs: decreased Pao_2 with clinical indications of hypoxemia; $Paco_2$ may be increased, decreased, or normal depending on ventilation
   b. Blood culture: positive for specific organism in bacteremia
   c. Sputum: may be induced or obtained through bronchoscopy with either protected specimen brush or bronchoalveolar lavage
      (1) Gram's stain
      (2) Acid-fast stain
      (3) Culture and sensitivity to identify specific organism if bacterial
      (4) Acid-fast: to rule out tuberculosis
      (5) Legionella
   d. Purified protein derivative skin test for tuberculosis
   e. Chest x-ray
      (1) Localization and pattern
         (a) Bronchopneumonia: inflammation of the bronchioles and alveoli
         (b) Interstitial pneumonia: inflammation of the tissue around alveoli
         (c) Alveolar pneumonia: inflammation of the alveoli; usually caused by a virus

(d) Necrotizing pneumonia: necrosis of a portion of lung tissue
(2) Viral pneumonias cause diffuse changes
(3) Pleural effusion may indicate empyema
f. Percutaneous needle aspiration of infiltrate: especially in immunocompromised patient not responding to antibiotics

Nursing Diagnoses

1. Impaired Gas Exchange related to V/Q mismatching and intrapulmonary shunt
2. Ineffective Breathing Pattern related to increased work of breathing and fatigue
3. Ineffective Airway Clearance related to retained secretions and increased viscosity of secretions
4. Risk for Deficient Fluid Volume related to increased sensible loss from hyperventilation, fever, oxygen therapy, and decrease fluid intake
5. Risk for Infection related to inadequate primary defenses, invasive procedures, chronic disease, and poor airway clearance
6. Imbalanced Nutrition: Less than Body Requirements related to lack of exogenous nutrients and increased nutrient requirements
7. Activity Intolerance related to imbalance between oxygen supply and oxygen demand and to dyspnea
8. Anxiety related to change in health status
9. Ineffective Individual Coping and Ineffective Family Coping related to hospitalization and critical illness

Collaborative Management

1. Prevent nosocomial pneumonia or spread of infection.
   a. Prevent cross-contamination.
      (1) Wash hands with soap and water or waterless antiseptic agent before and after ventilator contact or suctioning; also wear gloves.
      (2) Maintain universal precautions; other specific precautions may be indicated depending on the type of pneumonia.
   b. Prevent colonization.
      (1) Avoid unnecessary antibiotics (e.g., prophylactically administered antibiotics in situations where not warranted).
      (2) Avoid unnecessary stress ulcer prophylaxis, and use sucralfate (Carafate) rather than agents that reduce the acidity of gastric secretions.
      (3) Provide oral care.
         (a) Every 2 to 4 hours
            (i) Use suction foam swabs to clean teeth and tongue followed by moisturizing swabs and water-soluble lip balm.
               a) Avoid lemon glycerin swabs, which are drying to the oral mucosa.
            (ii) Suction secretions from the oropharynx.
               a) Rinse catheter (e.g., Yankauer) with sterile water or saline after each use.
               b) Store oropharyngeal suction catheter in a nonsealed bag when not in use.
               c) Replace oropharyngeal suction device, tubing, and suction canister every 24 hours.
         (b) Twice daily
            (i) Brush teeth to prevent dental plaque colonization.
               a) Use a soft-bristle pediatric toothbrush along with toothpaste, preferably with an alkaline pH.
               b) Remove and thoroughly clean removable partial dentures.
            (ii) Use 0.12% chlorhexidine gluconate (Peridex) by spray or rinse as prescribed.
               a) Chlorhexidine has been shown to be effective in the prevention of nosocomial pneumonia in some patient populations (e.g., cardiac surgery patients).
               b) Chlorhexidine is a broad-spectrum antibacterial agent that is not absorbed through the skin or mucous membranes.
               c) Initiate this oral care preoperatively for surgical patients.
      (4) Use aseptic preparation and maintenance of enteral feedings to prevent contamination and gastric colonization.
      (5) Selective decontamination of the digestive tract may be prescribed.
         (a) Topical antibiotics such as colistin (Colimycin) and amphotericin B (Fungizone)
         (b) Of questionable effectiveness and costly
         (c) May allow emergence of bacterial resistance
   c. Prevent aspiration of contaminated secretions.
      (1) Avoid intubation by using noninvasive positive pressure ventilation if possible.
      (2) Prevent accidental extubation by adequately securing endotracheal tube.
      (3) Avoid nasal tubes if possible: nasotracheal, nasogastric, or nasopharyngeal airways.
         (a) These may cause sinusitis and/or potentiate gastric reflux.
         (b) Orotracheal tube is preferred over nasotracheal tube.
         (c) Orogastric tube is preferred over nasogastric, but risk of gastric reflux is still present because it also causes incompetence of the gastroesophageal sphincter; percutaneous endoscopic gastrostomy tube is preferred if it is anticipated that the need for enteral feeding will be prolonged.
            (i) Remove nasogastric or orogastric tube as soon as possible.

(4) Limit the duration of intubation and mechanical ventilation if possible.
(a) Evaluate appropriateness for weaning at least daily by evaluating spontaneous ventilatory parameters after a "sedation vacation."
(b) Use weaning protocols.
(5) Maintain endotracheal or tracheostomy cuff pressure between 20 and 25 mm Hg (25 and 35 cm H_2O).
(6) Maintain continuous aspiration of subglottic secretions using a specialized endotracheal tube (e.g., Mallinckrodt's Hi-Lo Evac endotracheal tube [Figure 5-3]): a dorsal lumen allows continuous suctioning of pooled secretions above the cuff of the endotracheal tube.
(7) Suction secretions only as necessary, and avoid saline lavage during suctioning of endotracheal tube or tracheostomy.
(a) Ineffective in liquifying secretion
(b) Accentuates oxygen desaturation during suctioning
(c) Dislodges 5 times the number of bacterial colonies than suction catheter alone
(d) Incomplete removal with suctioning allows colonized saline to lie in lungs
(8) Rinse the suction catheter after suctioning (catheter pulled back to black line, saline injected into irrigation port while suction is maintained).
(9) Elevate the HOB to 30 to 45 degrees; turn and reposition patient every 2 hours.
(10) Prevent gastric distention and regurgitation.
(a) Ensure correct placement of tube.
(b) Evaluate gastric retention for patients receiving enteral feedings; duodenal or jejunal feedings may be beneficial in prevention of aspiration.
(c) Use gastric suction if necessary.
(11) Avoid unnecessary ventilator circuit changes/manipulation; change ventilator circuit and closed-suction systems when contamination of the circuit with blood, emesis, or purulent secretions is noted.
(a) Ventilator tubing changes more often than every 48 hours have been shown to increase the risk of nosocomial pneumonia.
(12) Empty water condensation in ventilator or nebulizer tubing into water trap, never back into humidifier reservoir.
(a) Use a heated wire ventilator circuit if possible to prevent this condensation (also referred to as *rainout*).
(13) Prevent aspiration of enteral feedings (see Aspiration Lung Disorder).

d. Encourage the patient to breathe deeply and to use incentive spirometry, especially in postoperative patients; adequate analgesia must be achieved so that the patient will breathe deeply.

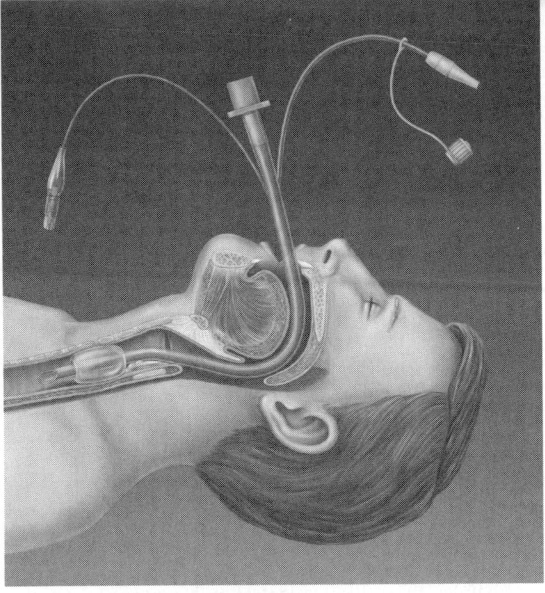

Figure 5-3 Specialized endotracheal tube used for continuous aspiration of subglottic secretions. (From Nellcor Puritan Bennett Inc. [2004]. *Hi-Lo Evac endotracheal tube with evacuation lumen.* Retrieved February 10, 2007, from http://www.nellcor.com/_Catalog/PDF/Product/Hi-LoEvac.pdf)

2. Maintain airway and improve ventilation.
   a. Position the patient for optimal ventilation.
      (1) Elevate HOB to 30 to 45 degrees.
      (2) Turn patient from "good lung down" to back; use of a 60-degree lateral rotation bed also is advocated.
   b. Administer antimicrobials as prescribed.
      (1) Antibiotics for bacterial infection
         (a) CAP: should be started within 4 hours of arrival to hospital; broad-spectrum antibiotic prescribed initially empirically (i.e., most likely organism[s] as determined by experience); antibiotic prescription is changed if necessary depending on patient response and/or culture
         (b) Critically ill patients usually put on a beta-lactam (e.g., amoxicillin, penicillin, or piperacillin [Pipracil]) and either a macrolide (azithromycin [Zithromax], clarithromycin [Biaxin], dirithromycin [Dynabac]) or a fluoroquinolone (levofloxacin [Levaquin], moxifloxacin [Avelox], sparfloxacin [Zagam])
         (c) VAP: possible antibiotic combinations
            (i) Early onset VAP: amoxicillin-clavulanate and gentamicin
            (ii) Late onset VAP: third-generation cephalosporin and amikacin

(iii) Methicillin-resistant staphylococci: vancomycin added
(2) Antivirals (e.g., amantadine [Symmetrel], zanamivir [Relenza], or oseltamivir [Tamiflu]) for viral infection
(3) Other antimicrobials as prescribed
c. Provide adequate hydration: 2 to 3 L per 24 hours unless contraindicated by cardiac or renal disease.
(1) Oral fluids: noncaffeinated
(2) IV fluids: usually D_5NS
d. Maintain bronchial hygiene and provide chest physiotherapy as indicated.
(1) Inspiratory maneuvers: deep breathing; incentive spirometry
(2) Humidified air and/or oxygen
(3) Encouragement to cough or suctioning if the patient is unable to clear airways
(4) Postural drainage, percussion, vibration if necessary
(5) Bronchodilators as prescribed
(6) Expectorants (e.g., guaifenesin [Robitussin] or potassium iodide [SSKI]) may be used, but hydration is most important; water is the best expectorant
(7) Mucolytics (e.g., acetylcysteine [Mucomyst]) may be used to decrease the tenacity of the mucus
(8) Sedatives: generally avoided unless patient is very agitated or on mechanical ventilation
(9) Antitussives: avoid use of antitussives unless the cough is nonproductive and is causing fatigue
e. Prepare the patient for bronchoscopy as requested: it may be necessary if airway clearance techniques are inadequate.
f. Ensure intubation and mechanical ventilation as indicated.
(1) If $Paco_2$ continues to rise and acidosis develops
(2) The goal of mechanical ventilation is to normalize the pH, not necessarily the $Paco_2$
3. Optimize oxygen delivery and decrease oxygen consumption.
a. Administer oxygen.
(1) Nasal cannula or mask; masks are contraindicated in chronically hypercapnic patients because the high concentration of oxygen provided by these delivery systems likely would eliminate the hypoxic drive
(2) Flow rate or oxygen concentration to keep Spo_2 approximately 95% unless contraindicated; in patients with chronic hypercapnia, adjust flow rate or oxygen concentration to keep Spo_2 approximately 90%
b. Provide rest periods especially after meals or activities.
c. Treat fever.
(1) Antipyretics (acetaminophen [Tylenol])
(2) Use of cooling blankets with attention to the prevention of shivering
4. Treat chest pain: analgesics in doses adequate to allow patient to deep breathe and cough as indicated.
5. Provide appropriate nutritional support.
6. Monitor for complications.
a. Acute respiratory failure
b. Pleural effusion
c. Empyema
d. Lung abscess
e. Septic shock
7. Provide instruction and counseling regarding lifestyle modification and need for pharmacologic therapy.
a. Importance of immunizations (e.g., influenza, pneumococcus, and *Haemophilus*)
b. Hydration
c. Nutrition
d. Smoking cessation
e. Hand-washing techniques, disposal of tissues, prevention of cross-contamination
f. Recognition of symptoms to report to the physician
g. Prescribed antimicrobials and the importance of taking the entire prescription

Severe Acute Respiratory Syndrome (SARS)

Definition

A virulent respiratory infection thought to be caused by a newly recognized coronavirus (SARS-CoV)

Etiology

1. Highly but selectively contagious (e.g., absence of transmission between some persons with very close contact, evidence of transmission between persons without very close contact)
a. Contact with an individual with SARS
b. Living in an area affected by SARS
c. Travel to an area affected by SARS
2. Transmission
a. Respiratory droplet
b. May be airborne
c. May be enteral (fecal droplets)
d. Though the virus may survive on inert surfaces for days, this is probably not a major route of spread

Pathophysiology

1. Stages
a. Phase 1: viral replication phase
(1) Progressive pneumonia and increasing oxygen dependence
(2) Clinically characterized by fever and myalgia
b. Phase 2: immune response phase
(1) Immunopathologic dysregulation and uncontrolled activation of the cytokine system may result in lung damage
(a) Diffuse alveolar damage and exudates
(b) Hyaline membrane formation

(c) Pneumocyte proliferation
(d) Lymphocytic interstitial infiltrates
(2) Clinically characterized by recurrence of fever, hypoxemia, and progression of pneumonia on chest x-ray
c. Phase 3: ARDS
(1) Clinically characterized by need for ventilatory support
2. Outcomes
a. Gradual improvement (approximately 75% of patients)
b. Recurrence of fever, further deterioration, ARDS (approximately 25% of patients)
c. Death occurs in approximately 8% to 15% of infected patients: the terminal event is usually severe respiratory failure, MODS, sepsis, or concurrent medical illness (e.g., myocardial infarction [MI] or stroke)

Clinical Presentation

Early diagnosis of SARS is based on clinical presentation and possible contact with known patient with SARS along with exclusion of known infectious and noninfectious processes that may mimic SARS.

1. Suspected or probable classification
a. Suspected
(1) Fever of greater than 38° C with cough or dyspnea
(2) History of close contact with a suspected or probable case of SARS, travel to an affected area, or living in an affected area
(a) Close contact is described as cared for, lived with, or had direct contact with respiratory secretions or body fluids
b. Probable
(1) As when suspected along with one of the following:
(a) Radiographic evidence of infiltrates consistent with pneumonia or ARDS
(b) Positive for SARS-CoV coronavirus by one or more assays
(c) Autopsy findings consistent with the pathology of ARDS without an identifiable cause
2. Subjective
a. Acute febrile illness after an incubation period of 2 to 10 days (but may be as long as 16 days)
(1) Fever
(a) Elderly may not present with high fever or other cardinal symptoms
(2) Chills
(3) Malaise
(4) Myalgia
(5) Nonproductive cough
(6) Dyspnea
(7) Headache
(8) Dizziness
(9) Nausea, vomiting, diarrhea
b. History of either living in an area affected by SARS, travel to an area affected by SARS, or contact with someone with suspected or probable SARS
3. Objective
a. Temperature greater than 38° C
b. Breath sound changes: crackles
4. Diagnostic
a. Laboratory
(1) Hematology
(a) Leukopenia
(b) Lymphopenia
(c) Mild thrombocytopenia
(2) Clotting profile
(a) Elevated D dimer
(b) Prolonged partial thromboplastin time
(3) Chemistry: elevated (LDH), creatine kinase, aspartate transaminase, and alanine transaminase
(4) ABGs: hypoxemia
b. Diagnostic tests for SARS-CoV
(1) Reverse transcription-polymerase chain reaction to detect RNA of SARS-CoV
(a) Positive result indicates that there is genetic material of the SARS-CoV in the sample
(b) Negative does not rule out SARS
(2) Antibody tests to detect antibodies to SARS-CoV: indirect fluorescent antibody yields positive results after approximately day 10 of illness, whereas enzyme-linked immunosorbent assay yields positive result after approximately day 21
(a) Positive indicates a previous infection with SARS-CoV
(b) Negative indicates no infection with SARS-CoV or that the test was completed too early for antibody development
(3) Cell culture to detect SARS-CoV: only means of showing the existence of a live virus
(a) Positive indicates the presence of live SARS-CoV in the sample
(b) Negative does not rule out SARS
c. Chest x-ray
(1) A normal chest x-ray does not rule out SARS, especially early in the course of the process
(2) Unilateral, bilateral, and/or multifocal consolidations frequently are seen
(3) Pleural effusions usually are not seen
d. Chest CT: ill-defined ground glass opacification especially in the lung periphery; peripheral alveolar opacities
5. Prognostic variables for critical care unit admission or death
a. Advanced age (older than 65 years is associated with a mortality of greater than 50%)
b. High peak level of LDH
c. High absolute neutrophil count at presentation

Nursing Diagnoses

1. Impaired Gas Exchange related to V/Q mismatching and intrapulmonary shunt

2. Ineffective Breathing Pattern related to increased work of breathing and fatigue
3. Ineffective Airway Clearance related to retained secretions and increased viscosity of secretions
4. Risk for Deficient Fluid Volume related to increased insensible loss from hyperventilation, fever, oxygen therapy, and decreased fluid intake
5. Risk for Infection related to inadequate primary defenses, invasive procedures, chronic disease, and poor airway clearance
6. Impaired Nutrition: Less than Body Requirements related to lack of exogenous nutrients and increased nutrient requirements
7. Activity Intolerance related to imbalance between oxygen supply and oxygen demand and to dyspnea
8. Anxiety related to change in health status
9. Ineffective Individual Coping and Ineffective Family Coping related to hospitalization and critical illness

Collaborative Management

1. Optimize oxygen delivery and decrease oxygen consumption.
   a. Administer oxygen as indicated: flow rate or oxygen concentration to keep Spo_2 at least 90%.
   b. Provide rest periods especially after meals or activities.
   c. Treat fever: antipyretics (acetaminophen [Tylenol]); use cooling blankets, taking care to prevent shivering.
2. Maintain airway and ventilation.
   a. Position patient for optimal ventilation: elevate HOB to 30 to 45 degrees; periodic prone positioning may be indicated.
   b. Provide adequate hydration: oral and/or IV fluids; however, avoid fluid overload.
   c. Ensure bronchial hygiene and provide chest physiotherapy as indicated.
      (1) Inspiratory maneuvers: deep breathing; incentive spirometry
      (2) Humidification of inspired air/oxygen
      (3) Encouragement to cough; suctioning of secretions if the patient is unable to clear airways
      (4) Postural drainage, percussion, vibration if necessary
      (5) Bronchodilators as prescribed
      (6) Bronchoscopy may be necessary if airway clearance techniques are inadequate
      (7) Nitric oxide by inhalation has been recommended in severe cases
   d. Ensure intubation and mechanical ventilation as indicated for acute respiratory failure.
      (1) Noninvasive positive pressure ventilation (e.g., bi-PAP) may be used initially.
      (2) Follow mechanical ventilation recommendations similar to ARDS.
         (a) Tidal volume limited to 6 mL/kg and plateau pressure limited to 30 cm H_2O
         (b) PEEP frequently required to maintain oxygen saturation
3. Prevent transmission of the highly contagious virus through diligent respiratory and contact precautions.
   a. Respiratory transmission from direct contact with respiratory particles is believed to be the main route of spread; evidence of viral shedding in stool samples suggests that the virus also may be spread by the fecal-oral route.
      (1) Negative pressure room if available; if not available, the patient should be placed in an area with an independent air supply/exhaust system
      (2) Disposable long sleeve gowns, gloves, eye protection, and disposable respirators with at least 95% (N95, P99, P100) filtering efficiency before entering the patient's room and removed before leaving the patient's room
      (3) Hand washing before putting on gloves and after removing gloves and other protective wear
      (4) Nebulization, noninvasive positive pressure ventilation, high-frequency oscillatory ventilation, and bronchoscopy should be avoided if possible
      (5) Visitors should be restricted or prohibited
      (6) Minimization of the number of health care workers who have contact with the patient
   b. Considerations
      (1) Patients treated in critical care units have a more severe illness that might be related to a higher viral burden; therefore they may be more infective.
      (2) Procedures frequently performed in critically ill patients, such as nebulization, noninvasive ventilation, endotracheal intubation, suctioning, and bronchoscopy, are associated with a higher risk of respiratory droplet transmission.
      (3) Patients continue to shed the virus in respiratory secretions, urine, and feces 3 weeks after the onset of the illness, though the period of infectivity is still unclear; patients are thought to remain infectious for up to 10 days after resolution of fever.
      (4) SARS-CoV survives for many days when dried on surfaces
4. Treat the viral infection and any secondary bacterial infections.
   a. Administer antivirals as prescribed; efficacy has not been established for SARS-CoV.
      (1) Ribavirin was used extensively during the 2003 outbreak of SARS but was ineffective and had serious side effects.
      (2) Interferon beta, which blocks the SARS virus from entering the cell, and cysteine protease inhibitors, which inhibit replication of SARS-CoV, are being investigated as possible treatments.

(3) Efforts to develop an effective vaccine to SARS-CoV are ongoing, but the ability of the virus to mutate complicates efforts.
b. Administer antibiotics as prescribed to cover usual causes of CAP and/or treat secondary bacterial infections.
c. Administer corticosteroids as prescribed, though their efficacy is unclear; they are recommended only in the most severe cases of SARS.
5. Provide instruction and counseling regarding lifestyle modification and need for pharmacologic therapy.
   a. Importance of immunizations (e.g., influenza, pneumococcus, and *Haemophilus*)
   b. Recognition of symptoms to report to the physician
   c. Pharmacologic agents: prescribed antimicrobials

Aspiration Lung Disorder

Definitions

1. Aspiration lung disorder: lung injury related to the inhalation of gastric contents, oropharyngeal secretions, food, or other foreign material into the tracheobronchial tree
2. Aspiration pneumonitis: chemical injury of the lung caused by aspiration of gastric contents, oropharyngeal secretions, or exogenous liquids
3. Aspiration pneumonia: lung infection caused by aspiration of material colonized with bacteria

Etiology (Risk Factors)

1. Altered consciousness and/or gag reflex
   a. Sedation
   b. Anesthesia especially when the patient has eaten recently
   c. CNS disorders
      (1) Cerebral infarction or hemorrhage
      (2) Seizures
      (3) Neuromuscular diseases
   d. Drug or alcohol intoxication
2. Altered anatomy
   a. Endotracheal tube keeps the epiglottis splinted open
   b. Tracheostomy tube impairs swallowing mechanism
   c. Nasogastric or orogastric tube causes incompetence of the gastroesophageal sphincter
   d. GI tamponade (e.g., Sengstaken-Blakemore tube)
   e. Facial, neck, or oral trauma
3. GI conditions
   a. Esophageal abnormalities (e.g., tracheoesophageal fistula or stricture)
   b. Gastroesophageal reflux
      (1) Obesity
      (2) Hiatal hernia
      (3) Pregnancy
   c. Decreased GI motility (e.g., diabetic gastroparesis)
   d. GI hemorrhage
   e. Vomiting
   f. Intestinal obstruction
      (1) Functional (e.g., ileus)
      (2) Structural (e.g., tumor or volvulus)
4. Enteral nutritional support
   a. Impaired gastric motility: a frequent problem in critically ill patients because of perfusion deficits, sepsis, and drugs (e.g., propofol and opioids)
   b. Improper positioning of patients especially if on enteral feedings
5. Drugs that decrease gastroesophageal sphincter tone: anticholinergics (e.g., atropine), adrenergics (e.g., dopamine), nitrates, caffeine, calcium channel blockers (e.g., nifedipine), estrogen

Pathophysiology

1. Oropharyngeal secretions are aspirated most commonly.
   a. Includes silent aspiration as oropharyngeal secretions leak around the cuff of an endotracheal tube
2. Aspiration of large particles can obstruct major airways and can cause asphyxia and potentially death.
3. Aspiration of smaller particles causes segmental atelectasis and subacute inflammatory pulmonary reaction with extensive hemorrhage.
   a. Clear acidic liquid causes chemical burn and destruction of the type II pneumocytes, frequently referred to as *aspiration pneumonitis*.
      (1) Fluid and blood accumulate in the interstitium and the alveoli
      (2) Decreased lung compliance and decreased alveolar ventilation
      (3) Hypoxemia, bronchospasm, and hemorrhage with pulmonary edema and necrosis
   b. Clear nonacidic liquid causes reflex airway closure, pulmonary edema, surfactant changes; contaminated material may cause massive infection.
   c. Aspiration of material colonized with bacteria potentially causes severe lung infections (e.g., pneumonia or lung abscess).
4. Aspiration into the right lung is more common than aspiration into the left lung because of the straighter angle of the right mainstem bronchus off the trachea.

Clinical Presentation

1. Subjective
   a. Dyspnea
   b. Cough
   c. Chest pain: pleuritic
   d. Anxiety
   e. May have history of witnessed vomiting and aspiration
2. Objective
   a. Tachycardia
   b. Tachypnea
   c. Fever
   d. Increased work of breathing: use of accessory muscles; intercostal retractions
   e. Productive cough or suctioned material

(1) Foul-smelling sputum
(2) Food and stomach contents may be seen in secretions suctioned from lungs
(a) If aspirated, enteral feedings will test positive for glucose.
(3) Pink, frothy sputum may occur with acidic aspiration

f. Breath sounds
(1) Stridor if obstruction of the upper airway occurs
(2) Diminished breath sounds
(3) Adventitious sounds: crackles; rhonchi; wheezing

g. Hypoxemia (decreased Spo_2, Sao_2, Pao_2) and clinical indications of hypoxia (Box 4-3)

h. Compliance: decreased static and dynamic compliance; increased peak inspiratory pressures

3. Diagnostic
a. Serum
(1) WBC count increased
(2) ABGs
(a) Pao_2 and Sao_2 decreased
(b) $Paco_2$ may be normal, decreased, or increased depending on ventilation pattern (e.g., may be low due to hyperventilation or high due to hypoventilation)

b. Tracheal aspirate: visualization or analysis to determine whether aspiration has occurred
(1) Dye: visual assessment of tracheal aspirate for discoloration caused by blue dye (usually blue food coloring) that was added to enteral feeding
(a) It is no longer recommended to add blue food coloring to enteral feedings for the following reasons:
(i) May result in generalized absorption of the dye from the GI tract; more likely in patients with multiple organ failure
a) Discoloration of body fluids and tissues
b) May cause fatal liver toxicity
c) Causes questionable specificity because discoloration of tracheal secretions may have occurred by systemic route
(ii) May result in infection because of contamination of the food coloring
(iii) Interferes with occult blood testing
(iv) Causes allergic reactions in some persons because of presence of FD&C yellow No. 5
(v) Has relatively low sensitivity
(2) Glucose: use of glucose oxidase reagent strips to detect presence of glucose
(a) More sensitive than dye method
(b) Some potential problems
(i) Blood in tracheal secretions may cause a positive test result (false positive)
(ii) Low glucose formulae may not cause a positive result
(iii) There are concerns regarding specificity because some patients not being enterally fed have had positive results
(iv) There are concerns about validity of using strips intended for blood or urine for tracheal aspirate
(3) Pepsin immunoassay: new method; may be most sensitive indicator of aspiration but limited validation at present

c. Sputum: presence of polymorphonuclear leukocytes
(1) Culture and sensitivity: infecting organism if pneumonia present

d. Chest x-ray
(1) Bilateral patchy infiltrates or atelectasis
(2) Pulmonary edema may be present

Nursing Diagnoses

1. Risk for Aspiration related to impaired swallowing ability, altered consciousness, impaired protective reflexes, delayed gastric emptying, and artificial airway
2. Impaired Gas Exchange related to V/Q mismatching, intrapulmonary shunt, and intraalveolar fluid
3. Ineffective Breathing Pattern related to airway obstruction and increased work of breathing and fatigue
4. Ineffective Airway Clearance related to retained secretion
5. Risk for Infection related to aspiration of foreign material, inadequate primary defenses, invasive procedures, chronic disease, and poor airway clearance
6. Imbalanced Nutrition: Less than Body Requirements related to lack of exogenous nutrients and increased nutrient requirements
7. Anxiety related to change in health status

Collaborative Management

1. Prevent aspiration of gastric contents.
a. Use appropriate positioning to reduce risk of aspiration, and reduce volume of aspiration should vomiting occur.
(1) Place unconscious patient in side-lying position; endotracheal intubation may be necessary.
(2) Avoid flat position especially in patients receiving enteral feedings; keep HOB elevated to 45 degrees continuously for patients on continuous feedings and for at least 30 minutes after intermittent feedings.
(a) Stop continuous enteral feedings at least 30 minutes before any procedure that requires that the HOB be lowered.
(b) If the HOB cannot be elevated, position the patient on his or her right side as much as possible to facilitate movement of gastric contents through the pylorus

and allow drainage of emesis out of the mouth rather than to be aspirated.

(3) Do not restrain in such a way that the patient cannot protect his or her airway if vomiting occurs.

b. Maintain proper functioning of nasogastric, orogastric, or intestinal tube used for gastric suctioning or enteral feeding.
   (1) Check placement by aspiration and testing the pH; gastric secretions have a pH of 4 or less unless the patient is receiving acid-suppressing medications or continuous feedings; x-ray is the most reliable indicator of tube placement; intestinal tubes have a pH of greater than 7.
   (2) Reassess placement if gastric secretions decrease in volume.
   (3) Use x-ray to confirm placement of small-lumen feeding tubes, for aspiration is difficult because of tube collapse
c. Prevent aspiration in patients with artificial airways.
   (1) Keep the cuff of endotracheal or tracheostomy tube inflated to 20 to 25 mm Hg (25 to 35 cm H_2O).
      (a) If the patient is not on a mechanical ventilator, inflate the cuff during meals and suction secretions from the mouth and oropharynx before deflating the cuff.
   (2) Suction secretions from the oropharynx to reduce oropharyngeal secretions that accumulate above the cuff of an endotracheal tube.
      (a) Subglottic suctioning is advocated to prevent pneumonia associated with this silent aspiration; involves specialized endotracheal tubing with a port above the cuff that allows continuous suction to remove accumulated secretions.
d. Select appropriate tube and site for enteral feeding.
   (1) Use intragastric feedings when GI motility is normal because they are easier and less expensive to place than small intestinal tubes.
      (a) Small-lumen feeding tubes cause less gastroesophageal incompetence than do larger-lumen nasogastric tubes.
      (b) Tubes that do not go through the gastroesophageal sphincter (e.g., percutaneous endoscopic gastrostomy or needle jejunostomy tubes) are best for long-term enteral feeding.
   (2) Use small intestinal tubes and feedings when GI motility is impaired.
      (a) Because these feedings increase gastric secretions and because duodenal feedings may reflux back into the stomach, aspiration is still possible; a nasogastric or orogastric tube may be inserted to monitor gastric volume or for gastric decompression.
e. Monitor for gastric retention in patients on gastric enteral feedings.
   (1) Check for retention before each feeding if intermittent enteral feedings are being administered and every 4 to 6 hours if continuous enteral feedings are being administered.
      (a) If more than 200 mL is aspirated, consider the following:
         (i) Changing to continuous feedings if bolus or intermittent feedings are being used
         (ii) Changing the enteral feeding site to the duodenum or jejunum (though this does not completely eliminate the risk)
         (iii) Administering metoclopramide (Reglan) or erythromycin as prescribed to increase gastric motility
         (iv) Continue to reassess
      (b) If more than 500 mL is aspirated, withhold feeding for 1 hour and then recheck for retention.
         (i) Holding or discontinuing feedings can result in malnutrition, so consider changes previously stated
   (2) Because aspiration of small-lumen feeding tubes is difficult since they tend to collapse with suction, increase in abdominal girth, absent bowel sounds, and nausea are indications of retention that indicate that the feeding should be stopped in patients with these tubes.
f. Monitor the secretions suctioned or expectorated: glucose testing may be performed to confirm presence of enteral feeding in sputum.
g. Keep appropriate equipment at bedside.
   (1) Airway suctioning equipment
   (2) Wire cutters for patients with wired jaws
   (3) Scissors for patient with Sengstaken-Blakemore tube
h. Prepare the patient for surgery for intractable aspiration as requested: tracheoesophageal diversion or laryngotracheal separation.

2. Maintain airway, ventilation, and oxygenation if aspiration does occur.
   a. Position the bed in a slight Trendelenburg position with the patient in a right lateral decubitus position.
   b. Suction secretions from the airway immediately; provide adequate oxygenation during suctioning.
      (1) Endotracheal intubation may be necessary
      (2) Bronchoscopy for removal of large particles if indicated
   c. Stop enteral feeding if it is being administered.
   d. Monitor ABGs and pulse oximetry: a decrease in Spo_2, Sao_2, and Pao_2 may indicate the development of ARDS.

e. Administer oxygen therapy if hypoxemia is present.
  (1) CPAP or PEEP may be necessary to maintain adequate oxygenation.
f. Initiate mechanical ventilation as prescribed if hypercapnia develops.
g. Administer bronchodilators as prescribed.
h. Administer antibiotics as prescribed (prophylactically administered antibiotics are not recommended, but antibiotics specific to positive sputum or blood cultures are indicated).
i. Prepare the patient for pulmonary resection if abscess develops.

3. Monitor for complications.
  a. Acute respiratory failure
  b. ARDS
  c. Pneumonia
  d. Lung abscess
  e. Empyema

Status Asthmaticus

Definitions

1. Asthma: a recurrent, reversible airway disease characterized by increased airway responsiveness to a variety of stimuli that produces airway narrowing
2. Status asthmaticus: exacerbation of acute asthma characterized by severe airflow obstruction that is not relieved after 24 hours of maximal doses of traditional therapy

Etiology

1. Extrinsic: when a specific allergy can be related to the attack
  a. Dust and dust mites
  b. Animal dander, feathers
  c. Pollen
  d. Mold
  e. Preservatives (e.g., bisulfites)
  f. Food such as nuts, legumes (e.g., peanuts), chocolate, eggs, shellfish
  g. Food additives
2. Intrinsic: when the attack is seemingly unrelated to a specific allergen
  a. Infection, such as bacterial or viral pneumonia, bronchitis, or sinusitis
  b. Stress
  c. Exercise
  d. Gastroesophageal reflux disease (GERD)
  e. Aspiration
  f. Fear, anger, crying, laughing
  g. Menstrual cycle
  h. Smoke
  i. Propellants
  j. Air pollution
  k. Changes in inspired air such as cold or hot air, very high or very low humidity
  l. Alcohol
  m. Medications
    (1) Aspirin
    (2) Nonsteroidal antiinflammatory drugs (NSAIDs)
    (3) Beta-blockers

Pathophysiology

1. Trigger
  a. Extrinsic triggers cause IgE to be released; IgE stimulates the mast cells in the pulmonary submucosa to release histamine and slow-reacting substance of anaphylaxis (SRS-A)
    (1) Mast cells, eosinophils, epithelial cells, neutrophils, macrophages, and T lymphocytes contribute to the pathophysiologic changes.
    (2) IgE combines with the antigen.
    (3) Mast cells degranulate and release mediators of the inflammatory process.
    (4) Mast cells release histamine and SRS-A.
    (5) Histamine attaches to the receptor sites in the large bronchi, causing swelling and inflammation.
    (6) SRS-A, composed of three types of leukotrienes, causes inflammation and edema of the smooth muscle of the smaller bronchi and release of prostaglandins that enhance the effects of histamine.
    (7) Inflammation causes epithelial damage and airway smooth muscle hyperresponsiveness.
  b. Intrinsic triggers affect the balance between sympathetic and parasympathetic branches of the autonomic nervous system.
2. Airway narrowing, caused by inflammation and bronchoconstriction, is greatest during expiration.
  a. The work of breathing is increased, and fatigue occurs, impairing ventilation.
  b. Air trapping causes hyperinflation of alveoli.
3. Mucus further narrows the airway lumen.
  a. Increased amounts of thick, tenacious mucus are caused by the following:
    (1) Increased number of goblet cells
    (2) Excessive secretion of mucus caused by histamine
    (3) Dehydration related to increased insensible water loss via respiratory tract during tachypnea
  b. Excessive mucus in smaller airways causes V/Q mismatching and shunt.
4. Deposition of collagen impairs diffusion of oxygen across the alveolar-capillary membrane.
5. Acute respiratory failure with hypoxemia and respiratory acidosis eventually occurs if the attack is not reversed promptly.
  a. Hypoxemia results from a V/Q mismatch following inflammation, bronchoconstriction, and mucous plugging.
  b. Hypercapnia and respiratory acidosis results from hypoventilation caused by respiratory muscle fatigue.
6. Intrathoracic pressures are elevated and venous return to the right ventricle is decreased, cardiac output falls, and cardiopulmonary arrest may occur.

Clinical Presentation

1. Subjective
  a. History of a slow, progressive worsening of airflow obstruction over the course of several days or weeks

Table 5-5 Asthma: Arterial Blood Gas Analysis

Stage	Pao_2	$Paco_2$	pH	Acid-Base Imbalance
I	Normal	Decreased	Increased	Respiratory alkalosis
II	Decreased	Decreased	Increased	Respiratory alkalosis Mild to moderate hypoxemia
III	Very low	Normal	Normal	Significant hypoxemia
IV	Extremely low	Elevated	Decreased	Respiratory acidosis Critical hypoxemia

b. Anxiety
c. Dyspnea
d. Chest tightness
e. Fatigue
f. Insomnia
g. Anorexia

2. Objective
   a. Tachycardia
   b. Tachypnea; inability to speak in full sentences because of dyspnea
   c. Cough with thick, tenacious sputum production
   d. Use of accessory muscles
   e. Intercostal retractions
   f. Prolonged expiration (more than 1 to 3 [I:E] ratio)
   g. Diaphoresis
   h. Peak expiratory flow rate (PEFR) below 80% of patient's personal or predicted best; frequently below 50% of patient's personal best
   i. Clinical indications of dehydration: poor skin turgor; dry mucous membranes; increased specific gravity of urine
   j. Clinical indications of hypoxemia (Box 4-3)
   k. Clinical indications of hypercapnia (Box 4-4)
   l. Breath sound changes: rhonchi, wheezing
   m. Indications of potential imminent respiratory arrest
      (1) Change in consciousness: drowsiness or confusion
      (2) Paradoxical thoracoabdominal movement
      (3) Absence of rhonchi and wheezes may occur in critical stages; indication of absence of airflow
      (4) Bradycardia
      (5) Pulsus paradoxus greater than 15 mm Hg
3. Diagnostics
   a. Serum
      (1) WBC count may be increased if infection is the cause.
      (2) Eosinophil count may be increased if patient if not receiving steroids.
      (3) Hematocrit may be increased because of dehydration.
      (4) Electrolytes: Potassium and/or magnesium may be low during an acute attack.
      (5) Theophylline level: if therapeutic, administer 10 to 20 mcg/dL; if patient has not been taking the drug, theophylline level will be less than therapeutic.
      (6) ABGs (Table 5-5)
   b. Sputum
      (1) Increased viscosity
      (2) May have positive culture
      (3) Eosinophil stain: increase in number of eosinophils indicates allergic reaction
   c. Pulmonary function studies (may be impossible to do during attack because the patient is so dyspneic)
      (1) Decreased tidal volume and vital capacity
      (2) Increased residual volume
      (3) Forced expiratory volume$_1$ (FEV_1) and forced expiratory volume$_3$ (FEV_3) are diminished with improvement after bronchodilators
         (a) Best FEV_1 is likely a better predictor of mortality than best peak expiratory flow in patients with asthma (Hansen et al., 2001)
   d. Electrocardiogram (ECG): sinus tachycardia
   e. Chest x-ray
      (1) Normal or hyperinflated lungs with flattened diaphragms
      (2) Helpful to rule out foreign body, aspiration, pulmonary edema, PE, pneumonia, or pneumothorax

Nursing Diagnoses

1. Ineffective Breathing Pattern related to increased airway resistance and increased work of breathing and fatigue
2. Impaired Gas Exchange related to alveolar hypoventilation
3. Ineffective Airway Clearance related to excessive mucus production, increased viscosity of mucus, and decreased ability to expectorate
4. Risk for Infection related to retained secretions
5. Risk for Fluid Volume Deficit related to increased insensible loss caused by hyperventilation
6. Risk for Infection related to inadequate primary defenses, invasive procedures, chronic disease, and poor airway clearance
7. Imbalanced Nutrition: Less than Body Requirements related to lack of exogenous nutrients and increased nutrient requirements
8. Activity Intolerance related to imbalance between oxygen supply and oxygen demand

9. Anxiety related to change in health status
10. Knowledge Deficit related to disease process, self-care, and prescribed therapies

Collaborative Management

1. Assess predisposing factors; eliminate and/or treat cause.
   a. Antibiotics to treat infection promptly
   b. Avoidance of exposure to pulmonary irritants and pollutants
   c. Avoidance of drugs or foods that may trigger an attack
   d. Cromolyn sodium (Intal) or nedocromil (Tilade) are inhaled mast cell stabilizers that prevent the release of histamine from the mast cells; these agents have no direct bronchodilation or antiinflammatory effect and are not helpful during an acute attack
2. Maintain airway and improve ventilation.
   a. Elevate HOB to 30 to 45 degrees; overbed table may be helpful for patient to lean on.
   b. Administer pharmacologic agents as prescribed.
      (1) Bronchodilators to relax bronchial smooth muscle
         (a) Leukotriene inhibitors/leukotriene receptor antagonists (e.g., zafirlukast [Accolate], zileuton [Zyflo], or montelukast sodium [Singulair]) may have been used as a preventive agent; they are not helpful for treatment of acute bronchospasm
         (b) $Beta_2$ stimulants
            (i) Action: stimulate $beta_2$ receptors to cause smooth muscle relaxation
            (ii) Long-acting agents (e.g., salmeterol [Serevent]) by metered-dose inhaler likely will have been used long-term by the patient with a diagnosis of asthma
            (iii) Short-acting $beta_2$ agonists (e.g., metaproterenol [Alupent, Metaprel], albuterol [Proventil, Ventolin], pirbuterol [Maxair], bitolterol [Tornalate], terbutaline [Brethaire], or epinephrine)
               a) Metered-dose inhaler usually is used and may be as effective as a nebulizer when used with a spacing device.
               b) Nebulizer frequently is used if the PEFR is less than 50% of the patient's personal best; the beta agonist is administer by nebulizer every 20 minutes or continuously for 1 hour.
                  i) Continuous use has been shown as effective with no more side effects than intermittent use and requires less clinician time.
               c) Intermittent positive pressure breathing (IPPB) system should be avoided except in patients with very poor inspiratory effort who cannot distribute medication adequately, because IPPB can cause pneumothorax, especially in this high-risk group.
               d) Intravenous beta agonists are not recommended if inhalation therapy is possible because they do not result in better results but increase adverse effects significantly.
            (iv) Monitor closely for adverse effects such as significant tachycardia, dysrhythmias, hypertension, headache, tremor, anxiety, and hypokalemia
         (c) Anticholinergics (e.g., ipratropium bromide [Atrovent]) may be used in severe attacks to augment the effects of $beta_2$ agonists.
            (i) Action: block parasympathetic stimulation (making sympathetic stimulation dominant) to cause smooth muscle relaxation
            (ii) May be especially helpful for asthma stimulated by an intrinsic trigger
            (iii) Administered by a metered-dose inhaler or nebulizer
            (iv) May be administered as a combination beta agonist (e.g., ipratropium bromide and albuterol sulfate [Combivent])
         (d) Xanthines (e.g., theophylline or aminophylline) may be given IV for refractory attack.
            (i) Actions
               a) Smooth muscle relaxation causing bronchodilation, though less effective than nebulized beta agonists; also more adverse effects than beta agonists
               b) Immune-modulating effects including inhibition of T lymphocytes and other inflammatory cells and inhibition of cytokine release
            (ii) No longer first-line agent primarily because of the narrow therapeutic window and interactions with other commonly prescribed drugs, but should be continued in patients taking xanthine therapy at home
               a) Obtain a theophylline level for patients who have been receiving xanthines at home.
               b) Monitor closely for indications of theophylline toxicity.
                  i) GI: anorexia; nausea, vomiting
                  ii) Cardiac: dysrhythmias
                  iii) Neurologic: restlessness; seizures

(iii) Administration orally for long-term therapy but usually by IV infusion in acute asthma

(e) Magnesium: used in acutely ill asthmatic patients with severe exacerbation

(i) Actions: smooth muscle relaxation, bronchodilation, improved airflow

(ii) Administered as IV infusion: usual dose is 1 to 2 g over 20 minutes

(iii) Contraindicated in hypotension or renal failure

(iv) Monitor blood pressure during infusion; note and report significant hypotension or loss of deep tendon reflexes

(2) Corticosteroids to reduce inflammation

(a) Actions

(i) Decrease mucosal swelling and release of histamine by the mast cells

(ii) Potentiates bronchodilators

(b) Administration

(i) Patient has usually already administered steroids (e.g., beclomethasone [Vanceril, Beclovent], flunisolide [AeroBid], triamcinolone [Azmacort], or fluticasone [Flovent]) via metered-dose inhaler before hospitalization.

a) Steroids by inhalation diminish (but do not completely avoid) the systemic effects of steroid administration.

(ii) Steroids initially may be administered IV (e.g., methylprednisolone [Solu-Medrol]) or orally (prednisone and prednisolone) in status asthmaticus.

a) Initial large doses are titrated downward over days to weeks.

b) Alternate day oral dosing decreases the potential for adrenal suppression.

(iii) Steroid-resistant asthma: IV immunoglobulin may be administered

(3) Expectorants (e.g., guaifenesin [Robitussin] or potassium iodide [SSKI]) may be used, but hydration is most important; water is the best expectorant

(4) Mucolytics (e.g., acetylcysteine [Mucomyst]) generally are contraindicated because of the adverse effect of bronchospasm

(5) Sedatives: generally avoided unless patient is very agitated

(6) Antitussives: avoid use of antitussives

c. Maintain bronchial hygiene.

(1) Abdominal (i.e., deep) breathing

(2) Effective coughing

(3) Suctioning only if coughing is ineffective

(4) Chest physical therapy generally is not recommended and may be unnecessarily stressful for a patient with status asthmaticus

d. Use noninvasive ventilatory methods (CPAP or bi-PAP) as prescribed.

(1) May be used with a mask if the patient is not intubated

(2) May prevent further deterioration and intubation and mechanical ventilation

e. Ensure intubation and mechanical ventilation as necessary

(1) Indicated if $Paco_2$ continues to rise and acidosis develops

(2) The goal of mechanical ventilation is to normalize the pH, not necessary the $Paco_2$

(a) Mode: assist-control or pressure-regulated volume-controlled ventilation

(b) Tidal volume: 4 to 8 mL/kg

(c) Respiratory rate: 10 to 14 breaths/min and adjust to normalize pH, though $Paco_2$ still may be elevated

(i) Permissive hypercapnia, expected and accepted hypercapnia, results from the deliberate attempt to decrease alveolar ventilation by reducing tidal volumes and alveolar pressures.

(ii) Sedation may be required.

(iii) Bicarbonate infusions may be used to keep the pH no less than 7.2.

(d) Flow rate: 60 to 100 L/min; higher inspiratory flow rate shortens inspiration to allow more time for expiration to reduce air trapping and auto–PEEP

(i) I:E ratio: 1:3 or 1:4 to allow longer expiratory times

(e) Peak inspiratory pressure should be kept under 40 cm H_2O, and plateau pressure should be kept below 30 cm H_2O if possible

(f) Fio_2: adjusted to maintain Spo_2 of approximately 90%

(g) PEEP should be avoided if possible because this patient is at high risk for barotrauma

(i) Monitor levels of auto–PEEP caused by air trapping

3. Optimize oxygen delivery and decrease oxygen consumption.

a. Administer oxygen as indicated.

(1) Uncontrolled high-flow oxygen should be avoided in acute asthma; oxygen concentration should be adjusted to keep Spo_2 ~90%.

b. Teach and encourage relaxation techniques.

c. Teach and encourage abdominal breathing, though this is difficult for the patient when dyspneic and tachypneic.

d. Provide rest periods especially after meals or activities.

e. Use Heliox as prescribed (controversial in acute asthma)

(1) Helium is a light gas that decreases the work of breathing when it replaces nitrogen in the inspired air
(a) Oxygen percentage is prescribed, and helium replaces nitrogen to make up the remainder (e.g., 80% helium/20% oxygen, 70% helium/30% oxygen, or 60% helium/40% oxygen)
(2) Actions
(a) Decreases airway resistance and work of breathing
(b) Decreases hypercapnia and need for intubation and mechanical ventilation
(3) Administration
(a) By face mask
(b) By mechanical ventilator: requires recalibration for this lighter gas
4. Provide adequate rehydration.
a. Oral fluids: noncaffeinated
b. IV fluids: usually D_5NS
5. Provide instruction and counseling regarding lifestyle modification and need for pharmacologic therapy.
a. Recognition and avoidance of triggers; allergy testing and desensitization may be needed
b. Symptom monitoring
(1) To measure PEFR twice daily
(2) When to call the physician
(a) PEFR drops by 20% or more below its usual level
(b) Indications of respiratory infection
c. Drug therapy
(1) Inhaled bronchodilators and corticosteroids
(a) How to use and clean a metered-dose inhaler or nebulizer
(b) To rinse mouth after inhaled corticosteroids to avoid oral fungal infection (e.g., candidiasis)
(2) Cromolyn may be prescribed
(3) Antimicrobials
d. Breathing exercises: slow abdominal breathing; pursed lip breathing
e. Importance of immunizations (e.g., influenza, pneumococcus, or *Haemophilus*)
f. Control of GERD
(1) H_2 receptor antagonists or PPIs (e.g., omeprazole [Prilosec], pantoprazole [Protonix], or rabeprazole)
(2) Avoidance of large meals and supine position after eating
(3) Normalization of body weight
6. Monitor for complications.
a. Acute respiratory failure
b. Barotrauma (e.g., pneumothorax)
c. Pneumonia
d. Dysrhythmias
e. Hypovolemia
f. Hypotension related to hypovolemia, lung hyperinflation decreasing venous return to the heart, tension pneumothorax, and oversedation

Pulmonary Embolism/Infarction

Definition

Obstruction of blood flow to one or more arteries of the lung by a thrombus lodged in a pulmonary vessel; other types of emboli include fat, air, amniotic fluid, tumor, and foreign body (e.g., catheter fragment)
1. Massive: more than 50% occlusion of pulmonary blood flow; caused by occlusion of a lobar artery or larger artery
2. Submassive: less than 50% occlusion of pulmonary blood flow; in patients with preexisting heart or lung disease, hemodynamic deterioration occurs with less than 50% pulmonary vascular obstruction

Etiology

1. Risk factors for thrombus formation (Virchow's triad)
a. Hypercoagulability
(1) Malignancy: especially breast, lung, pancreas, or GI or genitourinary (GU) tracts
(2) Estrogen, especially in smokers
(a) Oral contraceptives
(b) Postmenopausal hormone replacement therapy
(3) Dehydration and hemoconcentration
(4) Fever
(5) Sickle cell anemia
(6) Pregnancy and postpartum period
(7) Polycythemia vera
(8) Abrupt discontinuance of anticoagulants
(9) Sepsis
(10) Protein C, protein S, or antithrombin III deficiency
b. Alterations in the vessel wall
(1) Trauma
(2) IV drug use
(3) Aging
(4) Vasculitis
(5) Varicose veins
(6) Diabetes mellitus
(7) Atherosclerosis
(8) Inflammatory process
c. Venous stasis
(1) Prolonged bed rest or immobilization
(2) Obesity
(3) Advanced age
(4) Burns
(5) Pregnancy
(6) Postpartum period
(7) HF
(8) MI
(9) Bacterial endocarditis
(10) Recent surgery especially legs, pelvis, or abdomen
(11) Thrombus formation in heart (e.g., atrial fibrillation [AF])
(12) Cardioversion
2. Risk factors for fat embolism
a. Long bone (e.g., femur) fracture, pelvic fracture, multiple fractures

   b. Orthopedic surgery with intramedullary manipulation
   c. Trauma to adipose tissue or liver
   d. Osteomyelitis
   e. Sickle cell crisis
   f. Burns
   g. Acute pancreatitis
   h. Liposuction
3. Risk factors for air embolism
   a. Recent surgical procedure
   b. Insertion of deep vein catheter
   c. Cardiopulmonary bypass
   d. Hemodialysis
   e. Endoscopy

Pathophysiology

1. More than 90% of thrombi develop in the deep veins of the lower extremities; superficial thrombophlebitis poses little risk unless the associated clot extends into the major deep veins; this would be suggested by swelling of the leg.
2. Thrombus formation enhances platelet adhesiveness and causes release of serotonin (vasoconstrictor).
3. Factors contributing to dislodgment of the thrombi
   a. Intravascular pressure changes
      (1) Sudden standing (e.g., initial ambulation)
      (2) Valsalva maneuver (e.g., coughing, sneezing, or vomiting)
      (3) Fluid challenges
      (4) Massaging legs
   b. Natural mechanism of clot dissolution: 7 to 10 days after clot develops
4. Consequences
   a. The clinical spectrum of PE ranges from asymptomatic to life-threatening.
   b. A clot develops that moves to the pulmonary vessels, where it stops when it is too large to move through.
   c. Ventilation continues, but perfusion is decreased: V/Q mismatch; increased alveolar dead space.
   d. No gas exchange takes place, so there is decreased alveolar carbon dioxide which causes bronchoconstriction and alveolar shrinking so that less inspired air goes into nonperfused alveoli and more inspired air goes into perfused alveoli.
   e. Cessation of blood flow damages type II pneumocytes and leads to a decrease in surfactant.
   f. Loss of surfactant causes atelectasis, interstitial fluid movement into the alveolus, and decreased lung compliance.
   g. Increased airway resistance and decreased lung compliance increase work of breathing.
   h. Pulmonary infarction may occur, causing hemorrhage, consolidation, and necrosis.
      (1) Pleural effusion or lung abscess may occur.
      (2) Some degree of pulmonary fibrosis may occur as the lung heals.
      (3) Infarction occurs only in approximately 10% of cases of PE because of dual blood supply to the lung (pulmonary and bronchial).
   i. Pulmonary arterial obstruction and pulmonary vasoconstriction caused by hypoxemia and release of vasoconstrictive mediators increase PVR.
   j. Increased PVR causes pulmonary hypertension and increased right ventricular afterload.
   k. Increased right ventricular wall stress causes compression of the right coronary artery, decreased subendocardial perfusion, and potentially right ventricular microinfarction.
   l. Increased right ventricular workload and ischemia may lead to right ventricular hypokinesis and dilation, tricuspid regurgitation, and right ventricular failure (RVF) (acute cor pulmonale).
   m. Systemic hypotension and cardiac arrest may occur.
5. Fat emboli
   a. Most likely to develop 1 to 3 days after injury but may occur up to a week after injury
   b. Fat globules enter the bloodstream and form emboli
   c. Presence of fat emboli in the bloodstream causes interactions with platelets and free fatty acids along with release of vasoactive substances
   d. Cerebral ischemia
6. Air emboli
   a. Activation of the clotting cascade
   b. Interruption of circulation

Clinical Presentation

1. Small embolus: patient is asymptomatic
2. Small to medium embolus
   a. Anxiety
   b. Dyspnea
   c. Tachypnea
   d. Tachycardia
   e. Chest pain
   f. Cough
   g. Accentuated P_2 (pulmonic component of S_2; the second component of S_2)
   h. Right-sided S_3 or S_4 (audible at sternum)
   i. Breath sound changes: crackles
3. Large to massive: massive PE is when 50% of pulmonary artery bed is occluded
   a. Feeling of impending doom
   b. Dyspnea
   c. Tachypnea
   d. Tachycardia
   e. Chest pain
   f. Mental clouding and/or syncope
   g. Cyanosis
   h. Clinical indications of RVF: jugular venous distention (JVD); hepatomegaly; murmur of tricuspid regurgitation; right ventricular heave
   i. Hypotension or sudden shock
   j. May present as pulseless electrical activity

4. If pulmonary infarction develops (hours to days after embolism), the patient also will have the following:
   a. Fever
   b. Pleuritic chest pain
   c. Hemoptysis
   d. Pleural friction rub
5. Hemodynamic monitoring
   a. Elevated central venous pressure and right atrial pressure (RAP)
   b. Elevated pulmonary artery pressures with normal PAOP (increased diastolic pulmonary artery (PAd) pressure/PAOP gradient)
   c. Elevated PVR
   d. Decreased cardiac output/cardiac index in massive PE
6. Diagnostics
   a. Laboratory
      (1) D dimer
         (a) Elevated in almost all patients with PE because of endogenous fibrinolysis (i.e., high negative predictive value)
         (b) High sensitivity but low specificity; 99% negative predictive value
         (c) Indeterminate V/Q and a positive D dimer is an indication for pulmonary angiogram
      (2) Troponin I: may be elevated; indicates right ventricular microinfarction
      (3) Brain natriuretic peptide: may be elevated with right ventricular overload
      (4) ABGs
         (a) If thrombotic
            (i) Decreased Pao_2, Sao_2, Svo_2; Pao_2 less than 50 mm Hg in a patient with previously normal ABGs indicates greater than 50% obstruction of the pulmonary flow and that pulmonary hypertension is present
            (ii) Decreased $Paco_2$
            (iii) Respiratory alkalosis initially; may have metabolic acidosis if severe hypoxemia; respiratory acidosis may develop with significant atelectasis or fatigue
         (b) If fat or air embolism
            (i) Decreased Pao_2, Sao_2
            (ii) Increased $Paco_2$
            (iii) Respiratory acidosis; may have metabolic acidosis if severe hypoxemia
   b. ECG
      (1) Dysrhythmias
         (a) Sinus tachycardia
         (b) Atrial dysrhythmias, especially AF are common
         (c) Ventricular dysrhythmias may occur in hypoxemia
      (2) Blocks: new right bundle branch block (RBBB) may be seen
      (3) Tall, peaked P waves in lead II (P pulmonale)
      (4) Right axis deviation may be seen (QRS complex negative in I, positive in aVF)
      (5) Right ventricular strain: ST segment elevation in V_1 and V_2
      (6) Helpful to rule out MI as cause of signs/symptoms
   c. Chest x-ray
      (1) Almost always normal initially but may be helpful to rule out other sources of patient symptoms
      (2) If thrombotic
         (a) Initially normal
         (b) After 24 hours: small infiltrates may be seen following atelectasis; elevated hemidiaphragm on affected side; decreased pulmonary vascularity
         (c) If pulmonary infarction: infiltrates and pleural effusion may be seen
      (3) If fat embolism
         (a) Diffuse extensive interstitial and alveolar infiltrates
   d. Echocardiography
      (1) Usually normal but may show right ventricular dilation, hypokinesis, and tricuspid regurgitation
      (2) May show bulging of interventricular septum into left ventricle that reduces left ventricular size with D-shaped left ventricle
      (3) Also helpful to rule out cardiac tamponade, dissection of the aorta, and acute MI
   e. V/Q scan
      (1) Shows perfusion defect with normal ventilation
      (2) Positive predictive value of high probability V/Q scan is 96% when supported by high clinical suspicion of PE; negative predictive value of negative V/Q scan is also excellent, with a normal V/Q scan accurately ruling out PE 98% of the time; unfortunately, 75% of patients fall within the indeterminate category
      (3) Intermediate or low probability V/Q scan with positive D dimer is indication for pulmonary angiography
   f. Spiral (helical) CT
      (1) Widely available
      (2) Easier study to obtain than a V/Q scan or pulmonary angiogram
      (3) Capable of demonstrating a variety of thoracic pathologic conditions that can mimic PE
      (4) Sensitivity greatly affected by generation of scanner used; significantly better sensitivity with new scanners; excellent specificity
   g. Magnetic resonance angiography (MRA)
      (1) Gadolinium-enhanced MRA allows high-resolution angiography during a single breath
      (2) Fast but accurate test that does not involve nephrotoxic contrast agents
   h. Pulmonary angiography
      (1) Shows cutoff of a vessel or a filling defect within 24 to 72 hours
      (2) Continues to be the gold standard, but not without risks

(3) Indicated in patients with a high probability of having a PE and nondiagnostic noninvasive studies
(4) Excellent sensitivity and specificity
(5) Disadvantages: risk of significant bleeding, provides a relative contraindication for fibrinolytic therapy because of the risk of bleeding from the puncture site

7. If fat embolism: may have no symptoms for 12 to 48 hours
   a. Subjective
      (1) Restlessness, agitation, irritability, confusion
      (2) Dyspnea
      (3) Delirium
   b. Objective
      (1) Tachypnea
      (2) Tachycardia
      (3) Fever
      (4) Petechiae on conjunctivae, anterior chest, neck, axilla
      (5) Retinal hemorrhages with emboli present on the retina
      (6) Breath sound changes: stridor, wheezes, crackles
      (7) Lethargy, coma
      (8) Seizures
      (9) Hypoxemia: decreased Spo_2, Sao_2, Pao_2
      (10) Clinical indications of hypoxia (Box 4-3)
   c. Diagnostic
      (1) Serum
         (a) Elevated lipase
         (b) Elevated triglycerides
         (c) Increased free fatty acids
         (d) Elevated sedimentation rate
         (e) Decreased hemoglobin, hematocrit
         (f) Thrombocytopenia
         (g) Elevated fibrin split products
      (2) ABGs: hypoxemia
      (3) Urinalysis: fat globules in the urine
      (4) Sputum: fat globules in the sputum
8. If air embolism
   a. Subjective
      (1) Feeling of impending doom
      (2) Light-headedness
      (3) Weakness
      (4) Nausea
      (5) Chest pain
      (6) Dyspnea
      (7) Palpitations
      (8) Confusion
   b. Objective
      (1) Pallor
      (2) Tachypnea
      (3) Tachycardia
      (4) Hypotension
      (5) Churning noise ("mill wheel murmur") may be audible
      (6) Hypoxemia: decreased Spo_2, Sao_2, Pao_2
      (7) Clinical indications of hypoxia (Box 4-3)
      (8) Clinical indications of pulmonary edema: S_3, crackles
      (9) Seizures
   c. Diagnostic
      (1) Serum: ABGs: hypoxemia; hypercapnia
      (2) Chest x-ray: may show evidence of RVF and/or pulmonary edema
      (3) V/Q scan: similar to PE but may resolve within 24 hours
      (4) Echocardiography: shows air in right ventricle, right ventricular dilation, and/or pulmonary hypertension

Nursing Diagnoses

1. Impaired Gas Exchange related to V/Q mismatching and alveolar dead space
2. Ineffective Breathing Pattern related to increased work of breathing and fatigue
3. Decreased Cardiac Output related to acute pulmonary hypertension, right ventricular microinfarction, and RVF
4. Risk for Infection related to inadequate primary defenses, invasive procedures, chronic disease, and poor airway clearance
5. Imbalanced Nutrition: Less than Body Requirements related to lack of exogenous nutrients and increased nutrient requirements
6. Activity Intolerance related to imbalance between oxygen supply and oxygen demand
7. Altered Protection related to fibrinolytics and/or anticoagulants
8. Anxiety related to change in health status
9. Knowledge Deficit related to disease process, self-care, and prescribed therapies

Collaborative Management

1. Prevent emboli formation.
   a. All patients
      (1) Deep breathing exercises hourly for postoperative patients
      (2) Ambulation as soon as possible
      (3) Leg exercises, especially for patients who cannot ambulate; passive range of motion of all extremities for patients who cannot do leg exercises
      (4) Frequent repositioning; avoid extreme knee or hip flexion; instruct patient not to cross his or her legs
      (5) Adequate fluid intake to prevent dehydration and hypercoagulability
      (6) Careful venipuncture and IV care
         (a) Avoidance of venipunctures in legs
         (b) Atraumatic venipuncture; avoid multiple sticks
   b. Patients with moderate risk for deep venous thrombosis (DVT) also require elastic stockings or intermittent pneumatic compression devices
      (1) Elastic stockings: take care to prevent constriction and tourniquet effect of stockings
      (2) Intermittent pneumatic compression devices: also referred to as *sequential compression devices*

(a) Stimulate endogenous fibrinolytic activity in addition to direct physical stimulation of increased venous blood return

c. Patients with high risk for DVT are likely to have subcutaneous low-dose unfractionated heparin (UFH) or low-molecular-weight heparin (LMWH) prescribed if not contraindicated
  (1) UFH: 5000 units every 8 to 12 hours
  (2) Enoxaparin (Lovenox): 30 mg every 12 hours
  (3) Dalteparin sodium (Fragmin): 2500 units daily

d. Patients with documented DVT require low-dose UFH or LMWH

2. Prevent dislodgment of clot.
  a. Monitor patient closely for clinical indications of DVT.
    (1) Low-grade fever
    (2) Calf pain/tenderness
    (3) Unilateral edema, erythema, warmth, dilated collateral veins
    (4) Positive venography, venous duplex, and/or compression ultrasonography
  b. Instruct the patient regarding avoidance of Valsalva maneuver.
  c. Maintain steady IV flow rates.
  d. Avoid leg massage.

3. Maintain adequate airway, ventilation, and oxygenation.
  a. Administer oxygen to maintain Spo_2 greater than 90%.
    (1) Nasal cannula at 5 L/min unless contraindicated
    (2) High concentrations of oxygen via non-rebreathing mask may be required to maintain a Spo_2 greater than ~90%
  b. Administer analgesics as prescribed to prevent splinting and encourage deep breathing.
  c. Provide quiet, restful environment.
  d. Ensure intubation and mechanical ventilation if required.
    (1) The primary initial problem in PE is diffusion caused by the perfusion defect; the patient generally is ventilating adequately initially (frequently even excessively as evidenced by a low $Paco_2$) but may require intubation and mechanical ventilation as respiratory muscle fatigue occurs.

4. Arrest thrombosis and reestablish perfusion.
  a. Obtain baseline clotting profile.
  b. Administer fibrinolytic therapy as prescribed.
    (1) Indications
      (a) Hypodynamic instability
      (b) Acute RVF
      (c) Significant hypoxemia despite optimal oxygen therapy
    (2) Actions
      (a) Dissolves recent clots promptly to speed pulmonary tissue reperfusion
      (b) Reverses RVF
      (c) Improves pulmonary capillary blood volume
    (3) Agent: tissue plasminogen activator (TPA): alteplase (Activase) 100 mg over 2 hours
    (4) Contraindications and nursing management as in MI section of Chapter 3
    (5) Anticoagulation follows fibrinolytic therapy
  c. Administer anticoagulants as prescribed.
    (1) Action: prevents extension of the clot and reocclusion
    (2) Parenteral agents: usually maintained for 7 to 10 days
      (a) UFH
        (i) Dose: 70 to 80 units/kg initially, followed by 15 to 20 units/kg/hr to maintain activated partial thromboplastin time of 60 to 80 seconds; higher doses may be necessary initially because of low antithrombin III levels after PE
      (b) LMWH: may be prescribed in stable patients
        (i) Agent: enoxaparin (Lovenox): 1 mg/kg subcutaneously every 12 hours
        (ii) Advantages
          a) Longer plasma half-life than UFH
          b) More predictable anticoagulant response to weight-adjusted doses than UFH
          c) No need to monitor clotting studies, though monitoring is indicated in patients who are morbidly obese, who have renal insufficiency, or who weigh less than 50 kg
          d) Lower incidence of heparin-induced thrombocytopenia and thrombocytopenia (HITT)
        (iii) Potential disadvantage: longer half-life and lesser reversibility with protamine than UFH
      (c) For patients with HIT (also referred to as *heparin-associated thrombocytopenia* or *white clot syndrome*)
        (i) Lepirudin (Refludan)
        (ii) Argatroban
    (3) Oral agent: warfarin (Coumadin)
      (a) Started 3 to 4 days before parenteral anticoagulants are discontinued and continued for up to 6 months
      (b) Usual starting dose is 5 mg daily and adjusted to maintain international normalized ratio of 2 to 3
  d. Prepare patient for pulmonary embolectomy as requested: indicated for patient with massive PE with hemodynamic instability (e.g., cardiogenic shock) who cannot receive fibrinolytic therapy.
    (1) Surgical embolectomy
      (a) Complication rates for pulmonary embolectomy are relatively high
      (b) Requires cardiopulmonary bypass
    (2) Catheter embolectomy
      (a) Clot fragmentation using pigtail catheter
      (b) Rheolytic thrombectomy using high-velocity saline jet (e.g., AngioJet)

(c) Clot aspiration (e.g., transluminal extraction catheter)

e. Prepare patient for insertion of inferior vena cava filter as requested.
   (1) Indications
      (a) Recurrent PE despite effective anticoagulation
      (b) Anticoagulants are contraindicated
      (c) Note that these are effective in protecting the lung from successive emboli, but they do not do anything about the current PE
   (2) Types
      (a) Vena caval umbrella
      (b) Greenfield filter
      (c) Bird's nest filter (does not require precise axial orientation)

f. Provide treatment of pulmonary hypertension and acute RVF as prescribed.
   (1) First priority is elimination of the pulmonary vascular obstruction and reduction of PVR: fibrinolytics, embolectomy.
   (2) Inotropes (e.g., dobutamine [Dobutrex]) and fluids also may be prescribed to ensure adequate left ventricular contractility and filling volume.

g. Administer antibiotics as prescribed for septic emboli (rather than fibrinolytics and anticoagulants).

5. Monitor for complications.
   a. Pulmonary infarction
   b. Cerebral infarction
   c. MI
   d. RVF
   e. Dysrhythmias or blocks
      (1) Atrial dysrhythmias are common if RVF occurs.
      (2) Ventricular dysrhythmias may occur in hypoxemia.
      (3) RBBB may occur but is usually transient.
   f. Hepatic congestion and necrosis
   g. Pneumonia
   h. Pulmonary abscess
   i. ARDS
   j. DIC
   k. Shock
   l. Complications of therapy
      (1) Bleeding related to fibrinolytic or anticoagulant therapy
      (2) Oxygen toxicity related to high concentrations of oxygen

6. Specific to fat embolism
   a. Prevention: early immobilization of long bone fractures
   b. Treatment
      (1) Oxygen via nasal cannula at 5 L/min unless contraindicated; 100% oxygen by non-rebreathing mask may be necessary to maintain Spo_2 of at least 95%
      (2) Intubation and mechanical ventilation may be necessary
      (3) Steroids (e.g. hydrocortisone) to decrease inflammatory response (controversial)
      (4) Fluids to flush the fatty acids and prevent renal damage
      (5) Osmotic diuretics: if pulmonary edema is present
      (6) Red blood cells and/or platelets may be necessary

7. Specific to air embolism
   a. Prevention
      (1) Priming of IV tubings and central catheters with fluid to remove air before connection or insertion
      (2) Use of IV pumps with air detectors
      (3) Use of twist-lock type connections on central venous catheters to prevent accidental disconnections
      (4) Positioning of patient in Trendelenburg position for the insertion of central venous catheters or treatment of chest trauma unless contraindicated (e.g., head trauma)
      (5) Instruction of the patient to hold his or her breath and bear down (i.e., Valsalva maneuver) during tubing changes and catheter removal
      (6) Use of pressure dressing to central venous site at time of catheter removal
   b. Treatment
      (1) Left lateral decubitus position with head down (referred to as *Durant's maneuver*) if air embolism suspected
      (2) Attempt to aspirate the air embolus
      (3) External cardiac compressions push air out of the right ventricle into the pulmonary circulation, fragmenting the air bolus into smaller air bubbles
      (4) Oxygen via 100% non-rebreathing mask; hyperbaric oxygen is indicated for arterial embolization and clinical deterioration
      (5) Anticoagulants may be administered

Chest Trauma

General Information

1. Types of trauma
   a. Blunt trauma leaves the body surface intact.
   b. Penetrating trauma disrupts the body surface.
   c. Perforating trauma leaves entrance and exit wounds as an object passes through the body.
2. Etiology
   a. Motor vehicle collision
   b. Motorcycle collision
   c. Vehicle/pedestrian collision
   d. Fall
   e. Assault
   f. Explosion
   g. Projectiles: bullet, knives, impalement
3. Mechanisms of injury
   a. Blunt chest trauma
      (1) Rapid acceleration/deceleration: Shearing force causes stretching of tissue, organs, blood vessels with resultant tearing, leaking, or rupture.

(2) Direct impact: Object striking chest or chest striking object causes rib, sternal, or scapular fractures or injury to the heart or lung parenchyma.
(3) Compression: Force of rapid deceleration as tissues hit a fixed object such as the sternum or rib cage causes concussion, contusion, bleeding, or rupture of an organ.

b. Penetrating chest trauma
(1) Penetration of lung, heart, great vessel, or diaphragm causes bleeding and may cause loss of intactness of an organ or vessel.

Pulmonary Contusion

1. Definition: damage to the lung parenchyma that results in localized edema and hemorrhage
2. Etiology
   a. Blunt trauma: high-speed motor vehicle collision is most common
   b. Crush injuries
   c. Chest compressions during cardiopulmonary resuscitation
   d. Frequently associated with flail chest
3. Pathophysiology
   a. Blunt trauma causes deceleration injury to chest wall and compression of thoracic cavity.
   b. Diminished thoracic size compresses lung tissue, and decompression causes capillary rupture and subsequent hemorrhage.
   c. Initial hemorrhage is caused by bruising, pulmonary tears, and lacerations.
   d. Then interstitial and alveolar edema occur at site of contusion.
   e. Finally, massive interstitial edema occurs with general inflammation.
   f. Damaged or closed alveolar-capillary units cause V/Q mismatch and shunt.
   g. Increased PVR, decreased lung compliance, decreased pulmonary blood flow occurs.
   h. Atelectasis may occur because of retained secretions and infection.
   i. Severe pulmonary lacerations may cause concurrent hemothorax.
   j. Pulmonary contusion may accompany flail chest and may be masked by the obvious ventilation difficulties seen in flail chest.
4. Clinical presentation (may be delayed 24 to 48 hours)
   a. Subjective
      (1) Anxiety, restlessness
      (2) Dyspnea
      (3) Chest tenderness
   b. Objective
      (1) Tachycardia
      (2) Tachypnea
      (3) Increased work of breathing: use of accessory muscles; tripod position
      (4) Ecchymosis at site of impact
      (5) Ineffective cough, guarding
      (6) Hemoptysis
      (7) Dullness to percussion on affected side
      (8) Breath sound changes: crackles; wheezes
   c. Diagnostic
      (1) ABGs
         (a) Decreased Pa_{O_2}
         (b) Pa_{CO_2} may be normal or decreased depending on ventilation pattern (e.g., may be low because of hyperventilation)
      (2) Chest x-ray
         (a) Changes may take between 2 and 24 hours to develop on chest x-ray patchy, poorly defined areas of increased parenchymal density reflecting intraalveolar hemorrhage; linear and irregular infiltrates in the bronchioles
         (b) If severe, extensive areas of increased parenchymal density within one or both lungs
         (c) Diaphragm may be lower on affected side because injured lung is bigger
         (d) To differentiate ARDS from pulmonary contusion
            (i) Pulmonary contusion usually is localized and occurs near the site of external trauma.
            (ii) ARDS causes diffuse bilateral changes.
      (3) CT scan: assesses damage to pulmonary parenchyma and pleural cavity
5. Nursing diagnoses
   a. Impaired Gas Exchange related to V/Q mismatching and intrapulmonary shunt
   b. Ineffective Breathing Pattern related to chest pain
   c. Ineffective Airway Clearance related to retained secretions
   d. Risk for Fluid Volume Excess related to altered permeability of alveolar-capillary membrane
   e. Pain related to pleural injury, chest wall injury, rib fracture, and inflammation
   f. Risk for Infection related to inadequate primary defenses, invasive procedures, and poor airway clearance
   g. Imbalanced Nutrition: Less than Body Requirements related to lack of exogenous nutrients and increased nutrient requirements
   h. Activity Intolerance related to imbalance between oxygen supply and oxygen demand
   i. Anxiety related to change in health status
6. Collaborative management
   a. Establish and maintain airway, ventilation, and oxygenation.
      (1) Oxygen per nasal cannula at 2 to 5 L/min to achieve an Sp_{O_2} greater than 95% unless contraindicated; if patient has history of COPD, administer oxygen to achieve an oxygen saturation of ~90% by pulse oximetry
      (2) Analgesics in doses adequate to allow patient to deep breathe and cough as indicated
      (3) Chest physiotherapy
         (a) Suctioning if patient cannot cough adequately to clear airways
         (b) Bronchoscopy may be necessary if airway clearance techniques are inadequate

(4) Endotracheal intubation and mechanical ventilation with PEEP may be necessary
   (a) Synchronous independent lung ventilation may be necessary to prevent the detrimental effects of PEEP on the normal alveoli (e.g., increased alveolar pressure and decreased blood flow)
      (i) Requires double-lumen endotracheal tube and two mechanical ventilators
(5) Positioning with good lung down
(6) Careful fluid administration to prevent pulmonary edema
   (a) Goal is usually to maintain RAP at ~4 mm Hg and PAOP at ~10 mm Hg.
   (b) Diuretics also may be given.
(7) Steroids were given frequently in the past but are no longer recommended

b. Control pain.
   (1) Narcotics given on a regular schedule
   (2) Intercostal nerve block
   (3) Epidural analgesic
c. Monitor for complications.
   (1) Pneumonia: common complication
      (a) Prophylactically administered antibiotics are not recommended; antibiotics are indicated only if infection is present.
      (b) Culture sputum as indicated.
   (2) Lung abscess
   (3) Empyema
   (4) Pulmonary edema
   (5) PE
   (6) ARDS

Closed (Noncommunicating) Pneumothorax

(Also Called *Simple Pneumothorax*)
(Figure 5-4)

1. Definition: air enters the intrapleural space through the lung, causing partial or total collapse of the lung
   a. Small: 15% or less
   b. Medium: 15% to 60%
   c. Large: greater than 60%
2. Etiology

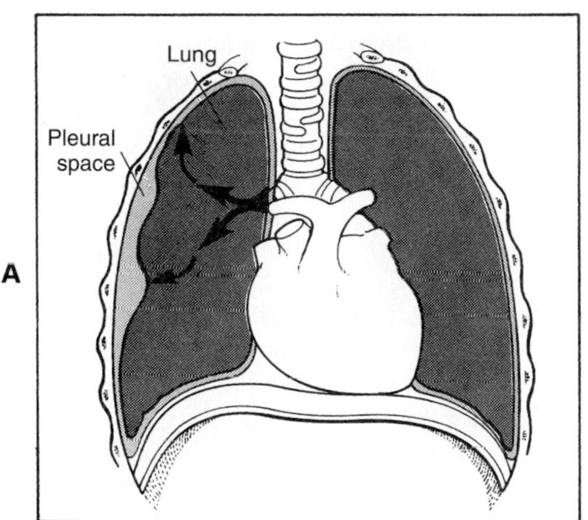

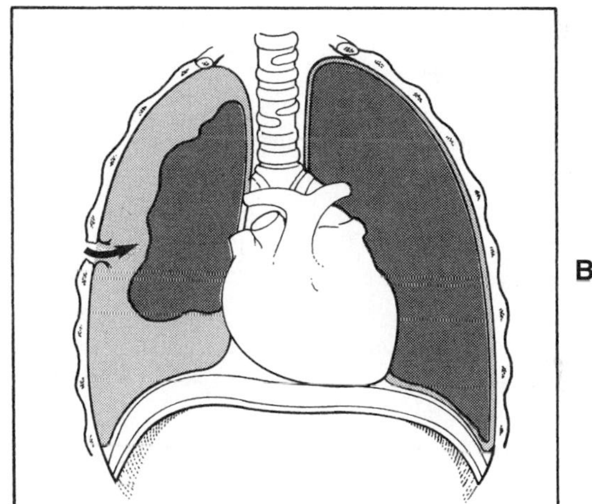

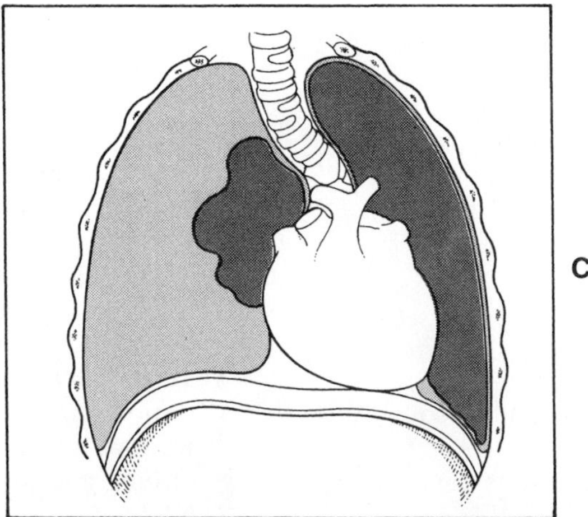

Figure 5-4 Pneumothorax. **A,** Closed. **B,** Open. **C,** Tension. (From Wilson, S. F., & Thompson, J. M. [1990]. *Respiratory disorders.* St. Louis, MO: Mosby-Year Book.)

a. Primary: related to congenital bleb (common in endomorphic males, age 20 to 40 years)
b. Secondary
   (1) Emphysematous bullous
   (2) Tuberculosis
   (3) Lung cancer
c. Traumatic
   (1) Blunt trauma caused by motor vehicle collision, falls, blows to chest, blast injuries
   (2) Cardiopulmonary resuscitation
   (3) Positive pressure mechanical ventilator
d. Iatrogenic causes: central venous catheterization via subclavian or low jugular vein puncture; intracardiac injection; thoracentesis; positive pressure ventilation

3. Pathophysiology
   a. Disruption of normal negative intrapleural pressure
      (1) Lung laceration by rib fracture or needle
      (2) Compression of the lung at the height of inspiration when alveolar pressure is high
      (3) Rupture of weak alveolus, bleb, or bulla
   b. Lung collapse
   c. Decreased surface area for exchange of gases
   d. Acute respiratory failure
4. Clinical presentation
   a. Subjective
      (1) Dyspnea
      (2) Chest pain: sudden, sharp, may be referred to corresponding shoulder, across chest, or abdomen
   b. Objective
      (1) Tachycardia
      (2) Tachypnea
      (3) Cough: dry, nonproductive
      (4) Asymmetric chest excursion with limited motion of affected hemithorax
      (5) Subcutaneous emphysema possible
      (6) Decreased fremitus on affected side
      (7) Hyperresonance to percussion on affected side
      (8) Diminished to absent breath sounds on affected side
      (9) Clinical indications of hypoxemia may be present
      (10) If patient on mechanical ventilator
         (a) Dramatic increase in peak inspiratory pressures
         (b) High pressure alarm
   c. Diagnostic
      (1) ABGs
         (a) Decreased $Pa{O_2}$
         (b) Increased $Pa{CO_2}$
      (2) Chest x-ray
         (a) Air in pleural space and lung collapse on affected side
         (b) May show mediastinal shift toward unaffected side
      (3) CT of thorax: better at detecting very small or anterior pneumothorax that may be missed on chest x-ray
5. Nursing diagnoses
   a. Impaired Gas Exchange related to alveolar hypoventilation
   b. Ineffective Breathing Pattern related to chest pain and decreased lung expansion
   c. Pain related to pleural injury, inflammation, and presence of chest tube
   d. Risk for Infection related to inadequate primary defenses, invasive procedures, chronic disease, and poor airway clearance
   e. Imbalanced Nutrition: Less than Body Requirements related to lack of exogenous nutrients and increased nutrient requirements
   f. Activity Intolerance related to imbalance between oxygen supply and oxygen demand
   g. Anxiety related to change in health status
6. Collaborative management
   a. Establish and maintain airway, ventilation, and oxygenation.
      (1) Oxygen per nasal cannula at 2 to 5 L/min to achieve an $Sp{O_2}$ greater than 95% unless contraindicated; if patient has history of COPD, administer oxygen to achieve an oxygen saturation of ~90% by pulse oximetry
      (2) Analgesics in doses adequate to allow patient to deep breathe and cough as indicated
      (3) Positioning patient for optimal ventilation: semi-Fowler or Fowler's position
      (4) If supine: position with good lung down
      (5) Chest tube (not necessary if less than 15% and asymptomatic)
         (a) Inserted into fourth to fifth intercostal space at midaxillary line
         (b) Connected to a Heimlich flutter valve or chest drainage system
   b. Control pain: narcotics given on a regular schedule.
   c. Monitor for complications.
      (1) Recurrent pneumothorax
         (a) Avoidance of IPPB in patients with COPD
         (b) If positive pressure mechanical ventilation: careful adjustment of tidal volume and PEEP: close monitoring of peak inspiratory pressures
         (c) Careful placement of subclavian or jugular venous catheters
         (d) Decortication may be performed for patients with recurrent spontaneous pneumothorax; involves the stripping of the parietal pleura from the apex of the lung to allow the visceral pleura to adhere to the chest wall
      (2) Atelectasis
      (3) Pneumonia, abscess

Tension Pneumothorax (See Figure 5-4)

1. Definition: accumulation of air in pleural space without means of escape, causing complete collapse of lung and potential mediastinal shift
2. Etiology
   a. Blunt or penetrating trauma
   b. Positive pressure mechanical ventilation: especially if patient

(1) Has emphysematous bullae or congenital blebs
(2) Is receiving large tidal volumes and/or PEEP
c. Nonfunctional (e.g., clotted or clamped) chest drainage system
d. Occlusive dressing on an open pneumothorax
3. Pathophysiology
a. Air rushes into, but not out of, the pleural space
b. Disruption of negative intrapleural pressure; creation of a positive pressure in the pleural space
c. Ipsilateral lung collapses
d. If tear does not seal, a one-way valve effect may be produced, allowing air to enter during inspiration but not to escape during exhalation
e. Increasing positive intrapleural pressure may cause mediastinal shift leading to compression of the contralateral lung, thoracic aorta, vena cava, and heart
f. Decreased right ventricular filling, decreased cardiac output
g. Acute respiratory failure and shock may occur
4. Clinical presentation
a. Subjective
(1) Dyspnea
(2) Chest pain
b. Objective
(1) Tachycardia
(2) Tachypnea
(3) Asymmetric chest excursion with limited motion of affected hemithorax
(4) Subcutaneous emphysema possible
(5) Decreased fremitus on affected side
(6) Hyperresonance to percussion on affected side; may even be tympanic
(7) Diminished to absent breath sounds on affected side
(8) Clinical indications of hypoxemia may be present
(9) If mediastinal shift:
(a) Tracheal shift away from affected side
(b) Point of maximal impulse shift away from affected side
(c) JVD
(d) Hypotension
c. Diagnostic
(1) ABGs
(a) Decreased Pa_{O_2}
(b) Increased Pa_{CO_2}
(2) Chest x-ray
(a) Absence of lung marking on the affected side
(b) Widening of the ICSs on the affected side
(c) Mediastinal shift (away from the affected side) may be present
5. Nursing diagnoses
a. Potential Decrease in Cardiac Output related to mediastinal shift, cardiac compression, and tearing of great vessels
b. Impaired Gas Exchange related to alveolar hypoventilation and lung compression
c. Ineffective Breathing Pattern related to chest pain and decreased lung expansion
d. Pain related to pleural injury, inflammation, and presence of chest tube
e. Risk for Infection related to inadequate primary defenses, invasive procedures, chronic disease, and poor airway clearance
f. Imbalanced Nutrition: Less than Body Requirements related to lack of exogenous nutrients and increased nutrient requirements
g. Activity Intolerance related to imbalance between oxygen supply and oxygen demand
h. Anxiety related to change in health status
6. Collaborative management
a. Establish and maintain airway, ventilation, and oxygenation.
(1) Oxygen per nasal cannula at 2 to 5 L/min to achieve an Sp_{O_2} greater than 95% unless contraindicated; if patient has history of COPD, administer oxygen to achieve an oxygen saturation of ~90% by pulse oximetry
(2) Emergency decompression with perpendicular insertion of a large-bore needle (or IV catheter [e.g., angiocath]) into second anterior interspace at the MCL on the affected side until a chest tube can be inserted; a flutter valve (e.g., Heimlich valve or finger cot with a slit cut at the end) may be placed on the needle to allow air to escape but prevent atmospheric air from entering the pleural space
(3) Chest tube and chest drainage system
(4) Analgesics in doses adequate to allow patient to deep breathe and cough as indicated
(5) Position patient for optimal ventilation: semi-Fowler or Fowler's position
(6) If supine: position with good lung down
b. Control pain: narcotics given on a regular schedule or by patient-controlled analgesia.
c. Monitor for complications.
(1) Shock
(2) Cardiopulmonary arrest
(3) Atelectasis
(4) Pneumonia, abscess

Open (Communicating) Pneumothorax

(Also Called *Sucking Chest Wound*)
(See Figure 5-4)

1. Definition: air enters the interpleural space through the chest wall
2. Etiology: penetrating trauma
3. Pathophysiology
a. Communication between the intrathoracic space and the atmosphere results in equilibrium between intrathoracic and atmospheric pressures.
b. Air movement occurs into and out of opening in chest wall.

c. If opening in chest wall is smaller than diameter of trachea, patient may tolerate condition well.
d. If opening is larger, more air enters pleural space than enters lungs through trachea.
e. During inspiration, the affected lung collapses, resulting in ineffective gas exchange.
f. Wound may cause tension pneumothorax.

4. Clinical presentation
   a. Subjective
      (1) Dyspnea
      (2) Chest pain
   b. Objective
      (1) Tachycardia
      (2) Tachypnea
      (3) Obvious wound with noise of air moving in and out of pleural space
      (4) Subcutaneous emphysema is usually present
   c. Other subjective, objective, and diagnostic findings as for closed pneumothorax
5. Nursing diagnoses
   a. Impaired Gas Exchange related to alveolar hypoventilation
   b. Ineffective Breathing Pattern related to chest pain and decreased lung expansion
   c. Pain related to pleural injury, inflammation, and presence of chest tube
   d. Risk for Infection related to inadequate primary defenses, invasive procedures, chronic disease, and poor airway clearance
   e. Imbalanced Nutrition: Less than Body Requirements related to lack of exogenous nutrients and increased nutrient requirements
   f. Activity Intolerance related to imbalance between oxygen supply and oxygen demand
   g. Anxiety related to change in health status
6. Collaborative management
   a. Establish and maintain airway, ventilation, and oxygenation.
      (1) Oxygen per nasal cannula at 2 to 5 L/min to achieve an SpO_2 greater than 95% unless contraindicated; if patient has history of COPD, administer oxygen to achieve an oxygen saturation of ~90% by pulse oximetry
      (2) Position patient for optimal ventilation: semi-Fowler or Fowler's position; good lung down or back
      (3) Closure of open sucking chest wound with gauze dressing taped on three sides so that air can escape during expiration
      (4) Chest tube and water-seal drainage
      (5) Analgesics in doses adequate to allow patient to deep breathe and cough as indicated
      (6) Surgical intervention may be needed to explore and débride the wound
   b. Control pain: narcotics given on a regular schedule.
   c. Monitor for complications.
      (1) Tension pneumothorax
      (2) Atelectasis
      (3) Pneumonia, abscess

Hemothorax

1. Definition: accumulation of blood in pleural space causing compression and collapse of the lung
2. Etiology
   a. Blunt or penetrating trauma to chest wall, lung tissue, or mediastinum
   b. Pleural or pulmonary neoplasm
   c. Anticoagulant therapy
   d. Iatrogenic causes: subclavian vein puncture (e.g., insertion of deep vein catheter), lung biopsy
3. Pathophysiology
   a. Hemorrhage into pleural space compresses and collapses lung.
   b. Ventilation and oxygenation are impaired.
   c. Hemorrhage may lead to shock.
4. Clinical presentation
   a. Subjective
      (1) Chest pain may be present
      (2) Dyspnea
   b. Objective
      (1) Tachycardia
      (2) Hypotension
      (3) Asymmetric chest excursion with limited motion of affected hemithorax
      (4) Dullness to percussion on affected side
      (5) Diminished or absent breath sounds on affected side
      (6) May have clinical indications of shock if greater than 400 mL
   c. Diagnostic
      (1) Serum
         (a) Hemoglobin and hematocrit: may be decreased, but remember that changes may occur for up to 6 hours after blood loss
         (b) ABGs
            (i) Decreased PaO_2
            (ii) Increased $PaCO_2$
      (2) Chest x-ray
         (a) Fluid in pleural space and lung compression
         (b) Blunting of costophrenic angle if greater than 250 mL
         (c) Hazy appearance over the lower chest
5. Nursing diagnoses
   a. Decreased Cardiac Output related to hemorrhage and loss of circulating volume
   b. Altered Tissue Perfusion related to loss of hemoglobin and oxygen-carrying capacity
   c. Impaired Gas Exchange related to alveolar hypoventilation and lung compression
   d. Ineffective Breathing Pattern related to chest pain and decreased lung expansion
   e. Pain related to pleural injury, inflammation, and the presence of a chest tube
   f. Risk for Infection related to inadequate primary defenses, invasive procedures, chronic disease, and poor airway clearance
   g. Imbalanced Nutrition: Less than Body Requirements related to lack of

exogenous nutrients and increased nutrient requirements

h. Activity Intolerance related to imbalance between oxygen supply and oxygen demand

i. Anxiety related to change in health status

6. Collaborative management
   a. Establish and maintain airway, ventilation, and oxygenation.
      (1) Oxygen per nasal cannula at 2 to 5 L/min to achieve an Spo_2 greater than 95% unless contraindicated; if patient has history of COPD, administer oxygen to achieve an oxygen saturation of ~90% by pulse oximetry
      (2) Chest tube with chest drainage system may be adequate treatment if bleeding is self-limiting
      (3) Indications for surgery for isolation and repair of source of hemorrhage
         (a) Initial drainage of more than 1500 mL of blood after placement of chest tube
         (b) Drainage of blood at rate greater than 250 mL/hr for more than 2 hours after placement of chest tube
         (c) Hemodynamic instability despite fluid resuscitation
      (4) Positioning for optimal ventilation
         (a) Semi-Fowler or Fowler's position unless patient has significant hypotension with HOB elevated
         (b) After thoracotomy, nonoperative ("good") lung down or supine with regular turning
   b. Maintain perfusion and adequate circulating volume.
      (1) Fluids and/or blood transfusion may be necessary.
      (2) Autotransfusion may be indicated if blood loss is greater than 400 mL.
   c. Control pain: narcotics given on a regular schedule.
   d. Monitor for complications.
      (1) Atelectasis
      (2) Shock

Flail Chest (Figure 5-5)

1. Definition: instability of chest wall as a result of multiple rib or sternal fractures causing paradoxical movement of the chest wall during ventilation
2. Etiology: blunt trauma such as from a motor vehicle collision or assault
   a. Two or more ribs broken in two or more places
   b. Fractured sternum
   c. Sternotomy that has not healed (patients with diabetes mellitus have this complication most often especially if the internal mammary artery has been used for the coronary artery bypass graft)
3. Pathophysiology
   a. Fractured segment is free of the bony thorax and moves independently in response to intrathoracic pressure.

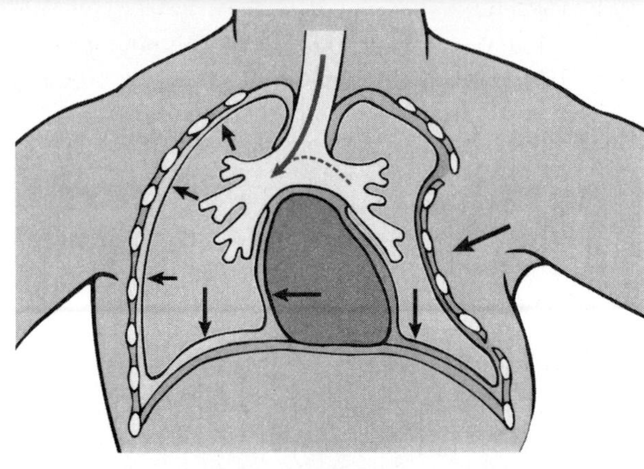

Inspiration

Expiration

Figure 5-5 Flail chest produces paradoxical chest excursion. On inspiration, the flail section sinks in. On expiration, the flail section bulges outward.

      (1) During inspiration, atmospheric pressure exceeds intrathoracic pressure on affected side, causing chest wall to move inward.
      (2) On expiration, intrathoracic pressure exceeds atmospheric pressure, causing chest wall to move outward until the thorax contracts.
   b. The bellows effect of the thorax is lost, and intrapleural pressure is less negative than normal.
   c. Ventilation is diminished; tidal volume is decreased, causing hypercapnia and resultant hypoxemia; atelectasis may occur.
   d. Increased work of breathing causes fatigue.
   e. Note related injuries: pulmonary contusion frequently accompanies flail chest; pneumothorax and pleural effusion also may be present.
4. Clinical presentation
   a. Subjective
      (1) Dyspnea
      (2) Chest pain: related to inspiration, movement
      (3) Chest tenderness to palpation
   b. Objective
      (1) Tachycardia
      (2) Tachypnea
      (3) Diminished air movement at mouth and nose
      (4) Ineffective cough

(5) Ecchymosis over thorax
(6) Paradoxical movement of flail segment
(7) Palpable detached segment, bony crepitation at fracture sites
(8) Subcutaneous emphysema possible
(9) Breath sound changes: diminished breath sounds on affected side
(10) Clinical indications of hypoxia (Box 4-3)

c. Diagnostic
(1) ABGs
(a) Decreased Pao_2
(b) Decreased Sao_2
(c) Increased $Paco_2$
(2) Spirometry: decreased tidal volume and vital capacity
(3) Chest x-ray: shows rib and/or sternal fractures

5. Nursing diagnoses
a. Impaired Gas Exchange related to alveolar hypoventilation
b. Ineffective Breathing Pattern related to chest wall splinting and loss of thoracic bellows effect
c. Ineffective Airway Clearance related to retained secretions
d. Pain related to pleural injury, chest wall injury, rib fracture, and inflammation
e. Risk for Infection related to inadequate primary defenses, invasive procedures, chronic disease, and poor airway clearance
f. Imbalanced Nutrition: Less than Body Requirements related to lack of exogenous nutrients and increased nutrient requirements
g. Activity Intolerance related to imbalance between oxygen supply and oxygen demand
h. Anxiety related to change in health status

6. Collaborative management
a. Establish and maintain airway, ventilation, and oxygenation.
(1) Oxygen per nasal cannula at 2 to 5 L/min to achieve an Spo_2 greater than 95% unless contraindicated; if patient has history of COPD, administer oxygen to achieve an oxygen saturation of ~90% by pulse oximetry
(2) Reestablishment of the thoracic bellows effect
(a) Stabilize flail segment with hand or tape (temporary); avoid binding or constricting chest excursion.
(b) Position patient on affected side if cervical spine fracture has been ruled out.
(c) Intubation and internal stabilization with mechanical ventilation may be necessary if patient cannot maintain adequate ventilation despite adequate analgesia.
(i) Indications: respiratory rate greater than 35 breaths/min, Pao_2 less than 60 mm Hg with supplemental oxygen; $Paco_2$ greater than 50 mm Hg
(ii) Mechanical ventilation may need to be maintained for 3 weeks or longer
(d) Surgical internal stabilization of rib and sternal fragments may be done especially if thoracotomy is needed for another reason.
(3) Chest physiotherapy
(a) Deep breathing and incentive spirometry
(b) Position patient for optimal ventilation: semi-Fowler or Fowler's position
(c) Postural drainage, percussion, vibration
(i) Do not percuss over fractured areas.
(d) Coughing, suctioning if coughing is ineffective and rhonchi are present
(e) Bronchoscopy may be necessary if airway clearance is inadequate

b. Provide adequate analgesia to encourage deep breathing (and coughing if indicated).
(1) Epidural analgesia
(2) IV narcotics
(3) Intercostal nerve blocks
(4) Intrapleural analgesia

c. Assist in insertion of chest tube and establish water-seal drainage if pneumothorax also is present.
d. Monitor for complications.
(1) Atelectasis
(2) Pneumonia, abscess

Diaphragmatic Rupture

1. Definition: rupture of the diaphragm allowing the movement of abdominal contents into the thorax
2. Etiology: injury below the nipple line, in flanks, or lateral chest wall
a. Blunt trauma from motor vehicle collision, assault, or fall against a immobile object
b. Penetrating injury such as from a gunshot or knife wound
c. There may be a latent period after the injury
3. Pathophysiology
a. Opening in the diaphragm
(1) Blunt trauma
(a) More common on the left side because the left hemidiaphragm is weaker than the right and the right hemidiaphragm is protected somewhat by the liver
(b) A sudden, dramatic increase in abdominal or thoracic pressure causes a tear in the diaphragm
(2) Penetrating trauma causes a perforation in the diaphragm
b. The intrathoracic pressure is negative, whereas the intraabdominal pressure is positive
c. The size of the rupture determines the extent to which the organs migrate upward: the stomach and/or loops of intestine may enter the chest and compromise lung expansion
d. Ventilation problems are most evident if the left hemidiaphragm is affected, because when the right hemidiaphragm is affected, the liver is fixed and cannot move upward into the thorax
(1) Abdominal contents compress the lung on the affected side and even may cause mediastinal shift.

(2) The decrease in the effectiveness of the diaphragm causes ineffective ventilatory excursion.

4. Clinical presentation
   a. Subjective
      (1) Dyspnea
      (2) Dysphagia
      (3) May have nausea and eructation
      (4) Abdominal pain and/or epigastric pain
         (a) May radiate to the left shoulder (as a result of injury to the phrenic nerve)
         (b) Exacerbated by supine position
   b. Objective
      (1) Tachypnea
      (2) Hypotension
      (3) Diminished or absent breath sounds on the affected side
      (4) Abdominal distention
      (5) Bowel sounds audible over the affected side of the chest
      (6) JVD if a mediastinal shift occurs
   c. Diagnostic
      (1) Chest x-ray
         (a) May be normal if no abdominal contents have been displaced into the thorax
         (b) May show hollow mass above the diaphragm (the stomach)
         (c) May show mediastinal shift
      (2) CT of the chest and abdomen
         (a) Confirms rupture of the diaphragm and any movement of abdominal contents into the thorax
         (b) Diagnostic study of choice
5. Nursing diagnoses
   a. Impaired Gas Exchange related to alveolar hypoventilation
   b. Ineffective Breathing Pattern related to loss of ventilatory muscle effectiveness
   c. Pain related to injury to chest, flank, and/or abdomen
   d. Imbalanced Nutrition: Less than Body Requirements related to disruption of the GI tract
   e. Activity Intolerance related to imbalance between oxygen supply and oxygen demand
   f. Anxiety related to change in health status
6. Collaborative management
   a. Establish and maintain airway, ventilation, and oxygenation.
      (1) Oxygen per nasal cannula at 2 to 5 L/min to achieve an Spo_2 greater than 95% unless contraindicated; if patient has history of COPD, administer oxygen to achieve an oxygen saturation of ~90% by pulse oximetry
      (2) Nasogastric tube placement to decompress the stomach
      (3) Surgical intervention to pull the abdominal organs back into the abdomen and repair the diaphragm; prophylactic antibiotics will be prescribed
   b. Provide adequate analgesia to encourage deep breathing (and coughing if indicated).
      (1) Epidural analgesia
      (2) IV narcotics
      (3) Intrapleural analgesia
   c. Monitor for complications.
      (1) Atelectasis
      (2) Pneumonia, abscess
      (3) Bowel strangulation
      (4) Tension viscerothorax: chest tube is indicated

LEARNING ACTIVITIES

1. **DIRECTIONS:** Complete the following crossword puzzle regarding thoracic surgery and trauma.

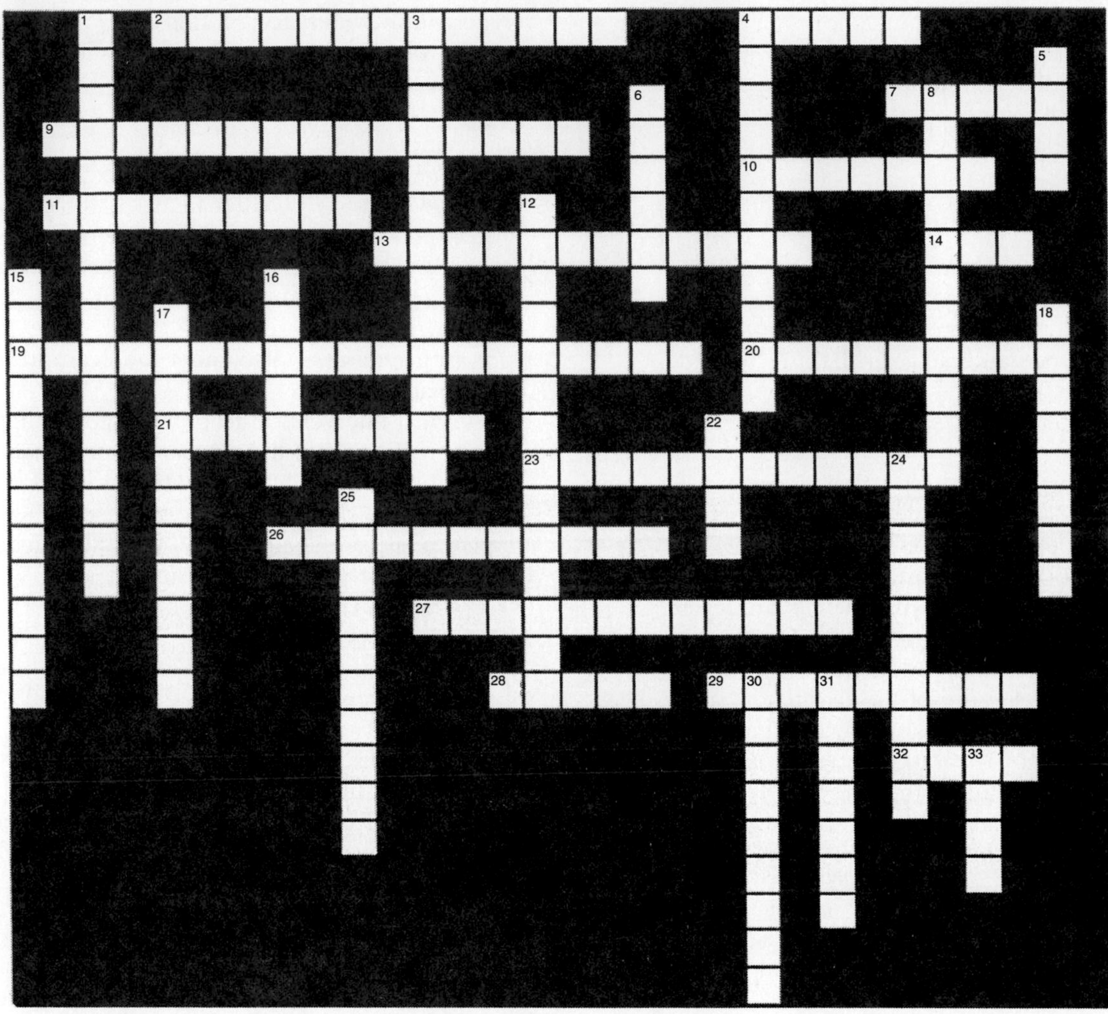

ACROSS

2. A surgical procedure to decrease the volume in a hemithorax after lung resection to prevent mediastinal shift
4. When two or more ribs are fractured or the sternum is fractured, a _____ chest results
7. To hold the chest tube with thumb and forefinger of one hand and then slide the other thumb and forefinger down the tube and then release the first thumb and forefinger
9. A method of collecting and reinfusing blood lost through a chest tube; may be used after chest trauma or surgery
10. The type of pneumothorax that results when pressure in the chest increases and the mediastinum shifts to the opposite side
11. Edema and hemorrhage of the lung parenchyma caused by trauma are referred to as a pulmonary _____
13. This type of analgesia involves injection of a local anesthetic through a thoracostomy tube or catheter
14. A chest tube that is placed anterior and superior is intended to remove _____
19. A surgical procedure for cancer of the esophagus
20. Postoperative pneumonectomy patients should be placed on their _____ side or back
21. A surgical procedure to remove a lobe of a lung
23. A surgical procedure to remove hyperinflated areas of the lung done for patients with COPD; also may be called lung volume reduction surgery
26. The process of fusing the two layers of the pleura by injecting an agent such as sterile

talc into the interpleural space
27. The process of inserting a chest tube; may be open or closed
28. A chest tube that is placed lateral and inferior is intended to remove _____
29. A surgical procedure to remove a segment of the lung is referred to as a segmental _____
32. Successively to squeeze and then release the chest tube to try to improve patency

DOWN

1. The presence of air and blood in the interpleural space; frequently surgically induced
3. A surgical procedure to remove an entire lung
4. _____ in the water-seal chamber indicates a patent chest tube with transmission of interpleural pressures to the chamber
5. The type of pneumothorax that creates a sucking sound as the patient breathes
6. Arm and shoulder exercises after thoracotomy are recommended to reduce the chance of _____ shoulder
8. A surgical procedure that opens the thorax
12. An internal air leak indicates _____ fistula
15. The presence of air in the interpleural space
16. The type of pneumothorax that is caused by rupture of a congenital bleb or a fractured rib
17. The presence of lymph fluid in the interpleural space
18. A type of valve that may be used for pneumothorax with little or no liquid drainage
22. Patients with unilateral lung conditions (except pneumonectomy) should be placed on their _____ lung or their back
24. A surgical procedure used in patients with myasthenia gravis
25. The presence of blood in the interpleural space
30. Crepitus around the chest tube insertion site indicates subcutaneous _____
31. The presence of pus in the interpleural space
33. Bubbling in the water-seal chamber indicates an air _____

2. DIRECTIONS: List 10 possible causes of acute respiratory failure.

1. ______
2. ______
3. ______
4. ______
5. ______
6. ______
7. ______
8. ______
9. ______
10. ______

3. DIRECTIONS: Match the cause of acute respiratory failure to the primary treatment.

a. Upper airway obstruction
b. Airway secretions
c. Overdosage of narcotics
d. Bronchospasm
e. Pneumothorax
f. Pneumonia
g. Postoperative pain
h. ARDS
i. Myasthenic crisis
j. Atelectasis

___ 1. Antimicrobials
___ 2. Deep breathing and incentive spirometry
___ 3. Chest tube
___ 4. Positioning and airway placement
___ 5. Cholinergic drugs and mechanical ventilator
___ 6. Encouragement of coughing, suctioning if patient cannot cough effectively
___ 7. PEEP
___ 8. Bronchodilators
___ 9. Naloxone (Narcan)
___ 10. Analgesics

4. DIRECTIONS: List five pulmonary and five nonpulmonary causes for ARDS.

Pulmonary	Nonpulmonary
a.	a.
b.	b.
c.	c.
d.	d.
e.	e.

5. DIRECTIONS: Match the treatment to the pathophysiology of ARDS. Choices may be used more than once.

a. PEEP
b. Nitric oxide
c. Fluid restriction and diuretics
d. High concentrations of oxygen
e. Prone positioning
f. Nonsteroidal antiinflammatory drugs

___ 1. Pulmonary hypertension
___ 2. Intrapulmonary shunt
___ 3. Mediator release
___ 4. Diffusion defect
___ 5. Pulmonary edema
___ 6. V/Q mismatch

6. **Directions:** Identify whether the following microorganisms are associated with CAP, HAP, or SARS. More than one may be listed.

Staphylococcus aureus	
Serratia marcescens	
Escherichia coli	
Legionella pneumophila	
Proteus mirabilis	
Bacteroides fragilis	
SARS-CoV	
Hantavirus	

7. **Directions:** List four nursing interventions to prevent aspiration in a patient receiving enteral feedings.
   1. ______
   2. ______
   3. ______
   4. ______

8. **Directions:** Complete the following table describing ABG changes in asthma using ↑ for increased, ↓ for decreased, or ↔ for no change.

Stage	PaO_2	$PaCO_2$	pH	Acid-Base Imbalance
I				
II				
III				
IV				

9. **Directions:** List five classifications of bronchodilators and an example of each.

Classification	Example
1.	
2.	
3.	
4.	
5.	

10. **Directions:** List three causes of PE in each of the following categories.

Hypercoagulability	Alteration in Blood Vessel	Venous Stasis

11. **Directions:** Match the treatment to the pathologic condition in PE. More than one may be used.

a. Embolectomy
b. Dobutamine
c. Heparin
d. Tissue plasminogen activator
e. Fluids

___ 1. Forward failure of left ventricle
___ 2. Pulmonary hypertension
___ 3. Occlusion of pulmonary blood supply
___ 4. Backward failure of right ventricle
___ 5. Low levels of antithrombin III

12. **Directions:** Identify whether the parameters in this case study are decreased, normal, or increased. Discuss implications and treatment goals.

Patient A is a 65-year-old woman admitted with a fractured hip. She had surgery 2 weeks ago. Earlier today she complained about chest pain, shortness of breath, and a feeling of doom. ABGs revealed respiratory alkalosis and hypoxemia. After she was transferred to the critical care unit, the physician inserted a pulmonary artery catheter to aid in diagnosis and evaluation of therapy. Her body surface area is 1.6 m^2.

Parameter	↑, ↓, or Normal	Parameter	↑, ↓, or Normal
BP: 112/84 mm Hg		SV: 40 mL/beat	
MAP: 93 mm Hg		SI: 25 mL/m^2/beat	
HR: 110 beats/min		SVR: 1364 dynes/sec/cm^{-5}	
RA: 18 mm Hg		SVRI: 2182 dynes/sec/cm^{-5}	
PA: 55/32 mm Hg		PVR: 618 dynes/sec/cm^{-5}	
PAm: 40 mm Hg		PVRI: 989 dynes/sec/cm^{-5}	
PAOP: 6 mm Hg		LVSWI: 30 g • m/m^2	
CO: 4.4 L/min		RVSWI: 7 g • m/m^2	
CI: 2.75 L/min/m^2		Svo_2: 58%	
Sao_2: 85% on 5 L/min by nasal cannula		Do_2I: 470 mL/min/m^2	

BP, Blood pressure; *CI*, cardiac index; *CO*, cardiac output; *Do_2I*, oxygen delivery index; *HR*, heart rate; *LVSWI*, left ventricular stroke work index; *MAP*, mean arterial pressure; *PA*, pulmonary artery pressure; *PAm*, mean pulmonary artery pressure; *PAOP*, pulmonary artery occlusive pressure; *PVR*, pulmonary vascular resistance; *PVRI*, pulmonary vascular resistance index; *RA*, right atrial pressure; *RVSWI*, right ventricular stroke work index; *Sao_2*, arterial oxygen saturation; *SI*, stroke index; *SV*, stroke volume; *Svo_2*, venous oxygen saturation; *SVR*, systemic vascular resistance; *SVRI*, systemic vascular resistance index.

Implications and treatment goals:

____

____

____

____

____

13. DIRECTIONS: Match the clinical presentation to the type of chest trauma.

a. Pulmonary contusion
b. Flail chest
c. Simple pneumothorax
d. Hemothorax
e. Tension pneumothorax
f. Diaphragmatic rupture

___ 1. Chest pain, dyspnea, diminished breath sounds on affected side, hyperresonance to percussion, tracheal shift from affected side

___ 2. Chest pain, dyspnea, diminished breath sounds on affected side, hyperresonance to percussion, may have tracheal shift away toward affected side

___ 3. Ecchymosis at site of impact, chest tenderness, dyspnea, hemoptysis

___ 4. Epigastric pain, dyspnea, dysphagia, bowel sounds audible over affected side of chest

___ 5. Chest pain, dyspnea, diminished breath sounds on affected side, dullness to percussion

___ 6. Chest tenderness, dyspnea, paradoxical chest movement

14. Directions: Complete the following crossword puzzle to review pulmonary drugs and therapies.

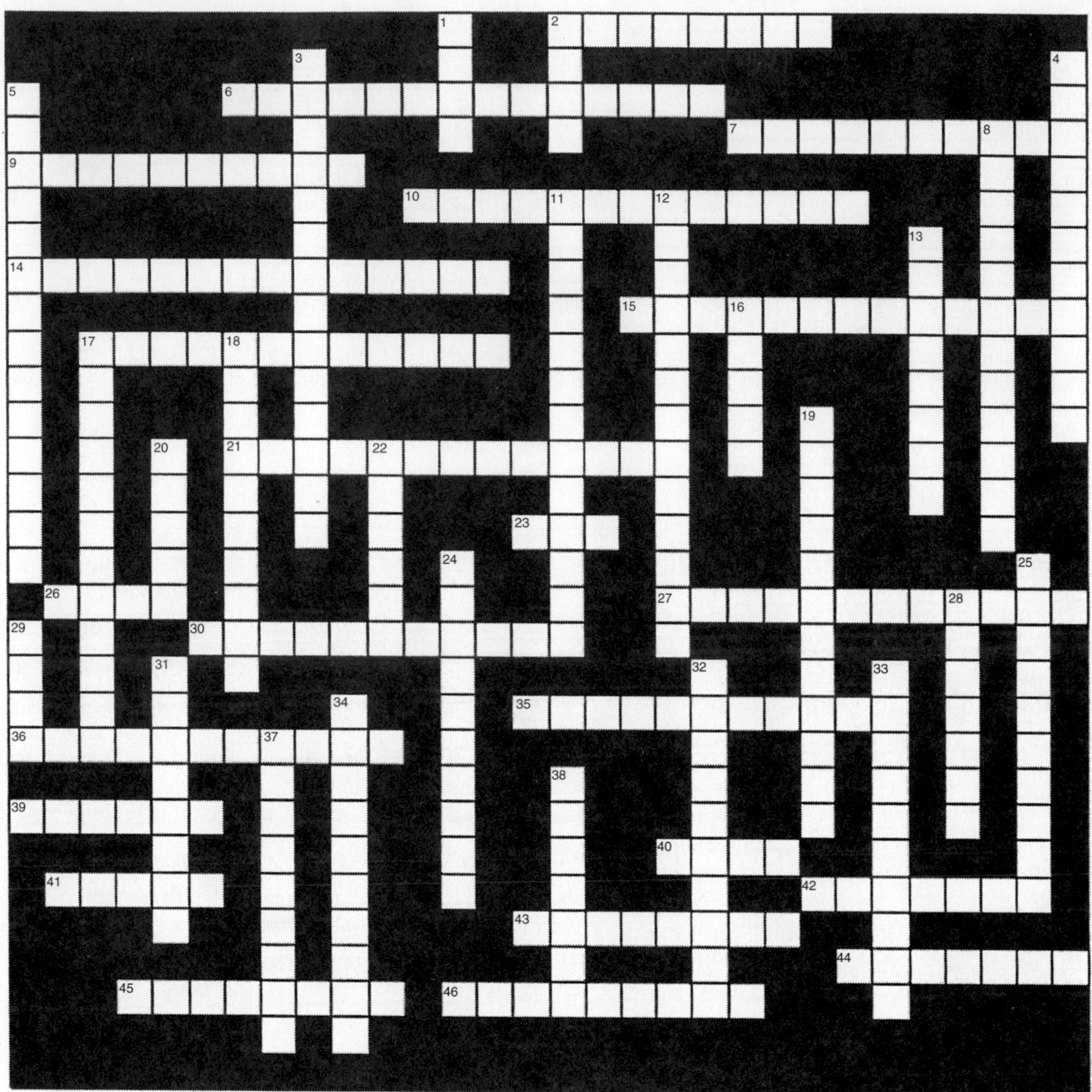

ACROSS

2. A drug that prevents the release of SRS-A from the mast cells; used prophylactically in patients with asthma
6. A steroid that frequently is given by inhalation in patients with asthma (generic)
7. A machine that pushes air into the lungs to inflate them
9. A drug used for stress ulcer prophylaxis that does not support gastric colonization (generic)
10. A diagnostic study to obtain fluid from the pleural space for analysis
14. A function normally performed by the upper airway that must be included in the care of a patient with an artificial airway
15. This type of airway should not be used in conscious patients because it would trigger the gag reflex
17. Pulmonary vasodilator (generic)
21. Xanthine bronchodilator; also dilates pulmonary vasculature (generic)
23. An inspiratory mode of mechanical ventilation; provides a number of mandatory breaths and then allows the patient to breathe between the mandatory breaths
26. Type of heparin that may be administered subcutaneously to prevent DVT and PE (abbreviation)
27. This type airway provides a relative seal to allow mechanical ventilation without the surgical risks of tracheostomy
30. Intubated patients identify their major stressor as the inability to _____
35. Respiratory equipment should not be rinsed in tap water because these bacteria frequently are found in tap water
36. This type of tracheostomy tube allows a leak across the vocal cords so that the patient can speak
39. A gas that may be used in place of nitrogen in inspired air for patients with increased airway resistance
40. One method of ensuring that cuff pressure is not excessive is the minimal _____ technique
41. The combination of pressure support ventilation and CPAP
42. This type of oxygen delivery system is comfortable for patients but only

provides up to 40% oxygen concentration
43. A risk of high concentrations of oxygen is oxygen _____
44. Placing a patient with an air embolism in a left lateral decubitus position with his or her head down is referred to as _____ maneuver (possessive)
45. A sedative frequently used in mechanically ventilated patients; need to consider fat calories (generic)
46. A drug used in patients with PE with acute RVF or refractory hypoxemia to break down the clot (generic)

DOWN

1. An expiratory maneuver used in a mechanically ventilated patient to decrease shunt and increase the driving pressure of oxygen (abbreviation)
2. An expiratory maneuver used in a spontaneously breathing patient to decrease shunt and increase the driving pressure of oxygen (abbreviation)
3. A drug that breaks down the disulfide bonds in mucus (generic)
4. A $beta_2$ stimulant that may be given orally, subcutaneously, or by inhalation (generic)
5. This type of airway may be used in conscious patients and frequently is used to prevent trauma to the nasal mucosa in patients who need nasotracheal suctioning
8. A surgical procedure to make an opening in the trachea
11. A drug that may be given in metabolic alkalosis; may cause metabolic acidosis
12. This type of oxygen mask delivers the highest oxygen concentration
13. Type of suction device used to suction the oropharynx
16. Patient position recommended to optimize V/Q matching in patients with ARDS
17. An antibiotic that may be used to increase gastric motility (generic)
18. This type of activity decreases stress and oxygen requirements; may include music, imagery, stretching, yoga
19. IV antifungal (generic)
20. A forceful expiration to expel mucus from the lungs
22. Indicated when Sao_2 is less than 90%
24. A method of airway clearance used if the patient cannot effectively cough; used only when indicated
25. A complication of mechanical ventilation; risk is increased when large tidal volumes or PEEP are used
28. A drug used to prevent extension or recurrence of a clot in patients with PE (generic)
29. A device attached to an endotracheal tube or tracheostomy that provides a relative seal for mechanical ventilation and airway protection
31. _____ drainage is a method of bronchial hygiene that uses gravity to drain secretions into the upper airway so that they can be coughed out
32. Group of drugs that should be administered to allow a patient to breathe deeply after thoracotomy
33. A muscle paralytic that may be administered by IV infusion in patients on mechanical ventilation (generic)
34. A method of airway clearance that uses tapping with cupped hands to loosen secretions
37. A $beta_2$ stimulant that is administered orally or by inhalation
38. Testing sputum for _____ is a common method to check for aspiration of enteral feeding

LEARNING ACTIVITIES ANSWERS

1.

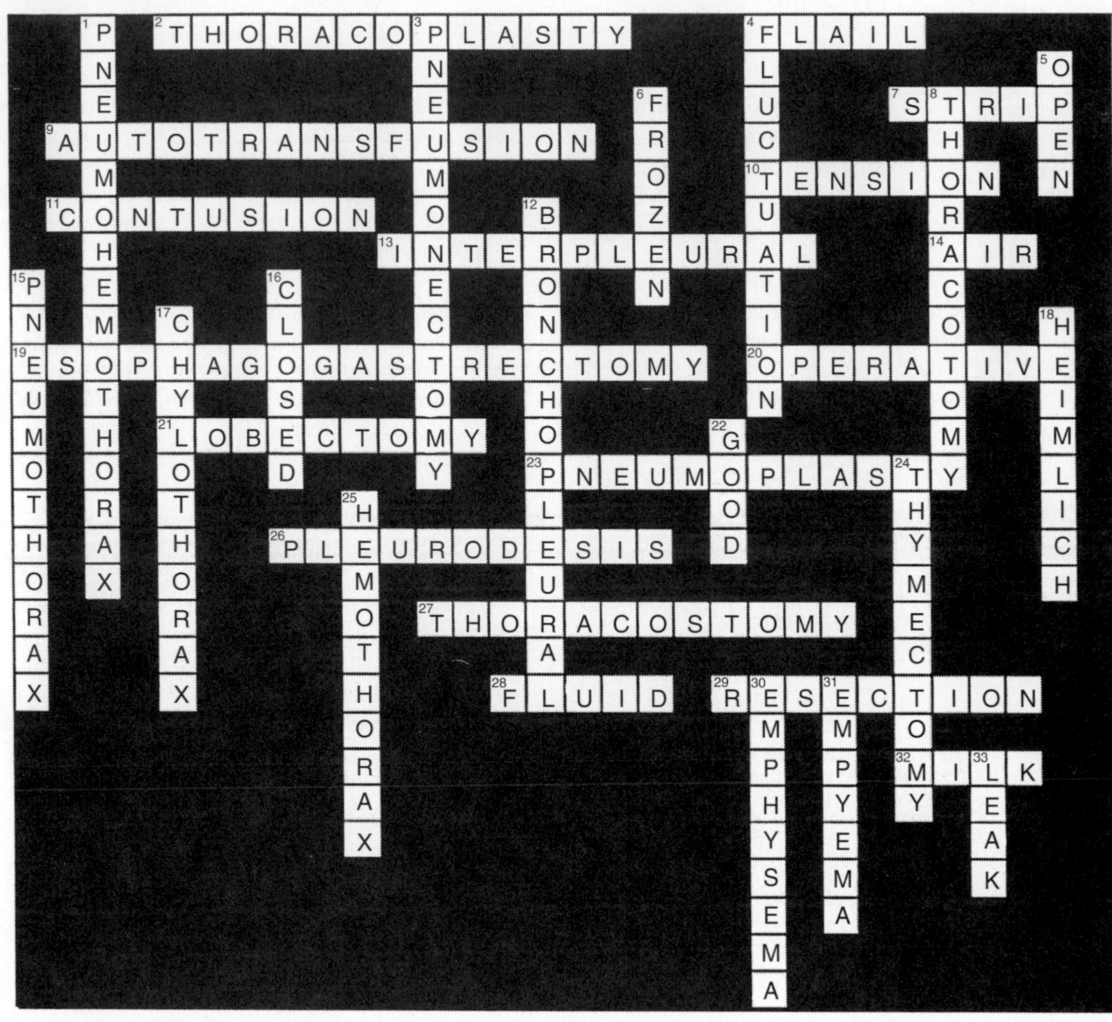

2. Any 10 of the following:
   ARDS (early)
   Aminoglycosides
   Amyotrophic lateral sclerosis
   Anesthesia
   Aspiration pneumonitis
   Asthma
   Atelectasis
   Chest trauma
   CNS depressant drugs
   COPD with acute exacerbation
   Cystic fibrosis
   Epiglottitis
   Fat embolism
   Guillain-Barré syndrome
   Head trauma
   Kyphoscoliosis
   Morbid obesity
   Multiple sclerosis
   Muscle paralytics
   Muscular dystrophy
   Myasthenia gravis
   Near drowning
   Neuromuscular blocking drugs
   Organophosphate poisoning
   Pleural effusion
   Pneumonia
   Pneumothorax

Poliomyelitis
Pulmonary edema
PE
Pulmonary fibrosis
Sleep apnea
Smoke inhalation
Spinal cord injury
Status asthmaticus
Surgery: especially thoracic, abdominal, flank incision
Tracheal obstruction

3.

f 1. Antimicrobials
j 2. Deep breathing and incentive spirometry
e 3. Chest tube
a 4. Positioning and airway placement
i 5. Cholinergic drugs and mechanical ventilator
b 6. Encouragement of coughing, suctioning secretions if patient cannot cough effectively
h 7. PEEP
d 8. Bronchodilators
c 9. Naloxone (Narcan)
g 10. Analgesics

4. Any five in each column.

Pulmonary	Nonpulmonary
Chest trauma: pulmonary contusion Near drowning Hypervolemia, pulmonary edema Inhalation of toxic gases and vapors Smoke Chemicals Oxygen toxicity Pneumonia: viral, bacterial, or fungal Aspiration pneumonitis Radiation pneumonitis PE: thrombotic; air; fat; amniotic fluid Radiation Drugs: bleomycin	Sepsis (No. 1 cause) Shock or prolonged hypotension Septic shock Hypovolemic shock Anaphylactic shock Cardiogenic shock Neurogenic shock Multisystem trauma Burns Cardiopulmonary bypass DIC Toxemia of pregnancy Acute pancreatitis Diabetic coma Head injury Drug overdosage: heroin; methadone; barbiturates; aspirin; thiazide diuretics Multiple blood transfusions

5.

b 1. Pulmonary hypertension
a 2. Intrapulmonary shunt
f 3. Mediator release
d, a 4. Diffusion defect
a, c 5. Pulmonary edema
e, b 6. V/Q mismatch

6.

Staphylococcus aureus	CAP, HAP
Serratia marcescens	HAP
Escherichia coli	HAP
Legionella pneumophila	CAP, HAP
Proteus mirabilis	HAP
Bacteroides fragilis	CAP
SARS-CoV	SARS
Hantavirus	CAP

7.
1. Elevate the HOB 45 degrees.
2. Ensure appropriate positioning of feeding tube.
3. Check for gastric residuals and hold feedings if indicated.
4. Keep cuff of endotracheal tube inflated to 20 mm Hg (25 cm H_2O).

8.

Stage	Pa_{O_2}	Pa_{CO_2}	pH	Acid-Base Imbalance
I	↔	↓	↑	Respiratory alkalosis
II	↓	↓	↑	Respiratory alkalosis and mild to moderate hypoxemia
III	↓	↔	↔	Moderate hypoxemia
IV	↓	↑	↓	Respiratory acidosis and critical hypoxemia

9.

Classification	Example
Leukotriene inhibitors/leukotriene receptor antagonists	Zafirlukast (Accolate) Zileuton (Zyflo) Montelukast sodium (Singulair)
Adrenergic agents	Salmeterol (Serevent) Metaproterenol (Alupent, Metaprel) Albuterol (Proventil, Ventolin) Pirbuterol (Maxair) Bitolterol (Tornalate) Terbutaline (Brethaire) Epinephrine
Anticholinergic agents	Ipratropium bromide (Atrovent)
Xanthines	Aminophylline Theophylline (Theobid, Quibron) Oxtriphylline (Choledyl SA)
Electrolyte	Magnesium

10. Any five in each column.

Hypercoagulability	Alterations in Blood Vessel	Venous Stasis
Malignancy: especially breast, lung, pancreas, or GI or GU tracts Oral contraceptives high in estrogen: especially in smokers Dehydration and hemoconcentration Fever Sickle cell anemia Pregnancy Polycythemia vera Thrombocytopenia Abrupt discontinuance of anticoagulants Sepsis	Trauma IV drug use Aging Vasculitis Varicose veins Diabetes mellitus Atherosclerosis Inflammatory process	Prolonged bed rest or immobilization Obesity Advanced age Burns Pregnancy Postpartum period Congestive heart failure MI Bacterial endocarditis Recent surgery especially legs, pelvis, or abdomen Thrombus formation in heart AF Cardioversion

11.

e 1. Forward failure of left ventricle
a, d 2. Pulmonary hypertension
a, d 3. Occlusion of pulmonary blood supply
b 4. Backward failure of right ventricle
c 5. Low levels of antithrombin III

12.

Parameter	↑, ↓, or Normal	Parameter	↑, ↓, or Normal
BP: 112/84 mm Hg	Normal	SV: 40 mL/beat	↓
MAP: 93 mm Hg	Normal	SI: 25 mL/m^2/beat	↓
HR: 110 beats/min	↑	SVR: 1364 dynes/sec/cm^{-5}	Normal
RAP: 18 mm Hg	↑	SVRI: 2182 dynes/sec/cm^{-5}	Normal
PAP: 55/32 mm Hg	↑	PVR: 618 dynes/sec/cm^{-5}	↑
PAm: 40 mm Hg	↑	PVRI: 989 dynes/sec/cm^{-5}	↑
PAOP: 6 mm Hg	Normal	LVSWI: 30 g • m/m^2	↓
CO: 4.4 L/min	Normal	RVSWI: 7 g • m/m^2	Normal
CI: 2.75 L/min/m^2	Normal	Svo_2: 58%	↓
Sao_2: 85% on 5 L/min by nasal cannula	↓	Do_2I: 470 mL/min/m^2	↓

Discussion: Patient A's hemodynamic parameters confirm pulmonary hypertension. Note the increase in PAd pressure with a normal PAOP. Remember that if the PAd pressure is more than 5 mm Hg above the PAOP, pulmonary hypertension exists. The increased PVR is further evidence of pulmonary hypertension. Sympathetic nervous system stimulation has caused the tachycardia and the high SVR. Considering her history, you would suspect PE as the cause. V/Q scan or spiral CT would be indicated to aid in the diagnosis of a PE. ABGs should be analyzed for degree of hypoxemia. Treatment goals for this patient include improving oxygenation (100% by non-rebreathing mask probably would be required, and the patient may need to be intubated if she fatigues and $Paco_2$ increases), reestablishing pulmonary perfusion (fibrinolytics are indicated in this patient because she has acute RVF and refractory hypoxemia), and preventing extension of the clot and reocclusion (heparin). Note that it has been 2 weeks since her surgery, which is long enough for the surgical clot to have been lysed by the natural fibrinolytic process, so fibrinolytics are not contraindicated on that basis. If fibrinolytics are contraindicated for other reasons, pulmonary artery catheter aspiration or fragmentation of the clot may be attempted. Surgical pulmonary embolectomy is associated with a relatively high mortality and should be avoided if possible.

13.

e 1. Chest pain, dyspnea, diminished breath sounds on affected side, hyperresonance to percussion, tracheal shift away from affected side

c 2. Chest pain, dyspnea, diminished breath sounds on affected side, hyperresonance to percussion, may have tracheal shift toward affected side

a 3. Ecchymosis at site of impact, chest tenderness, dyspnea, hemoptysis

f 4. Epigastric pain, dyspnea, dysphagia, bowel sounds audible over affected side of chest

d 5. Chest pain, dyspnea, diminished breath sounds on affected side, dullness to percussion

b 6. Chest tenderness, dyspnea, paradoxical chest movement

14.

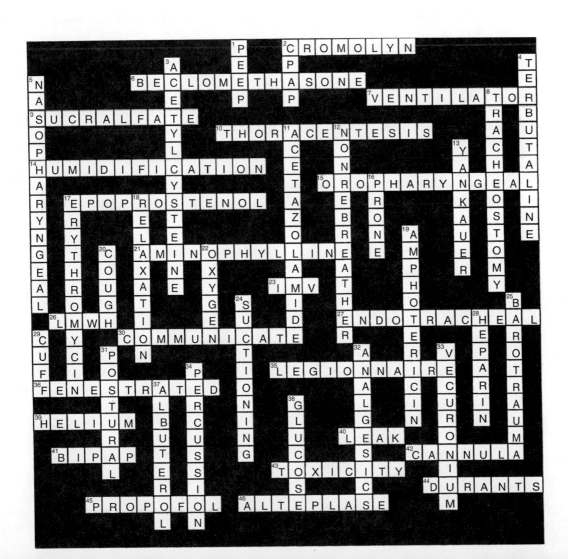

References

Bell, R. L., Ovadia, P., Abdullah, F., Spector, S., & Rabinovici, R. (2001). Chest tube removal: End-inspiration or end-expiration? *Journal of Trauma, 50*(4), 674-677.

Bernard, G. R., Artigas, A., Brigham, K. L., Carlet, J., Falke, K., Hudson, L., et al. (1994). Report of the American-European Consensus Conference on ARDS: Definitions, mechanisms, relevant outcomes and clinical trial coordination. The Consensus Committee. *Intensive Care Med, 20*(3), 225-232.

Daschner, F., Kappstein, I., Engles, I., Reuschenbach, K., Pfesterer, J., & Kreig, N. (1988). Stress ulcer prophylaxis and ventilation pneumonia: Prevention by antibacterial cytoprotective agents. *Infection Control and Hospital Epidemiology, 9,* 59-65.

Hagler, D. A., & Traver, G. A. (1994). Endotracheal saline and suction catheters: Sources of lower airway contamination. *American Journal of Critical Care, 3*(6), 444-447.

Hansen, E. F., Vestbo, J., Phanareth, K., Kok-Jensen, A., & Dirksen, A. (2001). Peak flow as predictor of overall mortality in asthma and chronic obstructive pulmonary disease. *Am J Respir Crit Care Med, 163*(3 Pt 1), 690-693.

Bibliography

Ahrens, T. A., Kollef, M. H., Stewart, J., & Shannon, W. (2004). Effect of kinetic therapy on pulmonary complications. *American Journal of Critical Care, 13*(5), 376-382.

Aklog, L., Williams, C. S., Byrne, J. G., & Goldhaber, S. Z. (2002). Acute pulmonary embolectomy: A contemporary approach. *Circulation, 105,* 1416-1419.

American Heart Association. (2005). Part 10.5: Near-fatal asthma. *Circulation, 112*(24 suppl), IV139-IV142.

American Thoracic Society. (2007). *Definitions.* Retrieved April 17, 2007, from http://www.thoracic.org/sections/copd/for-health-professionals/definition-diagnosis-and-staging/definitions.html

Aquila, A. M. (2001). Deep venous thrombosis. *Journal of Cardiovascular Nursing, 15*(4), 25-44.

Balas, M. C. (2000). Prone positioning of patients with acute respiratory distress syndrome: Applying research to practice. *Critical Care Nurse, 20*(1), 24-36.

Baumann, M. H. (2003). What size chest tube? What drainage system is ideal? And other chest tube management questions. *Current Opinion in Pulmonary Medicine, 9*(4), 276-281.

Behnia, M. M., & Garrett, K. (2004). Association of tension pneumothorax with use of small-bore chest tubes in patients receiving mechanical ventilation. *Critical Care Nurse, 24*(1), 64-65.

Brooks, J. A. (2001). Postoperative nosocomial pneumonia: Nurse-sensitive interventions. *AACN Clinical Issues, 12*(2), 305-323.

Combes, P., Fauvage, B., & Oleyer, C. (2000). Nosocomial pneumonia in mechanically ventilated patients, a prospective randomised evaluation of the Stericath closed suctioning system. *Intensive Care Medicine, 26*(7), 878-882.

DeRiso II, A. J., Ladowski, J. S., Dillon, T. A., Justice, J. W., & Peterson, A. C. (1996). Chlorhexidine gluconate 0.12% oral rinse reduces the incidence of total nosocomial respiratory infection and nonprophylactic systemic antibiotic use in patients undergoing heart surgery. *Chest, 109,* 1556-1561.

Duncan, C. R., & Erickson, R. S. (1982). Pressures associated with chest tube stripping. *Heart and Lung, 11*(2), 166-171.

El-Masri, M. M., Williamson, K. M., & Fox-Wasylyshyn, S. M. (2004). Severe acute respiratory syndrome: Another challenge for critical care nurses. *AACN Clinical Issues, 15*(1), 150-159.

Elpern, E. H., Stutz, L., Peterson, S., Gurka, D. P., & Skipper, A. (2004). Outcomes associated with enteral tube feedings in a medical intensive care unit. *American Journal of Critical Care, 13*(3), 221-227.

Esmond, G. (Ed.). (2001). *Respiratory nursing.* Edinburgh: Bailliere Tindall.

Evans, B. (2005). Best-practice protocols: VAP prevention. *Nursing Management, 36*(12), 10-16.

Farag, A., & Costello, P. (2001). CT of pulmonary thromboembolic disease. *Applied Radiology, 30*(2), 22-26.

Fox, W. J., & Hughes, T. A. (2002). Use of intercostal bupivacaine with epinephrine after surgery to decrease use of narcotics and duration of intubation. *American Journal of Critical Care, 11*(5), 433-435.

Gainner, M., Roch, A., Forel, J.-M., Thirion, X., Arnal, J.-M., Donati, S., et al. (2004). Effect of neuromuscular blocking agents on gas exchange in patients presenting with acute respiratory distress syndrome. *Critical Care Medicine, 32*(1), 113-119.

Gattinoni, L. (2001). Effect of prone positioning on the survival of patients with acute respiratory failure. *New England Journal of Medicine, 345*(8), 568-573.

Grap, M. J., Munro, C. L., Elswick, R. K., Sessler, C. N., & Ward, K. R. (2004). Duration of action of a single, early oral application of chlorhexidine on oral microbial flora in mechanically ventilated patients: A pilot study. *Heart and Lung, 33*(2), 83-91.

Grossman, S., & Grossman, L. C. (2005). Pathophysiology of cystic fibrosis: Implications for critical care nurses. *Critical Care Nurse, 25*(4), 46-51.

Harris, J. R., & Miller, T. H. (2000). Preventing nosocomial pneumonia: Evidence-based practice. *Critical Care Nurse, 20*(1), 51-68.

Houston, S., Hougland, P., Anderson, J. J., LaRocco, M., Kennedy, V., & Gentry, L. O. (2002). Effectiveness of 0.12% chlorhexidine gluconate oral rinse in reducing prevalence of nosocomial pneumonia in patients undergoing heart surgery. *American Journal of Critical Care, 11*(6), 567-570.

Huang, M., & Singer, L. G. (2005). Surgical interventions for COPD. *Geriatrics and Aging, 8*(3), 40-46.

Huffman, S., Pieper, P., Jarczyk, K. S., Bayne, A., & O'Brien, E. (2004). Methods to confirm feeding tube placement: Application of research in practice. *Pediatric Nursing, 30*(1), 10-13.

Hui, D. S. C., & Sung, J. J. Y. (2003). Severe acute respiratory syndrome. *Chest, 124*(1), 12-15.

Janson, S. (2000). Biologic markers of airway inflammation in asthma. *AACN Clinical Issues, 11*(2), 232-240.

Kaye, J., Ashline, V., Erickson, D., Zeiler, K., Gavigan, D., Gannon, L., et al. (2000). Critical care bug team: A multidisciplinary team approach to reducing ventilator-associated pneumonia. *American Journal of Infection Control, 28*(2), 197-201.

Kollef, M. H. (2004). Prevention of hospital-associated pneumonia and ventilator-associated pneumonia. *Critical Care Medicine, 32*(6), 1396-1405.

Kruse, J. A., Fink, M. P., & Carlson, R. W. (2003). *Saunders manual of critical care*. Philadelphia: Saunders.

Kunis, K. A., & Puntillo, K. A. (2003). Ventilator-associated pneumonia in the ICU. *American Journal of Nursing, 103*(8), 64AA-64GG.

Lam, S., & Chen, J. (2003). Changes in heart rate associated with nebulized racemic albuterol and levalbuterol in intensive care patients. *American Journal of Health-System Pharmacy, 60*(19), 1971-1975.

Lee, D. L., Chiang, H.-T., Lin, S.-L., Ger, L.-P., Kun, M.-H., & Huang, Y.-C. T. (2002). Prone-position ventilation induces sustained improvement in oxygenation in patients with acute respiratory distress syndrome who have a large shunt. *Critical Care Medicine, 30*(7), 1446-1452.

MacLaren, R., & Jung, R. (2002). Stress-dose corticosteroid therapy for sepsis and acute lung injury or acute respiratory distress syndrome in critically ill adults. *Pharmacotherapy, 22*(9), 1140-1156.

Manocha, S., Walley, K. R., & Russell, J. A. (2003). Severe acute respiratory syndrome (SARS): A critical care perspective. *Critical Care Medicine, 31*(11), 2684-2692.

Marini, J. J., & Gattinoni, L. (2004). Ventilatory management of acute respiratory distress syndrome: A consensus of two. *Critical Care Medicine, 32*(1), 250-255.

Marion, B. S. (2001). A turn for the better: 'Prone positioning' of patients with ARDS. *American Journal of Nursing, 101*(5), 26-35.

Mathews, P. J., & Mathews, L. M. (2000). Reducing the risks of ventilator-associated infections. *Dimensions of Critical Care Nursing, 19*(1), 17-21.

Maykel, J. A., & Bistrian, B. R. (2002). Is enteral feeding for everyone? *Critical Care Medicine, 30*(3), 714-716.

Meade, M. O., Jacka, M. J., Cook, D. J., Dodek, P., Griffith, L., & Guyatt, G. H. (2004). Survey of interventions for the prevention and treatment of acute respiratory distress syndrome. *Critical Care Medicine, 32*(4), 946-954.

Metheny, N. A., Chang, Y.-H., Ye, J. S., Edwards, S. J., Defer, J., Dahms, T. E., et al. (2002). Pepsin as a marker for pulmonary aspiration. *American Journal of Critical Care, 11*(2), 150-154.

Metheny, N. A., & Maloney, J. (2002). Controversy in using blue dye in enteral tube feedings as a method of detecting pulmonary aspiration. *Critical Care Nurse, 22*(5), 84-85.

Metheny, N. A., Schallom, M. E., & Edwards, S. J. (2004). Effect of gastrointestinal motility and feeding tube site on aspiration risk in critically ill patients: A review. *Heart and Lung, 33*(3), 131-145.

Miracle, V. A., & Winston, M. (2001). Take the wind out of asthma. *Dimensions of Critical Care Nursing, 20*(1), 2-9.

Munro, C. L., & Grap, M. J. (2004). Oral health and care in the intensive care unit: State of the science. *American Journal of Critical Care, 13*(1), 25-33.

Murray, T. A., & Patterson, L. A. (2002). Prone positioning of trauma patients with acute respiratory distress syndrome and open abdominal incisions. *Critical Care Nurse, 22*(3), 52-56.

Peiris, J. S. M., Yuen, K. Y., Osterhaus, A. D. M. E., & Stohr, K. (2003). The severe acute respiratory syndrome. *New England Journal of Medicine, 349*(25), 2431-2341.

Perozzi, K. J., & Englert, N. C. (2004). Amniotic fluid embolism: An obstetric emergency. *Critical Care Nurse, 24*(4), 54-61.

Pfeifer, L. T., Orser, L., Gefen, C., McGuinness, R., & Hannon, C. V. (2001). Preventing ventilator-associated pneumonia. *American Journal of Nursing, 101*(8), 24AA-24GG.

Puntillo, K. A., & Ley, S. J. (2004). Appropriately timed analgesics control pain due to chest tube removal. *American Journal of Critical Care, 13*(4), 292-304.

Resar, R., Pronovost, P., Haraden, C., Simmonds, T., Rainey, T., & Nolan, T. (2005). Using a bundle approach to improve ventilator care processes and reduce ventilator-associated pneumonia. *Joint Commision Journal on Quality and Patient Safety, 31*(5), 243-248.

Schlicher, M. L. (2001). Using liquid ventilation to treat patients with acute respiratory distress syndrome: A guide to a breath of fresh liquid. *Critical Care Nurse, 21*(5), 55-65.

Shorr, A. F., & O'Malley, P. G. (2001). Continuous subglottic suctioning for the prevention of ventilator-associated pneumonia: potential economic implications. *Chest, 119*(1), 228-235.

Smith-Sims, K. (2001). Hospital-acquired pneumonia. *American Journal of Nursing, 101*(1), 24AA-24EE.

Smulders, K., van Der Hoeven, H., Weers-Pothoff, I., & Vandenbroucke-Grauls, C. (2002). A randomized clinical trial of intermittent subglottic secretion drainage in patients receiving mechanical ventilation. *Chest, 121*(3), 858-862.

Swanson, R. W., & Winkelman, C. (2002). Exploring the benefits and myths of enteral feeding in the critically ill. *Critical Care Nursing Quarterly, 24*(2), 67-74.

Travers, A. H., Rowe, B. H., Barker, S., Jones, A., & Camargo, C. (2002). The effectiveness of IV beta-agonists in treating patients with acute asthma in the emergency department. *Chest, 122*(4), 1200-1207.

Urden, L., Stacy, K., & Lough, M. (2006). *Thelan's critical care nursing: Diagnosis and management* (5th ed.). St. Louis: Mosby.

Velmahos, G. (2001). Spiral CT inadequate for diagnosis of pulmonary embolism in critically ill surgical patients. Retrieved June 26, 2001, from http://criticalcare.medscape.com/reuters/prof/2001/05/05.30/20010529clin006.html

Ware, L. B., & Matthay, M. A. (2000). The acute respiratory distress syndrome. *New England Journal of Medicine, 342*(18), 1334-1346.

Wells, J. L., & Salyer, S. W. (2001). Diagnosing pulmonary embolism: A medical masquerader. *Clinician Reviews, 11*(2), 66-79.

Wenzel, S. E. (2000). Severe asthma: Defining, diagnosing, and treating. *Journal of Respiratory Diseases, 21*(3), 164-174.

Wilkins, R. L., Stoller, J. K., & Scanlan, C. L. (2003). *Egan's fundamentals of respiratory care* (vol. 8). St. Louis: Mosby.

Wong, G. W. K., & Hui, D. S. C. (2003). Severe acute respiratory syndrome. *Thorax, 58*(7), 558-660.

Yeaw, E. (1992). How position affects oxygenation: Good lung down? *American Journal of Nursing, 92*(3), 27-32.

Zack, J. E., Garrison, T., Trovillion, E., Clinkscale, D., Coopersmith, C. M., Fraser, V. J., et al. (2002). Effect of an education program aimed at reducing the occurrence of ventilator-associated pneumonia. *Critical Care Medicine, 30*(11), 2407-2412.

The Gastrointestinal System

CHAPTER 6

Selected Concepts in Anatomy and Physiology

General Information about the Gastrointestinal (GI) System

1. Functions of the GI system
   a. Digestion and absorption of nutrients
   b. Elimination of waste material
   c. Detoxification and elimination of bacteria, viruses, chemical toxins, and drugs
2. Processes of the GI system (Figure 6-1)
   a. Ingestion
   b. Digestion
   c. Absorption
   d. Elimination
3. Structures of the GI system (Figure 6-2)
   a. Alimentary canal: from the mouth to the anus
      (1) Oropharynx
      (2) Esophagus
      (3) Stomach
      (4) Small intestine: divided into duodenum, jejunum, and ileum
      (5) Large intestine: divided into cecum, ascending colon, transverse colon, descending colon, sigmoid colon, and rectum
   b. Accessory organs of digestion
      (1) Liver
      (2) Gallbladder
      (3) Pancreas
4. Cell layers (Figure 6-3)
   a. All areas of the GI tract have the same cell layers (external to internal).
      (1) Serosa: outermost layer that is frequently continuous with the peritoneum
      (2) Muscularis
      (3) Submucosa
      (4) Mucosa: innermost layer that is exposed to dietary mucosa

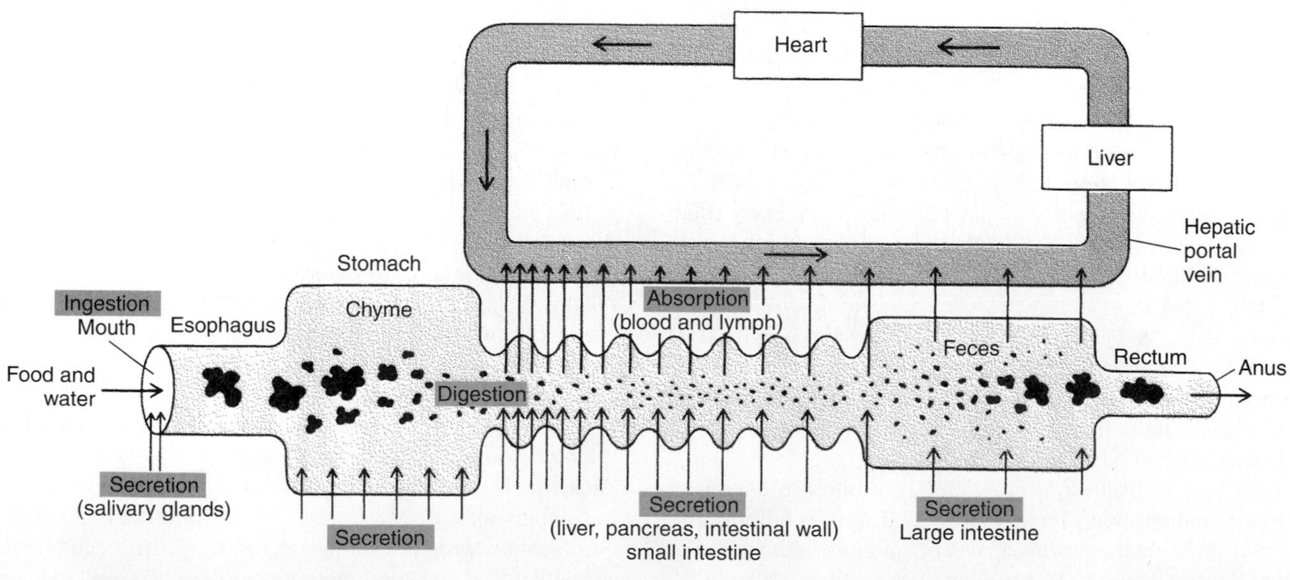

Figure 6-1 Summary of processes of the GI system. (From Kinney, M. R., Packa, D. R., & Dunbar, S. B. [1998]. *AACN's clinical reference for critical-care nursing* [4th ed.]. St. Louis: Mosby.)

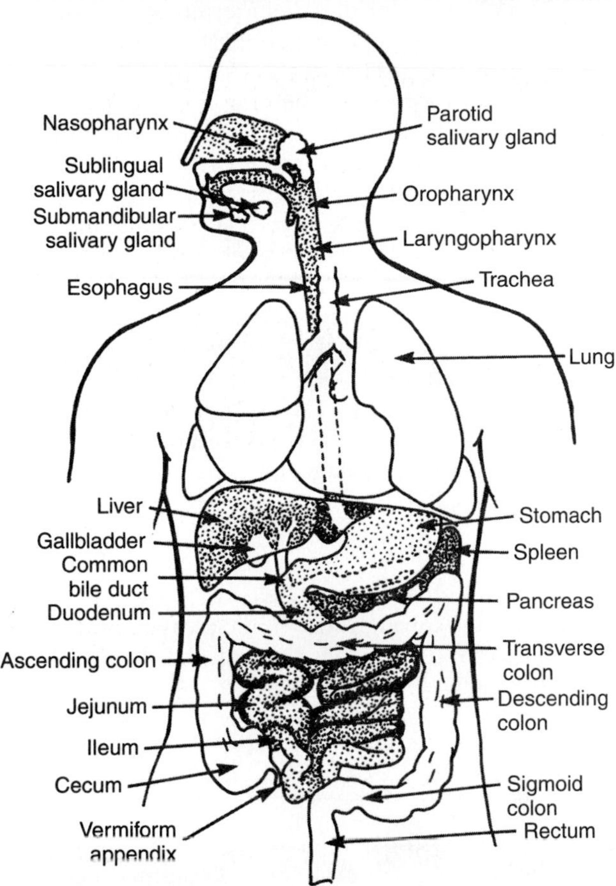

Figure 6-2 Structures of the GI system. (From Kinney, M. R., Packa, D. R., & Dunbar, S. B. [1998]. *AACN's clinical reference for critical-care nursing* [4th ed.]. St. Louis: Mosby.)

5. Peritoneum
   a. The abdominal viscera are covered by the peritoneum.
      (1) The parietal layer lines the abdominal cavity wall.
      (2) The visceral layer covers the abdominal organs.
      (3) The peritoneal cavity is a potential space between the parietal and visceral layers.
   b. The peritoneum has two folds.
      (1) The mesentery contains blood and lymph vessels and attaches the small intestine and part of the large intestine to the posterior abdominal wall.
      (2) The omentum contains fat and lymph nodes.
         (a) Lesser omentum from lesser curvature of stomach and upper duodenum to the liver
         (b) Greater omentum from stomach over the intestines

Alimentary Canal

1. Oropharynx
   a. Location: mouth to esophagus
   b. Description
      (1) Oral cavity
         (a) Lips
         (b) Cheeks
         (c) Palate
         (d) Teeth
         (e) Tongue
            (i) Mucus glands

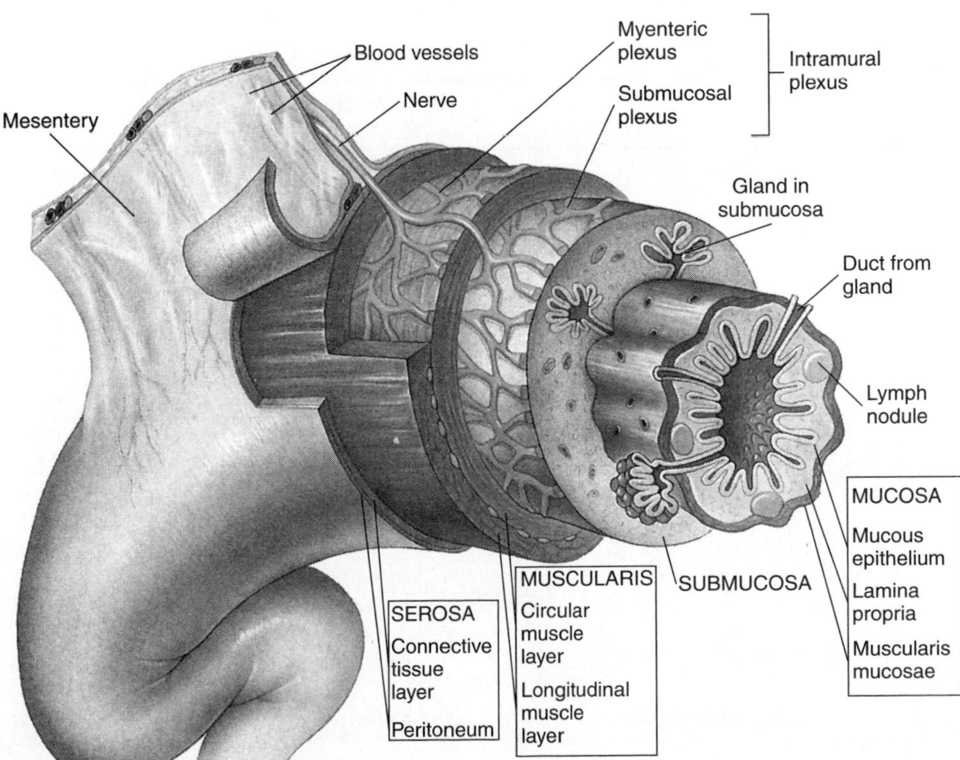

Figure 6-3 Cell layers of the GI tract. (From Doughty, D. B., & Jackson, D. B. [1993]. *Gastrointestinal disorders: Mosby's clinical nursing series.* St. Louis: Mosby.)

(ii) Serous glands
(f) Salivary glands
(i) Parotid glands (two)
(ii) Submandibular glands (two)
(iii) Sublingual glands (two)
(2) Muscles of mastication
(3) Pharynx
(a) Nasopharynx
(b) Oropharynx
(c) Laryngopharynx

c. Secretions: saliva (Table 6-1)
(1) Stimulated by the thought, sight, smell, or taste of food
(2) Consists of the following:
(a) Ptyalin (amylase): begins the breakdown of polysaccharides (starches) to disaccharides
(b) Mucus: provides lubricant
(3) Volume: 1500 mL/day

d. Process
(1) The teeth break up the food into smaller pieces to increase surface area for digestive enzymes to act.
(2) The masseter muscles are innervated by cranial nerve V (trigeminal).
(3) The tongue moves the food around in the mouth for better chewing and moves the food to the back of the throat to begin the process of swallowing.
(4) Swallowing (deglutition; Figure 6-4) consists of three stages; only stage one occurs in the mouth.
(a) Voluntary: The tongue forces the bolus of food into the pharynx.
(b) Pharyngeal: The bolus of food passes from the pharynx to the esophagus; the epiglottis closes to protect the larynx.
(c) Esophageal: The bolus of food passes from the esophagus to the gastroesophageal sphincter.

e. Functions: Table 6-2

2. Esophagus
a. Location
(1) Lies behind the trachea
(2) Passes through the thoracic cavity and the diaphragm; passes through the diaphragm at the diaphragmatic hiatus

Table 6-1 Digestive Enzymes

Source	Enzyme	What It Acts On	What Is Produced
Salivary glands (saliva) (1500 mL/day)	• Ptyalin (amylase)	• Polysaccharides (starches)	• Disaccharides
Stomach (gastric juice) (2500 mL/day)	• Pepsin	• Proteins	• Polypeptides
	• Gastric lipase	• Emulsified fats	• Fatty acids • Glycerol
	• Renin	• Soluble milk protein	• Insoluble form
Liver (bile) (500 mL/day)	• None	• Nonemulsified fats	• Emulsified fats
Pancreas (pancreatic juice) (1500 mL/day)	• Trypsin	• Denatured proteins • Polypeptides	• Peptides • Amino acids
	• Chymotrypsin	• Proteins • Polypeptides	• Peptides • Amino acids
	• Pancreatic lipase	• Emulsified fats	• Fatty acids • Glycerol
	• Pancreatic amylase	• Disaccharides	• Polysaccharides
	• Nucleases	• Nucleic acids	• Nucleotides
	• Carboxypeptidase	• Polypeptides	• Smaller polypeptides
Small intestine (1000 mL/day)	• Enterokinase	• Trypsinogen	• Trypsin
	• Aminopeptidase	• Polypeptides	• Smaller polypeptides
	• Dipeptidase	• Dipeptides	• Amino acids
	• Sucrase	• Sucrose	• Glucose • Fructose
	• Lactase	• Lactose	• Glucose • Galactose
	• Maltase	• Maltose	• Glucose
	• Nucleotidase	• Nucleotides	• Nucleosides • Phosphoric acid
	• Nucleosidase	• Nucleosides	• Purine • Pentose
	• Intestinal lipase	• Fat	• Glycerides • Fatty acids • Glycerol

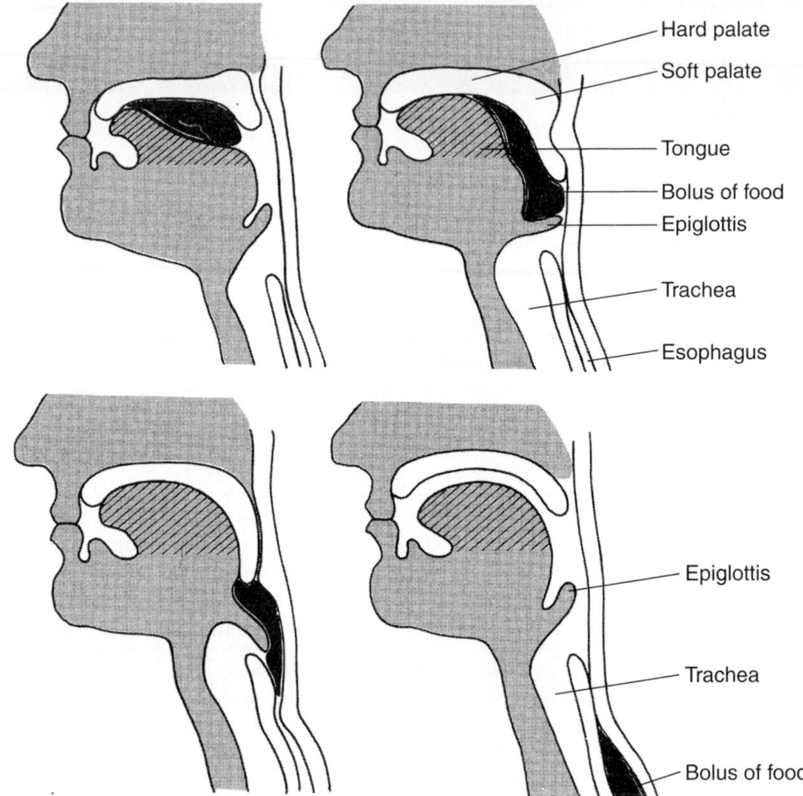

Figure 6-4 The swallowing mechanism. (From Abels, L. F. [1986]. *Critical care nursing*. St. Louis: Mosby.)

b. Description: hollow tube from the pharynx to the stomach; approximately 25 cm in length and 2 cm in diameter
c. Structure (Figure 6-5)
  (1) Cell layers (external to internal)
    (a) Does not have a serosal layer
    (b) Muscularis
      (i) Type of muscle
        a) Upper one third: skeletal muscle
        b) Lower two thirds: smooth muscle
      (ii) Direction of muscle
        a) Inner: circular
        b) Outer: longitudinal
    (c) Submucosa
    (d) Mucosa: lined with mucous membrane that secretes a protective mucoid substance
  (2) Sphincters
    (a) Hypopharyngeal
      (i) Also referred to as the *upper esophageal sphincter*
      (ii) Made of cricopharyngeal muscle
    (b) Gastroesophageal
      (i) Also referred to as the *lower esophageal sphincter*
      (ii) A physiologic rather than anatomic sphincter: consists of the last 2 to 4 cm of the esophagus
d. Secretions: mucus
e. Process: final phase of swallowing (involuntary)
  (1) When a bolus of food enters the esophagus, the hypopharyngeal sphincter opens.
  (2) Food is moved through the esophagus by gravity and peristaltic action; peristalsis is the alternating contraction and relaxation of muscle fibers that propels the substance in a wavelike motion through the esophagus, stomach, and intestines.
  (3) The gastroesophageal sphincter opens, and food enters the stomach.
  (4) The process takes 5 to 10 seconds.
f. Functions: Table 6-2

3. Stomach (Figure 6-6)
  a. Location: inferior to the diaphragm with approximately 80% to 85% of the organ to the left of midline
  b. Description
    (1) Largest dilation of the GI tract
    (2) From 25 to 30 cm in length and 10 to 15 cm at maximal diameter
    (3) Relatively little muscle tone, which permits increased distention
  c. Structure
    (1) Anatomic divisions
      (a) Cardia: portion of stomach that immediately adjoins the esophagus
      (b) Fundus: dome-shaped portion of stomach that extends left of the cardia

Table 6-2 Functions of the Components of the Gastrointestinal System

Component	Function
Oropharynx	• Salivation • Ingestion • Mastication • Lubrication and moistening of food • First and second stages of swallowing
Esophagus	• Third stage of swallowing • Lubrication of food • Provision of vent for increased gastric pressures
Stomach	• Secretion of gastric enzymes • Mixing of food with gastric enzymes • Reduction of osmolality of food • Absorption of water • Movement of food through the pylorus
Small intestine	• Receipt of chyme from the stomach and movement of the chyme forward to facilitate proper absorption of proteins, carbohydrates, fats, electrolytes, vitamins, minerals, drugs, and water • Receipt of bile and pancreatic fluid to aid in digestion • Movement of chyme via peristalsis and segmentation • Bacteria in the small intestine help break down and digest protein and, to some degree, fat
Large intestine	• Secretion of mucus to lubricate and protect intestinal lining • Movement of chyme through colon to rectum and initiation of urge to defecate • Storage of feces • Elimination of digestive wastes: defecation • Absorption of water and electrolytes • Synthesis of vitamins (folic acid, riboflavin, vitamin K, nicotinic acid) • Metabolism of blood urea to ammonia
Liver	• Secretion of bilirubin, bile salts, cholesterol, fatty acids, calcium, and other electrolytes into bile • Storage of amino acids, glucose, vitamins, minerals (copper, iron), and blood ◦ Vitamins: riboflavin, nicotinic acid, pyridoxine; vitamins A, D, E, K, and B_{12} • Conversion of complex sugars to simple sugars • Conversion of carbohydrates to fats • Conversion of stored glucose (glycogen) to glucose (process is called *glycogenolysis*) • Conversion of amino acids and fats to glucose (process is called *gluconeogenesis*) • Conversion of amino acids to fatty acids and triglycerides • Formation of phospholipids and cholesterol • Formation of lipoproteins from triglycerides and peptides • Conversion of amino acids to plasma proteins (e.g., albumin, fibrinogen, and globulins) • Phagocytosis of old red blood cells • Formation of clotting factors and heparin • Conversion of ammonia to urea • Conversion of creatine to creatinine • Conversion of vitamin D_3 to 25-hydroxycholecalciferol • Detoxification of bacteria • Biotransformation of drugs to active and/or inactive metabolites • Deactivation of certain hormones
Gallbladder	• Collection, concentration, and storage of bile • Passageway for bile from liver to intestine • Regulation of bile flow • Release of bile

Pancreas	• Exocrine function
	  ◦ Secretion of pancreatic juice for digestion of carbohydrates, proteins, and fats
	  ◦ Secretion of bicarbonate to neutralize chyme
	• Endocrine function
	  ◦ Secretion of insulin and glucagon

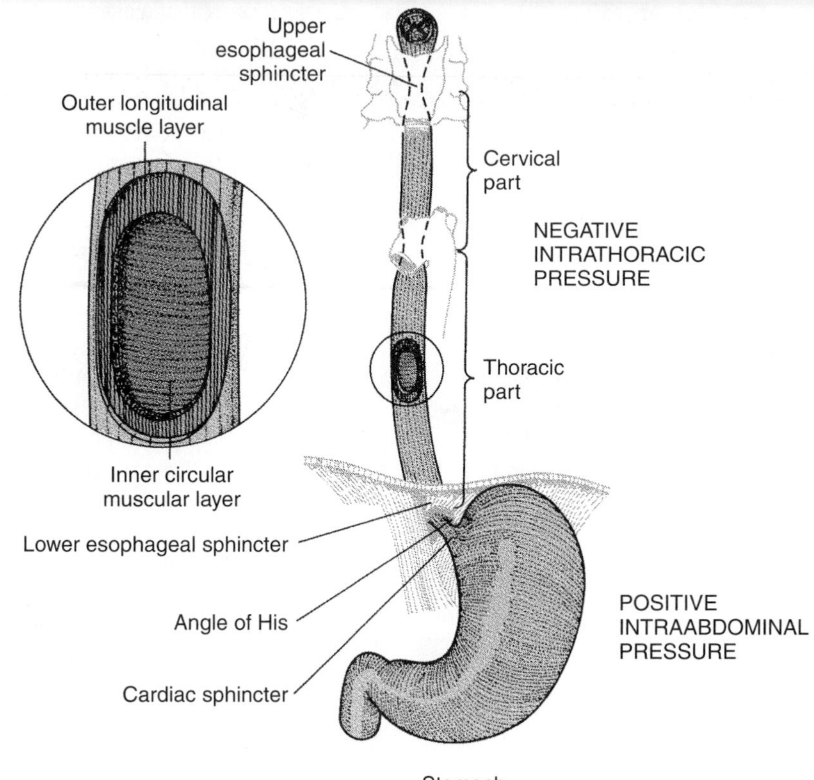

Figure 6-5 Anatomy of the esophagus. (From Beare, P. G., & Myers, J. L. [1994]. *Principles and practice of adult health nursing* [2nd ed.]. St. Louis: Mosby.)

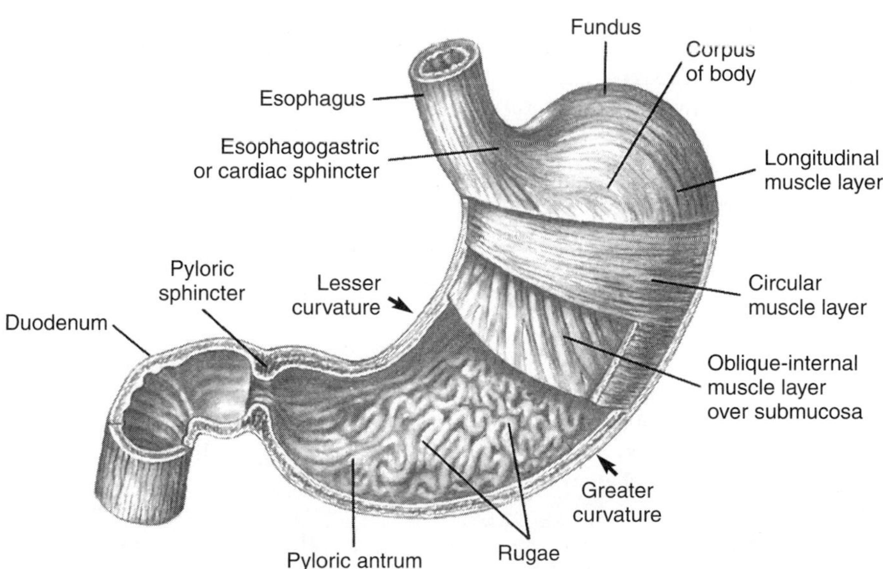

Figure 6-6 Anatomy of the stomach. (From Thompson, J. M., and others: *Mosby's clinical nursing* [3rd ed.]. St. Louis: Mosby.)

(c) Greater curvature: lateral, convex side
(d) Body: major area (belly) of stomach
(e) Lesser curvature: medial, concave side
(f) Antrum: lower portion close to pylorus

(2) Sphincters
(a) Cardiac: between esophagus and stomach
(b) Pyloric: between stomach and duodenum

(3) Layers of stomach wall (external to internal)
(a) Serosa: continuous with the peritoneum
(b) Muscularis
(i) Outer: longitudinal muscle fibers
(ii) Middle: circular muscle fibers
(iii) Inner: transverse muscle fibers

(c) Submucosa
(i) Blood vessels
(ii) Lymph vessels
(iii) Connective tissue
(iv) Fibrous tissues
(d) Mucosa: contains rugae that are thick folds on the interior of the stomach; rugae do all of the following:
(i) Increase surface area for exposure
(ii) Allow for distention
(iii) Contain the openings of the gastric glands
(e) Gastric glands
(i) Cardiac glands: just distal to the gastroesophageal junction; secrete pepsinogen and mucus
(ii) Oxyntic glands: fundic area
a) Mucous neck cells secrete mucus.
b) Chief cells secrete pepsinogen.
c) Oxyntic (also referred to as *parietal*) cells secrete the following:
i) Hydrochloric acid (HCl)
ii) Intrinsic factor
d) Enterochromaffin (endocrine) cells secrete serotonin.
(iii) Pyloric glands: antral area
a) Gastrin secreted by G cells
b) Serotonin secreted by enterochromaffin cells

d. Secretions: see Table 6-1
(1) Description: Gastric secretions are clear and contain water, salts, enzymes, and HCl.
(2) Gastric secretions are stimulated when a bolus of food enters the upper portion of the stomach.
(3) Gastric secretions contain the following:
(a) HCl
(i) Stimulated by histamine; acetylcholine; gastrin
(ii) Functions
a) Denature proteins and break intermolecular bonds
b) Activate a number of enzymes secreted by stomach
c) Kill bacteria
(b) Pepsinogen
(i) Activated by HCl to form pepsin
(ii) Function: pepsin catalyzes splitting of bonds between particular types of amino acids in protein chains
(c) Intrinsic factor: mucoprotein necessary for intestinal absorption of vitamin B_{12} in the ileum; deficiency of vitamin B_{12} causes pernicious anemia
(d) Mucus: contributes to the maintenance of the gastric mucosal barrier
(4) Control of gastric secretion
(a) Cephalic phase
(i) Mediated by parasympathetic nervous system (PNS)
(ii) Release of HCl when stimulated by thought, sight, smell, and taste of food
(b) Gastric phase
(i) Enhances acid secretion
(ii) Stimulated by distention of stomach and digestion products of food
(c) Intestinal phase
(i) Continuation of gastric acid secretion but in lesser amounts
(ii) Stimulated by distention, hypertonic solution, acid, and fats within duodenum

e. Process
(1) As food moves toward the pyloric sphincter at the distal end of the stomach, peristaltic waves increase in force and intensity.
(2) The food bolus becomes a substance known as *chyme*.
(3) Gastric motility is affected and controlled by various factors.
(a) Affected by the following
(i) Quantity and pH of contents
(ii) Degree of mixing
(iii) Peristalsis
(iv) Ability of the duodenum to accept the chyme
(b) Controlled by the following:
(i) Sympathetic nervous system (SNS) and PNS
(ii) Reflexes
(iii) Gastric hormones
(4) Chyme is pumped through the pyloric sphincter into the duodenum.
(5) The stomach empties as chyme moves through the pyloric channel.
(a) Rate of gastric emptying proportional to the volume of the contents of the stomach
(b) Regulation of gastric emptying affected by the following:
(i) Consistency of the fluid chyme; liquids selectively move through the pylorus before solids
(ii) Receptiveness of the duodenum
(c) Factors inhibiting gastric emptying
(i) Chyme with high lipid content
(ii) High acidity in antrum
(iii) Emotions: pain, anxiety, sadness, hostility
(iv) Hormones: secretin and cholecystokinin
(d) Food usually stays in the stomach 2 to 6 hours after ingestion.

f. Function: see Table 6-2

4. Small intestine
a. Description
(1) Length: 7 m; diameter: 2.5 cm

(2) Extends from pylorus to ileocecal valve

b. Structure

(1) Divisions

(a) Duodenum: short segment only 30 cm long

(b) Jejunum: the next two fifths after the duodenum

(c) Ileum: the last three fifths after the duodenum

(2) Layers of wall (external to internal)

(a) Serosa: continuous with the peritoneum

(b) Muscularis

(c) Submucosal

(d) Mucosal

(3) Sphincters

(a) Pylorus: from stomach to duodenum

(b) Ileocecal: controls flow of contents into large intestine and prevents reflux from the large intestine back into the ileum

(4) Villi (Figure 6-7)

(a) Fingerlike projections of mucosa and submucosa prominent in duodenum and jejunum increase surface area

(b) Contain a single lymph vessel called a *lacteal* and a dense capillary bed to aid in absorption

(c) Contain many different types of cells to absorb fats, carbohydrates (CHO), or proteins and/or secrete enzymes and mucus

(i) Brunner's glands: cells that secrete mucus; primarily in duodenum

(ii) Goblet cells: cells that secrete mucus

(iii) Crypts of Lieberkühn: cells that produce watery mucus called *succus entericus*, a carrier substance for absorption of nutrients when the villi come in contact with the chyme

(iv) Paneth cells: uncertain function but may regulate intestinal flora

(v) Peyer's patches

a) Cells in mucosa and submucosa

b) Lymphoid follicles that carry out antibody synthesis

c. Secretions

(1) Stimulated by the presence of chyme in the duodenum and release of gastric hormones

(2) See Table 6-1

d. Process

(1) Movement of chyme

(a) During fasting and sleeping states, muscle contraction moves from antrum to ileum to sweep the gut of contents.

(b) During eating state, the following occur:

(i) Concentric, segmenting contractions take place in the jejunum; these help to mix secretions of the small intestines with the chyme particles.

(ii) Slow, propulsive contractions (peristalsis) slowly push the chyme in the direction of the large intestine.

(iii) Continuous shortening and lengthening of the villi constantly stirs the intestinal contents.

(c) The movement of chyme from the small intestine to the large intestine is regulated by the gastroileal reflex; increased contractions in the ileum occur as the chyme nears the large intestine.

(d) Movement of chyme through small intestine takes approximately 3 to 10 hours.

e. Function: see Table 6-2

5. Large intestine

a. Description: length is 90 to 150 cm; diameter is 4 to 6 cm extending from ileum to anus

b. Structure

(1) Divisions (Figure 6-8)

(a) Cecum

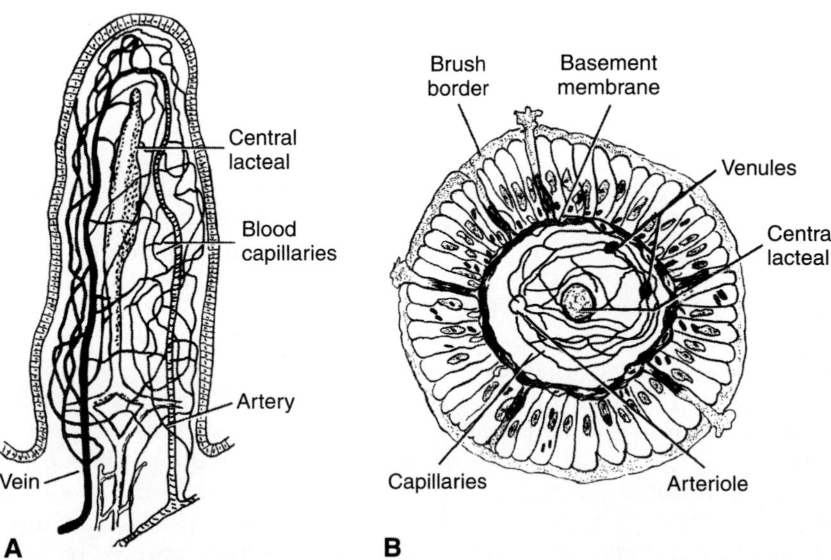

Figure 6-7 Villi. **A,** Longitudinal. **B,** Cross section. (From Abels, L. F. [1986]. *Critical care nursing*. St. Louis: Mosby.)

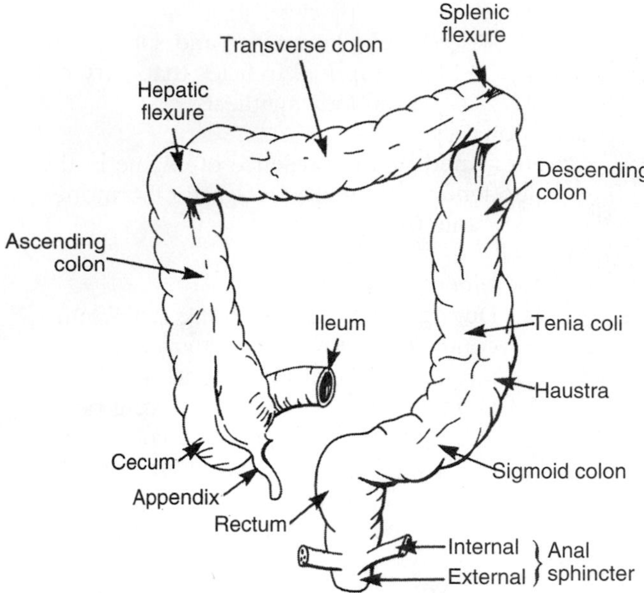

Figure 6-8 Anatomy of the colon. (From Kinney, M. R., Packa, D. R., & Dunbar, S. B. [1998]. *AACN's clinical reference for critical-care nursing* [4th ed.]. St. Louis: Mosby.)

(b) Colon
(i) Ascending colon
(ii) Transverse colon
(iii) Descending colon
(iv) Sigmoid colon
(c) Rectum
(2) Flexures
(a) Hepatic: bend at the liver; in the right upper quadrant (RUQ)
(b) Splenic: bend at the spleen; in the left upper quadrant (LUQ)
(3) Sphincters
(a) Ileocecal: from small intestine to cecum
(b) Anal: internal and external anal sphincters
(4) Layers of large intestinal wall
(a) Serosa: continuous with the peritoneum
(b) Muscularis
(c) Submucosa
(d) Mucosa
c. Process
(1) Movement of intestinal contents
(a) Haustral shuttling
(i) Periodic uncoordinated tonic contractions or segmentations of the longitudinal and circular muscles
(ii) Contents displaced short distances
(iii) Weak peristaltic contractions that move the chyme through the large intestine
(b) Phasic, random, nonpropulsive contractions
(i) Last 30 seconds to 2 minutes
(ii) Contents displaced short distances in both directions
(iii) Mixes the stool material and helps in the absorption of liquid contents without advancement toward the anus
(c) Spontaneous mass movements
(i) Fecal contents are pushed forward by mass movements that typically occur only a few times each day.
(ii) Mass movements are stimulated by gastrocolic reflexes initiated when food enters the duodenum from the stomach, especially after the first meal of the day.
(iii) These movements move feces into the rectum.
(iv) The defecation reflex occurs when feces enters the rectum; peristaltic waves in the rectum and relaxation of the internal and external anal sphincter occur.
(v) Afferent impulses are transmitted to the sacral segment of the spinal cord, from which reflex impulses are transmitted back to the colon and rectum, initiating relaxation of the internal anal sphincter.
(vi) Evacuation of the colon may be facilitated by the Valsalva maneuver.
(2) Factors that enhance colonic motility
(a) High-residue diets
(b) Fluids
(c) Irritation of colon (e.g., spicy foods)
(d) Irritant laxatives
(3) Factors that inhibit colonic motility
(a) Low-residue diet
(b) Anticholinergic drugs
(c) Opiates
(4) Movement of fecal contents through large intestine approximately 12 hours
d. Function: Table 6-2

Accessory Organs of Digestion
(Figure 6-9)

1. Liver
a. Location: in RUQ, fitting snugly against right inferior diaphragm
b. Description
(1) Largest organ in the body: 1.5 kg
(2) Attached to the abdominal wall by the falciform ligament, which also divides the left and right lobes
(3) Four main lobes
(a) Right: larger than left
(b) Left
(c) Caudate
(d) Quadrate
(4) Covered by a thick capsule of connective tissue (called *Glisson's capsule*); contains blood vessels and lymphatic vessels
(5) Capsule covered by a layer of serosa continuous with the peritoneum
c. Structure (Figure 6-10)

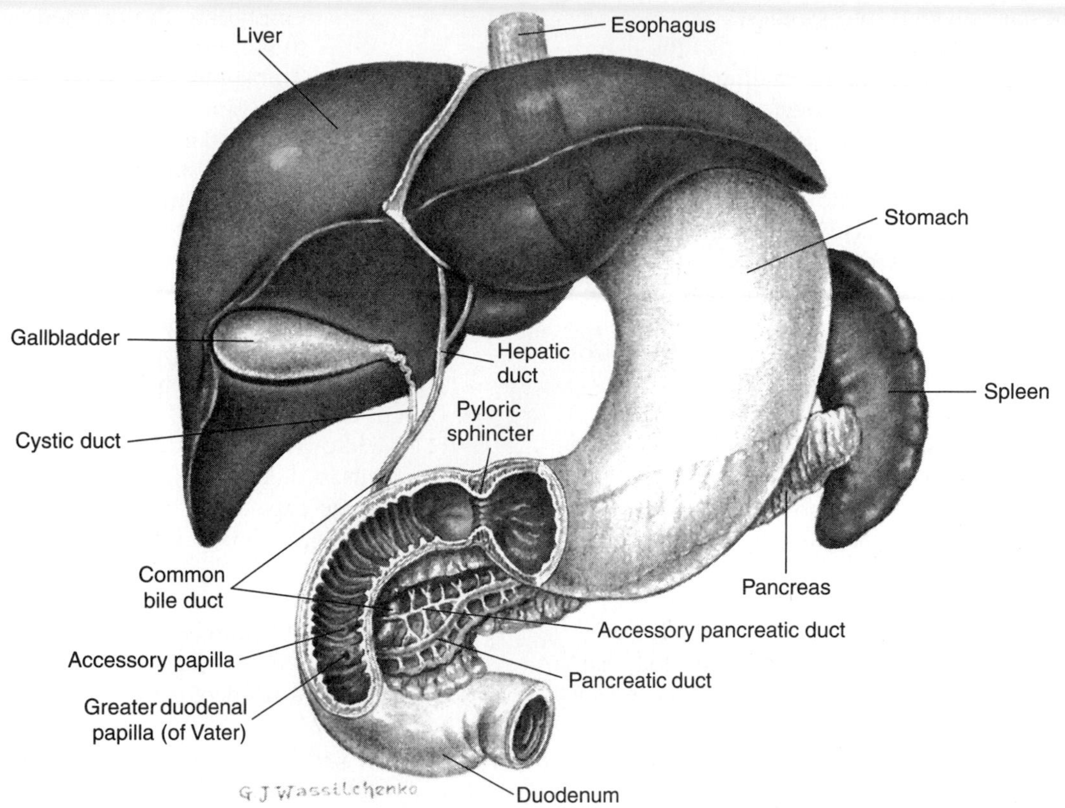

Figure 6-9 Accessory organs of the gastrointestinal system. (From Doughty, D. B., & Jackson, D. B. [1993]. *Gastrointestinal disorders: Mosby's clinical nursing series.* St. Louis: Mosby.)

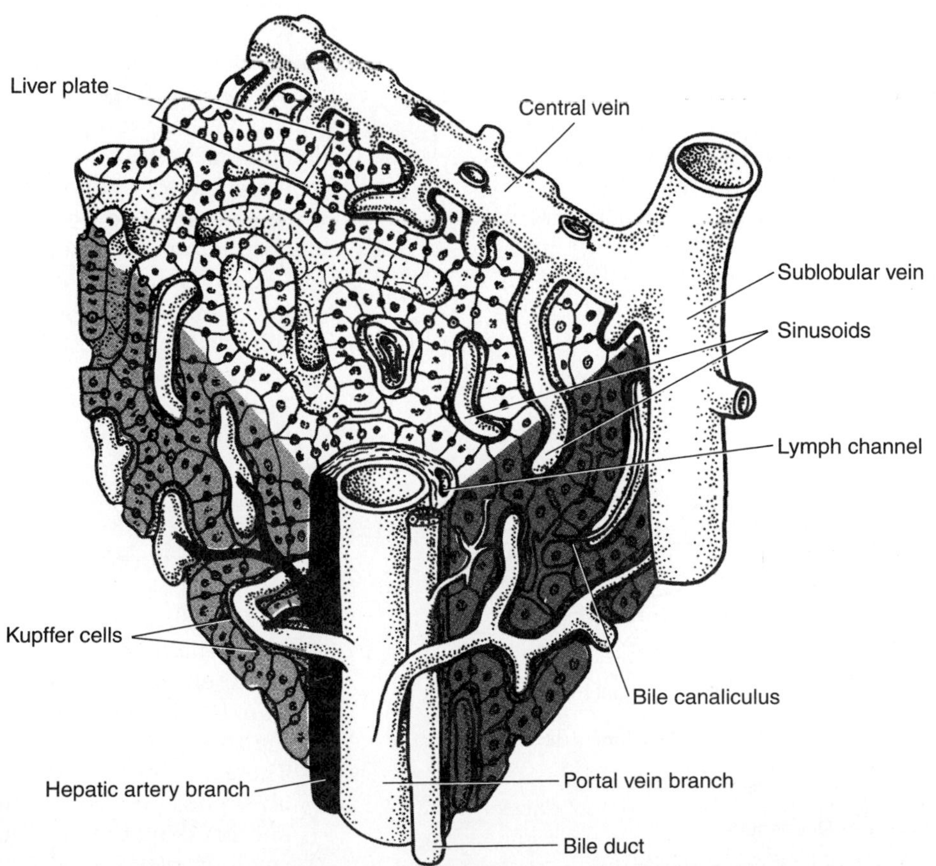

Figure 6-10 Microscopic structure of the liver lobule. (From Lewis, S. M., & Collier, I. C. [1992]. *Medical-surgical nursing* [3rd ed.]. St. Louis: Mosby.)

(1) Lobes are divided into lobules.
(2) Lobules are the functioning unit of the liver; the liver has more than 1 million lobules.
(a) Hepatic cells (hepatocytes) are arranged in chains around a central vein.
(b) Blood flows through sinusoids that separate the hepatic chains.
(c) The sinusoids receive oxygenated blood from branches of the hepatic artery and nutrient-rich blood from branches of the hepatic portal vein; the hepatic cells remove oxygen, nutrients, and toxins from the blood.
(d) Each lobule has its own hepatic artery, portal vein, and bile duct, collectively called the *portal triad*.
(e) The lobule is composed of branching plates of liver cells radiating from center to periphery.
(f) Kupffer cells, which are responsible for phagocytosis, line the sinusoids; Kupffer cells are a part of the reticuloendothelial system; they destroy old or defective red blood cells (RBCs) and remove bacteria and foreign particles from the blood.
(g) Ducts
(i) Bile canaliculi are located between the hepatic cells and empty bile into the small bile ducts.
(ii) Small bile ducts join to form the right and left hepatic ducts.
(iii) Left and right hepatic ducts merge to form the common hepatic duct.
(iv) Cystic duct from the gallbladder joins the common hepatic duct to form the common bile duct (Figure 6-11).
(v) The pancreatic duct joins the common bile duct, and together they empty into the duodenum through the ampulla of Vater.
(vi) The sphincter of Oddi is a valve in the common bile duct that regulates the passage of bile from the common bile duct into the duodenum.

d. Secretions: Bile is described under Gallbladder.
e. Function: see Table 6-2

2. Gallbladder
a. Location
(1) Attached to undersurface of liver
(2) Connected to the upper portion of the duodenum by the common bile duct
b. Description
(1) Saclike organ about 7 to 10 cm in length and 3 cm in diameter
(2) Storage capacity of 50 to 70 mL
(3) Layers (exterior to interior)
(a) Serous layer: continuous with the peritoneum
(b) Smooth muscle layer
(c) Mucous membrane layer (has rugae that allow an increase in gallbladder size)
c. Structure
(1) The gallbladder has four anatomic divisions:
(a) Fundus: distal portion of the body that forms a blind sac
(b) Body: connects the fundus to the infundibulum
(c) Infundibulum: connects the body to the neck
(d) Neck: narrows into the cystic duct
(2) The cystic duct merges with the common hepatic duct to form the common bile duct, which joins with the pancreatic duct to form the ampulla of Vater.
(3) The sphincter of Oddi is at the terminal end of the common bile duct, located at the entrance into the duodenum.
(a) Regulates the flow of bile and pancreatic juices into the intestine
(b) Inhibits the entry of bile into the pancreatic duct
(c) Prevents reflux of intestinal contents into the duct
d. Secretions
(1) See Table 6-1
(2) Bile
(a) Bile is produced by the liver and is stored in the gallbladder.
(b) The gallbladder contracts in response to the hormone cholecystokinin when food is present in the small intestine; release is stimulated when fatty food is present in the small intestine.
(c) The action of bile is to assist in the absorption of fats by emulsifying the fats and breaking down large fat droplets into small droplets.
(d) Bile is composed of the following:
(i) Water

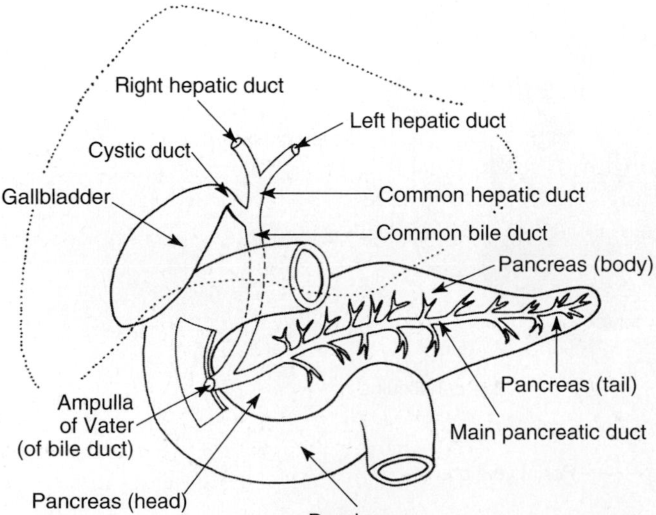

Figure 6-11 Ductal systems of the GI tract. (From Kinney, M. R., Packa, D. R., & Dunbar, S. B. [1998]. *AACN's clinical reference for critical-care nursing* [4th ed.]. St. Louis: Mosby.)

(ii) Bile pigments
(iii) Bile salts
(iv) High concentration of cholesterol
(v) Some neutral fats, phospholipids, and inorganic salts

(e) The major bile pigment is bilirubin, a breakdown product of hemoglobin.
(i) Metabolism (Figure 6-12)
a) The heme portion of the hemoglobin molecule is converted to bilirubin by reticuloendothelial cells, is released into bloodstream, and binds to albumin as fat-soluble, unconjugated bilirubin (indirect).
b) In the liver, indirect bilirubin is bound to glucuronic acid to form water-soluble conjugated (direct) bilirubin, which is excreted into the hepatic ducts.

e. Process
(1) Contraction of the gallbladder is stimulated by the hormone cholecystokinin.

f. Function: see Table 6-2

3. Pancreas
a. Location: lies in the posterior curvature of the stomach; lies behind the duodenum and spleen
b. Description
(1) Length: 15 to 20 cm; diameter: 5 cm
(2) Anatomic divisions
(a) Head: over the vena cava in the C-shaped curve of the duodenum
(b) Body: lies behind duodenum and extends across the abdomen behind stomach
(c) Tail: under the spleen
(3) Not surrounded by a capsule
c. Structure (Figure 6-13)
(1) Connected lobes are formed by lobules.
(2) Lobules are clustered cells.
(3) The acini are arranged around a small central lumen; they secrete their enzymes into the central lumen.
(4) These central lumina are drained into ductules.
(5) Ductules drain into intralobular ducts, which drain into interlobular ducts, which empty into the pancreatic duct (also called the *duct of Wirsung*).
(6) The pancreatic duct runs from the tail to the head of the pancreas and unites with the common bile duct to form the ampulla of Vater, which empties into the duodenum.
(7) Cells have exocrine and endocrine functions.
(a) Acinar cells have exocrine (through a duct) functions.
(b) Alpha and beta cells of the islets of Langerhans have endocrine (ductless) functions.
(i) Alpha cells secrete glucagon.
(ii) Beta cells secrete insulin.
(iii) Delta cells secrete somatostatin.

d. Secretions: see Table 6-1

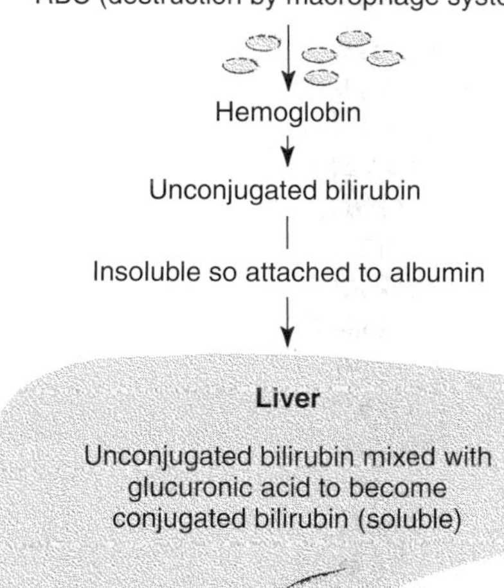

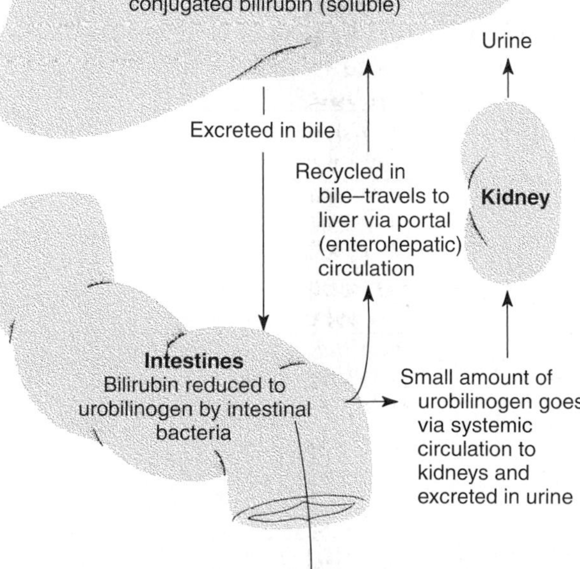

Figure 6-12 Bilirubin metabolism. *RBC,* Red blood cell. (From Lewis, S. M., & Collier, I.C. [1992]. *Medical-surgical nursing* [3rd ed.]. St. Louis: Mosby.)

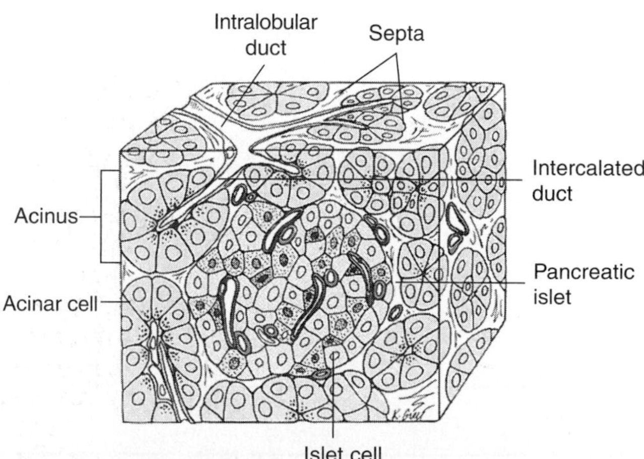

Figure 6-13 Pancreatic acini and ducts. (From Doughty, D. B., & Jackson, D. B. [1993]. *Gastrointestinal disorders: Mosby's clinical nursing series.* St. Louis: Mosby.)

(1) Pancreatic secretions are triggered by the presence of undigested food in the small intestine.
(2) Acinar cells secrete a high concentration of sodium bicarbonate, water, sodium, potassium, and digestive enzymes (lipase, amylase, trypsin, ribonuclease, deoxyribonuclease).
(a) Trypsinogen: secreted in inactive form; activated in contact with bile salts
(b) Chymotrypsinogen: secreted in inactive form; activated in contact with bile salts
(3) Secretions are controlled by the following:
(a) Vagus nerve and PNS
(b) Hormonal: secretin and cholecystokinin

e. Functions: see Table 6-2

Gastrointestinal Hormones

See Table 6-3.

Blood Supply (Figure 6-14)

1. Arterial: aorta → aortic arch → thoracic arch → abdominal aorta →
   a. Celiac artery: The following branches of the celiac artery supply these specified organs:
      (1) Left gastric: supplies stomach and esophagus
      (2) Hepatic to right gastric: supplies stomach
      (3) Gastroduodenal: supplies stomach and duodenum
      (4) Cystic: supplies gallbladder
      (5) Splenic: supplies stomach, pancreas, and spleen
   b. Superior mesenteric arteries supply the following:
      (1) Jejunum
      (2) Ileum
      (3) Cecum
      (4) Ascending colon
      (5) Part of transverse colon
   c. Inferior mesenteric arteries supply the following:
      (1) Transverse, descending, and sigmoid colon
      (2) Rectum
   d. Hepatic artery and vein supply the liver.
2. Venous
   a. Portal vein collects and delivers blood from entire venous drainage of the GI tract to the liver; branches: gastric; splenic; superior mesenteric; inferior mesenteric
   b. Portal vein subdivides into liver sinusoids, which then unite with branches from hepatic artery to form hepatic vein, which empties into inferior vena cava
   c. Partially metabolized digestive products are brought to liver sinusoids where hepatocytes complete the next stage of metabolism

Table 6-3 Gastrointestinal Hormone

Hormone	Source	Stimulus for Release	Action
Gastrin	Gastric mucosa of the antrum of the stomach and the pylorus	Partially digested proteins in pylorus	• Stimulates release of gastric juices
Secretin	Duodenal mucosa	Partially digested proteins, fats, acid in the intestine	• Inhibits gastric motility and acid secretions • Pancreatic bicarbonate secretion
Cholecystokinin	Duodenal mucosa	Fats in duodenum	• Increases gallbladder contraction • Decreases stomach tone
Gastric inhibitory peptide	Small intestine mucosa	Fats and carbohydrates in duodenum	• Stimulates secretion of insulin • Decreases motor activity of the stomach • Slows emptying of gastric contents into the small intestine
Vasoactive intestinal peptide	Small intestine mucosa	Acid in the duodenum	• Stimulates intestinal juice • Inhibits gastric secretion
Enterogastrone	Small intestine mucosa	Partially digested proteins, fats, and acids in intestine	• Inhibits gastric secretion and motility • Relaxation of sphincter of • Oddi and contraction of gallbladder
Villikinin	Small intestine mucosa	Chyme in intestine	• Stimulates movement of intestinal villi
Pancreozymin	Duodenal mucosa	Partially digested proteins, fats, and acids in duodenum	• Stimulates pancreatic juice

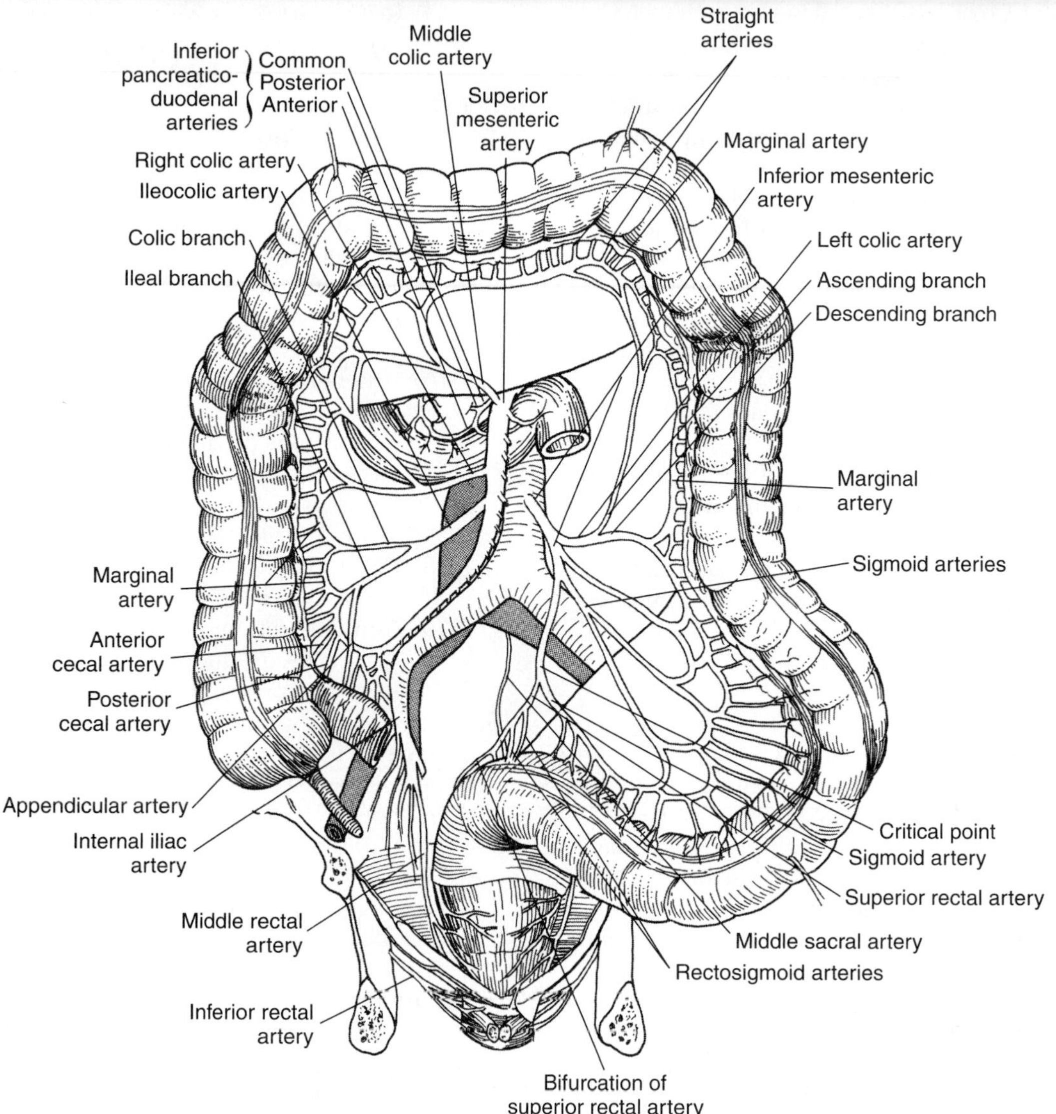

Figure 6-14 Arterial blood supply of the GI system. (From Society of Gastroenterology Nurses and Associates. [1993]. *Gastroenterology nursing: A core curriculum.* St. Louis: Mosby.)

Nervous Innervation

1. Extrinsic
   a. PNS: increases the activity of the GI tract; innervated via the vagus nerve
   b. SNS: decreases the activity of the GI tract; innervated via the SNS fibers, which run parallel to the major blood vessels of the GI tract
2. Intrinsic
   a. Located inside the wall of GI tract
   b. Consists of extensions from extrinsic nerves of the autonomic nervous system (ANS)
   c. Form two major and three minor networks of plexuses

Functions of the Gastrointestinal System

1. Ingestion
   a. Ingestion begins with the sensation of hunger, controlled by the feeding center of the hypothalamus
   b. Ingestion ends with the sensation of satisfaction provided by the satiety center also in the hypothalamus
   c. Food and liquids enter the alimentary tract at the mouth
2. Secretion: see Table 6-1
3. Digestion
   a. CHO: 4 kcal/g
      (1) Digestion begins in the mouth where polysaccharides (starch) are broken down to disaccharides (e.g., sucrose, lactose, and maltose) by the action of ptyalin (amylase)

(2) The process continues when the disaccharides are broken down to monosaccharides (e.g., glucose, galactose, and fructose) by the action of pancreatic amylase and intestinal enzymes (e.g., sucrase, lactase, and maltase)

b. Proteins: 4 kcal/g
   (1) Digestion begins in the stomach where pepsin breaks down proteins into polypeptides.
   (2) The process continues when the polypeptides are broken down into peptides and amino acids in the small intestine by the action of trypsin, chymotrypsin, and carboxypeptides from the pancreas and aminopeptidases and dipeptidase from the intestinal villi.

c. Fats: 9 kcal/g
   (1) Digestion of fats that already are emulsified (e.g., cream and butter) begins in the stomach by lipase.
   (2) Digestion of nonemulsified fats occurs in the small intestine with emulsification of the fats by bile and pancreatic lipase.
   (3) Fats are broken down into glycerol and fatty acids.

4. Absorption
   a. Basic absorption mechanisms
      (1) Active transport requires an energy source (e.g., adenosine triphosphate) to move substances into and out of the cell; substances absorbed by active transport include proteins, glucose, sodium, and potassium.
      (2) Passive diffusion is passive movement from an area of high solute concentration to an area of low solute concentration; substances absorbed by passive diffusion include free fatty acids and water.
      (3) Facilitated diffusion is movement that requires a carrier that moves into the cell, but energy is not required; a substance absorbed by facilitated diffusion is fructose.
      (4) Nonionic transport is movement of solutes freely into and out of the cell; substances absorbed by nonionic transport include unconjugated bile salts and drugs.
      (5) Solvent drag is flow of water to higher osmotic concentration; it contributes to absorption and reduction in osmolality that occurs in the jejunum.
   b. Specific absorption in small intestine
      (1) Electrolyte absorption: active transport from all areas of intestine
      (2) Water absorption: small and large intestine
         (a) Approximately 2 L of fluid is ingested daily.
         (b) Approximately 7 L of fluid is secreted by the GI tract daily.
         (c) Of these 9 L, 7500 mL are reabsorbed, with only 1500 mL reaching the cecum.
         (d) Additional fluid is reabsorbed in the large intestine, but only 200 mL is lost in the stool.
      (3) CHO absorption
         (a) Fructose by facilitated diffusion
         (b) Glucose and galactose by active transport
      (4) Protein absorption: amino acids absorbed by active transport in ileum and jejunum
      (5) Fat absorption
         (a) Micellar solubilization of fatty acid with bile salt to form micelle
         (b) Diffusion of micelle into jejunal cell
         (c) Delivery of fatty acids to circulation via lymphatic system
      (6) Water-soluble vitamin absorption: all areas of small intestine by passive diffusion (absorption of vitamin B_{12} requires intrinsic factor)
      (7) Fat-soluble vitamin absorption: absorbed in jejunum (bile salts required)
      (8) Calcium absorption: mainly in duodenum (vitamin D required)
      (9) Iron absorption: all areas of the intestine (especially in duodenum) by active transport; stored as protein-bound iron

5. Synthesis
   a. Bacteria in the large intestine produce vitamin K.
   b. Peyer's patches in the small intestine play a role in antibody synthesis.

6. Effect on fluid and electrolyte balance
   a. Gastric losses are acidic; increased gastric losses (e.g., nasogastric suction and vomiting) cause metabolic alkalosis, hypokalemia, hyponatremia, and hypovolemia.
   b. Intestinal losses are alkaline: increased intestinal losses (e.g., biliary losses, pancreatic fistula, intestinal suction, and diarrhea) cause metabolic acidosis, hypokalemia, hyponatremia, and hypovolemia.

Assessment of the Gastrointestinal System

Interview

1. Chief complaint: why the patient is seeking help and duration of the problem
   a. Nonspecific problems/complaints
      (1) Change in appetite
      (2) Fatigue or weakness
      (3) Unintentional weight loss or weight gain
      (4) Fever, chills
   b. Abdominal pain: describe PQRST (Table 6-4)
      (1) *P*rovocation: relationship to food, drugs, activity, position, bowel movements, breathing, and stress
      (2) *P*alliation
         (a) Ineffective or effective treatments
         (b) Alleviating factors (e.g., position)
      (3) *Q*uality: sharp, dull, tearing, cramping, burning, gnawing, stabbing, aching, colicky
         (a) Visceral pain
            (i) Dull, poorly localized

Table 6-4 **Differentiation of Abdominal Pain**

Condition	Location of Pain	Quality of Pain	Associated Symptoms
Gastritis	• Epigastric or slightly left of midline	• May be described as indigestion	• Nausea and vomiting • May have hematemesis • Abdominal tenderness
Peptic ulcer	• Epigastric or RUQ	• Gnawing, burning	• Abdominal tenderness • Hematemesis (gastric) or melena (duodenal)
Pancreatitis	• Epigastric or LUQ • May radiate to back, flanks, or left shoulder	• Boring • Worsened by lying down	• Nausea and vomiting • Mild fever • Abdominal tenderness • May have Cullen's sign (i.e., bluish discoloration at umbilicus) indicating intraperitoneal bleeding or Grey Turner's sign (i.e., bluish discoloration at flanks) indicating retroperitoneal bleeding
Cholecystitis	• Epigastric or RUQ • May be referred to *below right scapula* • Murphy's sign: pain with deep breath while the nurse palpates under the right costal margin	• Cramping	• Nausea and vomiting • Abdominal tenderness in RUQ
Appendicitis	• Epigastric or periumbilical pain; later localizes to RLQ • McBurney's sign: pain with palpation at McBurney's point (i.e., point at one third the distance between the right anterioriliac crest and the umbilicus) • Rovsing sign: pain in RLQ with palpation of LLQ indicates peritoneal irritation	• Dull to sharp	• Anorexia, nausea, vomiting • Fever • Diarrhea • Leukocytosis • Rebound tenderness indicates peritoneal irritation
Intestinal obstruction	• Epigastric or umbilical	• Spastic to dull	• Change in bowel habits • Melena or hematochezia • Hyperactive to hypoactive bowel sounds

LLQ, Left lower quadrant; *LUQ*, left upper quadrant; *RLQ*, right lower quadrant; *RUQ*, right upper quadrant.

(ii) May be caused by organic lesions or functional disturbance within the GI tract

(b) Somatic pain

(i) Sharp, well localized

(ii) May be caused by inflammation of abdominal organs that cause peritoneal irritation

(c) Referred pain

(i) Pain experienced at a distance from the disease process

(ii) May be explained by the embryologic origins of the structures involved

(4) *R*egion: location

(a) May be poorly localized

(b) May be referred pain (Figure 6-15)

(i) Pain may be felt in a remote area that is supplied by the same nerve as the diseased or damaged organ.

(ii) The pain is usually sharp and localized but not over area of injury.

(5) *R*adiation

(6) *S*everity: 0-to-10 scale

(7) *T*iming: constant, intermittent; duration

c. Abdominal distention

d. Change in bowel elimination

(1) Change in color of stools

(a) Clay-colored stools indicate biliary obstruction

(b) Tarry stools (melena) indicate upper GI bleeding

(c) Bloody stools (hematochezia) indicate lower GI bleeding

(2) Change in consistency of stools

(3) Change in frequency of stools

(4) Excessive flatus

(5) Use of laxative or enemas

(6) Relationship to food, drugs, and alcohol

e. Nausea/vomiting

(1) Onset, duration

(2) Frequency

(3) Character and color; presence of blood in vomitus (hematemesis)

(4) Palliation

(a) Ineffective or effective treatment

(b) Alleviating factors

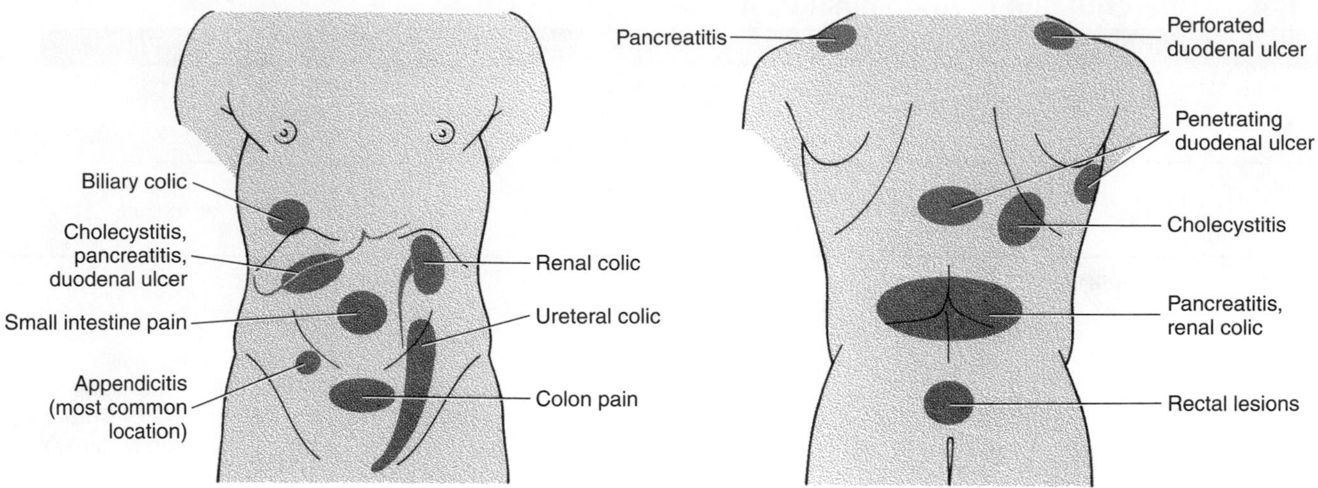

Figure 6-15 Common areas of referred abdominal pain. (From Beare, P. G., & Myers, J. L. [1994]. *Principles and practice of adult health nursing* [2nd ed.]. St. Louis: Mosby.)

- (5) Timing
  - (a) Time of day
  - (b) Relationship to food, odors, drugs, alcohol, activity, and bowel movements
- (6) Aggravating factors
- (7) Associated pain

f. Abdominal trauma
- (1) Gunshot entrance and exit wound
- (2) Knife wounds
- (3) Burns or abrasions
- (4) Ecchymotic areas associated with blunt trauma

g. Dentition problems
- (1) Caries
- (2) Gingivitis
- (3) Poor-fitting dentures

h. Painful swallowing
i. Dysphagia
j. Dyspepsia
k. Eructation
l. Flatulence
m. Edema
n. Abnormal bruising or bleeding
o. Jaundice
p. Change in color of urine: dark brown or orange urine may indicate biliary obstruction
q. Pruritus
r. Fecal incontinence
s. Rectal bleeding
t. Anal discomfort

2. History of present illness: use PQRST format
3. Medical history

a. Past illnesses
- (1) Jaundice
- (2) Anemia
- (3) Obesity: use of liquid diets, GI bypass, or gastric balloon
- (4) Eating disorders (e.g., bulimia and anorexia nervosa)
- (5) Alcoholism
- (6) Peptic ulcer disease
- (7) GI hemorrhage
- (8) Cholelithiasis
- (9) Hepatic disease
  - (a) Cirrhosis
  - (b) Hepatitis
  - (c) History of blood transfusion
- (10) Pancreatitis
- (11) Cancer
- (12) Irritable bowel syndrome
- (13) Inflammatory bowel disease (e.g., ulcerative colitis and Crohn's disease)
- (14) Diverticulitis
- (15) Polyps
- (16) Hemorrhoids
- (17) Renal disease
- (18) Cardiovascular disease
- (19) Diabetes mellitus
- (20) Chronic obstructive pulmonary disease (COPD) (high incidence of peptic ulcer disease)

b. Past injury: abdominal trauma
c. Past surgical procedures
d. Past diagnostic studies (e.g., endoscopy, x-ray, and stool exam for occult blood)
e. Food intolerances or allergies; type of reaction if allergy

4. Family history

a. Eating disorders (e.g., obesity, anorexia nervosa, or bulimia)
b. Anemia
c. Peptic ulcer disease
d. Pancreatic disease (e.g., pancreatitis or pancreatic cancer)
e. Diabetes mellitus
f. Liver disease (e.g., cirrhosis or hepatitis)
g. Malabsorption syndrome
h. Inflammatory bowel disease (e.g., ulcerative colitis or Crohn's disease)
i. Irritable bowel syndrome
j. Alcoholism
k. Cancer

5. Social history
   a. Relationship with spouse or significant other; family structure
   b. Occupation
   c. Educational level
   d. Stress level and usual coping mechanisms
   e. Recreational habits
   f. Exercise habits
   g. Dietary habits
      (1) Appetite
      (2) Usual foods
      (3) Number and time of meals and snacks
      (4) Fluid intake
      (5) Food restrictions
         (a) Intolerances
         (b) Prescribed restrictions
         (c) Religious restrictions
      (6) Change in eating habits
   h. Usual bowel habits
   i. Caffeine intake
   j. Tobacco use: record as pack-years (number of packs per day times the number of years the patient has been smoking)
   k. Alcohol use: record as alcoholic beverages consumed per month, week, or day
   l. Exposure to toxins or infectious disease
   m. Travel
6. Medication history
   a. Prescribed drug, dose, frequency, and time of last dose
   b. Nonprescribed drugs
      (1) Over-the-counter drugs
      (2) Substance abuse
   c. Patient understanding of drug actions and side effects
   d. Drugs causing potential problems for patients with GI problems
      (1) Antibiotics
      (2) Aspirin
      (3) Nonsteroidal antiinflammatory drugs (NSAIDs) (e.g., ketorolac [Toradol] and ibuprofen [Motrin])
      (4) Corticosteroids
      (5) Acetaminophen (Tylenol)
      (6) Many drugs have anorexia, nausea, and vomiting as side effects
      (7) Many drugs are hepatotoxic (Box 6-1)
   e. Drugs frequently used for GI problems
      (1) Antacids, H_2 receptor antagonists, proton pump inhibitors
      (2) Stool softeners
      (3) Laxatives
      (4) Cathartics
      (5) Anticholinergics
      (6) Corticosteroids
      (7) Antidiarrheals
      (8) Antiemetics
      (9) Tranquilizers
      (10) Sedatives
      (11) Barbiturates

BOX 6-1 Selected Hepatotoxic Agents

Acetaminophen (Tylenol)
Acetylsalicylic acid (A.S.A.)
Allopurinol (Zyloprim)
Amiodarone (Cordarone)
Amitriptyline (Elavil)
Ampicillin (Polycillin)
Carbamazepine (Tegretol)
Carbenicillin (Geopen)
Carbon tetrachloride
Chlorambucil (Leukeran)
Chlordiazepoxide (Librium)
Chlorpromazine (Thorazine)
Chlorpropamide (Diabinese)
Cimetidine (Tagamet)
Clindamycin (Cleocin)
Cyclosporine (Sandimmune)
Dantrolene (Dantrium)
Diazepam (Valium)
Doxepin (Sinequan)
Erythromycin estolate (Ilosone)
Ethanol
Ethrane
Ferrous sulfate
Haloperidol (Haldol)
Halothane (Fluothane)
Hydrochlorothiazide (HydroDIURIL)
Imipramine (Tofranil)
Indomethacin (Indocin)
Isoniazid
Ketoconazole
Meprobamate (Equanil)
6-Mercaptopurine (Purinethol)
Methotrexate
Methoxyflurane (Penthrane)
Methyldopa (Aldomet)
Miconazole
Monoamine oxidase inhibitors
Nicotinic acid
Oral contraceptives
Oxacillin (Prostaphlin)
Penicillin (Pen Vee K)
Phenazopyridine (Pyridium)
Phenobarbital (Luminal)
Phenylbutazone (Butazolidin)
Phenytoin (Dilantin)
Probenecid (Benemid)
Prochlorperazine (Compazine)
Promethazine (Phenergan)
Propoxyphene (Darvon)
Propylthiouracil (PTU)
Quinidine
Rifampin (Rifadin)
Sulfonamides (trimethoprim and sulfamethoxazole [Bactrim, Septra], sulfisoxazole [Gantrisin])
Tetracyclines (Achromycin)
Tolbutamide (Orinase)
Trimethobenzamide (Tigan)
Tripelennamine (Pyribenzamine)

Vital Signs

1. Blood pressure (BP): sitting; lying; standing especially in hemorrhaging patient; systolic BP less than 100 mm Hg and a heart rate greater than 100 beats/min indicates a blood loss of at least 20% reduction in blood volume
2. Heart rate
3. Respiratory rate
4. Temperature
5. Height
6. Weight

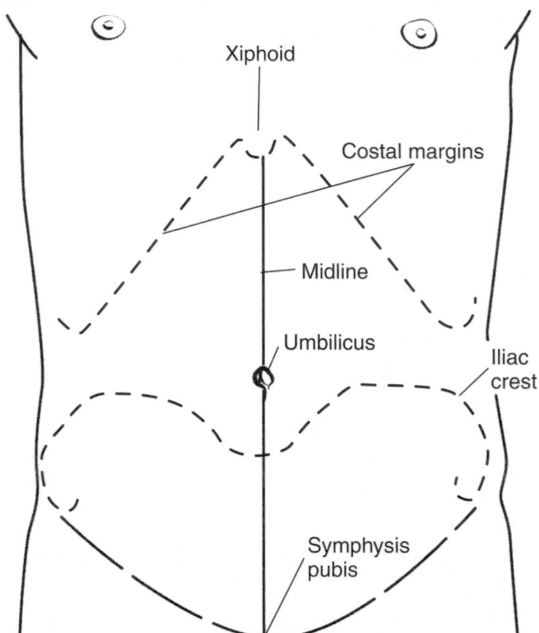

Figure 6-16 Landmarks of the abdomen.

Inspection

1. Landmarks (Figure 6-16)
   a. Xiphoid
   b. Costal margin
   c. Midline
   d. Umbilicus
   e. Anterior superior iliac crest
   f. Symphysis pubis
   g. The abdomen may be divided into
      (1) Four quadrants (Figure 6-17, *A* to *D*): horizontal and vertical lines intersect at the umbilicus
      (2) Nine regions (Figure 6-18, *A* to *I*)
2. General survey
   a. Apparent health status
   b. Apparent age relative to chronologic age
   c. Level of consciousness
   d. Gross deformity
   e. Nutritional status
   f. Stature/posture
      (1) Patient flexing his or her knees to relieve abdominal tension frequently is seen in peritonitis
      (2) Patient leaning forward to relieve abdominal pain frequently is seen in pancreatitis
   g. Gait
3. Mouth
   a. Lips: color; texture; lesions; swelling; symmetry

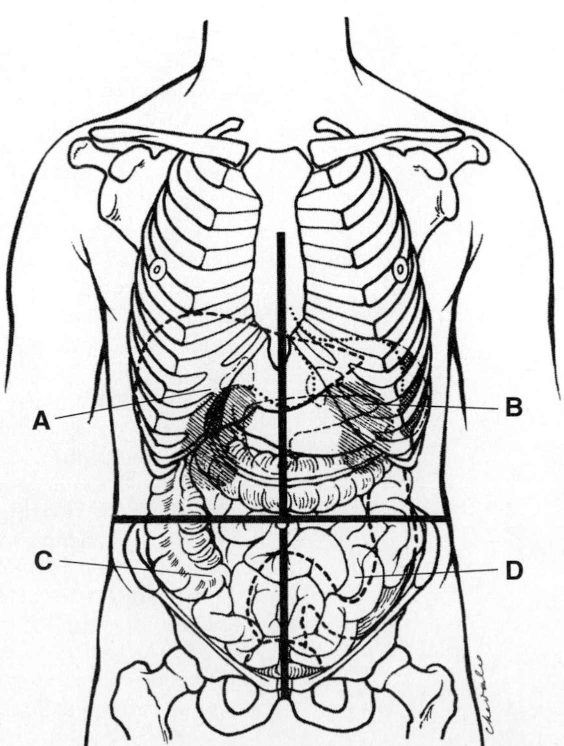

Figure 6-17 The abdomen divided into four quadrants. **A,** Left upper quadrant (LUQ); **B,** right upper quadrant (RUQ); **C,** right lower quadrant (RLQ); **D,** left lower quadrant (LLQ). (From Abels, L. F. [1986]. *Critical care nursing*. St. Louis: Mosby.)

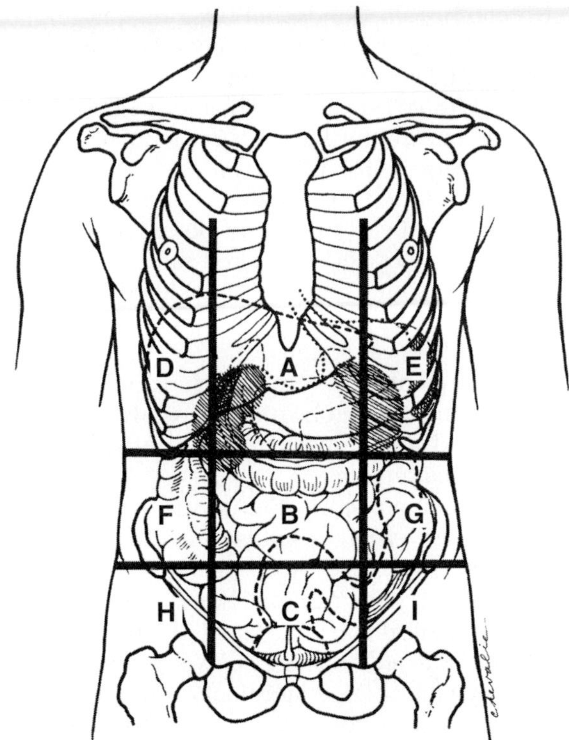

Figure 6-18 The abdomen divided into nine regions. *A*, Epigastric; *B*, umbilical; *C*, hypogastric; *D* and *E*, right and left hypochondriac; *F* and *G*, right and left lumbar; *H* and *I*, right and left inguinal. (From Abels, L. F. [1986]. *Critical care nursing*. St. Louis: Mosby.)

b. Gums: inflammation; retraction; hypertrophy; bleeding; lesions
c. Teeth: caries; state of repair; occlusion; dentures: fit; gum ulceration caused by ill-fitting dentures
d. Tongue: swelling; laceration; lesions; coating
e. Mucosa: moisture; lesions; color
f. Odor
   (1) Fetor hepaticus: sweet fecal odor caused by hepatic failure
   (2) Feculent breath: foul fecal odor caused by severe bowel obstruction
   (3) Severe halitosis: foul odor may be caused by poor dental hygiene or neoplasms of esophagus or stomach

4. Skin
   a. Color: should be homogenous over the entire abdomen
      (1) Pallor: anemia
      (2) Jaundice: occurs when bilirubin is greater than 3 mg/dL; associated with any of the following:
         (a) Liver disease
         (b) Biliary obstruction
         (c) Excessive hemolysis
      (3) Bluish: caused by infiltration of the abdominal wall with blood
         (a) Location
            (i) Grey Turner's sign: ecchymosis to flanks indicative of retroperitoneal bleeding (e.g., from pancreas, duodenum, kidneys, vena cava, or aorta)
            (ii) Cullen's sign: ecchymosis around umbilicus indicative of intraperitoneal bleeding (e.g., from liver or spleen)
         (b) Causes
            (i) Hemorrhagic pancreatitis
            (ii) Infarcted bowel
            (iii) Ruptured ectopic pregnancy
   b. Lesions or discoloration
      (1) Scars: trauma; surgical procedures
      (2) Striae
         (a) Usually vertical
         (b) Initially pinkish or bluish; become silvery with time
         (c) May be caused by pregnancy, obesity, or ascites
         (d) Purplish striae may be caused by Cushing's syndrome
      (3) Rash
      (4) Ecchymosis
      (5) Abrasions
      (6) Spider angioma: may be associated with:
         (a) Vitamin B_{12} deficiency
         (b) Liver disease
         (c) Pregnancy
      (7) Palmar erythema: seen in cirrhosis and hepatic failure
   c. Shiny, edematous abdomen
      (1) Ascites: intraperitoneal fluid frequently associated with cirrhosis, intraabdominal malignancy (e.g., liver or ovarian), or right ventricular failure
      (2) Anasarca: entire body edema that may be seen in end-stage heart failure or renal failure
   d. Superficial vascularity
      (1) May be caused by obstruction of inferior vena cava or portal vein
      (2) Caput medusae: pronounced dilation of the periumbilical veins radiating from the umbilicus; seen in severe portal venous hypertension
   e. Stoma: location; color; drainage; condition of peristomal skin
   f. Draining wounds: location; drainage; condition of surrounding skin
   g. Fistula: location; drainage; condition of surrounding skin

5. Contour of abdomen
   a. Profile
      (1) Normal: flat from xiphoid process to pubic symphysis
      (2) Scaffold: concave abdomen seen in malnutrition
      (3) Distention or protuberance
         (a) Diffuse and symmetric
            (i) Fat
            (ii) Flatus
            (iii) Fetus (i.e., pregnancy)
            (iv) Feces (i.e., obstruction)
            (v) Fluid (i.e., ascites)
            (vi) Fatal growths (i.e., malignancy)
            (vii) Fibroids

(b) Distention in upper quadrants: gastric dilation; pancreatic cyst or malignancy
(c) Distention in lower quadrants: pregnancy; uterine fibroid; distended bladder; ovarian tumor
(d) Distention in one quadrant: hernia; tumor; cyst; obstruction; organomegaly

6. Abdominal girth
   a. Measure abdominal girth at largest area
   b. Mark on either side of tape measure so that measurements are consistently at same location
   c. One inch increase is equal to an increase in intraabdominal volume of 500 to 1000 mL
7. Weakness of abdominal wall
   a. Diastasis recti abdominis: abnormal separation of the two abdominal rectus muscles when the patient tenses abdominal muscles by raising his or her head from the bed
   b. Hernia: abdominal, umbilical, or inguinal
8. Movement of abdomen
   a. Breathing: normal
      (1) Women generally breathe thoracically when upright
      (2) Men and women generally breathe abdominally when supine
   b. Peristalsis: abnormal to see waves of peristalsis across the abdomen: generally associated with intestinal obstruction
   c. Aortic pulsation: normally visible at the end of expiration in a supine patient especially if patient is thin; pulsatile swelling in the epigastrium suggests an abdominal aortic aneurysm or an epigastric solid tumor overlying the aorta
9. Umbilicus
   a. Color
      (1) Bluish (Cullen's sign): caused by infiltration of the abdominal wall with blood
      (2) Inflammation: may be seen with poor hygiene
   b. Contour
      (1) Deeply inverted: obesity
      (2) Everted: pregnancy or ascites
      (3) Nodular (Sister Mary Joseph's nodule): may indicate intraabdominal carcinoma (especially stomach) with metastasis to the navel

Auscultation

1. Auscultation is done before percussion or palpation to prevent "stirring up" the abdomen; order for physical assessment of the abdomen therefore is inspection, auscultation, percussion, and palpation
2. Preparation: may be helpful to put pillow under knees to relax abdominal muscles
3. Bowel sounds
   a. Method
      (1) Use diaphragm with light pressure for 1 minute in each of the four abdominal quadrants.
      (2) Disconnect nasogastric suction.
      (3) If bowel sounds are hypoactive, 5 minutes of auscultation without audible bowel sounds is required before documenting the absence of bowel sounds.
   b. Normal bowel sounds: bubbling or soft gurgling noises heard every 5 to 20 seconds in an irregular pattern; heard in all quadrants
      (1) Return of bowel motility after surgery
         (a) Small intestine: 4 to 24 hours
         (b) Stomach: 2 to 4 days
         (c) Colon: 3 to 7 days
      (2) Feeding before return of bowel sounds after surgery now is considered safe
      (3) Bowel sounds are not considered an indication of feeding tolerance
   c. Abnormal bowel sounds
      (1) Infrequent or absent bowel sounds
         (a) Functional obstruction: paralytic ileus
         (b) Advanced mechanical intestinal obstruction
      (2) Loud, hyperactive (but normal-pitched) bowel sounds: hyperperistalsis (e.g., diarrhea or catharsis caused by GI bleeding)
      (3) High-pitched "rushing" bowel sounds: early mechanical small intestinal obstruction
      (4) Low-pitched "rushing" bowel sounds: early mechanical large intestinal obstruction
4. Succussion splash: roll patient side to side while listening over left upper quadrant; indicative of pyloric obstruction
5. Vascular sounds
   a. Method: use bell over specified areas
   b. Bruits
      (1) Listen over midline and renal and femoral arteries.
      (2) If bruit is noted, check circulation to extremities; if decreased blood flow is noted, aneurysm should be suspected.
         (a) Notify physician.
         (b) Keep patient quiet.
         (c) Do not palpate abdomen
   c. Venous hum: hum of medium tone created by blood flow in a large, engorged vascular organ such as liver or spleen
6. Peritoneal friction rub: scratchy sound heard over inflamed spleen or neoplastic liver

Percussion

1. Percussion tones normally heard over abdomen
   a. Dull: liver, full sigmoid colon, full bladder
   b. Flat: bone
   c. Tympany: gastric bubble, bowel
2. Tests for ascites
   a. Fluid wave: Tap one side of the abdomen and feel for the wave to hit the hand on other side of abdomen; have a colleague or the patient place the ulnar surface of his or her hand at the midline of the abdomen to stop skin transmission.
   b. Shifting dullness: Percuss dullness indicating fluid at flanks while patient supine, mark fluid level, and turn patient on one side and note shift of dullness line (Figure 6-19).
   c. Midline dullness: Dullness at midline with the patient leaning forward in a standing position indicates intraabdominal fluid.

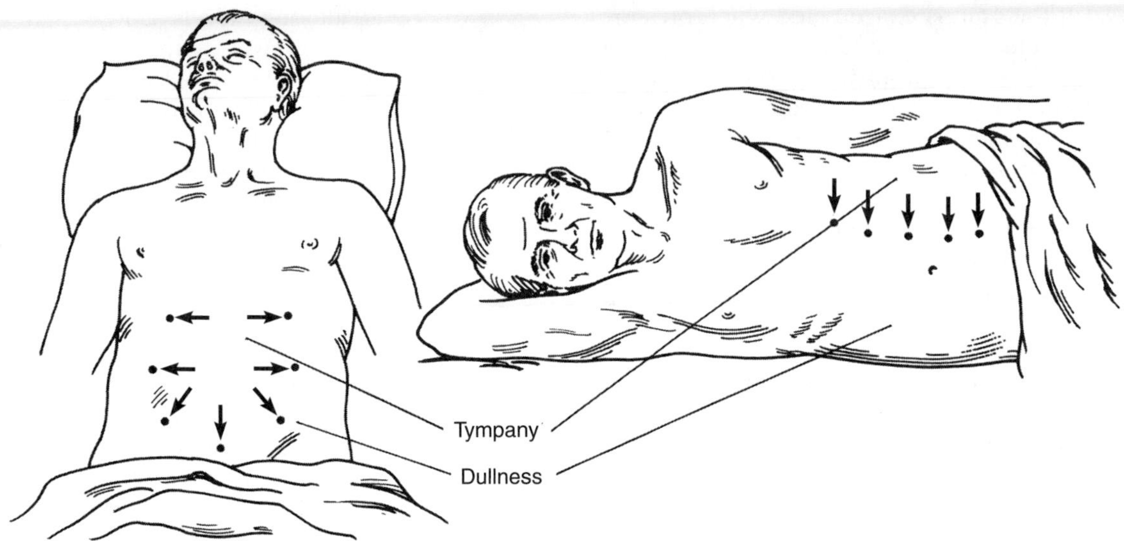

Figure 6-19 Test for ascites: shifting dullness. (From Beare, P. G., & Myers, J. L. [1994]. *Principles and practice of adult health nursing* [2nd ed.]. St. Louis: Mosby.)

3. Organ borders
   a. Liver (dullness between right lung resonance and bowel tympany)
      (1) Normal span 6 to 12 cm in the right midclavicular line
      (2) Enlarged and tender in right ventricular failure (RVF), hepatitis, and mononucleosis
      (3) May be large or small in cirrhosis
      (4) Absence of liver dullness: may indicate free air in peritoneum from bowel perforation
   b. Spleen (dullness under left diaphragm): if percussible, should be less than 7 cm at the left midaxillary line
   c. Stomach (tympany under left costal margin)
   d. Bladder (dullness above symphysis pubis): percussible only if enlarged
   e. Intestine (tympany over abdomen): may percuss dullness over LLQ if sigmoid colon is full

Palpation

1. Method
   a. Warm hands
   b. Examine each quadrant
   c. Always palpate tender areas last
   d. Carry on conversation with patient to keep patient (and patient's abdominal muscles) relaxed, and place a pillow under the knees and a pillow under the head
2. Light palpation: use fingertips to depress 1 to 2 cm; note the following:
   a. Temperature
   b. Moisture
   c. Superficial skin reflexes: movement of the umbilicus toward the quadrant that is stroked
   d. Voluntary guarding
      (1) Patient may splint abdominal muscles voluntarily, especially when sensitive spot is touched; watch for nonverbal indicators of pain during palpation.
   e. Involuntary guarding or rigidity
      (1) Diffuse rigidity suggests an infectious, neoplastic, or inflammatory process in the peritoneal cavity.
      (2) Rigid, boardlike abdomen is associated with acute perforation of a viscus with spillage of air or GI contents into the peritoneal cavity.
   f. Tender areas
   g. Large masses
      (1) If mass is pulsatile, refrain from additional abdominal palpation because this may be an abdominal aortic aneurysm.
      (2) If mass is not pulsatile, describe the following:
         (a) Size
         (b) Location
         (c) Consistency
         (d) Contour
         (e) Tenderness
         (f) Mobility
3. Deep palpation: Use one hand on top of the other to depress 4 to 5 cm.
   a. Do not use deep palpation in the following situations:
      (1) Polycystic kidneys
      (2) After renal transplant
      (3) Malignant tumor: may cause seeding
      (4) Recent surgery
   b. Note the following:
      (1) Direct tenderness
         (a) Associated with local inflammation of the abdominal wall, the peritoneum, or a viscus
      (2) Rebound (or indirect) tenderness (also referred to as *Blumberg's sign*)
         (a) Performed by pressing into the tender area and then letting go

(b) If the pain is exacerbated when pressure is released, rebound tenderness is present and peritoneal inflammation is suspected
(c) Rebound tenderness is especially significant when it occurs at a site away from the area of direct tenderness
(3) Organ size
(a) Liver edge: may be palpable
(i) Ask patient to take deep breath and move hand in and up to check for tenderness, smoothness of edge.
a) Tenderness frequently is caused by hepatitis or engorgement caused by RVF.
b) Hard, lumpy liver is associated with cancer or cirrhosis.
(ii) A normal size liver may be palpable especially in patients with COPD caused by hyperinflation of lungs; hepatomegaly exists only if liver span by percussion is greater than 12 cm.
(b) Gallbladder: palpable only if enlarged with stones; if palpable, located under liver edge in RUQ
(4) Splenic tenderness
(a) Palpate left side of abdomen with patient in lateral decubitus position.
(b) Note any tenderness.
(c) Spleen is palpable only if significantly enlarged (e.g., injury, leukemia, mononucleosis, or portal hypertension).
(5) Aortic pulsation: Check for lateral expansion that may indicate an aneurysm
4. Ballottement
a. Gentle repetitive bouncing of tissues against the hand
b. May be used to evaluate organ enlargement

Intraabdominal Pressure

1. Definitions
a. Intraabdominal pressure (IAP): the pressure within the abdominal cavity
b. Intraabdominal hypertension (IAH): elevation of IAP above normal
c. Abdominal compartment syndrome: pressure within the abdominal cavity increases to the point that perfusion is compromised and the viability and function of the tissues within the abdominal cavity are threatened
2. Values
a. Normal 0 to subatmospheric
b. Elevated pressures
(1) Mildly elevated (10 to 20 mm Hg): common after abdominal surgery
(2) Moderately elevated (21 to 40 mm Hg)
(3) Severely elevated (greater than 40 mm Hg)
c. Clinical implications
(1) A critical level of IAH has not been established: an IAP of 25 mm Hg traditionally has been considered a critical value, although levels as low as 10 mm Hg may cause organ dysfunction.
(2) There is a volume-pressure curve: the abdominal wall can compensate for increases in intraabdominal volume up to a point; then any additional increase in intraabdominal volume results in a rapid increase in IAP and compromised organ perfusion.
3. Methods of measurement
a. Assist with placement of an access for measuring IAP.
(1) Via a catheter (e.g., peritoneal dialysis catheter) inserted into peritoneal cavity and attached to a transducer
(2) Via a catheter inserted into the sample port of an indwelling urinary catheter and attached to a transducer (Figure 6-20)
(a) Accuracy of this method is affected by neurogenic bladder, abdominal packing, elevation of the head of the bed (HOB), pelvic fracture or hematoma, or intraperitoneal adhesions
b. Attach a pressure monitoring system with the air-fluid interface of the transducer leveled to the symphysis pubis.
c. Place the patient in supine position.
d. After drainage of the bladder, remove air from the system and then instill 50 to 100 mL of isotonic sterile saline into the bladder.
e. Measure the pressure at end expiration.
4. Conditions associated with risk for IAH and abdominal compartment syndrome include the following:
a. Abdominal or pelvic trauma
(1) Pelvic fractures
(2) Intraperitoneal or retroperitoneal hemorrhage or hematoma
(3) Visceral edema caused by ischemia and/or massive fluid resuscitation
b. Abdominal surgery
(1) Pneumoperitoneum during laparoscopic procedures
(2) Liver transplantation
(3) Postoperative bleeding
c. Intraabdominal infection
d. Ruptured abdominal aortic aneurysm
e. Pancreatitis
f. Intraabdominal neoplasm
g. Intestinal obstruction
h. Ascites
i. Circumferential full-thickness burns of the abdomen
j. Septic shock
k. Use of military antishock trousers or pneumatic antishock garments
l. Obstetric conditions
(1) Pregnancy
(2) Preeclampsia
(3) Pregnancy-related disseminated intravascular coagulation (DIC)

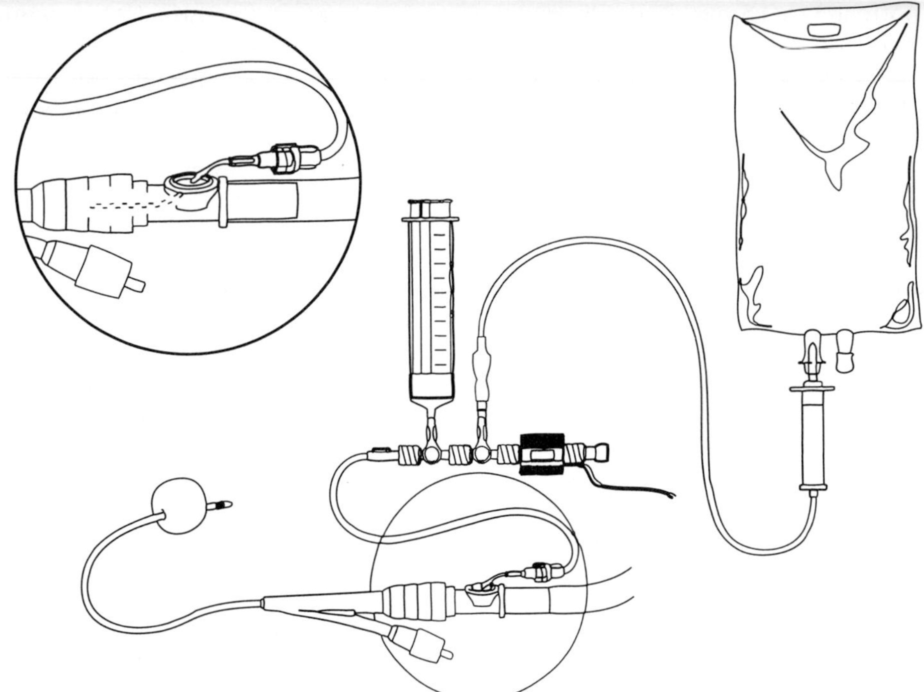

Figure 6-20 Measurement of IAP using a intravenous catheter into the specimen port of the urinary drainage tubing. (From Cheatham, M. L. [1999]. Intra-abdominal hypertension and abdominal compartment syndrome. *New Horizons,* 7[1], 96-115.)

5. Pathophysiologic consequences of IAH
   a. Increased heart rate, respiratory rate
   b. Decreased arterial oxygen saturation (Sao_2), oxygen saturation by pulse oximetry (Spo_2)
   c. Increased central venous pressure, pulmonary artery pressure, pulmonary artery occlusive pressure (PAOP), systemic vascular resistance
   d. Decreased cardiac output/cardiac index
   e. Normal or decreased BP
   f. Increased intrathoracic pressure
   g. Decreased lung compliance
   h. Decreased glomerular filtration rate and urine output
   i. Increased intracranial pressure (ICP)
   j. Decreased cerebral perfusion pressure
   k. Decreased portal, celiac, and mesenteric blood flow
   l. Metabolic acidosis
6. Treatment of IAH and abdominal compartment syndrome
   a. Elevate the HOB between pressure readings.
   b. Encourage the patient to take deep breaths to prevent atelectasis and encourage venous return to the heart.
   c. Assist with paracentesis if free fluid is cause.
   d. Decompress the GI tract as prescribed.
      (1) Prokinetic agents (e.g., metoclopramide)
      (2) Gastric and/or colonic tube
      (3) Enemas
   e. Reduce edema by diuresis, dialysis, and/or ultrafiltration.
   f. Prepare the patient for surgical decompression as requested in symptomatic patients with IAP of greater than or equal to 20 mm Hg or greater than 15 mm Hg with evidence of organ ischemia.
      (1) The abdomen is opened and excess fluid, blood, and blood clots are removed.
      (2) Recognize that reperfusion washes anaerobic metabolic byproducts from the viscera, which may cause hypotension; fluids, mannitol, and sodium bicarbonate may be used before and during decompression surgery.
      (3) The abdomen may be left open after surgery for repair after swelling has subsided (usually within 5 to 7 days).
         (a) Vacuum-assisted closure may be used after surgery to continue to reduce edema.

Diagnostic Studies

1. Serum chemistries
   a. Sodium: normal 136 to 145 mEq/L; elevated in dehydration from severe diarrhea or intestinal obstruction
   b. Potassium: normal 3.5 to 5.5 mEq/L; decreased in GI losses from upper or lower GI tract
   c. Chloride: normal 96 to 106 mEq/L
      (1) Elevated in dehydration
      (2) Decreased in vomiting, diarrhea, or intestinal obstruction
   d. Calcium: normal 8.5 to 10.5 mg/dL; decreased in acute pancreatitis

e. Phosphorus: normal 3 to 4.5 mg/dL
   (1) Elevated in intestinal obstruction
   (2) Decreased in malnutrition or malabsorption syndromes
f. Magnesium: normal 1.5 to 2.2 mEq/L; decreased in chronic diarrhea
g. Glucose: normal 70 to 110 mg/dL; elevated in diabetes mellitus and pancreatitis
h. Blood urea nitrogen (BUN): normal 5 to 20 mg/dL
i. Creatinine: normal 0.7 to 1.5 mg/dL
j. Gastrin: normal less than 200 ng/L; elevated in Zollinger-Ellison syndrome (gastrin-producing pancreatic tumor) or G cell hyperplasia that may cause peptic ulcer disease
k. Ammonia: by-product of protein metabolism
   (1) Normal 15 to 110 mOsm/dL
   (2) Elevated in hepatic failure, renal failure, and heart failure
l. Iron: normal 50 to 150 mcg/dL
m. Iron-binding capacity: 250 to 410 mcg/dL
n. Lactate: less than 1 mmol/L
o. Carcinoembryonic antigen (CEA): normal less than 2 ng/mL; elevated in cancer of the colon, lung, pancreas, stomach, breast, head, neck, and prostate
p. Bilirubin
   (1) Total: normal 0.3 to 1.3 mg/dL; elevated in hepatic disease, biliary obstruction, or excessive hemolysis
   (2) Direct: normal 0.1 to 0.3 mg/dL; elevated in biliary obstruction
   (3) Indirect: normal 0.1 to 1 mg/dL; elevated in hepatic disease or excessive hemolysis
q. Serum proteins
   (1) Total protein: normal 6 to 8 g/dL
   (2) Albumin: normal 3.5 to 4.5 g/dL; half-life is 19 to 20 days, so poor indicator of acute changes in nutritional status
   (3) Prealbumin: normal 15 to 35 mg/dL; half-life is only 2 to 3 days, so indicates changes in nutritional status better than albumin
   (4) Transferrin: normal 250 to 300 mg/dL; half-life is only 8 to 10 days, so indicates changes in nutritional status better than albumin
   (5) Globulin: normal 1.5 to 3 g/dL
   (6) Albumin/globulin ratio: normal 1.5/1 to 2.5/1; reverse in chronic hepatitis, chronic liver disease
   (7) Fibrinogen: normal 0.1 to 0.4 g/dL
r. Serum lipids
   (1) Cholesterol: normal 150 to 200 mg/dL
   (2) Triglycerides: normal 40 to 150 mg/dL
s. Pepsinogen: normal 200 to 425 units/mL
   (1) Elevated in hemoconcentration
   (2) Decreased in malnutrition or hemorrhage
t. Enzymes
   (1) Alkaline phosphatase: normal 30 to 85 units/L; elevated in cirrhosis, rheumatoid arthritis, biliary obstruction, liver tumor, and hyperparathyroidism
   (2) Amylase: normal 56 to 190 units/L; elevated in acute pancreatitis, pancreatic cancer, pancreatic pseudocysts, perforated peptic ulcer, mesenteric thrombosis, ectopic pregnancy, renal failure, and mumps
   (3) Lipase: normal up to 1.5 units/mL; elevated in acute or chronic pancreatitis, duodenal ulcer, biliary obstruction, cirrhosis, and hepatitis; stays elevated longer than amylase in pancreatitis
   (4) Alanine aminotransferase (ALT): normal 5 to 36 units/mL
      (a) Formerly called *SGPT*
      (b) Elevated in hepatitis, cirrhosis, liver tumor, hepatotoxic drugs, cholestasis, and infectious mononucleosis
   (5) Aspartate aminotransferase (AST): normal 15 to 45 units/mL
      (a) Formerly called *SGOT*
      (b) Elevated in hepatitis, cirrhosis, acute pancreatitis, skeletal muscle disease or trauma, and liver tumor
   (6) Gamma-glutamyl transferase: normal 5 to 38 units/L; elevated in hepatitis, cirrhosis, liver tumor, cholestasis, alcohol ingestion, and myocardial infarction
   (7) Lactate dehydrogenase (LDH): normal 90 to 200 units/L; elevated in hepatitis, hemolytic anemia, pancreatitis, muscular dystrophy, pulmonary infarction, myocardial infarction (MI), pernicious anemia, and renal disease
u. Serologic testing for viral hepatitis

2. Hematology
   a. Hematocrit (Hct): normal 40% to 52% for males; 35% to 47% for females
   b. Hemoglobin (Hgb): normal 13 to 18 g/dL for males; 12 to 16 g/dL for females
   c. White blood cells (WBCs): normal 3500 to 11,000 cells/mm^3
      (1) Differential: shift to left (increase in bands) indicates acute infection
   d. Erythrocyte sedimentation rate: normal up to 15 mm/hr for males; up to 20 mm/hr for females
3. Clotting profile: may be abnormal in liver disease
   a. Prothrombin time (PT): normal 12 to 15 seconds; therapeutic 1.5 to 2.5 times normal
   b. Activated partial thromboplastin time (aPPT): normal 25 to 38 seconds; therapeutic 1.5 to 2.5 times normal
   c. Activated clotting time: normal 70 to 120 seconds; therapeutic 150 to 190 seconds
   d. Thrombin time: normal 10 to 15 seconds
   e. Bleeding time: normal 1 to 9½ minutes
   f. International normalized ratio: normal less than 2
   g. Platelets: normal 150,000 to 400,000 per cubic millimeter
4. Urine
   a. Glucose: normal negative
   b. Ketones: normal negative
   c. Amylase: normal negative
   d. Bilirubin: normal negative

e. Urobilinogen: normal 0.3 to 3.5 mg/dL
   (1) Elevated in hepatocellular disease
   (2) Decreased in complete biliary obstruction
f. Specific gravity: 1.005 to 1.03
g. Osmolality: 50 to 1200 mOsm/L

5. Gastric contents
   a. Gastric analysis with a nasogastric (NG) tube
      (1) Histamine or insulin is administered before collection of a sample of gastric contents.
      (2) Gastric contents are analyzed for the presence of HCl.
      (3) Have antihistamine (e.g., diphenhydramine [Benadryl]) or 50% dextrose available.
   b. pH determination
      (1) Method
         (a) Flush NG tube with 20 mL of tap water, and then clear tube with air before aspirating.
         (b) Do not use the same syringe used to give antacids or H_2 receptor antagonist to obtain the sample for pH testing.
      (2) Used for the following:
         (a) To determine tube placement: stomach pH 1 to 3, intestine pH 6.5 or higher
         (b) To determine effectiveness of H_2 receptor antagonist and/or antacid therapy: pH of 3.5 to 5 is desirable
6. Stool
   a. Fecal occult blood test: normal negative
   b. Ova, parasites, blood: normal negative; specimen must be warm
   c. Fecal fat: normal 5 g per 24 hours
      (1) Elevated in cystic fibrosis, Crohn's disease, biliary tract obstruction, and pancreatic duct obstruction
      (2) Specimen must be sent to laboratory in a wax-free container
   d. Urobilinogen: normal 0 to 4 mg/day
      (1) Decreased in biliary obstruction
      (2) Specimen must be sent to laboratory in a light-resistant container
   e. Culture: normal intestinal flora
   f. Assay for *Clostridium difficile* toxin A or B: positive is diarrhea caused by *C. difficile*, an opportunistic infection caused primarily by suppression of normal flora by antibiotic therapy
7. Other diagnostic studies (Table 6-5)

Malnutrition

Definitions

1. Malnutrition: Dietary intake of essential nutrients is insufficient to meet the metabolic demands of the body.
   a. Macronutrients: CHO; proteins; fats
   b. Micronutrients: vitamins; minerals; water
2. Types of malnutrition
   a. Marasmus: gradual wasting of body fat and somatic muscle with preservation of visceral proteins as seen in prolonged starvation and chronic illness
   b. Kwashiorkor: visceral protein wasting with preservation of fat and somatic muscle as seen in poverty; the patient may appear as well-nourished, overweight, or obese, and edema may be present
   c. Mixed marasmus and kwashiorkor: type most commonly seen in hospitalized patients and associated with the highest mortality and morbidity

Table 6-5 Gastrointestinal Diagnostic Studies

Study	Evaluates	Comments
Angiography: celiac or mesenteric	• Evaluates portal vasculature • Diagnoses source of GI bleeding • Evaluates cirrhosis, portal hypertension, vascular damage resulting from trauma, intestinal ischemia, and tumors • May be used to treat GI bleeding using vasopressin	• Bowel preparation (e.g., cathartics) as prescribed • NPO for 8 hours before the study • Sedative usually is prescribed before the procedure • Contrast media used: ◦ Check for allergy to iodine before the study ◦ Monitor for allergic reaction following procedure ◦ Ensure hydration following procedure *Postprocedure* • Keep extremity in which catheter was placed immobilized in a straight position for 6-12 hours • Monitor arterial puncture point for hemorrhage or hematoma • Monitor neurovascular status of affected limb • Monitor for indications of systemic emboli

Continued

Table 6-5 Gastrointestinal Diagnostic Studies—cont'd

Study	Evaluates	Comments
Barium enema (also called *lower GI series*) NOTE: Meglumine diatrizoate (Gastrografin) may be used especially if bowel perforation is suspected.	• Visualizes the movement, position, and filling of various segments of the colon after instillation of barium by enema • Diagnoses colorectal lesions, diverticulitis, inflammatory bowel disease, strictures, fistulae • Evaluates colon size, length, and patency	• Low-fiber diet for 1 to 3 days before the study • Bowel preparation with bowel irrigation (e.g., GoLYTELY) and cathartics • NPO for 8-12 hours before study • Cathartics must be given after study • Contraindicated if bowel perforation or obstruction exists
Barium swallow, upper GI series, and small bowel follow-through NOTE: Tests are ordered according to which area or areas need to be evaluated, such as the upper GI with small bowel follow-through evaluates stomach, pylorus, duodenum; barium swallow with upper GI evaluates esophagus, stomach, pylorus NOTE: Meglumine diatrizoate (Gastrografin) may be used especially if bowel perforation is suspected.	• Visualizes the position, shape, and activity of the esophagus, stomach, duodenum, and jejunum • Diagnoses esophageal lesions, varices, or esophageal motility disorders, hiatal hernia, gastric ulcers and tumors, small bowel obstruction, small bowel lesions, Crohn's disease • Evaluates gastric and small bowel motility	• Bowel preparation with bowel irrigation (e.g., GoLYTELY) and cathartics • NPO for 8-12 hours before study • Cathartics must be given after study • Contraindicated if bowel perforation or obstruction exists
Cholecystography (oral, IV, intravenous, percutaneous transhepatic, or common bile duct)	• Assesses gallbladder function, patency of the biliary system, and presence of gallstones • Diagnoses extrahepatic or intrahepatic jaundice, biliary calculi, biliary obstruction, and common bile duct injury	• Percutaneous transhepatic cholangiography is contraindicated in patients with bleeding disorders • Fatty meal the day before the study, but the evening meal is fat free • Enema may be given the evening before the study • NPO 8-12 hours before the study • Contrast medium is administered orally the evening before the study, administered IV immediately before the study, injected percutaneously into the bile duct, or injected directly into the common bile duct during surgery ◦ Check for allergy to iodine before the study ◦ Monitor for allergic reaction following procedure ◦ Ensure hydration following procedure • Monitor for clinical indications of bile leakage, hemorrhage, or peritonitis after percutaneous transhepatic cholangiography
Computed tomography scan of abdomen	• Diagnoses tumors, pancreatic cancer or cysts, pancreatitis, biliary tract disorders, obstructive versus nonobstructive jaundice, cirrhosis, liver metastases, ascites, lymph node metastases, and aneurysm • Evaluates vasculature and focal points found on nuclear scans • Used to direct biopsy of tumors or aspiration of abscess	• No special preparation required • Contrast medium may be used; if used: ◦ Check for allergy to iodine before the study ◦ Monitor for allergic reaction postprocedure ◦ Ensure hydration postprocedure

Table 6-5 Gastrointestinal Diagnostic Studies—cont'd

Study	Evaluates	Comments
Endoscopic retrograde cholangiopancreatography	• Diagnoses biliary stones, ductal stricture, ductal compression, and neoplasms of the pancreas and biliary system • Evaluates patency of biliary and pancreatic ducts, jaundice, pancreatitis, cholecystitis, and hepatitis	• Same as for esophagogastroduodenoscopy • Contraindicated if patient is uncooperative or if bilirubin is greater than 3.5 mg/dL • Monitor for clinical indications of pancreatitis (most common complication) after study • Monitor for clinical indications of sepsis
Endoscopy • Esophagogastroduodenoscopy • Colonoscopy • Proctosigmoidoscopy	• Directly visualizes mucosa of areas of the GI tract • Esophagogastroduodenoscopy can be extended to visualize the pancreas and gallbladder • Esophagogastroduodenoscopy is used to diagnose esophagitis, esophageal ulcers, esophageal strictures, esophageal varices, hiatal hernia, gastritis, gastric ulcers, pyloric obstruction, pernicious anemia, foreign bodies, and duodenal inflammation or ulcers; it evaluates esophageal or gastric motility, bleeding, lesions, and status of surgical anastomoses • Esophagoscopy or gastroscopy also may be used therapeutically for sclerosis of varices • Proctosigmoidoscopy diagnoses rectosigmoid cancer, strictures, polyps, inflammatory processes, and hemorrhoids; it evaluates bleeding from rectosigmoid and surgical anastomoses • Colonoscopy diagnoses diverticular disease, obstruction, strictures, radiation injury, polyps, neoplasms, bleeding, and ischemia • Colonoscopy or sigmoidoscopy may be used therapeutically for removal of polyps • Biopsies may be taken during any endoscopy	• Sedation may be prescribed, especially for colonoscopy • Bowel preparation with gastric irrigation (e.g., GoLYTELY) and cathartics required before lower GI endoscopy • NPO 4-8 hours before study • Keep patient NPO until gag reflex returns if sedation used • Monitor closely after procedure for clinical indications of perforation or hemorrhage
Flat plate of abdomen (may also be referred to as *KUB*)	• Diagnoses perforated viscus, paralytic ileus, mechanical obstruction, and intraabdominal mass • Evaluates the distribution of visceral gas (and identifies free air in the peritoneum indicative of bowel perforation) • Evaluates organ size	• No preparation required
Liver biopsy	• Obtains tissue specimen for microscopic evaluation • Diagnoses liver disease or malignancy	• May be performed open or closed ◦ Open is done in surgery ◦ Closed biopsy may be done at bedside • Clotting profile is evaluated preprocedure ◦ Closed biopsy is contraindicated if platelet count is less than 100,000 platelets/mm^3 • Patient must be cooperative because he or she must take a deep breath and hold it for closed biopsy

Continued

Table 6-5 Gastrointestinal Diagnostic Studies—cont'd

Study	Evaluates	Comments
		• Type and crossmatch for two units of blood preprocedure • NPO for 4-8 hours before study *Postprocedure* • Position patient on right side for 2 hours • Pressure dressing is applied, and the patient is on bed rest for 24 hours • Observe for the following: ○ Hemorrhage: hypotension, dyspnea (subphrenic hematoma) ○ Pneumothorax: dyspnea; chest pain; diminished breath sounds on right; hypoxemia ○ Sepsis: fever; leukocytosis; rebound tenderness
Liver scan	• Diagnoses cirrhosis, hepatitis, tumors, abscesses, cysts, and tuberculosis	• No preparation required
Magnetic resonance imaging	• Evaluates liver, biliary tree, pancreas, and spleen • Differentiation between cyst and solid mass • Diagnoses hepatic metastasis • Evaluates abscesses, fistulae, and source of GI bleeding • Used for staging of colorectal cancer	• Cannot be used in patients with any implanted metallic device, including pacemakers • No special preparation required • Cannot be done on a patient being mechanically ventilated
Paracentesis	• Analysis of fluid removed during peritoneal tap • Diagnoses intraperitoneal bleeding with diagnostic peritoneal lavage	• Monitor for peritoneal leakage after tap • Monitor for clinical indications of infection or peritonitis after tap
Percutaneous transhepatic portography	• Diagnoses esophageal varices and visualizes portal venous circulation	• As for angiography
Percutaneous transhepatic cholangiography	• Diagnoses extrahepatic or intrahepatic jaundice, biliary calculi, bile duct obstruction, and bile duct injury • Evaluates the patency of the biliary ductal system	• Contraindicated in uncorrected coagulopathy, allergy to iodine, severe ascites, or cholangitis • Monitor closely for clinical indications of bleeding • Monitor closely for clinical indications of peritonitis
Radionuclide imaging (hepatobiliary scintigraphy) • HIDA scan • PIPIDA scan	• Diagnoses hepatocellular disease, hepatic metastasis, biliary disease, lower GI bleeding, gastric reflux	• NPO 2 hours before study
Schilling test	• Evaluates ileal absorption of vitamin B_{12} • Diagnoses pernicious anemia caused by intrinsic factor and inadequate ilial absorption of intrinsic factor-vitamin B_{12} complex	• Intramuscular injections of vitamin B_{12} and oral radioactive B_{12} are given, and 24-hour urine specimen is collected
Ultrasound of abdomen	• Evaluates the pancreas, biliary ducts, gallbladder, and liver • Identifies tumor, abdominal abscesses, hepatocellular disease, splenomegaly, and pancreatic or splenic cysts • Differentiates obstructive from nonobstructive jaundice	• All barium must have been cleared from the GI tract before ultrasonography • NPO for 8 hours before study • If for evaluation of gallbladder: fat-free meal the evening before study

GI, Gastrointestinal; *IV*, intravenous; *NPO*, nothing by mouth.

Etiology

1. Decreased nutrient intake
   a. Recent weight loss
   b. Recent change in diet; fad or limited diet
   c. Eating disorder (e.g., obesity, bulimia, or anorexia nervosa); note that obesity is not overnourishment and that many obese patients are protein malnourished
   d. Anorexia
   e. Nausea
   f. Difficulty chewing or swallowing (e.g., stomatitis or dysphagia)
   g. Depression
   h. Alcoholism or drug addiction
   i. Social history of poverty, disability, or living alone
   j. Loss of the sense of taste or smell
   k. Use of drugs known to alter dietary intake or food utilization (e.g., antacids, antibiotics, laxatives, and antineoplastics)
2. Decreased absorption
   a. Diseases of the GI tract
   b. Malabsorptions (e.g., diarrhea and steatorrhea)
   c. Parasites
   d. Pernicious anemia
   e. Intestinal bypass or resection
   f. Drugs (e.g., antacids, cholestyramine, neomycin, and alcohol)
3. Increased nutrient losses
   a. Recurrent vomiting, diarrhea
   b. GI disease such as peritonitis or inflammatory bowel disease
   c. Diabetes mellitus
   d. Hemorrhage
   e. Peritoneal dialysis or hemodialysis
4. Increased nutrient requirements
   a. Recent surgery or trauma
   b. Chronic illnesses such as malignancy or renal, liver, lung, or heart disease or diabetes mellitus
   c. Prolonged hypercatabolic state (e.g., multiple trauma, major surgery, sepsis, or burns)
   d. Hyperthyroidism
   e. Hypoxia
5. Nosocomial malnutrition: related to mismanagement or inattention to nutritional requirements of hospitalized patients
   a. Nothing-by-mouth (NPO) status for diagnostic studies or postoperatively
   b. Feedings not advanced
   c. Wait and see
      (1) If appetite improves
      (2) If nausea, vomiting resolves
      (3) If ileus resolves

Pathophysiology

1. Atrophy of mucosal cells in the small bowel can occur in as little as 72 hours without nutrient intake in individuals with even minor acute illness or injury; this cell atrophy is a major facilitator for bacterial translocation, a common cause of sepsis and multiple-organ dysfunction syndrome (MODS) in critically ill patients.
2. Inadequate calories causes glycogenolysis and gluconeogenesis.
3. Stress of critical illness occurs; the stress hormones cortisol and glucagon have catabolic functions.
   a. Hypermetabolism
   b. Glycogenolysis with increased glucose use
   c. Gluconeogenesis with increased protein and fatty acid use
   d. Insulin resistance
   e. Depletion of lean body tissue
4. Glycogenolysis, gluconeogenesis, and stress hormones lead to hyperglycemia.
   a. Level of serum glucose is related to the degree of illness/injury.
   b. Hyperglycemia requires treatment with insulin to keep serum glucose within normal levels because hyperglycemia interferes with immune function.
5. Malnutrition causes immunodeficiency, poor wound healing, or eventually organ failure.

Clinical Presentation

1. Subjective
   a. Anorexia
   b. Diarrhea
   c. Weakness, fatigue, apathy
   d. Irritability
   e. Headache
2. Objective
   a. Dull, brittle dry hair and hair loss
   b. Integumentary changes
      (1) Pale, dry, flaky skin
      (2) Poor skin turgor
      (3) Poor wound healing
      (4) Peripheral edema
      (5) Transverse ridging of fingernails
   c. Oral changes
      (1) Fissures at angles of lips (cheilosis)
      (2) Hyperemic tongue; papillae may be hypertrophic or atrophic
      (3) Gum and teeth problems: loss of teeth; dental caries; bleeding or receding gums
   d. Muscle wasting
   e. Ascites
   f. Hepatomegaly, splenomegaly
   g. Neurologic changes
      (1) Altered mental status
      (2) Loss of balance and coordination
   h. Weight loss
      (1) Degrees of loss: 10% loss is significant; 20% loss indicates malnutrition
      (2) Loss of more than 1 kg/week associated with primarily protein loss
      (3) Body mass index
         (a) Formula: Weight (kg)/[Height (m) × Height (m)]
         (b) Optimal: 20 to 25
         (c) Obesity: greater than 25
         (d) Underweight: less than 20

i. Diminished skinfold and arm circumference measurement (rarely used in critical care)
 (1) Triceps skinfold
  (a) Measurement of skinfold thickness with calipers
  (b) Reflects measurement of the subcutaneous fat reserves of the body; normal 7.5 to 16.5 mm; less than 3 mm indicates severely depleted fat stores
 (2) Midarm muscle circumference
  (a) Measurement of middle of upper nondominant arm
  (b) Reflects measurement of muscle stores of the body

3. Diagnostics
 a. Visceral protein measurements
  (1) Albumin: decreased
   (a) Reflects changes in nutritional status slowly because half-life is 10 to 20 days
    (i) Normal: 3.5 to 5 g/dL
    (ii) Mild depletion: 2.8 to 3.4 g/dL
    (iii) Moderate depletion: 2.1 to 2.7 g/dL
    (iv) Severe depletion: less than 2.1 g/dL
   (b) May result from liver disease, nephrotic syndrome, or hypercatabolism
   (c) May reflect overhydration
  (2) Prealbumin: decreased
   (a) More reliable than albumin for monitoring overall protein status in acute care setting; half-life 24 hours
  (3) Transferrin: decreased; half-life 8 to 10 days
  (4) Retinol-binding protein: decreased; half-life 10 hours; decreases with even minor stress; significance not fully understood
  (5) Hemoglobin/hematocrit: may be decreased
  (6) Tests for immunocompetence
   (a) Total lymphocyte count (TLC): decreased
    (i) Formula: TLC = WBCs (in cubic millimeters) × Percent of lymphocytes, where *WBC* is white blood cells
     a) Normal: 1500 to 2500 cells/mm^3
     b) Mild depletion: less than 1500 cells/mm^3
     c) Moderate depletion: less than 1200 cells/mm^3
     d) Severe depletion: less than 800 cells/mm^3
    (ii) May be decreased by stress, steroids, or renal failure
    (iii) May be increased by infection, leukemia, or myeloma
   (b) Cell-mediated immunity: skin tests for the following:
    (i) *Candida albicans*
    (ii) Mumps
    (iii) Purified protein derivative of tuberculin
 b. Somatic (skeletal) protein measurements
  (1) Midarm muscle circumference
  (2) 24-hour urine specimen for creatinine
 c. Nitrogen balance study may show negative nitrogen balance
  (1) Requires 24-hour dietary record to evaluate nitrogen intake and 24-hour urine collection to measure urine urea nitrogen and evaluate nitrogen loss
  (2) Reliable only when renal function is normal

Nursing Diagnoses

1. Imbalanced Nutrition: Less than Body Requirements related to inability to ingest, digest, absorb, or use nutrients or to hypermetabolism
2. Risk for Infection related to anergy, immunocompromise, or placement of central venous catheter
3. Risk for Aspiration related to enteral feeding, poor airway protective mechanisms, delayed gastric emptying, and gastroesophageal incompetence with NG and nasointestinal tubes
4. Risk for Deficient Fluid Volume related to hyperosmolar feedings and hyperglycemia
5. Diarrhea related to intermittent enteral feedings, lactose intolerance, hyperosmolality, medications, contaminated formula, low fiber formula, or *Clostridium difficile*
6. Impaired Tissue Integrity related to mechanical irritation of enteral tube or central venous catheter

Collaborative Management

1. Prevent/detect negative nitrogen balance and malnutrition.
 a. Weigh patient daily at same time on same scale.
 b. Monitor diagnostic studies reflective of visceral protein stores (e.g., albumin, transferrin, and prealbumin).
2. Ensure delivery of adequate and appropriate nutrients.
 a. Indication for nutritional support: when the patient is required to be NPO for more than 5 days or if patient unable to meet nutritional needs with oral feedings
  (1) Note that 1 L of 5% dextrose provides only 170 kcal/L; although this provides fluids and delays gluconeogenesis for a short time, catabolism occurs after approximately 5 days at basal metabolic rate and occurs earlier in a hypermetabolic patient.
 b. Nutritional support within 48 hours of injury or critical illness may lessen the hypercatabolic state; nutritional support does the following:
  (1) Promotes anabolism to prevent negative nitrogen balance and loss of visceral and somatic protein stores
  (2) Provides needed nutrients for cellular energy
  (3) Supports healing and the immune system
  (4) Enhances feeling of well-being
 c. Calculation of nutritional requirements
  (1) Proteins
   (a) Basal protein requirement is 0.8 g/kg/day.
   (b) Most critically ill patients require approximately 1.5 g/kg/day.

(c) Patients with direct protein loss (e.g., crush injuries, burns, or hemorrhage) require 2 to 3 g/kg/day.
(d) Note that too much protein is associated with azotemia.
(2) Calories: 25 to 80 kcal/kg/day; varies according to age, activity level, metabolic rate, nutritional status, severity of illness, and other factors
(a) Basal or minimal illness: 25 kcal/kg/day
(b) Moderate illness: 35 kcal/kg/day
(c) Sepsis or extensive trauma: 45 kcal/kg/day
(d) Burns: 80 kcal/kg/day
(e) Note that overfeeding is associated with electrolyte imbalance especially hypophosphatemia
(3) Fluids: 25 to 35 mL/kg/day with an additional 150 mL/day for each degree of body temperature above 37°C

d. Distribution of nutrients to ensure adequate nonprotein calories to prevent the protein catabolism
(1) Proteins: 15% to 20%
(2) CHO: 50% to 60%
(3) Fats: 20% to 30%
(a) Note that propofol (Diprivan) is delivered in a 10% lipid emulsion vehicle, and these fat calories need to be included in total calorie allotments; consult with the dietitian regarding the amount of propofol that the patient is receiving in a 24-hour period so that these fat calories are included in the nutritional support plan

e. New concepts in nutritional support (Table 6-6)
f. Administer enteral nutritional support (Table 6-7) to patients with a functioning GI tract requiring nutritional support; remember, "If the gut works, use it"

Text continued on p. 396

Table 6-6 New Concepts in Nutritional Support

Nutrient	Comments
Glutamine	• Nonessential neutral amino acid that plays an important role in maintaining normal intestinal structure and function • May be "conditionally" essential in critical illness; providing glutamine to stressed patients: ◦ Supports the integrity of the gut ◦ Decreases the rate of protein catabolism • Glutamine deficiency causes gut mucosal atrophy and, eventually, intestinal necrosis leading to bacterial translocation and sepsis • Glutamine supplementation provides enterocytes their preferred energy source and prevents gut-induced SIRS • Use of glutamine in patients with intracranial pathologic condition is questionable, especially if seizures are occurring, because glutamine is a predominant stimulatory neurotransmitter
Arginine	• Semiessential amino acid ◦ Promotes nitrogen retention ◦ Improves protein turnover ◦ Improves wound healing ◦ Enhances immune function ◦ Important for production of nitric oxide, a potent regulator of vascular tone and cardiac contractility • Arginine supplementation reduces the risk of infection and sepsis and promotes wound healing
Nucleotides	• Role in energy transfer • Enhances natural killer cell activity • Supports growth and function of metabolically active cells, such as lymphocytes and macrophages
Branched-chain amino acids	• Leucine, isoleucine, and valine • Have beneficial effects on nitrogen balance in patients under stress • May be especially helpful in patients with hepatic failure or encephalopathy, but temporary lowering of daily protein intake is likely to produce the same effect
Medium-chain triglycerides	• Less irritating and more easily absorbed by the small bowel mucosa • May be better than long-chain triglycerides for patients with compromised gastrointestinal function, SIRS, or sepsis
Essential polyunsaturated fatty acids	• Omega-6 (e.g., linoleic acid) and omega-3 (e.g., alpha-linolenic acid) fatty acids • Balance between these fatty acids aids in efficient functioning of the immune system
Dipeptide/tripeptide formulae	• May be used for patients with malabsorption (e.g., severe Crohn's disease, bowel edema, inflammation, or ischemia)

SIRS, Systemic inflammatory response syndrome.

Table 6-7 **Enteral Nutritional Support**

Consideration	Comments
Indication	Patient has functioning GI tract but is unable or unwilling to consume nutrients

Advantages	• Preferred route for patients with functional GI tract
	  ○ Maintenance of gut structure and absorptive ability
	  ○ Reduced incidence of sepsis by prevention of translocation of GI bacteria into blood or lymph
	  ○ Fewer complications than parenteral route
	  ○ Lower cost than parenteral route
	  ○ Early enteral

Disadvantages	• Decreased gastric and intestinal motility often accompanies critical illness and may lead to an inability to achieve adequate caloric intake and may increase the risk of gastroesophageal reflux with resultant aspiration

Contraindications	• Absolute contraindications
	  ○ Diffuse peritonitis
	  ○ Intestinal obstruction
	    — Functional obstruction (e.g., paralytic ileus)
	    — Structural obstruction (e.g., tumor, volvulus, or adhesion)
	  ○ Intestinal perforation
	• Relative contraindications
	  ○ GI ischemia
	  ○ Enterocutaneous fistula
	  ○ Severe acute pancreatitis especially if hemorrhagic
	  ○ Severe malabsorption

Routes (Figure 6-21) and choice of tubes	*Routes*
	• Gastric
	  ○ Advantages
	    — Maintains natural bactericidal quality of acid environment
	    — Provides some protection from stress ulceration
	  ○ Disadvantage: increases risk of aspiration especially in patients with gastric atony, which is common in critically ill patients
	    — PEG may decrease this risk because the tube does not cause gastroesophageal sphincter incompetence
	• Intestinal
	  ○ Advantage: reduces risk of aspiration (though this is questionable)
	  ○ Disadvantage: placing tube is frequently difficult because critically ill patients frequently have delayed gastric motility; placement methods may include the following:
	    — Blind insertion
	      • Turn patient to right side and twist tube during advancement after gastric confirmation
	      • Air insufflation technique: instillation of 350-500 mL of air into the stomach
	      • Use of metoclopramide (Reglan)
	    — Fluoroscopic or endoscopic placement (e.g., percutaneous endoscopic jejunostomy)
	    — Surgical (needle jejunostomy tube)
	Choice
	• Small-gauge tube or tube that is placed below the gastroesophageal sphincter (such as PEG) tube or jejunostomy tube (including needle jejunostomy that may be done at the conclusion of a laparotomy) is preferred
	• Short-term (less than 6 weeks)
	  ○ Nasogastric or orogastric tube
	  ○ Nasointestinal or orointestinal tube (this may be advanced to the duodenum or jejunum)
	  ○ Needle jejunostomy
	• Long-term (more than 6 weeks)
	  ○ Gastrostomy
	  ○ Jejunostomy

Types of formulae	• Monomeric (also referred to as *elemental*) diets (e.g., Vivonex, Vivonex HN, Criticare HN, Vital HN, Travasorb NH, Impact, and Stresstein) contain predigested nutrients: required when feeding is delivered distal to presence of digestive enzymes (distal jejunum); hyperosmolar • Polymeric formulae contain intact protein and require a functional GI system ○ Intact protein and lactose-free enteral diets (e.g., Sustacal, Ensure, Enrich, and Osmolite)

Table 6-7 Enteral Nutritional Support—cont'd

Consideration	Comments
	◦ Intact protein, lactose-free, high-density enteral diets (e.g., Magnacal, Isocal HCN, Sustacal HC, Ensure Plus, and Ensure Plus HN) ◦ Blenderized meat-based enteral diets (e.g., Vitaneed and Compleat B) ◦ Specialized enteral diets — Immune-boosting formulae (e.g., Immune-Aid, Impact, Perative, and Replete): contain glutamine, arginine, and/or nucleotides — Trauma (e.g., Traumacal, Traum-Aid HBC, and Vivonex TEN) — Hepatic (e.g., Travasorb Hepatic and Hepatic-Aid): increased branched-chain amino acids — Pulmonary (e.g., Pulmocare): higher proportion of fats, less CHO to reduce carbon dioxide production — Renal (e.g., Travasorb Renal and Amin-Aid): essential amino acids — Diabetic (e.g., Glucerna and Suplena) — Fiber-containing formulae (e.g., Ensure with fiber, Jevity, and Sustacal with fiber) Modular ◦ CHO (e.g., Polycose and Nutrisource Modular System [carbohydrate]) ◦ Proteins (e.g., ProMod and Nutrisource Modular System [protein]) ◦ Lipids—Medium Chain Triglycerides (e.g., MCT oil and Nutrisource Modular System [lipid]) ◦ Lipids—Long Chain Triglycerides (e.g., Nutrisource Modular System [lipid LCT]) • Note calorie concentration (most have 1 kcal/mL, but some critical care solutions have 2 kcal/mL; and Pulmocare, which is higher in fat, has 1.5 kcal/mL) • Note osmolality (isotonic is 250-350 mOsm/L; hypertonicity contributes to dehydration and diarrhea)
Pattern of delivery	• Intermittent (cannot be used below the pylorus) • Continuously • Cyclic: feeding may be discontinued for periods during the 24-hour period; infusion frequently is initiated during nighttime hours
Monitor	• Position of the feeding tube ◦ X-ray is the only reliable method for confirming placement of enteral tubes; x-rays should be obtained to confirm desired placement before administering formula or medication by the tube for the first time ◦ Other nondefinitive methods include the following: — pH of aspirate may be helpful but not definitive: pH of 1-3 in stomach without pH-altering drugs, pH of 3-5 in stomach with pH-altering drugs, and greater than 7 in small intestine — Color of aspirate may be helpful but not definitive • Stomach: green, cloudy, or colorless • Intestine: yellow or brown • Tracheobronchial tube: tan, white, pale yellow, or clear — Auscultation over stomach when air is injected through the tube (air insufflation) is NOT recommended; poor sensitivity • GI tolerance of enteral feeding ◦ Abdominal distention or complaints of discomfort or fullness ◦ Vomiting ◦ Excessive residual volumes • Intake and output totaled every 8-12 hours • Weight daily • Bedside glucose testing by fingerstick every 6 hours; serum glucose by laboratory daily • Electrolytes daily • Blood urea nitrogen daily • Proteins, trace elements, liver function studies weekly
General guidelines	• Use an infusion pump for continuous infusion • Do not add blue food coloring (or methylene blue) to the enteral feeding; it is no longer recommended to add blue food coloring to enteral feedings for the following reasons: ◦ May result in generalized absorption of the dye from the GI tract; more likely in patients with multiple organ failure — Discoloration of body fluids and tissues — May cause fatal liver toxicity — Causes questionable specificity because discoloration of tracheal secretions may have occurred by systemic route

Continued

Table 6-7 Enteral Nutritional Support—cont'd

Consideration	Comments
	◦ May result in infection because of contamination of the food coloring ◦ Interferes with occult blood testing ◦ Causes allergic reactions in some persons because of presence of FD&C yellow No. 5 ◦ Has relatively low sensitivity • Keep HOB elevated 30-40 degrees during and after intermittent feeding and continuously for continuous feeding • Check for residual volume every 4 to 6 hours or before next intermittent feeding ◦ Injection of 30 mL of air with a 60-mL syringe before aspiration may facilitate aspiration from a small-lumen feeding tube ◦ If residual greater than 200 mL delay feeding, stop continuous infusion for at least 1 hour, and then check again — Note that the volume identified here is controversial, not evidence-based, and frequent interruptions may compromise adequacy of nutritional support — Note that whether to reinstill or discard the aspirated residual volume is controversial, with one study showing more complications (e.g., clogging) with reinstilling the aspiration and no increase in the incidence of electrolyte imbalance when the aspirate was discarded (Booker, Niedringhaus, Eden, & Arnold, 2000) ◦ If large residual volumes continue to limit feeding and impair nutritional support, consider the following interventions: — Place the patient on the right side for 20 minutes before recheck — Consult with the physician regarding the use of a drug to increase gastric motility (e.g., metoclopramide [Reglan] or erythromycin) — Advance the tube to below the pylorus (intestinal motility usually not affected by same factors as gastric motility) — Consult with the dietitian regarding a more calorie-dense formula in order to reduce required volume — Monitor and treat hyperglycemia to avoid gastroparesis • Use strict aseptic technique in administration of enteral feedings; discard feeding system after 24 hours if an open system or after 48 hours if a closed system • Begin with one-fourth to one-half strength at slow rate; increase gradually • Administer free water in volume of 1 mL/kcal to prevent hyperosmolality
Complications of enteral alimentation	• Clogged feeding tube ◦ Recognize factors that increase risk of clogging the tube — Calorie-dense formula — Small-bore feeding tube — Gravity drip ◦ Prevent clogging — Use an infusion pump for continuous feedings and by flushing with water when indicated • Flush with 30 mL of water before and after medication administration via tube • Flush with 30 mL of water before and after intermittent feedings or every 4 hours with continuous feedings • Flush with 30 mL of water after checking for residuals — Use liquid-form medications when possible ◦ Attempt to reestablish patency of a clogged tube by flushing with warm water (note that cranberry juice or cola has not been shown to be more effective than water); tube replacement may be required • Tube displacement ◦ Tape tube securely and monitor for a change in external length ◦ Prevent vomiting with antiemetics • Nausea/vomiting ◦ Slow feeding ◦ Allow feeding to come to room temperature before infusion ◦ Reduce osmolality of the feeding by diluting with water ◦ Decrease amount of fat in feeding ◦ Administer lactose-free formula ◦ Consider the use of drugs to increase gastric motility (e.g., metoclopramide [Reglan] or erythromycin) ◦ Consider the need to move the tube from the stomach into the duodenum

Table 6-7 Enteral Nutritional Support—cont'd

Consideration	Comments
	• Endotracheal aspiration of tube feeding ◦ Elevate HOB 30-40 degrees at all times if feeding is continuous; during and for 60 minutes after intermittent feeding ◦ Keep cuff inflated during feeding if patient is intubated or has tracheostomy ◦ Check for residual volume in stomach every 4 to 6 hours • Diarrhea ◦ Caused by decreased plasma colloidal oncotic pressure resulting from low serum proteins — Maintain adequate nutritional support; diarrhea will resolve when plasma proteins are more normal — Administer intravenous albumin as prescribed ◦ Bacterial contamination — Wash hands before manipulation of equipment and use clean technique — Use a closed system — Change administration system daily or according to policy — Do not allow solutions to hang at room temperature for more than 12 hours if an open system or 24 hours if a closed system — Avoid antidiarrheals, which slow peristalsis and increase the risk of sepsis ◦ Hypertonicity — Initiate enteral feedings at a slow rate and/or half strength; gradually increase rate and/or strength — Use isotonic solutions if possible; dilute hyperosmolar feeding with free water ◦ Alteration in normal flora from antibiotics and proliferation of *Clostridium difficile* — Administer metronidazole (Flagyl) or vancomycin — Encourage ingestion of yogurt (with active cultures) or *Lactobacillus acidophilus* to restore normal flora ◦ Also: — Consider the addition of fiber (e.g., Jevity) — Use only lactose-free formulae — Consider discontinuance of causative medications (e.g., elixirs containing sorbitol and antacids) — Administer pancreatic enzymes for pancreatic insufficiency • Constipation ◦ Add fiber ◦ Increase free water ◦ Increase activity if possible ◦ Administer laxative as prescribed • Dehydration ◦ Monitor daily weight and intake and output ◦ Administer free water as indicated • Electrolyte imbalance ◦ Treat cause (e.g., diarrhea) ◦ Monitor serum electrolytes ◦ Replace electrolytes as prescribed ◦ Consult with the physician and dietitian regarding modification of formula • Hyperglycemia ◦ Monitor serum glucose every 6 hours ◦ Consult with physician and dietitian regarding modification of formula ◦ Administer insulin as prescribed • Overfeeding ◦ Monitor renal and liver function studies ◦ Monitor for fluid overload, hyperglycemia, hyperlipidemia, electrolyte imbalance ◦ Consult with the physician and dietitian regarding caloric and protein prescriptions • Refeeding syndrome ◦ Start feedings slowly especially in high-risk patients (e.g., NPO for several days, existing malnutrition, alcoholism, or sepsis); may take 24-48 hours to get intake to recommended level of nutrition ◦ Monitor glucose, potassium, and phosphorus; insulin and electrolyte replacement may be required

CHO, Carbohydrates; *GI*, gastrointestinal; *HOB*, head of bed; *NPO*, nothing by mouth; *PEG*, percutaneous endoscopic gastrostomy.

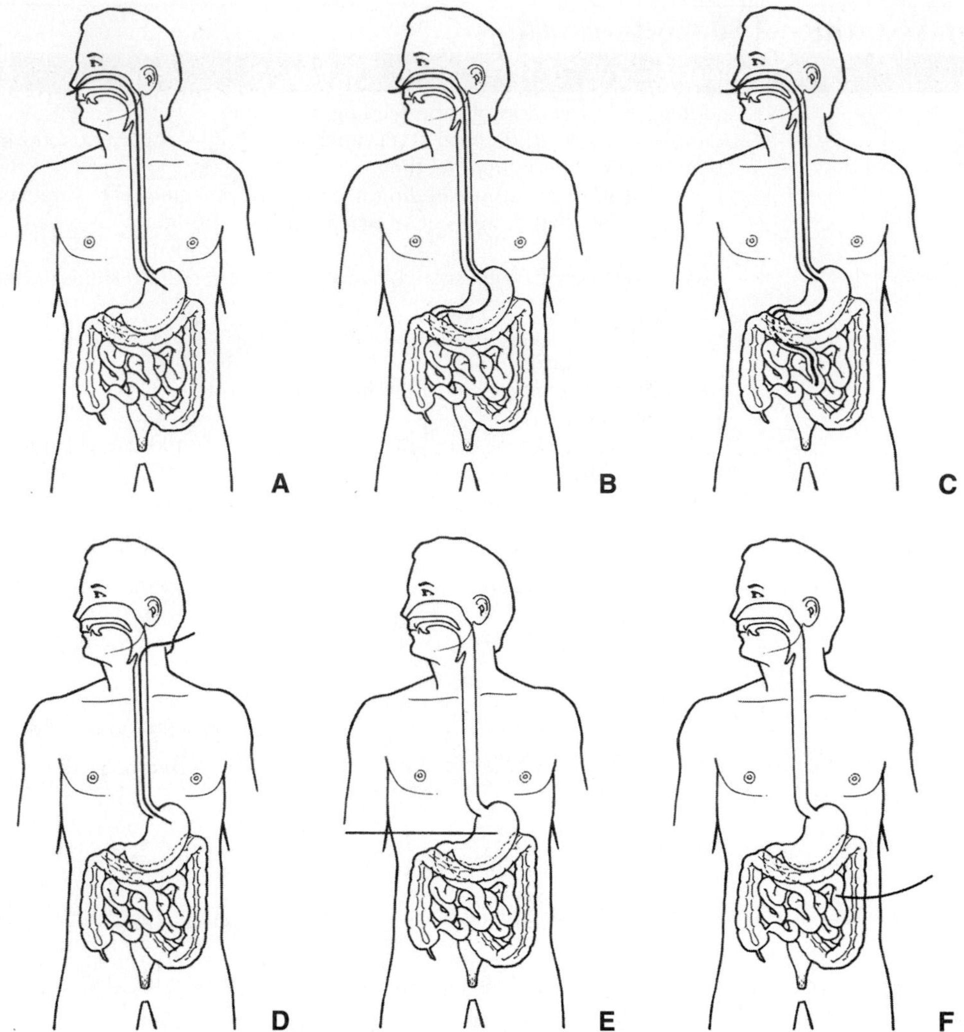

Figure 6-21 Enteral nutrition routes. **A,** Nasogastric. **B,** Nasoduodenal. **C,** Nasojejunal. **D,** Esophagostomy. **E,** Gastrostomy. **F,** Jejunostomy. (From Flynn, J. B. M., & Bruce, N. P. [1993]. *Introduction to critical care skills*, St. Louis: Mosby.)

g. Administer parenteral nutritional support (Table 6-8) to patients without a functioning GI tract who require nutritional support; also may be used with oral or enteral nutrition to increase the amount of nutrients provided in hypermetabolic patients
h. Ensure a smooth transition from enteral or parenteral feedings to oral nutrition
   (1) Consult with the dietitian and the physician regarding plans for this transition.
      (a) Parenteral to enteral feeding: total parenteral nutrition (TPN) rate is decreased by one half when one half to one third of the patient's total caloric requirements are met by enteral feeding and is discontinued when total caloric requirements are met by enteral feedings
      (b) Parenteral to oral diet
         (i) Start with clear liquids and advance to full liquids while observing for aspiration.
         (ii) Advance to solid food after 2 to 3 days of liquids and decrease TPN by one half if at least 500 kcal are consumed.
         (iii) Discontinue nutritional support when the patient is able to tolerate sufficient oral nutrition for 2 to 3 days.
         (iv) High-protein and high-calorie drinks, shakes, and puddings may be used as nutritional supplements to augment small, frequent meals.
      (c) Enteral to oral diet
         (i) Monitor oral intake and use nutritional supplements to boost caloric intake if needed.
         (ii) Cyclic enteral feeding may be considered if calorie intake is consistently inadequate; usually feedings are administered at night.

Table 6-8 Parenteral Nutritional Support

Consideration	Comments
Indications	• When the enteral route is contraindicated (see Table 6-7) • When the enteral route is ineffective (high caloric needs or shock)
Routes	• Central vein: referred to as *TPN* ◦ Allows the administration of hypertonic glucose solutions because of rapid dilution by blood as the solution enters the great vessel ◦ Subclavian or internal jugular usually used; percutaneously inserted central catheter also may be used • Peripheral vein: referred to as *PPN* ◦ Used for patients who cannot take in sufficient nutrition enterally for 5-7 days but who are not hypermetabolic ◦ Not usually adequate to provide sufficient calories for critically ill patient because of osmolality (and therefore calorie) limitations
Type of catheter	• Short term: peripheral or central venous catheter; multilumen catheter usually used to provide lumen for parenteral nutrition, lumen for blood and/or fluids, and lumen for parenteral drugs • Long-term: Hickman (Figure 6-22), Broviac, or Groshong catheter; Infuse-a-Port; Port-a-Cath
Solution: 1 L of standard TPN formula (25% dextrose and 8.5% amino acids) provides ~1000 kcal (1 kcal/mL)	• CHO: hypertonic dextrose ◦ Concentrations — TPN: usually 25% but may be as high as 35% dextrose — PPN: no more than 10% dextrose ◦ CHO and fats provide enough calories for maximal protein-sparing effect ◦ Dextrose provides 3.4 cal/g • Protein: crystalline amino acids 2.5%-8.5% (note that no more than 5% amino acid solution via parenteral line [i.e., PPN]); includes essential and nonessential amino acids and provides 4.3 calories/gram ◦ Specialized formulae are available for specific diseases — Hepatic failure (e.g., HepatAmine and Branch Amin): branched-chain amino acids — Renal failure (e.g., RenAmin and NephrAmine): essential amino acids • Fats: oil-in-water emulsions composed of soybean oil or a combination of soybean oil and safflower oil that provide fatty acids as long-chain triglycerides ◦ 30% to 50% of nonprotein calories should be supplied by lipids not exceeding 2.5 g/kg/day — Linoleic acid, the only essential fatty acid, should provide at least 4% of the total calorie intake to prevent deficiency of essential fatty acid — Excessive amounts of lipids may have a detrimental effect on pulmonary function and the reticuloendothelial system ◦ Concentrations — 10%; lipids provide 1.1 kcal/mL — 20%; lipids provide 2 kcal/mL — 30%; lipids provide 3 kcal/mL ◦ Medium-chain triglycerides are oxidized immediately for fuel and may be preferred in systemic inflammatory response syndrome and sepsis • Electrolytes: sodium chloride; potassium; calcium; magnesium; phosphate • Buffer: acetate or bicarbonate • Minerals: iron; zinc; copper; manganese; cobalt; iodine; chromium; selenium • Vitamins: multivitamins 1 ampule daily ◦ Vitamin K (10-20 mg) should be administered every week; may be given intramuscularly or subcutaneously or added to TPN solution as phytonadione (AquaMEPHYTON) ◦ Thiamine replacement should be considered especially when chronic alcohol ingestion is known or suspected to prevent Wernicke's encephalopathy • Three-in-one admixture has everything in one infusion rather than lipid piggybacked in separately ◦ Advantages: lower cost with less equipment, waste, and nursing time ◦ Disadvantage: risk of solution instability; monitor closely for a cream-colored layer (also referred to as *creaming*) or a complete emulsion crack with a separation of the oil and water and return to pharmacy if separation noted
Possible additives	• Regular insulin (note that sliding scale insulin still must be administered as needed) • Heparin • H_2 receptor antagonists • Metoclopramide (Reglan) • NOTE: All additives should be added under a laminar hood (in pharmacy department) rather than on nursing unit.

Continued

Table 6-8 **Parenteral Nutritional Support—cont'd**

Consideration	Comments
Monitor	• Vital signs and infusion rate at least every 4 hours (depending on patient acuity) • Intake and output totaled every 8-12 hours • Weight daily • Bedside glucose testing by fingerstick every 6 hours; serum glucose by laboratory daily • Electrolytes daily • Blood urea nitrogen daily • Complete blood count, proteins, trace elements, liver function studies, triglycerides, cholesterol, platelet count, prothrombin time weekly • Catheter site
General guidelines	• Use strict sterile technique during catheter insertion and management • Assess patient for central venous catheter insertion complications (pneumothorax, hemothorax, chylothorax, arterial puncture); request chest x-ray after insertion of central venous catheter; do not initiate fluids at a rate faster than keep-vein-open rate until chest x-ray confirms placement • Ensure a dedicated catheter or lumen of a multilumen catheter for TPN infusion ◦ Do not use a catheter or lumen that has been previously used for central venous pressure measurements or for the prolonged administration of crystalloid solution or blood products ◦ Do not use the catheter (or lumen) for drawing blood samples or infusing any other fluids • Assess the solution before infusion ◦ Examine expiration date, and discard any expired solutions ◦ Do not hang cloudy solutions ◦ Monitor closely for emulsion crack if hanging three-in-one solution (also called *total nutrient admixture* [TNA]); do not hang solution if a layer of fat is seen separated at top of bag • Initiate at 1200-2400 cal/day and increase to desired caloric intake as prescribed • Remove from refrigerator 30 minutes before infusing • Keep rate constant (volumetric pump required) • Use an inline filter; 0.22 μm if lipids are piggybacked in distal to filter; 1.2 μm if TNA is used because smaller filter will not allow lipids to flow through • Change dressing every 48 hours or according to hospital policy or anytime that the dressing becomes soiled ◦ Gauze and tape or semipermeable transparent dressing (e.g., Op-Site or Tegaderm); note that semipermeable transparent dressings have been associated with a higher rate of catheter-related infection and sepsis than standard gauze and tape probably because of inadequate permeability and infrequency of dressing change; they should not be used in patients with oily skin or acne near catheter insertion site • Change tubing every 24-72 hours or according to hospital policy; lipid tubing (including TNA tubing) should be changed every 24 hours • Do not allow a bag to hang more than 24 hours
Complications	• Allergic reaction (especially to lipids) ◦ Note fever, chills, shivering, and chest or back pain ◦ Stop infusion • Infection and sepsis ◦ Use meticulous aseptic technique with all aspects of catheter care; change dressing every 48 hours or whenever soiled; change tubing every 24-72 hours; minimize number of entries into the system ◦ Monitor for clinical indications of catheter-related sepsis: fever, leukocytosis, glucose intolerance, redness, swelling, tenderness, and purulent drainage at insertion site ◦ Obtain blood cultures (not through this catheter), remove catheter and culture tip • Hyperglycemia ◦ Monitor serum glucose levels ◦ Administer insulin therapy; usually administered as insulin drip if serum glucose greater than 500 mg/dL • Hyperosmolar nonketotic dehydration ◦ Monitor serum glucose levels ◦ Administer insulin therapy; usually administered as insulin drip if serum glucose greater than 500 mg/dL ◦ Administer 5% dextrose and hypotonic saline (one fourth or one half) or 5% dextrose in water (depending on patient's serum osmolality) to correct free water deficit ◦ Discontinue TPN until patient stable as prescribed

Table 6-8 Parenteral Nutritional Support—cont'd

Consideration	Comments
	• Hypoglycemia ◦ Prevent interruption of TPN infusion (e.g., catheter occlusion or accidental removal) ◦ Use infusion pump (mandatory) ◦ Never discontinue TPN abruptly unless for hyperglycemic hyperosmolar nonketotic coma • Electrolyte imbalances: hyperchloremic metabolic acidosis; hyponatremia; hypokalemia; hypocalcemia; hypomagnesemia; hypophosphatemia ◦ Adjust TPN solution concentration and/or alteration of infusion rate as prescribed • Refeeding syndrome: fluid imbalance; hypokalemia; hypophosphatemia; hypoglycemia or hyperglycemia ◦ Monitor fluid, electrolyte, glucose levels especially during the first 24-48 hours after TPN initiated ◦ Adjust TPN solution concentration and/or alteration of infusion rate as prescribed • Increased carbon dioxide production ◦ Monitor closely for clinical indications of hypercapnia; request arterial blood gases as indicated ◦ Decrease the percentage of calories supplied by CHO and increase percentage of calories supplied by fats if hypercapnia occurs or during weaning • Air embolism ◦ Prevent air embolus by the following: — Ask the patient to hold his or her breath or perform Valsalva maneuver during catheter insertion, tubing changes, and catheter removal — Purge all air from tubings before attachment to catheter — Use air-eliminating filters on central line tubings — Use Luer-Lok connections ◦ Note dyspnea, hypotension, churning murmur over precordium, confusion ◦ If clinical indications of air embolism do occur: ◦ Place patient in Trendelenburg's position on left side ◦ Aspirate air with a syringe attached to the central venous catheter ◦ Administer oxygen • Subclavian thrombosis (rare) ◦ Monitor for swelling of involved arm, face, neck, erythema, fever ◦ Remove catheter ◦ Administer fibrinolytic or anticoagulation therapy as prescribed

CHO, Carbohydrates; *PPN*, peripheral parenteral nutrition; *TNA*, total nutrient admixture; *TPN*, total parenteral nutrition.

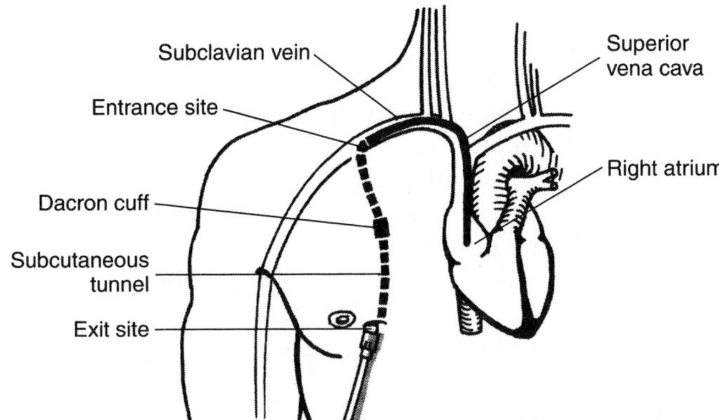

Figure 6-22 Hickman catheter for administration of TPN. (From Long, B. C., Phipps, W. J., & Cassmeyer, V. L. [1993]. *Medical-surgical nursing: A nursing process approach* [3rd ed.]. St. Louis: Mosby.)

(2) Continue to monitor weights and food intake daily during transition times

3. Provide frequent oral hygiene, and prevent skin breakdown.

Upper Gastrointestinal Hemorrhage

Definitions

1. Peptic ulcer: a sharply defined erosion in mucosa that may involve the submucosa and muscular layers of the esophagus (~5%), stomach (~15%), or duodenum (~80%)
2. Esophageal varices: dilation of the submucosal esophageal veins
3. Gastritis
4. Mallory-Weiss tear: acute longitudinal tear of the esophagus caused by forceful retching
5. Gastritis: a generalized inflammation of the gastric mucosa

Etiology

1. Peptic ulcer
   a. *Helicobacter pylori:* a bacterial infection that now has been identified as a common cause of recurrent ulcer disease
   b. Other predisposing factors
      (1) Genetic predisposition
      (2) Smoking
      (3) Diet
         (a) Coffee or tea
         (b) Carbonated beverages
         (c) Beer
      (4) Drugs and therapies
         (a) Antineoplastics
         (b) Radiation therapy
         (c) Drugs that alter the mucosal barrier
            (i) Alcohol
            (ii) NSAIDs (e.g., aspirin, ibuprofen, and indomethacin)
         (d) Drugs that decrease gastric mucosal renewal: corticosteroid, phenylbutazone
         (e) Drugs that increase acid stimulation
            (i) Coffee (because of peptides, not caffeine)
            (ii) Nicotine
            (iii) Reserpine
         (f) Hormones (e.g., estrogen)
      (5) High emotional stress (e.g., type A personality)
      (6) High physiologic stress situation
         (a) COPD
         (b) Multiple trauma
         (c) Major surgery
         (d) Myocardial infarction
         (e) Hepatic failure
         (f) Renal failure
         (g) Burns: referred to as *Curling's ulcer*
         (h) Neurologic trauma: referred to as *Cushing's ulcer*
            (i) Cerebral trauma
            (ii) Spinal cord injury
            (iii) Neurosurgery
         (i) Acute respiratory distress syndrome
         (j) Mechanical ventilation for more than 5 days
         (k) Coagulopathy
         (l) Sepsis
         (m) Shock
         (n) MODS
2. Cirrhosis: portal hypertension
   a. Cirrhosis
      (1) Alcoholic cirrhosis: most likely
      (2) Viral or toxic hepatitis
      (3) Chronic biliary obstruction
      (4) Chronic right ventricular failure
   b. Portal vein thrombosis
   c. Hepatic venous outflow obstruction
   d. Congenital hepatic fibrosis
   e. Schistosomiasis: a parasitic infection
3. Mallory-Weiss tear: forceful retching and vomiting (e.g., alcoholism or bulimia)
4. Gastritis
   a. Dietary intolerances especially milk intolerance
   b. Alcohol
   c. Drugs such as aspirin, steroids, NSAIDs
   d. Uremia
   e. Certain systemic diseases such as hepatitis
   f. Ingestion of strong acids or alkalis (referred to as *corrosive gastritis*)

Pathophysiology

1. Peptic ulcer
   a. Injury is caused by one or more of the following factors:
      (1) Presence of *Helicobacter pylori* bacteria
      (2) Increased acid production or inability to buffer acid
      (3) Impaired mucosal barrier to acid
      (4) Impaired gastric motility
      (5) Stress
         (a) Acid hypersecretion related at least in part to increased endogenous (or exogenous) glucocorticoids
         (b) Decreased mucosal pH
         (c) Ischemia
         (d) Altered mucosal defense mechanisms
   b. Ulceration occurs when there is injury to mucosa allowing acid to diffuse back through the broken barrier.
   c. Hemorrhage, perforation, or scarring with obstruction indicates the need for immediate treatment.
      (1) Gastric ulcers are more likely to occur with hematemesis or perforation.
      (2) Duodenal ulcers are more likely to occur with melena, perforation, or scarring with obstruction.
2. Esophageal varices
   a. Fibrotic liver changes and resistance to normal venous drainage of the liver to the portal vein (hepatic venous obstruction) causes increased pressure
   b. Portal hypertension
   c. Pressure transmitted to collateral circulation
   d. Dilation of the submucosal veins of the distal esophagus and stomach
   e. Predisposition to bleed (these vessels were not intended to tolerate this pressure), which leads to bleeding frequently triggered by the following:
      (1) Increased intraabdominal pressure (e.g., Valsalva maneuver)
      (2) Mechanical trauma (e.g., poorly chewed hard foods or insertion of NG tube)
      (3) Chemical trauma (e.g., gastroesophageal reflux)
      (4) Coagulopathy
   f. Massive bleeding from mouth (note that these patients do not truly vomit; they simply open their mouth and massive amounts of blood are emitted)

3. Mallory-Weiss tear: arterial bleeding that is usually self-limiting
4. Gastritis: irritants cause inflammation of the gastric mucosa and oozing of blood

Clinical Presentation

1. Peptic ulcer
   a. Subjective
      (1) History: epigastric pain, previous ulcer, previous GI bleeding, alcoholism, liver disease
      (2) Epigastric pain
      (3) Fatigue, weakness
      (4) Thirst
      (5) Anxiety
   b. Objective
      (1) Bleeding
         (a) Blood or coffee-ground material appears in vomitus if gastric ulcer
         (b) Black stools if duodenal
         (c) If bleeding is gradual, faintness, fatigue, and pallor may be only indications
      (2) Hyperactive bowel sounds
      (3) Patient may have signs of acute condition in the abdomen if ulcer perforated (Box 6-2); other terms for an acute condition in the abdomen include *surgical abdomen* or *"hot belly"*
   c. Diagnostic
      (1) Serum
         (a) Chemistry
            (i) Gastrin level: may be elevated in gastric ulcer
            (ii) Amylase: elevated if perforation causes penetration into the pancreas and causes acute pancreatitis
            (iii) Total proteins, albumin, transferrin: may be decreased because many of these patients are malnourished
         (b) Hematology
            (i) CBC: anemia
            (ii) Hgb, Hct: decreased but changes may take 4 to 6 hours after acute bleed
         (c) Clotting studies: PT and partial thromboplastin time (PTT) prolonged if liver is affected
      (2) Gastric analysis: may show hyperacidity; may show blood in the gastric secretions
      (3) Stools for occult blood: positive
      (4) Electrocardiogram (ECG): may show indications of ischemia (e.g., ST-T wave changes)
      (5) Flat plate of abdomen: may show free air under diaphragm, which indicates perforation
      (6) Gastroscopy: important in differentiating cause of upper GI bleeding; can determine ulcer presence, location, and stage of healing
      (7) Upper GI series: may show anatomic deformity created by ulcer crater; may show delayed gastric emptying if edema or scarring is present
      (8) Biopsy: may be done to rule out gastric cancer or malignant gastric ulcer
      (9) Angiography
         (a) Rarely performed
         (b) May reveal bleeding site or sites
         (c) May include the placement of a catheter for intraarterial administration of vasopressors (e.g., vasopressin)
2. Esophageal varices
   a. Subjective
      (1) History of precipitating causes (e.g., excessive or chronic alcohol intake)
      (2) Report of sudden, painless hemorrhage orally
   b. Objective
      (1) Bright, red blood gushing from mouth (average blood loss is 10 units)
      (2) Jaundice
      (3) Abdominal distention
      (4) Hyperactive bowel sounds
      (5) Melena
      (6) Hepatomegaly
      (7) Splenomegaly
      (8) Clinical indications of hypoperfusion: tachycardia; tachypnea; hypotension; cool, clammy skin; decreased urine output; agitation; confusion
   c. Diagnostic
      (1) Serum
         (a) Chemistry
            (i) BUN: elevated
            (ii) Bilirubin: may be elevated
            (iii) Albumin: decreased because of liver disease
            (iv) AST, ALT, LDH: elevated because of liver disease
         (b) Hematology: Hgb, Hct decreased
         (c) Clotting studies: PT and aPTT prolonged because of liver disease
         (d) Arterial blood gases: may reveal metabolic acidosis related to shock and hypoperfusion
      (2) Stool: positive for occult blood

BOX 6-2 Clinical Indications of an Acute Condition in the Abdomen

Abdominal distention
Abdominal pain
Diminished or absent bowel sounds
Fever
Leukocytosis
Nausea, vomiting
Rebound tenderness
Rigid, boardlike abdomen

(3) ECG: may show indications of ischemia (e.g., ST-T wave changes)
(4) Barium swallow: reveals the presence of esophageal varices
(5) Esophagogastroduodenoscopy: reveals the presence of esophageal varices
(6) Percutaneous transhepatic portography: reveals esophageal varices and measures pressure in the portal circulation
(7) Angiography
(a) Rarely performed
(b) May reveal bleeding site or sites
(c) May include the placement of a catheter for intraarterial administration of vasopressors (e.g., vasopressin)

3. Mallory-Weiss tear: hematemesis after forceful vomiting
4. Gastritis: coffee-ground hematemesis

Nursing Diagnoses

1. Deficient Fluid Volume related to hemorrhage and fluid shifts
2. Decreased Cardiac Output related to decreased preload
3. Ineffective Tissue Perfusion: Cerebral, Cardiopulmonary, Renal, Gastrointestinal, and Peripheral related to anemia, hypovolemia, and vasopressin therapy
4. Ineffective Airway Clearance related to displacement of esophageal balloon in balloon tamponade
5. Impaired Gas Exchange related to anemia, aspiration, and airway compromise from balloon tamponade
6. Risk for Aspiration related to hematemesis
7. Imbalanced Nutrition: Less than Body Requirements related to poor intake and altered food metabolism
8. Risk for Injury related to coagulopathy and altered consciousness
9. Interrupted Family Processes related to situational crisis, powerlessness, and change in role
10. Deficient Knowledge related to required lifestyle changes

Collaborative Management

1. Ensure airway, oxygenation, and ventilation.
a. Position patient for optimal ventilation and to prevent aspiration.
(1) Elevate head of the bed 30 to 45 degrees
(2) Turn to left side
b. Administer oxygen as necessary to maintain Sao_2 at 95% unless contraindicated; in patients with COPD, administer oxygen to achieve an Spo_2 of ~90%.
c. Assist with endotracheal intubation as requested.
(1) Before balloon tamponade for esophageal varices: recommended to prevent obstruction of airway in case of accidental dislodgment of the esophageal balloon
(2) Before endoscopy if indicated
2. Maintain hemodynamic stability.
a. Monitor blood loss and hemodynamic stability.
(1) Insert large-bore orogastric or NG tube and perform gastric lavage.
(a) Note that gastric lavage does not truly aid in clotting as previously believed and actually may dislodge clots; purposes of gastric lavage include the following:
(i) To monitor bleeding
(ii) To remove nitrogenous materials (blood) out of the gut so that they will not be converted to ammonia
(iii) Allow visualization during endoscopy
(b) Use room temperature saline for lavage; problems occur with the use of iced lavage.
(i) Less effective in cessation of bleeding
(ii) Prolongation of clotting times
(iii) Hypothermia
a) Causing the oxyhemoglobin dissociation curve to shift to the left, decreasing tissue delivery of oxygen
b) Causing the patient to shiver, increasing oxygen consumption
(2) Insert indwelling urinary catheter to evaluate hourly urine output.
(3) Assist with insertion of arterial catheter and pulmonary artery catheter in patients with severe hemorrhage.
b. Replace circulating blood volume.
(1) Insert at least two short (1¼-inch) large-gauge (16 or 18) peripheral IV catheters; two units of blood are drawn during catheter insertion for laboratory analysis and type and crossmatch.
(2) Administer crystalloids initially as prescribed; colloids also may be prescribed.
(a) Maintain urine output of 0.5 to 1 mL/kg/hr.
(b) Maintain PAOP of 12 to 15 mm Hg.
(c) Avoid lactated Ringer's solution in patients with liver disease.
(3) Administer blood and blood products as prescribed.
(a) Red packed cells should be given early if significant blood loss is suspected to prevent tissue hypoxia; indications include the following:
(i) Persistent hemodynamic instability after 2 L of crystalloid
(ii) Hematocrit less than 25%
(iii) Clinical indications of hypoperfusion (see Table 2-2)
(b) Fresh blood is preferred especially in patients with liver disease because it is lower in ammonia than banked blood.

(c) After multiple transfusions, consider replacing clotting factors, platelets, and calcium.

c. Control bleeding.

(1) Administer vasopressin IV as prescribed; vasopressin slows blood loss by constricting the splanchnic arteriolar bed and decreasing portal venous pressure.

(a) Administer through a central line at a dose of 0.2 to 0.6 unit/min for up to 36 hours; then slowly decrease the dose.

(b) Monitor for adverse effects of vasopressin: bradycardia; hypertension; water retention causing hyponatremia (syndrome of inappropriate antidiuretic hormone); chest pain; dysrhythmias; abdominal cramping and pain; and oliguria.

(i) Because vasopressin may cause constriction of coronary arteries, nitroglycerin infusion may be used concurrently to prevent chest pain.

(ii) Close monitoring of the BP blood pressure is essential because hypertension may increase bleeding.

(c) Vasopression also may be infused directly into the superior mesenteric artery by a catheter placed during angiography.

(2) Administer octreotide acetate (Sandostatin) as prescribed; octreotide reduces splanchnic blood flow, gastric acid secretion, GI mobility, and pancreatic exocrine function.

(a) Octreotide may be administered IV or subcutaneously.

(b) Usual dose in upper GI hemorrhage is a 100-mcg IV bolus followed by 50 mcg/hr IV for 48 hours and then 100 mcg subcutaneously every 8 hours for 72 hours.

(c) Monitor for adverse effects of octreotide: pain or burning at injection site, abdominal pain, and diarrhea.

(3) Assist with diagnostic/therapeutic endoscopy.

(a) Diagnostic: to identify the specific cause of the bleeding

(b) Therapeutic for peptic ulcer or Mallory-Weiss tear

(i) Endoscopic thermal therapy uses heat to cauterize the bleeding vessel.

(ii) Endoscopic injection therapy uses hypertonic saline, epinephrine, or dehydrated alcohol to cause localized vasoconstriction of the bleeding vessel.

(c) Therapeutic for esophageal varices

(i) Sclerotherapy

a) Sclerosing agent (ethanolamine oleate [Ethamolin], morrhuate sodium [Scleromate], sodium tetradecyl [Sotradecol]) is injected into the varix and surrounding tissue; the sclerosing agent causes variceal inflammation, venous thrombosis, and eventually scar tissue; repeated injections may be necessary to completely decompress the bleeding varix and decrease the risk of recurrent hemorrhage.

b) Varices are categorized as I to IV by their size; classes III and IV are at high risk to bleed if not already bleeding.

c) Monitor for complications of sclerotherapy.

i) Retrosternal pain

ii) Transient fever

iii) Transient dysphagia

iv) Local ulceration

v) Pulmonary symptoms including diminished breath sounds

vi) Bleeding

vii) Stricture

viii) Perforation

ix) Sepsis

d) Sclerotherapy is repeated in 4 to 7 days and every 6 to 8 months thereafter.

(ii) Esophageal variceal ligation: rubber bands or O-rings are placed on the target vessels at gastroesophageal junction

(4) Stop bleeding in esophageal varices through measures that lower venous pressure.

(a) Administer beta-blockers (e.g., propranolol) as prescribed.

(b) Assist in placement of a multiple-lumen tube for balloon tamponade (Figure 6-23 and Table 6-9) if bleeding cannot be controlled pharmacologically, endoscopically, or through use of transjugular intrahepatic portosystemic shunt (TIPS)

d. Correct coagulopathy, which is frequently significant in patients with esophageal varices and liver disease.

(1) Administer vitamin K as prescribed; recombinant clotting factors (e.g., rFVIIa) may be prescribed.

(2) Monitor closely for bleeding.

(3) Monitor clotting studies.

(4) Avoid invasive procedures and injections.

3. Prepare patient for surgery if necessary to control bleeding.

a. Peptic ulcer

(1) Indications for surgery

(a) Continuation of bleeding despite treatment

(b) Administration of more than 8 units of blood over 24 hours

(c) Hemorrhage to the point of hypotension or shock

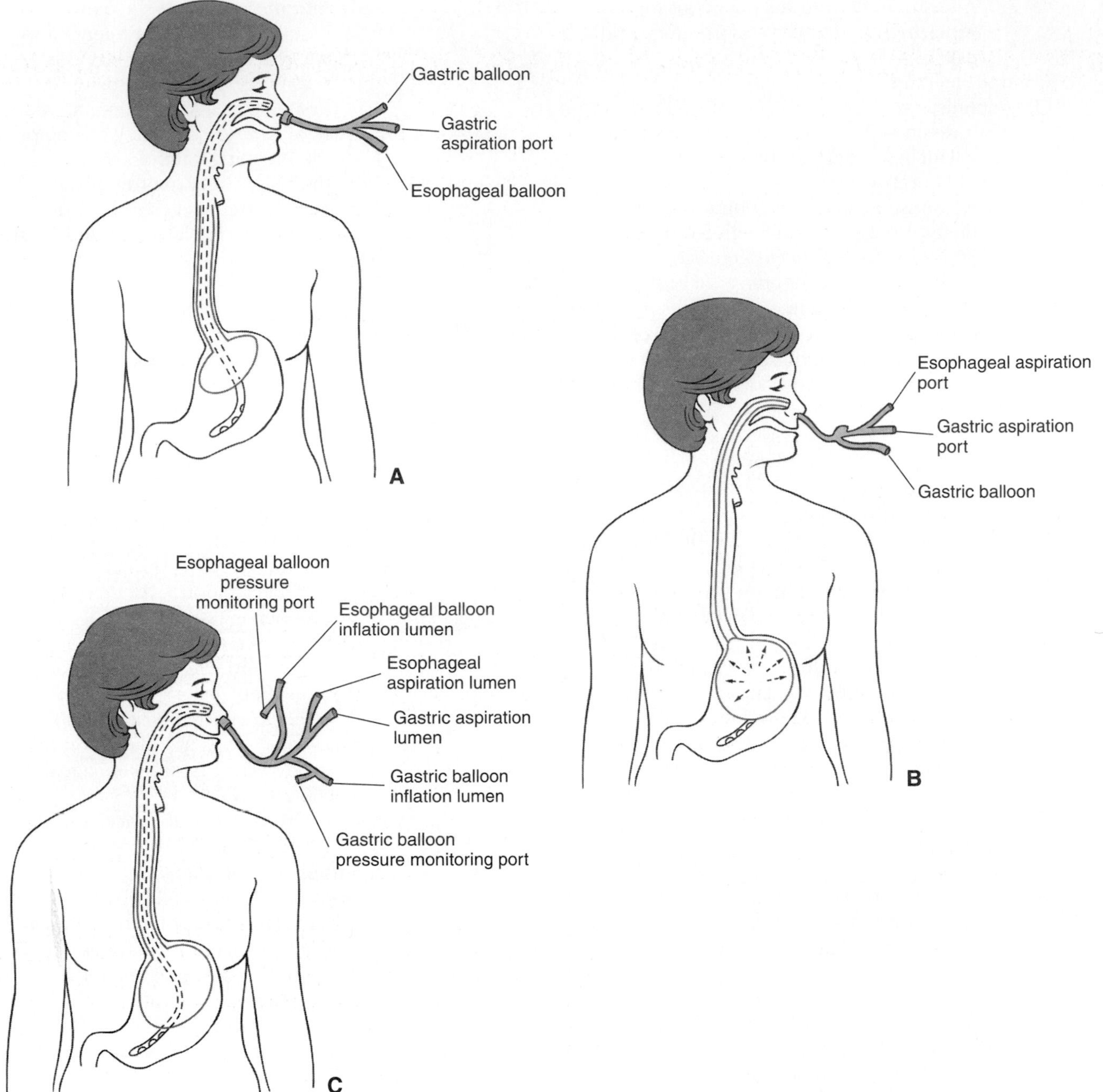

Figure 6-23 Esophageal tamponade tubes. **A,** Sengstaken-Blakemore tube. **B,** Linton tube. **C,** Minnesota tube. (From Thelan, L. A., Urden, L. D., Lough, M. E., & Stacy, K. M. [1998]. *Critical care nursing: Diagnosis and management* [3rd ed.]. St. Louis: Mosby.)

(d) Rebleeding after homeostasis achieved

(2) Surgical interventions
   (a) Oversewing of bleeding point
   (b) Pyloroplasty
   (c) Antrectomy: removal of the antrum; decreases acidity by removing antrum, which secretes gastric acid
   (d) Vagotomy: dividing the vagus nerve along the esophagus
      (i) Decreases acid secretion in the stomach
      (ii) If ulcer is prepyloric, vagotomy should be performed to prevent obstruction
   (e) Gastrectomy: partial or total
      (i) Types (Figure 6-24)
         a) Billroth I: antrectomy; vagotomy; and gastroduodenostomy
         b) Billroth II: antrectomy; vagotomy; and gastrojejunostomy
         c) Total gastrectomy: gastrectomy with anastomosis of esophagus to the duodenum or jejunum

Table 6-9 Balloon Tamponade for Esophageal Varices

Consideration	Comments
Action	• Applies pressure to esophageal and intragastric varices
Tubes	• SB tube (Figure 6-23): esophageal balloon; gastric balloon; gastric suction • L tube: gastric balloon; esophageal suction; gastric suction • M tube: esophageal balloon; gastric balloon; esophageal suction; gastric suction
Lumens	• Gastric balloon: 200-500 mL for SB tube; 450-500 mL for M tube; 700-800 mL for L tube • Esophageal balloon: usually 20 mm Hg (25 cm H_2O); but may be as high as 30-40 mm Hg to control bleeding • Gastric suction: nonvented • Esophageal suction: nonvented
Insertion	• Generally done by physician but may be done by specifically trained nurse • Check balloon for leaks before insertion by inflating with air and putting in a basin of saline • Use viscous lidocaine or Cetacaine* to anesthetize the nose and posterior pharynx • The catheter is advanced to ~50-cm mark • The gastric balloon is inflated to 200-300 mL; the lumen is double-clamped to prevent leakage • The catheter is pulled back until resistance is met, and then a nasal sponge is placed at the nose to keep the gastric balloon up against the gastroesophageal junction ○ A football helmet with face mask also may be used — If a helmet is used, check fit closely; skin breakdown frequently is caused by an ill-fitting helmet ○ 0.5-1 kg weight may be used hung over the end of the bed • The esophageal balloon is inflated to a pressure of 20-40 mm Hg until bleeding is controlled; the lumen is double-clamped to prevent leakage • The suction lumens are connected to intermittent low suction (these are nonvented) • Label all lumens; obtain chest x-ray check placement
Management	• Monitor and maintain airway ○ Elevate HOB to 45 degrees unless patient is unconscious; if patient is unconscious, elevated HOB 15 degrees on left side ○ Have suction equipment available ○ Intubation is desirable but not absolutely required ○ Suction secretions from the oropharynx and nasopharynx often because the patient cannot swallow with the tube in — Not as much of an issue with M tube because there is suction above the esophageal balloon — A small nasogastric tube may be inserted into the nostril opposite the SB tube to drain secretions that collect above the esophageal balloon • Maintain pressures at prescribed levels ○ Periodic deflation at specific intervals (e.g., every 4 hours) may be prescribed because the pressures required to control bleeding exceed the pressure of capillary filling, and ischemia or necrosis may occur — Monitor patient closely for bleeding during any time of deflation • Have scissors at bedside to release pressure from esophageal balloon if it accidentally moves into the pharynx and acute respiratory distress occurs ○ Keep second tube in the room for replacement if necessary • Maintain traction on tube to keep gastric balloon pulled up against the gastroesophageal junction • Note amount of pressure/volume in each part of tube; maintain inflation of balloons • Ensure patency of the gastric suction lumen and keep connected to low intermittent suction to prevent aspiration or retention of blood in the gut, which is likely to increase ammonia levels • Monitor patient closely for skin breakdown at mouth or nose; lubricate every 8 hours with water-soluble lubricant • Deflation of the esophageal balloon usually is done at 24 hours; deflation of the gastric balloon usually is done at 48 hours; monitor patient closely for recurrent bleeding when balloons are deflated
Complications	• Airway obstruction • Aspiration • Perforation of esophagus: sudden epigastric or substernal pain, respiratory distress, increased bleeding, shock • Dysrhythmias • Chest pain • Bronchopneumonia • Laceration, ulceration of stomach • Pressure necrosis of hypopharynx, esophagus, or upper stomach • Hiccups

*Combination of benzocaine, butamben, and tetracaine hydrochloride.
HOB, Head of bed; *L*, Linton; *M*, Minnesota; *SB*, Sengstaken-Blakemore.

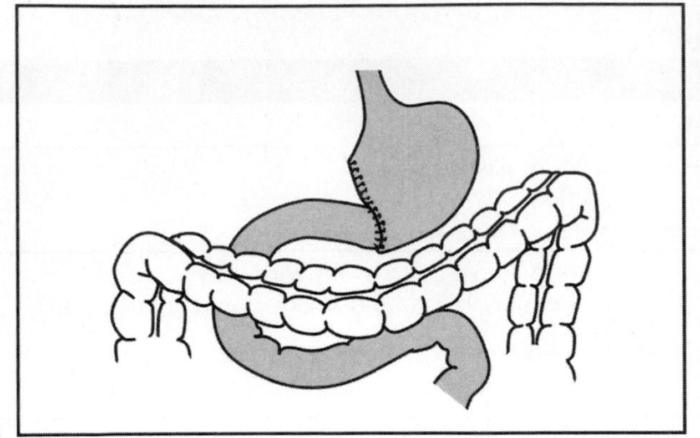

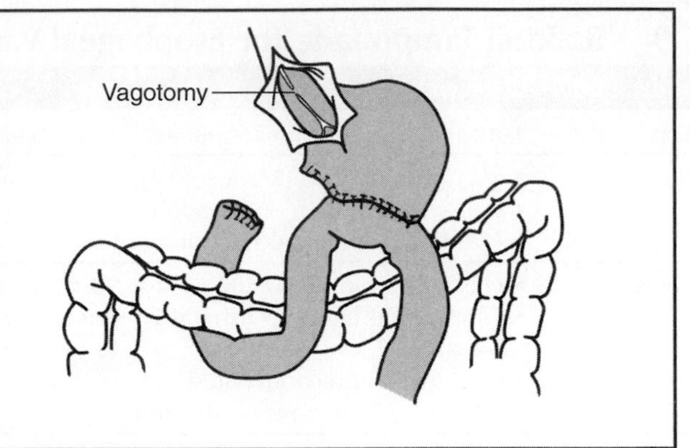

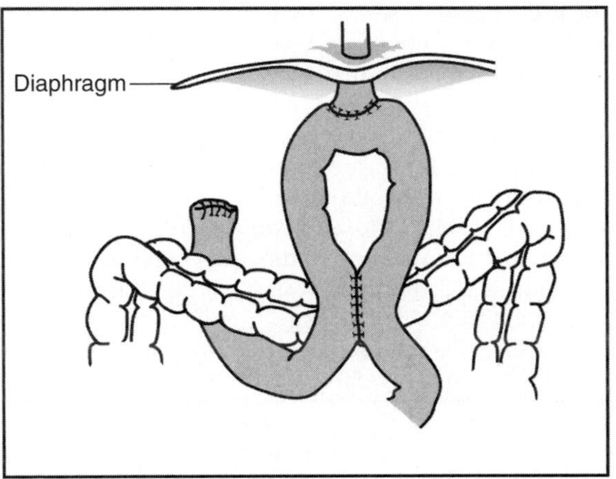

Figure 6-24 Gastric resection procedures. **A,** Billroth I. **B,** Billroth II. **C,** Total gastrectomy.

(ii) Monitor for the following:
  a) Early dumping syndrome (hyperosmolality effect related to a hyperosmolar bolus of food being "dumped" into the duodenum because of absence of pyloric valve and normal, more gradual gastric emptying): occurs within 30 minutes after eating; dizziness, weakness; tachycardia; cool, clammy skin
  b) Late dumping syndrome (hyperinsulinism effect related to an increase in insulin production by the pancreas in response to a large bolus of food causing an increase in blood glucose): occurs 2 hours after meal; complaints of dizziness, weakness, restlessness; tachycardia; cool, clammy skin; malabsorption
  c) Pernicious anemia: related to removal of parietal cells that make intrinsic factor necessary for the absorption of vitamin B_{12} in the ileum

b. Esophageal varices
  (1) Indications for surgery
    (a) Continuation of bleeding despite treatment
    (b) Administration of more than 8 units of blood over 24 hours
    (c) Hemorrhage to the point of hypotension or shock
    (d) Rebleeding after homeostasis achieved
  (2) Portosystemic shunt: portacaval, mesocaval, or splenorenal
    (a) Lowers portal pressure by diverting blood flow
    (b) Associated with a higher incidence of hepatic encephalopathy and avoided if possible
  (3) TIPS
    (a) Invasive angiographic method; less invasive than surgical shunt
    (b) Shunts blood between the portal and systemic venous systems entirely within the liver; connection is made between the hepatic and portal veins and a stent is placed in the tract
    (c) Complications: hemorrhage; renal failure; septic shock; shunt stenosis; hepatic encephalopathy

4. Prevent encephalopathy
  a. Remove nitrogenous materials from the GI tract.
    (1) Perform gastric lavage with room temperature saline so that bacteria in GI tract cannot digest the globin (i.e., protein).

(2) Administer osmotic laxatives (e.g., lactulose) as prescribed.
(3) Administer enemas as ordered.

b. Monitor patients with portacaval shunts closely for clinical indications of elevated ammonia levels (e.g., confusion, irritability, decreased attention span, apathy, and slurring of speech).

5. Prevent further damage to the gastric mucosa caused by gastric irritants, hyperacidity, and/or impaired mucosal barrier.
   a. Discontinue any gastric irritants.
   b. Administer pharmacologic agents that decrease gastric acidity and/or protect gastric mucosa.
      (1) Agents (See Chapter 13 for more information on these agents.)
         (a) Decrease gastric pH to between 3.5 and 5 (normal pH of gastric secretions is between 1 and 3)
            (i) Antacids (e.g., aluminum-magnesium complex [Riopan], magnesium hydroxide and aluminum hydroxide [Maalox, Mylanta], and calcium carbonate [Tums])
            (ii) Histamine (H_2) receptor antagonist (e.g., ranitidine [Zantac], famotidine [Pepcid], and nizatidine [Axid])
            (iii) Proton pump inhibitors (e.g., omeprazole [Prilosec], lansoprazole [Prevacid], and esomeprazole [Nexium])
         (b) Provide agents to improve the mucosal barrier to acid.
            (i) Prostaglandin E_1-analog (e.g., misoprostol [Cytotec])
            (ii) Mucosal protectant (aluminum hydroxide, sulfated sucrose): (e.g., sucralfate [Carafate])
      (2) Note the controversy regarding use of these agents *prophylactically*
         (a) Although a traditional goal has been to maintain the gastric pH at 3.5 or greater (normal pH of gastric secretions is 1 to 3) in critically ill patients, this has been shown to contribute to gastric bacterial colonization and nosocomial pneumonia.
         (b) Mucosal protectants do not change the gastric pH significantly, though they do provide a protective barrier to gastric acid in the protection of ulcers.
   c. Provide required nutritional support by enteral route if possible.
   d. Remove NG or orogastric tube after lavage is completed (and enteral nutritional support not required) because the gastric tube may increase acid production by stimulating gastric secretion.
   e. Administer drug therapy for *Helicobacter pylori;* any of the following combinations may be prescribed.
      (1) Bismuth subsalicylate + metronidazole + tetracycline + H_2 receptor antagonist
      (2) Omeprazole + clarithromycin
      (3) Ranitidine bismuth citrate + clarithromycin
      (4) Lansoprazole + amoxicillin + clarithromycin
      (5) Lansoprazole + amoxicillin
6. Decrease anxiety.
   a. Maintain a calm and reassuring approach.
   b. Administer anxiolytics as prescribed and indicated; avoid hepatotoxic agents if the patient has liver disease.
   c. Keep the patient and family informed regarding patient status.
   d. Encourage discussion of fears and concerns.
   e. Assess for alcohol withdrawal syndrome (Box 6-3); if present, do the following:
      (1) Administer central nervous system depressants (e.g., diazepam [Valium] or chlordiazepoxide [Librium]) as prescribed.
         (a) Most drugs used for this purpose, including diazepam (Valium) and chlordiazepoxide (Librium), have potential for liver toxicity; dosage is adjusted, and liver function studies are monitored.
      (2) Reorient patient frequently.
      (3) Encourage family attendance.
7. Maintain fluid and electrolyte balance: evaluate sodium, potassium, calcium, and magnesium and replace these as prescribed.
8. Maintain nutritional status by administering appropriate nutrients.
   a. Recommendations for patients with peptic ulcer
      (1) Provide bland proteins and fats in small, frequent meals.
      (2) Avoid stimulants of gastric secretions (e.g., coffee, tea, cola, spicy foods, and alcohol).
      (3) Progress to full diet as soon as possible.
   b. Recommendations for patients with esophageal varices
      (1) Give clear liquids initially; progress in dietary substance as indicated.

BOX 6-3 Alcohol Withdrawal Syndrome

Early
Anxiety, agitation
Diaphoresis
Mild hypertension
Mild tachycardia
Nausea, vomiting
Pruritus
Sleep disturbances
Time disorientation
Tremors
Visual disturbances

Late
Dehydration
Delirium
Delusions
Hallucinations
Hyperthermia
Marked hypertension
Marked tachycardia
Tonic-clonic seizures

(2) Avoid alcohol-containing mouthwash and drugs.
(3) Encourage thorough chewing of foods, especially hard, sharp foods such as crackers because they may injure the varices mechanically, causing recurrence of bleeding.

9. Monitor patient for complications.
   a. Aspiration pneumonitis
   b. Recurrent bleeding, hemorrhage
   c. Perforation
   d. Peritonitis
   e. Penetration into surrounding tissues (e.g., acute pancreatitis)
   f. Obstruction resulting from ulcer scarring at the pylorus
   g. MI
   h. Cerebral infarction
   i. DIC
   j. Sepsis
   k. Shock: hypovolemia or septic

Hepatic Failure/Encephalopathy

Definitions

1. Hepatic failure: inability of the liver to perform organ functions
2. Hepatic encephalopathy: neurologic failure as a result of hepatic failure

Etiology

1. Acute liver failure
   a. Viruses
      (1) Fulminant viral hepatitis (Table 6-10)
      (2) Herpes simplex
      (3) Herpes zoster
      (4) Epstein-Barr
      (5) Adenovirus
      (6) Cytomegalovirus
   b. Hepatotoxic drugs (Box 6-1; e.g., acetaminophen, halothane, methyldopa, isoniazid [INH], and 3,4-methylenedioxymethamphetamine [Ecstasy]) or toxins (*Amanita* mushrooms, carbon tetrachloride, sea anemone sting)
   c. Ischemia (e.g., shock and MODS)
   d. Trauma
   e. Reye's syndrome
   f. Budd-Chiari syndrome (i.e., hepatic vein obstruction)
   g. Acute fatty liver of pregnancy
   h. Acute hepatic vein occlusion

Table 6-10 Types of Viral Hepatitis

Type	Route	Incubation Period	Onset/Chronicity	Comments
A (HAV; infectious hepatitis)	Fecal-oral	2-6 weeks	Acute onset Chronicity does not develop	• 99% resolves, but 1% becomes fulminant • Treatment is supportive
B (HBV; serum hepatitis)	Parenteral Sexual Perinatal	4-24 weeks	Insidious onset Chronicity develops in less than 5%	• 1% becomes fulminant • 15%-25% develop liver cancer • Treatment includes interferon alfa-2b (Intron A); antivirals such as lamivudine (Epivir) or famciclovir (Famvir) also may be prescribed
C (HCV; non-A, non-B hepatitis; posttransfusion hepatitis)	Parenteral Sexual Perinatal	2-20 weeks	Insidious onset Chronicity develops in 50%-60%	• 20%-50% develop cirrhosis • 20% develop liver cancer • 20% develop liver failure • Treatment includes interferon alfa-2b (Intron A) or peginterferon alpha-2b (PEG-Intron) and ribavirin (Virazole); may also include corticosteroids
D (HDV; delta virus)	Superinfection or co-infection in patient with chronic hepatitis B	4-24 weeks	Acute onset Chronicity common with superinfection	• Up to 30% become fulminant • Most have worsening active hepatitis • Treatment is as for hepatitis B
E (HEV; enteric non-A, non-B hepatitis)	Fecal-oral Perinatal	2-8 weeks	Acute onset Chronicity does not develop	• Generally benign and self-limiting; however, 10%-20% mortality when occurs during pregnancy
F (HFV)	Parenteral Sexual Perinatal			• Now considered a variant of hepatitis B
G (HGV)				• Very little known

2. Chronic liver failure with an acute situation (e.g., peritonitis, GI hemorrhage, and catabolism)
   a. Cirrhosis
   b. Wilson's disease
   c. Primary or metastatic tumors of the liver

Pathophysiology

1. Cirrhosis
   a. Liver parenchymal cells are destroyed progressively and are replaced with fibrotic tissue, resulting in impaired hepatic function; three-quarters of the liver can be destroyed before symptoms appear.
   b. Distortion, twisting, and constriction of central sections cause impedance of portal blood flow and portal hypertension.
2. Fulminant hepatitis: liver cells fail to regenerate, and necrosis occurs
3. Portal hypertension and impaired hepatic function
   a. Esophageal varices may develop (see Upper Gastrointestinal Hemorrhage).
   b. Splenomegaly may occur, causing thrombocytopenia; thrombocytopenia and vitamin K deficiency cause clotting abnormalities.
   c. Liver is unable to produce adequate amounts of bile and is impaired in protein, carbohydrate, and fat metabolism.
      (1) Serum bilirubin levels become elevated since the liver is unable to conjugate the bilirubin and make bile
      (2) Deficiency of fat-soluble vitamins may occur since bile salts are required for absorption
      (3) Hypoglycemia may occur because the liver cannot perform the functions of glycogenolysis (i.e., breaking down stored carbohydrates to simple sugars) and gluconeogenesis (i.e., converting fats and proteins to simple sugars)
   d. Liver is unable to manufacture plasma proteins and inactivate hormones (e.g., aldosterone and estrogen).
      (1) Decreased plasma proteins (albumin being the most important) reduce the capillary oncotic pressure, so fluid shifts from the vascular space to third spaces such as the interstitial space (i.e., peripheral edema), the intraperitoneal space (i.e., ascites), and the interpleural space (i.e., pleural effusion).
      (2) Increased circulating levels of aldosterone cause continuing retention of sodium and water by the kidney along with increased excretion of potassium; fluid and electrolyte imbalances occur.
         (a) Hypokalemia
         (b) Hypocalcemia
         (c) Hypomagnesemia
         (d) Sodium levels may be increased, normal, or decreased depending on the intravascular volume and serum osmolality
      (3) Hepatorenal syndrome may develop.
         (a) Type of renal failure in which a gradual loss of function occurs but with no signs of tissue damage
         (b) Associated with cirrhosis of the liver and hepatitis
         (c) Cause not completely understood, but seems to result from decreased albumin and portal hypertension
   e. Liver is unable to detoxify toxins and drugs and to remove bacteria.
      (1) Toxins associated with hepatic failure: ammonia, cytokines, endotoxin, tumor necrosis factor alpha, bilirubin, and bile acids
      (2) Cumulative drug effects frequently occur because the liver is unable to biotransform drugs into inactive and, with some drugs, active metabolites; reduced intravascular volume impairs the ability of the kidney to excrete the active and inactive metabolites
      (3) Hepatic encephalopathy eventually may occur
         (a) Inability to convert ammonia, a by-product of protein metabolism, to urea causes increased serum ammonia levels.
         (b) Increased cerebral blood flow increases vasoactive peptides, which alter the blood-brain barrier, allowing neurotoxins (e.g., ammonia) to accumulate in the brain.
      (4) Increased susceptibility to increase and sepsis occurs due to:
         (a) Increased amounts of viable bacteria in the circulating blood
         (b) Neutrophil malfunction
         (c) Complement deficiency
         (d) Macrophage deficiency
   f. Liver is unable to store vitamins and manufacture clotting factors.
      (1) Fat-soluble vitamin (A, D, E, K) deficiencies may occur.
      (2) Clotting abnormalities occur because the liver manufactures all except two of the clotting factors.

Clinical Presentation

1. Subjective
   a. History of precipitating event
   b. Irritability
   c. Personality change
   d. Disorientation
   e. Weakness, fatigue
   f. Anorexia, nausea, vomiting
   g. RUQ dull abdominal pain
   h. Abdominal fullness
   i. Change in bowel habits
   j. Weight loss
2. Objective
   a. General: emaciation, cachectic appearance
   b. Cardiovascular
      (1) Tachycardia, dysrhythmias
      (2) Bounding pulses

(3) Hypertension or hypotension
(4) Flushed skin
(5) Spider angioma on upper trunk, face, neck, and arms
(6) Jugular venous distention
(7) Distended superficial vessels on abdomen (caput medusae)

c. Pulmonary
(1) Tachypnea or hyperpnea
(2) Decreased respiratory excursion

d. Neurologic
(1) Peripheral neuropathy
(2) Slow, slurred speech
(3) Asterixis
(4) Hyperactive reflexes
(5) Seizures
(6) Positive Babinski's reflex in encephalopathy
(7) Extreme lethargy or coma in encephalopathy

e. GI
(1) Fetor hepaticus
(2) Ascites
(3) Hematemesis
(4) Hepatomegaly early; liver atrophy occurs later
(5) Splenomegaly
(6) Ascites
(7) Bowel sounds: diminished
(8) Clay-colored (pale) stools if biliary obstruction
(9) Steatorrhea (i.e., excessive fat in stool)
(10) Esophageal varices and/or hemorrhoids

f. Renal
(1) Oliguria
(2) Dark amber urine

g. Hematologic/immunologic
(1) Abnormal bruising, bleeding
(2) Susceptibility to infection
(3) Poor wound healing

h. Integumentary
(1) Jaundice; usually noted in the sclera first
(2) Palmar erythema
(3) Petechiae
(4) Bruises
(5) Edema
(6) Pruritus
(7) Spider angioma

i. Endocrine changes
(1) Hypogonadism: testicular atrophy and reduced testosterone levels in men
(2) Gynecomastia in men
(3) Altered hair distribution

3. Diagnostic
a. Serum
(1) Chemistry
(a) Sodium: may be decreased or normal
(b) Potassium: may be decreased
(c) Calcium: may be decreased
(d) Magnesium: may be decreased
(e) BUN: may be elevated because of dehydration, hepatorenal syndrome, or GI bleeding
(f) Glucose: may be elevated or decreased
(g) Creatinine: may be elevated because of hepatorenal syndrome
(h) Cholesterol: elevated
(i) ALT, AST, LDH: elevated
(i) AST/ALT ratio greater than 1 suggests chronic liver failure or tumor
(ii) AST/ALT ratio less than 1 suggests hepatitis
(j) Alkaline phosphatase: elevated
(k) Bilirubin: elevated
(l) Ammonia: elevated in encephalopathy
(m) Total protein, serum albumin, fibrinogen: decreased
(2) Hematology
(a) Hgb, Hct: may be decreased if hemorrhage or hypersplenism
(b) WBC count: decreased; if normal or elevated, infection may be present
(c) Platelets: decreased in splenomegaly
(3) Clotting studies: prolonged PT and aPTT
(4) Arterial blood gases
(a) Respiratory alkalosis
(b) Hypoxemia may be seen

b. Urine
(1) Sodium: decreased
(2) Bilirubin: elevated in biliary obstruction
(3) Urobilinogen
(a) Elevated in hepatocellular disease
(b) Decreased in complete biliary obstruction

c. Chest x-ray: may show pleural effusion or atelectasis
d. Flat plate of abdomen: may reveal hepatosplenomegaly; abdominal haziness may be seen if ascites is present
e. Abdominal ultrasound: may reveal intraabdominal fluid if ascites is present
f. Barium swallow or esophagogastroduodenoscopy: may be done to identify presence of esophageal varices
g. Liver scan: may show diffuse changes of cirrhosis
h. Liver biopsy: may show fatty infiltration (early) or severe degeneration and scarring (advanced)
i. ERCP: may identify biliary obstruction
j. Paracentesis: cytologic examination may be done to rule out malignancy; ascites fluid has low specific gravity, low protein concentration, and cell counts
k. Electroencephalogram: shows abnormal and generalized slowing in patients with encephalopathy
l. Lumbar puncture: may be done to rule out neurologic cause of altered consciousness; cerebrospinal fluid shows increase in glutamine

4. Stages of encephalopathy (Table 6-11)

Table 6-11 Stages of Encephalopathy

Stage	Signs and Symptoms
I	• Mild confusion • Decreased attention span • Difficulty performing simple arithmetic computations (e.g., counting backward from 100 by sevens) • Decreased response time • Forgetfulness • Mood changes • Slurred speech • Personality changes • Irritability • Disruption in sleep-wake patterns • EEG normal
II	• Lethargy • Confusion • Apathy • Aberrant behavior • Tremor and asterixis (also referred to as *liver flap*) • Inability to reproduce simple designs (constructional apraxia) • Slowing of normal EEG
III	• Somnolent with diminished responsiveness to verbal stimuli • Severe confusion and incoherence following arousal • Speech incomprehensible • Tremor and asterixis • Hyperactive deep tendon reflexes • Hyperventilation • EEG abnormal
IV	• No response to stimuli or abnormal (e.g., decorticate or decerebrate) posturing to stimuli • Areflexia except for pathologic reflexes • Positive Babinski's reflex • Fetor hepaticus • EEG abnormal

EEG, Electroencephalogram.

Nursing Diagnoses

1. Impaired Gas Exchange related to ventilation/perfusion mismatching and intrapulmonary shunting
2. Ineffective Breathing Pattern related to diminished diaphragmatic excursion caused by ascites
3. Risk for Deficient Fluid Volume related to fluid sequestration (e.g., ascites, peripheral edema, and pleural effusion), hypoalbuminemia, and diuretic therapy
4. Decreased Cardiac Output related to decreased preload
5. Risk for Excess Fluid Volume related to altered regulatory mechanisms and increased circulating aldosterone
6. Sensory/Perceptual Alterations related to elevated toxins
7. Activity Intolerance related to fatigue, abnormal carbohydrate metabolism, and protein catabolism
8. Pain related to RUQ pain, pruritus, and ascites
9. Imbalanced Nutrition: Less than Body Requirements related to anorexia, nausea, and malabsorption
10. Risk for Injury related to coagulopathy, altered consciousness, and seizures
11. Impaired Skin Integrity related to skin fragility and pruritus
12. Risk for Infection related to hepatic dysfunction
13. Interrupted Family Processes related to situational crisis, powerlessness, and change in role
14. Deficient Knowledge related to required lifestyle changes

Collaborative Management

1. Identify and treat cause of hepatic failure.
   a. Administer *N*-acetylcysteine (Mucomyst) for acetaminophen toxicity; drug must be administered within 24 hours of acetaminophen ingestion.
   b. Administer antivirals (e.g., acyclovir or ganciclovir) as prescribed for viral causes; interferon also may be prescribed.
   c. Prevent further injury to the liver.
      (1) Avoid hepatotoxic drugs.
      (2) Avoid alcohol-containing mouthwash or medications.
   d. Monitor liver function studies.
2. Maintain airway, oxygenation, and ventilation.
   a. Elevate HOB 30 to 45 degrees, especially if ascites restricts diaphragmatic excursion.
   b. Monitor patient for and prevent aspiration.
      (1) Use artificial airways as necessary in patients with altered consciousness and airway protective mechanisms (e.g., gag reflex).
      (2) Intubation usually is required at stage III hepatic encephalopathy.

c. Administer oxygen as necessary to maintain Sao_2 at 95% unless contraindicated; in patients with COPD, administer oxygen to achieve an Spo_2 of ~90%.
d. Assist in management of ascites, which causes decreased diaphragmatic excursion and ventilation difficulties.
   (1) Monitor closely for clinical indications of atelectasis.
   (2) Assist with paracentesis as necessary; patient may need paracentesis if extremely dyspneic.
   (3) Administer aldosterone antagonists (also referred to as *potassium-sparing diuretics;* e.g., spironolactone [Aldactone]) as prescribed; loop diuretics also may be required because aldosterone antagonists tend to lose their effectiveness over time.
   (4) Restrict sodium to 500 mg/day, and restrict fluids to 1500 mL/day as prescribed; be alert to clinical indications of hypovolemia.
   (5) LeVeen or Denver shunt may be performed when patient is stable.
      (a) Surgical procedures that shunt ascites fluid into the superior vena cava
      (b) LeVeen shunt uses positive abdominal pressure caused by the diaphragm descent during inspiration to open a intraperitoneal valve and shunt fluid from the peritoneum to the superior vena cava
      (c) Denver shunt adds a subcutaneous pump that can be compressed manually to irrigate the intraperitoneal tubing
e. Control respiratory alkalosis associated with hyperammonemia.
   (1) Avoid assist-control mode because it will perpetuate the problem.
   (2) Use synchronized intermittent mandatory ventilation; muscle paralysis and sedation may be required to control $Paco_2$ levels.
f. Monitor patient closely for ARDS.
   (1) Monitor patient for clinical indications of respiratory distress and Spo_2.
   (2) Use mechanical ventilation strategies to prevent ventilator-induced lung injury: tidal volume ~6 mL/kg.

3. Maintain adequate circulating volume and fluid and electrolyte balance.
   a. Monitor patient closely for indications of fluid and electrolyte imbalances.
      (1) Monitor vital signs and hemodynamic parameters; invasive hemodynamic monitoring usually is indicated in stage III and IV hepatic encephalopathy.
      (2) Weigh patient daily at same time on the same scale.
      (3) Measure abdominal girth daily for patients with ascites.
      (4) Monitor serum osmolality, sodium, potassium, calcium, and magnesium.
   b. Maintain circulating blood volume.
      (1) Administer colloids as prescribed to improve capillary oncotic pressure and reduce third spacing; avoid protein-containing colloids (e.g., albumin) in hepatic encephalopathy.
      (2) Administer crystalloids as prescribed; avoid lactated Ringer's solution because the liver is responsible for converting lactate to bicarbonate.
   c. Maintain vascular tone: vasopressors may be necessary especially in stage III or IV hepatic encephalopathy.
   d. Administer electrolyte replacement as prescribed.
   e. Monitor for hepatorenal syndrome.
      (1) Observe urine output closely; note clinical indications of hepatorenal syndrome.
         (a) Oliguria
         (b) Low urinary sodium
         (c) Elevated BUN and serum creatinine
      (2) Administer diuretics as prescribed while monitoring closely for clinical indications of intravascular depletion and azotemia.
         (a) Avoid thiazide diuretics.
         (b) Use aldosterone antagonists (also frequently referred to as *potassium-sparing diuretics*; e.g., spironolactone [Aldactone]) as prescribed.
         (c) Use loop diuretics as prescribed; sometimes they are administered after albumin.
            (i) Albumin pulls fluid back into the intravascular space.
            (ii) Furosemide (Lasix) then eliminates fluids by preventing reabsorption of sodium and water in the renal tubules.
      (3) Prepare patient for hemodialysis or continuous renal replacement therapy (CRRT) as prescribed; unfortunately, frequently the patient is unresponsive to treatment.
         (a) CRRT is preferred because it is less likely to precipitate rapid osmolar shifts that can cause intracranial hypertension.
   f. Administer H_2 receptor antagonists and/or antacids as prescribed to maintain pH at 3.5 to 5 to reduce the risk of stress ulcer and GI hemorrhage.

4. Prevent and reduce elevated levels of toxins including ammonia.
   a. Stop nitrogen-containing drugs: ammonium chloride and urea.
   b. Administer neomycin (an aminoglycoside) orally or via NG tube as prescribed to kill the bacteria that convert nitrogenous wastes to ammonia.
      (1) Monitor for auditory or renal toxicity, because small amounts of neomycin are absorbed.

c. Administer lactulose (combination of galactose and fructose) orally or via NG tube as prescribed.
   (1) Acts as a chelating (bonds with) agent of ammonia by changing gut pH, which results in ammonia excretion
   (2) Changes gut flora to foster growth of non–ammonia-forming bacteria
   (3) Acts as an osmotic laxative; dose usually is adjusted for two semiformed stools per day
d. Administer magnesium citrate orally and/or tap water enemas as prescribed to remove nitrogenous wastes from the GI tract.
e. Prevent constipation with fiber, stool softeners, and enemas.
f. Assist with the use of liver support systems.
   (1) Hemodialysis: blood circulated through a porous filter for rapid removal of fluid and solutes
   (2) CRRT: blood circulated through a porous filter for slow removal of fluid and solutes
   (3) Hemoperfusion: hemodialysis or CRRT with a charcoal or resin exchange filter added
   (4) Therapeutic plasma exchange: plasma removed and replaced by donor plasma
   (5) Bioartificial liver support: blood flows through a hollow fiber cartridge loaded with cultured human or porcine hepatocytes
   (6) Extracorporal liver perfusion: blood circulated through a human or animal liver in vitro

5. Prevent, assess for, and treat intracranial hypertension and progression of hepatic encephalopathy.
   a. Perform frequent neurologic checks; invasive ICP monitoring may be used, especially in grade III and IV hepatic encephalopathy.
   b. Avoid hepatotoxic agents (Box 6-1).
   c. Avoid sedatives and analgesics and/or reduce dosage if necessary; diphenhydramine (Benadryl) or oxazepam (Serax) may be used for restlessness because they can be eliminated safely.
   d. Provide adequate rest; maintain bed rest in hepatic encephalopathy.
   e. Avoid activities that increase ICP (see Intracranial Hypertension in Chapter 7).
      (1) Teach the patient to avoid the Valsalva maneuver and other activities that increase intraabdominal or intrathoracic pressure.
      (2) Maintain normal $PaCO_2$ and hypoxemia, which increase ICP.
   f. Institute seizure precautions.
   g. Administer mannitol (Osmitrol) and/or drainage of cerebrospinal fluid (if ICP catheter in place) as prescribed for cerebral edema.

6. Decrease portal hypertension.
   a. Administer beta-blockers as prescribed.
   b. Prepare the patient for a shunt as requested.
      (1) Interventional radiologic procedure: TIPS (described under Upper Gastrointestinal Hemorrhage)
      (2) Surgical procedure (e.g., portacaval shunt): associated with higher incidence of hepatic encephalopathy than TIPS

7. Maintain normal serum glucose and nutritional status.
   a. Monitor serum glucose every 4 to 6 hours.
   b. Administer IV dextrose solution continuously; 10% dextrose may be required to prevent hypoglycemia.
   c. Increase dietary protein (0.6 to 1 g/kg/day) for patients with cirrhosis and hepatic failure, but restrict dietary protein (to less than 0.5 g/kg/day) in hepatic encephalopathy.
      (1) Ensure that adequate CHO are provided to prevent muscle (protein) catabolism and muscle wasting (caloric requirements 35 to 40 kcal/kg/day).
      (2) Add protein in 20-g increments during recovery from encephalopathy.
   d. Use appropriate route for nutritional support.
      (1) Oral: Administer antiemetics as prescribed before each meal and whenever indicated to prevent nausea (nausea is a significant impairment to oral nutritional intake in these patients).
      (2) Enteral
         (a) Necessary in patients with altered consciousness
         (b) Elemental formulae (e.g., Vivonex) frequently used while maintaining protein restrictions if indicated (i.e., hepatic encephalopathy)
      (3) Parenteral
         (a) Branched-chain amino acid formulae may be used in encephalopathy; dextrose and lipids are needed to prevent the metabolism of parenteral amino acids or somatic protein (i.e., catabolism) for energy requirements.
   e. Administer vitamins and minerals.
      (1) Fat-soluble vitamins (i.e., A, D, E, and K)
      (2) Thiamine and other B vitamins

8. Prevent and monitor for injury and infection.
   a. Prevent and monitor for skin breakdown.
      (1) Alleviate pruritus.
         (a) Cornstarch baths
         (b) Skin lubricating lotions
      (2) Apply cotton gloves to prevent scratching while sleeping.
      (3) Administer cholestyramine (Questran) as prescribed to reduce bile pigment accumulation in skin.
   b. Prevent and monitor for bleeding.
      (1) Avoid aspirin and NSAIDs.
      (2) Avoid invasive procedures, including injections, if possible.

(3) Administer vitamin K, fresh frozen plasma, and platelets as prescribed.
(4) Administer aminocaproic acid (Amicar) as prescribed.

c. Monitor patient closely for clinical indications of infection and sepsis.
(1) Administer antimicrobials as prescribed: antibiotics and antifungals.

9. Assess patient for clinical indications of alcohol withdrawal syndrome (Box 6-3).
   a. Administer sedatives as prescribed: most of these agents, including chlordiazepoxide (Librium) and diazepam (Valium), are hepatotoxic, so doses are adjusted and liver enzymes are monitored.
   b. Avoid alcohol-containing mouthwash or medications.
10. Participate in consideration of long-term treatment of hepatic failure.
    a. Early evaluation of candidacy for liver transplantation
11. Monitor for complications.
    a. Malnutrition resulting in immunosuppression, poor wound healing, and edema
    b. Coagulopathy
    c. Hemorrhage may be due to the following:
       (1) Esophageal varices
       (2) Coagulopathy
       (3) DIC
    d. Hypoglycemia
    e. Electrolyte imbalance
    f. Acute respiratory failure related to intrapulmonary shunt or noncardiac pulmonary edema
    g. Pancreatitis
    h. Infection, sepsis
    i. Acute renal failure related to hepatorenal syndrome, acute tubular necrosis, or hypovolemia
    j. Seizures
    k. Cerebral edema

Acute Pancreatitis

Definition

Acute inflammation of the pancreas; forms include the following:

1. Mild acute pancreatitis (previously referred to as *interstitial pancreatitis*): edematous pancreas with little necrosis damage; hypovolemia may occur as a result of fluid leak into peritoneal cavity
2. Severe acute pancreatitis (previously referred to as *necrotizing pancreatitis*); extensive necrosis of pancreas and peripancreatic tissue and fat; erosion into blood vessels; hemorrhage occurs; SIRS frequently occurs

B. Etiology

1. Obstruction of common bile duct
   a. Cholelithiasis
   b. Post-ERCP
2. Alcoholism
   a. Chronic alcohol intake leads to secretory and structural changes in the pancreas, contributing to duct obstruction.
   b. Alcohol increases the amount of trypsinogen.
3. Hypertriglyceridemia
4. Drugs
   a. Thiazide diuretics
   b. Furosemide
   c. Estrogen
   d. Procainamide
   e. Tetracycline
   f. Sulfonamides
   g. Corticosteroids
   h. Azathioprine (Imuran)
   i. Opiates
5. Peptic ulcer with perforation
6. Cancer, especially tumors of pancreas or lung
7. Injury to pancreas
   a. Trauma
   b. Surgical
      (1) Gastric
      (2) Biliary
      (3) Duodenal
   c. Iatrogenic
8. Radiation injury
9. Pregnancy: third trimester; ectopic pregnancy
10. Ovarian cyst
11. Hyperparathyroidism or other causes of hypercalcemia
12. Lupus erythematosus
13. Infections
    a. Mumps
    b. Coxsackievirus B
    c. *Mycoplasma*
    d. Infectious mononucleosis
    e. Viral hepatitis
    f. Human immunodeficiency virus
    g. Intestinal parasites (e.g., *Ascaris*)
14. Ischemia (e.g., shock and MODS)
15. Cardiopulmonary bypass
16. Infection, sepsis
17. Hereditary factors
18. Idiopathic (20% of cases)

Pathophysiology

1. Etiologic factor triggers activation of pancreatic enzymes and pancreatic cell injury
2. Autodigestion of pancreas is caused by the escape of prematurely activated proteolytic enzymes from the acinar space or cells into the periacinal tissue
   a. Trypsin causes edema, necrosis, and hemorrhage.
   b. Elastase causes hemorrhage.
   c. Phospholipase A causes fat necrosis and damages the pulmonary capillary endothelium; may lead to ARDS.
   d. Kallikrein causes edema, vascular permeability, smooth muscle contraction, and shock.
3. Damage to the acinar cells

4. Erosion into vessels may cause hemorrhage
5. Inflammatory process causes necrosis of fat in pancreas and exudates with high albumin content leading to hypoalbuminemia and ascites; fat necrosis results in precipitation of calcium, leading to hypocalcemia
6. Release of necrotic toxins may cause sepsis and/or SIRS

Clinical Presentation

1. Subjective
   a. Abdominal pain
      (1) Precipitation: may occur after a heavy meal or a drinking binge
      (2) Palliation: may be eased by leaning forward or by assuming fetal position
      (3) Quality: "boring"
      (4) Region: LUQ or epigastrium
      (5) Radiation: to back or flanks
      (6) Severity: moderate to severe
      (7) Timing: sudden onset; constant
   b. Associated symptoms
      (1) Abdominal tenderness, guarding
      (2) Nausea, vomiting, retching
      (3) Dyspepsia
      (4) Flatulence
      (5) Weight loss
      (6) Weakness
2. Objective
   a. Tachycardia
   b. Hypotension may be seen because of decreased circulating volume resulting from effusion or hemorrhage; may be decreased because of septic shock
   c. Fever: usually low grade (e.g., 37.8° to 39°C)
   d. Jaundice if biliary obstruction
   e. Vomiting
   f. Hematemesis
   g. Grey Turner's sign or Cullen's sign may be seen in hemorrhagic pancreatitis
   h. Abdominal distention
   i. Indications of peritoneal irritation: involuntary guarding during palpation of the abdomen and rebound tenderness
   j. Epigastric mass may be palpable
   k. Ascites may be present
   l. Decreased bowel sound
   m. Steatorrhea (bulky, pale, foul-smelling, floating)
   n. Breath sound changes: may be diminished because of atelectasis, pleural effusion, or ARDS; crackles also may be heard
   o. Chvostek's or Trousseau's signs may be positive in hypocalcemia
3. Diagnostic
   a. Serum
      (1) Chemistry
         (a) Potassium: decreased
         (b) Calcium: decreased
         (c) Magnesium: decreased
         (d) Glucose: elevated if endocrine function of the pancreas is compromised
         (e) Triglycerides: may be elevated
         (f) Amylase: usually elevated
            (i) Peaks at 4 to 24 hours after onset of symptoms; usually returns to normal within 4 days
            (ii) May not be elevated when pancreatitis is due to hypertriglyceridemia
         (g) Lipase: elevated
            (i) Stays elevated longer than amylase
            (ii) More specific than amylase
         (h) Albumin: decreased
         (i) BUN: may be elevated because of hypovolemia
         (j) AST, ALT, LDH, alkaline phosphatase, bilirubin: elevated in liver or biliary disease
      (2) Hematology
         (a) Hct: decreased with hemorrhage; elevated with hemoconcentration caused by third spacing
         (b) WBC count: usually elevated with shift to the left
      (3) Arterial blood gases
         (a) Metabolic acidosis
         (b) Respiratory complications may cause respiratory acidosis and hypoxemia
      (4) Urine: amylase usually elevated
      (5) Stool: increase in fecal fat
      (6) ECG: may suggest MI (e.g., ST-T wave elevations)
      (7) Chest x-ray
         (a) May show bilateral or only pleural effusion on left side, elevated left hemidiaphragm, and atelectasis of the left side
         (b) May show pulmonary complications of pancreatitis (e.g., atelectasis, pneumonia, ARDS, or pleural effusion)
      (8) Flat plate of abdomen
         (a) May show cause (e.g., cholelithiasis)
         (b) May show ileus and bowel dilation
         (c) May show calcified pancreatic stones
      (9) Upper GI
         (a) May show delayed gastric emptying
         (b) May show enlargement of duodenum
         (c) May show presence of dilated loop of smooth bowel adjacent to the pancreas
      (10) Abdominal ultrasound: may show pancreatic swelling, edema, gallstones, pseudocyst, or peripancreatic fluid collections
      (11) CT scan with contrast
         (a) May show enlargement, edema, or necrosis of the pancreas
         (b) May show complications of pancreatitis (e.g., pancreatic pseudocyst or abscess)

(c) Balthazar and Ranson's system for grading pancreatitis by CT findings
(i) Grade A: normal pancreas
(ii) Grade B: focal or diffuse enlargement of pancreas
(iii) Grade C: mild peripancreatic inflammatory changes
(iv) Grade D: fluid collection in a single location
(v) Grade E: multiple fluid collections or gas within the pancreas or peripancreatic inflammation
(12) MRI: shows inflammatory changes within the pancreas
(13) ERCP
(a) Contraindicated in acute pancreatitis; used more often in chronic pancreatitis
(b) Identifies ductal changes or calculi
(14) Hepatobiliary iminodiacetic acid scan: may identify hepatocellular disease from biliary obstruction as cause of pancreatitis
(15) Peritoneal lavage: positive for blood in hemorrhagic pancreatitis

4. Ranson's prognostic criteria
a. Scoring
(1) Each of the following criteria increases the severity (and mortality) in pancreatitis
(a) Only one to two criteria: mild pancreatitis; mortality approximately 1%
(b) More than six criteria: severe pancreatitis; predicted mortality greater than 60%
b. Criteria
(1) At the time of admission or diagnosis
(a) Age over 55 years
(b) WBC count more than 16,000 cells/mm^3
(c) Serum glucose greater than 200 mg/dL
(d) Serum LDH greater than 350 units/L
(e) Serum AST greater than 250 units/L
(2) After 48 hours
(a) Hct drop greater than 10%
(b) Increase in BUN greater than 5 mg/dL
(c) Calcium less than 8 mg/dL
(d) Base deficit greater than 4 mEq/L
(e) Estimated fluid sequestration greater than 6 L
(f) $Pa{O_2}$ less than 60 mm Hg

Nursing Diagnoses

1. Pain related to pancreatic inflammation and peritoneal inflammation
2. Deficient Fluid Volume related to vomiting, NG suction, hemorrhage, and fluid sequestration within peritoneum
3. Decreased Cardiac Output related to decreased preload
4. Impaired Gas Exchange related to diminished lung expansion, anemia, atelectasis, and ARDS
5. Impaired Nutrition: Less than Body Requirements related to poor intake, impaired digestion, NPO or dietary restrictions, and hypermetabolism
6. Risk for Infection related to peritonitis and abscess
7. Risk for Injury related to electrolyte imbalance
8. Interrupted Family Processes related to situational crisis, powerlessness, and change in role
9. Deficient Knowledge related to required lifestyle changes

Collaborative Management

1. Maintain airway, oxygenation, and ventilation.
a. Elevate HOB 30 to 45 degrees especially if ascites restricts diaphragmatic excursion.
b. Administer oxygen as necessary to maintain $Sa{O_2}$ of 95% unless contraindicated; in patients with COPD, administer oxygen to achieve an $Sp{O_2}$ of ~90%.
c. Monitor $Sp{O_2}$ closely, and evaluate work of breathing in detection of development of atelectasis and/or ARDS.
2. Maintain adequate circulating volume and fluid and electrolyte balance.
a. Administer crystalloids and colloids as prescribed to restore circulating blood volume.
b. Monitor sodium, calcium, potassium, magnesium, and phosphate.
(1) Administer calcium replacement orally or IV as prescribed.
(2) Administer potassium replacement as prescribed.
(3) Restrict sodium to 500 mg/day for patients with ascites.
c. Measure abdominal girth daily in patients with ascites.
d. Weigh daily at same time on same scale.
3. Decrease release of and destruction by pancreatic enzymes.
a. Maintain NPO status during acute phase.
b. Insert NG tube to decompress the stomach and decrease risk of vomiting until ileus is resolved.
c. Administer drugs as prescribed to decrease secretion of pancreatic enzymes (NOTE: no evidence of effectiveness)
(1) Octreotide acetate (Sandostatin) IV or subcutaneously
(2) Histamine$_2$ receptor antagonists IV
d. Keep environment free of food odors.
e. Perform mouth care with water or normal saline only; do not use alcohol-containing or flavored mouthwash or toothpaste.

4. Prevent and treat pain and discomfort.
   a. Maintain bed rest; encourage knee flexing while patient is in supine position to relax abdominal muscles.
   b. Maintain quiet environment, comfortable temperature, and dim lighting.
   c. Administer analgesics.
      (1) Opiates (e.g., morphine and hydromorphone) preferably administered via patient-controlled analgesia
         (a) NOTE: Though meperidine (Demerol) for years has been considered the analgesic of choice in acute pancreatitis, recent studies show no significant difference between morphine and meperidine in the degree of spasm of the sphincter of Oddi.
      (2) Neurolytic block of the celiac plexus for severe persistent pain.
   d. Use nonpharmacologic pain relief methods (e.g., imagery and distraction).
   e. Treat nausea with prescribed antiemetics.
   f. Ensure adequate sleep and rest.
5. Administer appropriate nutritional support considering restrictions.
   a. Administer nutritional support during acute phase of illness.
      (1) Parenteral nutrition initially
      (2) Enteral nutrition below the duodenum after ileus is resolved
         (a) Though enteral feeding traditionally has been thought to be contraindicated in acute pancreatitis, recent studies indicate that enteral feeding may be administered safely if the tube is below the ligament of Treitz (e.g., jejunostomy tube).
         (b) Advantages over parenteral nutrition include the following:
            (i) Maintains immune responsiveness and gut integrity
            (ii) Reduces risk of bacterial translocation
            (iii) Fewer complications
   b. Clear liquids or elemental diet (e.g., Vivonex) may be used after inflammation subsides (pain subsides, serum amylase is normal), progressing to low-fat, full liquids and eventually progressing to a regular diet.
   c. Avoid alcohol and food high in fats.
   d. Administer fat-soluble vitamins, thiamine, and folic acid as prescribed.
   e. Monitor serum glucose levels closely, and administer glucose or insulin as indicated.
6. Prevent and monitor for infection.
   a. Administer antibiotics prophylactically as prescribed.
      (1) Antibiotics are prescribed that effectively penetrate the pancreatic tissue and provide good coverage against gram-negative enteric and anaerobic organisms (e.g., imipenem/cilastatin [Primaxin], ofloxacin [Floxin], or metronidazole [Flagyl]).
      (2) If no improvement after 1 week, CT–guided aspiration may be performed; bacteria in aspirate suggest infected pancreatic necrosis and indicate the need for surgery.
   b. Monitor for clinical indications of abscess formation (e.g., increase in abdominal pain, vomiting, fever, and leukocytosis).
7. Prepare patient for surgical measures for relief of pancreatitis if necessary (during acute phase, surgery is performed only if absolutely necessary).
   a. Cholecystectomy if bile reflux is the cause of pancreatitis
   b. Drainage and removal of abscess or pseudocysts
   c. Pancreatic resection/total pancreatectomy
      (1) Used if pancreas and/or other organs are necrotic
      (2) After surgical débridement of necrotic tissue, the abdomen may be left open and packed or closed with drains in place
      (3) Total pancreatectomy; results in diabetes and other metabolic difficulties
         (a) Islet cell autotransplantation sometimes is performed
         (b) Segmental pancreatic autotransplantation sometimes is performed: part of viable pancreatic tissue reimplanted following total pancreatectomy
8. Maintain normal serum glucose levels.
   a. Monitor serum glucose levels closely.
   b. Administer insulin as indicated and prescribed.
   c. Maintain constant infusion of TPN solution or enteral feedings.
9. Assess patient for clinical indications of alcohol withdrawal syndrome (Box 6-3).
   a. If present, administer sedatives as prescribed; most of these agents, including chlordiazepoxide (Librium) and diazepam (Valium), are hepatotoxic; doses are adjusted and liver enzymes are monitored.
   b. Avoid alcohol-containing mouthwash or medications.
10. Monitor patient for complications.
   a. Hypoglycemia or hyperglycemia
   b. Hypocalcemia
   c. Pseudocysts
      (1) Description: a cavity containing inflammatory debris, pancreatic secretions, and necrotic tissue that does not have a lining membrane
      (2) Complications of a pseudocyst include peritonitis, hemorrhage, abscess, or intestinal obstruction
      (3) Collaborative management includes drainage of the pseudocyst by surgical, endoscopic, or percutaneous approach
   d. Pancreatic abscess
      (1) Caused by accumulation of pus in or near the pancreas
      (2) Clinical presentation includes fever, palpable mass, abdominal tenderness, nausea, vomiting, and leukocytosis

(3) Collaborative management includes surgery for drainage

e. Pancreatic fistula
   (1) Caused by a communication between the pancreas and the skin
   (2) Clinical presentation includes drainage of extremely alkaline pancreatic secretions onto the skin and severe excoriation
   (3) Collaborative management includes fluid and electrolyte replacement; octreotide acetate (Sandostatin) may be used

f. Hypovolemic shock
   (1) Caused by exudate of protein-rich fluid into retroperitoneal space or by erosion into the vascular bed and hemorrhage
   (2) Clinical presentation includes tachycardia, hypotension, oliguria, and other indications of hypoperfusion
   (3) Collaborative management includes volume resuscitation, including crystalloids, colloids, and blood administration for hemorrhagic pancreatitis

g. SIRS
h. ARDS
i. DIC
j. Sepsis
k. Acute renal failure
l. Perforation

Intestinal Infarction/Obstruction/ Perforation

Definitions

1. Intestinal infarction: necrosis of the intestinal wall resulting from ischemia
2. Intestinal obstruction: failure of the intestinal contents to progress forward through the lumen of the bowel
   a. Functional obstruction: caused by loss of peristalsis; usually referred to as *paralytic ileus*
   b. Structural (i.e., mechanical) obstruction: caused by factors that occlude the bowel lumen
      (1) Simple: luminal obstruction without compromise of blood supply
      (2) Strangulated: luminal obstruction with compromise of blood supply
3. Intestinal perforation: penetration of the lumen of the intestine with resultant spillage of intestinal contents into the peritoneal cavity

Etiology

1. Infarction
   a. Arteriosclerosis
   b. Vasculitis
   c. Mural thrombus, emboli: post-MI; atrial fibrillation; ventricular aneurysm; endocarditis
   d. Hypercoagulability (e.g., polycythemia and after splenectomy)
   e. Surgical procedures involving aortic clamping (e.g., abdominal aortic aneurysm repair)
   f. Vasopressors
      (1) Endogenous caused by sympathetic nervous system stimulation (e.g., shock)
      (2) Exogenous (e.g., norepinephrine and high-dose dopamine)
   g. Strangulated intestinal obstruction
   h. Intraabdominal infection
   i. Cirrhosis
2. Obstruction
   a. Functional (i.e., paralytic ileus): most common type of intestinal obstruction
      (1) Abdominal surgery
      (2) Hypokalemia
      (3) Intestinal distention
      (4) Peritonitis
      (5) Intestinal ischemia
      (6) Severe trauma
      (7) Spinal cord injury
      (8) Ureteral distention
      (9) Pneumonia
      (10) Pleuritis
      (11) Subphrenic abscess
      (12) Pancreatitis
      (13) Acute cholecystitis
      (14) Pelvic abscess
      (15) Narcotics (e.g., morphine)
      (16) Sepsis
   b. Structural (i.e., mechanical)
      (1) Small bowel: most obstructions occur in the small bowel, especially at the ileum
         (a) Adhesions: most common
         (b) Incarcerated hernia
         (c) Volvulus
         (d) Foreign body
         (e) Neoplasm
      (2) Large bowel: most often the sigmoid colon
         (a) Neoplasm: most common
         (b) Stricture
         (c) Intussusception
         (d) Diverticulitis
         (e) Fecal or barium impaction
3. Perforation
   a. Peptic ulcer
   b. Bowel obstruction
   c. Appendicitis
   d. Penetrating wound

Pathophysiology

1. Infarction
   a. Decrease in blood flow to major mesenteric vessels causes vasoconstriction and vasospasm.
   b. Prolonged ischemia increases the permeability of the bowel and edema of the intestinal wall.
      (1) Normal bowel flora (e.g., *Escherichia coli* and *Klebsiella*) may penetrate the bowel wall, causing peritonitis.
   c. Edema of intestinal wall may cause full-thickness necrosis and bowel perforation with leakage of normal bowel flora into the peritoneal cavity and peritonitis.

2. Obstruction
   a. Obstruction of bowel prevents adequate forward movement of bowel contents
   b. Impairment in digestion
   c. Sequestration of gas and fluids proximal to the obstruction
   d. Shifting of fluids from the bowel into the peritoneal cavity
   e. Dehydration, hypovolemia, shock
   f. Specific to small intestine
      (1) Increased intraabdominal pressure puts pressure on the diaphragm, causing atelectatic changes and, possibly, pneumonia
      (2) Reverse peristalsis occurs with nausea, vomiting, and malnutrition
      (3) Fluid and electrolyte imbalance
   g. Specific to large intestine
      (1) Gas and fluid accumulation above the obstruction
      (2) Fluid and electrolyte imbalance
      (3) Distention of the bowel eventually causes perforation with leakage of intestinal bacteria into the peritoneal cavity, peritonitis, and sepsis
3. Perforation
   a. Leakage of GI content into peritoneal cavity
      (1) Leakage of intestinal flora causes infection
      (2) Chemical irritation causes inflammation
   b. Peritonitis and potentially sepsis

Clinical Presentation

1. Infarction
   a. Subjective
      (1) May have history of precipitating event
      (2) Anorexia
      (3) Pallor
      (4) Abdominal pain
         (a) Severe cramping periumbilical or nonspecific diffuse
         (b) Abdominal pain related to mesenteric ischemia may be referred to as *abdominal angina*
      (5) Abdominal tenderness
      (6) Urgency to have a bowel movement
   b. Objective
      (1) Tachycardia
      (2) Hypotension
      (3) Tachypnea
      (4) Fever
      (5) Clinical indications of dehydration
      (6) Vomiting: persistent, may be bloody
      (7) Abdominal distention
      (8) Abdominal guarding and rigidity
      (9) Urgent and bloody diarrhea
      (10) Hypoactive or absent bowel sounds
      (11) Weight loss
   c. Diagnostic
      (1) Serum
         (a) Chemistry
            (i) BUN: elevated because of dehydration
            (ii) Alkaline phosphatase: elevated
            (iii) Amylase: elevated
         (b) Hematology
            (i) Hct: elevated
            (ii) WBC count: elevated
         (c) Arterial blood gases: metabolic acidosis
      (2) Stool: guaiac positive
      (3) Angiography: show occlusion of the arterial supply
      (4) Sigmoidoscopy: shows dusky, ischemic bowel
2. Obstruction
   a. Small bowel
      (1) Subjective
         (a) May have history of precipitating event
         (b) Severe, sharp, episodic pain; steady, severe, localized pain may signal strangulation
         (c) Changes in bowel habits
            (i) Partial bowel obstruction: normal stools or diarrhea
            (ii) Complete obstruction: absence of stools
      (2) Objective
         (a) Vomiting early: may be projectile and/or fecal
            (i) Clear gastric fluid: obstruction at the pylorus
            (ii) Gastric contents and bile
               a) Obstruction in the proximal small intestine
               b) Paralytic ileus
            (iii) Brown fecal: obstruction in the distal small intestine
         (b) Abdominal distention
         (c) Clinical indications of dehydration
         (d) Bowel sounds: high-pitched
            (i) Increased early
            (ii) Decreased late
      (3) Diagnostic
         (a) Serum
            (i) Chemistry
               a) Sodium: may be decreased, increased, or normal depending on hydration level and serum osmolality
               b) Potassium: decreased
               c) Chloride: decreased
               d) BUN: elevated because of dehydration
            (ii) Hematology
               a) Hct: elevated
               b) WBC count: elevated
            (iii) Arterial blood gases: usually metabolic acidosis, but metabolic alkalosis may be seen with proximal obstruction and gastric losses
         (b) Upper GI: may show point of obstruction
         (c) Flat plate of abdomen: shows dilated loops of gas-filled bowel

(d) CT: aids in differentiation of cause and location of obstruction
(e) MRI: aids in differentiation of cause and location of obstruction

b. Large bowel
(1) Subjective
(a) May have history of precipitating event
(b) Dull pain
(c) Change in bowel habits: thin, ribbonlike stools progressing to constipation to the absence of stools with watery discharge
(d) Decrease in flatus
(2) Objective
(a) Vomiting late
(b) Abdominal distention
(c) Bowel sounds: low pitched
(i) Increased early
(ii) Decreased late
(d) Melena may occur if large bowel obstruction is caused by ulcerative colitis, cancer, or diverticulitis
(3) Diagnostic
(a) Serum
(i) Chemistry
a) Sodium: may be decreased, increased, or normal depending on hydration level and serum osmolality
b) Potassium: decreased
c) Chloride: decreased
d) BUN: elevated because of dehydration
e) CEA: elevated if caused by cancer
(ii) Hematology
a) Hct: may be elevated because of dehydration or decreased because of hemorrhage; large intestinal tumor frequently causes slow bleeding
b) WBC count: elevated
(iii) Arterial blood gases: metabolic acidosis
(b) Stools: may be positive for occult blood in large bowel obstruction resulting from ulcerative colitis, cancer, or diverticulitis
(c) Flat plate of abdomen: shows dilated loops of gas-filled bowel
(d) Barium enema: may show point of obstruction
(e) Endoscopy: obstruction may be visible on sigmoidoscopy or colonoscopy

3. Perforation
a. Subjective
(1) Abdominal pain
(2) Abdominal tenderness
(3) Anorexia
(4) Nausea
b. Objective
(1) Tachycardia
(2) Tachypnea
(3) Fever
(4) Vomiting
(5) Rigid, boardlike abdomen
(6) Rebound tenderness
(7) Absence of liver dullness because of free air in peritoneum
(8) Bowel sounds: diminished or absent
(9) NOTE: Bolded clinical indications frequently are referred to as an *acute abdomen*.
c. Diagnostic
(1) Serum: WBC count is elevated
(2) Flat plate of abdomen: free air in peritoneum may be seen
(3) Upper GI: contraindicated

Nursing Diagnoses

1. Pain related to bowel ischemia, perforation, and peritonitis
2. Deficient Fluid Volume related to vomiting and fluid shifts
3. Impaired Gas Exchange related to diminished lung expansion
4. Risk for Infection related to bowel ischemia and perforation
5. Ineffective Tissue Perfusion: Mesenteric related to mesenteric arterial insufficiency
6. Impaired Nutrition: Less than Body Requirements related to poor intake and altered food metabolism
7. Risk for Constipation related to impaired bowel motility
8. Interrupted Family Processes related to situational crisis, powerlessness, and change in role
9. Deficient Knowledge related to required lifestyle changes

Collaborative Management

1. Maintain airway, oxygenation, and ventilation.
a. Elevate HOB 30 to 45 degrees.
b. Administer oxygen as necessary to maintain Spo_2 at 95% unless contraindicated; in patients with COPD, administer oxygen to achieve an Spo_2 of ~90%.
2. Maintain adequate circulating volume and fluid and electrolyte balance.
a. Assess fluid status.
(1) Obtain patient's weight daily at the same time on the same scale.
(2) Hemodynamic monitoring may be necessary during fluid resuscitation.
b. Administer crystalloids and colloids as prescribed to restore circulating blood volume.
c. Administer blood and blood products as needed; whole blood or packed RBCs should be given early if significant bleeding is suspected; after multiple transfusions, consider replacing clotting factors, platelets, and calcium.
d. Monitor sodium, calcium, potassium, and phosphate; administer electrolyte replacement as indicated.

e. Discontinue vasopressors if they are the cause of ischemia.
3. Prevent and treat pain and discomfort.
   a. Maintain bed rest.
   b. Maintain quiet environment, comfortable temperature, and dim lighting.
   c. Administer analgesics (e.g., morphine) (NOTE: Analgesics sometimes are withheld until the diagnosis is made.)
   d. Encourage knee flexing while patient is in supine position to relax abdominal muscles.
   e. Use nonpharmacologic pain relief methods (e.g., imagery, distraction, and music).
   f. Treat nausea with prescribed antiemetics.
   g. Perform mouth care after emesis.
4. Prevent perforation of bowel if obstruction present.
   a. Discontinue all oral intake.
   b. Insert an NG tube or orogastric tube as prescribed to decompress the stomach, prevent vomiting, and reduce the risk of aspiration.
   c. Administer drugs as prescribed to enhance GI motility in partial intestinal obstruction.
      (1) Erythromycin
      (2) Metoclopramide (Reglan)
      (3) Octreotide (Sandostatin)
   d. Assist in insertion of nasointestinal tube (e.g., Miller-Abbott or Cantor) for proximal decompression of the bowel if indicated; usually this is used if obstruction is thought to be reversible or when the patient is not a safe surgical candidate; the tube is not used in paralytic ileus or complete intestinal obstruction.
      (1) Do not tape at the nose because these tubes move through the GI tract by peristalsis.
      (2) Elevate the HOB 30 degrees and turn the patient every 1 to 2 hours to encourage movement of the tube; these tubes usually move 4 to 5 cm/hr.
      (3) Use pH of aspirate to assess movement of the tube through the pylorus: acidic pH in stomach, alkaline pH in intestine.
      (4) Get flat plate of abdomen as requested to assess final position, and then tape tube in place.
      (5) Provide frequent nose and mouth care while tube is in place.
      (6) Irrigate the tube with 30 mL of isotonic saline as required to maintain tube patency.
   e. Insert a rectal tube as prescribed to reduce trapped air in complete large bowel obstruction.
   f. Prepare patient for therapeutic colonoscopy as requested.
      (1) Air insufflation for intussusception
      (2) Cecal dilation or endoscopic balloon duodenal dilation for small bowel obstruction
   g. Assist with palliative procedures to enhance quality of life in patients with terminal disease associated with bowel obstruction.
      (1) Insertion of distal gastric or jejunal tubes
      (2) Colonic dilation
      (3) Insertion of intestinal stents
5. Prepare the patient for surgery as requested: surgery is indicated for vascular obstruction, complete bowel obstruction, and bowel perforation.
   a. Bowel preparation with cathartics, enemas, and sterilization before surgery
      (1) Nonabsorbable aminoglycoside (e.g., neomycin) usually is used for bowel sterilization.
      (2) Do not give cathartics or enemas for patients who are completely obstructed.
   b. Procedures
      (1) Infarction
         (a) Exploratory laparotomy and embolectomy and/or arterial reconstruction with resection of irreparably damaged bowel
      (2) Obstruction
         (a) Correction of cause
            (i) Laparoscopic adhesiolysis: for obstruction caused by adhesion
            (ii) Herniorrhaphy: for reduction of hernia
            (iii) Reduction of volvulus or intussusception
         (b) Bowel resection: may require temporary or permanent bowel diversion with colostomy
            (i) Right hemicolectomy: for tumors in the cecum and ascending colon
            (ii) Left hemicolectomy: for tumors of the descending and sigmoid colon; prepare patient for the possibility of colostomy (temporary or permanent) in cases of left-sided obstruction
            (iii) Transverse colectomy: for tumors of the middle or left transverse colon
            (iv) Low anterior resection: for proximal and midrectal tumors
            (v) Abdominoperineal resection: for malignant lesions of the lower sigmoid colon, rectum, and anus; requires permanent colostomy
      (3) Perforation
         (a) Repair of perforation may require bowel resection; a temporary bowel diversion may be performed to allow the anastomosis to heal.
         (b) Antibiotic lavage may be done during surgery.
   c. Answer the patient's questions about the planned procedures.
   d. Prepare the patient for adjuvant therapy if required for colon cancer.
      (1) Chemoembolization: the infusion of a concentrated dose of an antineoplastic agent into the hepatic artery to embolize the artery
      (2) Radiation therapy
      (3) Brachytherapy: the placement of radioactive seeds in the area where the tumor was removed

(4) Chemotherapy: the administration of an antineoplastic agent before, during, or after surgery
(5) Cryosurgery: the freezing of liver metastasis
6. Prevent and monitor for infection.
   a. Administer antibiotics as prescribed.
   b. Reduce leakage of intestinal bacteria and risk of peritonitis and sepsis if perforation has occurred.
      (1) Keep the patient immobilized to reduce the chemical irritation to the peritoneum.
      (2) Antibiotics are given preoperatively.
      (3) Antibiotic lavage may be done during surgery.
      (4) Antibiotics are given postoperatively.
   c. Monitor patient closely for clinical indications of infection and sepsis.
      (1) Measure temperature every 4 hours.
      (2) Assess heart rate and BP hourly.
      (3) Note changes in mental status.
      (4) Note changes in color and character of wound drainage.
      (5) Monitor changes in WBC count.
   d. Clean around drains aseptically, and protect skin around drains postoperatively.
7. Administer appropriate nutritional support considering restrictions.
   a. Administer nutritional support parenterally in the acute phase.
   b. Provide oral feedings and advance diet when condition and postoperative paralytic ileus have resolved.
   c. Administer vitamin and mineral supplements as prescribed.
8. Monitor for complications.
   a. Fluid and electrolyte imbalance
   b. Hemorrhage
   c. Sepsis
   d. Peritonitis
   e. Respiratory distress resulting from abdominal distention
   f. Shock: hypovolemic or septic
   g. Abscess
   h. Perforation

Abdominal Trauma

Definition

Trauma that occurs between the nipple line and midthigh

Etiology

1. Penetrating trauma (e.g., motor vehicle collision; assault; sharp instruments [e.g., knife, gunshot wound, or impalement])
2. Blunt trauma (e.g., motor vehicle collision, assault, fall, or sport injury)
3. Iatrogenic trauma
   a. Peritoneal tap
   b. Endoscopy
   c. Biopsy
   d. Cardiopulmonary resuscitation

Pathophysiology

1. Seldom a single-organ injury
2. High-velocity penetrating trauma
   a. Extensive destruction of contact tissue
   b. Severe associated blast effect on the surrounding tissues
   c. Liver most often affected by penetrating trauma
3. Blunt trauma
   a. Caused by direct injury, crushing force between two objects, acceleration/deceleration, shearing, or twisting
   b. Pressure injury
   c. Spleen most often affected by blunt trauma; pancreas frequently is injured with spleen

Clinical Presentation

1. Subjective
   a. Abdominal pain: may be poorly localized or referred
      (1) Kehr's sign: left shoulder pain indicative of splenic rupture caused by blood below diaphragm that irritates the phrenic nerve
      (2) Rovsing sign: pain in RLQ with palpation of LLQ indicates peritoneal irritation
   b. Abdominal tenderness
2. Objective
   a. Seat belt sign: ecchymosis across the lower abdomen caused by seat belt
   b. Hematoma: note location
      (1) Hematoma in flank area may be seen in renal injury
   c. Entrance and exit wounds
   d. Grey Turner's sign or Cullen's sign: may be seen
   e. Coopernail's sign (ecchymosis of scrotum or labia): indicative of fractured pelvis
   f. Rigid abdomen: may indicate intraabdominal bleeding
   g. Ballance's sign (i.e., resonance over right flank with patient on left side): indicative of ruptured spleen
   h. Diminished femoral pulses: may be seen in vascular injury
   i. Loss of liver dullness: indicates perforation with free air in peritoneum
   j. Bowel sounds: diminished or absent
   k. Clinical indications of hypoperfusion or shock
   l. Clinical indications of perforation
   m. Specifics related to organ injured (Table 6-12)
3. Diagnostic
   a. Serum
      (1) Glucose: elevated because of stress
      (2) Amylase: may be elevated if injury to pancreas or bowel
      (3) ALT, AST, LDH: may be elevated if liver injury
      (4) Hgb, Hct: decreased with hemorrhage
      (5) WBC count: may be elevated if infection is present or if spleen is ruptured

Table 6-12 Clinical Indications of Organ Injury

Organ	Suspect Injury to This Organ If:	Clinical Indications of Injury	Complications
Liver	• Seat belt sign • Local sign of injury (RUQ) • Lower right rib fracture • Blunt or penetrating trauma • Acceleration/deceleration MVC • Presence of other abdominal injuries	• RUQ pain, tenderness, and guarding • Referred pain to right shoulder • Increase in abdominal girth and rigidity • Increased pain on inspiration • Clinical indications of shock • Leukocytosis • Elevated alanine transaminase, aspartate transaminase, and lactate dehydrogenase • Decreased Hgb and Hct • Abnormal clotting studies • Chest x-ray: elevated diaphragm on right side • Injury evident on FAST • Positive peritoneal lavage if performed	• Shock • Infection, sepsis • Subdiaphragmatic abscess • Clotting abnormalities • Atelectasis, pneumonia, ARDS • Hepatic failure
Spleen	• Seat belt sign • Local sign of injury (LUQ) • Lower left rib fractures • Left pneumothorax • Blunt or penetrating trauma to abdomen • Acceleration/deceleration MVC • Presence of other abdominal injuries	• LUQ pain, tenderness, and guarding • Increased abdominal girth and rigidity • Kehr's sign • Ballance's sign • Increased pain on inspiration • Clinical indications of shock • Decreased Hgb and Hct • Injury evident on FAST • Positive peritoneal lavage • Shock	• Shock • Atelectasis, pneumonia, • ARDS • Infection, sepsis especially if splenectomy performed • Subdiaphragmatic abscess
Pancreas	• Seat belt sign • Presence of other abdominal injuries • MVC • Blunt or penetrating trauma to abdomen	• Epigastric, back, or shoulder pain • Abdominal tenderness and guarding • Increased abdominal girth • Diminished bowel sounds • Clinical indications of shock • Hyperglycemia or hypoglycemia • Elevated serum lipase • Leukocytosis • Positive peritoneal lavage for amylase but unreliable because the pancreas is located retroperitoneally	• Shock • Diabetes • Pancreatitis • Pancreatic abscess or pseudocyst • Pancreatic fistula • Atelectasis, pneumonia, • ARDS
Stomach	• Penetrating trauma to abdomen • Presence of other abdominal injuries	• Epigastric or LUQ pain and tenderness • Hematemesis or bloody aspirate from nasogastric tube • Rebound tenderness • Clinical indications of shock • Leukocytosis • Positive peritoneal lavage • Free air on flat plate of abdomen	• Atelectasis, pneumonia, • ARDS • Gastric fistula
Intestine	• Seat belt sign • Presence of other abdominal injuries • Blunt trauma with deceleration • Penetrating injury	• Local sign of injury (e.g., ecchymosis or abrasion) • Nausea, vomiting • Abdominal pain: may be referred or rebound • Absent bowel sounds • Leukocytosis • Positive peritoneal lavage for blood and fecal matter • Free air on flat plate of abdomen • Positive fecal occult blood test	• Ileus • Peritonitis, sepsis • Abscess • Intestinal ischemia, infarction, obstruction, perforation • Fistula

Continued

Table 6-12 Clinical Indications of Organ Injury—cont'd

Organ	Suspect Injury to This Organ If:	Clinical Indications of Injury	Complications
Abdominal vessels	• Other abdominal injuries • Blunt or penetrating abdominal injury • Sudden deceleration in MVC or fall	• Clinical indications of shock • Abdominal distention and guarding • Increased abdominal girth and rigidity • Abdominal bruit • Diminished femoral pulses if aorta or iliac injury • Mottled lower extremities • Cullen's sign • Decreased Hgb and Hct • Shock	• Shock • Mesenteric ischemia or infarction • Infection, sepsis

ARDS, Acute respiratory distress syndrome; *FAST*, focused abdominal sonography for trauma; *Hct*, hematocrit; *Hgb*, hemoglobin; *LUQ*, left upper quadrant; *MVC*, motor vehicle collision; *RUQ*, right upper quadrant.

(6) Platelets: elevated if spleen is injured
(7) PT, aPTT: may be prolonged
(8) Drug and alcohol screens: may be positive

b. Urine
  (1) May show hematuria if renal trauma
  (2) May show myoglobinuria if crush injury has occurred

c. Stool: may be positive for occult blood
d. Chest x-ray: used to rule out concurrent thoracic injury; identify free air under diaphragm
e. Flat plate of abdomen: may show free air in peritoneum if stomach or bowel is perforated
f. IVP: if hematuria is present to look for renal trauma
g. Angiography: may show vascular injury
h. CT scan or MRI: to identify areas of injury
i. Focused abdominal sonography for trauma (FAST)
  (1) Use: detects fluid or blood in the pericardium, abdomen, or pelvis and allows visualization of the spleen and liver
    (a) Although the test cannot reliably identify injury to intraabdominal organs (this requires CT), it can predict accurately the need for laparotomy in trauma patients; very good sensitivity and excellent specificity
  (2) Advantages over diagnostic peritoneal lavage (DPL)
    (a) More rapid: generally completed in less than 5 minutes
    (b) Requires no preparation
    (c) Noninvasive
    (d) No contraindications

j. DPL: may be done to assess for intraabdominal bleeding, though FAST is usually the preferred screening study
  (1) Assist with placement of peritoneal catheter; if gross blood is obtained with catheter insertion, immediate exploratory laparotomy is indicated.
  (2) Instill 1 L of normal saline over 15 to 20 minutes.
  (3) Move the patient side to side after fluid instillation to distribute the lavage fluid.
  (4) Drain the fluid.
  (5) Send the fluid for analysis.
    (a) Considered positive if lavage fluid is grossly bloody or contains the following:
      (i) RBCs: more than 100,000 cells/mm^3
      (ii) WBCs: more than 500 cells/mm^3
      (iii) Amylase: more than 175 units/dL
      (iv) Bile, bacteria, intestinal content
    (b) Considered positive if newsprint cannot be read through the lavage fluid (i.e., newsprint sign)
    (c) Major limitation of peritoneal lavage is that it does not detect diaphragmatic or retroperitoneal injuries

k. Specifics related to organ injured (Table 6-12)

Nursing Diagnoses

1. Risk for Deficient Fluid Volume related to hemorrhage or blood sequestration and to sepsis
2. Pain related to trauma and surgery
3. Imbalanced Nutrition: Less than Body Requirements related to altered food metabolism and hypermetabolism
4. Impaired Gas Exchange related to diminished lung expansion and splinting
5. Ineffective Breathing Pattern related to pain and pressure against diaphragm
6. Ineffective Tissue Perfusion related to injury to vascular structures and hypovolemia
7. Risk for Infection related to intestinal perforation, peritonitis, and immunosuppression after splenectomy
8. Impaired Skin Integrity related to trauma and surgery
9. Interrupted Family Processes related to situational crisis, powerlessness, and change in role
10. Deficient Knowledge related to required lifestyle changes

Collaborative Management

1. Maintain airway, oxygenation, and ventilation.
  a. Stabilize the cervical spine.
  b. Elevate the HOB 30 to 45 degrees to allow for optimal diaphragmatic excursion.

c. Administer oxygen as necessary to maintain SpO_2 95% unless contraindicated; in patients with COPD, administer oxygen to achieve an SpO_2 of 90% by pulse oximetry.
d. Place oropharyngeal or nasopharyngeal airway in patients with altered consciousness; assist with endotracheal intubation if required.

2. Detect bleeding and maintain adequate circulating volume.
   a. Detect bleeding by performing head-to-toe assessment and assisting with peritoneal lavage; peritoneal lavage is especially important in an unconscious patient because a subjective report of tenderness or pain is absent.
   b. Insert indwelling urinary catheter to evaluate hourly urine output unless contraindicated; contraindications include the following:
      (1) Blood around the urinary meatus
      (2) Perineal or scrotal hematoma
      (3) Displacement of the prostate gland noted during rectal exam by physician
   c. Assist with insertion of arterial catheter and pulmonary artery catheter in patient with hemodynamic instability.
   d. Insert two short (1¼ inch) large-gauge (16 to 18) peripheral IV catheters; draw blood samples for laboratory analysis, and type and crossmatch for blood.
   e. Administer IV fluids to restore circulating blood volume.
      (1) Crystalloids
      (2) Colloids
      (3) Blood and blood products
         (a) Whole blood or packed cells should be given early if significant bleeding is suspected.
         (b) Consider replacing clotting factors, platelets, and calcium after multiple transfusions.
   f. Control bleeding.
      (1) Apply pressure to overt bleeding site.
      (2) Prepare patient for exploratory laparotomy as indicated.
         (a) Penetrating injury invading the peritoneum
         (b) Clinical indications of perforation such as an acute condition in the abdomen
         (c) Free air in peritoneum on x-ray
         (d) Shock
         (e) GI hemorrhage
         (f) Massive hematuria
         (g) Evisceration
         (h) Positive peritoneal lavage
         (i) Surgical indications on CT scan or angiography
3. Prevent and treat pain and discomfort.
   a. Maintain bed rest.
   b. Maintain quiet environment, comfortable temperature, and dim lighting.
   c. Administer analgesics (e.g., morphine); these may be contraindicated until diagnoses are made.
   d. Encourage knee flexing while the patient is in supine position to relax abdominal muscles in patients with peritoneal irritation.
   e. Use nonpharmacologic pain relief methods (e.g., imagery, distraction, and music).
4. Maintain fluid and electrolyte balance.
   a. Monitor sodium, calcium, potassium, magnesium, and phosphate.
   b. Administer electrolyte replacement as indicated.
5. Decompress GI tract.
   a. Insert NG tube; use orogastric tube in patients with midface fractures.
   b. Monitor NG output for color, amount, and odor of drainage.
   c. Cover any eviscerated organs with saline-soaked pads.
6. Administer appropriate nutritional support considering restrictions.
   a. Administer nutritional support parenterally acutely.
   b. Provide oral feeding and advance diet when condition is resolved surgically.
   c. Administer vitamin and mineral supplements.
7. Prevent and monitor for infection.
   a. Observe for signs of peritonitis (e.g., fever, peritonitis, and leukocytosis).
   b. Monitor abdominal girth.
   c. Administer antibiotics as prescribed; antibiotic lavage may be performed during exploratory laparotomy if bowel perforation has occurred.
   d. Maintain asepsis of wounds and drains.
   e. Monitor bowel sounds.
   f. Evaluate tetanus immunization status, and administer tetanus toxoid if indicated for penetrating trauma, abrasion, and lacerations.
8. Monitor patient for complications.
   a. Obstruction
   b. Perforation
   c. Peritonitis
   d. Pancreatitis
   e. Infection, abscess, sepsis
   f. Hemorrhage
      (1) Retroperitoneal
      (2) Intraperitoneal
   g. Shock: hypovolemic or septic
   h. DIC
   i. Atelectasis, pneumonia, ARDS
   j. Organ failure
   k. Abdominal compartment syndrome

Gastrointestinal Surgery

Gastrointestinal Surgical Procedures Frequently Requiring Critical Care

See Table 6-13.

Table 6-13 Gastrointestinal Surgical Procedures Frequently Requiring Critical Care

Surgical Procedure	Description	Indication
Billroth I (also referred to as *gastroduodenostomy;* Figure 6-24, A)	• Resection of the antrum of the stomach and anastomosis of the remainder of the stomach to the duodenum	• Ulcer or malignancy
Billroth II (also referred to as a *gastrojejunostomy;* Figure 6-24, B)	• Resection of the antrum of the stomach and anastomosis of the remainder of the stomach to the jejunum leaving the duodenal stump and accompanied by a vagotomy	• Ulcer or malignancy
Complete gastrectomy (Figure 6-24, C)	• Removal of the stomach with anastomosis of the esophagus to the jejunum leaving the duodenal stump	• Ulcer or malignancy
Whipple procedure (also referred to as *radical pancreaticoduodenectomy;* Figure 6-25)	• Removal of the lower stomach and duodenum with anastomosis of the remaining stomach to the jejunum with partial or total pancreatectomy and a possible splenectomy	• Cancer of the pancreas • Also may be performed for resection of necrotic tissue as a result of pancreatitis
Esophagogastrostomy (Figure 6-26)	• Removal of all or a portion of the esophagus, possibly with a portion of the stomach, with anastomosis to the remaining portion of the stomach	• Cancer of the lower and middle thirds of the thoracic esophagus • Corrosive esophagitis
Esophagoenterostomy (also may be referred to as a *esophagogastrectomy with a colon interposition;* Figure 6-27)	• Removal of all or a portion of the esophagus along with replacement with a segment of the colon	• Cancer of the esophagus • Corrosive esophagitis
Colon resection with end-to-end anastomosis; may include colostomy (Figure 6-28)	• Removal of a portion of the colon; may include formation of a colostomy • Temporary colostomy may be developed to divert bowel contents to allow for healing of the anastomosis • May be performed laparoscopically	• Tumor, bleeding, inflammation, necrosis, or trauma of the large intestine
Total colectomy and ileostomy	• Removal of the entire large intestine and the formation of a stoma from the end of the ileum • Also may include surgical formation of a continent ileostomy (i.e., Kock pouch) or ileoanal reservoir	• Ulcerative colitis
Abdominoperineal resection	• Removal of the anus, rectum, and sigmoid colon with creation of a permanent colostomy	• Malignancy of the rectum
RESTRICTIVE PROCEDURES FOR MORBID OBESITY		
Vertical banded gastroplasty	• Partitioning of the stomach near the gastroesophageal junction to create a small gastric pouch and outlet • Less commonly performed today because of lack of sustained weight loss	• Morbid obesity
Gastric banding (Figure 6-29)	• Placement of a prosthetic device around the gastric cardia to limit oral intake • May be done laparoscopically	• Morbid obesity
MALABSORPTIVE PROCEDURES FOR MORBID OBESITY		
Intestinal bypass	• Formation of an anastomosis between the upper small intestine and the lower small intestine or large intestine • Less commonly performed today because of high complication rate	• Morbid obesity
Roux-Y gastric bypass (Figure 6-30)	• Combines gastric restriction and malabsorption; in addition to creating a gastric pouch, the small bowel is resected so that the upper jejunum is connected to the pouch and the lower jejunum is anastomosed to the biliopancreatic limb; because digestive juices do not come into the small bowel until the lower jejunum, absorption is decreased • Usually performed via laparoscopic technique	• Morbid obesity

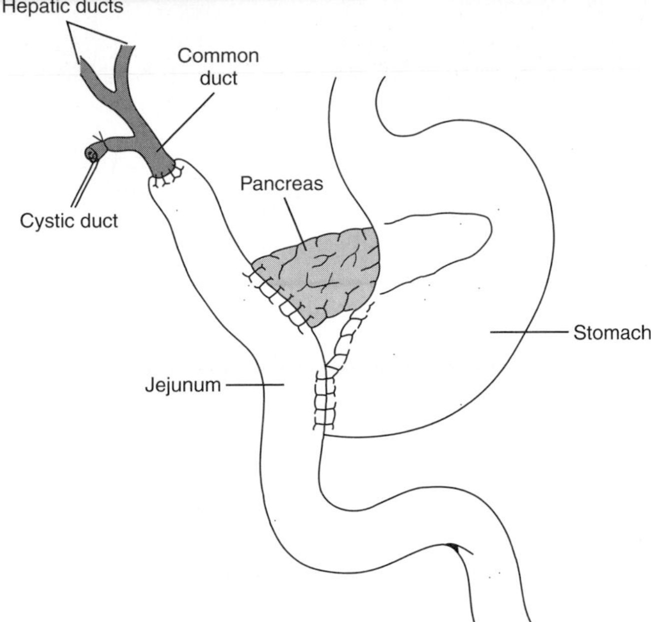

Figure 6-25 Whipple procedure (also referred to *radical pancreaticoduodenectomy*). (From Lewis, S. M., Heitkemper, M. M., & Dirksen, S. R. [2000]. *Medical-surgical nursing: Assessment and management of clinical problems* [5th ed.]. St. Louis: Mosby.)

Postoperative Management for Gastrointestinal Surgeries

1. Maintain airway, oxygenation, and ventilation.
   a. Monitor airway patency and use artificial airways as indicated; many of these patients still will be intubated and receiving mechanical ventilation.
   b. Monitor Spo_2, and administer oxygen to maintain it at 95% until contraindicated.
   c. Position the patient with HOB elevated to 30 to 40 degrees unless contraindicated; side-lying is frequently more comfortable for patients who have had rectal or perineal procedures.
   d. Use short-term breathing trials to evaluate the patient's ability to maintain spontaneous breathing so that weaning and extubation can be accomplished as soon as possible.
   e. Encourage deep breathing and incentive spirometry.
   f. Maintain hydration, encourage leg exercises, and have patient ambulate as soon as possible to prevent deep venous thrombosis (DVT) and pulmonary embolism.
2. Prevent and monitor for fluid volume deficit and/or electrolyte imbalance.
   a. Monitor vital signs, hemodynamics, urine output, daily weights, and laboratory values.
      (1) Use central venous pressure (CVP) or when CVP catheter is in place or PAOP when pulmonary artery catheter is in place to evaluate fluid status.
      (2) Evaluate electrolyte values as indicated.
      (3) Monitor Hgb and Hct as indicated.
      (4) Weigh patient daily.
   b. Administer fluids as prescribed: crystalloids and colloids.
   c. Monitor drains if in place for change in amount or character of drainage.
   d. Expect mobilization of third-spaced fluids and increase in urine output on second or third postoperative day; monitor for changes in electrolyte levels.
   e. Monitor for petechiae, ecchymosis, changes in clotting profile, and frank bleeding that may indicate a coagulopathy, such as DIC.
3. Prevent and/or treat pain.
   a. Administer narcotics (e.g., morphine, hydromorphone, or fentanyl) by patient-controlled analgesia as prescribed; epidural analgesia may be used.
   b. Administer NSAIDs as prescribed to augment the analgesic effect of narcotics by acting as antiprostaglandins.
      (1) Initially ketorolac (Toradol)
      (2) Oral agents (e.g., ibuprofen [Motrin] or naproxen [Naprosyn, Anaprox]) when patient is able to take drugs by mouth.
   c. Use noninvasive pain control measures.
   d. Teach the patient how to splint the incision during coughing; teach the family how to assist.
   e. Administer antiemetics for nausea; provide mouth care after each episode of vomiting and assess positioning of NG tube if still in place.
4. Prevent and monitor for infection.
   a. Monitor patient closely for clinical indications of infection.
      (1) Evaluate temperature at least every 4 hours.
      (2) Assess color, character, and odor of drainage from incision line, drains, and tubes.
      (3) Assess patient for clinical indications of peritonitis (e.g., abdominal pain; abdominal distention; rigid, boardlike abdomen; rebound tenderness; diminished or absent bowel sounds; nausea; vomiting; fever; and leukocytosis) caused by anastomotic leak.
      (4) Monitor patient for clinical indications of intraabdominal abscess (e.g., abdominal pain, fever, and leukocytosis).
   b. Administer antibiotics prophylactically and therapeutically as prescribed.
   c. Provide incision and drain care aseptically.
      (1) Protect the skin from excoriation by changing incisional dressing and dressings around drains as indicated.

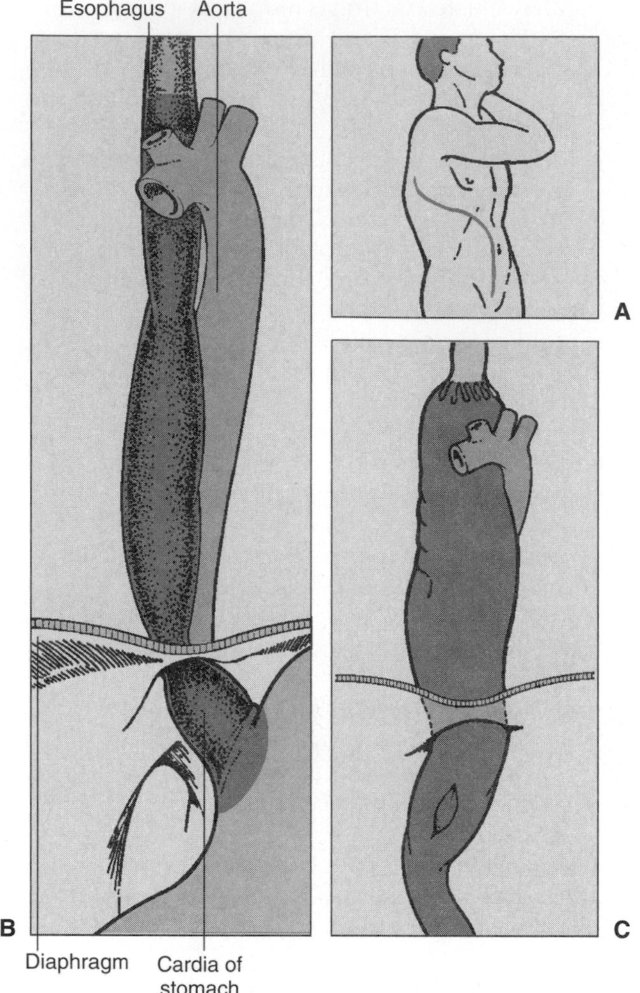

Figure 6-26 Esophagogastrectomy. **A,** Incision. **B,** Shaded portion to be resected. **C,** Completed reconstruction (From Beare, P. G., & Myers, J. L. [1998]. *Adult health nursing* [3rd ed.]. St. Louis: Mosby.)

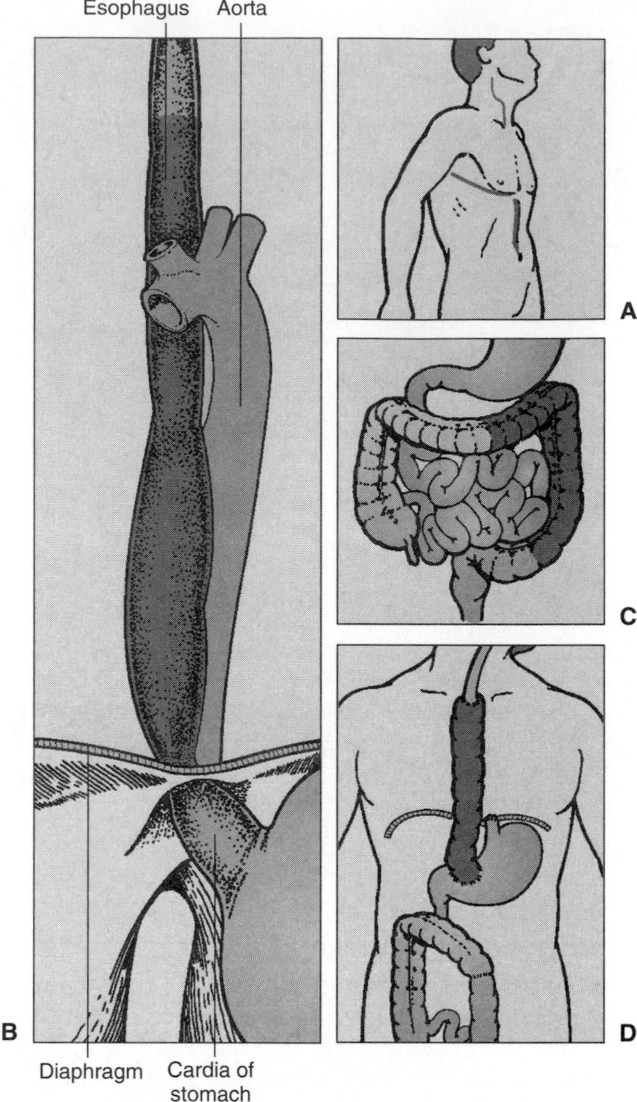

Figure 6-27 Esophagoenterostomy. **A,** Incision. **B,** Shaded portion to be resected. **C,** Portion of colon to be used. **D,** Completed reconstruction (From Beare, P. G., & Myers, J. L. [1998]. *Adult health nursing* [3rd ed.]. St. Louis: Mosby.)

(2) Change packing as prescribed.
 (a) Some patients may have wounds that are left open and are packed with saline-soaked dressings.
  (i) Do not use packing soaked in povidone-iodine (Betadine); known effects of Betadine on open wounds include the following:
   a) Toxic to fibroblasts
   b) Decreases epithelialization
   c) Increases susceptibility to infection
   d) Iodine may be absorbed and cause nephrotoxicity
 (b) Do not allow dressings to become dry (i.e., wet to dry); the dressings should still be moist (i.e., wet to moist) at the time of removal and replacement to prevent disruption of granulating tissue.

(3) Irrigate the wound with saline as prescribed.
 (a) Do not use hydrogen peroxide because it damages new epithelium.

(4) Monitor wound closely for a fistula tract.
 (a) Look for small openings along or near the incision or drain site; output is usually green or yellow.
 (b) Protect the skin from the potentially excoriating drainage by placing a wound drainage bag over the fistula; also allows measurement of fluid loss and collection of sample for electrolyte analysis to guide fluid and electrolyte replacement.

d. Monitor serum glucose, and administer insulin to keep serum glucose within normal limits.

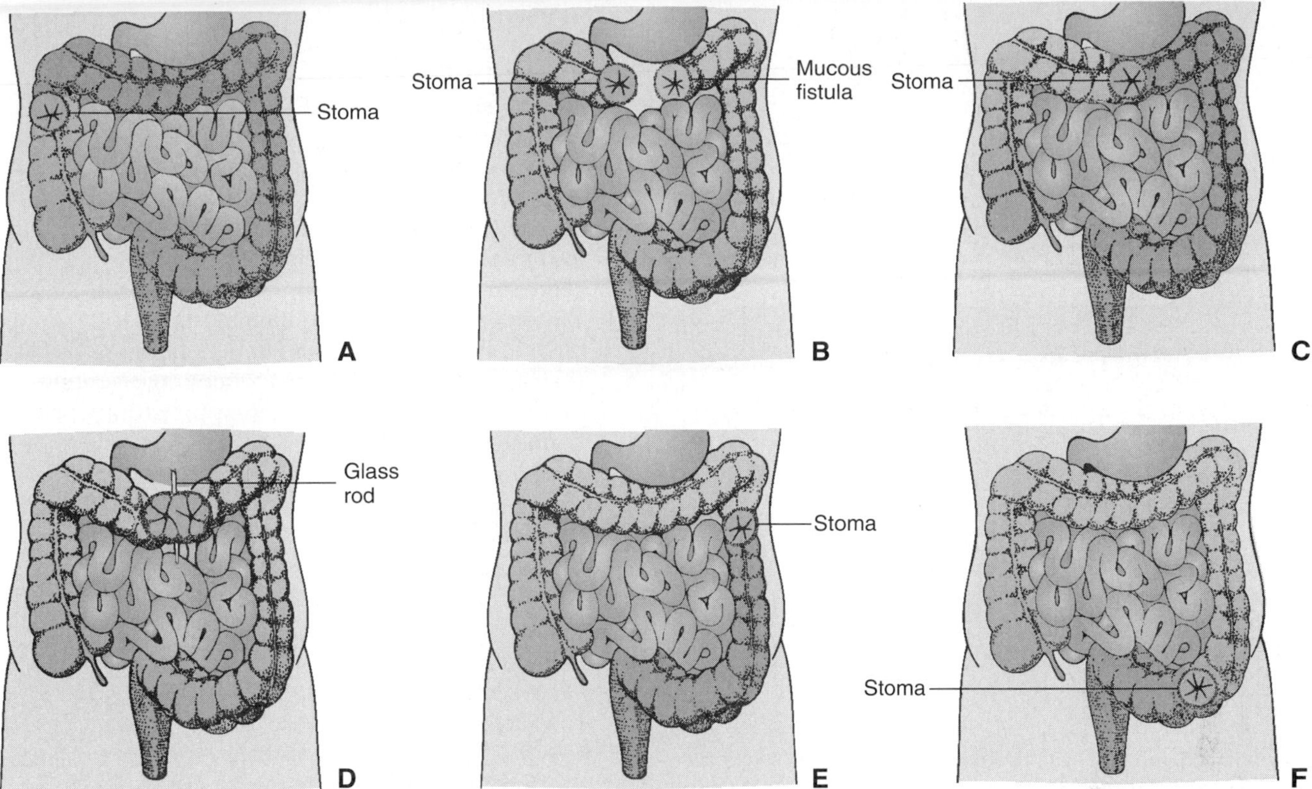

Figure 6-28 **A,** Ascending colostomy. **B,** Double-barrel colostomy. **C,** Transverse colostomy. **D,** Loop colostomy. **E,** Descending colostomy. **F,** Sigmoid colostomy. (From Beare, P. G., & Myers, J. L. [1998]. *Adult health nursing* [3rd ed.]. St. Louis: Mosby.)

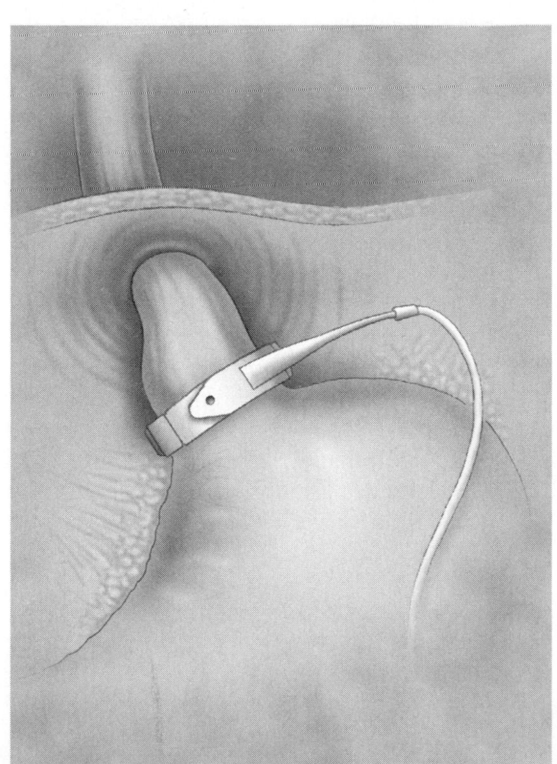

Figure 6-29 Example of gastric banding. (From American Association of Operating Room Nurses. [2004]. AORN bariatric surgery guideline. *AORN Journal, 79*[5], 1026-1052.)

e. Assess approximation of wound edges for indications of possible dehiscence or evisceration.

5. Reduce acidity of gastric secretions.
   a. Administer antacids, H_2 receptor antagonists, and/or proton pump inhibitors.
   b. Administer octreotide acetate (Sandostatin) as prescribed to suppress secretion of pancreatic peptides after Whipple procedure.
   c. Maintain NPO status while gastric suction required.
6. Maintain GI integrity.
   a. Monitor and maintain NG tube until return of bowel sounds.
      (1) Ensure proper tube placement; do not manipulate a tube placed during surgery without consulting surgeon.
   b. Monitor closely for indications of anastomotic leak.
   c. Monitor for return of bowel sounds, flatus, and bowel movement.
   d. Assess and provide bowel diversion care as indicated (bowel resection with formation of a temporary or permanent bowel diversion).
      (1) Maintain intactness of bowel diversion appliance.
      (2) Keep peristomal skin clean and dry.

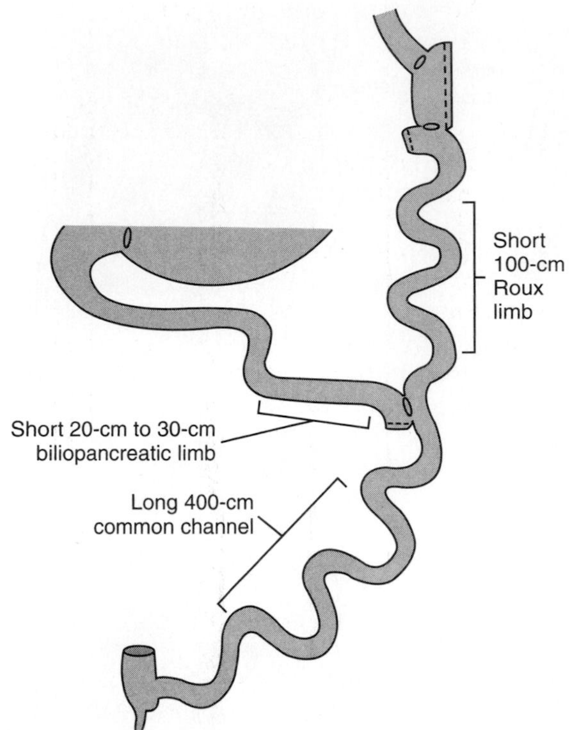

Figure 6-30 Example of gastric bypass: Roux-en-Y proximal gastric bypass. (From American Association of Operating Room Nurses. [2004]. AORN bariatric surgery guideline. *AORN Journal, 79*[5], 1026-1052.)

(3) Report any change in the drainage from the ileostomy/colostomy.
(a) Ileostomy: watery, excoriating, and continuous
(b) Ascending colostomy: watery or semisolid, excoriating, and continuous
(c) Transverse colostomy: pastelike or semisolid and occurs at unpredictable intervals; may be 3 to 5 days postoperative before any drainage
(d) Descending or sigmoid colostomy: formed stools that may be at predictable intervals (e.g., after breakfast) especially with irrigation routine; may be 3 to 5 days postoperative before any drainage
(4) Assess color of stoma and report any indications of ischemia.
(a) Stoma should be the same color as the oral mucosa, and it should be moist; report darkening such as burgundy or black.
(5) Report any stomal prolapse or retraction.

7. Maintain or improve nutritional status.
a. Assess nutritional status: weight; BUN; serum albumin; total protein; Hgb and Hct.
b. Administer TPN initially as prescribed, and follow diet progression as prescribed: usually small, frequent meals are indicated.
c. Administer enteral feedings as prescribed; a jejunostomy tube may be placed for nutritional support.
d. Monitor for diarrhea.
e. Administer oral pancreatic enzymes (pancrelipase [Creon, Pancrease, Viokase, or Cotazym]) with each meal as prescribed after the Whipple procedure.

8. Assist with adjustment to diagnosis of cancer.
a. Provide accurate information and clarification about the diagnosis, prognosis, and treatment plan when information is requested.
b. Be realistic, but do not eliminate hope.
c. Give patient and family members time to discuss their feelings and concerns; encourage venting.
d. Refer patient and family to support groups or for counseling as indicated.
e. Prepare the patient and family for additional treatments for malignancy if indicated, such as the following:
(1) Radiation therapy
(2) Antineoplastic drug therapy

9. Monitor patient for complications.
a. General
(1) Anastomotic leak
(2) Atelectasis, pneumonia, ARDS
(3) DVT, pulmonary embolism
(4) Infection, sepsis
(5) Prolonged ileus
(6) GI bleeding
(7) Stenosis or stricture
(8) Fistula
(9) Organ failure
(a) Cardiac
(b) Hepatic
(c) Pulmonary
(d) Renal
b. Specific to gastric resections
(1) Dumping syndromes
(a) Early: hyperosmolality causing hypovolemic effect
(b) Late: hypoglycemia caused by hyperinsulinemic response
(2) Pernicious anemia
(3) Diarrhea
(4) Chronic gastritis
c. Specific to Whipple procedure
(1) Delayed gastric emptying
(2) Pancreatic fistula
(3) Intraabdominal abscess
(4) Hemorrhage: usually caused by injury to portal vein or vena cava
(5) Wound infection
(6) Diabetes
(7) Pancreatic exocrine insufficiency
(8) Pancreatitis
(9) Marginal ulceration
d. Specific to esophagogastrectomy
(1) Esophageal stenosis or anastomotic stricture
(2) Chylothorax
(3) Myocardial ischemia
(4) Dysrhythmias

e. Specific to restrictive procedures for morbid obesity
   (1) Stomal outlet stenosis
   (2) Severe gastroesophageal reflux
   (3) Erosive esophagitis
   (4) Band erosion
   (5) Herniation of the stomach upward inside the band
   (6) Band migration
   (7) Regaining of weight
f. Specific to malabsorptive procedures for morbid obesity
   (1) Gastric pouch outlet stricture
   (2) Jejunojejunostomy obstruction
   (3) Dumping syndrome
   (4) Prolonged nausea and vomiting
   (5) Cholelithiasis
   (6) Anemia
   (7) Vitamin (A, D, E, K, B_{12}) and mineral (calcium, folic acid, iron) deficiencies
   (8) Electrolyte imbalance
   (9) Lactose intolerance
   (10) Anemia
   (11) Offensive, foul-smelling, soft bowel movements and flatus

10. Provide instruction to the patient and family regarding wound care, pharmacologic agents prescribed for home use, and signs/symptoms to report to the physician.

Learning Activities

1. **Directions:** Complete the following crossword puzzle related to GI anatomy and physiology.

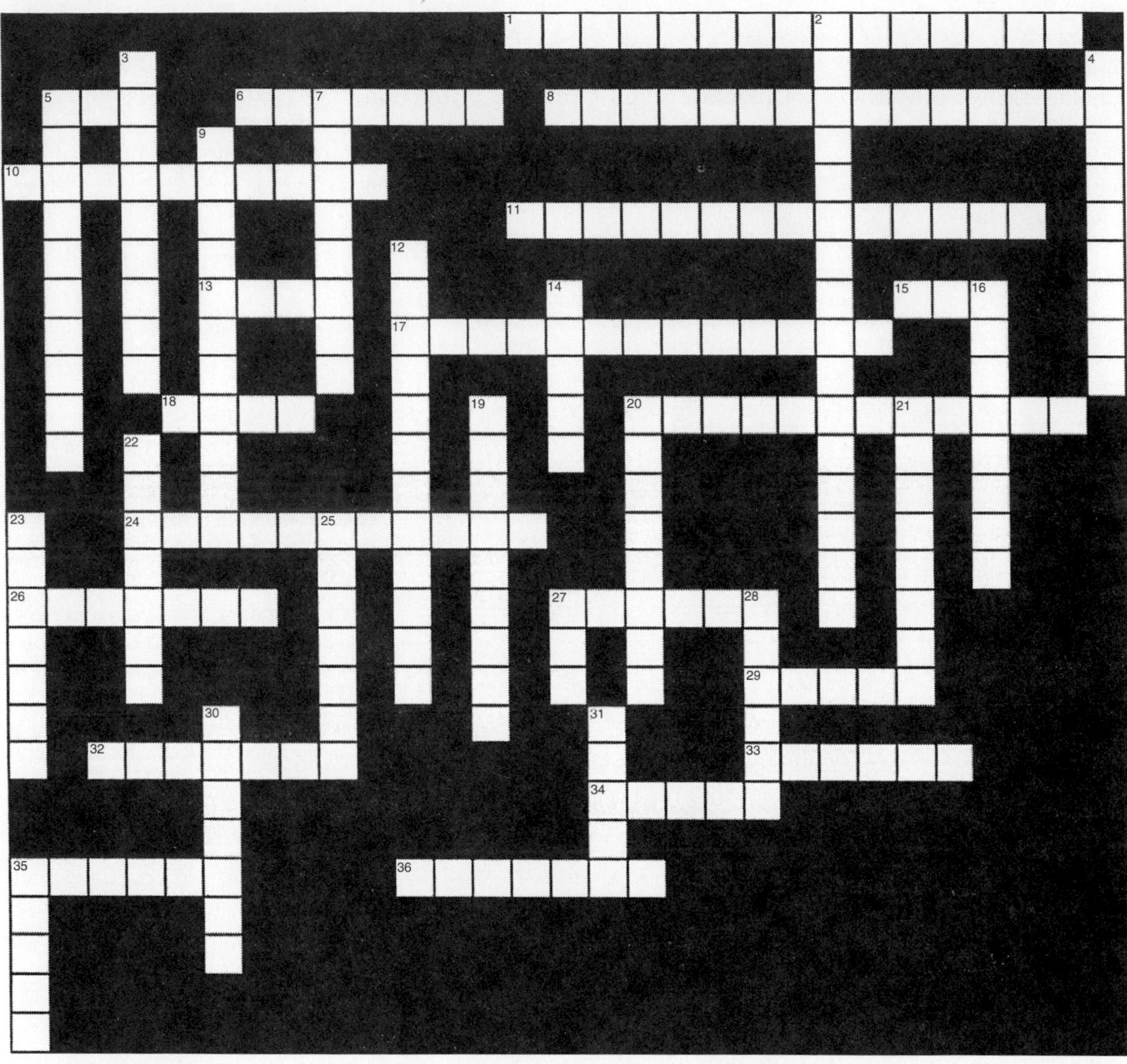

Across

1. The process of converting fats and proteins to glucose
5. The branch of the ANS that speeds gastric emptying (abbreviation)
6. The cells that line the sinusoids of the liver and are responsible for phagocytosis
8. The hormone that stimulates contraction of the gallbladder
10. The first portion of the alimentary canal
11. The process of breaking down stored CHO
13. A fluid produced by the liver and store in the gallbladder
15. The nutrient source that is broken down into fatty acids
17. Another term for swallowing
18. Sphincter of _____ is a valve in the common bile duct that regulates passage of bile
20. The nutrient source that is broken down into glucose, fructose, and galactose
24. The alternate contraction and relaxation of muscle fibers that propels food and chyme through the GI tract
26. One of these lymph vessels is located in each villi
27. The oral secretion stimulated by the thought, sight, smell, or taste of food
29. The last section of the small intestine
32. The nutrient source that is broken down into amino acids
33. Lower portion of the stomach, close to the pylorus
34. The accessory organ responsible for the conversion of ammonia to urea
35. The upper portion of the stomach
36. The hormone that is responsible for the secretion of HCl acid

Down

2. Sphincter that also is referred to as the lower esophageal sphincter
3. The hollow tube that passes through the thoracic cavity and the diaphragm
4. This factor is necessary for the intestinal absorption of vitamin B_{12}
5. The membrane that covers the abdominal viscera
7. The accessory organ with endocrine and exocrine functions
9. The accessory organ responsible for the storage and release of bile
12. The gastric acid that is stimulated by gastrin
14. Thick folds on the interior of the stomach that increase surface area
16. The vitamin that plays a chief role in the metabolic breakdown of glucose to yield energy in body tissue
19. The major bile pigment
20. The phase of gastric secretion that is stimulated by the thought, sight, smell, or taste of food
21. Shortest segment of the small intestine
22. The flexure of the large intestine that is in the RUQ
23. The flexure of the large intestine that is in the LUQ
25. The enzyme responsible for the breakdown of proteins into amino acids
27. This branch of the ANS slows gastric emptying (abbreviation)
28. These cells are in the pancreas and responsible for exocrine function
30. The largest dilation of the GI tract
31. Fingerlike projections of mucosa and submucosa in the duodenum and jejunum that increase surface area
35. Viscous, semifluid stomach contents that move through the pylorus into the small intestine

2. DIRECTIONS: Describe the following "signs" and identify what they indicate.

Sign	Description	Indicates
Ballance's		
Grey Turner's		
Cullen's		
Coopernail's		
Kehr's		
Chvostek's		
Trousseau's		

3. DIRECTIONS: List three general causes of jaundice.

a. ______________________
b. ______________________
c. ______________________

4. DIRECTIONS: Why is serum prealbumin a better assessment tool than albumin to evaluate improvement from nutritional support?

____
____

5. DIRECTIONS: Calculate the caloric intake for a patient receiving TPN with daily intake of 42 g of proteins, 250 g of CHO, and 140 g of fats.

____

6. DIRECTIONS: List four interventions for any patient with acute hemorrhage (regardless of location).

a. ______________________
b. ______________________
c. ______________________
d. ______________________

7. DIRECTIONS: List five possible reasons for upper GI hemorrhage.

a. ______________________
b. ______________________
c. ______________________
d. ______________________
e. ______________________

8. DIRECTIONS: List five methods to control bleeding in esophageal varices.

a. ______________________________
b. ______________________________
c. ______________________________
d. ______________________________
e. ______________________________

9. DIRECTIONS: List four classifications of drugs that are used to prevent ulcers and an example of each one.

Type	Example

10. DIRECTIONS: Match the following clinical manifestations of hepatic failure with the pathophysiologic change (answers may be used more than once).

a. Petechiae, purpura, bleeding
b. Jaundice
c. Third spacing
d. Testicular atrophy
e. Gynecomastia
f. Anemia, leukopenia, thrombocytopenia
g. Dull RUQ pain

___ 1. Splenic engorgement
___ 2. Stretching of the liver capsule
___ 3. Decrease in the metabolism of testosterone
___ 4. Decrease in metabolism of aldosterone
___ 5. Decrease in production of plasma proteins
___ 6. Decrease in metabolism of estrogen
___ 7. Decreased production of clotting factors
___ 8. Decrease in conjugation and excretion of bilirubin

11. DIRECTIONS: List one type of diuretic that is indicated and one type of diuretic that is contraindicated for ascites in hepatic failure.

Indicated	Contraindicated

12. DIRECTIONS: List five common causes of paralytic ileus.

a. ______________________________
b. ______________________________
c. ______________________________
d. ______________________________
e. ______________________________

13. DIRECTIONS: List five classic indications of an acute abdomen seen in intestinal perforation.

a. ______________________________
b. ______________________________
c. ______________________________
d. ______________________________
e. ______________________________

14. DIRECTIONS: Complete the following table. You may include more than one condition for each, but include only conditions discussed in this chapter.

Clinical Finding	Condition
Elevated lipase and amylase	
Sudden, painless hematemesis	
Decreased protein	
Rebound tenderness	
Jaundice	
Hypocalcemia	
Bleeding tendencies	
Elevated ammonia	
Bloody diarrhea	
Hyperbilirubinemia	
Fetor hepaticus	
High-pitched rushing bowel sounds	
Succussion splash	
Management	**Condition**
Irrigate NG tube until clear	
Neomycin and lactulose	
Sclerosis during endoscopy	
Aldosterone antagonist diuretics	
NPO status	
Sengstaken-Blakemore tube	
Volume and blood replacement	
Billroth I or II	

15. **Directions:** Complete the following crossword puzzle related to GI assessment, conditions, and treatments.

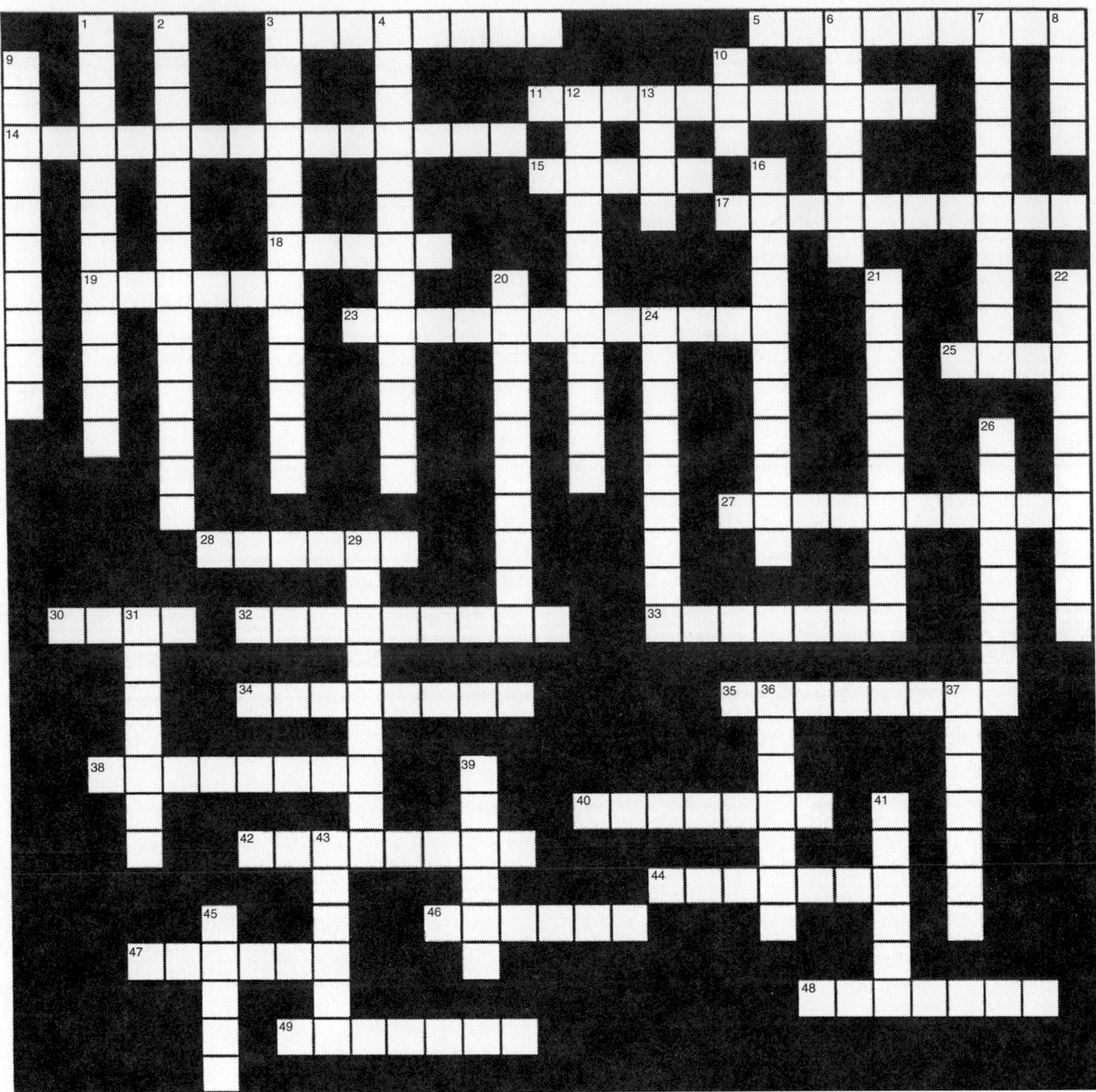

Across

3. The term for generalized, massive edema
5. An osmotic laxative frequently used in hepatic encephalopathy (generic)
11. The term for vomiting blood
14. A common cause of acute pancreatitis
15. A complication of vasopressin therapy that causes water intoxication (abbreviation)
17. This type of anemia is caused by a deficiency of intrinsic factor
18. Functional obstruction of the bowel
19. _____'s sign is a bluish discoloration around the umbilicus; indicative of intraabdominal bleeding
23. The gentle repetitive bouncing of tissues against the hand; used to evaluate organ enlargement
25. _____'s sign is caused by phrenic nerve irritation by subphrenic blood
27. An H_2 receptor antagonist (generic)
28. Hypertension of this circulatory system is seen in cirrhosis
30. A stent is placed between the hepatic and portal veins in this procedure performed in patients with esophageal varices (abbreviation)
32. This condition is manifested by coffee-ground gastric aspirate
33. The plasma protein most significant in maintaining capillary oncotic pressure
34. The type of drug frequently prescribed for patients with ascites
35. _____'s sign is indicative of splenic rupture
38. An IV proton pump inhibitor (brand name)
40. Elevated ______ levels cause neurologic changes in patients with hepatic encephalopathy
42. A "maneuver" that facilitates evacuation of the colon
44. The preferred method of nutritional support; should be used unless contraindications exist
46. This type of ulcer causes an erosion in the mucosa of the esophagus, stomach, or duodenum

47. The term for tarry stools
48. _____'s procedure also is called a pancreato-duodenectomy
49. _____ tenderness indicates that pain is more severe on release than with pressure

Down

1. An electrolyte imbalance seen in acute pancreatitis
2. Abnormal function of the brain
3. A drug commonly used for suicide gesture that is a major cause of hepatic failure in adolescents (generic)
4. A complication of hernia that may cause bowel ischemia or infarction
6. _____'s ulcer is a stress ulcer associated with cerebral trauma
7. A drug used in GI hemorrhage to suppress gastrin (generic)
8. This diagnostic study may cause pancreatitis (abbreviation)
9. A drug that acts as a mucosal barrier (generic)
10. A gastric feeding tube that is placed endoscopically (abbreviation)
12. The location of pain in acute pancreatitis
13. A serious pulmonary complication of acute pancreatitis (abbreviation)
16. A syndrome of renal failure associated with hepatic failure
20. The term for loud, hyperactive bowel sounds
21. The term for belching
22. The route of nutritional support used in functional or structural obstruction
24. This tube has four lumina and may be used for balloon tamponade in patients with esophageal varices especially if not controlled with therapeutic endoscopy
26. A deficiency of this vitamin is commonly seen in alcoholism
29. A flapping tremor seen in hepatic encephalopathy
31. An obstruction here is manifested by vomiting and a succussion splash
36. An abnormal accumulation of fluid in the peritoneal cavity
37. _____'s is a stress ulcer associated with burns
39. A type of shunt that is used for ascites
41. *Helicobacter* _____ is a bacterium associated with peptic ulcer
43. The most specific laboratory test for pancreatitis
45. The form of fluid replacement that is indicated for acute hemorrhage

Learning Activities Answers

1.

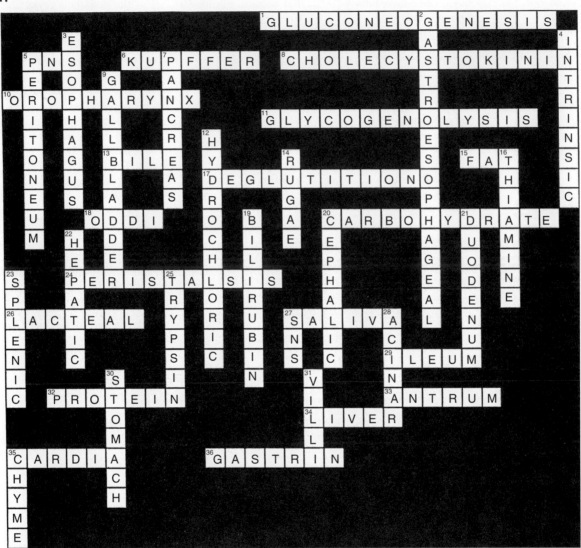

2.

Sign	Description	Indicates
Ballance's	Dullness over right flank with patient on left side	Ruptured spleen
Grey Turner's	Ecchymosis to flank	Retroperitoneal bleeding
Cullen's	Ecchymosis around umbilicus	Intraperitoneal bleeding
Coopernail's	Ecchymosis of scrotum or labia	Pelvic fracture
Kehr's	Left shoulder pain	Splenic rupture
Chvostek's	Spasm of the facial muscles elicited by tapping on the facial nerve	Hypocalcemia
Trousseau's	Carpal spasm induced by inflating a BP cuff on the upper arm to a pressure exceeding systolic BP	Hypocalcemia

3. a. Liver disease (e.g., cirrhosis or hepatitis)
b. Biliary obstruction (e.g., cholelithiasis)
c. Excessive hemolysis (e.g., hemolytic blood transfusion reaction)

4. The half-life of serum prealbumin is 2 to 3 days versus albumin with a half-life of 10 to 20 days. Therefore, serum transferrin shows improvement or decline more quickly.

5. 2428 calories

6. a. Administer oxygen (maintain Sa_{O_2} of at least 95%).
b. Insert at least two large-gauge (16 or 18) IV catheters.
c. Obtain blood samples for Hgb and Hct, and type and crossmatch.
d. Initiate normal saline infusion initially and then blood when prescribed and available.

7. a. Peptic ulcer
b. Esophageal varices
c. Mallory-Weiss tear
d. Gastritis
e. Vascular tumor

8. a. Sclerotherapy of varices
b. Ligation of varices
c. Intrahepatic (e.g., TIPS) or portosystemic shunt
d. Balloon tamponade
e. Octreotide (Sandostatin) or vasopressin (Pitressin)

9.

Type	Example
Antacids	Maalox Mylanta
Histamine (H_2) receptor antagonists	Cimetidine (Tagamet) Ranitidine (Zantac) Famotidine (Pepcid) Nizatidine (Axid)
Proton pump inhibitors	Omeprazole (Prilosec) Lansoprazole (Prevacid) Esomeprazole (Nexium)
Mucosal barrier	Sucralfate (Carafate)

10.
f, a 1. Splenic engorgement. Remember that splenic engorgement causes thrombocytopenia and, therefore, clotting abnormalities.
g 2. Stretching of the liver capsule
d 3. Decrease in the metabolism of testosterone
c 4. Decrease in metabolism of aldosterone
c, a 5. Decrease in production of plasma proteins. Remember that many plasma proteins are actually clotting factors.
e 6. Decrease in metabolism of estrogen
a 7. Decreased production of clotting factors
b 8. Decrease in conjugation and excretion of bilirubin

11.

Indicated	Contraindicated
Aldosterone antagonist (potassium sparing)	Thiazide

12. Any five of the following:
    Abdominal surgery
    Acute cholecystitis
    Hypokalemia
    Intestinal distention
    Intestinal ischemia
    Narcotics (e.g., morphine)
    Pancreatitis
    Pelvic abscess
    Peritonitis
    Pleuritis
    Pneumonia
    Sepsis
    Severe trauma
    Spinal cord injury
    Subphrenic abscess
    Ureteral distention

13. a. Abdominal pain
    b. Rebound tenderness
    c. Abdominal distention
    d. Rigid, boardlike abdomen
    e. Diminished bowel sounds
    f. Fever
    g. Leukocytosis
    h. Nausea, vomiting

14.

Sign/Symptom	Condition
Elevated lipase and amylase	Acute pancreatitis
Sudden, painless hematemesis	Esophageal varices
Decreased protein	Acute pancreatitis, liver disease, malnutrition
Rebound tenderness	Peritonitis
Jaundice	Liver disease, biliary obstruction, hemolysis
Hypocalcemia	Acute pancreatitis
Bleeding tendencies	Liver disease
Elevated ammonia	Hepatic failure, hepatic encephalopathy
Bloody diarrhea	Intestinal infarction
Hyperbilirubinemia	Liver disease, biliary obstruction, hemolysis
Fetor hepaticus	Hepatic failure
High-pitched rushing bowel sounds	Small bowel obstruction
Succussion splash	Pyloric obstruction
Management	**Condition**
Irrigate NG tube until clear	Upper GI bleed
Neomycin and lactulose	Hepatic failure; hepatic encephalopathy
Sclerosis during endoscopy	Esophageal varices
Aldosterone antagonist diuretics	Hepatic failure; hepatic encephalopathy
NPO status	Pancreatitis
Sengstaken-Blakemore tube	Esophageal varices
Volume and blood replacement	GI bleed
Billroth I or II	Gastric ulcer

15.

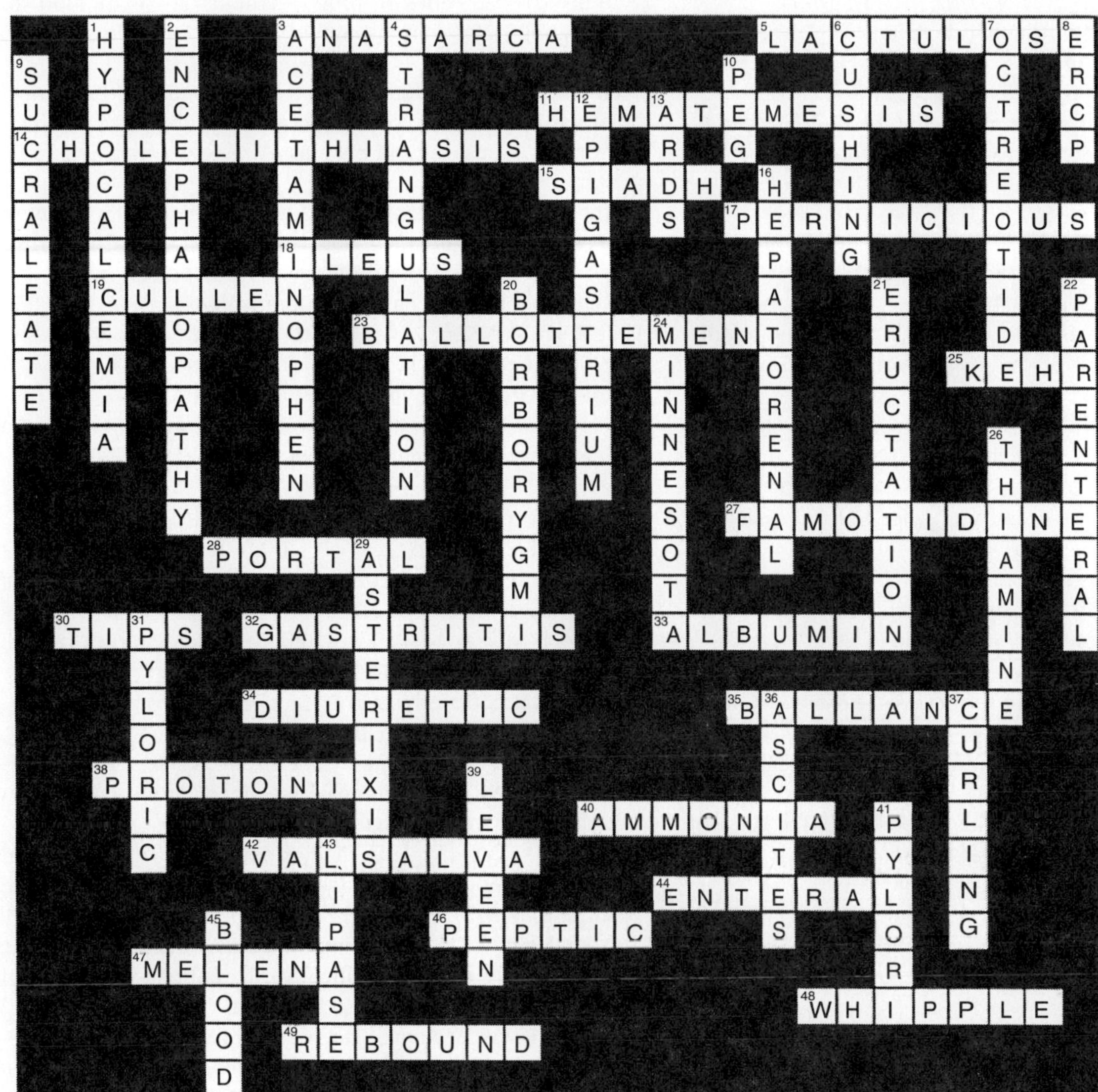

Reference

Booker, K. J., Niedringhaus, L., Eden, B., & Arnold, J. S. (2000). Comparison of 2 methods of managing gastric residual volumes from feeding tubes. *American Journal of Critical Care, 9*(5), 318-324.

Bibliography

Abir, F., & Bell, R. (2004). Assessment and management of the obese patient. *Critical Care Medicine, 32*(4), 587-591.

Abou-Assi, S., & O'Keefe, S. J. D. (2001). Nutrition in acute pancreatitis. *Journal of Clinical Gastroenterology, 32*(3), 203-209.

Abraham, S. C., Wilentz, R. E., Yeo, C. J., Sohn, T. A., Cameron, J. L., Boitnott, J. K., et al. (2003). Pancreaticoduodenectomy (Whipple resections) in patients without malignancy: Are they all 'chronic pancreatitis'? *American Journal of Surgical Pathology, 27*(1), 110-120.

Allen, M. E., Kopp, B. J., & Erstad, B. L. (2004). Stress ulcer prophylaxis in the postoperative period. *American Journal of Health-System Pharmacy, 61*(6), 588-596.

American Association of Operating Room Nurses. (2004). AORN bariatric surgery guideline. *AORN Journal, 79*(5), 1026-1052.

Case, K. O., Cuddy, P. G., & McGurk, E. P. D. (2000). Nutritional support in the critically ill patient. *Critical Care Nursing Quarterly, 22*(4), 75-89.

Charlebois, D., & Wilmoth, D. (2004). Critical care of patients with obesity. *Critical Care Nurse, 24*(4), 19-29.

Christou, N., Sampalis, J. S., Liberman, M., Look, D., Auger, S., McLean, A. P. H., et al. (2004). Surgery decreases long-term mortality, morbidity, and health care use in morbidly obese patients. *Annals of Surgery, 240*(3), 416-424.

Deshpande, K. S. (2003). Total parenteral nutrition and infections associated with use of central venous catheters. *American Journal of Critical Care, 12*(4), 326-327, 380.

Diaz, V., & Wyckoff, M. M. (2002). Surviving fulminant hepatic failure. *American Journal of Nursing, 102*(5 suppl.), 49-53.

DiMaria-Ghalili, R. A., & Amella, E. (2005). Nutrition in older adults. *American Journal of Nursing, 105*(3), 40-51.

Dudek, S. G. (2000). Malnutrition in hospitals: Who's assessing what patients eat? *American Journal of Nursing, 100*(4), 36-43.

Elpern, E. H., Stutz, L., Peterson, S., Gurka, D. P., & Skipper, A. (2004). Outcomes associated with enteral tube feedings in a medical intensive care unit. *American Journal of Critical Care, 13*(3), 221-227.

Foxworth, J. (2000). Stress ulcer prophylaxis in intensive care patients: An evidence-practice mismatch? *Critical Care Nursing Quarterly, 22*(4), 39-46.

Fritsch, D. E., & Steinmann, R. A. (2000). Managing trauma with abdominal compartment syndrome. *Critical Care Nurse, 20*(6), 48-58.

Gallagher, S. (2004). Taking the weight off with bariatric surgery. *Nursing2004, 34*(3), 58-64.

Garrett, K., Tsuruta, K., Walker, S., Jackson, S., & Sweat, M. (2003). Managing nausea and vomiting: Current strategies. *Critical Care Nurse, 23*(1), 31-52.

Grossman, S., & Bautista, C. (2001). A transitional feeding protocol for critically ill patients. *Dimensions of Critical Care Nursing, 20*(5), 46-51.

Hale, A. S., Moseley, M. J., & Warner, S. C. (2000). Treating pancreatitis in the acute care setting. *Dimensions of Critical Care Nursing, 19*(4), 15-21.

Holcomb, S. S. (2002). An update on hepatitis. *Dimensions of Critical Care Nursing, 21*(5), 170-177.

Huckleberry, Y. (2004). Nutritional support and the surgical patient. *American Journal of Health-System Pharmacy, 61*(7), 671-682.

Huffman, S., Pieper, P., Jarczyk, K. S., Bayne, A., & O'Brien, E. (2004). Methods to confirm feeding tube placement: Application of research in practice. *Pediatric Nursing, 30*(1), 10-13.

Hurst, S., Blanco, K., Boyle, D., Douglass, L., & Wikas, A. (2004). Bariatric implications of critical care nursing. *Dimensions of Critical Care Nursing, 23*(2), 76-83.

Kruse, J. A., Fink, M. P., & Carlson, R. W. (2003). *Saunders manual of critical care*. Philadelphia: Saunders.

Lenart, S., & Polissar, N. L. (2003). Comparison of 2 methods for postpyloric placement of enteral feeding tubes. *American Journal of Critical Care, 12*(4), 357-360.

Mackenzie, D. J., Popplewell, P. K., & Billingsley, K. G. (2004). Care of patients after esophagectomy. *Critical Care Nurse, 24*(1), 16-31.

Madsen, D., Sebolt, T., Cullen, L., Folkedahl, B., Mueller, T., Richardson, C., et al. (2005). Listening to bowel sounds: An evidence-based practice project. *American Journal of Nursing, 105*(12), 40-50.

Maykel, J. A., & Bistrian, B. R. (2002). Is enteral feeding for everyone? *Critical Care Medicine, 30*(3), 714-716.

McGinnis, C. (2002). Parenteral nutrition focus: Nutritional assessment and formula composition. *Journal of Infusion Nursing, 25*(1), 54-64.

Mechanick, J. I., & Brett, E. M. (2005). Nutrition and the chronically critically ill patient. *Current Opinion in Nutrition and Metabolic Care, 8*, 33-39.

Metheny, N. A., Chang, Y.-H., Ye, J. S., Edwards, S. J., Defer, J., Dahms, T. E., et al. (2002). Pepsin as a marker for pulmonary aspiration. *American Journal of Critical Care, 11*(2), 150-154.

Metheny, N. A., & Maloney, J. (2002). Controversy in using blue dye in enteral tube feedings as a method of detecting pulmonary aspiration. *Critical Care Nurse, 22*(5), 84-85.

Metheny, N. A., Schallom, M. E., & Edwards, S. J. (2004). Effect of gastrointestinal motility and feeding tube site on aspiration risk in critically ill patients: A review. *Heart and Lung, 33*(3), 131-145.

Metheny, N. A., & Titler, M. G. (2001). Assessing placement of feeding tubes. *American Journal of Nursing, 101*(5), 36-46.

Murray, D. (2003). Morbid obesity: Psychological aspects and surgical interventions. *AORN Journal, 78*(6), 990, 992-995.

Padula, C. A., Kenny, A., Planchon, C., & Lamoureaux, C. (2004). Enteral feedings: What the evidence says. *American Journal of Nursing, 104*(7), 62-70.

Parrish, C. R., & McCray, S. F. (2003). Nutritional support of the mechanically ventilated patient. *Critical Care Nurse, 23*(1), 77-80.

Powers, J., Chance, R., Bortenschlager, L., Hottenstein, J., Bobel, K., Gervasio, J., et al. (2003). Bedside placement of small-bowel feeding tubes in the intensive care unit. *Critical Care Nurse, 23*(1), 16-23.

Reising, D. L., & Neal, R. S. (2005). Enteral tube flushing. *American Journal of Nursing, 105*(3), 58-64.

Roberts, S. R., Kennerly, D. A., Keane, D., & George, C. (2003). Nutritional support in the intensive care unit: Adequacy, timeliness, and outcomes. *Critical Care Nurse, 23*(6), 49-57.

Sabol, V. K. (2004). Nutritional assessment of the critically ill adult. *AACN Clinical Issues, 15*(4), 595-606.

Spector, N. M., Hicks, F. D., & Pickleman, J. (2002). Quality of life and symptoms after surgery for gastroesophageal cancer. *Gastroenterology Nursing, 25*(3), 120-125.

Stechmiller, J. K., Childress, B., & Porter, T. (2004). Arginine immunonutrition in critically ill patients: A clinical dilemma. *American Journal of Critical Care, 13*(1), 17-23.

Swanson, R. W., & Winkelman, C. (2002). Exploring the benefits and myths of enteral feeding in the critically ill. *Critical Care Nursing Quarterly, 24*(2), 67-74.

Tisherman, S. A., Marik, P. E., & Ochoa, J. (2002). Promoting enteral nutrition 101. *Critical Care Medicine, 30*(7), 1653-1654.

Trujillo, E. B., Robinson, M. K., & Jacobs, D. O. (2001). Feeding critically ill patients: Current concepts. *Critical Care Nurse, 21*(4), 60-71.

Urden, L., Stacy, K., & Lough, M. (2006). *Thelan's critical care nursing: Diagnosis and management* (5th ed.). St. Louis: Mosby.

Vincent, J.-L., Dubois, M.-J., Navickis, R. J., & Wilkes, M. M. (2003). Hypoalbuminemia in acute illness: Is there a rationale for intervention? *Annuals of Surgery, 237*(3), 319-334.

Walker, J., & Criddle, L. M. (2003). Pathophysiology and management of abdominal compartment syndrome. *American Journal of Critical Care, 12*(4), 367-373.

Wiegand, D. L.-M. J., & Carlson, K. K. (2005). *AACN procedure manual for critical care* (5th ed.). Philadelphia: W. B. Saunders.

Wilkes, G. (2000). Nutrition: The forgotten ingredient in cancer care. *American Journal of Nursing, 100*(4), 46-51.

Zeigler, F. (2000). Managing patients with alcoholic cirrhosis. *Dimensions of Critical Care Nursing, 19*(2), 23-30.

The Neurologic System

CHAPTER 7

Selected Concepts in Anatomy and Physiology

General Information

1. Functions of the neurologic system
   a. Receiving stimuli from the internal and external environment over sensory pathways
   b. Communicating information between the body periphery and the central nervous system (CNS)
   c. Processing information received at reflex or conscious levels to determine appropriate responses
   d. Transmitting information over motor pathways to organs responsible for responding to the stimuli
2. Components of the neurologic system
   a. CNS
      (1) Brain
      (2) Spinal cord
   b. Peripheral nervous system
      (1) Cranial nerves
      (2) Spinal nerves
      (3) Peripheral nerves
   c. Autonomic nervous system (ANS)
      (1) Sympathetic nervous system (SNS)
      (2) Parasympathetic nervous system (PNS)

Microscopic Anatomy and Physiology

1. Nerve cells
   a. Neuroglia (also called *glial cells*)
      (1) Neuroglia are more numerous than neurons (85% of the cells in the CNS are neuroglial).
      (2) These cells provide support, nourishment, and protection to the neurons.
      (3) Most tumors of the CNS are neuroglial because the glial cells are mitotic and can replicate themselves.
      (4) Types
         (a) Microglia
            (i) Part of the reticuloendothelial system
            (ii) Rare in normal CNS tissue
            (iii) Become mobile and travel to the area of damage when the neurons become damaged; microglia then enlarge and phagocytize tissue debris
         (b) Oligodendroglia: responsible for myelin formation in the CNS
         (c) Astrocytes
            (i) May provide nutrients and regulate chemical environment for neurons
            (ii) Form the blood-brain barrier with the endothelium of the blood vessels
            (iii) Provide structure and support for nerve cells
            (iv) May have indirect role in synaptic transmission
         (d) Ependyma
            (i) Line the ventricles of brain and central canal of spinal cord
            (ii) Aid in secretion of cerebrospinal fluid (CSF)
   b. Neurons (Figure 7-1)
      (1) Transmit nerve impulses
      (2) Ten billion in CNS; most are in the cerebral cortex
      (3) Cannot regenerate in the CNS; can regenerate in peripheral nervous system by growing within the myelin if the cell body is intact
      (4) Components
         (a) Cell body (soma)
            (i) Nucleus: controls metabolic processes of cell
            (ii) Cytoplasm: contains organelles to carry out metabolic functions
         (b) Axons
            (i) Conduct impulses away from cell body to other neurons or to end-organs
            (ii) One axon per neuron
            (iii) May be myelinated or unmyelinated

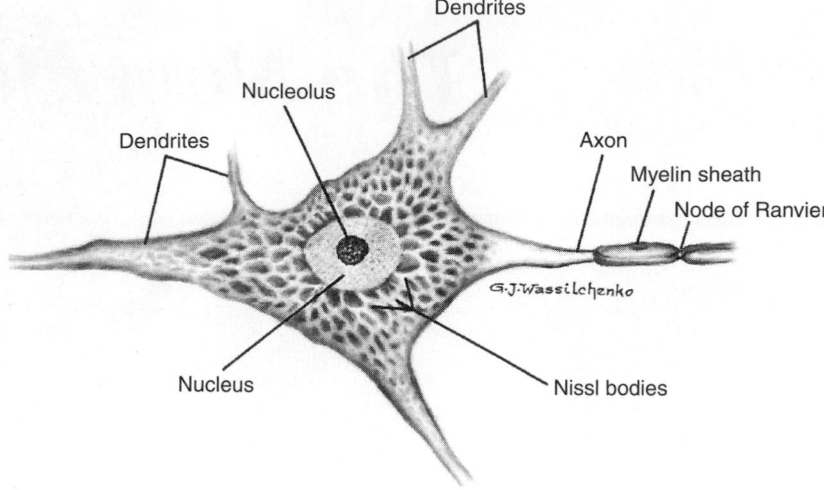

Figure 7-1 The neuron. (From Long, B. C., Phipps, W. J., & Cassmeyer, V. L. [1993]. *Medical-surgical nursing: A nursing process approach* [3rd ed.]. St. Louis: Mosby.)

(c) Dendrites
   (i) Conduct impulses toward cell body, which receives nerve impulses from the axons of other neurons
   (ii) May be more than one dendrite
(d) Neurofibrils: thin, threadlike fibers forming a network in the cytoplasm
(e) Nissl bodies
   (i) Specialize in protein synthesis with ribonucleic acid (RNA)
   (ii) Maintain and regenerate neuronal processes
(f) Myelin sheath
   (i) In some neurons, the axons covered with myelin, a white lipid substance, between the nodes of Ranvier
   (ii) Acts as insulation to speed conduction of impulses down the axon sheath
   (iii) Accounts for white color found in parts of brain and spinal cord
   (iv) Made by oligodendroglia in CNS and by Schwann cells in PNS
(g) Nodes of Ranvier
   (i) Constrictions occurring periodically along the axon where it is not covered by myelin
   (ii) Allows rapid conduction of impulses by saltatory conduction (node to node)
(h) Neurilemma
   (i) Outer coating of the neurons in the peripheral nervous system
   (ii) Provides for peripheral nerve regeneration
(i) Synaptic knobs: contain vesicles that store neurotransmitter substances

(5) Categorization
   (a) Direction of impulse formation
      (i) Afferent sensory neurons transmit impulses to the spinal cord or brain.
      (ii) Efferent motor neurons transmit impulses away from the brain or spinal cord.
      (iii) Remember SA ME (sensory afferent, motor efferent).
      (iv) Interneurons transmit impulses from sensory neurons to motor neurons.
   (b) Number of processes
      (i) Unipolar neurons have one process coming from the cell body; it bifurcates into an axon and a dendrite.
      (ii) Bipolar neurons have two processes (one axon and one dendrite) coming from the cell body.
      (iii) Multipolar neurons have one axon and more than one dendrite.
   (c) Location
      (i) Upper motor neurons (UMNs) originate above the brainstem.
      (ii) Lower motor neurons (LMNs) originate below the brainstem.

2. Neurophysiology
   a. Impulse transmission (Figure 7-2)
      (1) Initiated by a stimulus: chemical, electrical, mechanical, thermal
      (2) Change in permeability of the cell membrane to sodium
      (3) Depolarization of the cell caused by sodium influx; initiation of an action potential
      (4) Repolarization and return to normal resting polarized (ready) state occurs
      (5) Synaptic transmission (Figure 7-3)
         (a) Unidirectional conduction of an impulse from one neuron to the next
         (b) As the impulse nears the end of the axon, a release of neurotransmitter from the synaptic vesicles

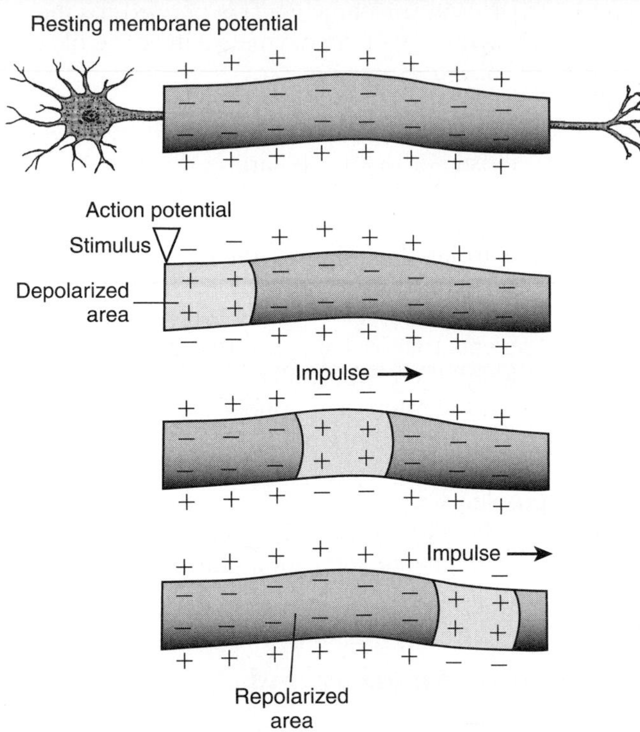

Figure 7-2 Transmission of a nerve impulse. (From Chipps, E. M., Clanin, N. J., & Campbell, V. G. [1992]. *Neurologic disorders: Mosby's clinical nursing series.* St. Louis: Mosby.)

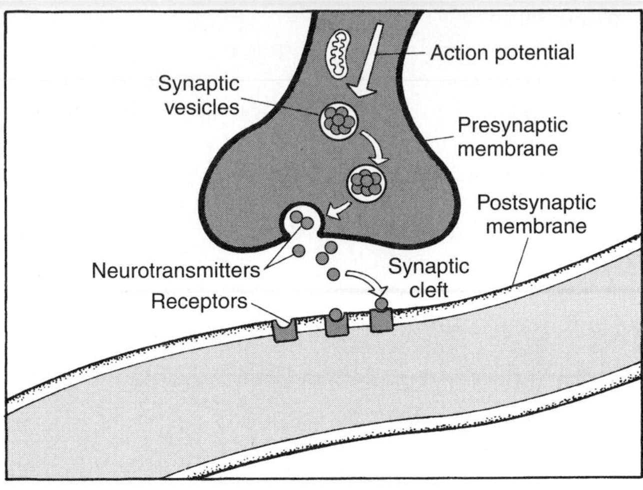

Figure 7-3 Synaptic transmission. (From Chipps, E. M., Clanin, N. J., & Campbell, V. G. [1992]. *Neurologic disorders: Mosby's clinical nursing series.* St. Louis: Mosby.)

(c) Diffusion of neurotransmitter across the synaptic gap changing the permeability of the cell membrane of the adjoining cell

(d) Continuation of the impulse to its end-organ or cell

(e) Types of synapses

(i) Axosomatic: the axon of one neuron synapses with the cell body of another neuron

(ii) Axodendritic: the axon of one neuron synapses with the dendrite of another neuron

(iii) Axoaxonic: the axon of one neuron synapses with the axon of another neuron

b. Refractory periods

(1) Absolute: period when the nerve cannot be stimulated again

(2) Relative: period when the nerve can be stimulated only by a strong impulse

3. Cerebral neurotransmitters (Table 7-1)

Table 7-1 Neurologic System Neurotransmitters

Name	Type	Region	Predominant Effect
Acetylcholine	Cholinergic	• Basal ganglia • Pyramidal cells • Parasympathetic branch of ANS	Excitatory
Norepinephrine	Amine	• Hypothalamus • Brainstem • Sympathetic branch of ANS	Inhibitory/excitatory
Dopamine	Amine	• Basal ganglia • Brainstem	Inhibitory
Serotonin	Amine	• Hypothalamus • Brainstem	Inhibitory
Gamma-aminobutyric acid	Amino acid	• Basal ganglia • Cerebellum • Spinal cord	Inhibitory
Glycine	Amino acid	• Spinal cord	Inhibitory
Beta-endorphins	Peptide	• Spinal cord	Inhibitory
Substance P	Peptide	• Pain fibers in spinal cord	Excitatory

ANS, Autonomic nervous system.

a. Function
   (1) Neurotransmitters are released from the presynaptic vesicles and act as a chemical bridge for the transmission of impulses from one neuron to another.
   (2) After synaptic transmission, the neurotransmitter is inactivated by an enzyme (e.g., cholinesterase deactivates acetylcholine).

b. Types
   (1) Excitatory neurotransmitters promote conduction of the impulse from one cell to the next.
   (2) Inhibitory neurotransmitters increase resistance to depolarization.

4. Cerebral metabolism
   a. Oxygen requirements
      (1) The brain weighs 2% of body weight but receives 20% of the cardiac output (CO) and uses 20% of oxygen delivered.
      (2) The brain, especially the cerebral cortex, is susceptible to change in oxygen delivery; the brainstem is the most resistant to hypoxic damage.
      (3) Anoxia causes brain edema and neuron death.
   b. Nutrient requirements
      (1) The brain has high metabolic energy needs.
      (2) Glucose is the main source of cellular energy (adenosine triphosphate [ATP]).
         (a) Triggered by the SNS, gluconeogenesis is an important process because it causes the conversion of protein and fat to glucose; the brain does not require insulin to use glucose.
         (b) Hypoglycemia is associated with neurologic symptoms.
            (i) Confusion usually occurs if blood glucose is less than 50 to 70 mg/dL.
            (ii) Coma occurs if blood glucose is less than 20 mg/dL.
         (c) Although hyperglycemia does not cause direct neurologic effects, the osmotic effect may cause hyperosmolality and brain dehydration (e.g., hyperglycemic hyperosmolar nonketotic coma).
      (3) Vitamins
         (a) Thiamine (B_1) is important in the Krebs cycle; deficiency of vitamin B_1 causes Wernicke's encephalopathy.
         (b) Vitamin B_{12} is important in the spinal cord and peripheral nervous system; deficiency of vitamin B_{12} causes pernicious anemia and gradual deterioration of the CNS and peripheral nerves.
         (c) Pyridoxine (B_6) is a coenzyme that participates in many enzymatic reactions in the CNS; deficiency of vitamin B_6 causes neuropathy and seizures.
         (d) Niacin (nicotinic acid) is needed for the synthesis of coenzymes; deficiency of niacin causes pellagra.

5. Blood-brain barrier
   a. Not a true structure but is a special permeability characteristic of brain capillaries and choroid plexus
   b. Functions
      (1) Acts to limit transfer of certain substances into extracellular fluid (ECF) or CSF of brain
      (2) Prevents toxic substances from readily entering the extracellular space of the nervous system; may hinder the effective use of certain drug therapies in the treatment of neurologic system problems
      (3) May be altered by trauma, induction of some toxic elements, intracranial tumor, or brain irradiation

Macroscopic Anatomy and Physiology

1. Scalp: skin covering the cranium
   a. Made of five layers
      (1) **S**kin: thicker than anywhere else in the body
      (2) **C**utaneous tissue
      (3) **A**dipose tissue
      (4) **L**igament layer referred to as *galea aponeurotica;* moves freely over the skull
      (5) **P**ericranium
   b. Blood vessels located in the subcutaneous tissue
      (1) The scalp is vascular
      (2) Blood vessels in the scalp do not contract well when injured
      (3) Scalp laceration can result in significant blood loss

2. Skull (Figure 7-4): bony structure of the head, consisting of the cranium and the skeleton of the face
   a. The skull is composed of an inner table and outer table separated by cancellous (spongy) bone; this structure allows for maximum strength and minimal weight.
   b. The cranium is a body vault that holds and protects the brain from external forces; volume capacity is approximately 1500 mL.
   c. The cranium consists of eight bones:
      (1) Frontal: one
      (2) Parietal: two
      (3) Temporal: two
      (4) Occipital: one
      (5) Ethmoid: one
      (6) Sphenoid: one
   d. The sphenoid bone divides interior of skull into three fossae (Figure 7-5).

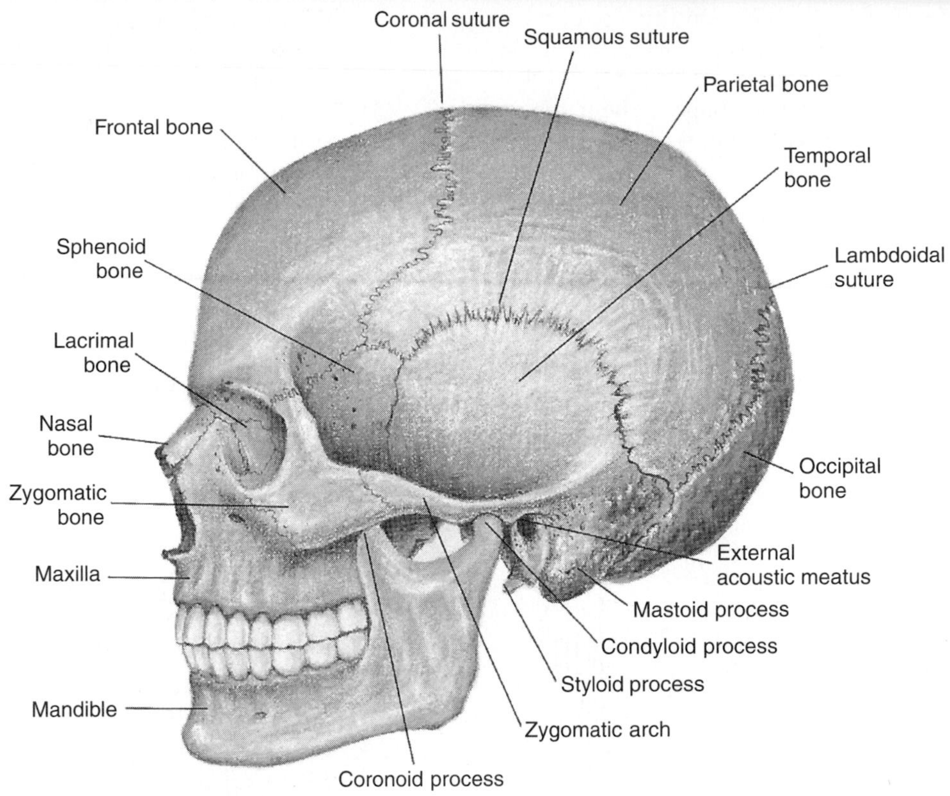

Figure 7-4 Lateral view of skull. (From Chipps, E. M., Clanin, N. J., & Campbell, V. G. [1992]. *Neurologic disorders: Mosby's clinical nursing series*. St. Louis: Mosby.)

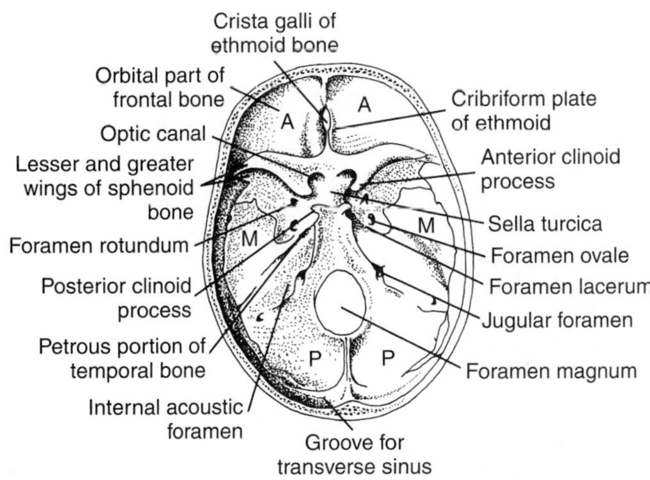

Figure 7-5 Bones that form the floor of the cranial cavity and the three fossae formed by these bones. (From Kinney, M. R., Packa, D. R., & Dunbar, S. B. [1998]. *AACN's clinical reference for critical-care nursing* [4th ed.]. St. Louis: Mosby.)

(1) Anterior fossa: contains the frontal lobes
(2) Middle fossa: contains the temporal, parietal, occipital lobes
(3) Posterior fossa: contains the cerebellum

e. The foramen magnum is a large oval-shaped opening at the base of the skull; this is the location of the connection of the brain and spinal cord.

3. Meninges (Figure 7-6): protective coverings of the brain and the spinal cord
   a. Pia mater
      (1) This is the delicate layer that adheres to surface of brain and spinal cord.
      (2) This layer follows sulci and gyri of brain and carries branches of cerebral arteries with it.
         (a) Sulci: shallow grooves or invaginations on the surface of the brain (deep sulci are referred to as *fissures*)
         (b) Gyri: convolutions on the surface of the brain
      (3) Blood vessels of pia form the choroid plexus.
   b. Arachnoid mater
      (1) This is the middle layer of the meninges.
      (2) The subarachnoid space is between the arachnoid mater and the pia mater.
         (a) Contains larger blood vessels of brain
         (b) Contains CSF
         (c) Contains arachnoid villi (projections of arachnoid mater that serve as channels for absorption of CSF into venous system)
   c. Dura mater
      (1) This is the outermost layer of meninges.
      (2) Meningeal arteries and venous sinuses lie within clefts formed by separation of inner and outer layers of dura.

(3) The epidural space is between the skull and the dura mater.
 (a) Only a potential space
 (b) Site of epidural hemorrhage or hematoma
(4) The subdural space is between the dura mater and the arachnoid mater.
 (a) Only a potential space
 (b) Site of subdural hemorrhage or hematoma
(5) The dura mater has several folds (Figure 7-7).
 (a) The falx cerebri separates the two cerebral hemispheres.

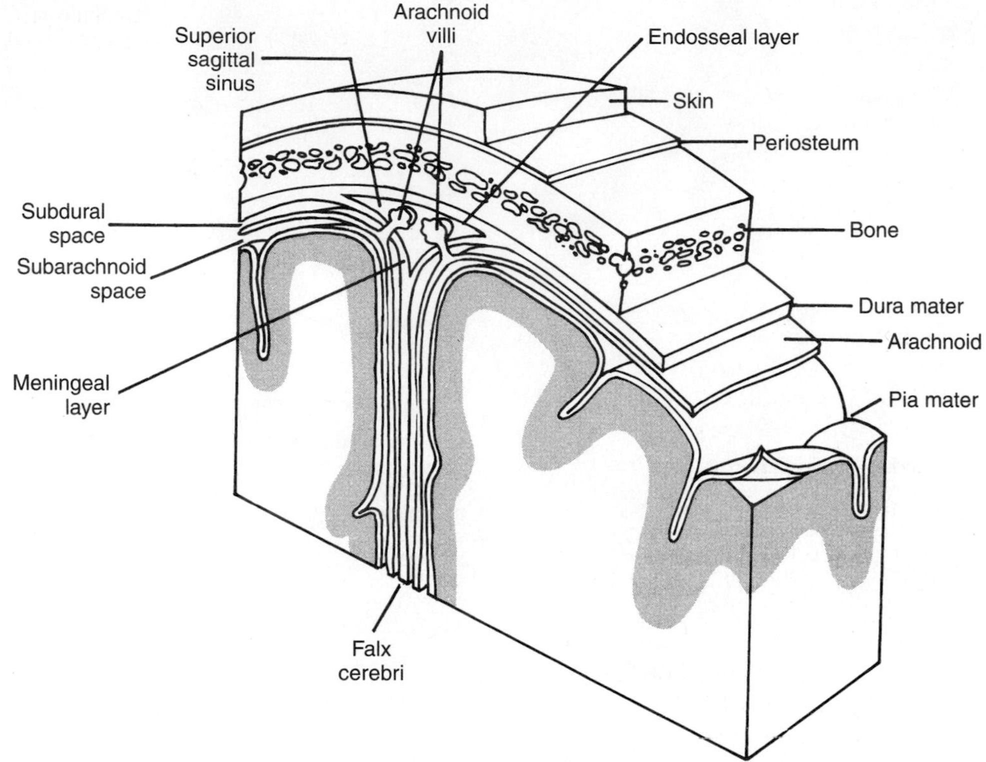

Figure 7-6 Coronal section of the skull and brain showing the relationship of the meninges. (From Barker, E. [1994]. *Neuroscience nursing*. St. Louis: Mosby.)

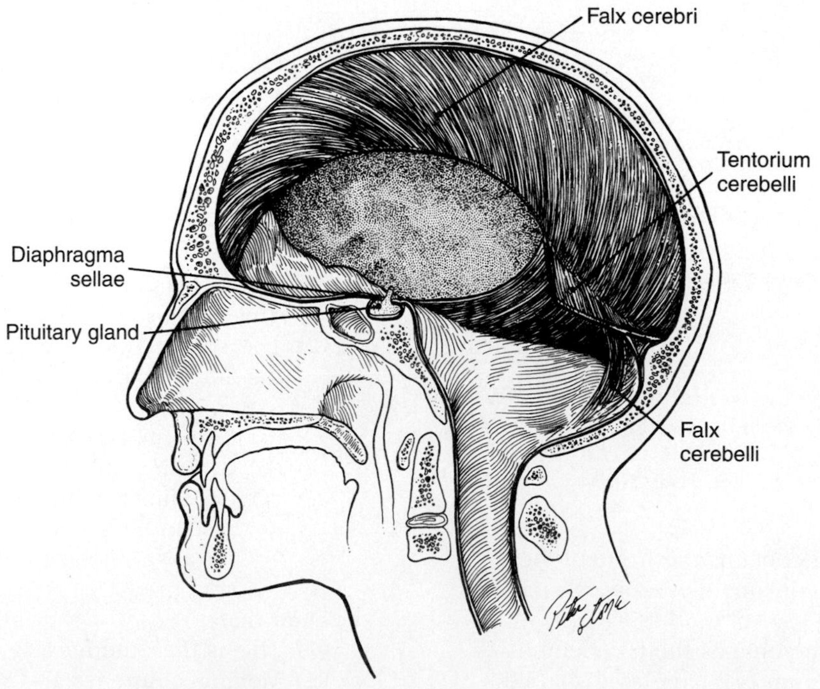

Figure 7-7 Folds of the dura. (From Kinney, M. R., Packa, D. R., & Dunbar, S. B. [1998]. *AACN's clinical reference for critical-care nursing* [4th ed.]. St. Louis: Mosby.)

(b) The falx cerebelli separates the two cerebellar hemispheres.
(c) The tentorium cerebelli separates the cerebral hemispheres from the cerebellum.
(d) The diaphragm sella canopies the sella turcica (where the pituitary gland is located) and encloses the pituitary gland.

4. Brain (Figure 7-8)
   a. General information
      (1) Weighs approximately 1.5 kg
      (2) Divided into cerebrum, brainstem, and cerebellum
   b. Telencephalon: two cerebral hemispheres connected by the corpus callosum
      (1) Cerebrum (Figure 7-9)
         (a) Structure
            (i) Outer layer of cerebral cortex is gray matter consisting of neuron cell bodies (six cell layers thick).
            (ii) Deeper layers of each hemisphere are white matter consisting of myelinated axons with four paired masses of gray matter known as *basal ganglia.*
            (iii) Fissures
               a) Longitudinal fissure (also referred to as *falx cerebri*): divides the left and right cerebral hemispheres
               b) Fissure of Rolando (also referred to as *central sulcus*): divides frontal lobe from parietal lobes; separates the motor and sensory strips
               c) Fissure of Sylvius (also referred to as *lateral sulcus*): divides frontal lobe from temporal lobes

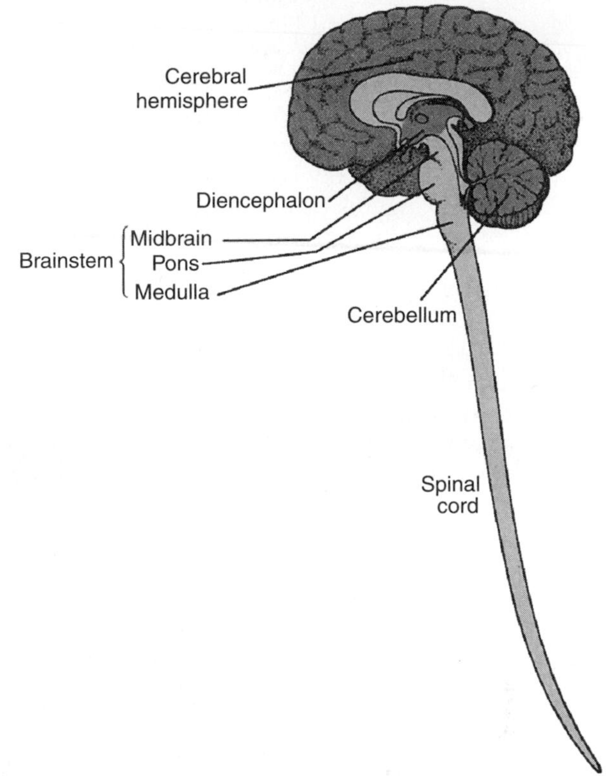

Figure 7-8 Major divisions of the CNS. (From Lewis, S. M., & Collier, I. C. [1992]. *Medical-surgical nursing* [3rd ed.] St. Louis: Mosby.)

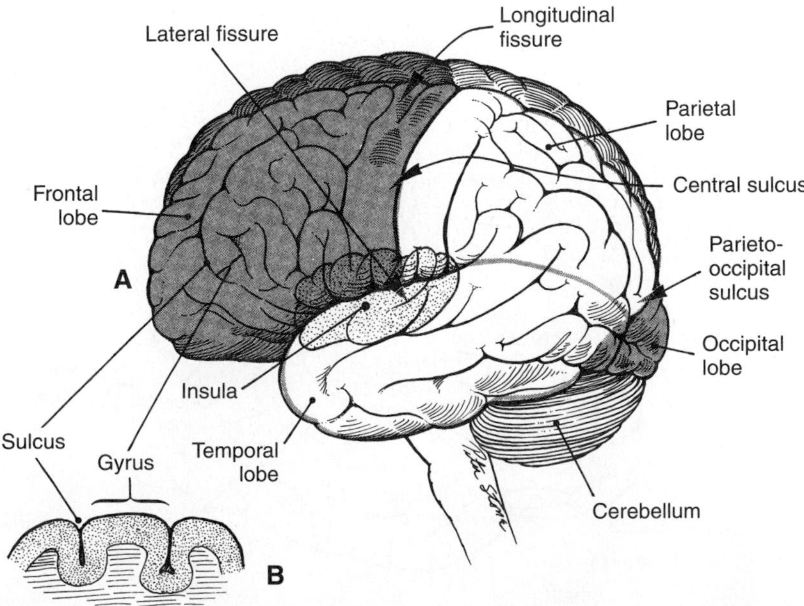

Figure 7-9 A, Lateral view of the cerebrum. **B,** Portion of the cortex in cross-section showing gyrus and sulcus.

(b) Cerebral cortical areas and functions (Table 7-2 and Figure 7-10)
- (i) Lobes
  - a) Frontal: contains the precentral gyrus (also referred to as the *motor strip*) (Figure 7-11)
  - b) Parietal: contains the postcentral gyrus (also referred to as the *sensory strip*) (see Figure 7-11)
  - c) Temporal
  - d) Occipital

Table 7-2 Cerebral Cortical Areas and Functions

Cerebral Cortical Area	Functions
Frontal lobe	• Personality • Behavior: ethical; moral; social • Intellectual functions ◦ Conscious thought ◦ Abstract thinking ◦ Judgment and foresight • Short-term memory • Voluntary motor function • Motor speech (Broca's area in dominant hemisphere)
Parietal lobe	• Localization of sensory information to the body surface • Sensory integration and discrimination • Object recognition • Position sense • Body awareness • Body image
Temporal lobe	• Emotion • Long-term memory • Processing of olfactory, gustatory, auditory input • Sensory speech (Wernicke's area in dominant hemisphere)
Occipital lobe	• Processing of visual input

- (ii) Cerebral hemispheres
  - a) Each hemisphere of the brain receives sensory information from the opposite side of the body and controls skeletal muscles of the opposite side.
  - b) Each hemisphere has specialization.
    - i) The left cerebral hemisphere is specialized for analysis, problem solving, language, mathematics, abstract reasoning, and interpretation of symbols.
    - ii) The right cerebral hemisphere is specialized for visuospatial patterns, nonverbal communication, music, and artistic ability.
  - c) Hemispheric dominance
    - i) Ninety percent of right-handed persons are left hemisphere dominant.
    - ii) Sixty percent of left-handed persons are right hemisphere dominant.
    - iii) Language centers are located in dominant hemisphere; lesions in dominant hemisphere frequently cause aphasia.

(c) Corpus callosum: path for fibers to cross from one cerebral hemisphere to the other

(d) Basal ganglia
- (i) Major center of the extrapyramidal system
- (ii) Functions
  - a) Regulates and controls motor integration
  - b) Influences posture
  - c) Allows fine voluntary movements

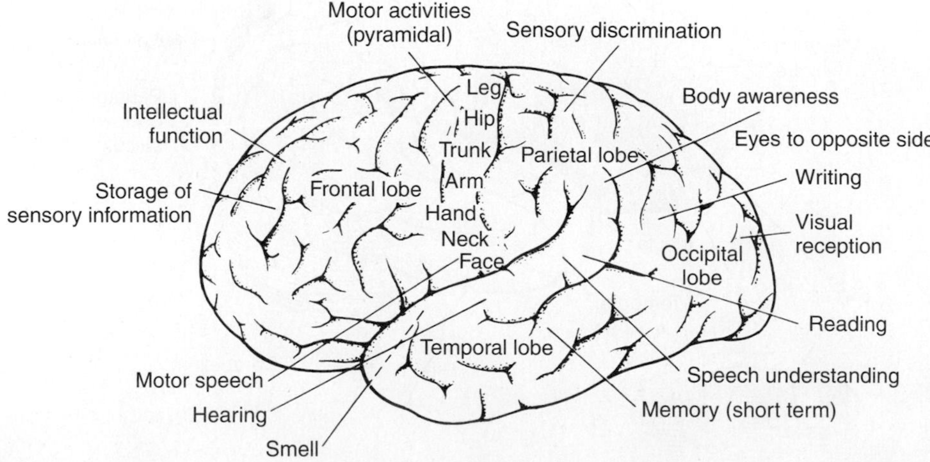

Figure 7-10 Functional areas of the cerebral cortex. (From Kinney, M. R., Packa, D. R., & Dunbar, S. B. [1998]. *AACN's clinical reference for critical-care nursing* [4th ed.]. St. Louis: Mosby.)

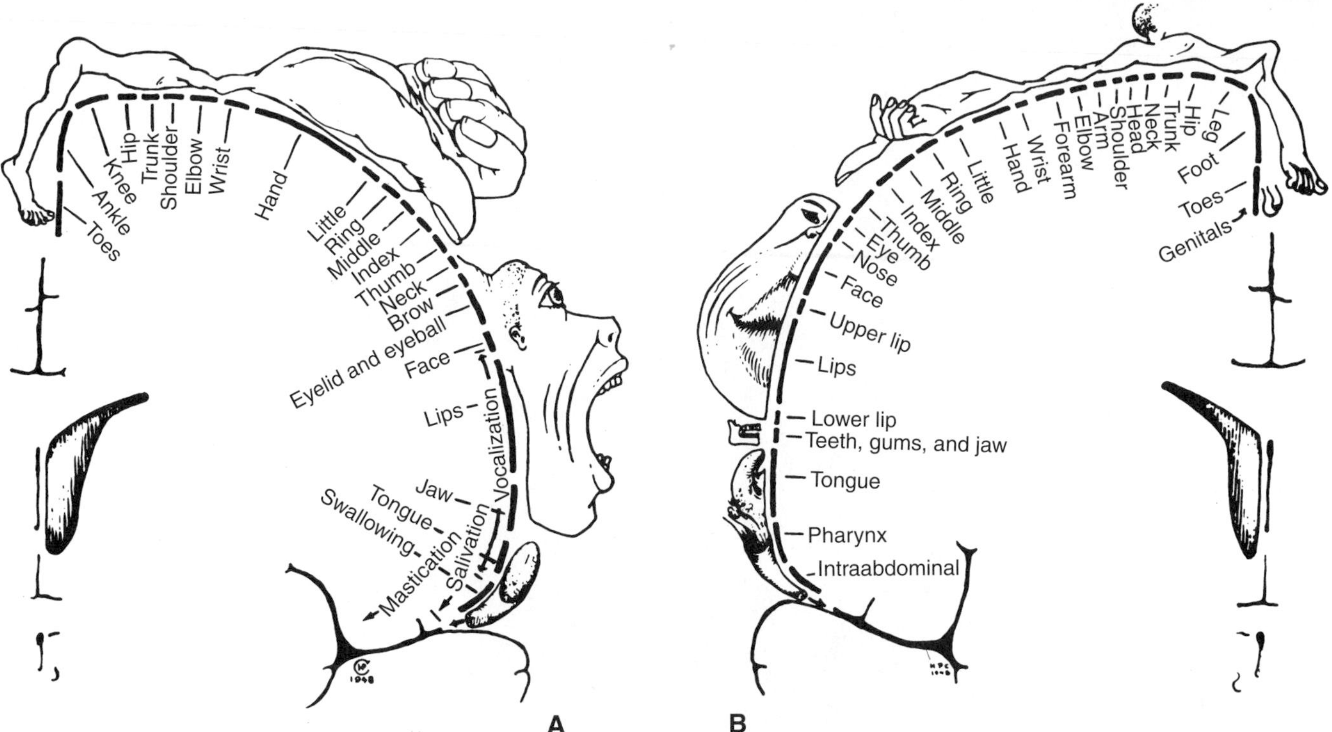

Figure 7-11 **A,** Motor homunculus showing areas of the motor strip devoted to specified areas of the body. **B,** Sensory homunculus showing areas of the sensory strip devoted to specified areas of the body. (From Urden, L., Stacy, K., & Lough, M. [2002]. *Thelan's critical care nursing: Diagnosis and management* [4th ed.]. St. Louis: Mosby.)

c. Diencephalon
   (1) Thalamus: relay of incoming messages to appropriate areas of the brain
   (2) Hypothalamus
      (a) Temperature regulation
      (b) Regulation of food and water intake
      (c) Sleep patterns
      (d) Autonomic responses
      (e) Control of hormonal secretion of pituitary gland
   (3) Limbic system
      (a) Self-preservation behaviors including aggression
      (b) Basic drives (e.g., food and sex)
      (c) Affective aspect of emotional behavior
      (d) Some aspects of memory

d. Brainstem
   (1) Functions
      (a) Relays messages between the brain and lower levels of the nervous system
      (b) Location of the origin of all cranial nerves except first and second
   (2) Divisions
      (a) Mesencephalon (midbrain)
         (i) Location of the origin of third and fourth cranial nerves
         (ii) Contains motor and sensory pathways
         (iii) Location of reticular activating system (RAS); responsible for arousal from sleep, wakefulness, and focusing of attention
      (b) Pons
         (i) Location of the origin of fifth, sixth, and seventh cranial nerves
         (ii) Connects cerebral cortex and cerebellum
         (iii) Contains motor and sensory pathways
         (iv) Contains respiratory centers
      (c) Medulla oblongata
         (i) Location of the origin of eighth, ninth, tenth, eleventh, and twelfth cranial nerves
         (ii) Connects motor and sensory tracts of spinal cord to medulla
         (iii) Contains cardiac and respiratory centers

e. Cerebellum
   (1) Coordinates muscle movement with sensory input
   (2) Controls balance
   (3) Influences muscle tone in relation to equilibrium
   (4) Affects locomotion and posture
   (5) Controls nonstereotyped movements
   (6) Synchronizes muscle action

5. Cerebral circulation (Table 7-3)
   a. The brain receives 20% of CO
   b. Arterial system (Figures 7-12 and 7-13)
      (1) External carotid system: arises from common carotid arteries
         (a) Occipital arteries: supply the posterior fossa
         (b) Temporal arteries: supply the temporal area
         (c) Maxillary arteries: form the middle meningeal arteries

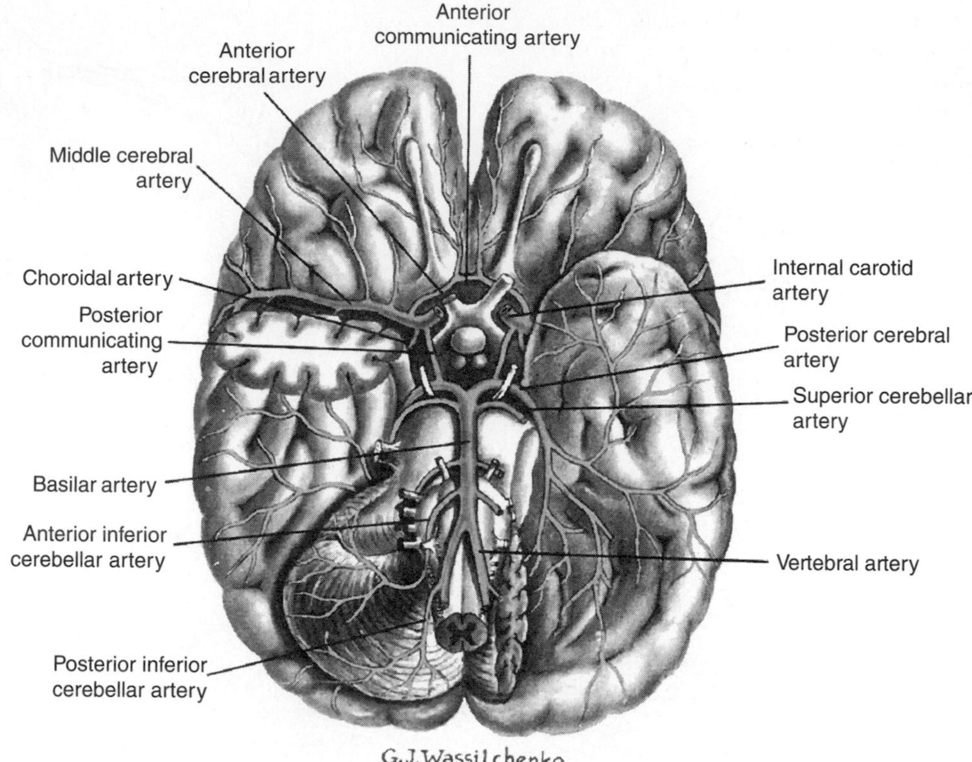

Figure 7-12 Arterial system of the brain. (From Urden, L., Stacy, K., & Lough, M. [2002]. *Thelan's critical care nursing: Diagnosis and management* [4th ed.]. St. Louis: Mosby.)

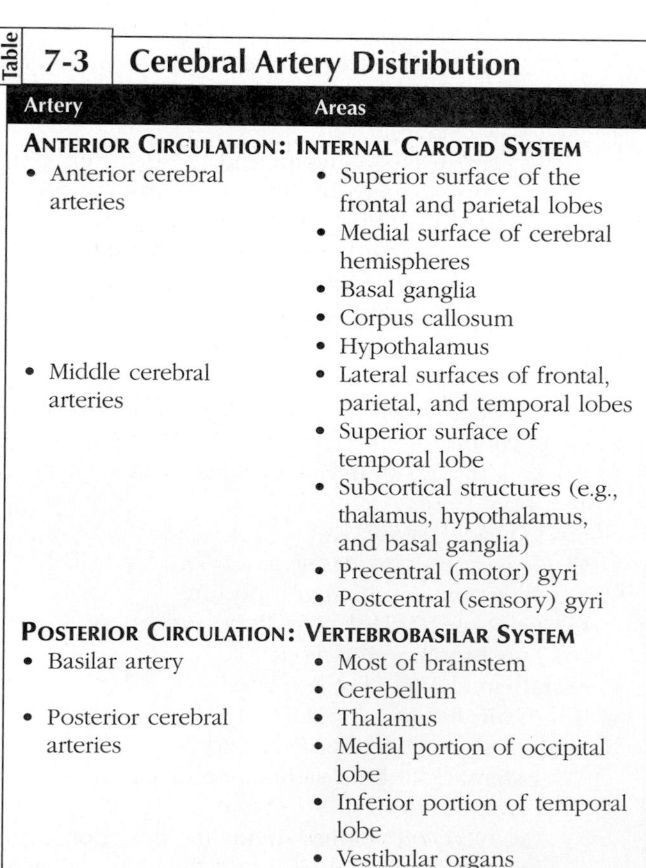

Table 7-3 Cerebral Artery Distribution

Artery	Areas
ANTERIOR CIRCULATION: INTERNAL CAROTID SYSTEM	
• Anterior cerebral arteries	• Superior surface of the frontal and parietal lobes • Medial surface of cerebral hemispheres • Basal ganglia • Corpus callosum • Hypothalamus
• Middle cerebral arteries	• Lateral surfaces of frontal, parietal, and temporal lobes • Superior surface of temporal lobe • Subcortical structures (e.g., thalamus, hypothalamus, and basal ganglia) • Precentral (motor) gyri • Postcentral (sensory) gyri
POSTERIOR CIRCULATION: VERTEBROBASILAR SYSTEM	
• Basilar artery	• Most of brainstem • Cerebellum
• Posterior cerebral arteries	• Thalamus • Medial portion of occipital lobe • Inferior portion of temporal lobe • Vestibular organs • Cochlear apparatus

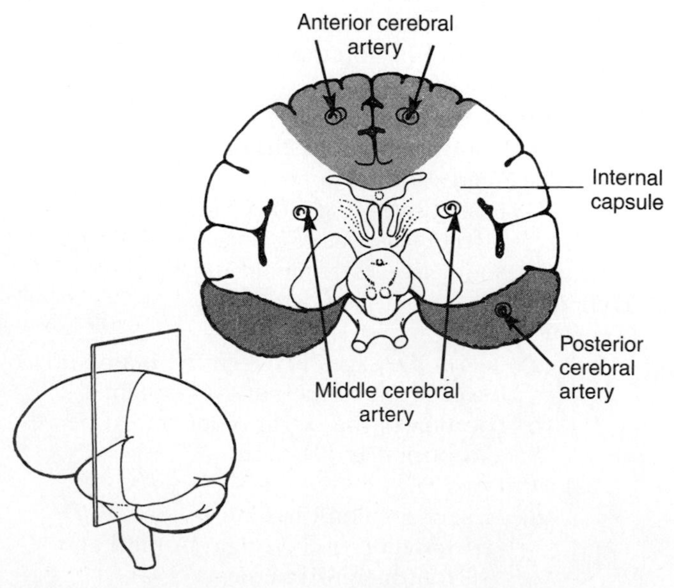

Figure 7-13 Distribution of the arterial blood supply. (From Urden, L., Stacy, K., & Lough, M. [2002]. *Thelan's critical care nursing: Diagnosis and management* [4th ed.]. St. Louis: Mosby.)

(d) Meningeal arteries: branches of external carotid arteries that supply dura mater (internal carotid and vertebral arteries supply pia and arachnoid mater)
(i) Anterior meningeal artery: supplies anterior portion of dura
(ii) Middle meningeal artery: supplies most of dura
(iii) Posterior meningeal artery: supplies occipital area of dura
(2) Anterior circulation: internal carotid system
(a) Arises from common carotid arteries
(b) Accounts for 80% of cerebral perfusion
(c) Includes the following:
(i) Anterior cerebral arteries
(ii) Anterior communicating artery
a) Connects right and left anterior cerebral arteries
b) Forms anterior section of circle of Willis
(iii) Middle cerebral arteries
(iv) Posterior communicating arteries
a) Connect posterior cerebral arteries with the anterior circulation
b) Form posterior portion of circle of Willis
(3) Posterior circulation: vertebrobasilar system
(a) Arises from subclavian arteries and joins at lower border of pons to form basilar artery
(b) Includes the following:
(i) Posterior cerebral arteries
(ii) Basilar artery
(iii) Anterior spinal artery: supplies anterior half of three quarters of spinal cord and medial aspect of brainstem
(iv) Posterior spinal arteries: traverses the cord along the dorsal roots
(4) Circle of Willis
(a) Formed by internal carotid and vertebral arteries
(b) Permits collateral circulation if one of the carotid or vertebral arteries becomes occluded; unfortunately, many persons have an incomplete circle of Willis, which prevents this collateral flow when injury or occlusion occurs
(c) Prone to aneurysmal formation because of multiple bifurcations

c. Cerebral blood flow (CBF)
(1) Brings oxygen and nutrients to the brain tissue for cellular energy production; waste products are removed from the blood
(2) CBF varies with changes in cerebral perfusion pressure (CPP) and diameter of the cerebrovascular bed
(a) Normal CBF is approximately 50 mL/100 g/min.
(b) Normal cerebral oxygen extraction ratio is between 25% and 35%; an oxygen extraction ratio greater than 40% indicates an imbalance between oxygen supply and demand and impending cerebral ischemia.
(i) Calculated by $(Sao_2 - Sjo_2)/Sao_2$, where Sao_2 is oxygen saturation of arterial blood measured by arterial blood gases (ABGs) or pulse oximetry and Sjo_2 is the saturation of the venous blood from the jugular vein measured by a fiberoptic catheter placed in the jugular bulb.
(3) CPP = MAP – mean ICP, where *CPP* is cerebral perfusion pressure, *MAP* is mean arterial pressure, and *ICP* is intracranial pressure
(a) Changes in MAP or ICP affect CPP.
(b) Normal MAP is 70 to 105 mm Hg; normal ICP is 5 to 15; so normal CPP is 60 to 100 mm Hg.
(c) CPP less than 50 mm Hg is associated with impaired neuronal functioning.
(4) Autoregulation is the ability of the brain to alter the diameter of the arterioles in order to maintain CBF at a constant level despite any changes in CPP
(a) When ICP approaches MAP, CPP decreases to the point at which autoregulation is impaired and CBF decreases.
(b) Limits of autoregulation are CPP between 50 and 150 mm Hg.
(i) CPP less than 50 mm Hg causes hypoperfusion (e.g., cardiopulmonary arrest or shock), causing anoxic encephalopathy.
(ii) CPP greater than 150 mm Hg causes hyperperfusion (e.g., hypertensive crisis), causing brain edema and hypertensive encephalopathy.
(5) Factors affecting CBF
(a) Increase in CBF
(i) Hypercapnia
(ii) Hypoxemia
(iii) Decreased blood viscosity
(iv) Hyperthermia
(v) Drugs: vasodilators
(b) Decrease in CBF
(i) Hypocapnia
(ii) Hyperoxemia
(iii) Increased blood viscosity
(iv) Hypothermia
(v) Intracranial hypertension
(vi) Drugs: vasopressors

(c) Drugs that often are used therapeutically to optimize CO, blood pressure (BP), and CPP and/or to minimize oxygen consumption may result in decreased CO, BP, CPP, and CBF when used inappropriately or in excess
(i) Negative inotropes (e.g., beta-blockers and barbiturates)
(ii) Vasodilators (e.g., nitroprusside and nitroglycerin)
(iii) Anesthetic agents

d. Venous system (Figure 7-14)
(1) The cerebrum has external veins that lie in subarachnoid space on surfaces of hemispheres and internal veins that drain the central core of cerebrum and lie beneath corpus callosum.
(2) External and internal venous systems empty into venous sinuses that lie between dural layers.
(a) Superior sagittal sinus drains venous blood from the anterior portions of the brain.
(b) Cavernous sinus drains venous blood from the inferior portions of the brain.
(c) Transvenous sinus drains venous blood from the posterior portion of the brain.
(3) The internal jugular veins collect blood from dural venous sinuses.

6. CSF
a. Characteristics
(1) Functions
(a) Cushions brain and spinal cord
(b) Allows for compensation for changes in ICP; displacement of CSF out of cranial cavity compensates for increases in intracranial volume to prevent increase in ICP
(2) Volume: 120 to 150 mL
(a) Distribution: 90 mL in lumbar subarachnoid space, 25 mL in ventricles, 35 mL in rest of subarachnoid space
(b) Daily synthesis: 500 mL
(3) Pressure: 80 to 180 mm H_2O, measured at lumbar level, with patient in side-lying position

b. CSF production and reabsorption
(1) CSF is a transudate of plasma formed by choroid plexus in ventricles.
(a) Choroid plexus: sheets of epithelial cells that project into the lumen of the ventricular spaces
(b) Majority (95%) of CSF produced in lateral ventricles
(2) CSF is absorbed via arachnoid villi, which return it to systemic circulation by the internal jugular veins; hydrostatic pressure gradient between CSF and venous sinus is one factor that determines CSF absorption.

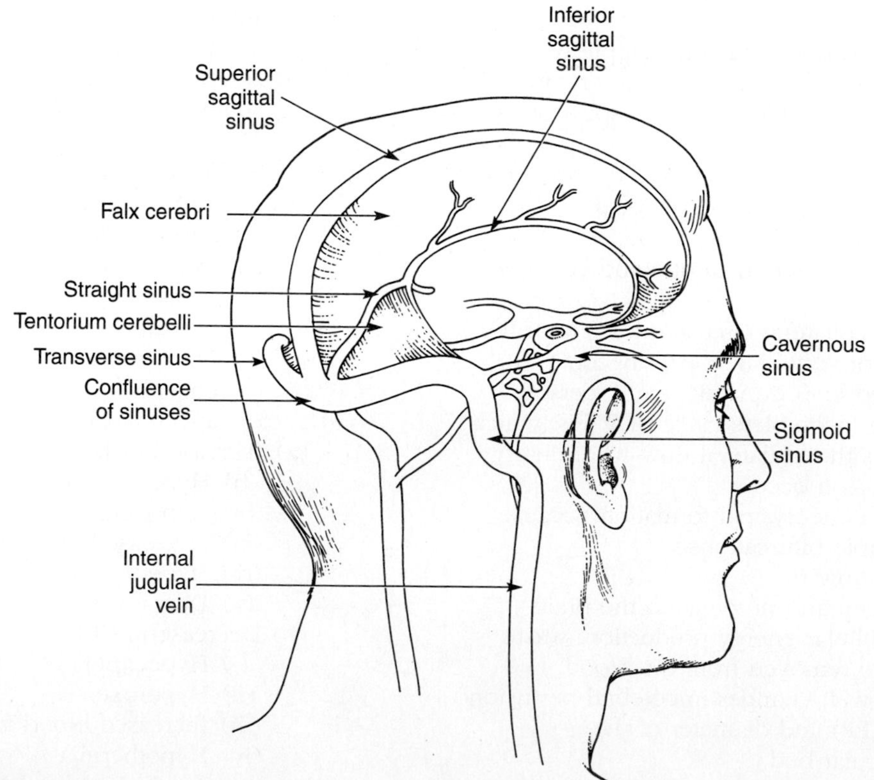

Figure 7-14 Venous system of the brain showing major dural venous sinuses and their connection to the internal jugular veins. (From Barker, E. [1994]. *Neuroscience nursing*. St. Louis: Mosby.)

c. CSF communication system within brain (Figure 7-15)
  (1) Ventricles: hollow spaces that are lined with ependyma; contain specialized epithelium called *choroid plexus* that produces CSF
    (a) The lateral ventricles are the largest of the ventricles; one lies in each cerebral hemisphere.
    (b) The third ventricle lies midline between the two lateral ventricles.
    (c) The fourth ventricle lies in posterior fossa.
  (2) Pathway of CSF circulation (Figure 7-16): lateral ventricles → foramen of Monro → third ventricle → aqueduct of Sylvius → fourth ventricle → cisterns and subarachnoid space, where arachnoid villi reabsorb CSF into the systemic circulation

7. Spine and spinal cord
  a. Structure
    (1) Vertebral column: composed of 7 cervical, 12 thoracic, 5 lumbar, 5 sacral, and 4 coccygeal vertebrae
    (2) Spinal cord: 42 to 45 cm extending from superior border of atlas to upper border of second lumbar vertebrae (L2); continuous with the brainstem
      (a) Meninges: pia mater, arachnoid mater, dura mater
      (b) Central canal: opening in the center of the spinal cord that contains CSF; communicates with the fourth ventricle
      (c) Central gray horns which form an H: contain mostly cell bodies (Figure 7-17)
        (i) The anterior (or ventral) horn of gray matter contains cell bodies of efferent or motor fibers
        (ii) The posterior (or dorsal) horn of gray matter contains cell bodies of afferent or sensory fibers
        (iii) The lateral horn of gray matter contains preganglionic fibers of autonomic system
      (d) Columns of white matter are fiber tracts that surround the gray matter: contain mostly myelinated axons (Figure 7-18)

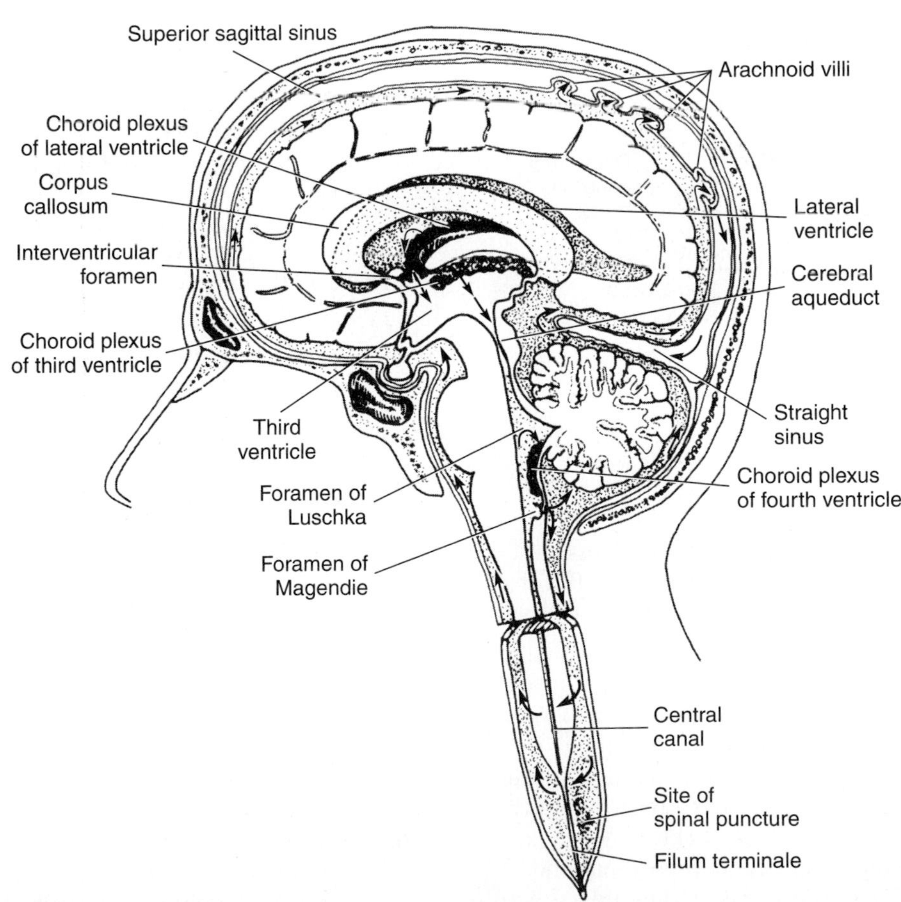

Figure 7-15 Lateral view of the ventricular system. Arrows show direction of CSF circulation. (From Kinney, M. R., Packa, D. R., & Dunbar, S. B. [1998]. *AACN's clinical reference for critical-care nursing* [4th ed.]. St. Louis: Mosby.)

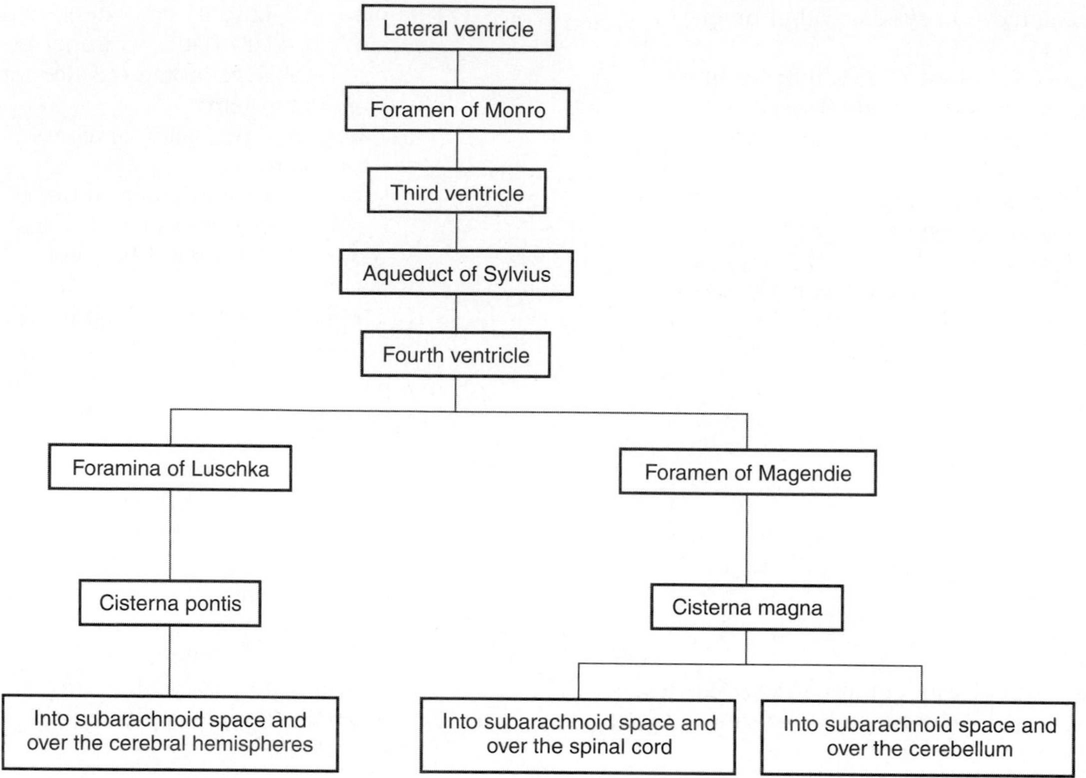

Figure 7-16 Circulation of CSF.

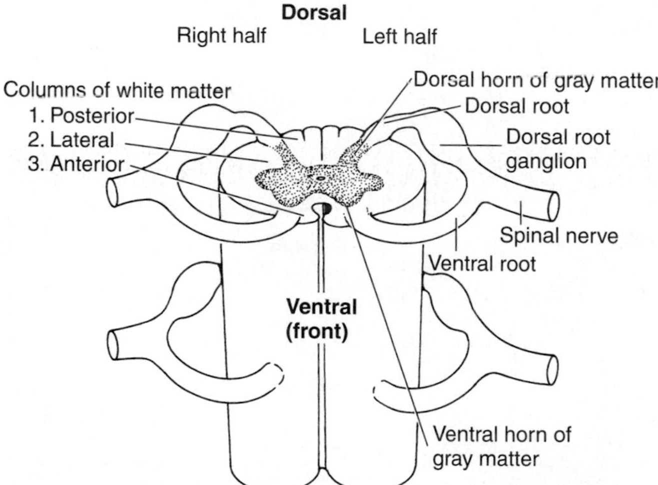

Figure 7-17 Segment of the thoracic spinal cord in cross-section. (From Kinney, M. R., Packa, D. R., & Dunbar, S. B. [1998]. *AACN's clinical reference for critical-care nursing* [4th ed.]. St. Louis: Mosby.)

(i) Posterior tracts (dorsal columns) and the anterior and lateral spinothalamic tracts are ascending tracts that conduct sensory impulses from the spinal cord to the thalamus and cerebral cortex.

(ii) Lateral tracts (the corticospinal and pyramidal) are descending tracts that conduct motor impulses from the brain to motor neurons in the anterior horn.

(iii) Spinal tracts are named by column, origin, and termination (e.g., lateral corticospinal tract is located in the lateral column, originates in the cortex, and terminates in the spine; it is therefore a descending tract [cortex to spine]); Table 7-4 describes clinically significant tracts.

(3) UMNs and LMNs
  (a) UMNs: located in the cerebral cortex and brainstem
    (i) Cell bodies lie in the motor area of the cerebral cortex.
    (ii) Axons pass through the spinal cord to synapse with the LMNs.
    (iii) Damage to UMN causes spastic paralysis and hyperactive reflexes.
  (b) LMNs: located in the spinal cord
    (i) Cell bodies lie in the anterior horn of gray matter in the spinal cord.
    (ii) Axons directly innervate striated muscle fibers.
    (iii) Damage to LMN causes flaccid paralysis and areflexia.

b. Function
  (1) Mediates the reflex arc (Figure 7-19)
    (a) An involuntary response to a stimulus (e.g., touching hot stove causes reflex withdrawal of hand)

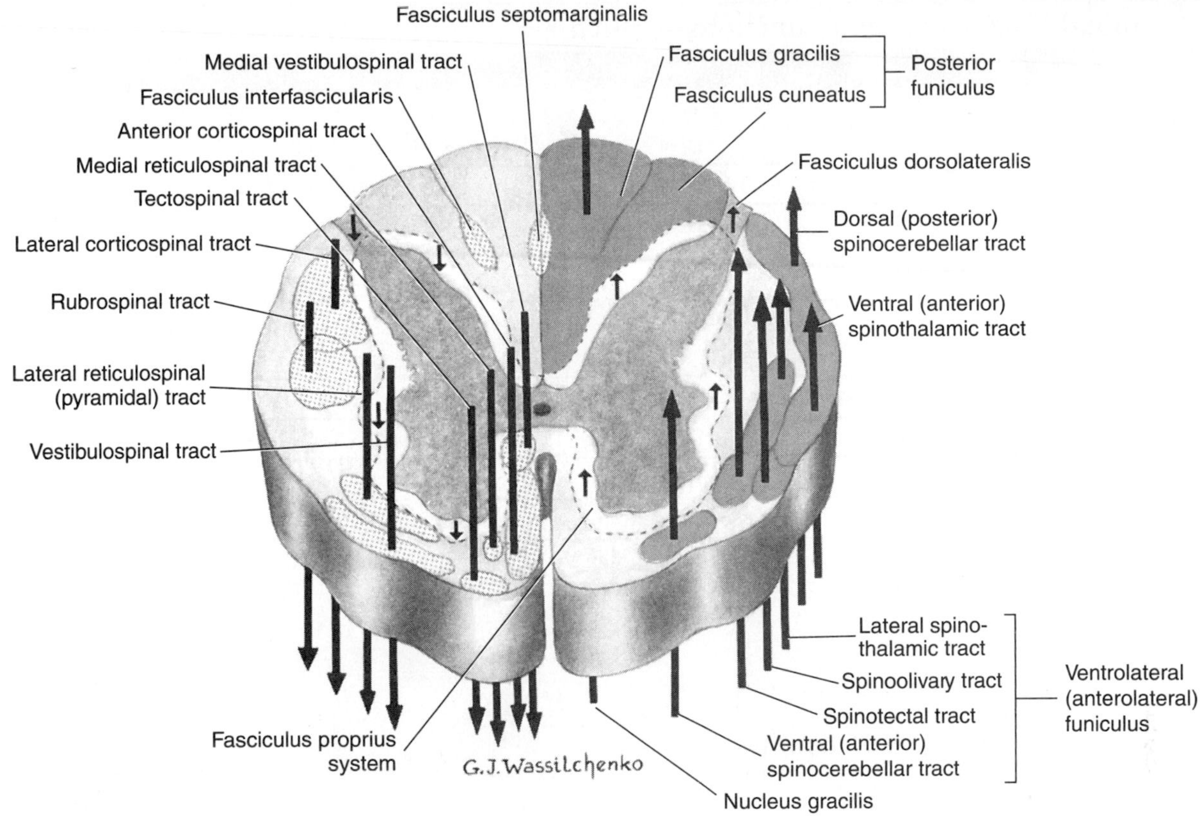

Figure 7-18 Spinal cord tracts of the white matter. (From Urden, L., Stacy, K., & Lough, M. [2002]. *Thelan's critical care nursing: Diagnosis and management* [4th ed.]. St. Louis: Mosby.)

Table 7-4 Spinal Cord Tracts and Functions

Tract	Column	Direction	Functions	Sidedness
Spinothalamic				
• Lateral spinothalamic	Lateral	Ascending	• Pain • Temperature	Contralateral
• Anterior spinothalamic	Anterior	Ascending	• Light touch • Pressure • Pain • Temperature	Contralateral
Spinotectal	Lateral	Ascending	• Tactile stimulation arousing consciousness	Contralateral
Spinocerebellar				
• Dorsal spinocerebellar	Lateral	Ascending	• Reflex proprioception • Muscle tone and synergy	Ipsilateral
• Ventral spinocerebellar	Lateral	Ascending	• Reflex proprioception • Muscle tone and synergy	Contralateral
Medial Lemniscal System				
• Fasciculus gracilis	Posterior	Ascending	• Position sense • Vibratory sense • Pressure • Tactile localization • Two-point discrimination	Ipsilateral
• Fasciculus cuneatus	Posterior	Ascending	• Position sense • Vibratory sense • Pressure • Tactile localization • Two-point discrimination	Ipsilateral

Continued

Table 7-4 Spinal Cord Tracts and Functions—cont'd

Tract	Column	Direction	Functions	Sidedness
PYRAMIDAL				
• Lateral corticospinal	Lateral	Descending	• Voluntary movement	Contralateral
• Ventral corticospinal	Lateral	Descending	• Voluntary movement	Ipsilateral
• Corticobulbar		Descending	• Facial expression • Swallowing • Speech	Contralateral
EXTRAPYRAMIDAL				
• Rubrospinal	Lateral	Descending	• Synergy and muscle tone	Contralateral
• Lateral vestibulospinal	Anterior	Descending	• Posture and equilibrium	Ipsilateral
• Medial vestibulospinal	Anterior	Descending	• Posture and equilibrium	Contralateral
• Lateral reticulospinal	Lateral	Descending	• Muscle tone	Ipsilateral
• Medial reticulospinal	Anterior	Descending	• Muscle tone	Ipsilateral
• Tectospinal	Anterior	Descending	• Vision and hearing	Contralateral

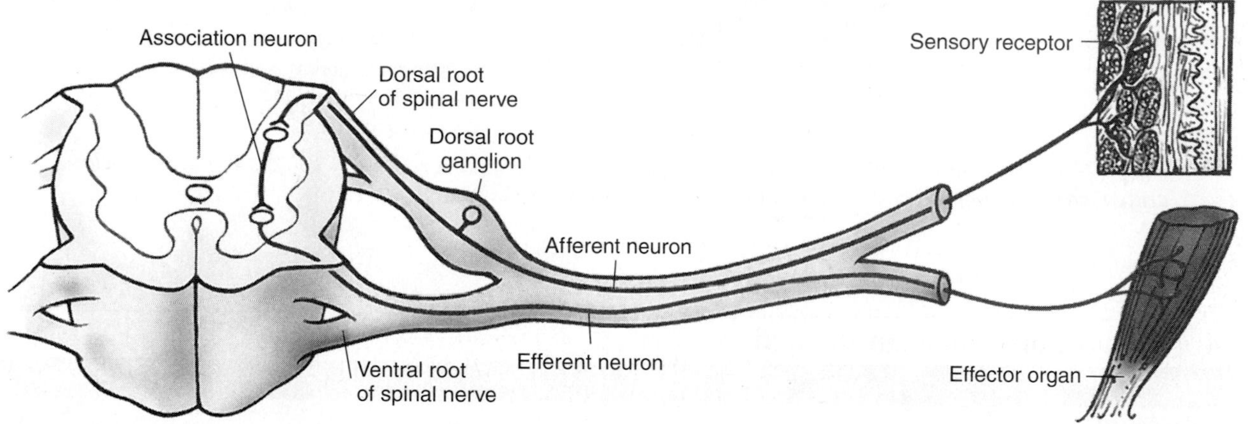

Figure 7-19 Basic diagram of a reflex arc, including the sensory receptor, afferent neuron, association neuron, efferent neuron, and effector organ. (From Lewis, S. M., & Collier, I. C. [1992]. *Medical-surgical nursing* [3rd ed.]. St. Louis: Mosby.)

(b) Does not go beyond the spinal cord to the brain; does not require cerebral interpretation

(c) Components

(i) Receptor organ

(ii) Afferent neuron

iii) Effector neuron

(iv) Effector organ

(2) Serves as the communicating pathway between the brain and the peripheral nervous system

8. Peripheral nervous system

a. Spinal segments consist of 31 pairs of spinal nerves: 8 cervical (C1 to C8), 12 thoracic (T1 to T12), 5 lumbar (L1 to L5), 5 sacral (S1 to S5), and 1 coccygeal.

(1) Fibers of spinal nerve

(a) Motor fibers

(i) Originate in anterior gray column of spinal cord

(ii) Form ventral root of spinal nerve and pass to skeletal muscles

(b) Sensory fibers

(i) Originate in spinal ganglia of dorsal roots

(ii) Peripheral branches distribute to visceral and somatic structures as mediators of sensory impulses to CNS

(2) Dermatomes: each spinal nerve innervates a specific portion of the skin identified as the dermatome for that spinal nerve (Figure 7-20 and Table 7-5)

(3) Spinal nerves form various nerve plexuses that innervate the skin and muscles throughout the body (Figure 7-20)

(a) Cervical plexus: C1 to C4

(b) Brachial plexus: C5 to C8, T1

(c) Lumbar plexus: L1 to L4

(d) Sacral plexus: L4 and L5, S1 to S4

b. Cranial nerves (Figure 7-21 and Table 7-6) consist of 12 pairs of nerves that carry impulses to and from the brain.

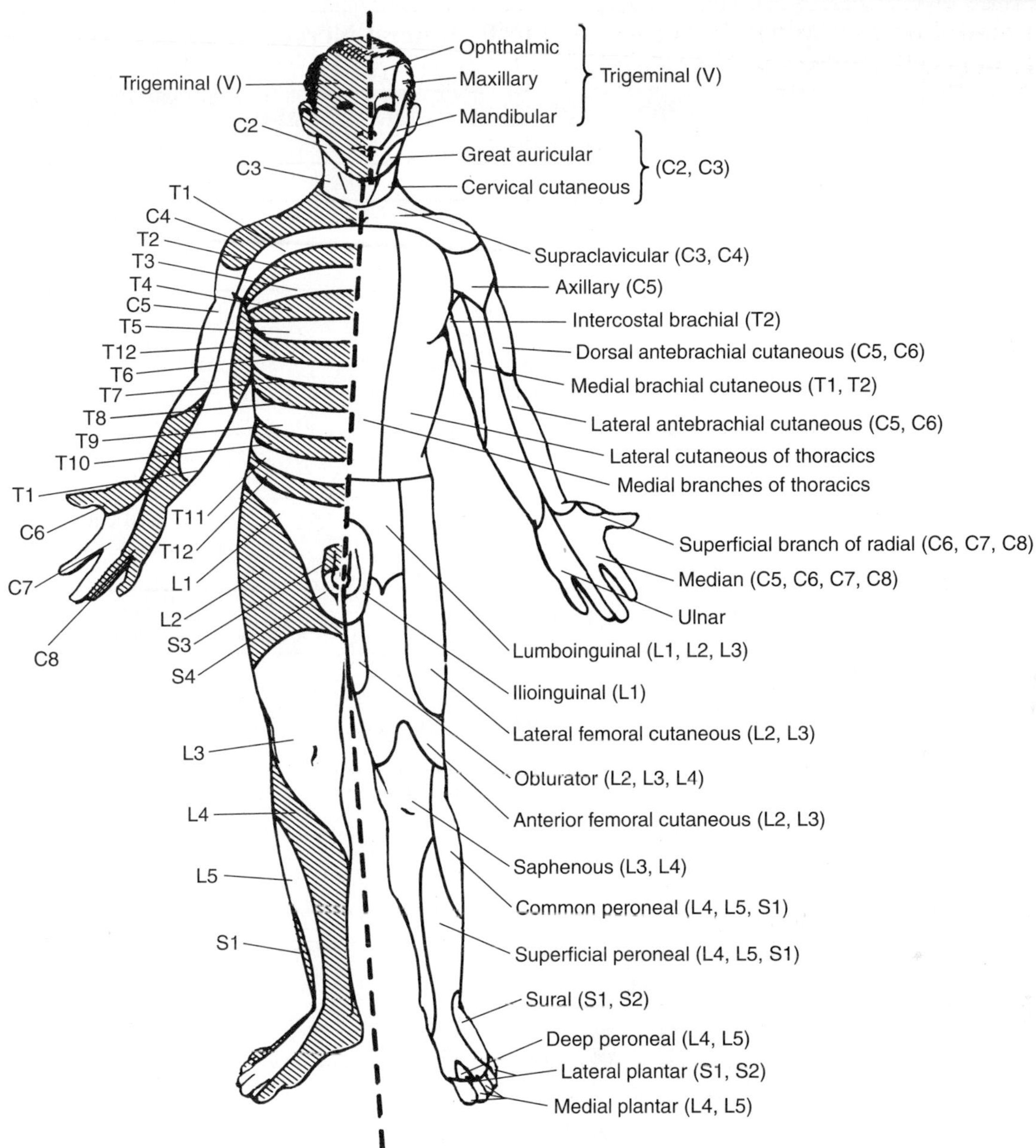

Figure 7-20 *Left:* Dermatome distribution. *Right:* Peripheral distribution of cutaneous nerves. (From Long, B. C., Phipps, W. J., & Cassmeyer, V. L. [1993]. *Medical-surgical nursing: A nursing process approach* [3rd ed.]. St. Louis: Mosby.)

9. ANS
   a. Structure
      (1) ANS consists of two neuron chains that carry information from the CNS to peripheral effector organs.
      (2) Preganglionic neuron has cell body in the CNS.
         (a) Sympathetic branch: Cell bodies are located in the spinal cord from T1 to L2.
         (b) Parasympathetic branch: Cell bodies are located in the nuclei of cranial nerves III, VII, IX, and X or in the spinal cord from S2 to S4.
      (3) The preganglionic neuron axon terminates on the postganglionic neuron cell bodies that are located throughout the body in autonomic ganglia.
      (4) The postganglionic neuron axon terminates and innervates the specific effector organs of the ANS.
      (5) Neurotransmitters form a chemical bridge in transmission of a nerve impulse.
         (a) Sympathetic branch: epinephrine; norepinephrine
         (b) Parasympathetic branch: acetylcholine
   b. Function
      (1) Controls activities of the viscera at an unconscious level
      (2) Consists of two parallel systems that regulate visceral organs by acting in opposing manners (Table 7-7)

Table 7-5 Relationship of Spinal Cord Segments to Peripheral Nerves, Muscles, and Functional Ability

Spinal Cord Segment	Peripheral Nerves	Muscles	Functional Ability
C3-C5	• Phrenic nerve	• Diaphragm	• Diaphragmatic chest excursion
C5	• Spinal accessory nerve	• Trapezius	• Shoulder shrug
C5-C6	• Axillary nerve • Musculocutaneous nerve • Radial nerve	• Deltoid • Biceps • Brachioradialis	• Arm elevation • Forearm flexion
C6-C8	• Radial nerve	• Triceps • Extensor carpi radialis and ulnaris • Flexor carpi radialis and ulnaris	• Forearm extension • Wrist extension • Wrist flexion
C8, T1	• Median nerve • Ulnar nerve	• Adductor pollicis • Dorsal interossei	• Handgrip • Finger spreading
T1-T12	• Thoracic and lumbosacral branches	• Intercostal muscles • Rectus abdominis and oblique muscles	• Intercostal chest excursion • Rotation at waist
L1-L3	• Femoral nerve	• Iliopsoas • Quadriceps	• Hip flexion • Knee extension
L2-L4	• Deep peroneal nerve • Sciatic nerve	• Extensor hallucis and digitorum • Biceps femoris and hamstrings	• Foot dorsiflexion • Knee flexion
L5-S2	• Inferior gluteal nerve • Tibial nerve	• Gluteus maximus • Gastrocnemius	• Hip extension • Plantar flexion

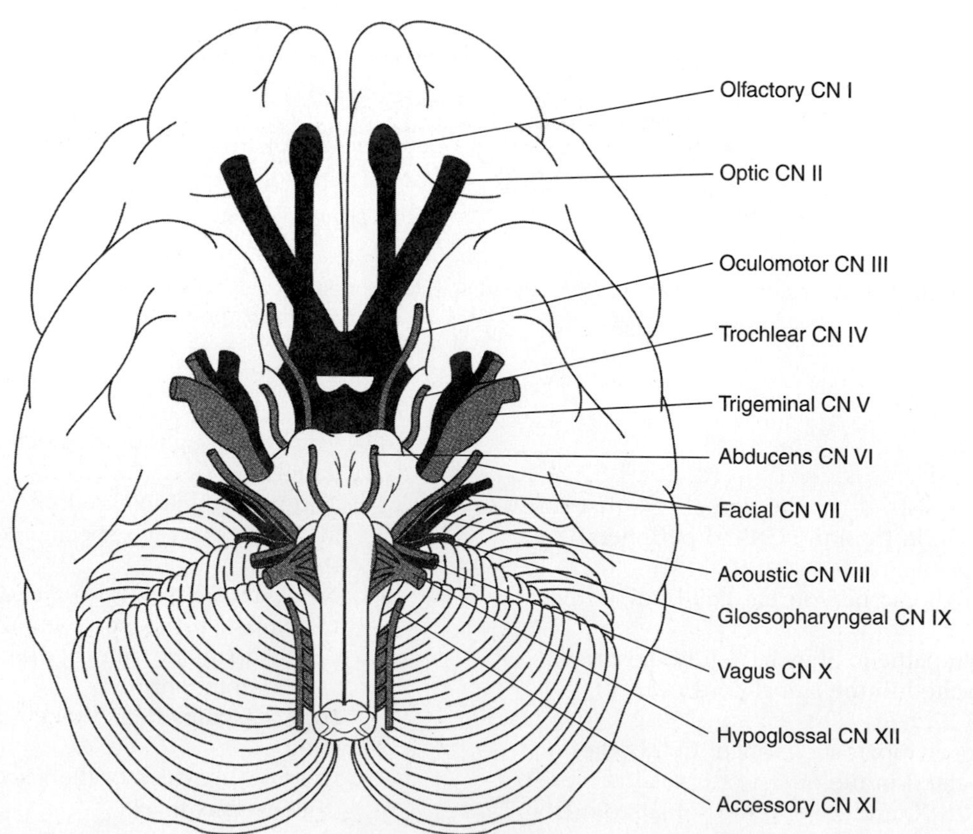

Figure 7-21 Diagram of the base of the skull showing entrance or exit of the cranial nerves. *CN,* Cranial nerve. (From Barkauskas, V. H., et al. [1994]. *Health and physical assessment.* St. Louis: Mosby.)

Table 7-6 **Cranial Nerve Summary**

Number	Name	Memory Jogger: Name	Memory Jogger: Motor/Sensory/Both	Functions
I	Olfactory	On	Some	Sensory • Smell
II	Optic	Old	Say	Sensory • Vision
III	Oculomotor	Olympus	Marry	Motor • Upward, lateral eye movement • Pupillary constriction • Eyelid elevation
IV	Trochlear	Towering	Money	Motor • Downward, medial eye movement
V	Trigeminal	Tops	But	Sensory • Sensation of scalp and face • Sensation of cornea of eye Motor • Temporal and masseter muscles
VI	Abducens	A	My	Motor • Lateral eye movement
VII	Facial	Fin	Brother	Sensory • Taste on anterior two thirds of tongue Motor • Muscles of facial expression • Eyelid closure • Lacrimal and salivary glands
VIII	Acoustic	And	Says	Sensory • Hearing • Equilibrium and balance
IX	Glossopharyngeal	German	Bad	Sensory • Taste on posterior one third of tongue • Pharynx Motor • Parotid gland
X	Vagus	Viewed	Business	Sensory • Pharynx, larynx, neck Motor • Palate, larynx, pharynx • Swallowing • Cardiac muscle • Secretory glands of pancreas and gastrointestinal tract
XI	Spinal accessory	Some	Marry	Motor • Shoulder and neck movement • Sternocleidomastoid and trapezius muscles
XII	Hypoglossal	Hops	Money	Motor • Tongue

(a) Sympathetic branch (also called *adrenergic*)
   (i) Dominates in crisis situations and often referred to as *fight or flight system*
   (ii) Innervated by physiologic or psychological stressors
   (iii) Promotes activities that prepare the body for crisis situations
(b) Parasympathetic branch (also called *cholinergic*)
   (i) Dominant in moments of calm or "steady state"
   (ii) Promotes activities that restore the energy sources of the body

Neurologic Assessment

Interview

1. Chief complaint: why the patient is seeking help and duration of the problem
   a. Symptoms related to neurologic problems
      (1) Head or spinal cord trauma
         (a) Sequence of events

Table 7-7 Autonomic Nervous System: Sympathetic and Parasympathetic Branch Function

	Sympathetic (Adrenergic)	Parasympathetic (Cholinergic)
Eyes	• Pupils dilate	• Pupils constrict
Heart	• Heart rate increases • Contractility increases • Coronary arteries dilate	• Heart rate decreases • Contractility decreases • No effect on coronary arteries
Lungs	• Bronchodilation	• Bronchoconstriction
Liver	• Glycogenolysis and lipolysis	• Glycogenesis
Gastrointestinal tract	• Salivary flow decreases • Gastric mobility and secretion decrease • Intestinal motility decreases	• Salivary flow increases • Gastric mobility and secretion increase • Intestinal motility increases
Urinary bladder	• Bladder relaxes • Sphincter closes	• Bladder contracts • Sphincter opens
Adrenal glands	• Secrete epinephrine, norepinephrine	• No effect
Skin	• Piloerection (goose pimples) • Increased perspiration	• No effect

(b) Mechanism of injury
(c) Elapsed time
(d) Extent of injury
(e) Previous treatment
(f) Current status
(2) Change in consciousness (e.g., difficulty staying awake)
(3) Headache
(a) Focal or generalized
(b) Unilateral or bilateral
(c) With or without fever
(i) Headache with fever: infectious process (e.g., meningitis or encephalitis)
(ii) Headache without fever: intracerebral hemorrhage or tumor
(d) Time of day: early morning headache suggestive of tumor
(4) Seizures
(a) New onset
(b) Increased frequency if patient has history of epilepsy
(5) Visual changes
(a) Loss of a portion of the visual field
(b) Diplopia
(c) Photophobia: may be experienced with increased ICP or meningitis
(d) Nystagmus
(6) Impaired speech (e.g., dysarthria or aphasia)
(7) Change in mood (e.g., depression, euphoria, or emotional lability)
(8) Change in thought processes (e.g., hallucinations, delusions, illusions, or paranoia) and cognition
(9) Change in behavior (e.g., hygiene habits, inappropriate laughter, or frequent crying)
(10) Change in motor function
(a) Tremor
(b) Paresis
(c) Paralysis
(11) Change in gait
(12) Dizziness, syncope, vertigo
(13) Change in sensory function
(a) Pain
(b) Paresthesia
(c) Anesthesia
(14) Memory changes
(15) Swallowing difficulties
(16) Difficulties with activities of daily living

2. History of present illness: determine PQRST
a. P
(1) Provocation: What provokes or worsens the pain?
(2) Palliation
(a) What relieves the pain?
(b) What was used but did not relieve pain?
b. Q
(1) Quality: What does the pain feel like?
c. R
(1) Region: Where is the pain located?
(2) Radiation: If the pain radiates, where does the pain radiate?
d. S
(1) Severity: How severe is the pain on a 0-to-10 scale, with 0 being no pain and 10 being the most severe pain?
e. T
(1) Timing
(a) Is the pain intermittent or continuous?
(b) What is the relationship of pain to other events or activities?
(c) When was the patient last seen functioning normally (important in stroke assessment and determination of candidacy for fibrinolytic therapy)?

3. Medical history
a. Congenital disorders
(1) Spina bifida
(2) Cerebral palsy
(3) Down syndrome

b. Childhood diseases: poliomyelitis
c. Epilepsy
d. Head trauma
e. Infectious neurologic conditions
   (1) Encephalitis
   (2) Meningitis
f. Neuromuscular disease
   (1) Multiple sclerosis
   (2) Myasthenia gravis
   (3) Amyotrophic lateral sclerosis (ALS)
   (4) Parkinson's disease
g. Spinal cord injury
h. Alzheimer's disease
i. Cancer
j. Cardiovascular disease
   (1) Coronary artery disease: angina; myocardial infarction
   (2) Valvular heart disease
   (3) Hypertension
   (4) Hyperlipidemia
   (5) Dysrhythmia especially atrial fibrillation
   (6) Ventricular aneurysm
   (7) Endocarditis
k. Cerebrovascular disease
   (1) Ischemic stroke
   (2) Hemorrhagic stroke
   (3) Carotid artery disease: bruit; prior carotid endarterectomy
l. Diabetes mellitus
m. Renal insufficiency/failure
n. Pulmonary embolism
o. Impairment of vision: use of eyeglasses, contact lenses, or prosthesis
p. Impairment of hearing: use of hearing aid

4. Family history
   a. Epilepsy
   b. Diabetes mellitus
   c. Cardiac disease
   d. Hypertension
   e. Cerebrovascular disease
      (1) Ischemic stroke
      (2) Hemorrhagic stroke
   f. Cancer
   g. Neurologic disorders
      (1) ALS
      (2) Huntington's disease
      (3) Muscular dystrophy
      (4) Neurofibromatosis
      (5) Tay-Sachs disease
      (6) Myasthenia gravis
      (7) Multiple sclerosis
      (8) Alzheimer's disease
      (9) Tremor
      (10) Dementia
   h. Psychiatric disorders
5. Social history
   a. Relationship with spouse or significant other; family structure
   b. Occupation: exposure to toxins (e.g., solvents, pesticides, arsenic, and lead)
   c. Educational level
   d. Stress level and usual coping mechanisms
   e. Recreational habits
   f. Exercise habits
   g. Dietary habits
   h. Caffeine intake
   i. Tobacco use: recorded as pack-years (number of packs per day times the number of years patient has been smoking)
   j. Alcohol use: record as alcoholic beverages consumed per month, week, or day
   k. Drug use or abuse
   l. Toxin exposure
   m. Travel
   n. Handedness: left or right
6. Medication history
   a. Prescribed drug, dose, frequency, and time of last dose
   b. Nonprescribed drugs
      (1) Over-the-counter remedies
      (2) Substance abuse
      (3) Herbs
   c. Patient understanding of drug actions and side effects
   d. Drugs frequently used for neurologic problems
      (1) Tranquilizers
      (2) Sedatives
      (3) Aspirin
      (4) Anticonvulsants
      (5) Antihypertensives
      (6) Platelet aggregation inhibitors
   e. Drugs that may cause neurologic problems
      (1) Tranquilizers
      (2) Sedatives
      (3) Aspirin
      (4) Anticoagulants
      (5) Alcohol

Vital Signs

1. Cushing's triad: increased systolic BP, decreased diastolic BP (widened pulse pressure), bradycardia; late sign of increased ICP
2. BP
   a. Hypotension
      (1) Hemorrhage
         (a) Because the cranium is an inexpansible vault, intracranial hemorrhage cannot result in hypotension because herniation would result before significant hypotension
         (b) Consider other sources of bleeding (e.g., lacerated liver, ruptured spleen, and thoracic trauma)
      (2) General neurologic deterioration
      (3) Of great concern because CPP = MAP − ICP
   b. Hypertension
      (1) Systolic hypertension may be seen as a component of Cushing's triad, a late sign of intracranial hypertension
      (2) May indicate a change in arterial resistance and associated with vessel occlusion (e.g., stroke)
   c. Pulse pressure: difference between systolic and diastolic

(1) Normal is 30 to 40 mm Hg.
(2) Increased pulse pressure is a component of Cushing's triad, a late sign of intracranial hypertension.

3. Pulse
   a. Sinus bradycardia: a component of Cushing's triad, a late sign of intracranial hypertension
   b. Sinus tachycardia
      (1) Hypoxia
      (2) Hemorrhage
      (3) General neurologic deterioration
   c. Atrial dysrhythmias (e.g., premature atrial contractions, atrial fibrillation, and atrial flutter) may be etiologic factor in ischemic stroke
4. Ventilatory rate and rhythm (Table 7-8)
5. Temperature
   a. Decreased (subnormal)
      (1) Shock
      (2) Drug overdose
      (3) Metabolic coma (e.g., myxedema coma)
      (4) Terminal stages of neurologic disease
   b. Increased
      (1) Infection
         (a) Systemic infection
         (b) CNS infection
      (2) Subarachnoid hemorrhage (SAH)
      (3) Seizures
      (4) Restlessness
      (5) Injury to hypothalamus: especially if inordinately elevated

General Appearance

1. Attire: appropriateness to age, environment
2. Grooming
   a. Hair
   b. Teeth
   c. Hygiene
   d. Nails
3. General behavior
   a. Demeanor
   b. Affect: facial expressions; body language
   c. Mood: euphoria; anger; depression; suicidal thoughts
4. Posture: gestures; fidgeting; restlessness; tremor; rigidity
5. Gait: ataxia is uncoordinated movements of the body
6. Obvious physical defects
   a. Hemiparalysis
   b. Facial asymmetry
   c. Ptosis
   d. Tremor
   e. Amputations
   f. Mass response: decorticate or decerebrate posturing

Mental Status and Cognition

1. Level of consciousness (LOC): the most sensitive clinical indicator of a change in neurologic status
   a. Consciousness is a state of awareness: self; environment; responses to environment
      (1) Arousal
         (a) Measure of being awake
         (b) Function of the RAS in the midbrain

Table 7-8 Ventilatory Rhythms

Rhythm	Description	Diagram	Significance
Eupnea	Regular rhythm at normal rate		• Normal
Bradypnea	Regular rhythm with rate less than 12 breaths/min		• CNS depression by injury, disease, or drugs
Cheyne-Stokes	Increasing rate and depth of ventilation followed by decreasing rate and depth of ventilation and then apnea		• Bilateral lesions of cerebral hemispheres • Lesion of basal ganglia • Cerebellar lesion • Lesion of upper brainstem • Metabolic condition
CNS hyperventilation	Sustained increased rate and depth of ventilation		• Lesions of lower midbrain or upper pons • May result from transtentorial herniation
Apneustic	Apnea with inspiration followed by exhalation		• Lesions of mid to lower pons
Cluster	Three to four breaths of identical rate and depth followed by apnea; sequence repeated		• Lesions of lower pons or upper medulla
Ataxic	No pattern to ventilation; completely irregular with mostly apnea		• Lesion of the medulla

CNS, Central nervous system.

(2) Awareness
  (a) Involves interpreting sensory input and giving an appropriate response
  (b) Requires an intact RAS and cerebral hemispheres

b. Evaluate the degree of stimulus to get a response
  (1) Verbal stimuli
    (a) Call the patient by name, speaking at normal voice volume.
    (b) Ask the patient to make a fist with his or her hand; when performed, ask the patient to open the fist.
    (c) Use increased volume ("yelling") if the patient does not respond to normal voice volume.
  (2) Tactile stimuli: Touch or shake the patient.
  (3) Painful stimuli: Use only if the other methods are unsuccessful; avoid trauma and bruising caused by pinching.
    (a) Techniques to elicit a pain response
      (i) Central: brain responds
        a) Pressure to trapezius muscle
          i) Squeeze large muscle mass between thumb and index finger; do not pinch skin.
        b) Pressure to Achilles tendon
          i) Squeeze large muscle mass between thumb and index finger; do not pinch skin.
        c) Supraorbital pressure
          i) Push up against the supraorbital ridge with thumb; exert gentle upward pressure.
          ii) Do not push into the eye socket; injury to the eye or vagal response may occur.
          iii) Do not use this technique in patients with facial fracture or cranial fracture.
        d) Sternal rub
          i) Rub sternum gently with knuckle.
          ii) If bruising results, discontinue using this technique.
      (ii) Peripheral: spine responds
        a) Nailbed pressure
          i) Apply pressure to the nailbed using the flat surface of a pen or pencil
          ii) Useful in determining sensory and motor function but should not be used as the only method of evaluation of pain response

c. LOC (Haymore, 2004)
  (1) Normal: arouses easily, maintains wakefulness, speaks coherently, responds appropriately to stimuli
  (2) Hypersomnia: prolonged sleeping time with normal sleep pattern
  (3) Lethargy, obtundation, stupor
    (a) These are confusing terms indicating diminishing levels of consciousness.
    (b) Description of the patient's response to stimuli and behavior rather than use of these labels is recommended.
  (4) Coma: absence of awareness and responsiveness caused by structural lesion or metabolic condition
  (5) Persistent vegetative state: unaware of self and surroundings
    (a) Sleep-wake patterns occur along with eye opening, but no response to stimuli occurs.
    (b) Brainstem and hypothalamic function are intact.
  (6) Locked-in syndrome: consciousness with near-complete paralysis
    (a) Able to answer questions with eye blink
    (b) Vision and hearing is preserved
    (c) Caused by lesion of midbrain or pons
  (7) Brain death: absence of all cortical and brainstem function

d. Glasgow Coma Scale (GCS) (Table 7-9)
  (1) Developed as a method to standardize observation of responsiveness in patients with traumatic brain injury
  (2) Best or highest response is recorded; E (eye), M (motor), V (verbal) may be recorded separately along with a quantitative score
  (3) Note if certain responses cannot be evaluated because of any of the following:
    (a) Endotracheal intubation or tracheostomy
    (b) Aphasia
    (c) Eyes swollen shut

Table 7-9 Glasgow Coma Scale

Parameter	Response	Score
Eye opening	Spontaneous	4
	To speech	3
	To pain	2
	None	1
	Untestable	U
Best motor response	Obeys commands	6
	Localizes pain	5
	Withdraws from pain	4
	Abnormal flexion (decorticate posturing)	3
	Abnormal extension (decerebrate posturing)	2
	None	1
	Untestable	U
Best verbal response	Oriented	5
	Confused	4
	Inappropriate	3
	Incomprehensible	2
	None	1
	Untestable	U

(4) Parameters
(a) Minimum: 3
(b) Maximum (normal): 15
(c) Clinically significant: change of 2 points or more

e. National Institutes of Health Stroke Scale (NIHSS) (Table 7-10)
(1) Used to assess the severity of presenting signs and symptoms
(2) Score over 22 indicates severe neurologic deficit
(3) Baseline assessment completed at admission; repeat assessments 2 hours after treatment, 24 hours after onset of symptoms, 7 to 10 days after onset of symptoms, and at 3 months after onset of symptoms

2. Cognitive function
a. Orientation: Patient may be alert but confused.
(1) Orientation to time
(a) Ability to give today's date (e.g., What is today's date?)
(b) Ability to state the year (e.g., What year is it?)

Table 7-10 National Institutes of Health Stroke Scale

Item/Domain	Response	Score
1A Level of consciousness	• Alert, keenly responsive	0
	• Obeys, answers, or responds to minor stimulation	1
	• Responds only to repeated stimulation or painful stimulation (excludes reflex response)	2
	• Responds only with reflex motor or totally unresponsive	3
1B Orientation Ask the month and patient age; must be exactly right	• Answers both correctly	0
	• Answers one correctly or patient unable to speak for any reason other than aphasia or coma	1
	• Answers neither correctly, or too stuporous or aphasic	2
1C Response to commands Ask patient to open and close eyes and then grip and release nonparetic hand	• Performs both tasks correctly	0
	• Performs one task correctly	1
	• Performs neither task correctly	2
2 Gaze Only horizontal movements tested	• Normal	0
	• Partial gaze palsy	1
	• Forced deviation or total gaze paresis not overcome by oculocephalic maneuver	2
3 Visual field Tested by confrontation	• No visual loss	0
	• Partial hemianopia	1
	• Complete hemianopia	2
	• Bilateral hemianopia (blind from any cause including cortical blindness)	3
4 Facial movement Encourage patient to smile and close eyes, or grimace symmetry	• Normal symmetrical movement	0
	• Minor paralysis (flattened nasolabial fold, asymmetry on smiling)	1
	• Partial paralysis (total or near total lower face paralysis)	2
	• Complete paralysis (absence of facial movement upper/lower face)	3
5a Left arm motor function Extend left arm palm down at 90 degrees (sitting) or 45 degrees (supine)	• No drift—holds for full 10 seconds	0
	• Drifts down before 10 seconds but does not hit bed/support	1
	• Some effort against gravity but cannot get up to 90 (or 45 if supine) degrees	2
	• No effort against gravity; limb falls	3
	• No movement	4
5b Right arm motor function Extend right arm palm down at 90 degrees (sitting) or 45 degrees (supine)	• No drift—holds for full 10 seconds	0
	• Drifts down before 10 seconds but does not hit bed/support	1
	• Some effort against gravity but cannot get up to 90 (or 45 if supine) degrees	2
	• No effort against gravity; limb falls	3
	• No movement	4
6a Left leg motor function Extend left leg and flex at hip to 30 degrees	• No drift—holds for full 5 seconds	0
	• Drifts down before 5 seconds but does not hit bed/support	1
	• Some effort against gravity	2
	• No effort against gravity; limb falls	3
	• No movement	4

Table 7-10 National Institutes of Health Stroke Scale—cont'd

Item/Domain	Response	Score
6b Right leg motor function Extend right leg and flex at hip to 30 degrees	• No drift—holds for full 5 seconds • Drifts down before 5 seconds but does not hit bed/support • Some effort against gravity • No effort against gravity; limb falls • No movement	0 1 2 3 4
7 Limb ataxia Finger/nose and heel/shin done on both sides. Not ataxia if hemiplegic or unable to comprehend. Ataxia must be out of proportion to any weakness present.	• Absent • Present in one limb • Present in two limbs	0 1 2
8 Sensory	• Normal • Pinprick less sharp or dull on affected side • Severe to total sensory loss; patient unaware of being touched	0 1 2
9 Best language Name items; read short sentences	• No aphasia • Some loss of fluency or comprehension • Severe aphasia—fragmentary communication; listener carries burden of communication • Mute, global aphasia; NO usable speech OR auditory comprehension	0 1 2 3
10 Dysarthria If not obviously present, have patient read	• Normal • Slurs some words • So slurred as to be unintelligible, or mute	0 1 2
11 Extinction/inattention	• No abnormality • Inattention to any sensory modality or extinction to bilateral simultaneous stimulation in one sensory modality • Profound hemi-inattention or hemi-inattention to more than one modality; does not recognize own hand	0 1 2

From National Institutes of Health. (2003). *NIH stroke scale*. Retrieved April 17, 2007, from http://www.ninds.nih.gov/doctors/NIH_Stroke_Scale_Booklet.pdf

(2) Orientation to place
(a) Ability to identify surroundings (e.g., Where are you now?)
(b) Ability to state address (e.g., Where do you live?)
(3) Orientation to person
(a) Ability to identify self by name (e.g., Who are you? What is your name?)
(b) Recognition of friends and family
(4) Orientation to situation: ability to identify why they are in the hospital (e.g., Why are you here?)

b. Memory
(1) How old are you?
(2) Remote memory: What is your birthday? Where were you born?
(3) Recent memory: What did you have for breakfast? What is your doctor's name?

c. Short-term recall: Can the patient repeat three or four objects after 3 to 5 minutes?

d. General knowledge: Ask a question about a current event.

e. Attention span: Is the patient able to stay on a subject?

f. Thought content: Note evidence of illusions, hallucinations, delusions, and paranoia.

g. Calculation skills: Can you count backward from 20 to 1?

h. Judgment: Why are you here? What would you do if there was a fire in the wastebasket?

i. Abstraction: Ask the patient to spell the word "world" backward.

3. Speech and language
a. Note punctuation, rhythm, stream of talk, sentence structure, appropriate use of words; speech should be fluent with expression of connected thoughts.
b. If patient cannot use or understand verbal communication, determine the following:
(1) Can the patient understand or use gestures?
(2) Can the patient understand written language or write messages?
c. Identify the presence of speech disorders.
(1) Dysphonia: difficulty producing sound
(2) Dysarthria: difficulty with articulation
(3) Dysprosody: lack of inflection while talking
(4) Aphasia: impaired understanding or expression of verbal and/or written language
(a) Receptive (sensory) aphasia: lesion in Wernicke's area in temporal area
(b) Expressive (motor) aphasia: lesion in Broca's area in frontal area
(c) Global: both

Motor Function

1. Muscle size
   a. Symmetry
   b. Atrophy or hypertrophy
2. Symmetric movement and strength of extremities
   a. Movement
      (1) Spontaneous movement and symmetry of movement
      (2) Assumption of a position of comfort
   b. Muscle strength (Table 7-11)
      (1) Arm strength
         (a) Test flexor and extensor muscle groups by evaluating strength against resistance
         (b) Pronator drift
            (i) Detection: Have patient hold his or her arms out in front with palms up and eyes closed.
            (ii) Normal: Patient should be able to hold arms even for at least 20 seconds.
            (iii) Abnormal: The weak arm begins to drift and pronate (turn palm downward).
      (2) Leg strength
         (a) Test flexor and extensor muscle groups by evaluating strength against resistance.
         (b) Ask the patient to raise legs one at a time to 30 degrees off the bed from supine position and hold in place for a count to 5; observe for drift.
      (3) Plegia positioning (Figure 7-22)

Table 7-11 Muscle Strength Grading Scale

Grade	Description
0/5	No movement or muscle contraction
1/5	Trace; no movement but evidence of muscle contraction
2/5	Not greater than gravity; movement with gravity eliminated
3/5	Greater than gravity; movement against gravity
4/5	Slight weakness; movement against some resistance
5/5	Normal; movement against full resistance

3. Muscle tone
   a. Flaccidity: no resistance to passive movement; flaccid paralysis generally is associated with LMN lesions but also may occur early in UMN lesions
   b. Hypotonia: little resistance to passive movement
   c. Hypertonia: increased muscle resistance to passive movement
   d. Rigidity: increased muscle resistance to passive movement of a rigid limb that is uniform through flexion and extension (paratonic rigidity may occur in coma and is a sign of diffuse cerebral dysfunction)
   e. Spasticity: gradual increase in tone causing increased resistance until tone suddenly is reduced
      (1) Clonus, continued rhythmic contraction of a muscle may be evident after the stimulus has been applied.
      (2) Spastic paralysis is associated with UMN lesions and emerges after resolution of the early flaccidity stage.
   f. UMN versus LMN (Table 7-12)
4. Coordination
   a. Point-to-point movements
      (1) Finger-nose test: Ask patient to touch his or her nose with a finger with eyes closed.
      (2) Finger-finger test: Ask patient to touch your finger with his or her finger with eyes closed.
      (3) Heel-knee test: Ask patient to run the heel of one foot down the opposite leg from thc knee to the foot.
   b. Rapid, rhythmic alternating movements
      (1) Pronation-supination test: Ask patient to rapidly pronate and supinate his or her hand.
      (2) Patting test: Ask patient to rapidly pronate and supinate his or her hand against a leg.
   c. Figure-of-eight test: ask patient to draw a figure-of-eight in the air with his or her great toe.
5. Gait
   a. Tandem gait: patient asked to walk heel to toe in a straight line
      (1) Normal: ability to walk heel to toe without difficulty
      (2) Abnormal: loss of balance indicates cerebellar dysfunction

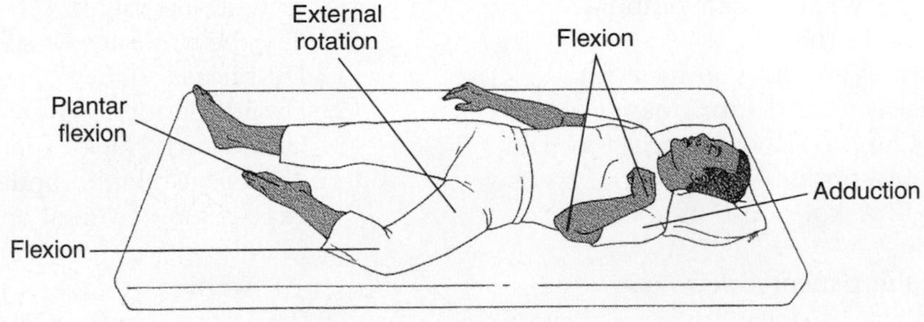

Figure 7-22 Plegia positioning. (From Beare, P. G., & Myers, J. L. [1994]. *Principles and practice of adult health nursing* [2nd ed.]. St. Louis: Mosby.)

Table 7-12 Locating Site of Motor Problems

		Upper Motor Neuron	
	Lower Motor Neuron	**Pyramidal Tract**	**Extrapyramidal Tract**
Effect	Flaccid paralysis Areflexia	• Spastic paralysis with hyperactive reflexes • Positive Babinski's reflex	• No paralysis • Altered muscle tone and abnormal movements
Muscle appearance	Atrophy Small muscular contractions (fasciculation)	Mild atrophy from disuse	Tremor when at rest
Muscle tone	Decreased	Increased	Increased
Muscle strength	Decreased or absent	Decreased or absent	Normal
Coordination	Absent or poor	Absent or poor	Slowed
Examples	• Poliomyelitis • ALS • Guillain-Barré syndrome	• Stroke • Spinal cord injury • Multiple sclerosis • ALS	• Parkinson's disease

ALS, Amyotrophic lateral sclerosis.

b. Abnormal gaits
  (1) Spastic: Leg is held stiff and moved slowly; toes and lateral aspect of foot scrape the floor as the leg is moved; this indicates corticospinal tract lesion.
  (2) Steppage: Foot is lifted very high for each step, with a distinctive slapping sound as it hits the floor; this indicates peripheral nerve injury.
  (3) Ataxic: Feet are broad-based, and steps are unsteady and staggering; this indicates cerebellar or dorsal column lesions.
  (4) Propulsive: Body is bent forward, steps are short, momentum is increased, and falls are common; this indicates basal ganglia dysfunction (e.g., Parkinson's disease).
  (5) Waddling: Pelvis opposite the weight-bearing hip drops and the trunk inclines, causing a waddle; this indicates proximal muscle weakness (e.g., muscular dystrophy).
  (6) Scissors: Thighs are held together and each foot alternately is brought forward; this indicates UMN lesion.

6. Station: tested by Romberg's test
  a. Method: patient asked to stand with feet together and arms extended in front with eyes closed
  b. Normal: patient able to stand erect and steady; slight swaying may be seen
  c. Abnormal: patient loses balance; this indicates loss of position sense and/or cerebellar dysfunction

7. Involuntary movements
  a. Posturing may occur spontaneously or to pain in comatose patients; also may be considered a "mass response"
    (1) Abnormal flexion (Figure 7-23, *A*)
      (a) Also called *decorticate posturing*
      (b) Arms are flexed toward the body; legs are extended
      (c) Indicates cerebral lesion
    (2) Abnormal extension (Figure 7-23, *B*)
      (a) Also called *decerebrate posturing*
      (b) Arms are extended, wrists are rotated externally, and legs are extended
      (c) Indicates midbrain or brainstem lesion
    (3) Opisthotonos
      (a) Also referred to as *arching*
      (b) Extension of arms and legs and arching of the back and neck
      (c) May indicate brainstem injury
    (4) Flaccid posture: Entire body is flaccid even with painful stimulation.
  b. Tremor
    (1) Resting: Parkinson's disease
    (2) Intentional: cerebellar disease

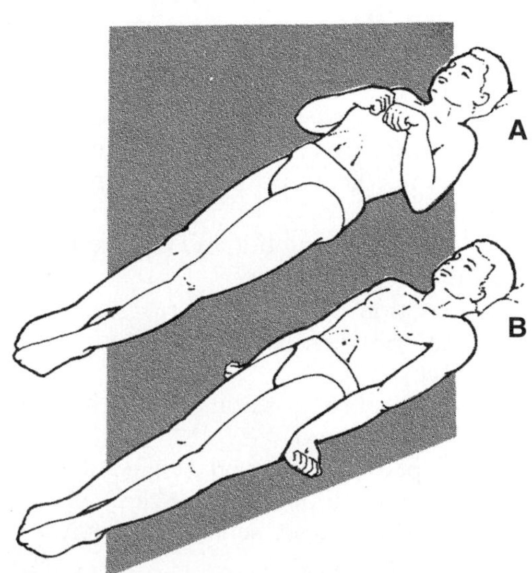

Figure 7-23 A, Abnormal flexion (decorticate) posturing. **B,** Abnormal extension (decerebrate) posturing. (From Urden, L., Stacy, K., & Lough, M. [2002]. *Thelan's critical care nursing: Diagnosis and management* [4th ed.]. St. Louis: Mosby.)

(3) Flapping: metabolic encephalopathy (e.g., hepatic or renal failure)
(4) Physiologic: stress induced
(5) Senile: age induced

c. Seizure: describe
(1) Preceding events: aura?
(2) Initial cry or sound
(3) Onset
(a) Initial body movements
(b) Deviation of head and eyes
(c) Chewing and salivation
(d) Posture of body
(e) Sensory changes
(4) Tonic and clonic phases
(a) Progression of movements of body
(b) Skin color and airway
(c) Pupillary changes
(d) Incontinence
(e) Duration of each phase
(5) LOC during seizure
(6) Postictal phase
(a) Duration
(b) General behavior
(c) Memory of events
(d) Orientation
(e) Pupillary changes
(f) Headache
(g) Aphasia
(h) Injuries
(7) Duration of entire seizure
(8) Medications given and response
(9) Findings on diagnostic studies
(a) Serum electrolytes
(b) Diagnostic imaging (e.g., computed tomography [CT] and magnetic resonance imaging [MRI])
(c) Electroencephalogram (EEG)

Sensory Function

1. Ability to perceive sensation
a. Superficial sensation
(1) Light touch: wisp of cotton on skin
(2) Superficial pain: light pinprick on skin (use sterile needle and discard appropriately after testing)
(3) Skin temperature: hot and cold test tubes on skin; rarely performed
b. Deep sensation
(1) Vibration: vibration of tuning fork on bony surface
(2) Position sense: position of great toe, thumb with eyes closed
(3) Deep pain: pressure on Achilles tendon, calf muscles, or upper arm muscles
c. Cortical/discriminatory sensation: requires cortical interpretation
(1) Two-point discrimination: ability to distinguish between one or two points; patient touch with two points at varying degrees of separation to see whether the patient feels only one point or two points
(2) Stereognosis: ability to distinguish common objects placed in the hand with eyes closed
(3) Topognosis: ability to distinguish which finger is being touched, with eyes closed
(4) Graphesthesia: ability to recognize numbers or letters traced on the skin with eyes closed
(5) Double simultaneous stimulation (tactile inattention testing): ability to differentiate between one point or two points when being touched by one or two points on opposite sides of the body in corresponding locations
d. Ability to recognize objects through the special senses; inability referred to as *agnosia*
(1) Visual: occipital lobe
(2) Auditory: temporal lobe
(3) Tactile: parietal lobe
(4) Body parts and relationships: parietal lobe
e. Distribution of sensory loss
(1) Entire side of body: parietal or thalamic lesion
(2) Dermatomal (Table 7-13 and Figure 7-20)
(a) Dermatome: skin area supplied by sensory fibers of a single spinal nerve
(b) Sensory loss below a dermatomal level: spinal cord lesion
(c) Sensory loss along a dermatome: spinal nerve lesion
(3) Peripheral nerve distribution (Figure 7-20)
f. Degrees of sensory loss
(1) Anesthesia: loss of sensation
(2) Dysesthesia: impaired sensation
(3) Hyperesthesia: increased sensation
(4) Hypoesthesia: decreased sensation
(5) Paresthesia: burning, tingling sensation

Cranial Nerve Function

1. Olfactory (I)
a. Test: patient's ability to identify familiar odors (e.g., coffee, cloves, tobacco, or alcohol) tested; each nostril tested separately with eyes closed; rarely performed in acute care

Table 7-13 Dermatomal Levels for Bedside Assessment

Anatomic Location	Spinal Level
Front of neck	C3
Thumb	C6
Ring and little fingers	C8
Nipple line	T4
Umbilicus	T10
Groin crease	L1
Knee	L3
Anterior ankle and foot	L5
Lateral foot and heel	S1
Genitalia	S3, S4

b. Normal: able to identify familiar odors
c. Abnormal: unable to identify familiar odors; referred to as *anosmia*

2. Optic (II)
   a. Visual acuity: test by the following:
      (1) Snellen chart
         (a) Ask patient to read lines of the Snellen chart from a distance of 20 feet or use a pocket Snellen card for patients who are bed-bound.
         (b) Record the number on the lowest line that the patient can read with 50% accuracy.
         (c) Test with glasses or contact lenses.
      (2) If patient cannot see well enough to read the Snellen chart, ask how many fingers you are holding up.
      (3) If the patient cannot see well enough to tell you how many fingers you are holding up, assess whether he or she blinks to visual threat.
   b. Visual fields
      (1) Test by confrontation: comparison of patient's visual field to examiner's visual field with eye on same side covered
      (2) Loss of vision or portion of visual field
         (a) Unilateral blindness: lesion of eye, retina, or optic nerve
         (b) Bitemporal hemianopsia: lesion of optic chiasm or lesion causing pressure on optic chiasm (e.g., pituitary tumor)
         (c) Left homonymous hemianopsia: lesion of right optic tract
         (d) Right homonymous hemianopsia: lesion of left optic tract
         (e) Left homonymous hemianopsia with macular sparing: lesion of right geniculocalcarine tract
         (f) Right homonymous hemianopsia with macular sparing: lesion of left geniculocalcarine tract
   c. Near vision
      (1) Test: Ask the patient to read newsprint at a distance of 12 inches or use pocket Snellen card.
      (2) Normal: Patient should be able to read newsprint at 1 foot.
   d. Funduscopic examination with ophthalmoscope to detect papilledema (Figure 7-24)
      (1) Optic disk is pushed forward
      (2) Disk margins are blurry
      (3) Indication of intracranial hypertension
         (a) May be late in acute intracranial hypertension
         (b) May be first sign in chronic intracranial hypertension (e.g., tumor)

3. Oculomotor (III), trochlear (IV), abducens (VI)
   a. Eyelids: elevation of the eyelid is controlled by cranial nerve III; ptosis may indicate cranial nerve III injury

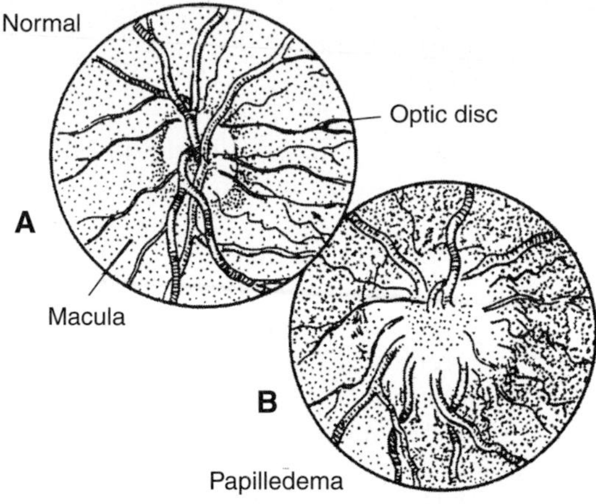

Figure 7-24 **A,** Normal fundus. **B,** Fundus showing papilledema. (From Hausman, K. A., et al. [1985]. *Analyzing neurological status.* St. Louis: Mosby.)

   b. Pupils
      (1) Size
         (a) Normal 2 to 6 mm
         (b) Abnormal: Clinically significant change is change of more than 1 mm.
            (i) Pinpoint (and nonreactive)
               a) Pontine lesion
               b) Medication effect
                  i) Opiates (e.g., morphine)
                  ii) Miotics (e.g., pilocarpine)
            (ii) Midsize (2 to 6 mm) but nonreactive: midbrain lesion
            (iii) Unilateral large (greater than 6 mm) and nonreactive (may be referred to as *blown* or *hutchinsonian pupil*): pressure on oculomotor nerve on same side
            (iv) Bilateral large (greater than 6 mm) and nonreactive
               a) Brainstem lesion
               b) Medication effect
                  i) Parasympatholytics (e.g., atropine)
                  ii) Sympathomimetics (e.g., epinephrine)
      (2) Equality
         (a) Normal: equal
         (b) Abnormal: unequal (referred to as *anisocoria*)
            (i) Normal variation: 15% to 20% of the population has slightly unequal pupils (1 mm or less difference)
            (ii) Abnormal: difference of more than 1 mm or change from baseline
            (iii) Injury effects
               a) Injury to parasympathetic fibers of the oculomotor nerve: ipsilateral (same side) pupil dilation
               b) Injury to sympathetic fibers of the sympathetic fibers of the oculomotor nerves (e.g., Horner syndrome: ipsilateral pupil constriction)

(3) Shape
  (a) Normal: round
  (b) Abnormal
    (i) Oval
      a) May precede dilated pupil as a sign of pressure on the oculomotor nerve
      b) Associated with ICP of 18-35 mm Hg
    (ii) Irregular (e.g., keyhole shaped may be seen in patients after cataract removal due to concurrent iridectomy)
(4) Position
  (a) Normal: midposition
  (b) Abnormal
    (i) Both eyes deviated toward one side
      a) Unilateral pontine lesion
      b) Fixed lesion such as tumor, stroke, or hemorrhage: toward the lesion and away from the hemiparesis
      c) Seizure: away from the seizure focus and toward the hemiparesis
    (ii) Downward deviation of both eyes (frequently with inward convergence): thalamic lesion
    (iii) Downward deviation of 1 eye: oculomotor (III) nerve palsy
    (iv) Medial deviation of 1 eye: trochlear (IV) nerve palsy
(5) Reactivity to light
  (a) Test
    (i) Darken the room if pupils are small
    (ii) Use a small, bright penlight in front of each eye
    (iii) Note pupil constriction as the direct reaction
    (iv) Note pupil constriction of the opposite pupil as consensual reaction
  (b) Normal: brisk bilateral direct and consensual reaction to light
  (c) Abnormal
    (i) Sluggish or absent reaction; indicative of any of the following:
      a) Cranial nerve III pressure or injury
      b) Hypothermia
      c) Barbiturate intoxication
    (ii) Hippus: pupil initially reacts briskly and then follows an exaggerated rhythmic contraction and dilation of the pupil; may be normal but may be indicative of any of the following:
      a) Early cranial nerve III pressure or injury
      b) Midbrain injury
      c) Barbiturate intoxication
(6) Accommodation
  (a) Test: Ask the patient to focus on a distant object and accommodate as the object moves closer.
  (b) Pupils dilate when focusing on a far object.
  (c) Pupils constrict when focusing on a near object.
(7) Ciliospinal reflex
  (a) Test: Squeeze trapezius muscle and observe reaction of pupil on same side.
  (b) Normal: ipsilateral pupil dilation with trapezius squeeze
  (c) Abnormal: no response; indicative of interruption of sympathetic fibers of oculomotor nerve

c. Extraocular movements
  (1) Test: Ask patient to keep head straight and follow your finger with eyes; move your finger in the direction of the six cardinal positions of gaze (Figure 7-25)
  (2) Normal: Both eyes move conjugately in the direction of your finger.
  (3) Abnormal: One or both eyes do not move to follow finger; this is indicative of cranial nerve injury or isolated muscular dysfunction.

d. Abnormal eye movements
  (1) Nystagmus: jerky eye movement that oscillates the eye back and forth quickly; may be seen in lesions of vestibular system or brainstem
  (2) Dysconjugate eye movement: may indicate damage to the brainstem
  (3) Conjugate eye movement: may indicate cerebral hemispheric damage

4. Trigeminal (V)
  a. Sensory branch
    (1) Test
      (a) Three branches (ophthalmic, maxillary, mandibular) tested on both sides with a wisp of cotton (light touch) and pinprick (superficial pain)
        (i) Normal: detection of touch and pain
        (ii) Abnormal: no detection of touch or pain
      (b) Corneal blink reflex
        (i) Detection: corneal touched with a wisp of cotton
        (ii) Normal: bilateral blink; indicates intactness of trigeminal (V) and facial (VII) cranial nerves

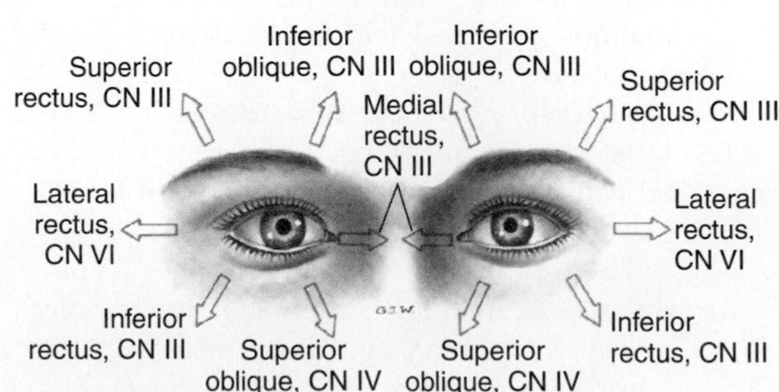

Figure 7-25 The six cardinal positions of gaze. *CN,* Cranial nerve. (From Seidel, H. M., and others: [1991]. *Mosby's guide to physical examination* [2nd ed.]. St. Louis: Mosby.)

(iii) Abnormal: decreased or absent blink; may indicate cranial nerve V injury (NOTE: Contact lens wearers have diminished corneal blink reflex.)

b. Motor branch
   (1) Test: face inspected for muscle atrophy and tremor; the masseter muscle palpated while the patient clenches teeth; the temporal muscles palpated as the patient squeezes eyes closed
   (2) Normal: symmetry of muscle strength, no atrophy or tremor
   (3) Abnormal: asymmetry of muscle strength; may indicate cranial nerve V injury

5. Facial (VII)
   a. Motor branch
      (1) Test: symmetry of facial expressions noted while patient raises eyebrows, frowns, smiles, and closes eyelids tightly
      (2) Abnormal: asymmetry of facial expression; loss of nasolabial fold, eye remaining open; indicates cranial nerve VII injury (Bell's palsy)
   b. Sensory branch
      (1) Test: ability to taste sour and bitter on posterior tongue tested; rarely performed in acute care
      (2) Normal: ability to taste
      (3) Abnormal: inability to taste; indicates cranial nerve VII injury

6. Acoustic (VIII)
   a. Cochlear branch: hearing keenness
      (1) Whisper test
         (a) Test: Turn face away and whisper to see whether patient can hear what is whispered.
         (b) Test each ear separately.
         (c) This test differentiates between hearing and lip reading.
      (2) Weber test
         (a) Test: Place a tuning fork at the midline vertex of skull.
         (b) Normal: Patient hears equally well on both sides.
         (c) Abnormal: Patient indicates difference between the two ears and will hear the sound better with the "good" ear.
      (3) Rinne test
         (a) Test: Place tuning fork on the mastoid; when the patient can no longer hear the sound by bone, move the tuning fork in front of the ear.
         (b) Normal: Air conduction is usually better than bone conduction, so the patient should still be able to hear the sound when the tuning fork is moved in front of the ear after the patient reports not being able to hear the sound any longer by bone.
         (c) Abnormal: Patient has inability to hear the sound by air after the cessation of the sound by bone; diminished air conduction is associated with middle ear infection or disease.
   b. Vestibular branch
      (1) Not tested directly; problems may be detected by symptoms such as nystagmus, vertigo, nausea, vomiting, pallor, sweating, and hypotension
      (2) Reflexes: vestibular branch of cranial nerve VIII and connections with cranial nerves III and VI provide information regarding integrity of the brainstem
         (a) Oculocephalic reflex (also called *doll's eyes reflex*) (Figure 7-26, *A* and *B*)
            (i) Prerequisites
               a) Cervical spine has been cleared radiologically.
               b) Patient is unconscious.
               c) Eyes are held open so that eye movement can be observed.
            (ii) Test: Rotate patient's head side to side.
            (iii) Normal: Eye move in the opposite direction of the head (presence of doll's eyes: like an expensive china doll) indicates supratentorial cause for the coma.
            (iv) Abnormal: Eyes that stay midline or turn to the same direction as the head (absence of doll's eyes) indicate compression in the midbrain-pontine area.
         (b) Oculovestibular reflex (also called *caloric testing*; Figure 7-26, *C* and *D*)
            (i) Prerequisites
               a) Intact tympanic membrane
               b) Absence of basal skull fracture
            (ii) Test
               a) Elevation of the head of bed (HOB) 30 degrees
               b) Injection of 20 to 50 mL of iced water into the ear canal and against the tympanic membrane
            (iii) Normal: nystagmus with deviation toward the irrigated ear
            (iv) Abnormal
               a) No eye movement
               b) Dysconjugate eye movement

7. Glossopharyngeal (IX), vagus (X)
   a. Phonation
      (1) Test: patient asked to say "Ah"
      (2) Normal: bilateral elevation of palate
      (3) Abnormal: no elevation of palate on one side
   b. Speech
      (1) Test: speech assessed; any hoarseness detected
      (2) Normal: voice clear with ability to change volume and pitch
      (3) Abnormal: hoarseness; indicates damage to the laryngeal branch of cranial nerve X

c. Taste
   (1) Test: ability to taste sour and bitter on posterior tongue tested; rarely performed in acute care
   (2) Normal: ability to taste
   (3) Abnormal: inability to taste sour or bitter

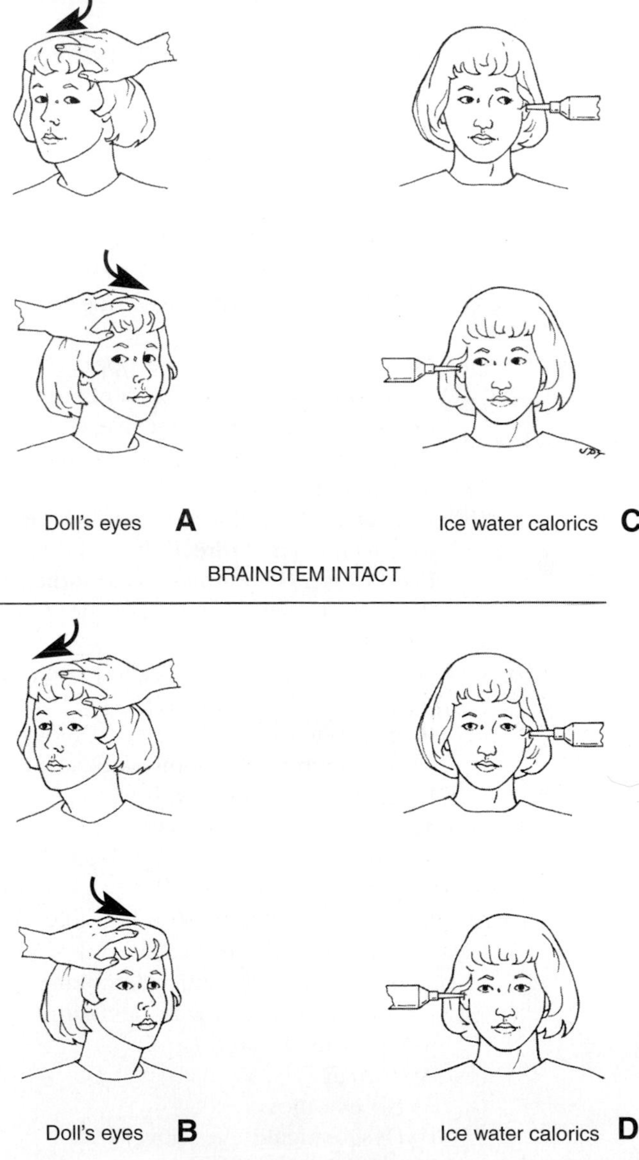

Figure 7-26 **A,** Oculocephalic (doll's eyes) reflex with normal response: eyes move in the direction opposite the direction that the head is turned. **B,** Oculocephalic (doll's eyes) reflex with abnormal response: eyes move in the same direction as the head is being turned or stay midline. **C,** Oculovestibular (caloric) reflex with normal response: nystagmus is present, and there may be conjugate movement toward the irrigated ear. **D,** Oculovestibular (caloric) reflex with abnormal response: no nystagmus or dysconjugate movement of the eyes. (From Beare, P. G., & Myers, J. L. [1994]. *Principles and practice of adult health nursing* [2nd ed.]. St. Louis: Mosby.)

d. Swallowing
   (1) Test
      (a) Hold tongue down with a tongue blade and touch each side of the pharynx with a cotton swab
      (b) Palpate elevation of larynx with swallow
      (c) If patient is conscious, give sip of water
   (2) Normal: involuntary swallow or gag when palate is stroked, elevation of larynx with swallow; and effective swallow; indicates intactness of ninth and tenth cranial nerves
   (3) Abnormal
      (a) No swallow or gag; do not give fluids; position on side; have suction equipment available
      (b) Cough on water swallow: request evaluation by speech and language pathologist

e. Gag
   (1) Test: palate stroked with a tongue blade (NOTE: Do not perform this test within 2 hours after eating.)
   (2) Normal: involuntary gag; indicates intactness of ninth and tenth cranial nerves
   (3) Abnormal: no gag (NOTE: Do not give fluids; position patient on side; have suction equipment available.)

f. Cough
   (1) Test: touch hypopharynx with suction catheter
   (2) Normal: involuntary cough; indicates intactness of ninth and tenth cranial reflexes
   (3) Abnormal: no cough

8. Spinal accessory (XI)
   a. Test
      (1) Sternocleidomastoid and trapezius muscles inspected for size and symmetry
      (2) Patient asked to shrug shoulders as you push down with your hands on patient's shoulders
      (3) Patient asked to turn head to each side against resistance
   b. Normal: symmetry; adequate muscle strength
   c. Abnormal: asymmetry; poor muscle strength

9. Hypoglossal (XII)
   a. Test
      (1) Tongue inspected for atrophy, fasciculations, and alignment
      (2) Tongue strength tested with your index finger when the patient pushes his or her tongue against a cheek
   b. Normal: no atrophy, fasciculations, midline alignment when protrudes, normal strength
   c. Abnormal: atrophy, fasciculations, or deviation from midline; decreased strength

Reflexes

1. Deep tendon (also called *muscle-stretch reflexes*)
   a. Test: tendon tapped with a reflex hammer
   b. Normal: contraction of the muscle and a jerk of affected limb

c. Abnormal
   (1) Hyporeflexia
      (a) Less than normal contraction
      (b) May be seen in hypocalcemia, hyperphosphatemia, hypomagnesemia, and LMN lesion
   (2) Hyperreflexia
      (a) More than normal contraction; may be associated with clonus
      (b) May be seen in hypercalcemia, hypophosphatemia, hypermagnesemia, and UMN lesion
d. Grading scale (Table 7-14)
e. Locations and spinal levels
   (1) Jaw: cranial nerve V (trigeminal)
   (2) Biceps: elbow flexion; C5 to C6
   (3) Brachioradialis: wrist extension; C5 to C6
   (4) Triceps: elbow extension; C7 to C8
   (5) Patellar: knee extension; L2 to L4
   (6) Achilles: foot extension; S1 and S2

2. Superficial reflexes
   a. Abdominal reflexes
      (1) Test: abdomen stroked toward umbilicus with blunt end of cotton-tipped applicator
      (2) Normal: umbilicus moves toward the quadrant that is stroked
      (3) Abnormal: no response; indicates lesion at T7 to T9 for upper abdomen; T11 to T12 for lower abdomen

Table 7-14 Grading Scale for Deep Tendon Reflexes

Grade	Description
0	Absent
1+	Diminished
2+	Normal
3+	More brisk than average but may be normal
4+	Hyperactive with clonus

   b. Cremasteric reflex
      (1) Test: inner thigh stroked
      (2) Normal: testis on stimulated side elevates
      (3) Abnormal: no response: indicates lesion at L1 to L2
   c. Plantar reflex
      (1) Test: sole of the foot stroked with a blunt instrument (Figure 7-27)
      (2) Normal: toes curl downward
      (3) Abnormal (Babinski's reflex): extension of great toe and fanning of other toes; indicates UMN lesion

3. Pathologic reflexes
   a. Babinski's: see Plantar reflex (above)
   b. Grasp
      (1) Test: something (frequently finger) placed in the patient's hand
      (2) Normal: releases grasp on command
      (3) Abnormal: will not release grasp on command; infantile reflex: indicates diffuse cerebral dysfunction
   c. Sucking
      (1) Test: corner of the patient's mouth touched
      (2) Normal: no response
      (3) Abnormal: patient purses lips and starts to suck; infantile reflex: indicates diffuse cerebral dysfunction
   d. Glabellar
      (1) Test: patient's forehead tapped
      (2) Normal: no response
      (3) Abnormal: patient repeatedly blinks; indicates diffuse cerebral dysfunction

Miscellaneous

1. Clinical indications of neurologic trauma
   a. Scalp: tears or swelling
   b. Head and face
      (1) Palpate face, maxilla, and mandible for fractures.
      (2) Note Battle's sign: bruising of mastoid (behind ear), which is indicative of basal skull fracture (Figure 7-28).

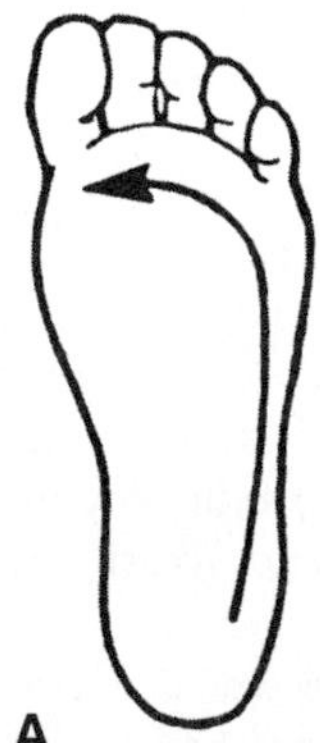

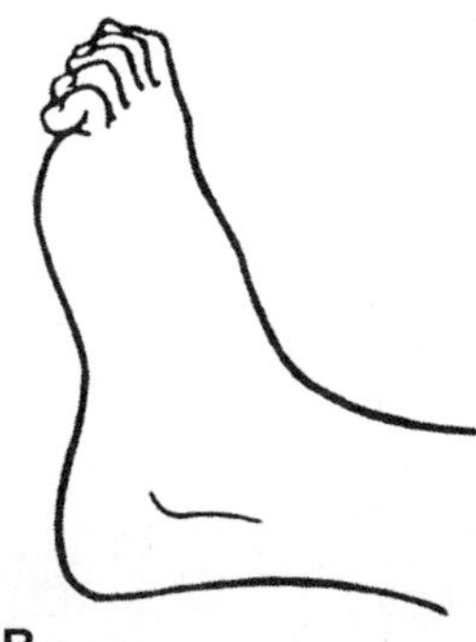

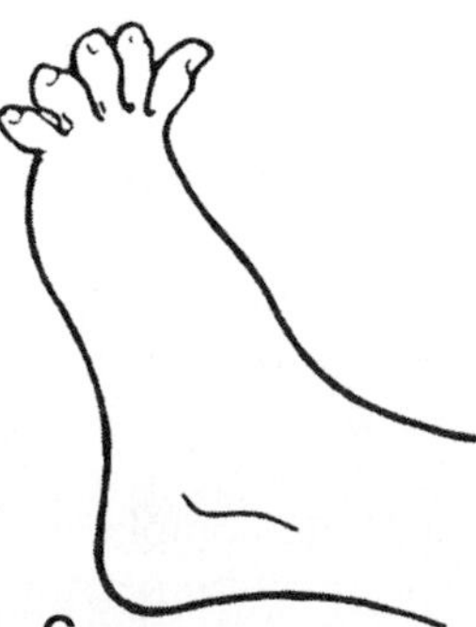

Figure 7-27 Babinski's reflex. **A,** Method of stroking sole of foot. **B,** Normal response (absence of Babinski's reflex). **C,** Abnormal response (presence of Babinski's reflex).

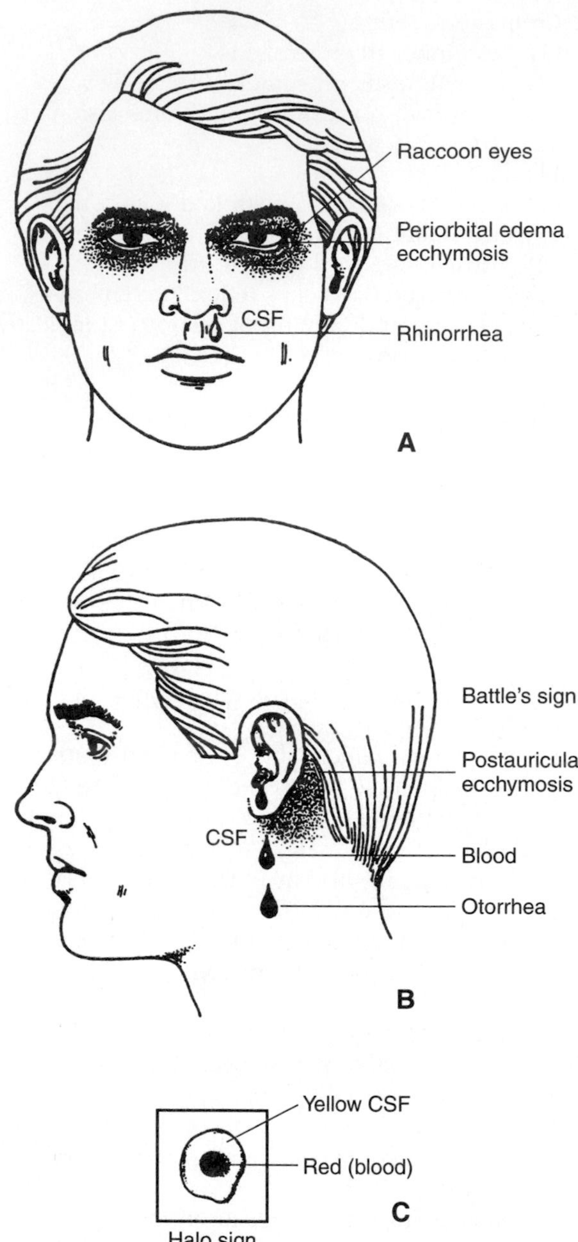

Figure 7-28 **A,** Raccoon eyes and rhinorrhea. **B,** Battle's sign with otorrhea. **C,** Halo sign. *CSF,* Cerebrospinal fluid. (From Barker, E. [1994]. *Neuroscience nursing*. St. Louis: Mosby.)

c. Eyes
 (1) Palpate eye orbits; note complaints of pain.
 (2) Evaluate visual acuity if corneal burn or trauma has occurred.
 (3) Note raccoon eyes: bruising around eyes indicative of basal skull fracture (Figure 7-28, *A*)

d. Nose
 (1) Palpate nose; note complaints of pain.
 (2) Note CSF leak: may be seen in basal skull fracture; referred to as *rhinorrhea.*
  (a) Differentiation of CSF from mucus by testing for significant glucose
   (i) CSF glucose is normally 60% of serum glucose.
   (ii) Low levels of glucose may be seen with mucus.
  (b) CSF also leaves a "halo" on 4 × 4-inch guaze or linens; this refers to blood settling in the middle with a lighter-colored concentric ring around the blood (Figure 7-28, *C*)

e. Ears
 (1) Note edema and trauma to external ear or ear canal.
 (2) Note blood in external ear canal or blood behind ear drum: seen in basal skull fracture.
 (3) Note CSF leak from ear: seen in basal skull fracture; referred to as *otorrhea* (Figure 7-28, *B*).

f. Injury to teeth, tongue, gums, mucosa

g. Alteration in consciousness

h. Clinical indications of intracranial hypertension (see Intracranial Hypertension)

2. Clinical indications of meningeal irritation
 a. Nuchal rigidity: indicative of meningeal irritation (e.g., infection or hemorrhage)
 b. Brudzinski's sign (Figure 7-29, *A*)
  (1) Prerequisite: cervical spine must be cleared radiologically
  (2) Detection: chin brought toward chest and head moved forward
  (3) Normal: absence of neck pain and absence of involuntary adduction and flexion of knees toward body
  (4) Abnormal: neck pain and involuntary adduction and flexion of legs with attempts to flex the neck; indicates irritation of the meninges by infection or blood
 c. Kernig's sign (Figure 7-29, *B*)
  (1) Detection: patient placed on his or her back and assisted to flex thigh toward his or her chest until hip is at 90 degree angle; then leg extended at knee
  (2) Normal: ability fully to extend leg without pain
  (3) Abnormal: inability to fully extend leg when thigh is flexed toward abdomen; neck pain also may occur; indicates irritation of the meninges by infection or blood

3. Clinical indications of brain death
 a. Criteria: irreversible cessation of all functions of the entire brain, including the brainstem; note that specific requirements for declaration of brain death may be affected by state law and hospital policy
  (1) Recognizable cause of coma (e.g., severe traumatic brain injury, intracranial hemorrhage or infarction, anoxic encephalopathy following cardiac arrest, drowning, or asphyxiation)
  (2) Exclusion of potentially reversible causes of coma (sedative drugs including alcohol, neuromuscular blocking agents, hypothermia, or metabolic or endocrine disturbance)

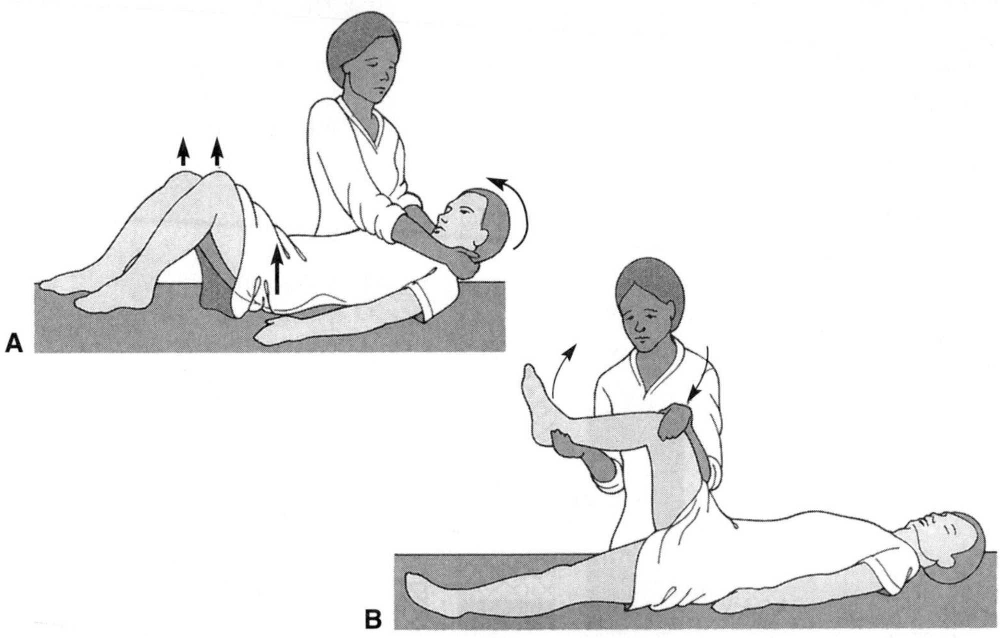

Figure 7-29 **A,** Brudzinski's sign. **B,** Kernig's sign. (From Barker, E. [1994]. *Neuroscience nursing*. St. Louis: Mosby.)

(a) BP greater than 90 mm Hg
(b) Temperature greater than 32° C (90° F)

(3) Clinical examination
   (a) Absence of responsiveness to noxious stimuli
   (b) Absence of movement, including posturing, shivering, and seizures, spontaneously or to central pain stimulation in the absence of sedation and neuromuscular blockade; spinal reflexes and Babinski's reflex may be present even in the presence of brain death
   (c) Absence of brainstem function
      (i) No pupillary light reflex
      (ii) No corneal reflex
      (iii) No oculocephalic reflex (doll's eyes)
      (iv) No oculovestibular reflex (caloric)
      (v) No gag or cough reflexes
   (d) Absence of spontaneous ventilation when tested for a sufficient time; usually 3 to 5 minutes of $Paco_2$ of greater than 60 mm Hg; apnea testing is performed by doing the following:
      (i) Disconnect the mechanical ventilator.
      (ii) Deliver 100% oxygen.
      (iii) Monitor for ventilatory effort.
      (iv) Measuring ABGs to confirm $Paco_2$ greater than 60 mm Hg.
      (v) Reconnecting the ventilator

(4) Diagnostic and laboratory studies
   (a) EEG: no electrical activity during a period of at least 30 minutes
   (b) Cerebral angiography: no intracerebral filling in circle of Willis or at carotid bifurcation
   (c) CBF scan: no uptake of radionuclide in brain parenchyma, indicating no CBF
   (d) Transcranial Doppler ultrasound: reverberating flow signals

b. Repeat evaluation in 6 hours is recommended
c. Signature of two physicians required for determination of brain death with one of the physicians not involved in the care of the patient; note that neither of the two physicians should be involved in organ transplantation

Neurologic Monitoring

1. ICP
   a. Indications
      (1) The need for ICP monitoring usually correlates with a GCS score of 8 or less.
      (2) All of the following are potential diagnoses when ICP monitoring may be needed:
         (a) Severe head trauma especially if abnormal findings on admission CT scan
         (b) Intracerebral masses
         (c) SAH
         (d) Intracerebral hemorrhage (e.g., massive stroke)
         (e) Infectious processes (e.g., encephalitis or meningitis)
         (f) Encephalopathy

(i) Anoxic encephalopathy (e.g., after cardiac arrest)
(ii) Reye's syndrome
(g) Hydrocephalus
(h) After craniotomy
(3) ICP monitoring should be used if deep sedation, paralysis, or barbiturate coma is being used, because LOC as an assessment parameter is eliminated

b. Purposes
(1) Diagnose intracranial hypertension
(2) Allow drainage of CSF to maintain pressure
(3) Observe effects of medical or nursing management
(4) Predict outcomes: Patients who sustain an ICP greater than 50 mm Hg for longer than 20 minutes have a poor prognosis.

c. General information
(1) CSF is considered the most accurate indication of ICP.
(a) The most accurate devices are measuring the pressure of CSF and are in contact with CSF.
(b) This contact with CSF creates an infection risk.
(c) Intraparenchymal devices show a linear relationship between intraventricular and intraparenchymal pressure measured with fiberoptic transducer-tipped probe.
(2) Several types of ICP measuring devices are available (Figure 7-30 and Table 7-15).
(a) Insertion of all of these devices is during craniotomy or through a small burr hole made with a twist drill using strict aseptic technique.
(3) Three types of monitoring systems are available.
(a) Fluid-filled system
(i) Sensor: fluid-filled catheter or bolt that communicates the subarachnoid or interventricular space and the transducer
(ii) Closed fluid-filled system between the sensor and the transducer
a) Prime the system using preservative-free isotonic saline.

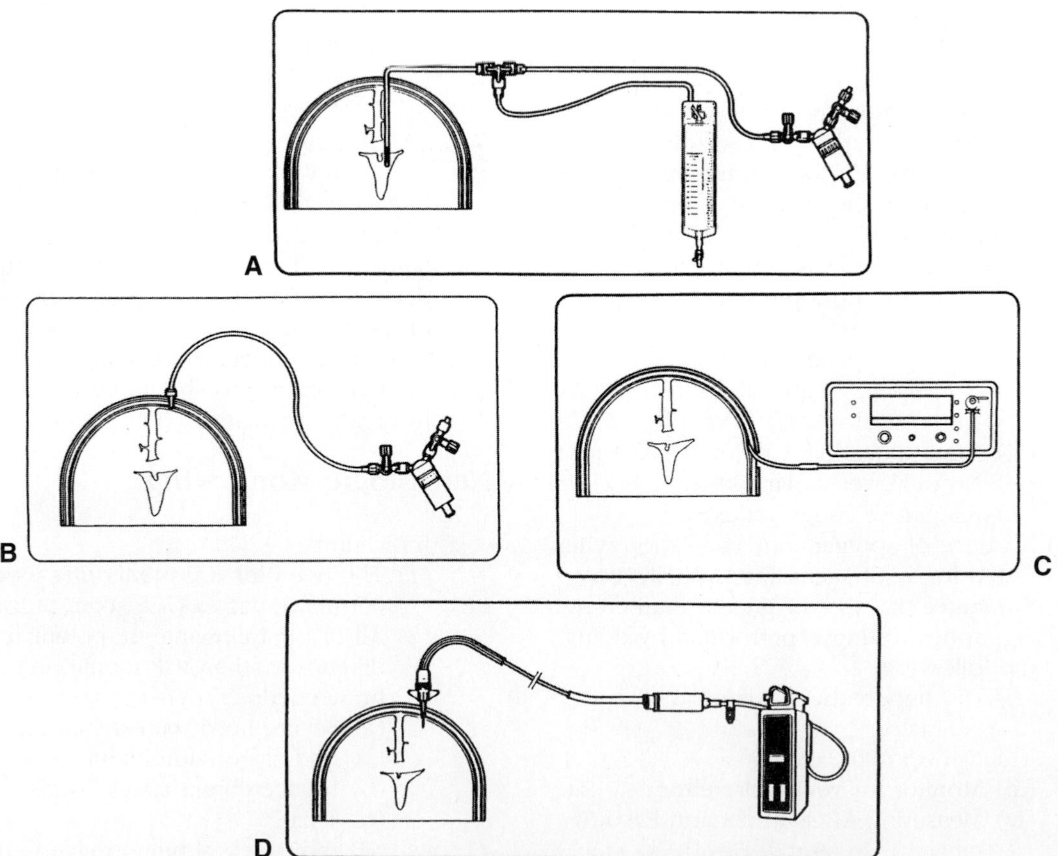

Figure 7-30 Devices for the measurement of ICP. **A,** Intraventricular catheter and system. **B,** Subarachnoid screw or bolt and system. **C,** Epidural transducer and system. **D,** Intraparenchymal transducer and system. (From Urden, L., Stacy, K., & Lough, M. [2002]. *Thelan's critical care nursing: Diagnosis and management* [4th ed.]. St. Louis: Mosby.)

Table 7-15 Intracranial Pressure Measuring Devices

Device	Location	Accuracy	Comments
Intraventricular catheter	Lateral ventricle Nondominant hemisphere is used if possible, but location of skull fracture and trauma may limit placement possibilities	Excellent Can test VPR	• Preferred because most accurate and reliable, low cost, and provides opportunity to drain CSF for specimen or treatment of intracranial hypertension • May be difficult to insert especially if ventricles are small or displaced • Therapeutic or diagnostic removal of CSF possible • Provides access for determination of VPR • May permit CSF leakage, but rapid CSF drainage may result in collapsed ventricle or subdural hematoma • May cause intracerebral bleeding or edema at cannula track • Infection rate 2%-5% • Fluid-filled system used if intraventricular catheter if placed
Subarachnoid bolt	Subarachnoid space	Fair; unreliable at high intracranial pressure	• Easy to insert; especially useful if ventricles are small • Inexpensive • Does not penetrate brain • Requires intact skull • Bolt can become occluded with clots or tissue; may require irrigation • Needs to be recalibrated frequently • Unable to drain CSF or to test VPR • Infection rate 1%-2% • Fluid-filled system used
Epidural sensor or transducer	Between the skull and the dura	Variable	• Easy to insert • Least invasive (does not penetrate dura) • Does not penetrate brain or dura • Unable to drain CSF or to test VPR • Infection rate less than 1% • Head position has no effect on pressure reading • Cannot be re-zeroed once in place • Epidural pressure is slightly higher than intraventricular pressure
Intraparenchymal transducer	1 cm into brain tissue	Excellent	• Easy to insert • Unable to drain CSF or to test VPR • Catheter relatively fragile; avoid sharp kinks or pulls • Head position has no effect on pressure reading • Cannot be re-zeroed once in place • Risk of intracerebral bleeding and infection

CSF, Cerebrospinal fluid; *VPR,* volume-pressure response.

b) Do not add heparin; do not use a pressure bag or intermittent flush device.
c) Use Luer-Lok connections.
d) Do not routinely irrigate; subarachnoid bolts may be irrigated if specifically ordered with approximately 0.1 mL every 2 hours; dilute antibiotic solution may be prescribed as irrigation solution.

(iii) Transducer: converts the pressure signal to an electrical signal that can be recorded

a) Position the transducer at the level of the foramen of Monro; this correlates externally to the tragus of ear.
b) Connect the transducer cable to the pressure module of the bedside monitor.

(b) Continuous drainage system (Figure 7-31)

(i) Place the drip chamber at the prescribed height above the foramen of Monro; height is based on the desired upper limit for controlling the ICP.

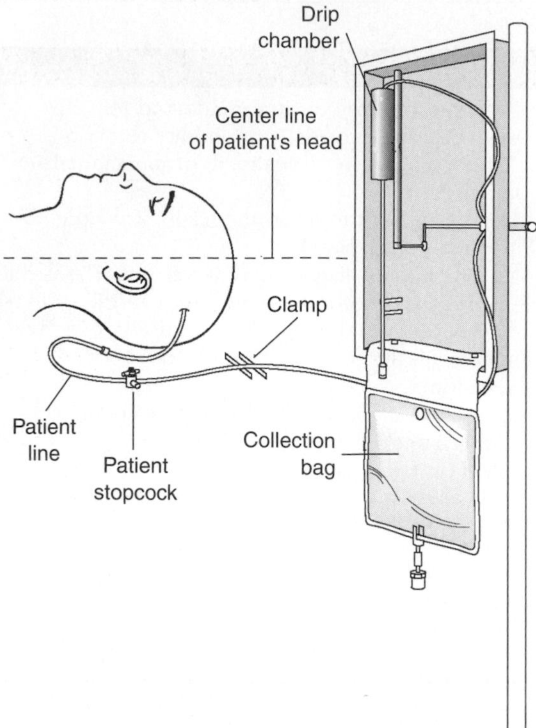

Figure 7-31 Continuous drainage system. Continuous drainage involves placing the drip chamber of the drainage system at a specified level above the foramen of Monro (usually 15 cm). The system is left open to allow continuous drainage of CSF into the chamber (which drains into a collection bag) against a pressure gradient that prevents excessive drainage and ventricular collapse. (Courtesy Codman/Johnson & Johnson Professional Inc., Raynham, MA.)

(ii) Use commercial systems that have one-way flow valves and micropore filters on air vents.

(c) Fiberoptic transducer
  (i) A fluid-filled system is not necessary.
  (ii) The catheter is plugged directly into the monitor.
  (iii) This system requires a special monitor module.

d. Measurement guidelines
  (1) Explain procedure to patient and/or family.
  (2) Re-zero the monitor with each head position change if fluid-filled system.
  (3) Do not stimulate patient before measurements.
  (4) Evaluate trends instead of one measurement.
  (5) Assist with volume-pressure response (VPR) test (or *pressure-volume index*) as requested.
    (a) Inject 1 mL of preservative-free isotonic saline in 1 second into an intraventricular catheter
    (b) Normal: increase in ICP of 2 mm Hg or less
    (c) Low compliance: increase in ICP of 3 mm Hg or more
  (6) If the ICP does not return to normal within 4 minutes after activity, compliance if poor.

e. ICP values
  (1) Normal: 5 to 15 mm Hg
  (2) Slightly elevated: 16 to 20 mm Hg
  (3) Moderately elevated: 21 to 40 mm Hg
  (4) Severely elevated: greater than 40 mm Hg

f. ICP waveforms (Table 7-16)
  (1) Normal waveform (Figure 7-32)
    (a) P1: upward spike with a systolic or percussion wave
    (b) P2: tidal wave
      (i) Most clinically significant; reflect elastic recoil during reduced systolic ejection phase of the cardiac cycle and arterial compliance within the brain
      (ii) As ICP rises so does the P2; this gives the waveform a rounded appearance
      (iii) When the amplitude of P2 is greater than that of P1 or becomes lost in the tracing, it is indicative of a decrease in compliance
    (c) P3: small superimposed notch that represents the pulsation of the arterial vessels in contact with the CSF
  (2) C waves (Figure 7-33)
    (a) Rapid, rhythmic oscillation of pressure without any relevance
    (b) Small spikes as high as 20 mm Hg at six per minute
    (c) Associated with changes in arterial BP and ventilation
  (3) B waves (Figure 7-33)
    (a) Sharp, sawtooth appearance waves
    (b) Pressures as high as 50 mm Hg lasting 30 seconds to 2 minutes
    (c) Related to changes in CBF
    (d) Though not significant alone, may precede A waves
  (4) A waves (Figure 7-33)
    (a) Elevations on top of baseline elevation of ICP
    (b) Pressures reach 50 to 100 mm Hg and last 5 to 20 minutes
    (c) Pathologic waves produced by secondary changes in cerebral blood volume
    (d) Require immediate treatment

g. Prevent, detect, and treat complications of ICP monitoring
  (1) Infection (e.g., bacterial meningitis or bacterial ventriculitis)
    (a) Risk factors associated with ICP monitoring–related infection
      (i) Intracerebral hemorrhage with intraventricular blood
      (ii) Open head trauma
      (iii) After craniotomy

Table 7-16 **Intracranial Pressure Waveforms**

Waveforms	Description	Significance	Comments
Normal	• Low amplitude fluctuations in ICP with pressure less than 15 mm Hg	• Normal	
C waves	• Rapid, rhythmic oscillation of pressure • Small spikes as high as 20 mm Hg at six per minute	• Not significant • Associated with changes in arterial blood pressure and ventilation	
B waves	• Sharp, sawtooth appearance waves • Pressures as high as 50 mm Hg lasting 30 seconds to 2 minutes	• Probably not clinically significant but may precede A waves	• Do not perform any activities that may further increase ICP • Assess for reversible causes of increased ICP (e.g., jugular vein compression by cervical collar or tight tracheostomy ties, compromised airway, or restlessness) • May indicate decreased brain compliance
A waves or plateau waves	• Elevations on top of baseline elevation of ICP • Pressures reach 50 to 100 mm Hg and last 5-20 minutes	• Most significant • Pathologic waves produced by secondary changes in cerebral blood volume • Ominous sign of decreasing cerebral compliance and rapidly progressing decompensation • Usually occur only in advanced stages of intracranial hypertension	• Requires treatment • Irreversible brain damage will occur if not resolved within 15 minutes
Terminal wave	• Flat wave with pressure 50-100 mm Hg	• Mean arterial pressure equals ICP, and cerebral blood flow ceases • Indicative of brain death	
Dampened waveform	• Low-voltage wave with pressure notches	• May be caused by tubing kinks, blood in line, or stopcock positioned incorrectly	

ICP, Intracranial pressure.

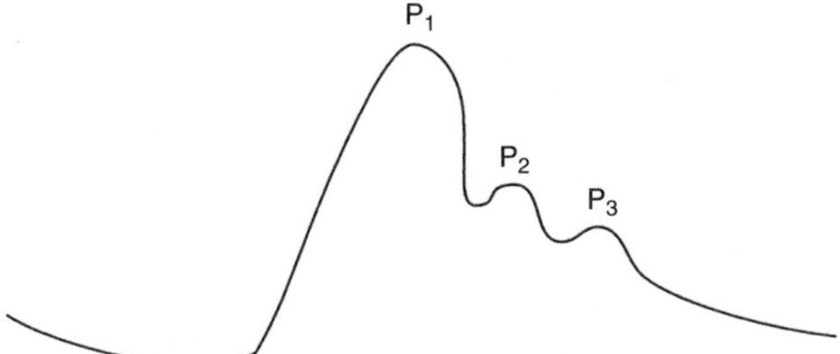

Figure 7-32 Components of a normal ICP waveform. (From Barker, E. [1994]. *Neuroscience nursing.* St. Louis: Mosby.)

(iv) ICP greater than 20 mm Hg
(v) Elderly patient
(vi) Burr hole larger than necessary
(vii) Nonsterile technique for insertion
(viii) Device that penetrates dura
(ix) Monitoring for more than 3 to 5 days
(x) Irrigation of ICP monitoring system
(xi) Opening of system for CSF specimen collection, VPR testing, or irrigation

(b) Prevention
(i) Change dressing daily or according to hospital policy using sterile technique.
(ii) Maintain closed system; limit irrigation; use strict aseptic technique if system must be interrupted (e.g., VPR test).
(iii) Monitoring should be maintained no longer than 3 to 5 days; if longer monitoring is required, device should be removed and replaced.

(c) Detection: monitor for clinical indications of infection.
(i) Fever
(ii) Leukocytosis
(iii) Cloudy CSF

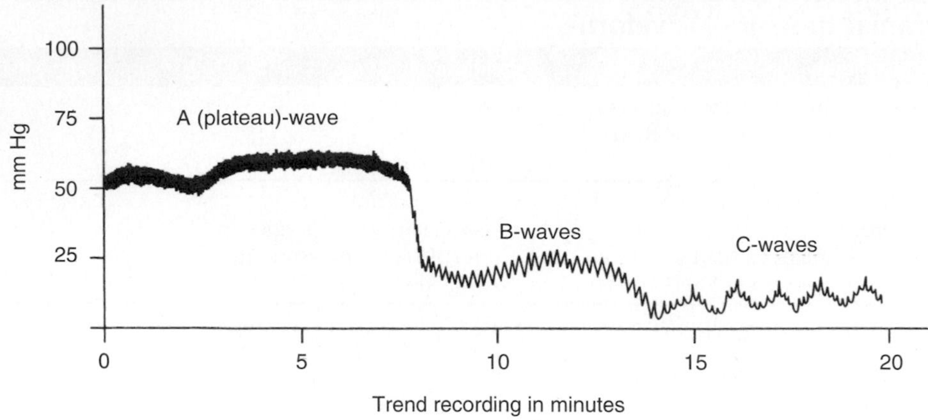

Figure 7-33 Abnormal ICP waveforms. (From Barker, E. [1994]. *Neuroscience nursing*. St. Louis: Mosby.)

(d) Treatment: Administer antibiotics as prescribed.
(i) Intravenous (IV) antibiotic
(ii) Intrathecal antibiotic (usually aminoglycosides)
(iii) Irrigation of ICP catheter with very small volume (e.g., 0.1 to 0.2 mL) of antibiotic solution
(2) Intercerebral hemorrhage, hematoma
(a) Monitor for change in color of CSF and change in neurologic status.
(b) Maintain the air-fluid meniscus of the transducer at the level of the foramen of Monro; do not allow drainage bag to be lowered below the head.
(3) CSF leak
(a) Use Luer-Lok connections.
(b) Maintain closed system.
(4) CSF overdrainage
(a) Do not drain CSF below a pressure of 15 to 20 mm Hg unless specifically instructed.
(b) Ventricular collapse may cause hemorrhage.
(5) Dislodgment or occlusion of catheter
(6) CSF leakage around insertion site
(7) Pneumoencephalopathy

2. CBF
a. Techniques
(1) Diagnostic tests that provide a snapshot in time
(a) Stable-xenon-enhanced CT
(b) Perfusion CT
(c) Perfusion MRI
(d) Single-photon emission computed tomography
(e) Positron emission tomography
(f) All provide excellent regional information about CBF
(2) Continuous monitoring methods
(a) Laser flowmetry
(i) A laser light probe is placed over the brain area of interest during craniotomy or by burr hole
(ii) The light deflection is transformed into a CBF measurement
(iii) Risks: infection, bleeding, displacement
(iv) Advantage: small size allows the probe to be placed in an ICP monitor
(b) Thermal diffusion flowmetry
(i) A catheter with a heat source and a thermistor is placed over the brain area of interest during craniotomy or by burr hole
(ii) CBF is determined by the difference between the temperature of the heat source and the thermistor; the greater the temperature difference, the lower the blood flow
(iii) Risks: infection, bleeding, displacement
(c) Disadvantage: CBF is measured in a local area of the brain, which may not reflect the global state of the brain or a specific region of interest.
(3) Intermittent measurement of CBF: transcranial Doppler ultrasound
(a) Doppler ultrasound probe placed over the skin on the cranium in temporal window that allows assessment of blood flow velocity through the anterior and middle cerebral arteries
(b) Normal flow velocity: less than 120 cm/sec
(i) Increase in flow velocity indicates that blood is flowing through a restricted area (e.g., vasospasm or stenosis) upstream from the probe.

(ii) Decrease in flow velocity indicates obstruction downstream (e.g., carotid stenosis) from the probe.
(c) Disadvantage: need for technical expertise
b. CBF values
(1) Normal: 50 to 60 mL/100 g/min
(2) Altered LOC and EEG: 20 to 25 mL/100 g/min
(3) Isoelectric EEG and neurotransmitter failure: 15 to 20 mL/100 g/min
(4) Ion pump failure and cytotoxic brain edema: 10 to 15 mL/100 g/min
(5) Calcium channels open, activation of intracellular enzymes, alterations of cell membrane: less than 10 mm Hg
3. Brain tissue oxygenation monitoring
a. Provides information about cerebral oxygen delivery to detect cerebral ischemia, a potential cause of secondary brain injury; secondary cerebral ischemia may occur even though ICP and CPP are normal
b. Indication: severe brain injury with risk of cerebral ischemia
c. Technique: a probe is placed into the white matter of the brain for global brain assessment or the penumbra of an injury for regional assessment
d. Normal value: 20 to 50 mm Hg in uninjured tissue; less than 15 mm Hg is correlated with a poor outcome and increased chance of death
e. Risks: infection, hematoma
4. SjO_2 monitoring
a. Provides a global measure of oxygen reserve for the brain as a whole
b. Technique
(1) Fiberoptic catheter placed into the jugular vein bulb to monitor continuously the oxygen saturation of the blood returning from the brain and intermittently sample venous blood gases
(2) Comparison between SaO_2 and SjO_2 allows calculation of arteriovenous (AV) oxygen difference
c. Normal value: 55% to 70%; saturation less than 55% indicates brain ischemia
d. Limitations
(1) May not be reliable if performed unilaterally because the oxygen content of each jugular bulb may differ
(2) Normal values do not ensure adequate perfusion to all brain areas
5. In-vivo optical spectroscopy
a. Technique
(1) A sensor is placed on the forehead to right or left of midline.
(2) Low-intensity near-infrared light is passed into the patient's forehead, where it penetrates the skull and passes through the cerebral cortex.
(3) The returned light at two distances from the light source allows determination of the rSO_2, which is a measure of the oxygen saturation of the mixed arterial and venous blood in the brain cortex.
b. Interpretation: used for trending
(1) Change in rSO_2 of 12 to 20 points or 20% to 30% correlates with changes in the neurologic status.
(2) rSO_2 index less than 50 is associated with poor outcomes.
6. Continuous EEG monitoring
a. Detects ischemia, severe metabolic and anoxic encephalopathy, drug intoxication, and seizures, including subclinical seizures
b. Technique: five electrodes are used to monitor two EEG leads
7. Bispectral index: an EEG parameter developed specifically to measure patient's response to sedation and anesthesia
a. Electrodes are placed across the patient's forehead to detect electrical activity in the brain; changes reflect changes in the effects of sedative and anesthetic agents
b. Values
(1) Value of close to 100 corresponds to an awake state
(2) Value of 70 to 90 corresponds to light to moderate sedation
(3) Value of 40 to 70 corresponds to a moderate to deep level of sedation
(4) Value of 40 or less corresponds to a deep hypnotic state or barbiturate coma
c. Advantage over traditional sedation scales (e.g., Ramsay or Riker): provides objective and reproducible data

Diagnostic Studies

1. Serum
a. Chemistries
(1) Sodium: normal 136 to 145 mEq/L
(2) Potassium: normal 3.5 to 5.5 mEq/L
(3) Chloride: normal 96 to 106 mEq/L
(4) Calcium: normal 8.5 to 10.5 mg/dL
(5) Phosphorus: normal 3 to 4.5 mg/dL
(6) Magnesium: normal 1.5 to 2.2 mEq/L or 1.8 to 2.4 mg/dL
(7) Glucose: normal 70 to 110 mg/dL
(8) Blood urea nitrogen (BUN): normal 5 to 20 mg/dL
(9) Serum osmolality: normal 285 to 295 mmol/kg
(10) Creatinine: normal 0.7 to 1.5 mg/dL
(11) Lactate: less than 1 mmol/L
(12) Enzymes
(a) Total creatine kinase: normal 55 to 170 units/L for males; 30 to 135 units/L for females
(b) Lactate dehydrogenase: 90 to 200 units/L

b. ABGs
 (1) pH: normal 7.35 to 7.45
 (2) $Paco_2$: normal 35 to 45 mm Hg
 (3) HCO_3: normal 22 to 26 mM
 (4) Pao_2: normal 80 to 100 mm Hg
 (5) Sao_2: greater than 95%
c. Hematology
 (1) Hematocrit: normal 40% to 52% for males; 35% to 47% for females
 (2) Hemoglobin: normal 13 to 18 g/dL for males; 12 to 16 g/dL for females
 (3) White blood cell (WBC) count: normal 3500 to 11,000 cells/mm^3
 (4) Erythrocyte sedimentation rate: normal up to 15 mm/hr for males; up to 20 mm/hr for females
d. Clotting profile
 (1) Prothrombin time (PT): normal 12 to 15 seconds; therapeutic 1.5 to 2.5 times normal
 (2) Partial thromboplastin time (PTT): normal 60 to 90 seconds; therapeutic 1.5 to 2.5 times normal
 (3) Activated partial thromboplastin time: normal 25 to 38 seconds; therapeutic 1.5 to 2.5 times normal
 (4) Activated clotting time: normal 70 to 120 seconds; therapeutic 150 to 190 seconds
 (5) Thrombin time: normal 10 to 15 seconds
 (6) Bleeding time: normal 1 to 9½ minutes
 (7) International normalized ratio: normal less than 2
  (a) Therapeutic range for atrial fibrillation: 1.5 to 2.5
  (b) Therapeutic range for deep venous thrombosis or pulmonary embolus: 2 to 3
  (c) Therapeutic range for prosthetic valves: 2.5 to 3.5
 (8) Platelets: normal 150,000 to 400,000/mm^3
e. Toxicology
 (1) Alcohol: normal 0 mg/dL
 (2) Dilantin: therapeutic 10 to 20 mcg/mL

2. Urine
 a. Glucose: normal negative
 b. Ketones: normal negative
 c. Specific gravity: normal 1.005 to 1.03
 d. Osmolality: normal 50 to 1200 mOsm/L
3. CSF analysis
 a. Properties
  (1) Colorless, odorless; cloudy in bacterial meningitis
  (2) Specific gravity: normal 1.007
  (3) pH: normal 7.35
  (4) Chlorides: normal 120 to 130 mEq/L
  (5) Sodium: normal 140 to 142 mEq/L
  (6) Glucose: normal 60% of serum glucose value; decreased in bacterial meningitis
 b. Protein: elevated in meningitis
  (1) By lumbar puncture (LP): normal 15 to 45 mg/dL
  (2) By cisternal puncture: normal 10 to 25 mg/dL
  (3) By ventricular puncture or catheter: normal 5 to 15 mg/dL
 c. Cells
  (1) Leukocytes: normal 0 to 5 cells/mm^3
  (2) Erythrocytes: normal 0 cells/mm^3
   (a) NOTE: Test tubes must be numbered to differentiate between traumatic puncture; if first test tube is bloody but others are clear, consider trauma; SAH would cause all test tubes to be equally bloody.
4. Other diagnostic studies (Table 7-17)

Table 7-17 Neurologic Diagnostic Studies

Study	Purposes	Comments
Angiography	• Visualizes extracranial and intracranial vasculature • Identifies aneurysm, AVM, vasospasm, and vascular tumors • Detects arterial occlusion and allows delivery of intraarterial therapy to restore blood flow	• May cause local hematoma, vasospasm, vessel occlusion, allergic reaction to contrast media, and transient or permanent neurologic dysfunction • Before test: ◦ Keep patient NPO for 4 hours and provide sedation before the study ◦ Check for allergy to iodine ◦ Evaluate renal function • After the test: ◦ Ensure hydration postprocedure (contrast medium used) ◦ Maintain bed rest for 8-12 hours ◦ Monitor arterial puncture point for hemorrhage or hematoma ◦ Monitor neurovascular status of affected limb ◦ Monitor for indications of systemic emboli ◦ Reevaluate renal function

Table 7-17 Neurologic Diagnostic Studies—cont'd

Study	Purposes	Comments
Cisternogram	• Views CSF flow • Identifies hydrocephalus • Evaluates CSF leakage through a dural tear • Evaluates abnormality of structures at the base of the brain and upper cervical cord region	• Contraindicated in intracranial hypertension
CT computerized axial tomography	• Views intracranial structures: size, shape, location, shifts • Differentiates between tumors, hemorrhage, and infarction • Identifies hydrocephalus, brain edema, infectious processes, trauma, aneurysm, hematoma, AVM, brain atrophy, and subacute and old brain infarction • Evaluates arterial system if CT angiography studies performed	• Patient must be cooperative • Contrast media may be used; contrast media may be used after a noncontrast CT • Check for allergy to iodine or seafood before study • Patient will be NPO for 4-8 hours before the study • Sedation may be given • Monitor for signs of allergic reaction • Encourage fluid intake • Evaluate renal function when contrast media used
Digital subtraction angiography: brain; spine	• Visualizes the vasculature, especially carotid and larger cerebral arteries • Evaluates occlusive vascular disease • Identifies tumors, aneurysms, AVM, vascular abnormalities	• May be done IV or intraarterially • If IV, is less invasive with fewer complications than cerebral angiography • If intraarterially, care as for angiogram • Contrast media are used • Check for allergy to iodine, seafood before study • Patient will be NPO for 4-8 hours before the study • Monitor for signs of allergic reaction • Encourage fluid intake
Electroencephalography	• Differentiates epilepsy from mass lesion • Detects focus of seizure activity • Evaluates drug intoxication • Evaluates electrical function of the brain, which may be abnormal in the presence of cerebrovascular alterations • Localizes tumor, abscess, and other mass lesions • May be used in designation of brain death	• Stimulants, anticonvulsants, tranquilizer, and antidepressants may be withheld for 24-48 hours before the study • Hair shampooed before and after study
Electromyography; nerve conduction velocity studies	• Detects muscle disease • Identifies peripheral neuropathies, nerve compression • Identifies nerve regeneration and muscle recovery	• Patient must be cooperative • Contraindicated in patients taking anticoagulants, with bleeding disorders, or skin infection • May be uncomfortable for patient
Electronystagmography	• Detects nystagmus, which may aid in identification of cerebellar or vestibular problem	
Evoked potential studies	• Evaluate electrical potentials (responses) of brain to external stimuli; evaluate sensory and somatosensory neurologic pathways • Identify neuromuscular disease, cerebrovascular disease, spinal cord injury, traumatic brain injury, peripheral nerve disease, and tumors • Determine prognosis in traumatic brain injury • Contribute to diagnosis of multiple sclerosis and brainstem injury	• Hair shampooed before and after study

Continued

Table 7-17 **Neurologic Diagnostic Studies—cont'd**

Study	Purposes	Comments
Isotope ventriculography	• Visualizes CSF circulation system	• No CSF withdrawn • May cause meningeal irritation and aseptic meningitis
LP or cisternal puncture	• Obtains CSF for analysis • Measures CSF opening pressure (roughly equivalent to intracranial pressure for most patients if done recumbent and no blockage is present	• Cisternal puncture is higher risk but may be used if scar tissue prevents LP • Patient must be cooperative • Contraindicated in patients with intracranial hypertension because herniation may occur • Contraindicated in bleeding disorders and in patients receiving anticoagulants • Patient kept flat for 4-8 hours to prevent headache • May cause headache, low back pain, meningitis, abscess, CSF leak, or puncture of spinal cord
Magnetic resonance angiography/magnetic resonance imaging	• As for CT • Visualizes tissue state (diffusion and perfusion) so that early ischemic changes are apparent (CT cannot visualize most early changes) • Identifies vascular lesions, tissue abnormalities, hemorrhage, infarction, epileptic foci, and multiple sclerosis • Identifies patency of large veins and venous sinuses • Identifies brainstem abnormalities • Identifies type, location, and extent of brain injury	• Patient must be cooperative • Contraindicated in patients with any implanted metallic device, including pacemakers • Tends to overestimate degree of stenosis
Myelography	• Visualizes spinal subarachnoid space • Detects spinal cord lesions and cord or nerve root compression • Detects pressure on spinal nerve roots	• If done with oil-based iophendylate (Pantopaque), patient must lie flat for 4-8 hours after study • May cause headache, nerve root irritation, allergic reaction, or adhesive arachnoiditis • If done with water-soluble metrizamide (Amipaque), patient should have head of bed elevated • May cause headache, nausea, vomiting, backache and neck ache, chest pain, seizures, hallucinations, speech disorders, dysrhythmias, or allergic reaction • Encourage fluid intake with either type of dye
Nerve conduction velocity studies	• Identifies peripheral neuropathies and nerve compression	• Needle electrodes are used
Oculoplethysmography	• Indirectly measures ocular artery pressure • Reflects adequacy of cerebrovascular blood flow in the carotid artery	• Contraindicated in patients who have undergone eye surgery within the last 6 months, who have had lens implants or cataracts, or who have had retinal detachment • May cause conjunctival hemorrhage, corneal abrasions, or transient photophobia
Pneumoencephalography	• Visualizes ventricular system and subarachnoid space • Identifies intracranial tumors • Identifies brain atrophy	• Care as for LP • Contraindicated in patients with intracranial hypertension • May cause headache, nausea, vomiting, autonomic dysfunction, herniation, subdural hematoma, air embolus, or seizures • Keep patient flat for 12-24 hours after the study

Table 7-17 Neurologic Diagnostic Studies—cont'd

Study	Purposes	Comments
Positron emission tomography or single-photon emission computed tomography	• Evaluates oxygen and glucose metabolism • Measures cerebral blood flow, which may be altered by traumatic brain injury, seizure, ischemia, stroke, or neoplasm • Also used to evaluate dementia, depression, schizophrenia, and Alzheimer's disease	• Patient must be cooperative • Contraindicated in pregnant and breast-feeding patients
Radioisotope brain scan	• Identifies tumors, cerebrovascular disease, infarction, trauma, infectious processes, and seizures	• Generally replaced by CT scan • Reassure patient that amount of radioactive material is minimal • Patient must be cooperative • Contraindicated in pregnant and breast-feeding patients
Regional cerebral blood flow (xenon [^{133}Xe] inhalation)	• Evaluates blood flow to the cerebral cortex • Identifies cerebrovascular disease • Detects regions of increased or decreased perfusion • Determines presence of collateral blood flow • Evaluates the effect of vasospasm on tissue perfusion	• Assure patient that amount of radioactive material is minimal • Contraindicated in pregnant and breast-feeding patients
Skull x-rays	• Detects skull fracture, facial fracture, tumor, bone erosion, cranial anomalies, air-fluid level in sinuses, abnormal intracranial calcification, and radiopaque foreign bodies	• Linear and basal fractures frequently missed by routine x-rays • Contraindicated in pregnant patients
Somnography	• Records electroencephalogram during sleep • Evaluates sleep and sleep disorders	
Spinal cord arteriography	• Differentiates between spinal AVM, angioma, tumor, and ischemia	• As for skull x-rays • May cause thrombosis of spinal vessels and allergy to contrast agent
Spine x-rays	• Detects vertebral dislocation or fracture, degenerative disease, tumor, bone erosion, or calcification • Identifies structural spinal deficits and rules out associated cervical spine injuries	• Care must be taken to prevent fracture displacement and spinal cord injury • C1-C2 view best obtained via open mouth; C6-C7 best obtained with arms pulled down
Suboccipital puncture	• Obtains CSF for analysis • Measures CSF pressure • Rarely performed but may be useful when LP is contraindicated	• May cause trauma to the medulla
Transcranial Doppler ultrasonography	• Measures blood flow velocity through the cerebral arteries • Identifies vasospasm, emboli, vascular stenosis, and brain death	• Quality of findings and interpretation vary with user • Transtemporal window required (lacking in 14% of general population)
Ventriculography	• Obtains CSF for analysis • Measures CSF pressure • Is used especially when intracranial hypertension contraindicates LP	• May cause meningeal irritation, seizures, herniation, intracerebral or intraventricular hemorrhage

AVM, Arteriovenous malformation; *CSF,* cerebrospinal fluid; *CT,* computed tomography; *IV,* intravenous; *LP,* lumbar puncture; *NPO,* nothing by mouth.

Intracranial Hypertension

Etiology

1. Mass lesion
   a. Hematoma
      (1) Epidural
      (2) Subdural
      (3) Intracerebral
   b. Neoplasm
      (1) Primary brain tumor
      (2) Metastatic tumor
   c. Abscess
   d. Trauma: caused by local edema (e.g., contusion may act as a mass lesion)
2. Brain edema: most common cause of intracranial hypertension; may be localized or generalized
   a. Cytotoxic edema
      (1) Intracellular swelling of neurons and glial cells
      (2) Caused by any of the following:
         (a) Hypoosmolality (e.g., low serum osmolality and sodium)
         (b) Hypoxia (decreases ATP production, which impairs sodium-potassium pump)
         (c) Cardiac arrest (cause of anoxic encephalopathy)
   b. Vasogenic edema
      (1) Increase in ECF caused by breakdown of blood-brain barrier; increased vascular permeability and leakage of plasma protein
      (2) Begins locally, becomes generalized
      (3) Caused by any of the following:
         (a) Trauma (e.g., contusion)
         (b) Tumors
         (c) Hemorrhage
         (d) Abscesses
         (e) Surgical trauma (e.g., craniotomy)
3. Cerebrovascular alterations
   a. Arterial vascular occlusions with cytotoxic and vasogenic edema
   b. Venous outflow obstruction: caused by decreased venous return from head
      (1) Neck rotation, hyperextension, hyperflexion
      (2) Tracheostomy ties or cervical collar
      (3) Increased intrathoracic pressure
         (a) Valsalva maneuver (e.g., coughing, vomiting, or straining at stool)
         (b) Positive pressure mechanical ventilation
         (c) Positive end-expiratory pressure (PEEP)
   c. Increase in CPP (caused by hypertensive crisis)
   d. Vasodilation (caused by hypercapnia, hypoxia, hyperthermia, or vasoactive drugs)
4. Increase in CSF volume (hydrocephalus)
   a. Increase in production of CSF (e.g., choroid plexus disease)
   b. Decrease in reabsorption of CSF
      (1) Communicating hydrocephalus (e.g., SAH or meningitis)
      (2) Noncommunicating hydrocephalus (e.g., tumor, surgical, or traumatic edema; hemorrhage or infarction obstructing outflow of CSF)

Pathophysiology

1. Intracranial volumes (Figure 7-34)
   a. Brain tissue: approximately 80% to 88%
      (1) NOTE: Elderly patients and alcohol or drug abusers may have cerebral atrophy; traction on bridging vessels increases the risk of intracranial bleeding; hemorrhage or hematoma may be very large before becoming symptomatic.
   b. Circulating blood: approximately 2% to 10%
   c. CSF: approximately 10%
2. ICP: the pressure exerted by brain tissue, blood, and CSF against the inside of the skull
   a. Measured as the pressure exerted by CSF within the ventricles of the brain
   b. Normal: 5 to 15 mm Hg
   c. Under normal circumstances, only slight fluctuation
3. Monro-Kellie hypothesis
   a. The cranium is an inexpansible vault.
   b. Inside the cranium is a closed system with three fluctuating volumes.
      (1) Compensation is the ability of the contents of the cranium to change or rearrange; compensation is more effective when volume increase is slower.
      (2) If the volume of one of the constituents of the intracranial cavity increases, a reciprocal decrease in volume of one or both of the others will occur.

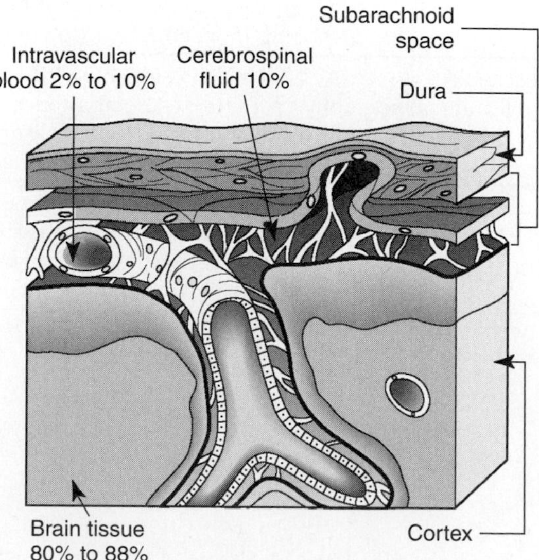

Figure 7-34 Intracranial volumes.

(a) Displacement of CSF from the cranium to the lumbar cistern
(b) Increased CSF reabsorption
(c) Compression of low pressure venous system; blood is shunted to venous sinuses

c. As successive units of any of the three volumes are added to the cranium, a critical point is reached where each additional unit of volume added increases ICP dramatically and herniation occurs.

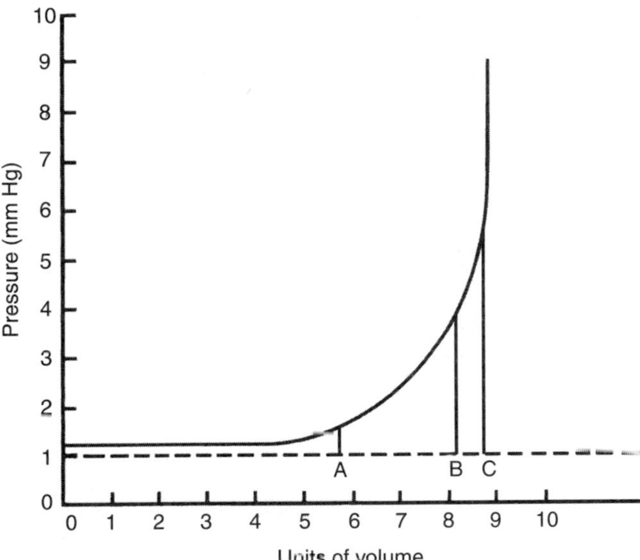

Figure 7-35 Intracranial volume-pressure curve. *A,* Pressure is normal, and increases in intracranial volume are tolerated without a resultant increase in ICP. *B,* Increases in volume can cause increases in pressure. *C,* Small increases in volume result in significant increases in pressure. (From Urden, L., Stacy, K., & Lough, M. [2002]. *Thelan's critical care nursing: Diagnosis and management* [4th ed.]. St. Louis: Mosby.)

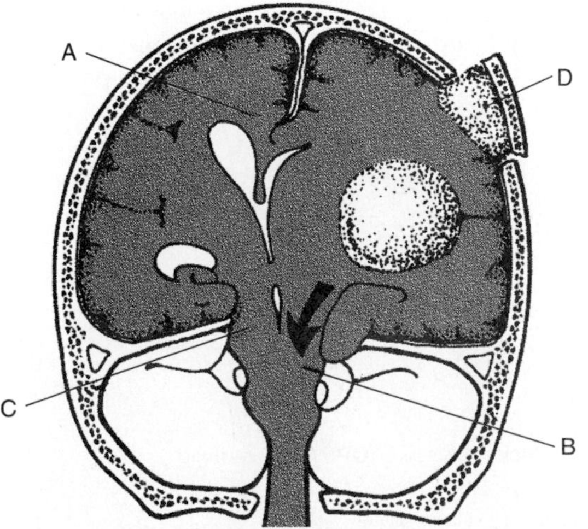

Figure 7-36 Supratentorial herniation. *A,* Cingulate. *B,* Uncal. *C,* Central. *D,* Transcalvarial. (From Thelan, L. A., Urden, L. D., Lough, M. E., & Stacy, K. M. [1998]. *Critical care nursing: Diagnosis and management.* [3rd ed.]. St. Louis: Mosby.)

(1) A volume-pressure relationship exists (Figure 7-35).
(2) When the critical point is reached, herniation syndromes occur (Figure 7-36 and Table 7-18).

4. Compliance
   a. The ability of the brain to tolerate increases in volume without a corresponding increase in pressure
   b. Compliance is poor; a small increase in volume causes a large increase in pressure
5. CPP
   a. Pressure at which the brain tissue is perfused; used to estimate adequacy of CBF
   b. Calculated by subtracting ICP from MAP; MAP – ICP (Figure 7-37)
   c. Normal CPP: 60 to 100 mm Hg; a CPP of greater than 60 mm Hg is considered a minimum desirable CPP in brain-injured patients
   d. Abnormal CPP
      (1) CPP greater than 150 mm Hg disrupts the blood-brain barrier and causes hyperperfusion and potentially brain edema.
      (2) CPP less than 50 mm Hg causes hypoperfusion and brain ischemia (although CPP of 70 mm Hg is required in most brain-injured patients, and some require an even higher CPP to perfuse the brain).
      (3) CPP less than 40 mm Hg is associated with CBF that is 25% of normal.
      (4) CPP less than 30 mm Hg causes irreversible ischemia.
      (5) As ICP approaches MAP, CBF decreases; when they equalize, CBF ceases and brain death is inevitable.
6. Autoregulation: the intrinsic ability of the cerebral blood vessels to dilate or constrict in response to changes in the environment of the brain
   a. Enables the cerebral blood vessels to maintain CBF in response to wide fluctuation in MAP
   b. Autoregulation fails if CPP is less than 50 mm Hg or greater than 150 mm Hg
7. CBF
   a. Varies with changes in CPP and diameter of cerebrovascular bed
   b. Normal CBF: 50 mL/min/100 g of brain
   c. Increased ICP and decreased CPP decreases CBF; the brain receives less oxygen and fewer nutrients, eventually causing neuronal death
8. Decompensation: brain loses its ability to compensation
   a. Pressure on cerebral vessels slows blood flow to the brain.
   b. Diminished circulation produces ischemia and an accumulation of carbon dioxide and lactic acid.

Table 7-18 Herniation Syndromes

Type of Herniation	Description	Clinical Indications	Comments
		SUPRATENTORIAL	
Cingulate (or subfalcine) herniation	Expanding lesion of one hemisphere shifts laterally and forces the cingulate gyrus under the falx cerebri; compression of vessels causes cerebral edema, ischemia, and intracranial hypertension	• No specific clinical indications • May have altered LOC or plegia • Cheyne-Stokes respiratory pattern may be seen	• Not life-threatening but a sign of brain decompensation • If condition not controlled, uncal or central herniation will occur
Uncal herniation	Expanding lesion in middle fossa or temporal lobe causes a lateral displacement, which pushes the uncus of the temporal lobe over the edge of the tentorium; uncus may be lacerated by sharp edge of tentorium	• First indication is unilateral (ipsilateral) pupil dilation with sluggish reaction to light; progresses to fixed, dilated pupils • Decreased LOC • Respiratory pattern change • Contralateral hemiplegia progressing to posturing	• Most common herniation syndrome • Life-threatening when hemorrhage or brainstem compression occurs
Central (or transtentorial) herniation	Expanding lesions of the frontal, parietal, or occipital lobes or severe generalized edema cause downward displacement of the basal ganglia and diencephalon through the tentorial notch, causing pressure on the midbrain	• First indication is change in LOC • Small, reactive pupils to fixed, dilated pupils • Respiratory pattern changes to apnea • Decorticate posturing to flaccidity	• May be preceded by cingulate or uncal herniation • Life-threatening
Transcalvarial herniation	Extrusion of cerebral tissue through the cranium	• No specific clinical indications	• May occur through an opening from a skull fracture, craniotomy site, burr hole • Risk of infection
		INFRATENTORIAL	
Upward transtentorial herniation	Expanding mass lesion of cerebellum, brainstem, or fourth ventricle causes protrusion of the central area of the cerebellum and the midbrain upward through the tentorial notch	• First symptom is unilateral (ipsilateral) pupil dilation • Obstructive hydrocephalus occurs with rapid deterioration of neurologic status	• May be life-threatening
Downward cerebellar (or tonsillar) herniation	Expanding lesion of the cerebellum exerts downward pressure, sending cerebellar tonsils through the foramen magnum; compression and displacement of the medulla oblongata occur	• Coma • Flaccid paralysis • Respiratory and cardiac arrest occur	• May be a complication of LP when LP is performed in presence of high intracranial pressure • Causes death

LOC, Level of consciousness; *LP,* lumbar puncture.

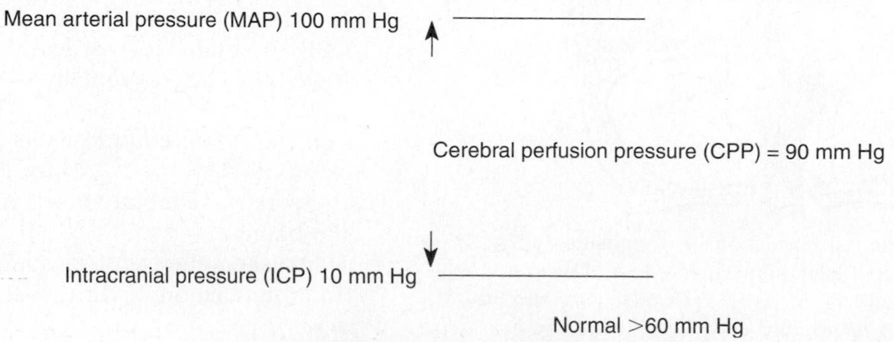

Mean arterial pressure (MAP) 100 mm Hg

Cerebral perfusion pressure (CPP) = 90 mm Hg

Intracranial pressure (ICP) 10 mm Hg

Normal >60 mm Hg

Figure 7-37 Calculation of CPP.

c. Hypoxia and hypercapnia trigger vasodilation, which increases blood volume and brain edema.
d. Brain edema increases ICP further.
e. Compression of cerebral vessels occurs and causes further ischemia.
f. Eventually cerebral circulation stops, and brain death occurs.

Clinical Presentation

1. Stages of intracranial hypertension (Figure 7-38)
2. Change in LOC
   a. Early: yawning, restlessness; confusion
   b. Late: diminishing LOC; posturing
3. Cranial nerve changes
   a. Oculomotor (III)
      (1) Early
         (a) Ipsilateral pupil changes
            (i) Change in size and shape (oval)
            (ii) Sluggish reaction to light
         (b) Conjugate eye deviation
      (2) Late
         (a) Ipsilateral pupil changes
            (i) Dilated, nonreactive to light pupil or pupils
            (ii) Ptosis
            (iii) Dysconjugate eye movement with brainstem lesions
   b. Optic (II): visual changes
      (1) Diplopia; blurring; decreased visual acuity; visual field deficit
      (2) Papilledema: more likely to occur when ICP rises slowly rather than quickly
   c. Trigeminal (V): impaired corneal reflex
   d. Glossopharyngeal (IX) and vagus (X): impaired gag and swallowing
4. Motor changes: contralateral
   a. Caused by compression or pressure on the corticospinal tracts
   b. Early: paresis, plegia
   c. Late: posturing
5. Vomiting: may occur, especially with lesions below the tentorium
   a. Pressure on the vomiting center in the brainstem causes projectile vomiting without nausea
6. Headache: increasing severity but inconsistent symptom
7. Seizures may occur
8. Reflexes: decrease in or absence of reflexes (e.g., cough, gag, or corneal reflexes)
9. Vital sign changes
   a. Cushing's triad
      (1) Caused by pressure on or ischemia of vasomotor center in brainstem

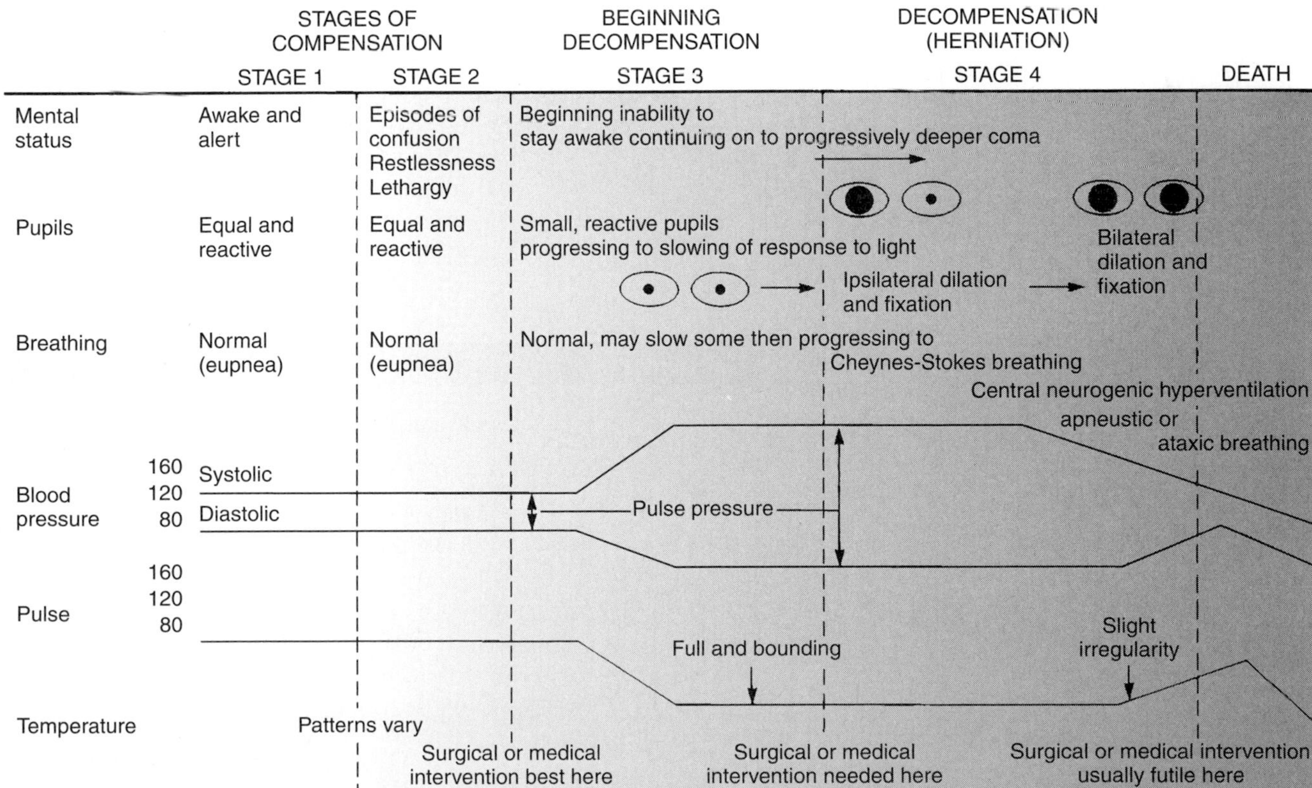

Figure 7-38 Clinical correlates of compensated and decompensated phases of intracranial hypertension. (From Beare, P. G., & Myers, J. L. [1994]. *Principles and practice of adult health nursing* [2nd ed.]. St. Louis: Mosby.)

    (2) Components
        (a) Increased systolic BP
        (b) Widening pulse pressure caused by diastolic BP being normal or decreased along with increased systolic BP
        (c) Bradycardia
  b. Respiratory pattern changes dependent on location of injury (Table 7-8)
  c. Temperature: central hyperthermia may occur late in intracranial hypertension because of pressure on the thermoregulatory center in the hypothalamus
10. ICP monitoring: elevated ICP
11. Diagnostic studies
  a. LP: contraindicated; may cause downward cerebellar herniation with medullary herniation and death
  b. CT scan: may show cause of intracranial hypertension or intracerebral shifts
  c. Cerebral angiography: may show cause of intracranial hypertension
  d. Skull x-ray: may show cause of intracranial hypertension and/or shift of pineal gland or sella turcica; rarely performed
  e. EEG: evaluates brain wave activity
  f. Evoked potentials: assesses brainstem integrity
  g. Electrocardiogram (ECG)
    (1) May show prolonged QT interval
    (2) Dysrhythmias: especially with SAH

Nursing Diagnoses

1. Decreased Adaptive Capacity: Intracranial related to failure of normal intracranial compensatory mechanisms
2. Ineffective Cerebral Tissue Perfusion related to intracranial hypertension
3. Ineffective Breathing Pattern related to brainstem herniation
4. Risk for Infection related to invasive procedures, traumatic wounds, and surgical wounds
5. Risk for Injury related to seizure activity and inadequate protective reflexes
6. Interrupted Family Processes related to situational crisis, powerlessness, and change in role
7. Deficient Knowledge related to required lifestyle changes

Collaborative Management

1. Monitor patient closely for clinical indications of intracranial hypertension; assist with insertion of ICP monitoring device if patient requires continuous monitoring.
2. Recognize factors that increase ICP (Box 7-1); prevent as many of these factors that you can; space activities that increase ICP that cannot be eliminated.
3. Prevent intracranial hypertension.
  a. Assess neurologic status frequently.
  b. Maintain adequate venous drainage from head.
    (1) Assess patient's response to elevation of the HOB by using CPP, ICP, CO, and BP and adjust accordingly; elevation of the HOB promotes venous drainage from the brain but may decrease CBF by decreasing BP.
    (2) Maintain head and neck in straight alignment to prevent compression of jugular veins.
    (3) Prevent compression of jugular veins by tracheostomy ties or cervical collar; loosen if necessary.
  c. Maintain patent airway and ventilation.
    (1) Endotracheal intubation
        (a) Necessary if protective reflexes are absent
        (b) Indicated when GCS score is less than 8 even in the absence of typical signs of acute respiratory failure

BOX 7-1 Causes of Intracranial Pressure Elevations

Ventilation and/or Oxygenation Problems
- Airway obstruction
- Deep breathing
- Hypercapnia
- Hypoxia
- Suctioning without hyperoxygenation

Position Changes
- Extreme hip flexion (greater than 90 degrees)
- Prone position
- Trendelenburg's position

Decreased Venous Return from Head
- Coughing
- Increased intrathoracic pressure
- Isometric exercise
- Neck flexion, hyperextension, or rotation
- Positive end-expiratory pressure
- Positive pressure mechanical ventilation
- Straining at stool
- Suctioning
- Tight tracheostomy ties or cervical collar
- Valsalva maneuver
- Vomiting

Increased Metabolic Rate
- Hyperthermia
- Rapid eye movement sleep
- Seizure activity

Stress
- Bright lights
- Disturbing conversation
- Noise
- Pain or noxious stimuli

(2) Mechanical ventilation may be necessary
(a) Recognize that positive pressure mechanical ventilation increases ICP; use of lower tidal volumes may minimize this effect.
(b) Recognize that PEEP increases ICP; use of only enough PEEP to maintain adequate Pao_2 may minimize this effect.

d. Prevent the increase in ICP caused by Valsalva maneuver.
(1) Instruct the patient to do the following:
(a) Exhale when turning in bed
(b) Cough with mouth open if coughing is necessary
(c) Avoid straining, bending, and sneezing
(d) Avoid hip flexion greater than 90 degrees
(2) Discourage isometric exercise.
(a) Do not use footboard to prevent footdrop.
(b) Use hightop tennis shoes, on for 2 hours and off for 2 hours.
(3) Administer stool softeners as indicated.
(4) Treat nausea with antiemetics to prevent vomiting.
(5) Prevent increase in ICP associated with suctioning.
(a) Suction only if necessary.
(b) Limit suctioning to 10 seconds.
(c) Limit suction to less than 120 mm Hg.
(d) Ensure that the catheter occludes no more than one half the diameter of the endotracheal tube.
(e) Hyperoxygenate the patient before and after suctioning.
(f) Lidocaine may be administered IV before suctioning to eliminate cough reflex.
(i) Dosage: 0.5 to 1.5 mg/kg
(ii) Disadvantage: may lower seizure threshold
(g) Do not suction via nose if there is evidence of head or facial trauma.

e. Monitor ICP during nursing care activities (e.g., turning, suctioning, and enteral feedings); space activities to allow ICP to return to normal before performing another activity that may increase ICP.

f. Monitor ventilation and oxygenation: hypercapnia and/or hypoxemia may cause vasodilation and increase ICP.
(1) ABGs
(2) Pulse oximetry (functional oxygen saturation [Spo_2]: oxygenation only)
(3) Capnography ($Paco_2$: ventilation only)

g. Maintain euvolemia.
(1) Hemodynamic monitoring may be necessary: maintain pulmonary artery occlusive pressure (PAOP) at 10 to 15 mm Hg.
(2) Administer IV fluids as prescribed: avoid hypotonic fluids (e.g., 5% dextrose in water), which may contribute to brain edema.

h. If CSF leakage is noted: do not pack nose or ears; apply mustache dressing under nose or 4 × 4-inch gauze over ear.

i. Reduce anxiety.
(1) Reorient patient frequently to person, place, date, and time.
(2) Explain procedures thoroughly.
(3) Do not conduct or allow emotionally disturbing conversations at bedside.
(4) Encourage family members to touch and talk to patient; let them know that many patients report an awareness during altered LOC.

j. Monitor ICP and calculate CPP; notify physician of significant changes or deteriorating trend.

4. Treat intracranial hypertension.
a. Provide therapy aimed at reducing volume of one of the three components of ICP
(1) *CSF*: drainage of CSF if intraventricular catheter in place
(a) Drainage usually is initiated when the ICP is greater than 20 mm Hg.
(b) Do not drain to ICP of less than 15 mm Hg unless specifically instructed: rapid CSF drainage may cause the brain to pull away from the dura, rupturing bridging veins and possibly causing SDH.
(c) Record volume of drainage.
(d) Maintain closed system and asepsis during fluid drainage; high risk for infection exists.
(2) *Circulating blood volume*
(a) Hyperventilation (with an manual resuscitation bag or mechanical ventilator) to maintain $Paco_2$ 30 to 35 mm Hg
(i) Should be performed only in the presence of acute neurologic deterioration suggesting herniation because it works by causing alkalosis, which constricts cerebral arteries and reduces intracranial volume and pressure but also potentially reduces CBF and causes brain ischemia; there is a delicate balance between vasoconstriction to decrease intracranial volume and pressure and vasoconstriction causing ischemia
(ii) Intended for short-term treatment only because renal compensation through excretion of sodium bicarbonate corrects pH within 2 to 3 days
(iii) Sjo_2 monitoring is recommended to identify the $Paco_2$ level that does not cause brain ischemia

(b) Barbiturate-induced coma
  (i) Actions
    a) Decreases ICP by decreasing CBF and metabolism
    b) Decreases metabolic rate and oxygen consumption of the brain
    c) May shunt blood from healthy brain tissue to ischemic areas
  (ii) Preferred agent: pentobarbital (Nembutal)
    a) Usually prescribed as 10 mg/kg IV over 30 minutes as a loading dose followed by 1 mg/kg/hr
    b) Maintain barbiturate level of 2.5 to 4 mg/dL
  (iii) Indications and expectations
    a) Indicated when ICP greater than 40 mm Hg despite aggressive therapy
    b) Expect 10 mm Hg decrease in ICP within 10 minutes
    c) Discontinued when the ICP has been normal for at least 24 to 72 hours; patient should be receiving anticonvulsants before discontinuance because seizures may occur
  (iv) Considerations
    a) Monitor hepatic and renal function.
    b) Monitor cardiac status and daily weight; may decrease cardiac contractility.
    c) Patient must be intubated and mechanically ventilated.
    d) Patient must have an ICP monitor; systemic arterial and pulmonary arterial pressure monitoring is recommended.
    e) Protect the corneas by instilling artificial tears and taping eyes shut or applying moisture chamber (plastic wrap taped in place over eyes).

(3) *Brain mass*
  (a) Maintenance of euvolemia
    (i) Actions
      a) Maintains CO, MAP, and CPP
      b) Prevents hyperosmolality and increased blood viscosity, which slows blood flow and may precipitate ischemia and occlusion
      c) Prevents brain edema caused by excess fluid administration
    (ii) Goals
      a) PAOP of 10 to 15 mm Hg or central venous pressure (CVP) of 5 to 10 mm Hg
      b) Serum osmolality less than less than 320 mmol/kg
      c) CPP greater than 60 mm Hg
    (iii) Considerations
      a) Isotonic crystalloids or colloids
        i) Colloids (e.g., dextran or albumin) frequently used but no evidence that they are superior to isotonic crystalloids, and isotonic crystalloids are much more cost-effective
      b) Hypertonic saline may be used
      c) Blood and/or blood products may be needed if there has been significant blood loss
      d) Hypotonic solutions (e.g., 5% dextrose in water) should be avoided because they reduce serum osmolality and contribute to brain edema
  (b) Administration of diuretics
    (i) Osmotic diuretics (e.g., mannitol [Osmitrol])
      a) Actions
        i) Increases plasma osmolality, which pulls fluid from brain tissue and decreases brain edema (this increase in intravascular volume then is eliminated by the kidneys)
        ii) May decrease blood viscosity and increase CBF without raising ICP
        iii) May have a neuroprotective effect (under investigation)
      b) Dosage: usually prescribed as 0.25 to 1 gm/kg IV; must be given with a 0.45 μm in-line filter
      c) Onset and duration: starts to work within 15 minutes; lasts 2 to 6 hours; may be repeated every 1 to 4 hours
      d) Considerations
        i) Indwelling bladder catheter is recommended.
        ii) Monitor for clinical indications of fluid overload initially especially in patients with history of cardiovascular disease.
        iii) Monitor for fluid deficit.
        iv) Osmotic diuretics may mask diabetes insipidus (DI).
        v) Monitor for electrolyte imbalance.
        vi) Monitor serum osmolality; should be less than 320 mmol/kg.

vii) Rebound intracranial hypertension may be seen 8 to 12 hours after mannitol administration; furosemide is given with mannitol to reduce the incidence of rebound.

(ii) Loop diuretics (e.g., furosemide [Lasix])
a) Actions
i) Reduces intracranial volume by reducing overall body fluid
ii) Decreases CSF production (unknown mechanism)
b) Dosage: usually prescribed as 0.5-1 mg/kg IV

(iii) Replacement of circulating volume must be ensured to prevent hyperviscosity and dehydration

(c) Surgical removal of brain mass: cerebral lobectomy may be performed as last resort (usually nondominant temporal lobe)

b. Prepare patient for surgery if indicated.
(1) Débride open wounds and suture scalp laceration.
(2) Elevate depressed skull fracture and repair dural tears.
(3) Evacuate epidural or subdural hemorrhage or hematoma.
(4) Control intracranial hemorrhage or hematoma.

5. Decrease metabolic requirements of the brain.
a. Administer anticonvulsants prophylactically as prescribed; usually no longer than 7 days.
b. Maintain normothermia (less than 38° C); hypothermia (~33° C), although experimental, may be ordered to lower metabolic and oxygen requirements further.
(1) Treat hyperthermia aggressively because a 1° C temperature elevation is associated with a 7% increase in metabolic rate and oxygen consumption.
(2) Central fever is attributed directly to brain injury and reflects hypothalamic dysfunction.
(a) Characterized by lack of sweating, absence of tachycardia, and may persist for days
(b) Controlled best by external cooling but avoid shivering; use hypothermia blanket
(i) Turn blanket off when the temperature reaches 38° C because the temperature of a neurologic patient tends to drift downward after a hypothermia blanket is turned off.
(ii) Do not allow the patient to shiver; small doses of meperidine (Demerol) or promethazine (Phenergan) may be used to decrease shivering.
(3) Peripheral fever is associated with infection.
(a) Characterized by sweating and tachycardia
(b) Controlled best by antipyretics (e.g., acetaminophen [Tylenol])
(4) Large-bore central IV catheters may be placed for cooled solutions; less shivering is noted.
c. Administer sedatives, muscle paralytic agents, and/or barbiturates as prescribed; preferred agents are short-acting and/or reversible.
(1) Analgesics and sedatives (e.g., morphine, propofol [Diprivan], or midazolam [Versed])
(a) Actions: reduces restlessness or agitation to decrease metabolic rate and oxygen consumption
(b) Considerations
(i) Monitor ventilatory status
(ii) May cause hypotension, which decreases CPP; fluid administration may be necessary to maintain preload
(2) Muscle paralysis (e.g., pancuronium [Pavulon], atracurium [Tracrium], or vecuronium [Norcuron])
(a) Actions
(i) Reduces skeletal muscle activity, metabolic rate, and oxygen consumption
(ii) Controls shivering and posturing, decreasing metabolic rate and oxygen consumption
(b) Considerations
(i) Patient must be mechanically ventilated.
(ii) Protect the corneas by instilling artificial tears and taping eyes shut.
(iii) Always administer sedative with muscle paralytic agents.
(3) Barbiturate-induced coma
d. Maintain calm, quiet environment.
(1) Prevent loud noises and disturbing conversations.
(2) Encourage family to touch the patient and speak to the patient encouragingly; a high percentage of patients remember things that were said or read to them while they were "unconscious."

6. Maintain MAP and CPP.
a. Assess for bleeding from chest, abdomen, pelvis, and extremities.
b. Control scalp bleeding by applying pressure until sutured.
c. Administer IV fluids as prescribed.
d. Administer inotropes and/or vasopressors as prescribed to maintain MAP and CPP; maintain systolic BP ~140 mm Hg.
e. Calcium channel blockers (e.g., nimodipine [Nimotop]) and/or hypervolemic hemodilution may be used for vasospasm.

7. Monitor patient for complications.
a. Permanent neurologic residual deficits
b. Herniation
c. Brain death

Craniotomy

Surgical Procedures

1. Craniotomy: opening of the cranium to allow access to the brain (Figure 7-39)
   a. Supratentorial craniotomy is used to access the cerebral hemispheres and accomplish any of the following:
      (1) Remove intracranial tumors, hematomas, abscesses, or epileptic foci
      (2) Clip or ligate aneurysm or AVMs in the anterior circulation
      (3) Place ventriculovenous, ventriculopleural, or ventriculoperitoneal shunt
      (4) Débride fragments and necrotic tissue; elevate and realign bone fragments
   b. Infratentorial craniotomy is used to access the brainstem and cerebellum to allow removal of cerebellar tumors and hemorrhages, acoustic neuromas, tumors of the brainstem or cranial nerves, and abscesses.
   c. Transsphenoidal approach (Figure 7-40) frequently is used to remove the pituitary gland; referred to as a *transsphenoidal hypophysectomy.*
      (1) A horizontal incision is made at the junction of the inner aspect of the upper lip and gingiva and extends laterally to the canine tooth on each side.
      (2) The sella turcica is entered through the floor of the nose and the sphenoid sinus.
      (3) Transsphenoidal hypophysectomy is indicated for pituitary tumor or to control pain associated with metastatic cancer.
2. Craniectomy: removal of a portion of the cranium
3. Cranioplasty: repair of the cranium usually with a synthetic material
4. Burr holes: small holes drilled through the cranium to allow access to underlying structures; frequently used for any of the following:
   a. Evacuation of EDH or SDH
   b. Insertion of intraventricular catheter for CSF drainage
   c. Insertion of another form of ICP monitoring device (e.g., subarachnoid screw)

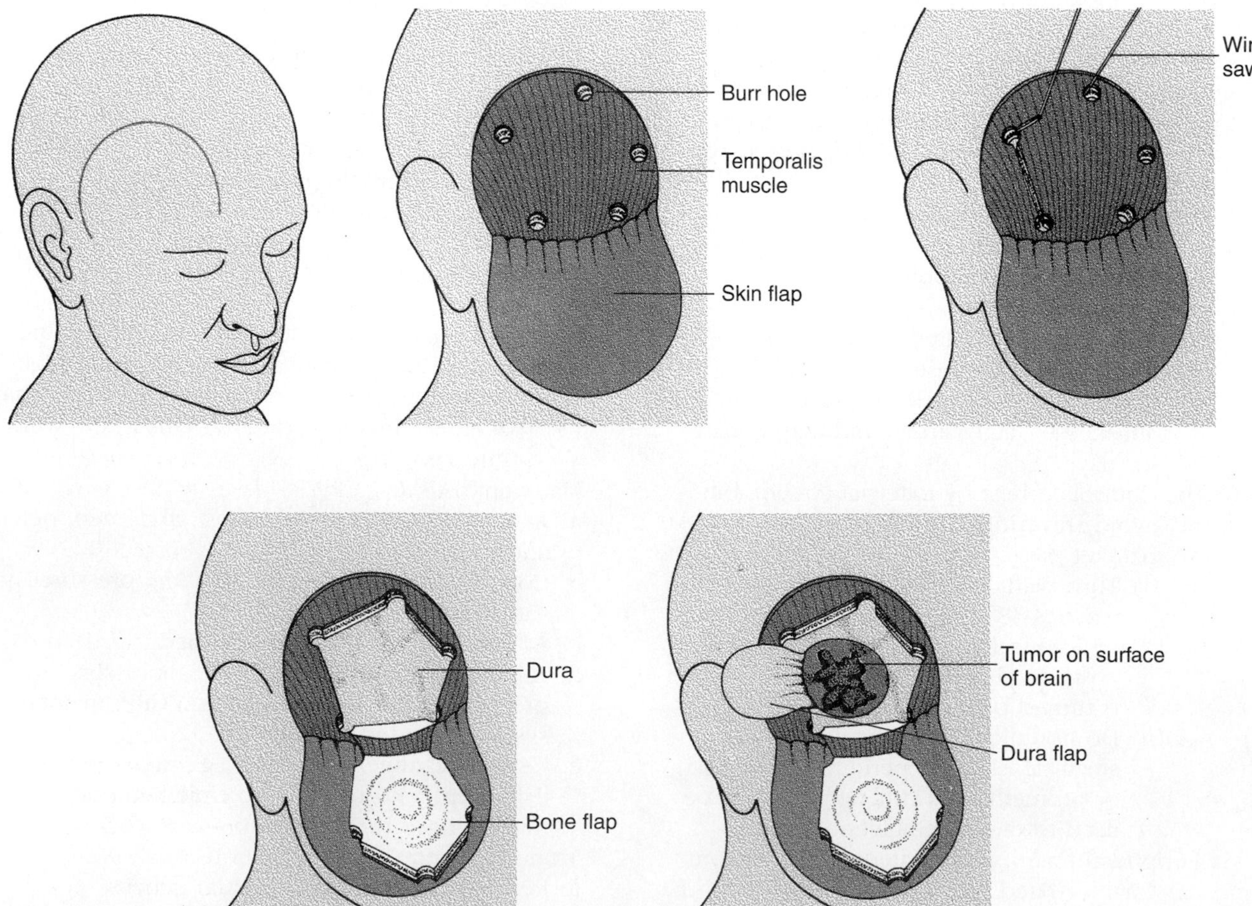

Figure 7-39 Craniotomy. (From Beare, P. G., & Myers, J. L. [1994]. *Principles and practice of adult health nursing* [2nd ed.]. St. Louis: Mosby.)

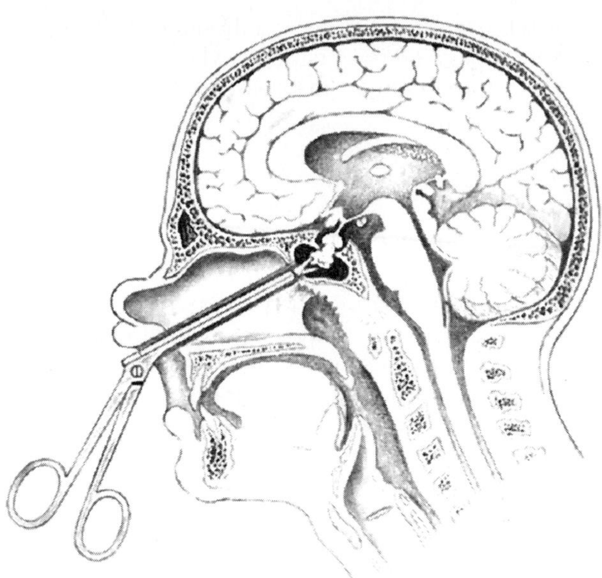

Figure 7-40 Transsphenoidal hypophysectomy. (From Urden, L., Stacy, K., & Lough, M. [2002]. *Thelan's critical care nursing: Diagnosis and management* [4th ed.]. St. Louis: Mosby.)

Nursing Diagnoses

1. Anxiety related to surgical procedure and surgical outcome
2. Ineffective Cerebral Tissue Perfusion related to intracranial hypertension and hydrocephalus
3. Decreased Adaptive Capacity: Intracranial related to brain edema caused by surgical trauma
4. Ineffective Airway Clearance related to increased secretions, diminished LOC, and inadequate protective reflexes
5. Impaired Gas Exchange related to inactivity and neurogenic pulmonary edema
6. Risk for Deficient Fluid Volume Deficit related to decreased fluid intake, increased fluid loss, and DI
7. Risk for Excess Fluid Volume related to syndrome of inappropriate antidiuretic hormone (SIADH)
8. Risk for Infection related to invasive procedures, traumatic wounds, and surgical wounds
9. Risk for Injury related to seizure activity, inadequate protective reflexes, and stress ulcer
10. Interrupted Family Processes related to situational crisis, powerlessness, and change in role
11. Deficient Knowledge related to required lifestyle changes

Preoperative Collaborative Management

1. Control pain and discomfort.
   a. Small doses of codeine or morphine may be prescribed.
   b. Take care to avoid oversedation because it eliminates LOC, the most important assessment parameter.
2. Prepare patient for surgery.
   a. Anticonvulsants (e.g., phenytoin [Dilantin]) may be initiated preoperatively.
   b. Hair is washed with an antimicrobial shampoo the night before surgery; the operative area usually is shaved in the operating room or the operating room holding area.
   c. Carefully record baseline neurologic status.
      (1) LOC
      (2) GCS score
      (3) Communication deficits
      (4) Cognitive deficits
      (5) Motor deficits
      (6) Sensory deficits
      (7) Cranial nerve deficits
   d. Inform the patient and family what to expect after surgery.
      (1) Equipment: IV catheter(s); oxygen therapy and possibly mechanical ventilation; indwelling bladder catheter; sequential compression stockings; possibly intraventricular catheter and ICP monitor
      (2) Mild to moderate headache
      (3) Photophobia
      (4) Periorbital edema and bruising
      (5) Head dressing and drain

Postoperative Collaborative Management

1. Prevent and monitor for clinical indications of and treat intracranial hypertension.
   a. Perform frequent neurologic assessments.
      (1) Compare results with preoperative status.
      (2) Check vision in patients having hypophysectomy.
   b. Monitor for clinical indications of intracranial hypertension (NOTE: This patient may have an intraventricular catheter in for monitoring ICP).
   c. Teach patient to avoid causes of intracranial hypertension (Box 7-1).
   d. Prevent twisting of head or neck or flexion of neck to allow jugular vein drainage; support head, neck, shoulders when turning patient in bed.
   e. Control conditions that increase cerebral metabolic rate.
      (1) Anticonvulsants for seizures
      (2) Antipyretics and cooling blankets for hyperthermia
      (3) Sedation as indicated for restlessness
      (4) Muscle paralytic agents, barbiturates to decrease the oxygen requirements of the brain (ICP monitoring is required because the most important assessment parameter [LOC] is eliminated)
   f. Administer treatments for intracranial hypertension as prescribed.
   g. Prevent and treat hypertension and hypotension to maintain CPP of 60 to 100 mm Hg.

h. Position patient appropriately.
   (1) If supratentorial craniotomy
      (a) Elevate HOB 30 degrees
      (b) If large mass removed, do not allow the patient to lie on operative side
   (2) If infratentorial craniotomy
      (a) Position patient flat with small pillow under nape of neck
      (b) Do not allow on back for 48 hours
   (3) If transsphenoidal craniotomy (e.g., hypophysectomy): elevate HOB 30 degrees
   (4) If insertion of interventricular shunt: position flat on nonoperative side
   (5) Other specific positioning may be prescribed by the surgeon

2. Maintain airway, oxygenation, and ventilation.
   a. Encourage deep breathing; if coughing is indicated (rhonchi are audible), instruct the patient to cough with mouth open.
   b. Administer oxygen to maintain Spo_2 of greater than or equal to 95% unless contraindicated.
   c. Assess swallow competency; have suction equipment available.
3. Maintain adequate hydration and electrolyte balance.
   a. Administer isotonic fluids as prescribed; avoid 5% dextrose in water and other hypotonic solutions.
   b. Prevent overhydration, which can predispose the patient to brain edema.
   c. Monitor patient closely for indications of overhydration or dehydration; evaluate urine output and urine specific gravity hourly.
   d. Assess head dressing hourly; notify surgeon if large amounts of drainage are noted.
4. Relieve headache.
   a. Inform patient to notify the nurse at the onset of headache; severe pain is not normal; notify physician.
   b. Administer small doses of morphine or codeine to avoid oversedation; when the patient can take oral medications, acetaminophen with codeine usually is used.
   c. Decrease environmental stimuli.
   d. Apply cool compresses to decrease periorbital edema; dressing may be clipped if too tight (clip on side opposite surgical site).
5. Prevent injury.
   a. Institute seizure precautions.
      (1) Have suction equipment available.
      (2) Have extra pillows available that can be placed between patient and side rails.
      (3) Assess onset, progression, and postictal period if seizure occurs.
      (4) Administer anticonvulsants as prescribed.
   b. Perform passive range of motion, and reposition the patient every 2 hours.
   c. Perform skin assessment frequently.
   d. Instill artificial tears every 2 hours to prevent corneal abrasions in patients who do not blink; a moisture chamber may be created using plastic wrap.
   e. Orient patient to time and place often; encourage family participation in reality orientation.
   f. Apply restraints only if indicated for self-protection.
6. Prevent and monitor for infection.
   a. Administer prophylactic and/or therapeutic antibiotics as prescribed.
   b. Monitor head dressing and drains for purulent drainage; assess wound during aseptic dressing changes for redness, swelling, induration, and drainage.
   c. Do not put tubes (e.g., suction catheter or nasogastric tube) into nose if patient has transsphenoidal approach; warn the patient not to blow or pick nose.
   d. Note drainage of CSF (CSF leak increases the risk of intracranial infection).
      (1) Assessment
         (a) Rhinorrhea
         (b) Otorrhea
         (c) Excessive swallowing
      (2) Management
         (a) Mustache dressing for rhinorrhea
         (b) 2 × 2-inch dressing over ear for otorrhea; sterile uribag also may be used.
   e. Monitor for and control hyperthermia: treat temperatures of greater than 38° C with hypothermia blanket and/or acetaminophen.
7. Monitor for complications.
   a. Intracranial hypertension: brain edema usually peaks about 48 to 72 hours
   b. Brain ischemia, infarction
   c. Cerebral hemorrhage
   d. CSF leak (NOTE: CSF leak is normal for up to 72 hours after transsphenoidal hypophysectomy.)
   e. CNS infection: encephalitis; meningitis
      (1) Clinical indications of CNS infection: headache; photophobia; nuchal rigidity; positive Kernig's and Brudzinski's signs; fever
      (2) Treatment: antibiotics
   f. Seizures
   g. Fluid and electrolyte imbalance
      (1) DI
         (a) Pathophysiology
            (i) Central or neurogenic DI: decrease in production of antidiuretic hormone (ADH) or brain edema causes blockage in the pathway from the hypothalamus (where ADH is produced) to the posterior pituitary (where ADH is stored and released)

(ii) Nephrogenic DI: decrease in the responsiveness of the renal tubule to ADH
(b) Clinical indications: thirst; polydipsia; polyuria (4 to 20 L/day); specific gravity of urine 1.005 or less; increased serum sodium; hyperosmolality
(c) Treatment: fluid replacement and vasopressin (ADH) for central DI; drugs to increase the responsiveness of the renal tube to ADH (e.g., chlorpropamide [Diabinese]) for nephrogenic DI
(2) SIADH
(a) Pathophysiology
(i) Increase in production or release of ADH, ectopic (e.g., tumor) source of ADH, or increase in responsiveness of the renal tubule to ADH
(ii) Increase in renal retention of water causes hyponatremia by dilution
(b) Clinical indications: decreased urine output; weight gain; confusion and lethargy; specific gravity of urine 1.035 or greater; decreased serum sodium (high potential for seizures)
(c) Treatment: fluid restriction; diuretics; hypertonic (3%) saline may be necessary if sodium level very low
(3) Cerebral salt-wasting syndrome (CSWS)
(a) Pathophysiology
(i) Poorly understood: hypotheses include the following:
a) Increased activity of the SNS causing exaggerated renal pressure and natriuresis
b) Presence of circulating natriuretic factors (e.g., atrial natriuretic peptide)
(ii) Renal loss of sodium leads to hyponatremia
(b) Clinical indications: hyponatremia, hypovolemia, high or normal serum osmolality, high urine sodium
(i) Frequently confused with SIADH, which would cause hypervolemia, low serum osmolality, and dilutional hyponatremia
(c) Treatment: fluid and sodium replacement, possibly requiring hypertonic (3% or 5%) saline
(i) As opposed to SIADH, which requires primarily fluid restriction and possibly sodium replacement

h. Hydrocephalus: frequently transient because of swelling
i. DVT: prevention methods include the following:
(1) Use sequential compression devices rather than graduated elastic stockings because these patients are at high risk for DVT; may be applied before surgery
(2) Low-dose heparin may be prescribed; low-molecular-weight heparin may be used
j. Stress ulcer (frequently referred to as *Cushing's ulcer*): prophylaxis with H_2 receptor antagonists or proton pump inhibitors usually is prescribed

Traumatic Brain Injuries

Etiology

Blunt or penetrating trauma (risk is decreased by helmets, airbags, seat belts, alcohol, and drugs)
1. Motor vehicle collision
2. Falls
3. Violence: assault; gunshot or knife wound
4. Sports-related accidents (e.g., boxing or football)
5. Industrial accidents

Pathophysiology

1. Focal injury (i.e., contusion)
   a. Partial or complete dysfunction of CNS functioning that persists for less than 24 hours
   b. Trauma causes the brain to strike the internal surfaces of the skull and orbital roof, resulting in bruising and petechial hemorrhages
   c. Laceration of the brain may occur
   d. Areas of infarction and necrosis may occur as a result of vascular injury, leading to oozing of blood into the injured area
   e. Subpial and intracerebral extravasation of blood
   f. Hemorrhage and edema may act as intracranial mass and cause intracranial hypertension
   g. Injury may be at site of impact (coup) and/or opposite site (contrecoup)
2. Diffuse injury (e.g., concussion or diffuse axonal injury)
   a. Widespread axonal disruption throughout the cerebral hemispheres
   b. Anatomic interruption of neuronal pathways
3. Secondary injury (NOTE: remember that the actual physical damage that occurs at the time of injury cannot be changed, so optimal outcome depends on avoiding or minimizing secondary injury to the brain attributed to these systemic or intracranial causes); brain ischemia is the most important cause of secondary brain injury
   a. Systemic causes
      (1) Hypotension
      (2) Hypoxia

(3) Anemia
(4) Hyperthermia
(5) Hypercapnia or hypocapnia
(6) Electrolyte imbalance
(7) Hyperglycemia or hypoglycemia
(8) Acid-base imbalance
(9) Systemic inflammatory response syndrome

b. Intracranial causes
(1) Intracranial hypertension
(2) Mass lesions
(3) Brain edema
(4) Vasospasm
(5) Hydrocephalus
(6) Infection
(7) Seizures

Clinical Presentation

1. Classification of head injuries
   a. Mild: GCS score of 13 to 15
   b. Moderate: GCS score of 9 to 12
   c. Severe: GCS score of 3 to 8
2. Concussion: may show focal neurologic deficit or alteration in LOC that clears within 6 to 12 hours or less
   a. Subjective
      (1) History of precipitating event
      (2) Unconsciousness for 10 to 15 minutes
      (3) Headache
      (4) Scalp tenderness or pain at injury site
      (5) Dizziness
      (6) Visual changes
      (7) Sluggishness
      (8) Nausea/vomiting
      (9) Memory loss
         (a) Retrograde or antegrade amnesia may occur
         (b) Posttraumatic amnesia, related to the events of the injury and events immediately preceding the injury, usually lasts less than 5 minutes
   b. Objective
      (1) Confusion, restlessness, irritability
      (2) Disorientation
3. Contusion: signs vary depending on severity of trauma and area of brain involved; neurologic deficit persists less than 24 hours
   a. Subjective
      (1) History of precipitating event
      (2) Memory loss
   b. Objective
      (1) Change in LOC
      (2) Motor or sensory dysfunction
      (3) Cranial nerve dysfunction
      (4) Focal neurologic signs (e.g., hemiparesis or hemiplegia may be seen)
      (5) Seizures
      (6) Clinical indications of intracranial hypertension may be seen
4. Diffuse axonal injury
   a. Subjective
      (1) History of precipitating event
   b. Objective
      (1) LOC may last days to weeks and usually is followed by long periods of retrograde and posttraumatic amnesia
      (2) May have purposeful movements, withdrawal from pain, restlessness
      (3) Posturing (i.e., decorticate or decerebrate) may be present
      (4) Permanent residual deficits in memory and cognitive and intellectual functioning occur; permanent residual psychological or personality changes are common
      (5) Death rates are high, and many of these patients may persist in a vegetative state; vegetative state is characterized by return of wakefulness (eyes open and sleep patterns observed) but without observable signs of cognition
      (6) Profound residual deficits
5. Diagnostic
   a. CT scan, MRI, magnetic resonance angiography (MRA)
      (1) May show brain edema, areas of petechial hemorrhages with severe contusions, and hemispheric shift
      (2) May detect presence of associated injuries such as carotid or vertebral dissection as may occur with acceleration/deceleration mechanism of injury
   b. EEG: may show brain wave abnormalities
   c. Evoked potentials: may show prolongation of transmission of impulses through the brainstem

Nursing Diagnoses

1. Decreased Adaptive Capacity: Intracranial related to failure of normal intracranial compensatory mechanisms
2. Ineffective Cerebral Tissue Perfusion related to intracranial hypertension or local arterial disruption
3. Ineffective Airway Clearance related to increased secretions, altered LOC, and inadequate protective reflexes
4. Ineffective Breathing Pattern related to inadequate airway and altered LOC
5. Pain related to injury
6. Risk for Deficient Fluid Volume related to decreased fluid intake, increased fluid loss, DI, and osmotic diuretics
7. Risk for Excess Fluid Volume related to fluid resuscitation and SIADH
8. Risk for Infection related to invasive procedures, traumatic wounds, and surgical wounds
9. Risk for Injury related to seizure activity and inadequate protective reflexes
10. Impaired Physical Mobility related to injury, paresis or plegia, bed rest, and altered LOC

11. Interrupted Family Processes related to situational crisis, powerlessness, and change in role
12. Deficient Knowledge related to required lifestyle changes

Collaborative Management

1. Perform a complete assessment for primary and secondary injuries.
   a. Remember that an adult head injury patient is not hypotensive because of blood loss from a closed head injury, so look for other causes of hypotension.
   b. Remember that hypotension decreases CPP, increases mortality dramatically, and contributes to secondary brain injury.
2. Maintain airway, ventilation, oxygenation.
   a. Assume that the patient has a spinal injury until radiologic clearance of spine: do not tilt or hyperextend the head; use jaw-thrust technique to maintain an open airway.
   b. Use oral or nasopharyngeal airway until lateral spine x-rays rule out fracture.
      (1) Do not use nasopharyngeal airway or nasal suctioning if facial or skull fracture is present.
      (2) Do not use oral airways in conscious patients because they stimulate the gag reflex.
   c. Assist with rapid sequence intubation if intubation is required.
   d. Administer oxygen as needed to maintain Spo_2 greater than or equal to 95% unless contraindicated.
   e. Prevent aspiration: position patient on side and have suction equipment available.
3. Prevent and monitor for clinical indications, and treat intracranial hypertension (see Intracranial Hypertension).
4. Maintain CPP of at least 60 mm Hg.
   a. Identify cause of hypotension if present.
   b. Maintain euvolemia: fluid resuscitation.
   c. Use therapies to decrease ICP if elevated.
   d. Use therapies to increase MAP.
      (1) Isotonic crystalloids, colloids, blood and blood products as prescribed; hypertonic saline also may be prescribed
      (2) Vasopressors may be required in low systemic vascular states (e.g., septic shock and neurogenic shock)
5. Prepare patient for surgery if indicated.
6. Prevent and monitor for complications.
   a. Vasogenic brain edema
   b. Neurogenic pulmonary edema
      (1) Pathophysiology: thought to be due to massive sympathetic discharge
      (2) Clinical presentation: pulmonary edema with normal PAOP
      (3) Treatment
         (a) Elevate HOB 30 degrees, avoiding hip flexion.
         (b) Administer codeine as prescribed for sedation.
         (c) Administer osmotic diuretics (e.g., mannitol) and beta-blockers (e.g., propranolol) as prescribed.
         (d) Use mechanical ventilation as necessary to maintain ventilation.
         (e) Use oxygen and PEEP as necessary to maintain oxygenation.
            (i) Weigh the benefits of PEEP (i.e., improves oxygenation by increasing the driving pressure of oxygen) against the risks (i.e., may increase ICP by reducing venous return)
   c. Sympathetic storm
      (1) Pathophysiology: an immediate sympathetic surge as an attempt to compensate for the effects of the injury
      (2) Clinical presentation: tachycardia, hypertension, hyperthermia, pupillary dilation, dysrhythmias, profuse sweating, hyperglycemia, agitation
      (3) Treatment: sedatives, opiates, beta-blockers
   d. Seizures
   e. Fluid and electrolyte imbalance: DI, SIADH, CSWS (see Craniotomy)
   f. Stress ulcers (frequently referred to as *Cushing's ulcers*)
   g. Postconcussion syndrome: persistent headache; inability to concentrate, memory problems, decreased problem-solving ability, irritability, emotional lability, depression, decreased libido, dizziness, tinnitus, diplopia, photophobia, decreased energy level, equilibrium disturbances
   h. Residual neurologic deficits
   i. Persistent coma

Skull Fractures

Etiology

1. Motor vehicle collision
2. Falls
3. Violence: assault; gunshot wounds; knife wounds
4. Sports-related accidents (e.g., boxing or football)
5. Industrial accidents

Pathophysiology (Figure 7-41)

1. Linear fractures (account for 80% of skull fractures)
   a. Fracture with no displacement of bone
   b. May interrupt major vascular channels
      (1) Linear fractures of the temporal-parietal bones may tear the middle meningeal artery, leading to epidural hematoma.
      (2) Linear fractures of the occipital bone may tear the occipital artery, leading to EDH.

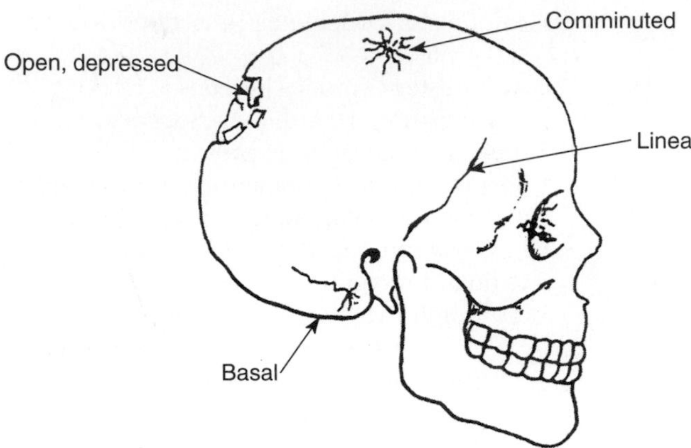

Figure 7-41 Types of skull fractures. (From Barker, E. [1994]. *Neuroscience nursing*. St. Louis: Mosby.)

2. Depressed
   a. Fracture that depresses outer table of the skull
   b. May cause brain laceration
   c. May cause intracranial hematoma
3. Basal
   a. Fracture of base of skull
   b. May cause injury to one or more cranial nerves or cause tearing of the dura with CSF leak

Clinical Presentation

1. Linear
   a. Subjective
      (1) History of precipitating event or condition
      (2) Scalp tenderness
   b. Objective
      (1) Swollen, ecchymotic area on scalp
      (2) May have scalp laceration (NOTE: Because of the mobility of the scalp, the laceration may not lie directly beneath laceration.)
2. Depressed
   a. Subjective
      (1) History of precipitating event or condition
      (2) Headache
   b. Objective
      (1) May have altered LOC with focal neurologic deficits
      (2) May have scalp laceration
         (a) Open fracture: scalp laceration present
         (b) Closed fracture: no scalp laceration present
      (3) Hemiparesis, hemiplegia
      (4) Seizures
      (5) Depressed frontal fracture may cause cranial nerve I (olfactory) deficit (loss of the sense of smell is referred to as *anosmia*)
      (6) Depressed temporal may cause cranial nerve VII (facial) or VIII (acoustic) deficits; may see ipsilateral facial paralysis (VII) or hearing or equilibrium problems (VIII)
3. Basal
   a. Subjective
      (1) History of precipitating event or condition
   b. Anterior fossa
      (1) May have rhinorrhea; usually lasts 2 to 3 days
      (2) May have bilateral ecchymotic eyes (referred to as *raccoon eyes*); takes 3 to 4 hours to develop after injury
      (3) May have injury to cranial nerve I (olfactory) causing anosmia
      (4) May have facial fractures
   c. Middle fossa
      (1) May have otorrhea or rhinorrhea
      (2) May have CSF or blood behind the tympanic membrane if the tympanic membrane remains intact; may cause hearing deficit
      (3) May have ecchymosis over mastoid bone (referred to as *Battle's sign*); takes 4 to 6 hours to develop after injury
      (4) May have cranial nerve injuries
   d. Posterior fossa
      (1) May have EDH, which may result in signs of intracranial hypertension
      (2) May have cerebellar, brainstem, or cranial nerve signs
         (a) Visual changes
         (b) Tinnitus
         (c) Facial paralysis
         (d) Conjugate eye deviation
4. Diagnostic
   a. Skull x-ray
      (1) Linear or depressed skull fractures may be seen on plain films
      (2) Basal skull fracture is difficult to confirm on x-ray; pneumocephalus, opacity of the mastoid or sphenoid sinus, or an air-fluid level in one of the sinuses may be seen
   b. CT, MRI: may visualize depressed fractures

Nursing Diagnoses

1. Decreased Adaptive Capacity: Intracranial related to failure of normal intracranial compensatory mechanisms
2. Ineffective Cerebral Tissue Perfusion related to intracranial hypertension
3. Ineffective Airway Clearance related to increased secretions, altered LOC, and inadequate protective reflexes
4. Ineffective Breathing Pattern related to inadequate airway and altered LOC
5. Pain related to injury
6. Risk for Deficient Fluid Volume related to scalp laceration, decreased fluid intake, increased fluid loss, and DI
7. Risk for Excess Fluid Volume related to fluid resuscitation and SIADH
8. Risk for Infection related to invasive procedures, traumatic wounds, surgical wounds, and dural defect
9. Risk for Injury related to seizure activity, inadequate protective reflexes, and altered LOC

10. Impaired Physical Mobility related to injury, paresis or plegia, bed rest, and altered LOC
11. Interrupted Family Processes related to situational crisis, powerlessness, and change in role
12. Deficient Knowledge related to required lifestyle changes

Collaborative Management

1. Prevent and monitor for clinical indications, and treat intracranial hypertension (see Intracranial Hypertension).
2. Maintain airway, ventilation, and oxygenation.
   a. Assume that the patient has a spinal injury until radiologic clearance of spine: do not tilt or hyperextend the head; use jaw-thrust technique to maintain open airway.
   b. Use oral or nasopharyngeal airway until lateral spine x-rays rule out fracture; do not use nasopharyngeal airway or nasal suctioning if facial or skull fracture is present.
   c. Do not use oral airways in conscious patients because they stimulate the gag reflex.
   d. Assist with rapid sequence intubation if intubation is required.
   e. Administer oxygen as needed to maintain Spo_2 greater than or equal to 95% unless contraindicated.
   f. Prevent aspiration: position patient on side and have suction equipment available.
3. Linear
   a. Monitor for clinical indications of intracranial hypertension or neurologic deficit.
   b. No specific treatment is required in the absence of neurologic symptoms.
4. Depressed
   a. Monitor for clinical indications of intracranial hypertension or neurologic deficit.
   b. Protect brain under cranial defect from injury; position patient away from cranial defect.
   c. Prevent and monitor for intracranial infection from open fracture.
      (1) Ensure meticulous cleansing and débridement of associated scalp laceration.
      (2) Surgical intervention is indicated if the depression of the skull is greater than the thickness of the skull (5 to 7 mm) and should be done emergently if scalp laceration or brain laceration is present.
      (3) Note indications of infection: fever; leukocytosis; redness, swelling, purulent drainage from wound.
      (4) Obtain culture if appropriate.
   d. Monitor for hemorrhage; removal of bone fragment from a venous sinus may result in hemorrhage; blood must be available.
5. Basal
   a. Prevent CNS infection.
      (1) Detect rhinorrhea/otorrhea; if present:
         (a) Do not obstruct flow: use mustache dressing
         (b) Elevate the HOB 30 degrees
      (2) Avert further tearing of dura by discouraging sneezing, blowing of the nose, and the Valsalva maneuver; instruct patient to cough with mouth open and to exhale when turning rather than holding the breath.
      (3) Do not use nasal oxygen, nasogastric tube, nasopharyngeal tube, or nasotracheal tube.
6. Monitor for complications.
   a. Linear: EDH
   b. Depressed
      (1) Laceration of brain tissue by brain fragments
      (2) Intracerebral hemorrhage or contusion
      (3) CNS infection (e.g., meningitis and encephalitis)
   c. Basal
      (1) Intracerebral hemorrhage
      (2) CNS infection (e.g., meningitis and abscess)
      (3) Cranial nerve injury
      (4) Carotid cavernous fistula
         (a) Rare but serious complication
         (b) Occurs when blood escapes from the carotid artery into the cavernous sinus
         (c) Clinical indications include bruit and pulsation of orbit over affected eye, exophthalmos, headache, and visual disturbances

Intracranial Hematomas

Etiology

Usually trauma

1. SDH (15% to 30% of patients with head trauma and 50% to 70% of all hematomas)
   a. May occur spontaneously, particularly if patient has coagulation disorder or is taking anticoagulants
   b. Is prevalent in older patients with cerebral atrophy and in alcoholics; may be bilateral
   c. Also may be due to purulent effusion
2. EDH (5% to 8% of patients with head trauma and 20% to 30% of all hematomas): often associated with linear skull fractures that cross major vascular channels
3. Intracerebral hematoma (ICH) (2% to 20% of patients with head trauma)
   a. May occur as result of gunshot wound or stab wound, laceration of brain from a depressed skull fracture, severe acceleration-deceleration injury
   b. Intracerebral bleeding caused by aneurysm, AVM, vascular tumor, or rupture of a vessel because of hypertension is described as a *hemorrhagic stroke* and is discussed in under Hemorrhagic Stroke

Pathophysiology (Figure 7-42)

1. SDH
   a. Usually venous bleeding; arterial origin is rare
   b. Accumulates below dura mater

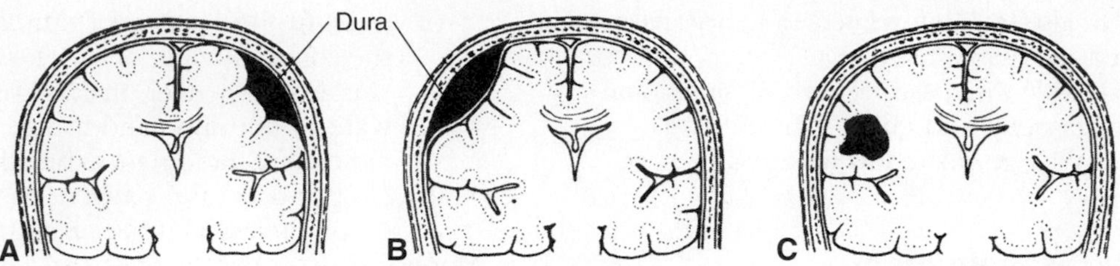

Figure 7-42 Types of hematomas. **A,** Subdural. **B,** Epidural. **C,** Intracerebral. (From Chipps, E. M., Clanin, N. J., & Campbell, V. G. [1992]. *Neurologic disorders: Mosby's clinical nursing series*. St. Louis: Mosby.)

c. Classification
   (1) Acute SDH: signs/symptoms occur within 48 hours after injury
   (2) Subacute SDH signs/symptoms occur within 2 weeks after injury
   (3) Chronic SDH: signs/symptoms may occur weeks to months after injury
      (a) Fibroblasts accumulate around the hematoma and encapsulate it.
      (b) Hemolysis of the clot liberates plasma proteins; this causes the encapsulated area to have a high osmotic pressure.
      (c) This causes an influx of water and swelling of the mass.

2. EDH
   a. Usually arterial bleeding; associated with tearing of arteries from skull fractures
      (1) Linear fractures of the temporal-parietal bones may tear the middle meningeal artery, leading to EDH.
      (2) Linear fractures of the occipital bone may tear the occipital artery, leading to EDH.
   b. May be due to venous bleeding; associated with fractures that cross major vascular channels such as the superior sagittal or transverse sinus (posterior fossa EDHs are usually of venous origin)
   c. Accumulates above the dura mater
3. ICH: hematoma into brain mass itself: may be due to bleeding caused by missile injury (e.g., gunshot wound or knife) or severe acceleration-deceleration force that causes bleeding into deep cerebral tissues

Clinical Presentation

1. SDH
   a. Subjective
      (1) History may include precipitating event or condition (in chronic SDH the patient may not be able to link to any particular event either because they cannot remember or because there is no true precipitating event [spontaneous])
      (2) Headache
      (3) Increasing irritability progressing to confusion progressing to decreased LOC
   b. Objective
      (1) Decreased LOC
      (2) Ipsilateral oculomotor paralysis
      (3) Contralateral hemiparesis/hemiplegia
2. EDH
   a. Subjective
      (1) History of precipitating event or condition
      (2) History of short period of unconsciousness followed by lucid interval and then rapid deterioration; lucid interval may be absent if initial blow is significant
      (3) Headache
   b. Objective
      (1) Increasing irritability progressing to confusion progressing to decreased LOC
      (2) Ipsilateral oculomotor paralysis
      (3) Contralateral hemiparesis/hemiplegia
3. ICH
   a. Subjective
      (1) History of precipitating event or condition
   b. Objective
      (1) Varies with area of brain involved, size of hematoma, and rate of blood accumulation
      (2) May or may not show clinical indications of intracranial hypertension
4. Diagnostic
   a. Skull and cervical spine x-rays: may reveal associated skull or spine fractures
   b. LP: *contraindicated* by intracranial hypertension
   c. CT scan: will show an area of increased density; may show midline shift
   d. MRI: shows hematoma
   e. Cerebral angiogram (rarely performed): may reveal avascular area with displacement or stretching of vessels

Nursing Diagnoses

1. Decreased Adaptive Capacity: Intracranial related to failure of normal intracranial compensatory mechanisms
2. Ineffective Cerebral Tissue Perfusion related to intracranial hypertension and hydrocephalus
3. Ineffective Airway Clearance related to increased secretions, altered LOC, and inadequate protective reflexes

4. Ineffective Breathing Pattern related to inadequate airway and altered LOC
5. Pain related to injury
6. Risk for Deficient Fluid Volume related to decreased fluid intake, increased fluid loss, and DI
7. Risk for Excess Fluid Volume related to fluid resuscitation and SIADH
8. Risk for Infection related to invasive procedures, traumatic wounds, and surgical wounds
9. Risk for Injury related to seizure activity and inadequate protective reflexes
10. Impaired Physical Mobility related to injury, paresis or plegia, bed rest, and altered LOC
11. Interrupted Family Processes related to situational crisis, powerlessness, and change in role
12. Deficient Knowledge related to required lifestyle changes

Collaborative Management

1. Detect and treat cranial, intracranial, and extracranial injuries.
2. Prevent and monitor for clinical indications, and treat intracranial hypertension (see Intracranial Hypertension).
3. Maintain airway, ventilation, and oxygenation.
   a. Assume that the patient has a spinal injury until radiologic clearance of spine: do not tilt or hyperextend the head; use jaw-thrust technique to maintain open airway.
   b. Use oral or nasopharyngeal airway until lateral spine x-rays rule out fracture; do not use nasopharyngeal airway or nasal suctioning if facial or skull fracture is present.
   c. Do not use oral airways in conscious patients because they stimulate the gag reflex.
   d. Assist with rapid sequence intubation if intubation is required.
   e. Administer oxygen as needed to maintain Spo_2 greater than or equal to 95% unless contraindicated.
   f. Prevent aspiration: position patient on side; have suction equipment available.
4. Prevent further bleeding; osmotic diuretics generally are not used because the tamponade effect of the hematoma helps to stop the bleeding.
5. Prepare patient for surgery.
   a. EDH and SDH
      (1) Usually burr hole and clot evacuation though small hematomas may be observed through serial CT scans to verify the gradual reabsorption of the hematoma.
      (2) Mortality increases dramatically if surgery is delayed.
   b. ICH
      (1) Surgery is indicated if ICH is large or there is a deteriorating neurologic status
      (2) Alternative treatment to surgery: stereotactic aspiration
         (a) Stereotactic placement of a small catheter into the center of the hematoma
         (b) Urokinase is injected and catheter sealed for 6 hours
         (c) Application of gentle suction to aspirate any liquefied hematoma
         (d) Repeat of cycle 8 times over 2 days
6. Detect and treat postoperative rebleed and/or brain edema; monitor patient closely for clinical indications of intracranial hypertension or deterioration of neurologic status.
   a. Usually elevate the HOB 20 to 30 degrees for acute and subacute SDH and EDH.
   b. Physician may request that the HOB be flat on side after surgery for removal of chronic SDH.
7. Prevent seizure activity: administer anticonvulsants prophylactically or therapeutically as prescribed.
8. Monitor for complications.
   a. Intracranial hypertension
   b. Hydrocephalus
   c. CNS infection
   d. Fluid and electrolyte imbalance: DI, SIADH, CSWS (see Craniotomy)
   e. SIADH
   f. Seizures

Hemorrhagic Stroke

Definition

Neurologic deficit caused by interruption of blood flow to the brain caused by vessel rupture

Etiology

1. Intraparenchymal brain hemorrhage
   a. Trauma: described in section on intracranial hematomas
   b. Hypertensive rupture of a cerebral vessel
   c. Also may be caused by vascular intracerebral tumor, fibrinolytic agents, anticoagulants, bleeding disorders, and spontaneous hemorrhagic conversion of an ischemic infarct
2. Subarachnoid hemorrhage: hemorrhage into the subarachnoid space
   a. Cerebral aneurysm: weakened bulging area on an intracranial blood vessel; account for the majority of subarachnoid hemorrhage
      (1) Most cerebral aneurysms are small (2 to 6 mm) and saccular and occur at bifurcations in circle of Willis.
         (a) Saccular (berry) aneurysms: usually congenital defects
         (b) Fusiform aneurysms: from atherosclerosis
         (c) Mycotic aneurysms: from necrotic vasculitis and septic emboli (rare)

(d) Traumatic aneurysms: from skull fracture disrupting vessel (rare)

b. AV malformation
  (1) A tangle of abnormal arteries and veins: arteries feed directly into veins without a capillary bed
  (2) Always congenital
  (3) May occur in other circulatory systems including the spinal cord

Pathophysiology

1. Aneurysm
  a. Two contributing factors are these:
    (1) Congenital weakness
    (2) Stress (e.g., hypertension)
  b. The aneurysm may act as mass lesion if intact and large.
  c. Weakness of an artery and high pressure (90% of ruptured aneurysms are associated with hypertension) leads to hemorrhage; hemorrhage is most likely when aneurysm is 8 to 10 mm in size.
  d. A clot initially forms in and around rupture site and temporarily inhibits continuing hemorrhage; increase in ICP and pressure from local tissues may stop bleeding.
  e. Blood leakage into subarachnoid space and in contact with meninges causes meningeal irritation.
  f. Cerebral vascular spasm often occurs and contributes to ischemia or infarction.
    (1) Increased constrictor mechanisms and decreased dilator functions
    (2) Hemolysis of erythrocytes trapped in the subarachnoid cisterns causes the release of oxyhemoglobin, bilirubin, methemoglobin, and other by-products of cell lysis to circulate within the subarachnoid space and increase the influx of calcium into the vascular smooth muscle, causing prolonged contraction and vessel constriction
    (3) Release of free radicals and peroxidation of lipids promote synthesis of vasoactive eicosanoids and endothelin and inhibit relaxation of the arterial wall
    (4) Failure of nitric oxide–dependent vascular relaxation may be a factor
    (5) Inflammatory mediators including prostaglandins, thromboxane A_2, leukotrienes, and histamine also may be a factors, because blood in the subarachnoid space causes inflammation and these mediators have been shown to be present in the CSF after SAH
  g. Communicating hydrocephalus can develop because of obstruction of CSF outflow through the arachnoid villi.
  h. As the clot around the aneurysm is broken down by natural fibrinolytic processes, rebleeding may occur.
  i. Intraparenchymal hemorrhage causes pressure on cerebral tissues and nerves and may lead to loss of function and death of neurons.
2. AV malformation
  a. Congenital tangle of arteries and veins
  b. Steals blood from other areas because it is an area of low resistance
  c. Causes ischemia of surrounding tissue
  d. Hemorrhage may occur

Clinical Presentation

1. Subjective
  a. History
    (1) Hypertension present in 90% of cases of ruptured aneurysm
    (2) Most patients have had a “warning leak” days or weeks before bleed
      (a) Headache
      (b) Generalized, transient weakness
      (c) Fatigue
      (d) Ptosis, diplopia, blurred vision
  b. Sudden, severe headache
    (1) Frequently described as “the worst headache of my life”
    (2) Sudden: described as a “thunder clap” or “like being hit in the head”
    (3) Localized progressing to generalized
    (4) May radiate to neck and back
  c. Nausea and vomiting may be present if severe bleed
2. Objective
  a. Restlessness progressing to altered LOC
    (1) Loss of consciousness is common in hemorrhage from aneurysm
    (2) Loss of consciousness is uncommon in hemorrhage from AVM
  b. If hemorrhage into ventricles
    (1) Nuchal rigidity
    (2) Photophobia
    (3) Kernig’s sign, Brudzinski’s sign
    (4) Hyperthermia
  c. Neurologic deficit
  d. Seizures
  e. Site and size determine specific clinical presentation
  f. Hunt and Hess aneurysm grading system (Table 7-19)
3. AVM specifically
  a. Patient may have bruit and report a constant swishing sound in the head with each heartbeat
  b. Motor/sensory defects
  c. Aphasia
  d. Dizziness, syncope
4. Diagnostic
  a. Serum
    (1) Hyponatremia may be present because of SIADH or CSWS.
    (2) PT and aPTT may be abnormal.

Table 7-19 Hunt and Hess Aneurysm Grading System

Grade	0	I	II	III	IV	V
Description	No bleed	Minimal bleed	Mild bleed	Moderate bleed	Moderate → severe bleed	Severe bleed
Level of consciousness	Alert	Alert	Awake	Drowsy	Stupor	Coma; moribund appearance
Headache	None	Minimal	Mild → moderate	Moderate → severe	Moderate → severe	Moderate → severe
Nuchal rigidity	None	Slight	Yes	Yes	Yes	Yes
Neurologic deficit	None	No	Minimal (e.g., cranial nerve palsy)	Mild (e.g., hemiparesis)	Moderate (e.g., hemiplegia)	Severe (e.g., posturing)

From Hunt, W. E., & Hess, R. M. (1968). Surgical risks as related to time of intervention in the repair of intracranial aneurysms. *Journal of Neurosurgery 28,* 14.

b. ECG
   (1) Changes that may occur with SAH
      (a) Flattened, peaked, or inverted T wave
      (b) Presence of U wave
      (c) QT prolongation
   (2) Dysrhythmias are common; torsades de pointes has been associated with SAH
c. Echocardiography: may show decreased ejection fraction caused by a "stunned" myocardium; mechanism unknown
d. LP: performed only if CT is nondiagnostic and there are no clinical indications of intracranial hypertension
   (1) Reveals bloody CSF, elevated protein in acute SAH; it is important to number the test tubes
      (a) If only test tube No. 1 is bloody: traumatic tap
      (b) If all test tubes are bloody: bloody tap
   (2) Reveals xanthochromic (dark amber) CSF if hemorrhage occurred several days (more than 5 days) ago
e. Transcranial Doppler ultrasonography: aids in diagnosing vasospasm
f. CT: identifies extent of SAH or intraparenchymal brain hemorrhage that may be suspicious of aneurysm; detects presence of hydrocephalus
g. MRI/MRA
   (1) May reveal small aneurysms that are not visualized with CT
   (2) May reveal ICH and intraventricular blood
   (3) May show vasospasm
h. Cerebral arteriogram: will illustrate size, shape, and location of aneurysm; may show vasospasm

Nursing Diagnoses

1. Decreased Adaptive Capacity: Intracranial related to failure of normal intracranial compensatory mechanisms
2. Ineffective Cerebral Tissue Perfusion related to hemorrhage, vasospasm, rebleed, intracranial hypertension, and hydrocephalus
3. Ineffective Airway Clearance related to increased secretions, altered LOC, and inadequate protective reflexes
4. Ineffective Breathing Pattern related to inadequate airway and altered LOC
5. Pain related to meningeal irritation by blood
6. Risk for Deficient Fluid Volume related to decreased fluid intake, increased fluid loss, and DI
7. Risk for Excess Fluid Volume related to volume expansion with triple H therapy, SIADH
8. Risk for Infection related to invasive procedures, traumatic wounds, and surgical wounds
9. Risk for Injury related to seizure activity and inadequate protective reflexes
10. Impaired Physical Mobility related to injury, paresis or plegia, bed rest, and altered LOC
11. Interrupted Family Processes related to situational crisis, powerlessness, and change in role
12. Deficient Knowledge related to required lifestyle changes

Collaborative Management

1. Maintain airway, ventilation, and oxygenation.
   a. Maintain airway.
      (1) Oropharyngeal or nasopharyngeal airway may be needed to hold tongue away from hypopharynx in obtunded patient.
      (2) Endotracheal intubation may be needed in patients without airway protective reflexes; sedation is recommended before intubation to avoid hypertension.

b. Maintain oxygenation and ventilation.
   (1) Administer oxygen as needed to maintain Spo_2 greater than or equal to 95% unless contraindicated.
   (2) Initiate mechanical ventilation as needed for hypoventilation.
c. Prevent aspiration.
   (1) Position patient on side.
   (2) Have suction equipment available.

2. Minimize potential for rebleed and promote stabilization of patient: rebleed occurs most often within 10 days after hemorrhage.
   a. Maintain BP within 10% of prehemorrhage levels; hypotension is associated with hypoperfusion, and hypertension is associated with rebleeding.
      (1) Alpha-blocker and beta-blocker (e.g., labetalol [Normodyne]) or vasodilators (e.g., hydralazine [Apresoline]) usually are used for hypertension
      (2) Vasopressors (e.g., phenylephrine [Neo-Synephrine]) for hypotension
   b. Decrease environmental stimuli (these interventions may be referred to as *aneurysm precautions*).
      (1) Provide a quiet, dimly lit private room.
      (2) Enforce bed rest with the HOB elevated 15 to 30 degrees
      (3) Instruct patient regarding how to avoid the Valsalva maneuver (e.g., cough with mouth open, exhale when turning in bed, and use stool softeners).
      (4) Instruct visitors that the patient should not be upset in any way; limit number of visitors and duration of visits.
      (5) Do not perform any rectal procedures (e.g., rectal temperature or enemas).
      (6) Provide sedation (usually phenobarbital) if patient is restless.
      (7) Treat fever with acetaminophen.
   c. Administer analgesics for headache, but avoid oversedation that would impair assessment.
      (1) Use short-acting narcotics (e.g., morphine, fentanyl, or codeine).
      (2) Avoid benzodiazepines.
   d. Prepare patient for surgery or interventional neuroradiologic procedures.
      (1) Aneurysm (Figure 7-43)
         (a) Indications
            (i) Surgery is indicated within 48 hours for grade I, II, or III aneurysm.
            (ii) Surgery usually is delayed for patients with grade IV or V aneurysm.
         (b) Surgical
            (i) Clipping: occlusion of the neck of the aneurysm with a ligature or metal clip; most common treatment especially if there is a well-defined neck
            (ii) Wrapping or coating: reinforcement of the sac with muscle, fibrin foam, or solidifying polymer
            (iii) Ligation: proximal ligation of a feeding vessel

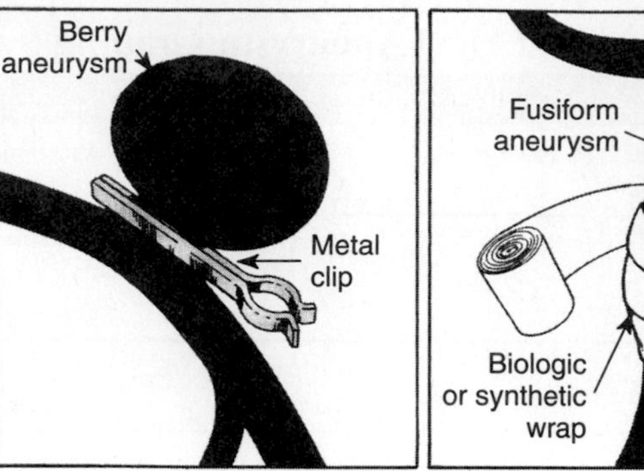

Figure 7-43 Clipping and wrapping of aneurysms. (From Chipps, E. M., Clanin, N. J., & Campbell, V. G. [1992]. *Neurologic disorders: Mosby's clinical nursing series*. St. Louis: Mosby.)

         (c) Endovascular procedures
            (i) Detachable coils: made of soft platinum; the device molds itself into the inner diameter of the aneurysmal dilation to cause thrombosis; an average of five coils are need to occlude the aneurysm; a clot forms and eventually the base of the aneurysm endothelializes and is cut off
            (ii) Intravascular balloon placement: silicone microballoon is placed into the aneurysm and detached
      (2) AVM
         (a) Surgical excision
         (b) Stereotactic radiosurgery if AVM may not be excised safely
         (c) Glue embolization: injection of glue into the arterial pedicle to cause thrombosis and block blood flow into the malformation
         (d) Embolization of the AVM with Silastic beads
         (e) Preoperative embolization followed by surgical excision
      (3) Intraparenchymal brain hemorrhage
         (a) Surgical removal of the clot depends on the size and location of the clot, the patient's ICP, and neurologic status.
            (i) Massive hematoma (greater than 3-cm diameter) with brainstem compression or intracranial hypertension
            (ii) Evidence of hydrocephalus
            (iii) Surgical accessibility
      (4) Provide postoperative management as described under Craniotomy; monitor for clinical indications of intracranial hypertension or rebleeding

3. Prevent and monitor for clinical indications, and treat intracranial hypertension (see Intracranial Hypertension)

4. Prevent and monitor for ischemia related to vasospasm following SAH caused by aneurysm.
   a. Recognize risk factors that increase the risk of the occurrence and severity of vasospasm.
      (1) Concomitant conditions
         (a) Hyperglycemia: controlling serum glucose may reduce the risk of vasospasm following SAH
      (2) CT: diffuse, thick blood in the subarachnoid space on CT scan especially if around the base of the brain
      (3) Location: hemorrhage in one of the vessels of the circle of Willis
      (4) Time frame: vasospasm occurs anytime from the third day after bleeding to 2 to 3 weeks after the initial bleed (peak incidence 5 to 12 days)
   b. Monitor for clinical indications of vasospasm.
      (1) Headache or worsening of headache
      (2) Visual changes
      (3) Change in LOC
      (4) Confusion
      (5) Pupil change
      (6) Focal neurologic deficit (e.g., hemiparesis and aphasia)
      (7) Seizures may occur
      (8) Increase in ICP if being monitored; blood may be visible in CSF if intraventricular catheter in place
      (9) Transcranial Doppler ultrasonography
         (a) Performed daily after SAH or more often if indicated
         (b) Note trends in flow velocity; intracranial blood flow velocities greater than 100 to 120 cm/sec suggests vasospasm; greater than 200 cm/sec suggests severe vasospasm
         (c) Correlate with clinical assessment
      (10) Angiography
         (a) Definitive study for diagnosis of cerebral vasospasm
         (b) Narrowing of arterial vessels may be seen on angiography before clinical indications of vasospasm are noted
   c. Provide therapies for the prevention and treatment of cerebral vasospasm.
      (1) Early clipping with flushing of excess blood and clots from the basal cisterns
      (2) Calcium channel blockers to prevent and/or reduce vasospasm
         (a) Nimodipine (Nimotop) is the preferred agent because it is lipid-soluble and therefore is able to cross the blood-brain barrier.
            (i) Dosage: 60 mg every 4 hours for 21 days after hemorrhage
            (ii) Adverse effects: hypotension; dose may be reduced to 30 mg every 2 to 4 hours
         (b) Prolonged-release nicardipine implants may be placed parallel to the ruptured artery and adjacent to the clot.
      (3) Triple-H therapy (hypertension, hypervolemia, hemodilution)
         (a) Goals: to increase CPP and CBF and to decrease risk of brain ischemia
         (b) Components
            (i) Hypertension
               a) The most debated of the three; some physicians use only hypervolemia and hemodilution especially before clipping
               b) Goal
                  i) Maintain systolic BP of 120 to 150 mm Hg if before the aneurysm has been clipped or otherwise secured.
                  ii) Maintain systolic BP of 160 to 200 mm Hg after clipping.
               c) Vasopressors (e.g., phenylephrine [Neo-Synephrine] or dopamine [Intropin]) may be needed if patient hypotensive; dobutamine (Dobutrex) also may be used to augment the CO
            (ii) Hypervolemia and hemodilution
               a) Isotonic crystalloids and/or colloids (e.g., albumin, dextran, and hetastarch)
               b) Hypervolemia: goal is to maintain a PAOP of 14 to 20 mm Hg and/or CVP of 10 to 12 mm Hg
               c) Hemodilution: goal is to maintain a hematocrit of 30% to 33%; patients with hematocrit levels of less than 25% require blood transfusion to optimize cerebral oxygenation
         (c) Usually maintained for 14 days after hemorrhage
         (d) Controversies related to triple-H therapy
            (i) Not every patient responds
            (ii) Significant costs
            (iii) Potential complications: pulmonary edema, myocardial ischemia, coagulopathy, electrolyte imbalance, rebleeding
      (4) Cerebral balloon angioplasty
         (a) Goal: widening of the stenotic segment with a balloon-tipped catheter
         (b) Limitation: can be used only with larger, accessible vessels
         (c) Complications
            (i) Vessel rupture
            (ii) Restenosis rarely occurs

(5) Intraarterial injection of papaverine
(a) Goal: relief of spasm of vessels too distal for the use of angioplasty but also may be used during angioplasty
(b) Complications: intracranial hypertension, brain ischemia

5. Provide instruction and counseling regarding lifestyle modification and need for pharmacologic therapy.
   a. Nonpharmacologic therapies
      (1) Weight normalization
      (2) Cessation of tobacco use
      (3) Limitation of alcohol consumption to one to two alcoholic beverages daily
      (4) Regular aerobic exercise in moderation
      (5) Complementary therapies: relaxation; imagery, biofeedback
      (6) Stress reduction
      (7) Yearly flu and pneumococcal vaccine
      (8) Recognition of symptoms of recurrence and when to call the physician
   b. Pharmacologic agents
      (1) Control of hypertension, hyperlipidemia, and diabetes mellitus
6. Monitor for complications.
   a. Vasospasm (in aneurysms)
   b. Rebleeding
   c. Brain edema and intracranial hypertension
   d. Hydrocephalus: may require ventriculoperitoneal shunt
   e. Fluid and electrolyte imbalance: DI, SIADH, CSWS (see Craniotomy)
   f. Seizures: anticonvulsants frequently are prescribed prophylactically because the increase in BP, increase in metabolic rate and oxygen demand, and compromised ventilation and oxygenation during seizure activity could be devastating
   g. Dysrhythmias (e.g., prolonged QT interval and torsades de pointes)
   h. DVT and pulmonary embolism: use sequential compression devices

Ischemic Stroke

Definitions

1. Transient ischemic attack (TIA): episode of neurologic impairment attributed to focal cerebral ischemia; resolves within 24 hours (Box 7-2)
2. Ischemic stroke: sudden, severe disruption of the cerebral circulation with a subsequent loss of neurologic function caused by thrombus or embolus
3. Lacunar stroke: special subset of thrombotic stroke seen almost exclusively in hypertensive patients; small perforating vessel thrombosis

Etiology

1. Thrombosis
   a. Intracranial arteriosclerosis
   b. Extracranial (i.e., carotid) atherosclerosis
   c. Hypertension
   d. Hypercoagulability (e.g., polycythemia)
2. Embolism
   a. Mural thrombi
      (1) Dysrhythmia (e.g., atrial fibrillation)
      (2) Ventricular aneurysm
   b. Carotid artery atherosclerosis
   c. Bacterial endocarditis
   d. Valvular heart disease
   e. Prosthetic cardiac valves
   f. DVT with patent foramen ovale
   g. Air or fat embolism (see Chapter 5)

BOX 7-2 Symptoms Occurring during Transient Ischemic Attacks

Anterior Circulation
- Aphasia (if dominant hemisphere affected)
- Contralateral sensory or motor defects
- Ipsilateral headache
- Ipsilateral monocular visual defect (amaurosis fugax) or homonymous hemianopsia
- Seizure activity

Posterior Circulation
- Bilateral visual defect; diplopia
- Bilateral sensory or motor defects
- Dysphagia
- Occipital headache
- Vertigo, syncope (drop attack), dizziness, ataxia

Pathophysiology

1. Risk factors include the following:
   a. Family history
   b. Hypertension
   c. Smoking
   d. Diabetes mellitus
   e. Valvular heart disease
   f. Coronary artery disease
   g. Heart failure
   h. Hyperlipidemia
   i. Obesity
   j. Sedentary lifestyle
   k. Drugs
      (1) Alcohol, especially heavy episodic consumption
      (2) Stimulants (e.g., cocaine and phenylpropanolamine)
      (3) Oral contraceptives
   l. Dysrhythmias, especially atrial fibrillation
   m. Hypercoagulability
2. Occlusive vascular disease (thrombosis or embolus) causes decreased oxygen to brain tissue causing ischemia and leading to infarction
3. Brain edema develops slowly usually over the first 72 hours; brain edema and persistent ischemia cause progressive damage to the penumbra, the ischemic brain tissue surrounding the infarction

Clinical Presentation

1. Subjective
   a. May have history of any of the following:
      (1) TIA
      (2) Hypertension
      (3) Cardiovascular disease
      (4) Arteriosclerosis
      (5) Diabetes mellitus
   b. Sudden onset of signs and symptoms
      (1) Thrombotic stroke usually occurs at night and often is discovered on awakening; likely caused by decrease in CO and BP with less flow through an area of critical stenosis
      (2) Embolic stroke is more likely to occur when the patient is active
2. Objective
   a. Varies depending on area of vessel involved and extent of injury (Box 7-3)
3. Diagnostic
   a. Serum
      (1) Lipids: may be elevated
      (2) Glucose
         (a) Hypoglycemia may mimic stroke.
         (b) Hyperglycemia frequently is seen in stroke.
      (3) Clotting profile: baseline before fibrinolytic agents
   b. ECG: may show dysrhythmias as a possible cause of cerebral emboli; Holter monitor may identify dysrhythmia
   c. Echocardiography: may show intracardiac source for cerebral emboli (e.g., ventricular aneurysm and bacterial endocarditis)
   d. LP: may be done to differentiate hemorrhagic from thrombotic stroke if there are no signs of intracranial hypertension
   e. Doppler carotid studies: may show carotid artery stenosis
   f. Transcranial Doppler ultrasonography: may be used to localize vessel occlusions and experimentally to assist with clot lysis
   g. CT
      (1) Normal early in ischemic stroke
      (2) Identifies the location and characteristics of subacute and old infarctions, the presence or absence of gross hemorrhage, and the presence or absence of a mass lesion
      (3) May show distortion or shift of ventricles
      (4) CT performed 24 hours after fibrinolytic administration to rule out intracranial hemorrhage
   h. MRI
      (1) Shows presence of early ischemic changes when a CT scan still looks normal
      (2) Identifies changes in the cranial or spinal structures
   i. Cerebral angiography: identifies occlusion, stenosis, aneurysms, hemorrhage in arterial system

Nursing Diagnoses

1. Decreased Adaptive Capacity: Intracranial related to failure of normal intracranial compensatory mechanisms
2. Ineffective Cerebral Tissue Perfusion related to thrombus, embolus, vasospasm, or intracranial hypertension
3. Risk for Aspiration related to impaired swallowing and inadequate protective reflexes
4. Ineffective Airway Clearance related to increased secretions, altered LOC, and inadequate protective reflexes
5. Ineffective Breathing Pattern related to inadequate airway and altered LOC

BOX 7-3 Clinical Indications Related to Vascular Occlusion

Anterior Cerebral Artery
- Contralateral paralysis of leg and foot
- Impaired gait
- Mental impairment
- Personality changes: flat affect; inappropriate emotional responses

Middle Cerebral Artery
- Aphasia if dominant hemisphere affected
- Apraxia, agnosia, neglect if nondominant hemisphere affected
- Contralateral sensory deficit
- Dysarthria
- Dysphagia
- Hemiplegia of face and arm on contralateral side
- Homonymous hemianopsia

Posterior Cerebral Artery
- Cortical blindness
- Homonymous hemianopsia
- Perseveration (abnormal persistence of a response)

Vertebral or Basilar Artery
- Ataxia
- Dizziness
- Dysarthria
- Dysphagia
- Ipsilateral facial numbness and weakness
- "Locked-in" syndrome (quadriplegia and mutism with intact consciousness)
- Nystagmus
- Weakness of tongue

6. Risk for Deficient Fluid Volume related to decreased fluid intake, increased fluid loss, and DI
7. Risk for Excess Fluid Volume related to fluid resuscitation and SIADH
8. Risk for Infection related to invasive procedures, traumatic wounds, and surgical wounds
9. Risk for Injury related to seizure activity and inadequate protective reflexes
10. Impaired Swallowing related to neuromuscular impairment
11. Imbalanced Nutrition: Less Than Body Requirements related to decreased protein/calorie intake and hypermetabolism
12. Impaired Physical Mobility related to injury, paresis or plegia, bed rest, and altered LOC
13. Impaired Verbal Communication related to dysphasia, aphasia, and intubation
14. Disturbed Body Image related to actual change in body function and appearance
15. Interrupted Family Processes related to situational crisis, powerlessness, and change in role
16. Deficient Knowledge related to required lifestyle changes

Collaborative Management

1. Maintain airway, ventilation, and oxygenation.
   a. Maintain airway.
      (1) Oropharyngeal or nasopharyngeal airway may be needed to hold tongue away from hypopharynx in obtunded patient.
      (2) Endotracheal intubation may be needed in patients without airway protective reflexes.
   b. Maintain oxygenation and ventilation.
      (1) Administer oxygen as needed to maintain Spo_2 greater than or equal to 95% unless contraindicated.
      (2) Turn patient frequently; 60-degree lateral rotation therapeutic bed is helpful to prevent pneumonia in these patients.
      (3) Initiate mechanical ventilation as needed for acute respiratory failure.
   c. Prevent aspiration.
      (1) Position patient on side.
      (2) Have suction equipment available.
2. Detect changes in neurologic status and restore or maintain CBF (Figure 7-44).
   a. Use the NIHSS (Table 7-10) to assess changes in neurologic status.
   b. Correct possible causes and contributing factors.
      (1) Assist in electrical or pharmacologic conversion of atrial fibrillation or administer anticoagulants to prevent mural thrombi.
      (2) Administer antihypertensives to control BP only if BP is greater than 220/120 mm Hg or cardiac ischemia, heart failure, or aortic dissection exist, fibrinolytic therapy is planned, or intracerebral hemorrhage is identified on CT.
         (a) Hypotension *must* be avoided because cerebral autoregulation is lost in the area of ischemia/infarction.
         (b) Labetalol (Normodyne) generally is used, but nitroprusside (Nipride) or hydralazine (Apresoline) also may be used.
      (3) Control hyperglycemia with IV insulin infusion.
   c. Administer fibrinolytic agents as prescribed.
      (1) Goal: lysis of an occluding clot to restore blood flow to the compromised but potentially viable penumbra
      (2) Indications
         (a) Presentation within 3 hours of acute ischemic stroke symptoms (or 6 hours if intraarterial fibrinolytic agents to be used)
            (i) Seven *D*'s of stroke care (American Heart Association, 2005)
               a) *D*etection of early indications and determination of time of onset
               b) *D*ispatch of emergency medical care
               c) *D*elivery of the patient to the nearest facility capable of implementing the most current stroke guidelines
               d) *D*oor and rapid triage in the emergency department
               e) *D*ata collected to aid in decision making
                  i) Baseline CT and/or MRI to exclude intracranial hemorrhage and other risk factors for intracranial hemorrhage
                  ii) History, physical examination, laboratory
               f) *D*ecision made regarding whether the patient meets criteria for fibrinolytic agents and does not have contraindications; as in Table 3-17 with the following additions:
                  i) Awakening with symptoms of stroke because the time of onset cannot be determined
                  ii) Seizure at the onset of stroke
                  iii) Age greater than 75 years
                  iv) NIHSS score greater than 22
                  v) Hypodensities on CT
                  vi) Subacute bacterial endocarditis
               g) *D*rug within 3 hours of the onset of symptoms
      (3) Dosage and routes
         (a) IV administered alteplase (Activase)
            (i) Total dose: 0.9 mg/kg with maximum dose of less than or equal to 90 mg
            (ii) Bolus: 10% of this total dose over 1 minute
            (iii) Infusion: remaining 90% of this total dose administer over 60 minutes

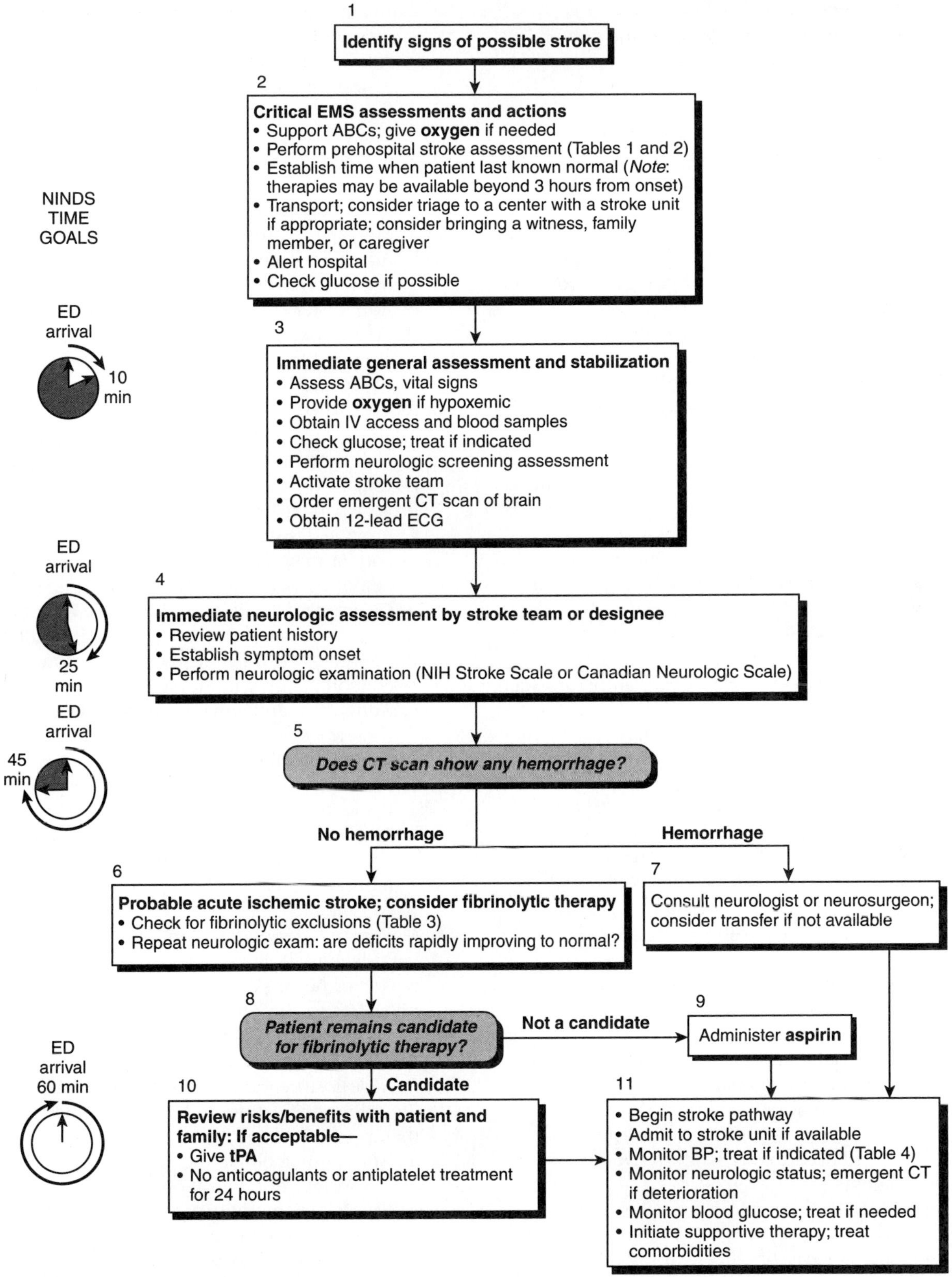

Figure 7-44 Algorithm for goals of management of patients with suspected stroke. (From American Heart Association. [2005]. Part 9: Adult stroke. *Circulation.* 112[24 suppl.], IV111-IV120.)

(b) Intraarterial
(i) Catheter is placed into the cerebral circulation under fluoroscopy.
(ii) Dose of alteplase (Activase) is approximately one half of IV dose.
(4) Management
(a) Monitor vital signs and neurologic status.
(b) Maintain BP less than or equal to 185 mm Hg systolic and less than or equal to 110 mm Hg diastolic; labetalol (Normodyne) usually is used.
(c) Do not administer anticoagulants or platelet aggregation inhibitors for 24 hours after IV fibrinolytic administration, but these may be used after intraarterial fibrinolytic administration.
(d) Repeat CT at 24 hours after fibrinolytic administration.
(e) As in Table 3-17

d. Administer anticoagulants and platelet aggregation inhibitors as prescribed if fibrinolytic agents are contraindicated or after 24 hours after IV administration of fibrinolytic agents.
(1) Anticoagulants (e.g., heparin) are especially important if emboli are of cardiac origin, such as in atrial fibrillation
(a) Low-molecular-weight heparin administered subcutaneously may be used for DVT prophylaxis.
(2) Platelet aggregation inhibitors
(a) Oral agents (e.g., aspirin and dipyridamole (Aggrenox), ticlopidine [Ticlid], or clopidogrel [Plavix]) or IV agents (abciximab [ReoPro], eptifibatide [Integrilin], or tirofiban [Aggrastat]) as prescribed
(i) IV agents are being study for primary use within 24 hours of stroke symptoms
(b) Especially important in patients with carotid, intracranial, or vertebrobasilar artery stenosis
(c) Contraindicated for 24 hours after IV administration of fibrinolytic agents

e. Prepare patient for surgical procedures as requested.
(1) Endarterectomy or carotid artery angioplasty with or without stenting for patients with signs of cerebrovascular insufficiency who have not had completed stroke (see Vascular Disease in Chapter 3)
(2) Evacuation of clot depending on size, location, and neurologic status

3. Prevent and monitor for clinical indications, and treat intracranial hypertension (see Intracranial Hypertension), especially during the first 72 hours.
4. Maintain fluid and electrolyte balance and nutritional status.
   a. Administer IV fluids as prescribed.
   b. Assess gag and swallow reflexes before giving fluids by mouth.
   c. Initiate early enteral feedings within 24 to 48 hours if patient is unable to take food by mouth.
5. Decrease metabolic requirements.
   a. Enforce bed rest initially.
   b. Administer minor tranquilizers as prescribed, but do not oversedate.
   c. Administer stool softeners as prescribed.
   d. Treat hyperthermia with antipyretics and cooling blankets; hypothermia therapy may be initiated.
6. Assess patient's ability to communicate, and establish means of communication; consult speech therapist as soon as possible in aphasic patients.
7. Protect patient from injury.
   a. Provide assistance during ambulation because patient may have postural imbalance related to hemiparesis/hemiplegia.
   b. Orient patient often, and provide explanations of care because confusion and disorientation, as well as memory deficits, may occur concomitantly with aphasia.
   c. Administer anticonvulsants prophylactically as prescribed.
8. Prevent deformities, decubitus ulcers, and hazards of immobility.
   a. Reposition patient every 2 hours.
   b. Perform passive range of motion exercises every 2 hours; assist with active range of motion exercises when patient is able to participate.
9. Maximize independence in activities of daily living; allow the patient to do whatever he or she can for himself or herself.
10. Provide emotional support, and encourage participation in support groups.
11. Provide instruction and counseling regarding lifestyle modification and need for pharmacologic therapy.
   a. Nonpharmacologic therapies
(1) Weight normalization
(2) Dietary modifications
(a) Low saturated fat
(b) Low (2 to 3 g) sodium
(c) American Diabetic Association diet for control of blood glucose for patient with diabetes mellitus
(3) Cessation of tobacco use
(4) Limitation of alcohol consumption to one to two alcoholic beverages daily
(5) Regular aerobic exercise in moderation
(6) Complementary therapies: relaxation; imagery, biofeedback
(7) Stress reduction

(8) Yearly flu and pneumococcal vaccine
(9) Recognition of symptoms of TIA or stroke and when to call the physician

b. Pharmacologic agents
(1) Control of hypertension, hyperlipidemia, and diabetes mellitus
(2) Platelet aggregation inhibitors and/or anticoagulants
(3) Discontinuance of oral contraceptive agents in premenopausal females and hormone replacement therapy in postmenopausal females

12. Monitor for complications.
a. Persistent neurologic trauma
b. Brain edema
c. Seizures: prophylactic anticonvulsants
d. Fluid and electrolyte imbalance: DI, SIADH, CSWS (see Craniotomy)
e. Spastic paralysis may cause contractures
(1) Range of motion
(2) Splints
f. Pneumonia
g. DVT, pulmonary embolism
(1) Subcutaneous low-molecular-weight heparin or unfractionated heparin usually is used prophylactically.
(2) Sequential compression devices also may be used.
h. Urinary tract infection, urosepsis
i. Pressure ulcers

Brain Tumor

Etiology

Multifactorial or unknown

1. Congenital
2. Hereditary factors

Pathophysiology

1. Although half of brain tumors are benign, death may occur because they exert pressure on vital centers.
   a. Malignant tumors cause progressive deterioration of the patient's condition, leading to death; they may be primary or metastatic.
   b. Benign CNS tumors may produce malignant effects because of their anatomic location and surgical inaccessibility.
      (1) Benign CNS tumors may cause death because they take up space in the cranial vault and cause intracranial hypertension and herniation.
      (2) Some benign CNS tumors may convert to malignant.
2. Space-occupying lesions destroy brain tissue and nerve structures and produce intracranial hypertension.
3. They may cause brain ischemia or edema, intracranial hypertension, seizures, focal neurologic deficits, hydrocephalus, and hormonal changes.
4. Primary brain tumors are categorized by their cell type; metastatic brain tumors are of the cell type of the primary tumor (Table 7-20).

Table 7-20 Types of Brain Tumors

Type	Comments
Gliomas • Astrocytomas (initially benign but prone to become malignant) • Oligodendrogliomas (usually benign but may become malignant) • Ependymomas (usually benign but may become malignant) • Medulloblastomas (highly malignant) • Glioblastoma multiforme (highly malignant)	• Most in cerebrum, but medulloblastoma in cerebellum and ependymomas in ventricular system • Most grow rapidly, but medulloblastoma is rapidly invasive • Most nonencapsulated; cannot be incised completely
Meningioma	• Benign, slow growing • Usually encapsulated; surgical cure possible • Recurrence possible
Pituitary adenoma	• Usually benign • Surgical approach usually successful
Acoustic neuroma	• Benign or low-grade malignancy • Arise from sheath of Schwann cells found on eighth cranial nerve • Will regrow if not completely excised • Surgical resection often difficult because of location
Metastatic tumor	• Malignant • Cancer cells spread to the brain via the circulatory system usually from lung, breast, or prostate cancer • Surgical resection difficult and prognosis poor

Clinical Presentation

1. Subjective
   a. Headache
      (1) Occurs at night after retiring
      (2) Present and worse on awakening
      (3) May be relieved by midmorning
   b. Visual changes
2. Objective
   a. Seizures: new onset
   b. Personality changes
   c. Vomiting without preceding nausea
      (1) More common in morning
   d. Papilledema
   e. Change in LOC
   f. Hormonal changes if pituitary involved
   g. Specific to affected area of brain (Table 7-21)
3. Diagnostic
   a. Hormone levels: may be abnormal if pituitary tumor
   b. Chest x-ray: may show primary tumor of lung
   c. Skull x-ray: may show shift of pineal gland
   d. EEG: aids in identification of seizure activity
   e. Brain scan: identifies the tumor
   f. Bone scan: may show bone cancer
   g. CT: identifies the tumor
   h. MRI: identifies the tumor and effect on surrounding tissue
   i. Angiography: may show vascular shifts caused by tumor or may show vascularity of tumor
   j. Biopsy: classifies tumor cell type

Table 7-21 Clinical Manifestations of Tumors Specific to Affected Area of Brain

Area	Clinical Manifestations
Frontal lobe	• Personality changes • Inappropriate behavior: loss of social behavior • Inappropriate affect: quiet, flat • Inattentiveness, inability to concentrate • Emotional lability • Recent memory loss • Decreased intellectual ability • Motor changes: hemiparesis, hemiplegia • Seizure activity possible • If dominant hemisphere: expressive aphasia
Parietal	• Sensory changes: hyperesthesia, paresthesia, loss of two-point discrimination • Constructional apraxia • Loss of right-left discrimination • Homonymous hemianopsia • Seizure activity possible
Temporal	• Poor judgment • Irritability • Regressive behavior • Auditory disturbances • Olfactory, visual, and gustatory hallucinations • Psychomotor seizures • If dominant hemisphere: receptive aphasia
Occipital lobe	• Visual disturbances: visual field defects • Visual hallucinations • Seizure activity possible: visual aura
Pituitary or hypothalamus	• Visual disturbances • Hormone imbalance: hypopituitarism or hyperpituitarism • Temperature regulation problems • Changes in sleep patterns
Brainstem	• Dysphagia • Vomiting • Ataxia • Nystagmus • Vomiting: with or without nausea • Decreased corneal reflex • Ventilatory pattern changes
Cerebellum	• Ataxia • Nystagmus • Unsteady gait • Decreased coordination • Vomiting: with or without nausea • Intentional tremors • Seizure activity possible

Nursing Diagnoses

1. Decreased Adaptive Capacity: Intracranial related to failure of normal intracranial compensatory mechanisms
2. Impaired Cerebral Tissue Perfusion related to intracranial hypertension
3. Pain related to intracranial hypertension and stretching of dura at tumor site
4. Ineffective Airway Clearance related to increased secretions, diminished LOC, and inadequate protective reflexes
5. Risk for Deficient Fluid Volume related to decreased fluid intake, increased fluid loss, and DI
6. Risk for Excess Fluid Volume related to fluid resuscitation and SIADH
7. Risk for Infection related to invasive procedures, traumatic wounds, and surgical wounds
8. Risk for Injury related to seizure activity and inadequate protective reflexes
9. Imbalanced Nutrition: Less Than Body Requirements related to decreased protein/calorie intake, hypermetabolism
10. Impaired Verbal Communication related to dysphasia, aphasia, and intubation
11. Impaired Physical Mobility related to injury, paresis or plegia, bed rest, and altered LOC
12. Self-Care Deficit related to decreased motor function resulting from tumor growth and pressure
13. Interrupted Family Processes related to situational crisis, powerlessness, and change in role
14. Deficient Knowledge related to required lifestyle changes
15. Anticipatory Grieving related to diagnosis of cancer

Collaborative Management

1. Prevent and monitor for clinical indications, and treat intracranial hypertension (see Intracranial Hypertension); glucocorticoids frequently are used to reduce brain edema
2. Maintain airway, oxygenation, and ventilation.
   a. Maintain airway.
      (1) Oropharyngeal or nasopharyngeal airway may be needed to hold tongue away from hypopharynx in obtunded patient.
      (2) Endotracheal intubation may be needed in patients without airway protective reflexes.
   b. Maintain oxygenation and ventilation.
      (1) Administer oxygen as needed to maintain Spo_2 greater than or equal to 95% unless contraindicated.
      (2) Initiate mechanical ventilation as needed for hypoventilation.
   c. Prevent aspiration.
      (1) Position patient on side.
      (2) Have suction equipment available.
3. Prepare patient for surgery, radiation, and/or chemotherapy.
   a. Surgery
      (1) Purposes of craniotomy for brain tumor
         (a) Debulk tumor to relieve pressure
         (b) Resect and remove tumor (usually followed by radiation)
         (c) Insert shunt for hydrocephalus
      (2) Postcraniotomy care (see Craniotomy)
   b. Radiation: after surgery for incompletely excised tumor or for nonsurgically accessible tumor
      (1) Whole-brain radiation therapy in high doses or superfractionated therapy
      (2) Brachytherapy or interstitial irradiation: placement of a radioactive source in contact with or implanted into the brain tumor
   c. Radiosurgery: closed-skull destruction of an intracranial target with ionizing beams of radiation; an intracranial guiding device aids in focusing the beams of radiation
      (1) Bragg peak proton beam
      (2) Linear accelerator radiosurgery
      (3) Gamma knife therapy
   d. Chemotherapy
      (1) Used after debulking in combination with radiotherapy, after irradiation, or for tumor recurrence
      (2) Antineoplastic agent determined by tumor type; more than one agent may be used
4. Monitor for complications.
   a. Fluid and electrolyte imbalance: DI, SIADH, CSWS (see Craniotomy)
   b. Brain ischemia
   c. Hydrocephalus
   d. Brain edema
   e. Seizures
   f. Herniation

Status Epilepticus

Definitions

1. Seizure: sudden, paroxysmal episode of exaggerated activity or abnormal behavior caused by excessive discharge of cerebral neurons; Table 7-22 describes types of seizures
2. Status epilepticus: seizure activity of 30 minutes or more duration caused by a single seizure or a series of seizures in which there is no return of consciousness between seizures
   a. Note that a more current definition is seizure activity lasting at least 10 minutes because treatment generally is initiated within 10 minutes, preventing the continuation of seizure activity for 30 minutes.

Etiology

1. Preexisting history of seizure disorder
   a. Withdrawal from anticonvulsant medications
   b. Acute alcohol or withdrawal
   c. Acute withdrawal from chronically used drugs that have sedative or depressant effects (e.g., barbiturates)
   d. Acute condition that lowers the seizure threshold
2. No preexisting history of seizure disorder
   a. Brain trauma
   b. Stroke: ischemic or hemorrhagic
   c. CNS infection: meningitis; encephalitis: abscess
   d. Brain tumors
   e. Encephalopathy: anoxic (e.g., cardiac arrest), hypertensive, or metabolic
      (1) Hypoglycemia
      (2) Hepatic failure
      (3) Uremia
      (4) Hyperosmolality
   f. Electrolyte imbalance
      (1) Hyponatremia
      (2) Hypocalcemia
      (3) Hypomagnesemia
   g. Drug or alcohol withdrawal
   h. Drug toxicity: lidocaine, meperidine, theophylline, salicylates, cyclic antidepressants, cocaine
   i. Sepsis

Pathophysiology

1. Prolonged grand mal seizures may deplete the brain of oxygen and glucose, which may produce hypoxia and neuronal death
2. Early: hypersympathetic phase
   a. CBF increases
   b. Tachycardia, hypertension
   c. Blood pH falls, Pao_2 falls, $Paco_2$ rises
   d. Glucose and potassium rise
3. Late: after 25 to 30 minute of seizure activity
   a. CBF is unable to keep up with cerebral metabolic demands
   b. Bradycardia, hypotension, dysrhythmias, hypoglycemia

Table 7-22 Types of Seizures

Type	Features	Duration
GENERALIZED: LOSS OF CONSCIOUSNESS		
Absence (petit mal)	• Momentary loss of consciousness • Blank stare, cessation of activity • Eye blinking, lip smacking may occur • May lose muscle tone	Seconds
Tonic-clonic (grand mal)	• May be preceded by an aura and a cry from forced expiration • Loss of consciousness • Symmetric tonic-clonic extremity movements • May experience apnea with cyanosis until tonic phase ends • May bite tongue, may be incontinent • Postictal fatigue, muscle soreness, confusion, lethargy, and/or headache	3-5 minutes
Myoclonic	• Short, abrupt muscle contractions of arms, legs, and torso • Contractions may be symmetric or asymmetric	Seconds
Clonic	• Muscle contraction and relaxation but slower than with myoclonic seizure	Several minutes
Tonic	• Abrupt increase in muscle tone of torso and face • Flexion of arms; extension of legs	Seconds
Atonic	• Abrupt loss of muscle tone • May cause falling and injuries related to fall	Seconds
PARTIAL: FOCAL AT ONSET BUT MAY EVOLVE INTO A GENERALIZED SEIZURE		
Simple partial	• Consciousness not impaired • Abnormal unilateral movement of arm, leg, or both • Patient may sense abnormal smell, sound, or sensation, such as numbness, tingling, or burning • Tachycardia or bradycardia, tachypnea, skin flushing, epigastric discomfort	Seconds to minutes
Complex partial	• Loss of consciousness, but eyes may be open • Lip smacking, chewing, picking at clothing • Mumbling, speaking in repetitive phrases • Posturing or jerking movements • Postictal confusion, amnesia common	Minutes

c. Marked elevations of creatine kinase and potassium
d. Ventricular fibrillation may occur
e. Rhabdomyolysis-induced renal failure

Clinical Presentation

1. Subjective
   a. History may include precipitating event or condition
      (1) History of epilepsy
      (2) History of noncompliance in taking anticonvulsant drugs
      (3) History of chronic drug or alcohol use
2. Objective
   a. Alteration in LOC
   b. Tonic and/or clonic body movements
   c. Incontinence of urine or stool
   d. Involuntary motor activities: lip smacking, swallowing, chewing
3. Diagnostic
   a. Evaluation of cause
      (1) BUN: increased in uremia, hyperosmolality
      (2) Liver function studies: increased in hepatic failure
      (3) Drug and alcohol levels
      (4) Anticonvulsant drug levels: subtherapeutic in noncompliance
   b. Serum
      (1) Electrolytes: hyperkalemia
      (2) Glucose: increased early; decreased late
      (3) Creatine kinase: increased
      (4) Lactic acid: increased
      (5) ABGs: may show hypercapnia and hypoxemia
   c. Urine: may show myoglobinuria
   d. Skull x-rays: may show cause
   e. EEG: will show seizure activity
   f. CT, MRI, MRA: may indicate pathologic conditions (e.g., mass lesions)
   g. LP: may show meningitis as cause

Nursing Diagnoses

1. Decreased Adaptive Capacity: Intracranial related to failure of normal intracranial compensatory mechanisms
2. Ineffective Cerebral Tissue Perfusion related to intracranial hypertension

3. Ineffective Airway Clearance related to increased secretions, diminished LOC, and inadequate protective reflexes
4. Ineffective Breathing Patterns related to obstruction of airway by tongue
5. High Risk for Infection related to invasive procedures, traumatic wounds, and surgical wounds
6. Hyperthermia related to seizure activity
7. Risk for Injury related to seizure activity and inadequate protective reflexes
8. Pain related to meningeal irritation
9. Hyperthermia related to infection
10. Interrupted Family Processes related to situational crisis, powerlessness, and change in role
11. Deficient Knowledge related to required lifestyle changes

Collaborative Management

1. Establish and maintain airway and adequate ventilation.
   a. Insert artificial airway if ventilation and oxygenation inadequate.
      (1) Use nasopharyngeal airway or nasotracheal intubation if mouth cannot be opened; do not try to force mouth open.
      (2) Monitor ABGs and pulse oximetry.
   b. Maintain oxygenation and ventilation.
      (1) Administer oxygen as needed to maintain Spo_2 greater than or equal 95% unless contraindicated.
      (2) Initiate mechanical ventilation as needed for hypoventilation.
   c. Prevent aspiration.
      (1) Position patient on his or her side: do not just turn head to the side; turn body on the side.
      (2) Have suction equipment available; suction secretions as indicated.
2. Protect patient from injury and prevent complications during seizure.
   a. Call for help.
   b. Do not leave patient.
   c. Loosen constrictive clothing.
   d. Remove pillow from under head.
   e. Turn patient to the side and maintain an open airway.
   f. Do not restrain, but gentle guiding of extremities is acceptable.
   g. Pad side rails with blankets or pillows.
   h. Maintain privacy.
   i. Assess for injury.
3. Assess for and eliminate causes or contributing factors.
   a. Analyze serum for glucose, sodium, potassium, calcium, phosphorus, magnesium, and BUN.
   b. Screen patient for drugs.
      (1) Barbiturates
      (2) Tricyclic antidepressants
      (3) Alcohol
   c. Obtain anticonvulsant drug levels.
   d. Obtain blood cultures if patient is hyperthermic.
   e. Correct contributing factors that lower seizure threshold (e.g., hypoxemia, acid-base imbalance, electrolyte imbalance, hyperthermia, and hypermetabolism).
4. Stop seizure activity.
   a. Initiate IV.
   b. Administer 100 mg thiamine and 50 mL of 50% dextrose in water if alcohol ingestion or hypoglycemia is suspected (thiamine is given with the dextrose to prevent Wernicke's encephalopathy, especially if patient has chronic malnutrition).
   c. Administer benzodiazepine or other drugs if seizures persist after dextrose and thiamine administration.
      (1) Benzodiazepine to stop the seizure
         (a) First choice: lorazepam (Ativan) (Table 7-23)
         (b) Second choice: diazepam (Valium) (Table 7-23)
      (2) Agents to prevent recurrence to be given after benzodiazepine
         (a) Phenytoin (Dilantin) (Table 7-23)
         (b) Fosphenytoin (Cerebyx) (Table 7-23)
         (c) Phenobarbital (Table 7-23)
      (3) Other agents for refractory status epilepticus
         (a) Pentobarbital (Nembutal)
         (b) Midazolam (Versed)
         (c) Propofol (Diprivan)
         (d) Rarely used IV agents: thiopental, valproic acid, etomidate, paraldehyde, lidocaine
         (e) Rarely used inhalation anesthetics: halothane, isoflurane, nitrous oxide
      (4) Monitor patient closely for hypotension; administer fluids as prescribed
      (5) Monitor patient for respiratory depression; ventilation with manual resuscitation bag and mask may be required; endotracheal intubation may be required
      (6) Reduce the infusion rate as prescribed after at least 12 hours without seizures
      (7) Monitor serum drug concentrations and adjust drug dosages as prescribed to maintain optimal levels
   d. Prepare patient for surgical procedures that may be required for removal of tumor, hematoma, or abscess.
5. Monitor patient and document duration of seizure activity, patient's LOC, and drugs.
   a. Aura: presence or absence; nature if present
   b. Cry: presence or absence
   c. Onset: site of initial body movements; deviation of head and eyes; chewing and salivation; posture of body; sensory changes
   d. Tonic and clonic phases: movement of body during progression; skin color and airway; pupillary changes; incontinence; duration of each phase

Table 7-23 Anticonvulsant Drugs

Drug	Intravenous Dosage	Time to Stop Seizure; Duration of Anticonvulsant Effect	Adverse Effects
Lorazepam (Ativan)	0.1 mg/kg (not to exceed 8 mg/kg) at a rate no faster than 2 mg/min	6-10 minutes; 12-24 hours	• Respiratory depression • Tachycardia • Hypotension • Dysrhythmias
Diazepam (Valium)	0.15-0.25 mg/kg at a rate of no faster than 5 mg/min	1-3 minutes; 30 minutes	• Respiratory depression • Tachycardia • Hypotension • Dysrhythmias
Phenytoin sodium (Dilantin)	10-20 mg/kg at rate no faster than 50 mg/min; must be mixed in saline	30 minutes; 24 hours	• Hypotension • Dysrhythmias; blocks • Hepatitis • Nephritis • Blood dyscrasias
Fosphenytoin (Cerebyx)	15-20 mg/kg phenytoin equivalent at rate no faster than 150 mg/min; may be administered intramuscularly	15 minutes; 24 hours	• Hypotension (less risk than phenytoin) • Dysrhythmias (less risk than phenytoin) • Nephritis • Blood dyscrasias
Phenobarbital (Luminal)	20 mg/kg at rate no faster than 50 mg/min (not actively seizing) or 100 mg/min (actively seizing)	20-30 minutes; 48 hours	• Respiratory depression • Hypotension • Angioedema • Thrombophlebitis

e. Relaxation phase: duration and behavior
f. Postictal phase: duration; ability to remember anything about the seizure; orientation; pupillary changes; headache; injuries
g. Duration: from aura to relaxation
h. Drugs administered

6. Monitor and assess condition closely to prevent complications.
   a. Insert nasogastric tube to prevent vomiting and aspiration.
   b. Monitor cardiac rate and rhythm and blood pressure.
   c. Have cardiovascular drugs available.
   d. Assess neurologic status frequently.
7. Provide reassurance and comfort during postictal period.
   a. Elevate HOB 30 degrees.
   b. Reassure and reorient patient on awakening.
   c. Provide privacy and calm environment.
   d. Discreetly clean patient if he or she was incontinent.
   e. Allow the patient to sleep.
8. Maintain fluid and electrolyte balance.
   a. Assess electrolytes, calcium and magnesium, and renal and hepatic function.
   b. Monitor for indications of myoglobinuria (e.g., cola-colored urine); administer treatment for myoglobinuria as prescribed (fluids and osmotic diuretics [e.g., mannitol]).
9. Monitor for complications.
   a. Injury during seizure
   b. Acute respiratory failure
   c. Aspiration
   d. Acid-base imbalance, electrolyte imbalance
      (1) Respiratory or metabolic acidosis
      (2) Hyperkalemia
   e. Hypoglycemia: Monitor serum glucose and administer parenteral dextrose as required.
   f. Hyperthermia: Treat body temperature greater than 40° C with antipyretics and/or hypothermia blanket.
   g. Renal failure related to myoglobinuria
      (1) Monitor serum creatine kinase to detect rhabdomyolysis, and note change in urine color (i.e., cola-colored) to detect myoglobinuria.
      (2) Treat myoglobinuria with fluids, mannitol, and sodium bicarbonate as prescribed.
   h. Residual neurologic deficits

Central Nervous System Infections

Definitions

1. Meningitis: acute inflammation of the brain and spinal cord that may involve all meningeal membranes; may be bacterial, fungal, or viral
2. Encephalitis: acute inflammation of the parenchyma of the brain and meninges

3. Brain abscess: accumulation of pus within the brain tissue; surrounded by inflamed tissue

Etiology

1. Meningitis
   a. Bacterial
      (1) Associated factors
         (a) Otitis media
         (b) Sinusitis, upper respiratory infection, or pneumonia
         (c) Penetrating head injury
         (d) Basal skull fracture
         (e) Intracranial surgery
         (f) ICP monitoring
         (g) Septicemia, septic embolus
      (2) Organisms
         (a) *Haemophilus influenzae*
         (b) *Neisseria meningitidis* (meningococcal)
         (c) *Diplococcus pneumoniae* (pneumococcal)
         (d) *Streptococcus pneumoniae*
         (e) *Escherichia coli*
         (f) *Enterobacter* species
         (g) *Klebsiella* species
         (h) *Pseudomonas* species
         (i) *Serratia*
         (j) *Salmonella*
         (k) Gonococcus
   b. Fungal
      (1) Associated factors
         (a) Immunosuppression
            (i) Acquired immunodeficiency syndrome
            (ii) Histoplasmosis
            (iii) After organ transplantation
            (iv) Steroid therapy
            (v) Cancer
         (b) Contaminated needles or syringes from drug abuse
      (2) Organisms
         (a) Cryptococcosis
         (b) Coccidioidomycosis
         (c) Mucormycosis
         (d) Candidiasis
         (e) Aspergillosis
   c. Viral
      (1) Associated factors
         (a) Immunosuppression
      (2) Organisms
         (a) Coxsackievirus
         (b) Echovirus
         (c) Adenovirus
         (d) Arbovirus
         (e) Poliovirus
         (f) Herpes simplex virus
         (g) Myxovirus (e.g., influenza, mumps, and measles)
         (h) Western equine encephalomyelitis virus *(Alphavirus)*
   d. Parasitic
      (1) *Plasmodium* (malaria)
      (2) *Toxoplasma gondii*
2. Encephalitis (almost always viral)
   a. Associated factors
      (1) Mosquito or tick bite (arbovirus)
      (2) Recent viral infection
      (3) Recent vaccination: measles; mumps; rubella
      (4) Immunocompromise
   b. Organisms
      (1) Arbovirus (e.g., West Nile virus and eastern equine encephalitis)
      (2) Herpes simplex
      (3) Rubella
      (4) Rubeola
      (5) Mumps
      (6) Mononucleosis
3. Brain abscess
   a. Associated factors
      (1) Middle ear and mastoid infection
      (2) Sinus infection
      (3) Penetrating head injuries, skull fractures
      (4) Compound fractures
      (5) Osteomyelitis of the skull
      (6) Neurosurgical or oral surgical procedures
      (7) Metastatic abscess
   b. Organisms
      (1) Streptococci
      (2) Staphylococci
      (3) Pneumococci

Pathophysiology

1. Meningitis
   a. Pathologic organisms gain access to subarachnoid space and meninges.
   b. Exudate forms in subarachnoid space, and inflammation of meninges occurs.
   c. Congestion of tissues and blood vessels occurs.
   d. Hyperemia of meningeal vessels occurs.
   e. Intracranial hypertension may result from hydrocephalus or brain edema.
2. Encephalitis: Virus acts as an intracellular parasite damaging the nervous system by destroying selected neuronal cells.
3. Brain abscess
   a. Bacteria are introduced into the brain tissue.
   b. Local edema, hyperemia, infiltration by leukocytes, and softening of the parenchyma occur.
   c. Surrounding brain tissue becomes necrotic and edematous.
   d. Central liquefaction occurs and becomes encapsulated.
   e. The abscess acts as a mass lesion and may cause intracranial hypertension.

Clinical Presentation

1. Meningitis
   a. Subjective
      (1) History of precipitating event or condition
      (2) Headache that gets progressively worse
      (3) Chills
      (4) Nausea, vomiting
      (5) Photophobia, pain when moving eyes

b. Objective
   (1) Infectious signs
      (a) Fever
      (b) Tachycardia
      (c) Chills
      (d) Skin rash: most likely with meningococcal meningitis
   (2) Meningeal irritation
      (a) Headache
      (b) Nuchal rigidity
      (c) Brudzinski's sign
      (d) Kernig's sign
   (3) Neurologic abnormalities
      (a) Change in LOC
      (b) Confusion, delirium
      (c) Cranial nerve involvement (e.g., pupil changes)
      (d) Focal neurologic signs
      (e) Seizures
c. Diagnostic
   (1) Serum
      (a) Blood cultures: may be positive for causative organism
      (b) WBC count: elevated
   (2) LP
      (a) Elevated CSF pressure (normal LP pressure is 80 to 180 cm H_2O, measured at lumbar level, with patient in side-lying position)
      (b) Increased WBC count in CSF
      (c) Elevated protein in CSF in most cases
      (d) Decreased glucose content in CSF in bacterial meningitis (glucose in CSF is normally 60% of serum glucose)
      (e) CSF is cloudy in bacterial meningitis
      (f) Glucose content in CSF is normal, and CSF is clear in viral meningitis
      (g) Culture: may identify organism
   (3) CT: normal, but CT scan of the head frequently and routinely is obtained before the performance of an LP to identify occult intracranial abnormalities and avoid the risk of brainstem herniation resulting from the LP

2. Encephalitis
   a. Subjective
      (1) History may include precipitating event or condition (e.g., mosquito or tick bite or contact with dead or sick bird)
      (2) Headache
      (3) Blurred vision, diplopia, photophobia
      (4) Weakness
      (5) Dysphagia
      (6) Gastrointestinal symptoms may occur
   b. Objective
      (1) Change in LOC: lethargy, coma
      (2) Fever
      (3) Nuchal rigidity
      (4) Dysphasia, aphasia
      (5) Hemiparesis
      (6) Nystagmus
      (7) Facial muscle weakness
      (8) Seizures
      (9) Hallucinations
      (10) Parkinsonian-like rigidity in tick-borne viral encephalitis
   c. Diagnostic
      (1) LP
         (a) Elevated or normal pressure
         (b) Elevated protein
         (c) Increased WBC count
         (d) Normal or low glucose
         (e) Culture: may identify organism
      (2) Brain biopsy: required for diagnosis of herpes simplex encephalitis
      (3) EEG: may show seizure activity
      (4) CT: normal early in course; later low-density lesions may be seen
      (5) MRI: may be more definitive than CT scan
      (6) Immunoglobulin M antibody to West Nile virus for West Nile encephalitis in serum or CSF

3. Brain abscess
   a. Subjective
      (1) History may include precipitating event or condition
      (2) Headache: constant and severe; increased with straining
      (3) Malaise
      (4) Irritability
      (5) Chills
      (6) Nausea, vomiting
      (7) Muscle weakness
      (8) Symptoms vary according to location of brain
   b. Objective
      (1) Change in LOC
      (2) Confusion
      (3) Hemiplegia
      (4) Fever
      (5) Nuchal rigidity may be present
      (6) Dysphasia/aphasia
      (7) Seizures
      (8) Signs vary according to location of brain
   c. Diagnostic
      (1) CT scan: may show localized changes in brain density
      (2) EEG: may show electrical silence at abscess location
      (3) LP
         (a) Increased pressure
         (b) Increased WBC count
         (c) Elevated protein
         (d) Normal glucose
      (4) Brain biopsy: may identify organism
      (5) Brain scan: locates abscess greater than 1 cm in size
      (6) Arteriogram: locate temporal lobe and cerebellar abscesses

Nursing Diagnoses

1. Decreased Adaptive Capacity: Intracranial related to failure of normal intracranial compensatory mechanisms

2. Ineffective Cerebral Tissue Perfusion related to intracranial hypertension
3. Pain related to injury
4. Ineffective Airway Clearance related to increased secretions, diminished LOC, and inadequate protective reflexes
5. Risk for Deficient Fluid Volume related to decreased fluid intake, increased fluid loss, and DI
6. Risk for Excess Fluid Volume related to fluid resuscitation and SIADH
7. Risk for Infection related to invasive procedures, traumatic wounds, and surgical wounds
8. Risk for Injury related to seizure activity and inadequate protective reflexes
9. Interrupted Family Processes related to situational crisis, powerlessness, and change in role

Collaborative Management

1. Maintain airway, ventilation, and oxygenation.
   a. Maintain airway.
      (1) Oropharyngeal or nasopharyngeal airway may be needed to hold tongue away from hypopharynx in obtunded patient.
      (2) Endotracheal intubation may be needed in patients without airway protective reflexes.
   b. Maintain oxygenation and ventilation.
      (1) Administer oxygen as needed to maintain Spo_2, greater than or equal to 95% unless contraindicated.
      (2) Initiate mechanical ventilation as needed for hypoventilation.
   c. Prevent aspiration.
      (1) Position patient on side.
      (2) Have suction equipment available.
2. Treat infection.
   a. Administer antibiotics (need to be fat-soluble to cross blood-brain barrier) to treat bacterial infection as prescribed.
   b. Administer antivirals to treat herpes simplex encephalitis as prescribed.
   c. Prepare patient for surgical excision and drainage of brain abscess.
3. Prevent and monitor for clinical indications, and treat intracranial hypertension (see Intracranial Hypertension).
   a. Steroids may be prescribed to decrease inflammation in bacterial meningitis: dexamethasone (Decadron) usually is prescribed before or with the first dose of antibiotics.
4. Maintain fluid and electrolyte balance.
   a. Administer fluids IV as prescribed.
   b. Monitor for overhydration and DI.
5. Control body temperature to less than 38° C.
   a. Administer antipyretics.
   b. Use hypothermia blanket.
   c. Use drugs (e.g., meperidine [Demerol]) as prescribed to control shivering.
6. Prevent, and monitor for, and control seizures.
   a. Institute seizure precautions.
   b. Administer anticonvulsant therapy as prescribed.
7. Treat headache with nonsedating analgesics (e.g., codeine).
8. Prevent transmission of disease.
   a. Universal precautions are adequate for most patients with CNS infections.
   b. Droplet precautions.
      (1) *Haemophilus influenzae* and *Neisseria meningitidis* (meningococcal) may be transmitted by droplets generated during coughing, sneezing, talking, intubation, and bronchoscopy, so initiate droplet precautions if there is a clinical suspicion of one of these pathogens.
      (2) Continue these precautions for 24 hours after the start of effective antibiotic therapy until another organism is confirmed.
   c. Antibiotic prophylaxis for close contacts is indicated for *Haemophilus influenzae* and *Neisseria meningitidis* (meningococcal).
   d. Vaccination
      (1) Vaccination for *Haemophilus influenzae* now is incorporated into the routine immunization schedule for children.
      (2) Vaccination for four serogroups of meningococcus (i.e., quadrivalent meningococcal vaccine) is recommended for high-risk populations, including military recruits, people traveling to an area with high risk of meningococcal disease, college students living in dormitories, and patients after splenectomy.
      (3) Pneumococcal vaccine is thought to be about 50% effected in preventing pneumococcal meningitis.
9. Monitor for complications.
   a. Seizures: prophylactic anticonvulsant may be prescribed
   b. Disseminated intravascular coagulation
   c. Fluid and electrolyte imbalance: DI, SIADH, CSWS (see Craniotomy)
   d. Brain edema and intracranial hypertension
   e. Subdural effusions
   f. Hydrocephalus
   g. Cranial nerve deficits
   h. Waterhouse-Friderichsen syndrome
      (1) A major complication of meningococcal meningitis
      (2) Overwhelming bacteremia with massive bilateral adrenal hemorrhage
      (3) Causes acute adrenal crisis and potentially death
   i. Residual neurologic deficits (e.g., motor or cognitive deficits, memory loss, hearing or vision loss, and seizure disorder)

LEARNING ACTIVITIES

1. Complete the following crossword puzzle related to neurologic anatomy and physiology.

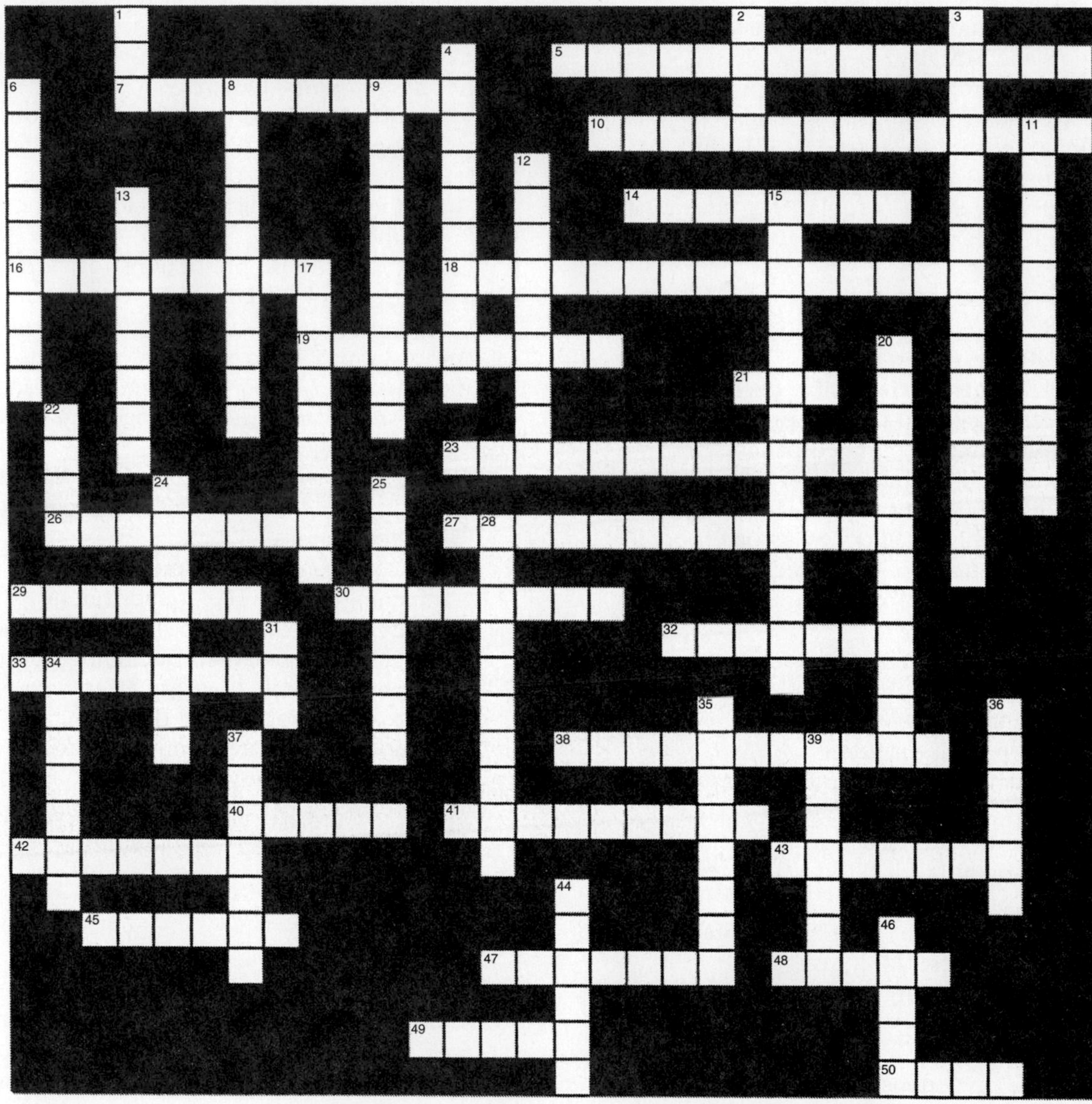

Across

5. The "steady state" branch of the ANS
7. A synapse between an axon of one neuron and the cell body of another neuron
10. The enzyme that breaks down acetylcholine
14. The cranial nerve that controls lateral eye movement
16. These nerve cells provide support, nourishment, and protection of the neurons
18. Neurons responsible for myelin formation in the CNS
19. The fold of the dura mater that separates the cerebral hemispheres from the cerebellum
21. Acts as a cushion for the brain and the spinal cord (abbreviation)
23. The division of the brain that contains the cerebral hemispheres
26. Neurons that transmit impulses to the spinal cord or brain
27. The primary neurotransmitter for the PNS
29. Unidirectional conduction of an impulse from one neuron to the next
30. The component of the neuron that conducts impulses toward the cell body
32. This portion of the brainstem contains the cardiac and respiratory centers
33. These neurons transmit impulses away from the spinal cord or brain
38. A neurotransmitter for the SNS
40. The cranial nerve that controls visual acuity
41. This nervous system contains sympathetic and parasympathetic branches

42. The nodes of _____ allow rapid conduction of impulses by saltatory conduction
43. Four paired masses of gray matter in the deeper layers of each hemisphere are called the basal _____
45. The coating or sheath that speeds transmission along the axon
47. The fissure that divides the frontal lobes from the temporal lobes
48. The foramen of _____ connects the lateral ventricles with the third ventricle
49. The shallow grooves on the surface of the brain
50. The component of the neuron that conducts impulses away from the cell body to other neurons or to end-organs

Down

1. The innermost layer of the meninges is the _____ mater
2. Convolutions on the surface of the brain
3. A chemical that acts as a bridge for transmission of impulses
4. The cranial nerve that controls the pupillary reaction
6. The middle layer of the meninges is the _____ mater
8. This structure extends from the brainstem to L2 (second lumbar) _____ (two words)
9. The cranial nerve that controls sensation on the face
11. The "fight or flight" branch of the ANS
12. These lobes control vision
13. These lobes control sensory function
15. The pathway between the two cerebral hemispheres (two words)
17. This type of cell forms the blood-brain barrier
20. The division of the brain that contains the thalamus, hypothalamus, and limbic system
22. The outermost layer of the meninges is the _____ mater
24. The lobes that control long-term memory
25. The bat-shaped bone that divides the interior of the cranium into three fossae
28. The part of the brain that coordinates muscle movement with sensory input
31. Cellular energy (abbreviation)
34. The posterior portion of these lobes controls voluntary motor function
35. Protective coverings of the brain and spinal cord
36. The cranial nerve that allows a smile
37. CSF is produced in capillary networks called _____ plexuses
39. The fissure that divides the frontal lobes from the parietal lobes
44. The circle of blood vessels that is formed by the internal carotid and vertebral arteries
46. _____'s area in the dominant frontal lobe is responsible for motor speech

2. Your patient has had a traumatic brain injury. His BP is 80/50 mm Hg, and his ICP is 20 mm Hg. Calculate his CPP. Should you be concerned? Why?

____

____

____

3. Identify the following physiologic alterations as being associated with either sympathetic or parasympathetic innervation.

	Sympathetic	Parasympathetic
Bronchodilation		
Coronary artery dilation		
Hypersalivation		
Increased blood glucose		
Increased perspiration		
Increased intestinal motility		
Pupil constriction		
Tachycardia		

4. Describe the following ventilatory patterns, and identify the site of a lesion that would cause them.

Pattern	Site of Lesion
CNS hyperventilation	
Cheyne-Stokes	
Cluster	
Ataxic	
Apneustic	

5. Name and identify how to assess the cranial nerves.

Number	Name	Method of Testing
I		
II		
III		
IV		
V		
VI		
VII		
VIII		
IX		
X		
XI		
XII		

6. List 10 factors that can increase ICP and that can be eliminated.

1. ______
2. ______
3. ______
4. ______
5. ______
6. ______
7. ______
8. ______
9. ______
10. ______

7. Identify six interventions that can decrease ICP, and identify whether they decrease brain mass, CSF, or blood.

Intervention	What Is Decreased?
1.	
2.	
3.	
4.	
5.	
6.	

8. Match the following sign or symptom associated with the neurologic condition.

a. Kernig's sign
b. Babinski's reflex
c. Absence of doll's eyes (oculocephalic reflex)
d. Change in LOC, pupillary changes, respiratory pattern changes, Cushing's triad
e. Periorbital edema
f. Battle's sign
g. Rhinorrhea
h. Personality change
i. "Worst headache of my life"
j. Myoglobinuria

___ 1. Brainstem lesion
___ 2. Chronic SDH
___ 3. SAH
___ 4. Status epilepticus
___ 5. Dural tear
___ 6. After craniotomy
___ 7. UMN lesion
___ 8. Meningeal irritation
___ 9. Intracranial hypertension
___10. Basal skull fracture

9. Your patient has had a hemorrhagic stroke. She has nuchal rigidity and decerebrate posturing. She does not vocalize at all and will not open her eyes even to pain. What is her GCS score? What grade bleed is this on the Hunt and Hess aneurysm grading scale?

______
______

10. Identify the following factors as being associated with which complication of SAH: vasospasm or rebleed.

	Vasospasm	Rebleed
Occurs most often immediately after the bleed or between 7 and 10 days after the bleed		
Caused by calcium influx into the vessel		
Occurs anytime after 3 days		
Treated by hypervolemic hemodilution and calcium channel blockers		
Caused by lysis of the protective clot		
Prevented by early clipping if the patient is stable enough		

11. List five ways that the use of fibrinolytic agents for ischemic stroke is different from use of fibrinolytic agents for myocardial infarction.

1. ______________________
2. ______________________
3. ______________________
4. ______________________
5. ______________________

12. Describe CSF changes in the following conditions.

Bacterial meningitis	
Viral meningitis	
SAH	

13. List five observations to make and interventions to perform during a seizure.

Observations to Make	Interventions
1.	
2.	
3.	
4.	
5.	

14. Complete the following crossword puzzle dealing with neurologic assessment, conditions, and treatment.

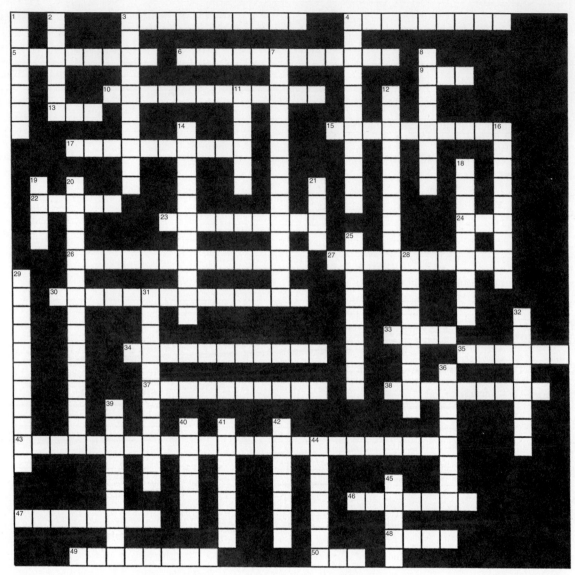

Across

3. The change in pressure for a given change in volume
4. A common oral anticonvulsant (generic)
5. The most common type of aneurysm
6. Rupture of an aneurysm sometimes is referred to as a _____ hemorrhage because the blood vessels are located in this area
9. This focal cerebral ischemia resolves within 24 hours (abbreviation)
10. This type of drug is used to lyse the clot in ischemic stroke
13. The most important assessment parameter in a patient with a neurologic condition (abbreviation)
15. CSF drainage from the nose
17. The calcium channel blocker most frequently used for cerebral vasospasm (generic)
22. This type of herniation is seen with unilateral conditions such as an EDH
23. The complication of cerebral aneurysm
24. This diagnostic study evaluates the electrical activity of the brain (abbreviation)
26. This reflex also is referred to as doll's eyes
27. Loss of sensation
30. This class of drug is used initially in status epilepticus
33. _____'s respiratory pattern is associated with a lesion of the lower pons or upper medulla
34. This type of posturing also is referred to as abnormal flexion
35. _____'s sign indicates meningeal irritation and is tested by extending the leg
37. This type of aphasia also is referred to as motor aphasia
38. Loss of motor function
43. A common cause of secondary injury in neurologic trauma patients
46. The type of paralysis seen with an LMN lesion
47. Basal skull fractures involving this fossa may cause rhinorrhea and injury to the olfactory nerve
48. A subjective sensation that often precedes a seizure
49. An abnormal weakness of an artery; most common intracranial location is in the circle of Willis
50. A severe injury to the brain that causes prolonged unconsciousness, brainstem dysfunction, and profound residual deficits (abbreviation)

Down

1. _____'s triad of vital sign changes is associated with intracranial hypertension
2. This type of rigidity is associated with meningeal irritation
3. The surgical procedure of opening the cranium
4. An abnormal sensitivity to light
7. The intrinsic ability of the cerebral vessels to dilate or constrict to maintain adequate CBF
8. CSF drainage from the ear
11. This type of fracture may interrupt major vascular channels and cause EDH
12. Inflammation of the meninges
14. Uncal herniation causes dilation of the _____ pupil
16. This diagnostic procedure uses injection of a radiopaque dye to visualize the cerebrovascular system
18. This respiratory pattern is associated with a lesion in the mid to lower pons
19. This type of hole is drilled into the cranium to allow access for aspiration of a clot or placement of an intracranial catheter
20. Testing for this reflex is also referred to as caloric testing
21. A state of unconsciousness in which the patient cannot be awakened
25. Diabetes _____ is a complication of craniotomy or brain trauma that causes polyuria and hemoconcentration
28. This type of herniation occurs when the brainstem is pushed downward through the foramen magnum
29. The two types of stroke are ischemic and _____
31. This type of posturing also is referred to as abnormal extension
32. A common IV osmotic diuretic (generic)
36. This pathologic reflex indicates an UMN lesion
39. This type of aphasia also is referred to as sensory aphasia
40. Basal skull fracture of this fossa causes otorrhea and Battle's sign
41. The common scoring system used to standardize observations of responsiveness in neurologic patients
42. This type of paralysis is seen with an UMN lesion
44. This complication of cerebral aneurysm is most likely to occur about 7 to 10 days after the initial bleed
45. This type of skull fracture is associated with raccoon eyes or Battle's sign

LEARNING ACTIVITIES ANSWERS

1.

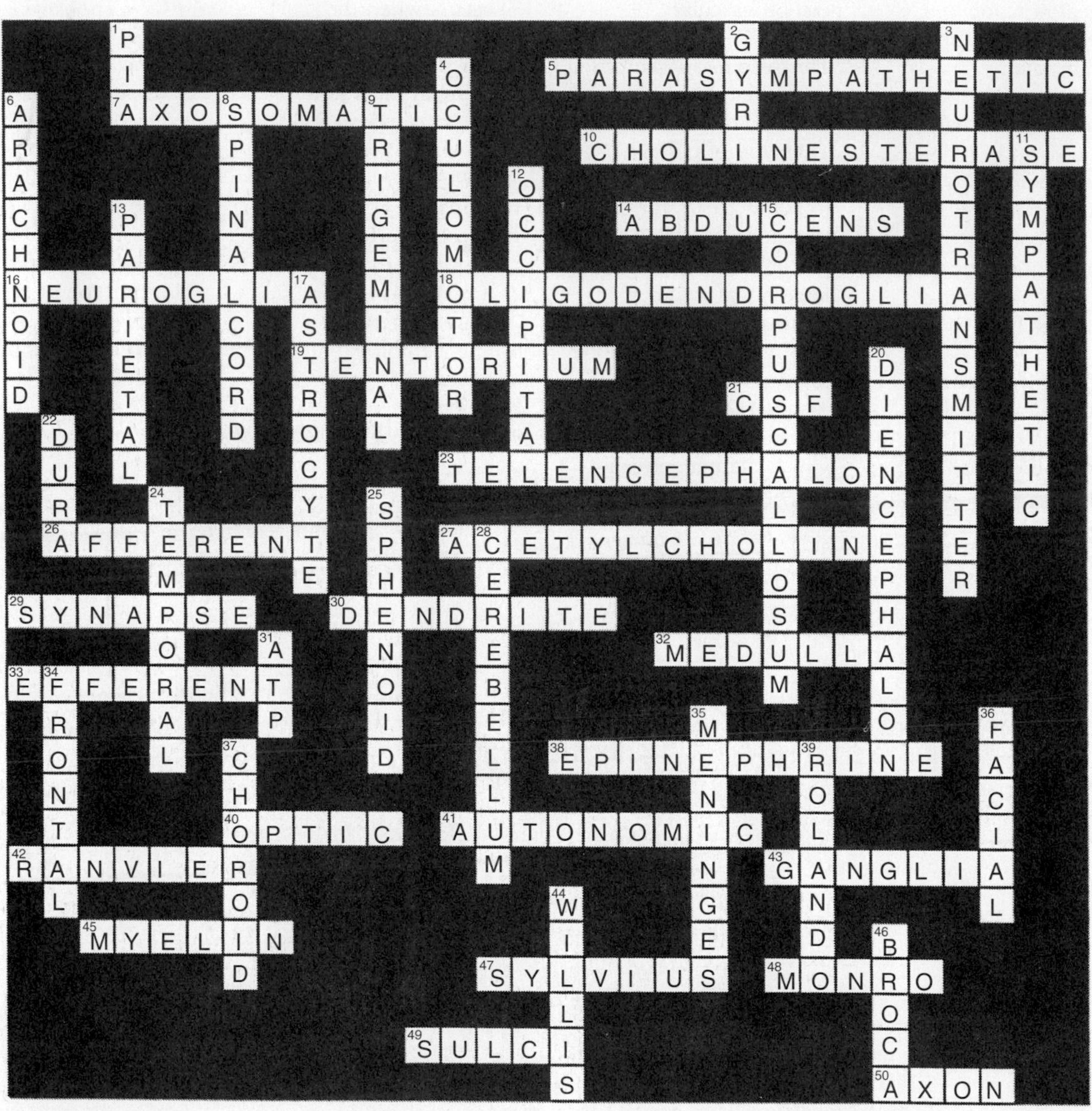

2.

To calculate MAP, use the following formula: [SBP + (DBP × 2)] ÷ 3. 80 + (2 × 50) = 180; then divide by 3, which gives 60 (where *SBP* is systolic blood pressure and *DBP* is diastolic blood pressure)

To calculate CPP, use the following formula: MAP − ICP: 60 − 20 = 40 mm Hg (where *MAP* is mean arterial pressure and *ICP* is intracranial pressure)

Should you be concerned? YES! CPP less than 50 mm Hg is associated with loss of autoregulation, hypoperfusion of the brain, and anoxic encephalopathy.

3.

	Sympathetic	Parasympathetic
Bronchodilation	x	
Coronary artery dilation	x	
Hypersalivation		x
Increased blood glucose	x	
Increased perspiration	x	
Increased intestinal motility		x
Pupil constriction		x
Tachycardia	x	

4.

Pattern	Site of Lesion
CNS hyperventilation	Lower midbrain or upper pons
Cheyne-Stokes	Cerebral hemispheres, basal ganglia, cerebellar lesion, or upper brainstem
Cluster (or Biot's)	Lower pons or upper medulla
Ataxic	Medulla
Apneustic	Mid to lower pons

5.

I	Olfactory	Evaluate the patient's ability to identify familiar odors
II	Optic	Evaluate visual acuity using Snellen chart or newsprint Evaluate the optic disk during funduscopic examination
III	Oculomotor	Evaluate the ability to open eyes widely Check size, shape, position, and reactivity of the pupils Have patient follow your finger with their eyes through the six cardinal positions of gaze Look for abnormal eye movement
IV	Trochlear	Have patient follow your finger with their eyes through the six cardinal positions of gaze
V	Trigeminal	Evaluate ability of the patient to detect light touch, superficial pain, and temperature on forehead, cheeks, and jaw Touch the cornea with a wisp of cotton and check for bilateral blink Palpate the strength of the masseter muscles with the patient clenching his teeth and the strength of the temporal muscles with the patient squeezing his eyes shut
VI	Abducens	Have patient follow your finger with their eyes through the six cardinal positions of gaze
VII	Facial	Ask the patient to smile and assess symmetry Test the patient's ability to taste salt and sugar on the anterior tongue
VIII	Acoustic	Evaluate ability of the patient to hear when speaking at normal voice tones Note any vertigo, nystagmus, nausea, vomiting, pallor, sweating, or hypotension
IX	Glossopharyngeal	Evaluate patient's ability to speak; note any hoarseness Look for bilateral elevation of the palate with phonation Test the patient's ability to taste sour and bitter on the posterior tongue Evaluate the patient's ability to swallow Test the gag reflex by stroking the palate with a tongue blade and looking for gag reflex Evaluate cough reflex by touching the hypopharynx with a suction catheter
X	Vagus	Tested with glossopharyngeal
XI	Spinal accessory	Ask the patient to shrug his or her shoulders as you push down on them with your hands Palpate the sternocleidomastoid and trapezius muscles for size and symmetry
XII	Hypoglossal	Look for midline alignment when the patient protrudes his or her tongue Look for fasciculations of the tongue

6.

1. Neck twisting or flexion
2. Valsalva maneuver
3. Airway obstruction
4. Pain or noxious stimuli
5. Disturbing conversation
6. Noise
7. Bright lights
8. Tight tracheostomy ties or cervical collar
9. Seizure activity
10. Hyperthermia

7.

Intervention	What Is Decreased?
1. Hyperventilation to cause respiratory alkalosis	Blood
2. Maintenance of euvolemia	Brain edema
3. Mannitol	Brain edema
4. Furosemide	Brain edema, CSF
5. Ventriculostomy and CSF drainage	CSF
6. Barbiturate coma	Blood

8.

c 1. Brainstem lesion
h 2. Chronic SDH
i 3. SAH
j 4. Status epilepticus
g 5. Dural tear
e 6. After craniotomy
b 7. UMN lesion
a 8. Meningeal irritation
d 9. Intracranial hypertension
f 10. Basal skull fracture

9.

GCS score: 4
Hunt and Hess aneurysm grade: V

10.

	Vasospasm	Rebleed
Occurs most often immediately after the bleed or between 7 and 10 days after the bleed		x
Caused by calcium influx into the vessel	x	
Occurs anytime after 3 days	x	
Treated by hypervolemic hemodilution and calcium channel blockers	x	
Caused by lysis of the protective clot		x
Prevented by early clipping if the patient is stable enough		x

11. List five ways that the use of fibrinolytic agents for ischemic stroke is different from use of fibrinolytic agents for myocardial infarction.

1. Dose: 0.9 mg/kg with maximum dose of less than or equal to 90 mg, with the initial bolus being 10% of this total dose over 1 minute and the remaining 90% of this total dose being infused over 60 minutes
2. Time frame: within 3 hours of the initial symptoms
3. Adjuvant therapy: no anticoagulants or platelet aggregation agents for the first 24 hours
4. Additional contraindications: awakening with symptoms (eliminates ability to determine time of onset of symptoms) and seizure at onset of symptoms (increases risk that the stroke is hemorrhagic rather than ischemic)
5. Additional contraindications including seizure at symptom onset and awakening with symptoms

12.

Bacterial meningitis	Elevated pressure Increased WBC count Normal or elevated protein Decreased glucose Cloudy appearance
Viral meningitis	Elevated pressure Normal or increased WBC count Normal or elevated protein Clear appearance
SAH	Elevated protein Bloody appearance if acute Dark amber (xanthochromic) if more than 5 days old

13.

Observations to Make	Interventions
Preceding events: Was there an aura?	Do not leave patient; provide privacy
Onset: • Body movements • Deviation of head and eyes • Chewing and salivation • Posture of body • Sensory changes	Loosen clothing
Tonic and clonic phases: • Progression of movements of the body • Skin color and airway • Pupillary changes • Incontinence • Duration of each phase	Open airway but do not try to pry mouth open; nasopharyngeal or nasotracheal airways may be used if necessary
LOC during seizure	Turn patient to side
Postictal phase • Duration • General behavior • Memory of events • Orientation • Pupillary changes • Headache • Aphasia • Injuries	Administer oxygen
Duration of entire seizure	Do not restrain; gentle guiding of extremities is acceptable
Medications given and response	Pad side rails with blankets or pillows Administer anticonvulsants such as diazepam or phenytoin Reorient patient after seizure Clean patient if incontinence has occurred Allow patient to sleep

14.

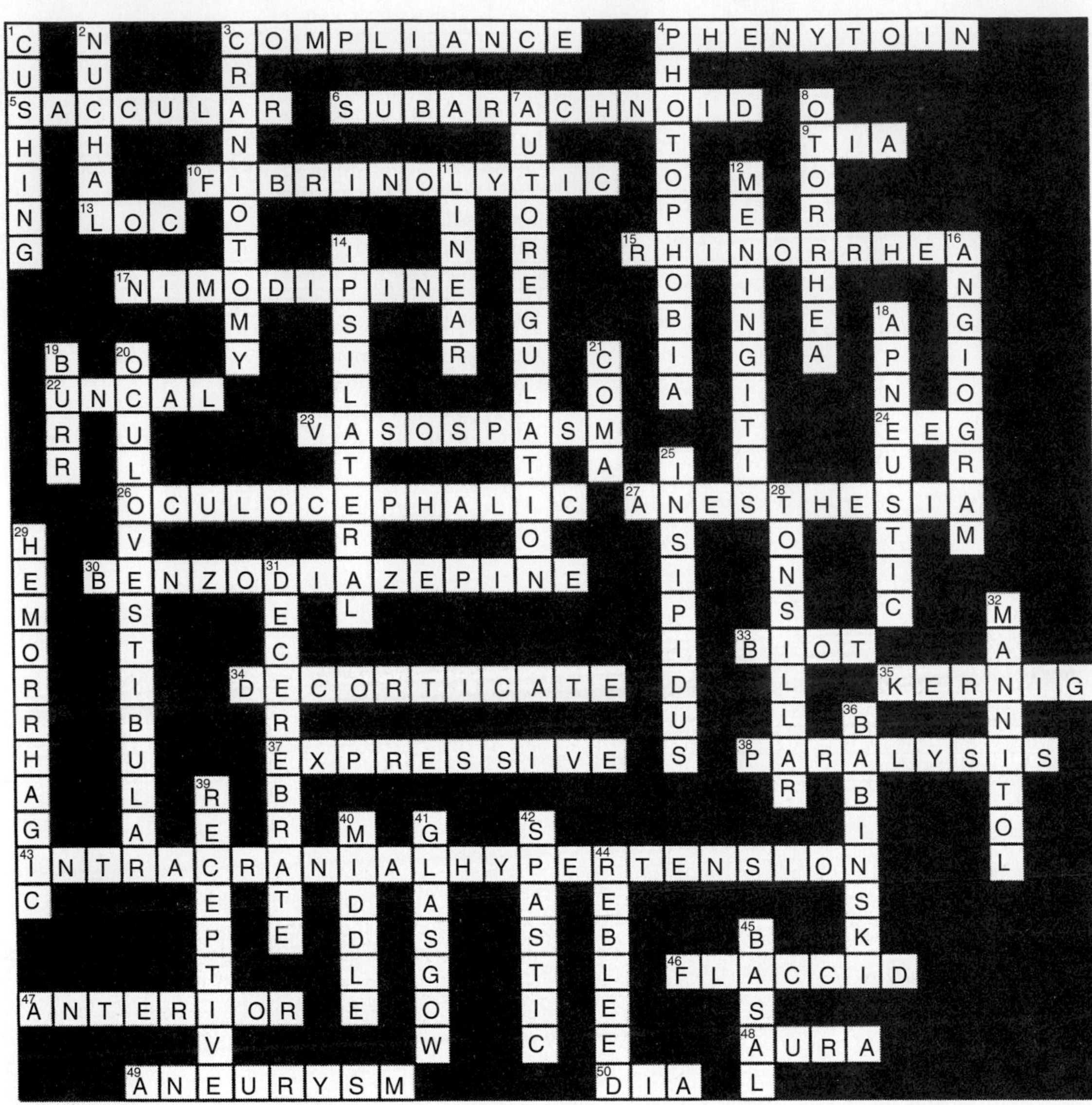

References

American Heart Association. (2005). Part 9: Adult stroke. *Circulation, 112*(24 suppl.), IV111-IV120.

Haymore, J. (2004). A neuron in a haystack: Advanced neurologic assessment. *AACN Clinical Issues, 15*(4), 568-581.

Bibliography

Albers, G. W., Amarenco, P., Easton, J. D., Sacco, R. L., & Teal, P. (2001). Antithrombotic and thrombolytic therapy for ischemic stroke. *Chest, 119*(Suppl.), 300S-320S.

Arbour, R. (2004). Intracranial hypertension: Monitoring and nursing assessment. *Critical Care Nurse, 24*(5), 19-34.

Aronin, S. I., & Quagliarello, V. J. (2003). Bacterial meningitis. *Infectious Medicine, 20*(3), 142-153.

Balas, M. C., Gale, M., & Kagan, S. H. (2004). Delirium doulas: An innovative approach to enhance care for critically ill older adults. *Critical Care Nurse, 24*(4), 36-46.

Barker, E. (2002). *Neuroscience nursing: A spectrum of care.* St. Louis, MO: Mosby.

Bender, K., & Thompson, F. E., Jr. (2003). West nile virus: A growing challenge. *American Journal of Nursing, 103*(6), 32-40.

Bond, A. E., Draeger, C. R. L., Mandleco, B., & Donnelly, M. (2003). Needs of family members of patients with severe traumatic brain injury: Implications for evidence-based practice. *Critical Care Nurse, 23*(4), 63-72.

Clay, H. D. (2000). Validity and reliability of the SjO_2 catheter in neurologically impaired patients: A critical review of the literature. *Journal of Neuroscience Nursing, 32*(4), 194-203.

Coles, J. P., Minhas, P. S., Fryer, T. D., Smielewski, P., Aigbirihio, F., Donovan, T., et al. (2002). Effect of hyperventilation on cerebral blood flow in traumatic head injury: Clinical relevance and monitoring correlates. *Critical Care Medicine, 30*(9), 1950-1959.

Fedorov, E. (2001). Helping patients with aphasia. *American Journal of Nursing, 101*(1), 24GG-24KK.

Friedman, J. A., Anderson, R. E., & Meyer, F. B. (2000). Techniques of intraoperative cerebral blood flow measurement. *Neurosurgical Focus, 9*(5), 1-5.

Harrington, C. (2003). Managing hypertension in patients with stroke: Are you prepared for labetalol infusion? *Critical Care Nurse, 23*(3), 30-38.

Henneman, E. A., & Karras, G. E. (2004). Determining brain death in adults: A guideline for use in critical care. *Critical Care Nurse, 24*(5), 50-56.

Hilton, G. (2001). Acute head injury: Distinguishing subdural from epidural hematoma. *American Journal of Nursing, 101*(9), 51-52.

Hinkle, J. L. (2002). SPECT: A powerful imaging tool. *American Journal of Nursing, 102*(3), 24A-24G.

Hinkle, J. (2005). An update on transient ischemic attacks. *Journal of Neuroscience Nursing, 37*(5), 243-248.

Johnson, A. L., & Criddle, L. M. (2004). Pass the salt: Indications for and implications of using hypertonic saline. *Critical Care Nurse, 24*(5), 36-48.

Kidd, K. C., & Criddle, L. M. (2001). Using jugular venous catheters in patients with traumatic brain injury. *Critical Care Nurse, 21*(6), 16-24.

Kruse, J. A., Fink, M. P., & Carlson, R. W. (2003). *Saunders manual of critical care.* Philadelphia: Saunders.

LeJeune, M., & Howard-Fain, T. (2002). Caring for patients with increased intracranial pressure. *Nursing 2002, 32*(11), 32cc31-32cc35.

Lemke, D. M. (2004). Riding out the storm: Sympathetic storming after traumatic brain injury. *Journal of Neuroscience Nursing, 36*(1), 4-9.

Littlejohns, L. R., & Bader, M. K. (2001). Guidelines for the management of severe head injury: Clinical application and changes in practice. *Critical Care Nurse, 21*(6), 48-65.

Littlejohns, L. R., Bader, M. K., & March, K. (2003). Brain tissue oxygen monitoring in severe brain injury: I. Research and usefulness in critical care. *Critical Care Nurse, 23*(4), 17-44.

March, K. (2000). Intracranial pressure monitoring and assessing intracranial compliance in brain injury. *Critical Care Nursing Clinics of North America, 12*(4), 429-436.

Mihailoff, G., & Briar, C. (2005). *Crash course: Nervous system.* Philadelphia: Elsevier.

Murphy, J. (2003). Pharmacological treatment of acute ischemic stroke. *Critical Care Nursing Quarterly, 26*(4), 276-282.

Nasraway, S. A., Jr., Wu, E. C., Kelleher, R. M., Yasuda, C. M., & Donnelly, A. M. (2002). How reliable is the bispectral index in critically ill patients? A prospective, comparable, single-blinded observer study. *Critical Care Medicine, 30*(7), 1483-1487.

Nolan, S., Naylor, G., & Burns, M. (2003). Code gray: An organized approach to inpatient stroke. *Critical Care Nursing Quarterly, 26*(4), 296-302.

Oropello, J. M. (2004). Determination of brain death: Theme, variations, and preventable errors. *Critical Care Medicine, 32*(6), 1417-1418.

Oyama, K., & Criddle, L. M. (2004). Vasospasm after aneurysmal subarachnoid hemorrhage. *Critical Care Nurse, 24*(5), 58-67.

Pena, C. G. (2003). Seizure: A calm response and careful observation are crucial. *American Journal of Nursing, 103*(11), 73-81.

Schretzman, D. (2001). Acute ischemic stroke. *Dimensions of Critical Care Nursing, 20*(2), 14-20.

Singh, S., Bohn, D., Carlotti, A. P. C. P., Cusimano, M., Rutka, J. T., & Halperin, M. L. (2002). Cerebral salt wasting: Truths, fallacies, theories, and challenges. *Critical Care Medicine, 30*(11), 2575-2579.

Sole, M. L., Klein, D. G., & Moseley, M. J. (2005). *Introduction to critical care nursing* (4th ed.). Philadelphia: Elsevier Saunders.

Sommargren, C. E. (2002). Electrocardiographic abnormalities in patients with subarachnoid hemorrhage. *American Journal of Critical Care, 11*(1), 48-56.

Stillwell, S. B. (2000). When you suspect epidural hematoma. *American Journal of Nursing, 100*(9), 68-75.

Sullivan, J. (2000). Positioning of patients with severe traumatic brain injury: research-based practice. *Journal of Neuroscience Nursing, 32*(4), 204-209.

Urden, L., Stacy, K., & Lough, M. (2006). *Thelan's critical care nursing: Diagnosis and management* (5th ed.). St. Louis, MO: Mosby.

Vance, D. L. (2001). Treating acute ischemic stroke with intravenous alteplase. *Critical Care Nurse, 21*(4), 25-34.

Weiss, J. (2001). Assessing and managing the patient with headaches. *Dimensions of Critical Care Nursing, 20*(3), 15-23.

Wiegand, D. L.-M. J., & Carlson, K. K. (2005). *AACN procedure manual for critical care* (5th ed.). Philadelphia: W. B. Saunders.

Winkelman, C. (2000). Effect of backrest position on intracranial and cerebral perfusion pressures in traumatically brain-injured adults. *American Journal of Critical Care, 9*(6), 373-382.

Wojner, A. W., El-Mitwalli, A., & Alexandrov, A. V. (2002). Effect of head positioning on intracranial blood flow velocities in acute ischemic stroke: A pilot study. *Critical Care Nursing Quarterly, 24*(4), 57-66.

Wong, F. W. H. (2000). Prevention of secondary brain injury. *Critical Care Nurse, 20*(5), 18-26.

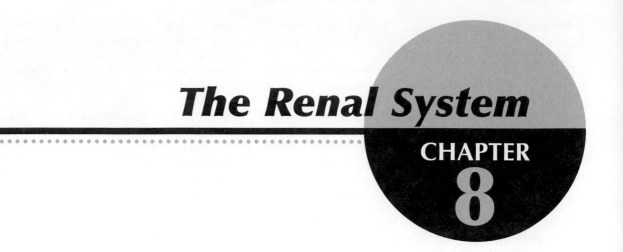

Selected Concepts in Anatomy and Physiology

General Information

1. Functions of the renal system
   a. Regulation of homeostasis and the internal environment of the body
      (1) Regulation of extracellular fluid volume
      (2) Regulation of extracellular fluid osmolality
      (3) Regulation of electrolyte balance
      (4) Excretion of metabolic wastes
      (5) Regulation of acid-base balance (in conjunction with the pulmonary system)
   b. Production and release of hormones
      (1) Regulation of blood pressure (BP) influenced by aldosterone and antidiuretic hormone (ADH)
      (2) Stimulation of red blood cell (RBC) production via erythropoietin
      (3) Synthesis and release of prostaglandins
   c. Participation in activation of vitamin D
2. Components of the renal system (Figure 8-1)
   a. Two kidneys
   b. Two ureters
   c. Urinary bladder
   d. Urethra

Functional Anatomy

1. General characteristics of the kidney
   a. Location of kidney
      (1) Posterior abdominal wall behind peritoneum
      (2) Opposite last thoracic and first three lumbar vertebrae on each side of spine
      (3) Right kidney slightly lower than left as a result of liver location
   b. Size, shape, weight of the kidney
      (1) Size: approximately $10 \times 5 \times 2.5$ cm or approximately fist sized
      (2) Shape: beanlike with convex lateral border and convex and concave medial border; long axis approximately vertical
      (3) Mass: 120 to 170 g per kidney
2. Extrarenal structures
   a. Renal capsule
      (1) Thin, smooth layer of fibrous membrane that surrounds each kidney
      (2) Acts as a protective layer
      (3) Prevents kidney swelling
      (4) Contains pain receptors
   b. Perirenal fat and renal fascia
      (1) Support and protect the kidney
      (2) Hold kidney in place
   c. Adrenal gland (also referred to as the *suprarenal gland*): rests on top of each kidney
   d. Hilum
      (1) Concave notch of medial aspect of kidney
      (2) Entry site for renal artery and nerves
      (3) Exit site for renal vein and ureter
   e. Ureters
      (1) Fibromuscular tubes located behind peritoneum; extend from kidney to posterior part of bladder floor
      (2) Ureter walls composed of smooth muscle with mucosa lining and fibrous outer coat
      (3) Collect urine from the renal pelvis and propel it to the bladder by peristaltic waves
      (4) Ureters enter the superior, posterior bladder at an oblique angle; this angle and the peristaltic action of the ureters prevent reflux of urine
   f. Bladder
      (1) Located behind symphysis pubis and below peritoneum
      (2) Collapsible bag of smooth muscle
      (3) Acts as a reservoir for urine until sufficient amount accumulates for elimination; expels urine from body by way of urethra
         (a) Adults void approximately 5 to 9 times per day
         (b) Volume of each voiding usually 100 to 300 mL but may be as much as 1 L
   g. Urethra
      (1) Located behind symphysis pubis, anterior to the vagina in females; extends through the prostate gland and penis in males
      (2) Acts as passageway for expulsion of urine from the urinary bladder to the urinary meatus, where it is expelled from the body

3. Renal structures (Figure 8-2)
   a. Renal parenchyma
      (1) Cortex
         (a) Approximately 1 cm wide, reddish-brown and granular appearance
         (b) Metabolically active portion of kidney where aerobic metabolism occurs and ammonia and glucose are formed
         (c) Site of glomerulus and proximal and distal tubules
      (2) Medulla
         (a) Approximately 5 cm wide, darker than cortex and striated
         (b) Composed of 6 to 10 pyramids formed by collecting tubules and ducts
            (i) Pyramids are triangular wedges of medullary tissue and are composed of collecting tubules
            (ii) Columns are inward extensions of cortical tissue between the pyramids; many of the blood vessels and nerves of the kidney are in these columns
            (iii) Renal lobe is composed of a pyramid and surrounding cortical tissue
         (c) Site of deepest part of Henle's loop
   b. Renal sinus: spacious cavity filled with adipose tissue, the renal pelvis, minor and major calyces, and the origin of the ureter
      (1) Calyces
         (a) Calyces are cuplike structures that drain the papillae.
         (b) Eight to 12 minor calyces open into 2 to 3 major calyces that form the renal pelvis.
      (2) Renal pelvis
         (a) Papillae are at the apices of the renal pyramids; collecting tubules drain into minor calyces at papillae.
         (b) Renal pelvis is like a small funnel tapering into the ureter and is formed by the union of several calyces.
         (c) Urine flows from collecting duct to renal pelvis and into the ureter.
   c. Nephron: microscopic functional unit of kidney (Figure 8-3)
      (1) Approximately 1 million in each kidney
      (2) Able to compensate for significant degree of nephron destruction by the following:
         (a) Filtering a greater solute (dissolved substances) load
         (b) Hypertrophy of remaining functional nephrons
      (3) Types of nephrons
         (a) Cortical (85% of nephrons are cortical nephrons)
            (i) The glomerulus is located in outer cortex.
            (ii) Cortical nephrons contain short loops of Henle that dip into the outer edge of the medulla.
         (b) Juxtamedullary (15% of nephrons are juxtamedullary nephrons)
            (i) The glomerulus is located in inner cortex.
            (ii) Juxtamedullary nephrons contain long loops of Henle that penetrate deep into medulla.
            (iii) These nephrons are important in the ability of the kidney to concentrate the urine.

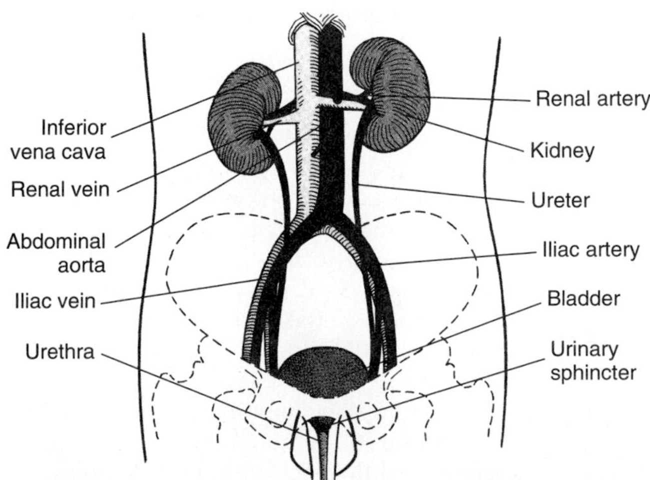

Figure 8-1 The kidneys and other structures of the urinary tract. (From Long, B. C., Phipps, W. J., & Cassmeyer, V. L. [1993]. *Medical-surgical nursing: A nursing process approach* [3rd ed.]. St. Louis: Mosby.)

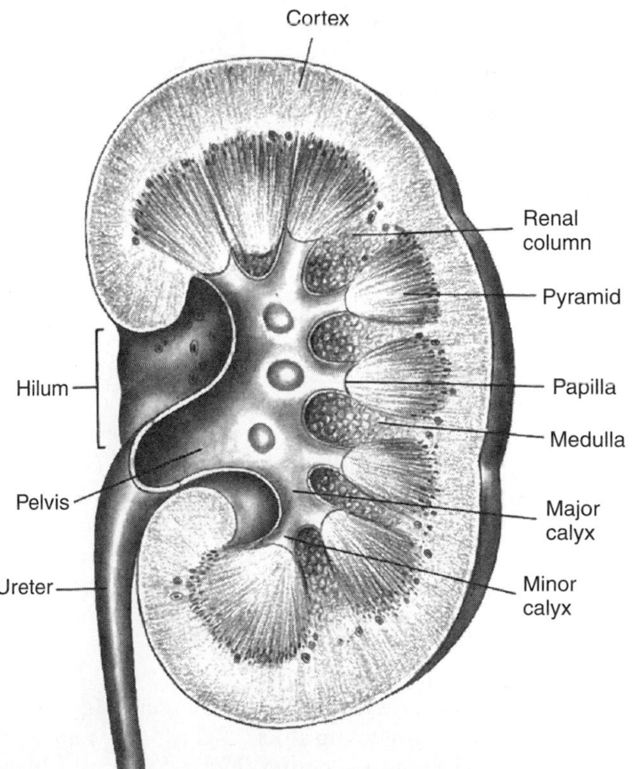

Figure 8-2 Cross-section of the kidney. (From Thompson, J. M., McFarland, G. K., Hirsch, J. E., & Tucker, S. M. [2002]. *Mosby's clinical nursing* [5th ed.]. St. Louis: Mosby.)

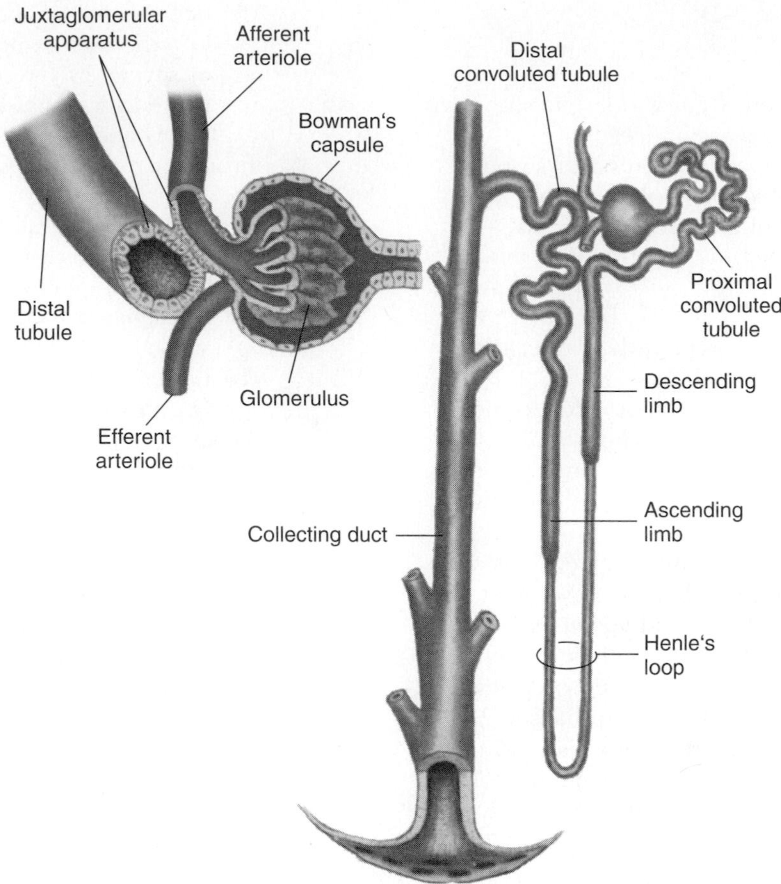

Figure 8-3 Components of the nephron. (From Urden, L. D., Stacy, K. M., & Lough, M. E. [2006]. *Thelan's critical care nursing: Diagnosis and management* [5th ed.]. St. Louis: Mosby.)

(4) Functional segments
  (a) Renal corpuscle: consists of Bowman's capsule and glomerulus
    (i) The glomerulus is a cluster of tightly coiled capillaries that produces an ultrafiltrate; a portion of this ultrafiltrate eventually becomes urine.
    (ii) Bowman's capsule is the funnel-shaped upper end of the proximal tubule.
  (b) Renal tubules
    (i) Segmentally divided into proximal convoluted tubule, loop of Henle, distal convoluted tubule
    (ii) Responsible for reabsorption and secretion, which alter the volume and composition of the ultrafiltration to form the final urine volume and composition
  (c) Collecting duct
    (i) Several nephrons converge into a collecting duct.
    (ii) The collecting duct relays the urine from the tubules to the minor calyx.

d. Renal vasculature
  (1) Pathway of blood supply
    (a) Renal arteries branch from the aorta.
    (b) The renal arteries branch into interlobar arteries, then arcuate arteries, and then interlobular arteries.
    (c) The interlobular arteries become the afferent arteriole, which forms the glomerulus.
    (d) The efferent arteriole leads out of the glomerulus and forms the peritubular capillary network.
    (e) The efferent arteriole from the juxtamedullary nephron forms a different capillary network called the *vasa recta*.
      (i) The vasa recta is a complex of long, straight capillary loops that run parallel to the ascending and descending loop of Henle.
      (ii) The vasa recta plays an important role in concentrating interstitial fluid found in the medulla.
      (iii) Blood flow through the vasa recta is sluggish.
    (f) The peritubular capillary network leads to the interlobular vein, which leads to the arcuate vein.

(g) The arcuate vein leads to the interlobar vein, which leads to the renal vein.
(h) The renal vein empties into the inferior vena cava.

(2) Renal blood flow
(a) The kidneys receives 20% to 25% of the cardiac output (CO), or approximately 1200 mL/min (600 mL/min for each kidney).
(b) Autoregulation maintains constancy in glomerular filtration rate (GFR).
(i) Systemic arterial pressure between 80 and 180 mm Hg prevents large changes in GFR because of the ability of the afferent arteriole to constrict or dilate.
a) Increases in mean arterial pressure (MAP) cause constriction of the afferent arteriole, which prevents the increased arterial pressure from raising the pressure in the glomerulus.
b) Decreases in MAP cause dilation of the afferent arteriole, so more blood is allowed to flow into the glomerulus.
(ii) Autoregulation fails at MAP of 80 mm Hg or less.

(3) Juxtaglomerular apparatus consists of the macula densa and the juxtaglomerular cells
(a) The macula densa is a part of the distal tubule that lies close to the afferent and efferent arterioles.
(b) Juxtaglomerular cells produce and store the enzyme renin, which is secreted in response to hypotension.

e. Lymphatics
(1) There is an abundant supply of lymphatic vessels to the kidney.
(2) Lymphatic vessels from the kidney drain into thoracic duct.

f. Nervous innervation
(1) The autonomic nervous system supplies the primary innervation of the kidney and the urinary tract.
(2) The renal plexus is formed by the superior splanchnic and inferior splanchnic nerves and enters the kidney at the hilum; the bladder, ureters, and urethra are supplied by the inferior mesenteric plexus, the hypogastric plexus, and the pudic nerve from the sacral region.
(3) The sympathetic nervous system (SNS) and parasympathetic nervous system innervate the kidney, but the SNS has the prominent effect on the kidney; SNS fiber endings are found in the afferent and efferent arterioles and in all sections of the tubule; effects on the kidney include the following:
(a) Low level: increased sodium reabsorption within the proximal tubule
(b) Moderate level: constriction of afferent and efferent arterioles decreases renal blood flow and GFR
(c) High level: predominant effect of afferent arteriole constriction; extreme reduction in renal blood flow and potential cessation of GFR

Physiology

1. Formation of urine involves three processes: filtration, reabsorption, and secretion (Figure 8-4); major functions of each portion of the nephron (Figure 8-5)

a. Glomerular filtration: the pressure of the blood within the glomerular capillaries causes blood to be filtered into Bowman's capsule, where it begins to pass down to the tubule
(1) Filtration is the transfer of water and dissolved substances through a permeable membrane from a region of high pressure to low pressure
(2) Filtration depends on hydrostatic pressure, which may be affected by the following:
(a) Diminished renal perfusion from hypovolemia
(b) Occlusion of the glomeruli from diabetic neuropathy
(c) Alteration in the plasma protein concentration from hypoproteinemia
(d) Alterations in the basement membrane from an autoimmune disorder
(e) Arteriolar constriction from SNS stimulation or vasopressors
(3) GFR
(a) Depends on the following:
(i) Permeability of the capillary walls
(ii) Vascular pressure
(iii) Filtration pressure
(b) Clearance: complete removal of a substance from the blood

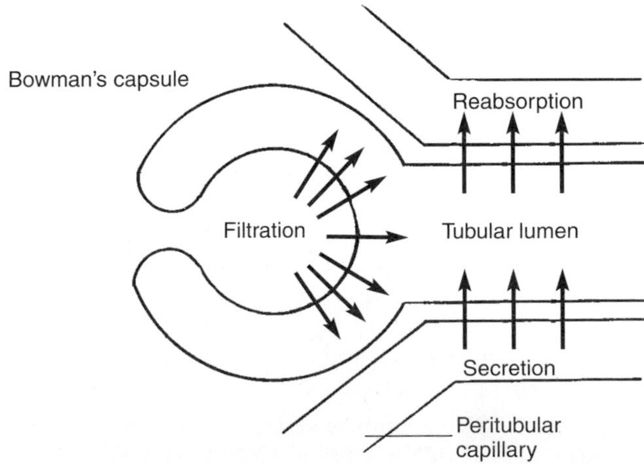

Figure 8-4 Processes of filtration, secretion, and reabsorption in the formation of urine. (From Richard, C. [1987]. *Comprehensive nephrology nursing*. Boston: Little, Brown.)

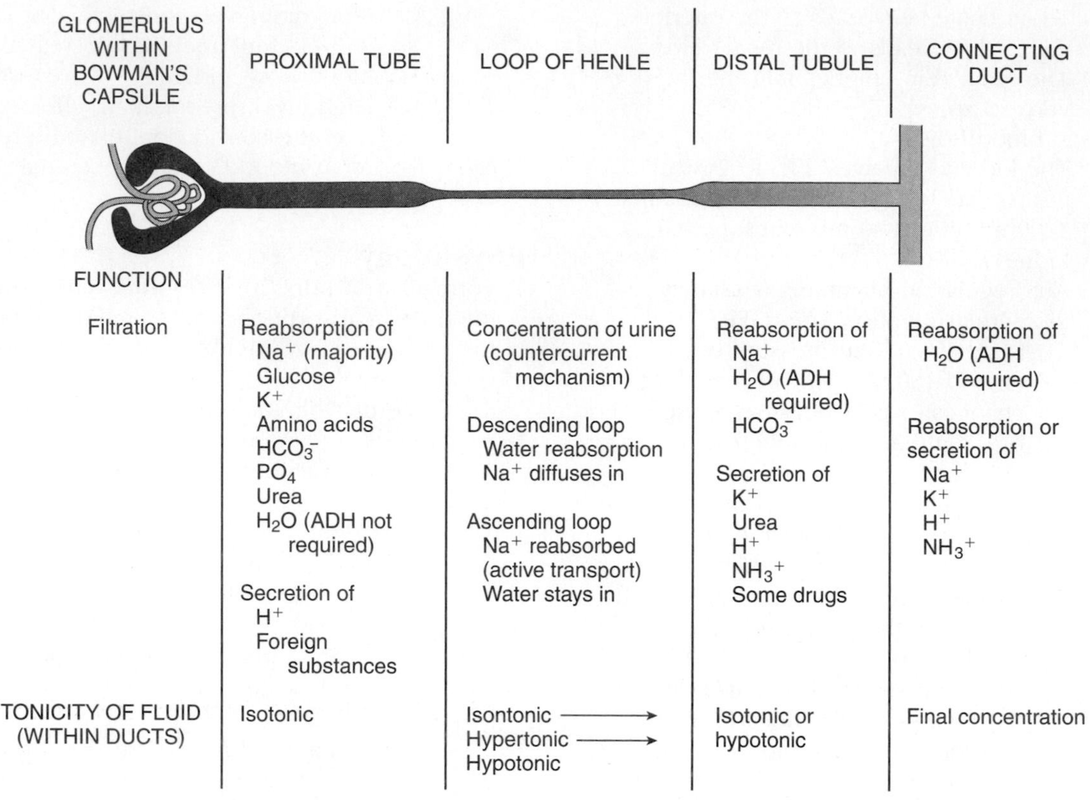

GLOMERULUS WITHIN BOWMAN'S CAPSULE
PROXIMAL TUBE
LOOP OF HENLE
DISTAL TUBULE
CONNECTING DUCT
FUNCTION
Filtration
Reabsorption of Na^+ (majority) Glucose K^+ Amino acids HCO_3^- PO_4 Urea H_2O (ADH not required)
Secretion of H^+ Foreign substances
Concentration of urine (countercurrent mechanism)
Descending loop Water reabsorption Na^+ diffuses in
Ascending loop Na^+ reabsorbed (active transport) Water stays in
Reabsorption of Na^+ H_2O (ADH required) HCO_3^-
Secretion of K^+ Urea H^+ NH_3^+ Some drugs
Reabsorption of H_2O (ADH required)
Reabsorption or secretion of Na^+ K^+ H^+ NH_3^+
TONICITY OF FLUID (WITHIN DUCTS)
Isotonic
Isontonic
Hypertonic
Hypotonic
Isotonic or hypotonic
Final concentration

Figure 8-5 Major functions of each portion of the nephron. *ADH*, Antidiuretic hormone. (From Sole, M. L., Klein, D. G., & Moseley, M. J. [2005]. *Introduction to critical care nursing* [4th ed.]. Philadelphia: Elsevier Saunders.)

(i) Clearance of a substance equals GFR if the tubules neither reabsorb nor secrete the substance.
(ii) Clearance of a substance is less than GFR if the tubules reabsorb the substance.
(iii) Clearance of a substance is greater than GFR if the tubules secrete the substance.

(c) Clinically measured by creatinine clearance because creatinine is filtered by the glomeruli and is not reabsorbed by the tubules
(i) Formula for GFR:

$$GFR = \frac{Ux \times v}{Px}$$

where x is substance freely filtered through glomerulus and not secreted or absorbed by tubules (e.g., creatinine), P is plasma concentration of x (e.g., creatinine), v is urine flow rate per minute, and U is urine concentration of x (e.g., creatinine)
(ii) Creatinine clearance is a calculation of GFR by comparing serum creatinine with the amount of creatinine excreted in the urine over a 24-hour period
(iii) GFR must be maintained at a constant rate, and autoregulation ensures this constant rate; systemic MAP must be maintained between 80 and 180 mm Hg to maintain autoregulation

(4) The glomerular membrane is a porous but semipermeable membrane
(a) Glomerular filtrate (also called *ultrafiltrate*) is similar in composition to blood except that it lacks blood cells, platelets, and large plasma proteins; water, sodium, glucose, potassium, chloride, phosphate, urea, uric acid, creatinine, ammonia, phenol, calcium, and magnesium pass through the glomerular membrane.
(b) Glomerular filtrate volume is usually 120 mL/min, but 99% of this will be reabsorbed in the renal tubule.

b. Reabsorption: passage of a substance that the body needs from the lumen of the tubules through the tubular cells and into the capillaries
(1) Processes
(a) Active transport
(i) The force used when the cell membranes must move molecules "uphill" against a concentration gradient

(ii) Requires the use of energy and a carrier substance; the substance combines with a "carrier" and diffuses through the tubular membrane where they reenter the bloodstream
(iii) Substances moved by active transport include glucose, protein, amino acids, and phosphate
(b) Passive transport: processes of osmosis and diffusion
(i) Diffusion: the passive movement of solute from an area of higher concentration to an area of lower concentration; urea and electrolytes are moved by diffusion
(ii) Osmosis: the passive movement of water from an area of lower solute concentration to an area of higher solute concentration
(2) Maximal tubular transport capacity: maximum amount of a substance that can be reabsorbed completely in 1 minute and reflects the renal threshold of a substance; if this threshold is exceeded, the substance appears in the urine (e.g., glucosuria)
c. Tubular secretion: passage of a substance not needed by the body from the capillaries through the tubular cells into the lumen of the tubule
d. Countercurrent mechanism uses the juxtamedullary nephrons with their long loops of Henle and occurs within the renal medullary interstitium
(1) Countercurrent multiplication is the mechanism that enables the body to excrete urine with an osmolality higher than the osmolality of serum.
(a) Sodium chloride is transported out of the filtrate as it moves up the ascending limb of the loop of Henle, but water is not able to follow because this limb is impermeable to water.
(b) Some of sodium chloride enters the peritubular capillaries and is removed from the kidney, but some reenters the descending limb of the loop of Henle, making the filtrate more concentrated than the blood from which it was derived.
(c) This process increases the osmotic pressure in the capillaries and tubules of the papillary region of the kidney until it is 4 times stronger than that of the blood in the afferent arteriole.
(2) Countercurrent *exchange* is the maintenance component of the countercurrent mechanism.
(a) The vasa recta minimizes the loss of solute from the interstitium by passive diffusion, maintaining the osmotic gradient necessary for the countercurrent multiplication process.
e. Total of 99% of the glomerular filtrate is reabsorbed from the tubules (especially the proximal limb); the remaining 1% is excreted as urine output
(1) Normal urine output is approximately 1500 mL/day
(2) Urine composition
(a) Water
(b) Nitrogenous wastes: urea; uric acid; creatinine; ammonia
(c) Ions: potassium; sodium; calcium; chloride; bicarbonate; hydrogen; phosphate; sulfate
(d) Hormones and their breakdown products
(e) Vitamins: particularly water-soluble B vitamins and vitamin C
(f) Toxins
(g) Drugs
(3) Abnormal constituents: glucose; albumin; RBCs; calculi; casts
2. Excretion of metabolic waste products
a. Urea
(1) Protein (ingested or borrowed from protein stores) is broken down into amino acids and nitrogenous wastes.
(2) Urea nitrogen is the end product of protein metabolism; it circulates in the bloodstream and is excreted in the urine.
(3) Blood urea nitrogen (BUN) varies with protein intake and hydration status, so BUN provides an unreliable evaluation of renal function.
b. Creatinine
(1) Creatinine is a waste product of muscle metabolism.
(2) The normal kidney excretes creatinine at a rate equal to the blood flow of the kidney or GFR.
(3) Serum creatinine is a better test for evaluation of renal function than BUN; urine creatinine clearance, which provides a comparison of serum creatinine and 24-hour urine creatinine, is an even better evaluation of renal function.
3. Renal regulation of acid-base balance (for more on acid-base balance, see Chapter 4)
a. Tubular excretion of H^+ ions in exchange for sodium reabsorption
b. Bicarbonate reabsorption into the circulation or excretion into the urine
c. Excretion of H^+ ions in the urine as NH_4Cl, H_2PO_4, and H_2O
d. Renal response to acidosis
(1) Increased H^+ ion secretion
(2) Increased bicarbonate reabsorption
(3) Production of ammonia to accommodate H^+ ion excretion
e. Renal response to alkalosis
(1) Decreased H^+ ion secretion
(2) Increased bicarbonate excretion
(3) Decreased production of ammonia

4. Fluid balance
   a. Body fluids are dilute solutions of water and solutes
   b. Measurement methods
      (1) Milliliter: the unit of measure for fluid volume
      (2) Milliequivalent (mEq): the unit of measure for chemical combining activity of an electrolyte
      (3) Milliosmole (mOsm): the unit of measure for osmotic pressure based on the number of dissolved particles in solution
         (a) Osmolality and osmolarity: frequently used interchangeably, though most calculations of body fluids are based on osmolality
            (i) Osmolality: number of osmoles per kilogram of solution; expressed as mOsm/kg
               a) Blood
                  i) Normal: 280 to 295 mOsm/kg H_2O
                  ii) Main constituent: sodium
               b) Urine
                  i) Normal: 50 to 1200 mOsm/kg H_2O
                  ii) Main constituents: urea, sodium
            (ii) Osmolarity: number of osmoles per liter of solution
               a) Isotonic: the tonicity of body fluids; osmolarity of 280 to 295 mOsm/L
               b) Hypotonic: lower tonicity than body fluids
               c) Hypertonic: higher tonicity than body fluids
   c. The human body is mostly water
      (1) Volume
         (a) Adult males: 60% of total body weight in adult males is water
         (b) Adult females: slightly less water at 55% of total body weight because of a higher percentage of body fat
         (c) Older adults: less water at 45% to 55% of total body weight
         (d) Obesity: body water decreases with increasing body fat
      (2) Distribution (Figure 8-6, *A*)
         (a) Intracellular
            (i) Fluid contained within the cells
            (ii) Accounts for 40% of total body weight
         (b) Extracellular
            (i) Fluid outside the cells
            (ii) Accounts for 20% of total body weight
            (iii) Distribution
               a) Interstitial
                  i) Fluid surrounding the cells
                  ii) Accounts for 15% of total body weight
               b) Intravascular
                  i) Fluid contained within the blood vessels
                  ii) Accounts for approximately 4% of total body weight
               c) Transcellular
                  i) Fluid contained within specialized cavities of the body (e.g., cerebrospinal, pericardial,

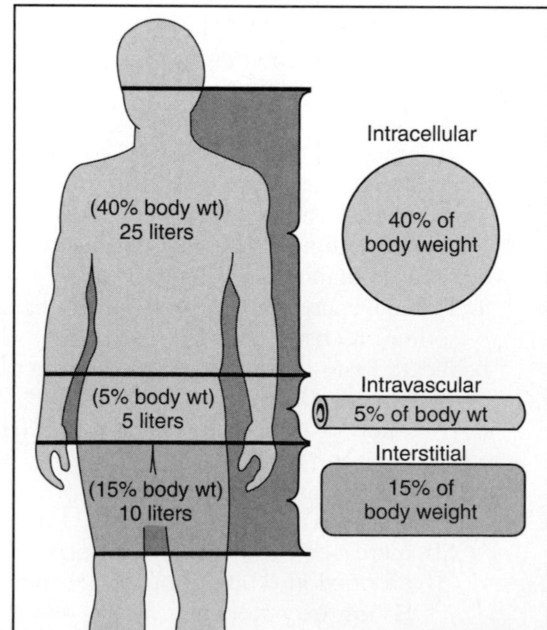

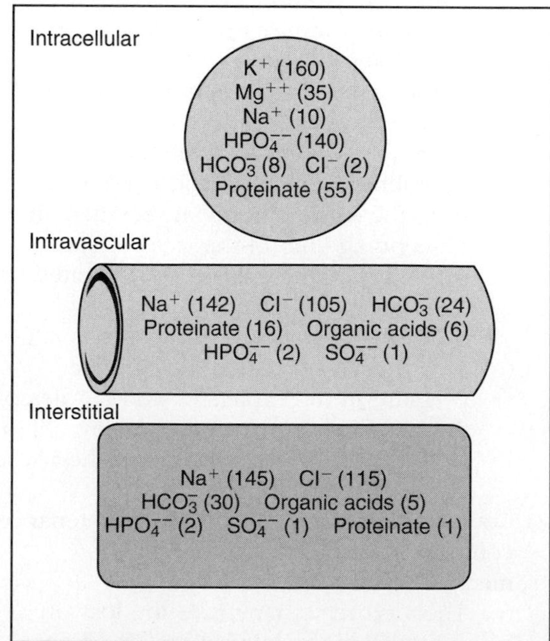

Figure 8-6 A, Distribution of body fluids. **B,** Electrolytes by fluid compartment. (From Urden, L. D., Stacy, K. M., & Lough, M. E. [2006]. *Thelan's critical care nursing: Diagnosis and management* [5th ed.]. St. Louis: Mosby.)

pleural, synovial, intraocular, and digestive fluids)
ii) Accounts for approximately 1% of total body weight

d. Homeostasis is the state of internal equilibrium within the body; fluid, electrolyte, and acid-base are in balance
   (1) Water and solutes are in constant movement and are exchanged continuously.
      (a) Most of the membranes of the body are semipermeable, allowing free movement of water and many nonelectrolytes and selective movement of electrolytes according to concentration gradients.
      (b) Movement of fluids, electrolytes, and other solutes occurs by the following processes:
         (i) Diffusion: solutes move from an area of higher solute concentration to an area of lower solute concentration
         (ii) Osmosis: solutions move from an area of lower solute concentration to an area of higher solute concentration
         (iii) Active transport: use of an energy source to move solutes from an area of lower solute concentration to an area of higher solution concentration
         (iv) Filtration: use of the pushing pressure of hydrostatic pressure to move water and selective solutes through a semipermeable membrane
      (c) Movement into and out of the cell occurs by diffusion, osmosis, and active transport.
         (i) Hydrostatic pressures push.
            a) Capillary hydrostatic pressure pushes fluid out of capillary and into interstitium.
            b) Interstitial hydrostatic pressure pushes fluid out of interstitium and into the capillary.
         (ii) Colloidal oncotic pressures pull.
            a) Capillary colloidal oncotic pressure pulls and holds fluid in the capillary.
            b) Interstitial colloidal oncotic pressure pulls and hold fluid in the interstitium.
         (iii) Starling's law of the capillaries describes the movement of fluid into and out of the capillaries (for more on capillary dynamics, see Chapter 2).
            a) Pressure differences at the venous and arterial ends of the capillaries influence the direction and rate of water and solute movement.
            b) Pressures pushing fluid out of the capillary dominate at the arterial end; pressures pushing fluid back into the capillary dominate at the venous end.
      (d) Pathology
         (i) Third spacing: fluid accumulation in any space that is not intravascular or intracellular (e.g., interstitial edema, ascites, pleural effusion, and pericardial effusion)
            a) Heart failure (HF): Peripheral edema is caused by venous congestion and excessive hydrostatic pressure at the venous end.
            b) Malnutrition: Decrease in plasma proteins decreases capillary colloidal oncotic pressure and allows excessive fluid to leak out of the capillary.
            c) Fluid resuscitation with hypotonic solutions (e.g., 5% dextrose in water): Fluids with osmolality less than serum cause movement of fluid out of the vascular bed into the interstitium.
   (2) Normal functioning of cells requires constancy of the bodily compartments; imbalances disrupt homeostasis.

e. Water exchanges occur continuously
   (1) Loss of water: total ~2400 mL per 24 hours
      (a) Lungs (400 mL)
      (b) Skin (400 mL)
      (c) Kidneys (1500 mL)
      (d) Intestines (100 mL)
      (e) Losses are increased by any of the following:
         (i) Increased respiratory rate
         (ii) Fever
         (iii) Hot, dry environment
         (iv) Injury to the skin (e.g., burns)
   (2) Gains of water: total ~2400 mL per 24 hours
      (a) Liquids (1500 mL)
      (b) Food (500 mL)
      (c) Oxidation of food and body tissues (400 mL)

f. Body fluid is regulated by the following mechanisms:
   (1) Thirst
      (a) Thirst mechanism is located in the anterior hypothalamus; osmoreceptor cells sense changes in serum osmolality and initiate impulses to produce the thirst sensation and the release of ADH.
      (b) The mechanism is stimulated by any of the following:
         (i) Intracellular dehydration
         (ii) Hypertonic body fluids
         (iii) Extracellular fluid loss
         (iv) Hypotension or decreased cardiac output
         (v) Angiotensin
         (vi) Dry mouth

(c) The effect of thirst is the conscious desire to drink fluids (NOTE: Thirst is unreliable in the elderly or confused).

(2) ADH
(a) ADH is produced by the hypothalamus and is stored in and released by the posterior pituitary gland; release may be altered by intracranial processes (e.g., head injury, tumors, or craniotomy) and extracranial processes (e.g., mechanical ventilation or tuberculosis).
(b) ADH is stimulated by any of the following:
(i) Hyperosmolality of extracellular fluid
(ii) Decrease in extracellular fluid volume
(iii) Hyperthermia
(c) Effects of ADH include the following:
(i) Acts on distal and collecting tubules, causing more water to be pulled from the tubule back into the blood
(ii) Increases total volume of body fluid by decreasing urine volume

(3) Renin-angiotensin-aldosterone (RAA) system (Figure 2-22)
(a) RAA system is stimulated by any of the following:
(i) Decreased BP stimulating stretch receptors in juxtaglomerular cells
(ii) SNS stimulation
(iii) Hyponatremia, hyperkalemia
(iv) Increased adrenocorticotropic hormone levels
(b) Effects of the RAA system include the following:
(i) Angiotensin II causes vasoconstriction and secretion of aldosterone, a mineralocorticoid produced by the adrenal cortex.
(ii) Aldosterone stimulates the renal tubules to reabsorb more sodium and water, which causes sodium retention, water retention, and decreased urine volume.
(iii) Vasoconstriction and sodium and water retention increases BP, which decreases renin secretion.

(4) Atrial natriuretic peptide (ANP)
(a) ANP is a hormonelike substance that is synthesized and stored by specialized atrial muscle cells.
(b) ANP secretion is stimulated by the following:
(i) Volume expansion
(ii) Elevated cardiac filling pressures
(c) Effects of ANP include the following:
(i) Increased excretion of sodium and water by the kidney
(ii) Decreased synthesis of renin and decreased release of aldosterone

(5) Countercurrent mechanism of kidney: mechanism for concentration and dilution of urine

5. Electrolyte balance
a. Solutes are substances dissolves in a solution and may be electrolytes or nonelectrolytes
(1) Nonelectrolytes (e.g., glucose, proteins, lipids, oxygen, carbon dioxide, urea, creatinine, and bilirubin) are solutes without an electrical charge; they stay intact in solution.
(2) Electrolytes are solutes that dissociate into positive or negative ions when in solution and will generate an electrical charge when in solution.
(a) Electrical charge
(i) Cations are positively charged ions.
a) Major intracellular cation is potassium
b) Major extracellular cation is sodium
c) Other cations: calcium; magnesium; hydrogen
(ii) Anions are negatively charged electrolytes.
a) Major intracellular anion is chloride
b) Major extracellular anion is phosphate
c) Other anion: bicarbonate
(iii) In each fluid compartment, the various cations and anions balance each other to achieve electrical neutrality; there is no net charge within a fluid compartment (Figure 8-6, *B*)

b. Renal regulation of electrolytes
(1) Excretion and/or retention of electrolytes
(2) Filter and reabsorb about one half of unbound serum calcium and activate vitamin D_3, a compound that promotes intestinal calcium absorption
(3) Regulates phosphorus excretion

c. Summary of electrolyte normal values, roles, regulation, and foods sources (Table 8-1)

6. Renal role in regulation of BP
a. Juxtaglomerular apparatus is a combination of specialized cells located near the glomerulus at the junction of the afferent and efferent arterioles; juxtaglomerular cells contain granules of inactive renin
b. RAA system as depicted in Figure 2-22

7. RBC synthesis and maturation
a. Erythropoietin secretion
(1) Stimulates production of RBCs in bone marrow
(2) Prolongs life of RBC

Table 8-1 Electrolyte Summary

Electrolyte	Functions	Regulation and Factors Affecting Serum Level	Food Sources
Sodium: normal 136-145 mEq/L	• Maintains extracellular osmolality and volume • Maintains active transport mechanism in conjunction with potassium • Influences the regulation of water and electrolyte status in the body by the kidney • Promotes the irritability of nerve tissue and the conduction of nerve impulses • Facilitates muscle contraction • Aids in some enzyme activities • Combines with bicarbonate and chloride to help regulate acid-base balance	• Aldosterone: causes sodium and water retention • GFR: sodium excretion is increased when GFR is high; decreased when GFR is low • "Third factor": promotes sodium excretion by inhibiting sodium reabsorption; suppression of this factor ensures sodium reabsorption • Increase in sodium concentration stimulates water retention by antidiuretic hormone release, diluting sodium back to normal level • Some excretion through skin in perspiration	• Bouillon • Celery • Cheeses • Dried fruits • Frozen, canned, or packaged foods • Monosodium glutamate • Mustard • Olives • Pickles • Preserved meat • Salad dressings, prepared sauces • Sauerkraut • Snack foods • Soy sauce
Potassium: normal 3.5-5.5 mEq/L	• Promotes transmission of nerve impulses • Maintains intracellular osmolality • Activates several enzymatic reactions • Helps regulate acid-base balance • Influences kidney function and structure • Promotes myocardial, skeletal, and smooth muscle contractility	• Aldosterone: increase in intracellular potassium or decrease in serum sodium causes aldosterone release and potassium excretion • GFR: potassium excretion is directly related directly to GFR in a normal kidney • Obligatory loss: the kidneys are unable to conserve potassium; it may be flushed out by diuresis even in the presence of a body deficit; 40-50 mEq lost each day • Renal failure: if kidneys fail to excrete potassium normally from the body (e.g., renal failure), toxic levels can occur pH: potassium shifts into the cell in alkalosis (causing hypokalemia) and out of the cell in acidosis (causing hyperkalemia)	• Apricots • Artichokes • Avocado • Banana • Cantaloupe • Carrots • Cauliflower • Chocolate • Dried beans, peas • Dried fruit • Mushrooms • Nuts • Oranges, orange juice • Peanuts • Potatoes • Prune juice • Pumpkin • Spinach • Sweet potatoes • Swiss chard • Tomatoes, tomato juice, tomato sauce
Calcium: normal 8.5-10.5 mg/dL or 4.5-5.8 mEq/L (NOTE: Calcium is affected by albumin levels; to correct calcium, add 0.8 mg/dL for each 1 g/dL decrease in albumin.)	• Hardens and strengthens bones and teeth • Aids in blood coagulation • Transmits neuromuscular impulses • Maintains cellular permeability • Serves essential role in cardiac contractility	• PTH: stimulated by a decrease in serum calcium; promotes calcium transfer from bone to plasma and aids in renal and intestinal absorption • Phosphorus: inhibits calcium absorption; calcium and phosphorus have an inverse relationship; if calcium goes up, phosphorus goes down and vice versa • Vitamin D: necessary for GI absorption; promotes calcium absorption • Calcitonin: aids transfer of calcium from plasma to bone, which directly lowers serum calcium • Albumin: 50% of serum calcium is bound to serum albumin; therefore a decrease in serum albumin will lower the total calcium level but not the ionized calcium level, and the patient will not have symptoms of hypocalcemia	• Brazil nuts • Broccoli • Cheese • Collard, mustard, turnip greens • Cottage cheese • Eggnog • Ice cream • Milk and cream • Milk chocolate • Molasses • Oat flakes • Rhubarb • Seafood, especially sardines with bones • Sesame seeds • Soy flour • Spinach • Yogurt

Continued

Table 8-1 Electrolyte Summary—cont'd

Electrolyte	Functions	Regulation and Factors Affecting Serum Level	Food Sources
		• pH: alkalosis increases binding between albumin and calcium so that the patient will exhibit symptoms of hypocalcemia though total body calcium is normal; acidosis decreases binding between albumin and calcium so that the patient may exhibit symptoms of hypercalcemia • Corticosteroids: contribute to demineralization of the bone and calcium loss; large doses decrease calcium absorption in GI tract • Diuretic effect: calcium is lost along with potassium and magnesium in patient taking diuretics	
Phosphorus: normal 3-4.5 mg/dL	• Aids in structure of cellular membrane • Essential for glucose metabolism in red blood cells; produces 2,3-DPG as an end product • Regulates the delivery of oxygen to the tissues; 2,3-DPG encourages unloading between hemoglobin and oxygen • Essential for adenosine triphophate or high-energy phosphate formation • May be connected with DNA, RNA, and genetic coding • Helps maintain bone hardness • Aids in enzyme regulation (adenosine triphosphatase) • Used by kidney to buffer hydrogen ions (phosphate)	• PTH: inhibits renal reabsorption of phosphates; calcium and phosphorus have an inverse relationship; if calcium goes up, phosphorus goes down and vice versa • Alterations in GFR affect phosphate excretion; increased GFR decreases reabsorption of phosphorus; decreased GFR increases reabsorption of phosphorus	• Dried beans and peas • Eggs and egg products • Fish, poultry • Meats, especially organ meats • Milk and milk products • Nuts • Seeds • Whole grains
Magnesium: normal 1.5-2.5 mEq/L	• Aids in neuromuscular transmission • Aids in cardiac contractility • Activates enzymes for cellular metabolism of carbohydrates and proteins • Aids in maintaining the active transport mechanism at the cellular level • Aids in the transmission of hereditary information to offspring	• Not completely understood • Factors that influence calcium and potassium balance also affect magnesium • Deficiencies of these electrolytes usually occur together (e.g., diuretics cause the loss of all three) • Availability of sodium: sodium is necessary for the absorption of magnesium • Diuretics: cause the excessive loss of magnesium • PTH: affects magnesium reabsorption as it does calcium	• Bananas • Chocolate • Coconut • Grapefruit • Green, leafy vegetables • Legumes • Milk • Molasses • Nuts and seeds • Oranges • Refined sugar • Seafood • Soy flour • Wheat bran

2, 3-DPG, 2, 3-diphosphoglyceric acid; *GFR*, glomerular filtration rate; *GI*, gastrointestinal; *PTH*, parathyroid hormone.

Table 8-1 **Electrolyte Summary—cont'd**

Electrolyte	Functions	Regulation and Factors Affecting Serum Level	Food Sources
Chloride: normal 96-106 mEq/L	• Maintains serum osmolality (along with sodium) • Combines with major cations to form important compounds (e.g., NaCl, HCl, KCl, CaCl) • Helps maintain acid-base balance through HCl production	• Indirectly affected by aldosterone • Changes almost always linked to sodium • pH: acidosis causes bicarbonate to be reabsorbed while chloride is excreted; alkalosis causes bicarbonate to be excreted while chloride is reabsorbed	• Bananas • Celery • Cheese • Dates • Eggs • Fish • Milk • Spinach • Table salt • Turkey

b. Postulated methods of erythropoietin synthesis and stimulus for secretion
   (1) Normal kidneys produce erythropoietin or synthesize an enzyme that catalyzes its formation.
   (2) Stimulation for formation is believed to be decreased Po_2 in renal blood.
c. Interference in this process causes anemia in patients with chronic renal failure

8. Prostaglandin synthesis
   a. Process occurs primarily in the medulla.
   b. Types of prostaglandins are as follows:
      (1) Vasodilators: prostaglandin E_2, prostaglandin D_2, prostaglandin I_2
      (2) Vasoconstrictors: prostaglandin A_2
   c. Release is stimulated by vasoactive substances (e.g., angiotensin, norepinephrine, or bradykinins).
   d. Effects of prostaglandins include the following:
      (1) Modulate the vasoconstrictive effects of angiotensin and norepinephrine; interference with this process may be one factor contributing to hypertension in patients with renal failure
      (2) Increase renal blood flow, which results in arterial vasodilation, inhibition of the distal tubule response to ADH, and promotion of sodium and water excretion
9. Renal role in bone mineralization
   a. Vitamin D is metabolized by the kidney from an inactive form to an active metabolite, 1,25-dihydroxycholecalciferol, which is necessary for the absorption of calcium and phosphorus from the intestine.
   b. Interference in this process causes osteodystrophy in patients with chronic renal failure.

Assessment of Fluid, Electrolyte, and Renal Status

Interview

1. Chief complaint: common symptoms of fluid, electrolyte, or renal conditions
   a. Flank or costovertebral angle (CVA) pain
      (1) Unilateral or bilateral
      (2) Constant or intermittent
      (3) Aggravated by CVA percussion
      (4) Dull ache to stabbing or throbbing pain
      (5) Relieved only by analgesics or treatment of underlying disease
      (6) Accompanying findings: hematuria; pyuria; change in urine volume
      (7) Possible causes: renal calculi; bladder cancer; bacterial cystitis; acute glomerulonephritis; obstructive uropathy; perirenal abscess; polycystic kidney disease; acute pyelonephritis; renal infarction; renal cancer; renal trauma; renal vein thrombosis; acute pancreatitis
   b. Changes in pattern of urination
      (1) Frequency: frequent voiding
      (2) Nocturia: getting up at night to void (more than twice)
      (3) Dysuria: painful urination
      (4) Urgency: a feeling of the need to void immediately
      (5) Hesitancy: difficulty starting the flow of urine
      (6) Change in stream
      (7) Retention: incomplete emptying of the bladder
      (8) Incontinence: inability to control urination
      (9) Enuresis: incontinence of urine in bed at night
   c. Change in urine output: increased or decreased amount
   d. Change in appearance of urine
      (1) Dilute: clear to light yellow
      (2) Concentrated: dark, amber
      (3) Pyuria: cloudy
      (4) Hematuria: pink to red
      (5) Bilirubinemia: orange to brown
      (6) Myoglobinuria: tea or cola colored
      (7) Hemoglobinuria: wine colored
   e. Neurologic
      (1) Visual changes: may be associated with uremia, fluid overload, or electrolyte imbalance
      (2) Paresthesias: may be associated with hypocalcemia
      (3) Headaches: may be associated with fluid overload or uremia
      (4) Seizures: may be associated with uremia, electrolyte imbalances, or fluid overload

(5) Decreased ability to concentrate: may be associated with uremia, electrolyte imbalance, or fluid overload
(6) Apathy: may be associated with uremia

f. Cardiovascular
(1) Palpitations: may be seen with dysrhythmias in electrolyte imbalance
(2) Chest pain: may be seen with uremia or electrolyte imbalance
(3) Edema: may be associated with uremia, fluid overload, or hypoproteinemia

g. Pulmonary
(1) Dyspnea: may be seen in renal failure patients as a result of left ventricular failure or pleural effusion
(2) Hemoptysis: seen in Goodpasture's syndrome

h. Gastrointestinal (GI)
(1) Halitosis: foul odor to breath; urinelike odor to breath may be associated with uremia; metallic taste in mouth
(2) Anorexia: may be associated with uremia
(3) Nausea, vomiting: may be associated with uremia, electrolyte imbalance, or fluid overload
(4) Constipation or diarrhea: may be related to fluid imbalance

i. Musculoskeletal
(1) Joint pain: may be associated with uremia, fluid imbalance, or electrolyte imbalance
(2) Muscle weakness: may be associated with electrolyte imbalance
(3) Muscle pain or cramps: may be associated with uremia or electrolyte imbalance

j. Dermatologic
(1) Pruritus: may be associated with uremia
(2) Bruising: may be associated with uremia
(3) Delayed healing: may be associated with uremia

k. Sexual
(1) Impotence: may be related to uremia
(2) Diminished libido: may be related to uremia
(3) Infertility: may be related to uremia

l. Other general symptoms
(1) Fatigue: may be associated with uremia
(2) Fever: may be associated with infection or dehydration
(3) Thirst: may be associated with fluid imbalance
(4) Change in body weight: may be associated with uremia or fluid imbalance

2. History of present illness
a. PQRST (provocation, palliation, quality, quantity, region, radiation, severity, timing)
b. Accompanying symptoms

3. Medical history
a. Renal/urinary tract
(1) Urinary tract infection (UTI)
(2) Calculi
(3) Renal insufficiency/failure
(a) Dialysis
(b) Renal transplantation
(4) Surgical procedures

b. Cardiovascular
(1) Hypertension
(2) Arteriosclerosis/atherosclerosis
(3) HF
(4) Bacterial endocarditis

c. Pulmonary: tuberculosis

d. Endocrine/metabolic
(1) Diabetes mellitus
(2) Gout

e. Immunologic/hematologic
(1) Connective tissue disorders
(a) Lupus erythematosus
(b) Scleroderma
(2) Goodpasture's syndrome: hemoptysis with glomerulonephritis
(3) Hemophilia
(4) Disseminated intravascular coagulation
(5) Sickle-cell disease
(6) Malignancy
(7) Blood transfusion

f. Gynecologic: toxemia of pregnancy

g. Infection
(1) Recent beta-hemolytic streptococcal infection
(2) UTI

4. Family history
a. Renal
(1) Inherited glomerulonephritis
(2) Polycystic disease
(3) Inherited nephritis (Alport's syndrome)
(4) Amyloidosis
(5) Malignancy
b. Cardiovascular
(1) Hypertension
(2) Coronary artery disease
c. Immunologic/hematologic
(1) Hemophilia
(2) Sickle cell disease
d. Endocrine: diabetes mellitus

5. Social history
a. Occupational exposure to toxins: lead; mercury; pesticides; methanol; radiation; carbon tetrachloride; phenol
b. Exercise habits: strenuous exercise in an unconditioned person may cause rhabdomyolysis
c. Fluid intake: type of fluids
d. Smoking: increased incidence of bladder cancer
e. Use of saccharine: increased incidence of bladder cancer

6. Medication history
a. Potentially nephrotoxic agents
(1) Antimicrobials
(a) Aminoglycosides
(b) Cephalosporins
(c) Sulfonamides
(d) Amphotericin B
(e) Bacitracin
(f) Rifampin
(2) Nonsteroidal antiinflammatory drugs (NSAIDs) (e.g., ibuprofen, indomethacin, or aspirin)
(3) Angiotensin-converting enzyme (ACE) inhibitors (e.g., captopril or enalapril)

(4) Antineoplastics (e.g., cisplatin or methotrexate)
(5) Analgesics containing phenacetin
(6) Cyclosporin A
(7) Methanol, ethylene glycol
(8) Carbon tetrachloride
(9) Contrast media
(10) Heavy metals (e.g., lead, arsenic, mercury, or uranium)
(11) Insecticides and fungicides
(12) Phencyclidine (PCP) and other street drugs

b. Diuretics
c. Antihypertensives
d. Anticoagulants
e. Electrolyte replacement therapy
f. Immunosuppressives
   (1) Corticosteroids
   (2) Azathioprine (Imuran)
   (3) Cyclophosphamide (Cytoxan)

Vital Signs

1. BP
   a. Increased: seen in fluid overload, renal disease, and hypertension
   b. Decreased: must be fluid loss of 15% to 25% before systolic BP falls
   c. Postural drop (tilt positive): decrease of 15 mm Hg in systolic pressure when patient sits or stands may be earlier change of hypovolemia
2. Pulse
   a. Increased: seen in SNS stimulation as may be seen in fluid overload or dehydration; response blunted or eliminated by beta-blockers
   b. Postural: increases of pulse by 20 beats/min when the patient sits or stands may be earlier change of hypovolemia
3. Respiratory rate and rhythm
   a. Tachypnea: seen in SNS stimulation as may be seen in fluid overload or dehydration
   b. Kussmaul's respirations: rapid, deep, gasping breaths seen in metabolic acidosis
4. Temperature: hyperthermia may be seen in dehydration
5. Weight changes
   a. Change of 1 lb is equal to 500 mL; change of 1 kg is equal to 1 L
   b. Evaluate weight before and after hemodialysis; evaluate weight after drainage of dialysate in patients on peritoneal dialysis
   c. Weight loss resulting from generalized debilitation may be seen in renal failure

Inspection and Palpation

1. Skin
   a. Color
      (1) Yellowish-gray color is seen in renal failure.
      (2) Pallor may indicate anemia.
      (3) Petechiae and bruising may be seen in renal failure as a result of platelet dysfunction.
   b. Skin texture
      (1) Rough, dry skin is seen in renal failure.
      (2) Uremic frost, a filmy coating over the skin, is seen in untreated uremia.
   c. Lesions: scratch marks may be seen as a result of pruritus in renal failure
   d. Skin turgor
      (1) Recoil should be immediate; decrease in skin turgor indicates interstitial dehydration but is not an early sign.
      (2) Evaluation of skin turgor to determine hydration status is not reliable in elderly patients because of poor elasticity.
   e. Edema
      (1) Late change of overhydration because patient may gain 3 to 4 kg before edema is noticeable
      (2) Location
         (a) Edema related to renal disease is frequently facial initially.
         (b) Anasarca (generalized, massive edema and does not pit) may be seen in end-stage renal disease (ESRD).
2. Mouth
   a. Halitosis: uremic fetor (urinelike odor to the breath) noted in renal failure
   b. Mucous membranes: stickiness of the oral mucous membranes and tongue is the preferred indicator of dehydration in the elderly; use a tongue blade to evaluate stickiness
3. Eyes
   a. Periorbital edema seen in nephrotic syndrome and other forms of renal disease
   b. Cataract formation common in renal failure
4. Ears: nerve deafness common in renal failure
5. Neurologic status
   a. Change in level of consciousness may indicate azotemia or electrolyte imbalance.
   b. Confusion may be indicative of uremia.
   c. Seizures may indicate hyponatremia and cerebral edema.
   d. Neuromuscular irritability and changes in muscle strength may reflect electrolyte imbalance.
6. Cardiovascular
   a. Dysrhythmias are common in electrolyte imbalance
   b. Jugular venous distention (JVD) (see Figure 2-29 in Chapter 2 for illustration)
      (1) To evaluate JVD
         (a) Place patient in a 45-degree angle.
         (b) Identify the angle of Louis, the raised notch that is created where the manubrium and the body of the sternum join (also called *manubriosternal junction* or *sternal angle*).
         (c) Measure height of neck vein distention.
         (d) Normal height of neck vein distention is 1 to 2 cm above the angle of Louis; neck vein distention of greater than 2 cm above the angle of Louis may be indicative of hypervolemia.

7. Abdomen
   a. Generalized edema and/or ascites: may be seen in renal failure
   b. Kidney
      (1) The kidney may be palpated by "capture" technique; put one hand under the patient below the costal margin and the other hand on the abdomen below the costal margin; ask the patient to take a deep breath and move hands together to try to "capture" the kidney.
      (2) The lower pole of a normal right kidney may be palpable because it is lower than the left kidney (pushed down by the liver).
      (3) A normal left kidney is not palpable.
      (4) If kidney is palpable, evaluate the following:
         (a) Size: normal size is 10 × 5 × 2.5 cm or about the size of a fist
            (i) Increased size may be seen in acute renal disease, polycystic disease, obstructive uropathy, pyelonephritis, and renal abscess or tumor.
            (ii) Decreased size may be seen in advanced chronic renal failure.
         (b) Pain or discomfort during palpation may indicate infection, calculi, tumor, hydronephrosis, or glomerulonephritis
   c. Bladder
      (1) The bladder is palpable in suprapubic area only when full.
      (2) If palpable, the bladder should be felt as a smooth, round, firm organ that is sensitive to palpation.
8. Extremities
   a. Asterixis: a hand-flapping tremor induced by extending the arm and dorsiflexing the wrist; indicative of increased ammonia levels; seen in renal failure and hepatic encephalopathy
   b. Vascular access (e.g., fistula, arteriovenous [AV] graft, or shunt): thrill over access indicates patency

Percussion

1. Thorax: flatness at lung bases may indicate pleural effusion that frequently is seen in renal failure
2. Abdomen
   a. Elicitation of a fluid wave: indicative of ascites, which frequently is seen in end-stage renal failure
   b. CVA (Figure 8-7): tap over CVA with ulnar surface of hand
      (1) CVA tenderness may be seen in pyelonephritis, renal calculi, renal abscess or tumor, glomerulonephritis, or intermittent hydronephrosis.
      (2) Bruising over CVA may indicate renal trauma.
   c. Bladder
      (1) The bladder is percussible in suprapubic area only when it contains at least 150 mL.
      (2) Dullness is audible above the symphysis pubis if the bladder is full of urine.
      (3) Pain during percussion may indicate cystitis.

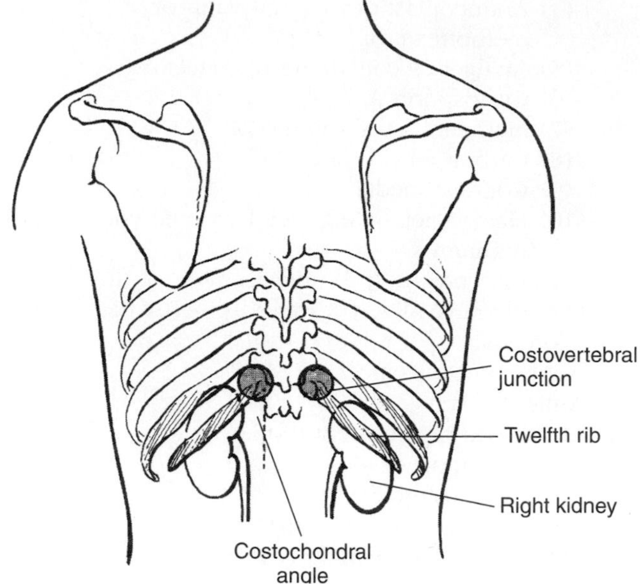

Figure 8-7 The costovertebral angle (From Barkauskas, V. H., et al. [2002]. *Health and physical assessment* [3rd ed.]. St. Louis: Mosby.)

Auscultation

1. Vascular sounds
   a. Renal bruit: may be audible to the left or right of midline in periumbilical region in renal vascular disease or renal vascular trauma
   b. Vascular access (e.g., fistula, AV graft, or shunt): bruit over access indicates patency
2. Heart sounds
   a. Rate and rhythm: dysrhythmias may be seen in electrolyte imbalance
   b. S_3: indicates heart failure
   c. Flow murmur: mitral regurgitation murmur (systolic murmur heard best at apex with diaphragm) may be heard with fluid overload
   d. Pericardial friction rub: may indicate pericarditis, a common complication of renal failure
3. Breath sounds: crackles may indicate fluid overload, heard initially at bases
4. Bowel sounds: changes may indicate electrolyte imbalance
   a. Hypoactive bowel sounds in hypokalemia
   b. Hyperactive bowel sounds in hyperkalemia

Urine Output

1. Important indicator of GFR
2. Decreased with diminished CO or dehydration
3. Increased in overhydration
4. Volume parameters
   a. Normal output is 1500 mL per 24 hours or at least 0.5 mL/kg/hr
   b. Polyuria: greater than 2500 mL per 24 hours
   c. Oliguria: 100 to 400 mL per 24 hours
   d. Anuria: 0 to 100 mL per 24 hours

Bladder Volume by Portable Ultrasound Bladder Scanner

1. Uses
   a. Differentiate between an empty bladder and urinary retention, thereby avoiding unnecessary catheterization.
   b. Evaluate residual urine in the bladder after voiding.
2. Technology
   a. Portable, ultrasound bladder scanner automatically computes the bladder volume based on cross-sectional images of the bladder
   b. Components
      (1) Instrument box with screen for digital display of bladder volume
      (2) Handheld ultrasound transducer
3. Methodology
   a. Indicate patient gender.
   b. Wash the transducer tip and apply ultrasound gel.
   c. Position the tip of the transducer of above the symphysis pubis and toward the bladder.
   d. Press the transducer button and hold until the machine beeps, indicating that scanning is complete.
   e. May be repeated once or twice more to evaluate consistency (to indicate a reliable reading.)
   f. Wash gel from patient's abdomen and transducer tip.
4. Implication: catheterization is generally indicated if bladder volume is greater than 300 mL

Hemodynamic Monitoring

1. Right atrial pressure (RAP) (from proximal port of pulmonary artery catheter) or central venous pressure (CVP) (from catheter in superior vena cava): normal 2 to 6 mm Hg
   a. Increased in hypervolemia
   b. Decreased in hypovolemia
2. Pulmonary artery occlusive pressure (PAOP): normal 8 to 12 mm Hg
   a. Increased in hypervolemia
   b. Decreased in hypovolemia

Diagnostic Studies

1. Serum
   a. Osmolality: normal 280 to 295 mOsm/kg
      (1) Measures particles exerting osmotic pull per unit of water
      (2) May be calculated: (Na × 2) + (BUN/2.6) + (Serum glucose/18), where *BUN* is blood urea nitrogen
      (3) Reflects total body hydration
         (a) Increased in dehydration
         (b) Decreased with fluid overload
   b. BUN: normal 5 to 20 mg/dL
      (1) Reflects difference between rate of urea synthesis and its excretion by the kidneys
         (a) Formed in the liver through enzymatic breakdown of protein
         (b) Not as accurate an indicator of renal failure as is creatinine because BUN levels fluctuate greatly with protein intake but creatinine levels are relatively unchanged by protein intake and hydration level
      (2) Abnormal values
         (a) Increased with decreased renal blood flow or urine production, dehydration, some neoplasms, and certain antibiotics; increased BUN also is referred to as *uremia*
         (b) Decreased in pregnancy, overhydration, severe liver disease, and malnutrition
      (3) BUN/creatinine ratio: normal ~10:1
         (a) When BUN is elevated disproportionately to the creatinine (e.g., BUN/creatinine ratio 20:1), consider an extrarenal cause such as one of the following:
            (i) Volume depletion (i.e., prerenal)
               a) Insufficient fluid intake
               b) Excessive fluid loss
                  i) Diuresis
                  ii) Vomiting
            (ii) Poor renal perfusion
               a) Shock
               b) Sepsis
               c) Decreased CO
               d) Renovascular disease
            (iii) Protein catabolism
               a) Starvation
               b) Blood in the GI tract
               c) Corticosteroids
         (b) When BUN and creatinine are elevated, maintaining the normal 10:1 ratio, consider a renal cause such as acute or chronic renal failure.
         (c) When BUN/creatinine ratio is lower than normal, consider the following:
            (i) Decreased protein intake
            (ii) Liver dysfunction
   c. Creatinine: normal 0.7 to 1.5 mg/dL
      (1) Nonprotein end product of muscle metabolism
         (a) More accurate than BUN in evaluating renal function because creatinine normally is filtered by the glomerulus and is not reabsorbed by the tubule
         (b) Unaffected by diet and fluid intake
      (2) Abnormal values
         (a) Increased
            (i) A twice-normal (~3 mg/dL) creatinine level suggests 50% nephron loss
            (ii) If more than 10 mg/dL, indicates ESRD with less than 10% of nephrons still functioning
         (b) Decreased: muscular dystrophy

Table 8-2 Anion Gap

Consideration	Comments
Calculation of anion gap	(Na + K) − (Cl + HCO_3 or CO_2 content)
Normal value	5-15
Causes of metabolic acidosis with normal anion gap: bicarbonate loss	Intestinal loss of bicarbonate • Diarrhea • Pancreatic fistula • Ureterosigmoidostomy Renal loss of bicarbonate • Carbonic anhydrase inhibitors (e.g., acetazolamide [Diamox]) • Aldosterone-antagonists (also referred to as *potassium-sparing diuretics*; e.g., triamterene [Dyrenium] and spironolactone [Aldactone]) • Renal tubular acidosis • Adrenal insufficiency • Primary hypoaldosteronism Excessive gain of chloride • Large quantities of normal saline • Ammonium chloride • Arginine hydrochloride
Causes of metabolic acidosis with increased anion gap: metabolic acid gain	Renal failure Lactic acidosis • Shock • Hypoxemia/hypoxia • Severe anemia • Status epilepticus • Cyanide poisoning Ketoacidosis • Diabetic ketoacidosis • Starvation • Alcohol Drugs and toxins • Salicylates • Methanol • Ethylene glycol • Paraldehyde • High-dose carbenicillin Rhabdomyolysis

d. Electrolytes
   (1) Sodium: normal 136 to 145 mEq/L
   (2) Potassium: normal 3.5 to 5.5 mEq/L
   (3) Chloride: normal 96 to 106 mEq/L
   (4) Calcium: normal 8.5 to 10.5 mg/dL
   (5) Phosphorus: normal 3 to 4.5 mg/dL
   (6) Magnesium: normal 1.5 to 2.2 mEq/L
e. Anion gap: a calculated parameter (Table 8-2)
   (1) Calculated by subtracting the anion from the cations
      (a) (Sodium + Potassium) − (Chloride + Carbon dioxide content or Bicarbonate)
      (b) Normal: 5 to 15
   (2) Helpful in determination of cause of metabolic acidosis
      (a) A normal anion gap indicates that the reason for the metabolic acidosis is bicarbonate loss.
      (b) An elevated anion gap indicates that the reason for the metabolic acidosis is an acid gain (e.g., lactic acid, ketoacid, or toxins).
f. Glucose: normal 70 to 110 mg/dL
g. Arterial blood gases (ABGs)
   (1) pH: normal 7.35 to 7.45
   (2) $Paco_2$: normal 35 to 45 mm Hg
   (3) HCO_3: normal 22 to 26 mEq/L
   (4) Pao_2: normal 80 to 100 mm Hg
h. Hematology
   (1) Hematocrit (Hct): normal 40% to 52% for males; 35% to 47% for females
      (a) Measures portion of blood volume occupied by RBCs
      (b) Increased in dehydration or polycythemia
      (c) Decreased with low RBCs or with normal hemoglobin (Hgb) and water overload
   (2) Hgb: normal 13 to 18 g/dL for males; 12 to 16 g/dL for females
   (3) White blood cells: 3500 to 11,000 cells/mm^3
i. Clotting profile
   (1) Prothrombin time: normal 12 to 15 seconds
   (2) Partial thromboplastin time: normal 25 to 38 seconds
   (3) Thrombin time: normal 10 to 15 seconds
   (4) Bleeding time: normal 1 to 9½ minutes
   (5) Platelets: normal 150,000 to 400,000/mm^3
j. Serum proteins
   (1) Total protein: normal 6 to 8 g/dL
   (2) Albumin: normal 3.5 to 4.5 g/dL
k. Serum lipids
   (1) Cholesterol: 150 to 200 mg/dL
   (2) Triglycerides: 40 to 150 mg/dL

2. Urine
   a. Visual examination: clear, yellow
   b. Glucose: normal negative; glycosuria occurs when renal threshold for glucose is exceeded; renal threshold is variable and patient-specific, so there is no accurate method to predict serum glucose
   c. Ketones: normal negative; ketonuria is seen in catabolism (e.g., starvation or diabetic ketoacidosis [DKA])
   d. Protein: normal 0 to 8 mg/dL
      (1) Proteinuria may occur after ingestion of a high-protein meal or can accompany renal changes of pregnancy
      (2) Consistent proteinuria suggests compromise of the glomerular membrane (e.g., nephrotic syndrome or glomerulonephritis)
   e. Myoglobin: normal negative or less than 20 ng/mL; myoglobinuria indicates muscle breakdown
   f. Hgb: normal negative; hemoglobinuria indicates free Hgb in the urine such as occurs in hemolytic blood transfusion reaction, hemolytic or sickle cell anemia, freshwater drowning, burns, disseminated intravascular coagulation
   g. Bilirubin: normal negative; urobilinogen indicates biliary obstruction or liver disease

h. Specific gravity: 1.005 to 1.030
  (1) Increased with any condition causing hypoperfusion of kidneys leading to oliguria (e.g., shock, severe dehydration, proteinuria, glycosuria, or contrast media)
  (2) Decreased in diabetes insipidus, overhydration, and when renal tubules lose their ability to reabsorb water and concentrate urine as in early pyelonephritis
i. Osmolality: 50 to 1200 mOsm/kg
  (1) Measures number of particles per unit of water in urine
  (2) Depends on the circulating titer of ADH and the rate of urinary solute excretion; should be 1.5 times that of serum osmolality
  (3) Increased in fluid volume deficit because of retention of fluid by the body
  (4) Decreased in fluid volume excess because of fluid being excreted by the kidney
j. Creatinine clearance
  (1) Estimate of GFR
  (2) Urine specimen for 24-hour period and a serum creatinine required
  (3) Normal: 85 to 135 mL/minute
k. Culture and sensitivity: normally no bacteria present; if bacteria are present, appropriate antibiotic therapy is identified
l. pH: normal 4 to 8 with average of 6
  (1) Increased urinary acidity indicates that the body is retaining bicarbonate.
  (2) Decreased urinary acidity (more alkaline) indicates that the kidney is retaining sodium and acids.
    (a) Alkaline urine may be associated with UTI.
    (b) Alkaline urine and serum acidosis are associated with renal tubular acidosis.
m. Spot urine electrolytes
  (1) Evaluates the ability of the kidney to conserve sodium and concentrate urine
  (2) Measures sodium, potassium, and chloride concentrations in the urine
    (a) Sodium: normal 40 to 220 mEq/L/day
    (b) Potassium: normal 25 to 120 mEq/L/day
    (c) Chloride: normal 110 to 250 mEq/L/day
n. Sediment
  (1) Casts: precipitation from the kidney that takes the shape of the tubule where it was formed; normally none or occasional hyaline casts
    (a) Hyaline casts: small amounts normal, but if large amounts, indicative of significant proteinuria
    (b) Erythrocyte casts: indicative of glomerulonephritis or vasculitis
    (c) Leukocyte casts: indicative of infectious process
    (d) Granular casts: indicative of acute tubular necrosis, interstitial nephritis, acute or chronic glomerulonephritis, chronic renal failure
    (e) Fatty casts: indicative of lipoid nephrosis or nephrotic syndrome
    (f) Renal tubular casts: indicative of acute renal failure
  (2) Bacteria: abnormal in catheterized specimen
  (3) Erythrocytes: small numbers normal; large numbers indicative of glomerulonephritis, interstitial nephritis, malignancy, infection, calculi, cystitis, or trauma
  (4) Leukocytes: small numbers normal; large numbers indicative of infection, interstitial nephritis
  (5) Renal epithelial cells: indicative of acute tubular necrosis, glomerulonephritis, interstitial nephritis
  (6) Crystals: indicative of stone formation
  (7) Eosinophils: indicative of allergic reaction in kidney

3. Other diagnostic studies (Table 8-3)

Table 8-3 Renal Diagnostic Studies

Study	Purposes	Comments
CT scan	• Provides a view of kidneys, retroperitoneal space, bladder, and prostate • Evaluates kidney size • Evaluates the kidney for tumors, abscesses, and obstruction	• No special preparation required • Can be used safely in patients with renal failure • Contrast medium may be used
Cystometrogram	• Evaluates the pressure exerted against the wall of the bladder to evaluate bladder tone	• No special preparation required • Urinary catheter inserted and saline instilled into bladder *Postprocedure* • Monitor for clinical indications of UTI

Continued

Table 8-3 Renal Diagnostic Studies—cont'd

Study	Purposes	Comments
Cystoscopy	• Visualizes bladder and urethra for identification of pathologic condition	*Preprocedure* • NPO after midnight if general anesthesia is to be used • Administer sedative if prescribed • No special preparation required *Postprocedure* • Pink-tinged urine is normal, but gross hematuria is abnormal; monitor urine output • Encourage fluid intake
IVP	• Evaluates position, size, shape, and location of kidneys • Provides visualization of internal kidney (parenchyma, calyces, pelvis) • Evaluates filling of renal pelvis • Outlines ureters and bladder • Identifies presence of cysts and tumors • Identifies obstruction and congenital abnormality	• Also called *excretory urogram* • Contraindicated in renal insufficiency, multiple myeloma, pregnancy, congestive heart failure, and sickle cell disease • Bowel preparation (e.g., cathartics) as prescribed • NPO for 8 hours before the test • Contrast media used ◦ Check for allergy to iodine before the study ◦ Monitor for allergic reaction postprocedure ◦ Ensure hydration postprocedure
Kidneys, ureters, and bladder (KUB)	• Outlines kidneys, ureters, and bladder • Evaluates size, shape, and position of kidneys • Identifies location of calculi	• Also called *flat plate of abdomen* • Bowel preparation (e.g., cathartics) may be prescribed if to be followed by IVP
Magnetic resonance imaging	• Differentiation between cyst and solid mass • Identifies infarction, trauma, and obstruction	• More specific than renal ultrasonography or CT scan because it shows subtle density changes • Cannot be used in patients with any implanted metallic device, including pacemakers • No special preparation required
Nephrotomogram	• Evaluates segments of the kidney at different levels • Differentiates cysts from solid masses	• Bowel preparation (e.g., cathartics) as prescribed • NPO for 8 hours before the test • Contrast media used ◦ Check for allergy to iodine before the study ◦ Monitor for allergic reaction postprocedure ◦ Ensure hydration postprocedure
Renal angiography	• Evaluates renal vasculature • Identifies renal artery stenosis • Identifies cysts, tumors, infarction, and trauma	• Bowel preparation (e.g., cathartics) as prescribed • NPO for 8 hours before the test • Sedative if usually prescribed before the • Contrast media used ◦ Check for allergy to iodine before the study ◦ Monitor for allergic reaction ◦ Ensure hydration postprocedure *Postprocedure* • Keep extremity in which catheter was placed immobilized in a straight position for 6 to 12 hours • Monitor arterial puncture point for hemorrhage or hematoma • Monitor neurovascular status of affected limb • Monitor for indications of systemic emboli

Table 8-3 Renal Diagnostic Studies—cont'd

Study	Purposes	Comments
Renal biopsy	• Obtains tissue specimen for microscopic evaluation	• May be performed open or closed • Clotting profile is evaluated preprocedure • Type and crossmatch for two units of blood preprocedure • Usually not performed if patient has only one functioning kidney (unless being done to evaluate possible transplant rejection) • Closed biopsy contraindicated in bleeding abnormalities, polycystic disease, hydronephrosis, neoplasm, UTI, and uncooperative patient *Postprocedure* • Pressure dressing is applied, and the patient is on bed rest for 24 hours • Observe for hematuria, flank pain, or hypotension
Renal radionuclide scan (renogram)	• Evaluates position, size, shape, and location of kidneys • Identifies obstruction, abscesses, cysts, and tumors • Evaluates renal perfusion • Evaluates glomerular filtration, tubular function, and excretion • Assesses status of renal transplant	• Assure patient that the amount of radioactive material is minimal • Do not schedule within 24 hours after IVP • Ask patient to void before scan • Encourage fluid intake after the procedure
Retrograde pyelogram	• Evaluates position, size, shape, and location of kidneys • Outlines ureters and bladder • Identifies presence of cysts and tumors • Identifies obstruction	• Does not require the kidney to excrete the dye, so may be used in patients with renal insufficiency • Bowel preparation (e.g., cathartics) as prescribed • NPO for 8 hours before the test • Contrast media used ◦ Check for allergy to iodine before the study ◦ Monitor for allergic reaction postprocedure ◦ Ensure hydration postprocedure • Monitor patient for clinical indications of UTI or sepsis
Ultrasonography	• Evaluates fluid versus solid mass • Identifies obstructions • Identifies cysts, abscesses, tumors, and polycystic kidney disease • Identifies hemorrhage • Identifies urinary tract obstruction and leaks	• No special preparation required • Can be used safely in patients with renal failure • Contrast media may be used
Voiding cystourethrography	• Identifies abnormalities of lower urinary tract to determine presence of reflux and residual urine	• No special preparation required • Encourage fluid intake postprocedure

CT, Computed tomography; *IVP*, intravenous pyelogram; *NPO*, nothing by mouth; *UTI*, urinary tract infection.

Fluid and Electrolyte Imbalances

Hypovolemia

1. Etiology
   a. Insufficient intake
   b. Inadequate replacement following excess fluid loss
   c. Excessive fluid losses
      (1) Hemorrhage
      (2) GI losses
         (a) Nasogastric or intestinal suction
         (b) Vomiting
         (c) Diarrhea
         (d) Fistula
      (3) Renal losses
         (a) Diuretics
         (b) Aldosterone insufficiency
         (c) Diuretic phase of acute renal failure
         (d) Osmotic diuresis caused by hyperglycemia

(4) Increased insensible losses
(a) Diaphoresis
(b) Tachypnea
(5) Draining wounds
d. Intravascular to extravascular shift (also called *third spacing*)
(1) Ascites
(2) Intestinal obstruction
(3) Peritonitis
(4) Burns
2. Clinical presentation
a. Subjective
(1) Weakness
(2) Anorexia, nausea, vomiting, constipation
(3) Thirst
(4) Syncope
b. Objective
(1) Tachycardia
(2) Orthostatic hypotension
(3) Low-grade fever
(4) Flushed skin (fluid loss) or cool, clammy skin (blood loss)
(5) Flat jugular veins
(6) Dry, sticky tongue and mucous membranes
(7) Poor skin turgor
(8) Lethargy, disorientation, coma
(9) Oliguria
(10) Weight loss more than 5% of body weight
(11) Hemodynamic changes: decreased CVP, PAOP, CO, increased SVR
c. Diagnostic
(1) Hct and serum osmolality increased if fluid lost; Hct decreased if blood lost
(2) Urine specific gravity greater than 1.030 if ADH osmoreceptor mechanism is intact
(3) BUN increased with normal creatinine (i.e., prerenal)
3. Nursing diagnoses
a. Deficient Fluid Volume related to excessive fluid losses, inadequate intake or replacement, and third spacing
b. Decreased Cardiac Output related to decreased preload
c. Ineffective Tissue Perfusion related to decreased Hgb and cardiac output
4. Collaborative management
a. Monitor urine output, intake and output (I&O), daily weight, and laboratory studies.
b. Treat the cause.
(1) Antiemetics for vomiting
(2) Antidiarrheals for diarrhea
(3) Control of hemorrhage: local pressure, prepare patient for surgery
(4) Antibiotics for infection
c. Replace fluids carefully to prevent hypervolemia.
(1) Oral fluids for mild deficits
(2) Parenteral fluids for moderate or severe deficits; replace fluids lost with similar fluids (e.g., blood for hemorrhage and normal saline with electrolytes for excessive diuresis)
(3) Monitor for clinical indications of fluid overload (e.g., S_3 and crackles)
d. Provide frequent oral and skin care.

Water Loss Syndromes

Serum osmolality greater than 295 mOsm/kg (may be referred to as *hyperosmolar hypernatremia*)
1. Etiology: water loss without sodium loss
a. Inadequate water intake
b. Hypertonic fluids or enteral feedings
c. Diabetes insipidus
d. Diabetes mellitus
e. Excess total parenteral nutrition (TPN)
f. Watery diarrhea
2. Clinical presentation
a. Subjective
(1) Weakness
(2) Thirst
(3) Syncope
b. Objective
(1) Tachycardia
(2) Hypotension
(3) Low-grade fever
(4) Flushed skin
(5) Dry, sticky tongue and mucous membranes
(6) Poor skin turgor
(7) Thirst
(8) Mental irritability, confusion
(9) Oliguria to anuria (except diabetes insipidus)
c. Diagnostic
(1) Hct and serum osmolality increased
(2) Serum sodium increased (concentration effect)
3. Nursing diagnoses
a. Deficient Fluid Volume related to excessive fluid losses, inadequate intake or replacement, and third spacing
b. Decreased Cardiac Output related to decreased preload
c. Ineffective Tissue Perfusion related to decreased Hgb and CO
4. Collaborative management
a. Monitor urine output, I&O, daily weight, and laboratory studies.
b. Treat the cause.
(1) Vasopressin for central diabetes insipidus; chlorpropamide (Diabinese) for nephrogenic diabetes insipidus
(2) Insulin for diabetes mellitus and hyperglycemia
(3) Antidiarrheals for diarrhea
(4) Antiemetics for nausea and vomiting
c. Provide appropriate volume replacement and normalize serum osmolality: administer water in excess of sodium (e.g., 5% dextrose in water or one-half normal saline).
d. Maintain adequate urine output with adequate volume replacement.
e. Provide frequent oral and skin care.

Hypervolemia

1. Etiology
   a. Excessive intake of fluid
      (1) Excess oral or parenteral fluids
      (2) Excess use of saline enemas
   b. Retention of sodium and water
      (1) Steroid therapy
      (2) HF
      (3) Liver disease (e.g., cirrhosis)
      (4) Stress response via ADH secretion and RAA system
      (5) Nephrotic syndrome
      (6) Acute or chronic renal failure
   c. Interstitial to intravascular shift
      (1) Remobilization of fluids after treatment of burns
      (2) Administration of hypertonic or hyperosmolar solutions (e.g., 3% saline and albumin)
2. Clinical presentation
   a. Subjective
      (1) Dyspnea
      (2) Headache
   b. Objective
      (1) Tachycardia
      (2) Increased BP
      (3) JVD
      (4) Tachypnea, dyspnea, crackles
      (5) Peripheral edema
      (6) Ascites
      (7) Increased urine output
      (8) Muscle weakness
      (9) Confusion, apathy, lethargy, coma
      (10) Hemodynamic changes: increased CVP and PAOP
      (11) Weight gain more than 5% of body weight
      (12) Clinical indications of pulmonary or cerebral edema
   c. Diagnostic
      (1) Hct and serum osmolality decreased
      (2) BUN decreased
      (3) Urine specific gravity less than 1.01 if ADH osmoreceptor mechanism is intact
      (4) Chest x-ray may show pulmonary vascular congestion
3. Nursing diagnoses
   a. Excess Fluid Volume related to decreased fluid elimination and excessive fluid intake or replacement
   b. Impaired Gas Exchange related to intraalveolar fluid
   c. Decreased Adaptive Capacity: Intracranial related to cerebral edema
4. Collaborative management
   a. Monitor urine output, I&O, daily weight, and laboratory studies.
   b. Prevent hypervolemia by closely monitoring intravenous (IV) fluids; volumetric or controller pumps should be used for patients predisposed to hypervolemia.
   c. Decrease excess volume.
      (1) Restrict fluids and/or sodium.
      (2) Administer diuretics as prescribed.
      (3) Hemodialysis or continuous renal replacement therapy may be used especially if renal insufficiency is present.
   d. Provide frequent oral and skin care.

Water Excess Syndromes

May be referred to as *hypoosmolar hyponatremia*

1. Etiology: water increased in excess of sodium
   a. Replacement of isotonic body fluids with hypotonic solution (e.g., 5% dextrose in water)
   b. Excess use of tap water enemas
   c. Psychogenic polydipsia
   d. GI or genitourinary (GU) irrigation with hypotonic fluids (e.g., tap water or distilled water)
   e. Excessive use of ice chips
   f. Syndrome of inappropriate antidiuretic hormone (SIADH)
   g. Administration of oral hypoglycemic agents and tricyclic antidepressants
2. Clinical presentation
   a. Subjective
      (1) Anorexia, nausea, vomiting
      (2) Abdominal and muscle cramps
      (3) Headache
      (4) Weakness
   b. Objective
      (1) Edema
      (2) Lethargy
      (3) Muscle twitching, seizures
      (4) Confusion
   c. Diagnostic
      (1) Serum osmolality less than 280 mOsm/kg
      (2) Serum sodium decreased (dilution effect)
      (3) Hct decreased
3. Nursing diagnoses
   a. Excess Fluid Volume related to decreased fluid elimination and excessive fluid intake or replacement
   b. Impaired Gas Exchanged related to intraalveolar fluid
   c. Decreased Adaptive Capacity: Intracranial related to cerebral edema
4. Collaborative management
   a. Monitor urine output, I&O, daily weight, and laboratory studies.
   b. Decrease water intake and normalize osmolality.
      (1) Restrict fluids.
      (2) Administer diuretics as prescribed.
      (3) Administer hypertonic (3%) saline as prescribed for severe hyponatremia.
         (a) Usually administered no more rapidly than 100 mL/hr and no more than 400 mL per 24 hours.
         (b) Monitor closely for clinical indications of fluid overload because hypertonic saline pulls fluid into the vascular space.
      (4) Initiate continuous renal replacement therapy (CRRT) as prescribed.

(5) Administer demeclocycline or lithium as prescribed for nephrogenic SIADH.
c. Provide frequent oral and skin care.
d. Monitor patient for clinical indications of cerebral or pulmonary edema: institute seizure precautions.

Hyponatremia

1. Etiology: decrease in sodium and water
   a. Decreased sodium intake
      (1) Sodium-restricted diet
      (2) Alcoholism
   b. Increased sodium excretion
      (1) Skin losses
         (a) Diaphoresis
         (b) Burns
      (2) GI losses
         (a) GI suctioning
         (b) Vomiting
         (c) Diarrhea
         (d) Draining wound or fistula
         (e) Laxative abuse
      (3) Renal losses
         (a) Diuretics: thiazide, loop
         (b) Adrenal insufficiency
         (c) Cerebral salt-wasting syndrome
2. Clinical presentation
   a. Subjective
      (1) Anorexia, nausea, vomiting, abdominal cramps
      (2) Apprehension
      (3) Headache
      (4) Weakness, fatigue
   b. Objective
      (1) Tachycardia
      (2) Postural hypotension
      (3) Diarrhea
      (4) Weight loss
      (5) Decreased skin turgor
      (6) "Fingerprinting" over sternum
      (7) Personality changes
      (8) Mental confusion, disorientation
      (9) Lethargy progressing to coma
      (10) Muscle cramps, muscle twitching, increased deep tendon reflexes (DTR)
      (11) Tremors, seizures
      (12) Oliguria
   c. Diagnostic
      (1) Serum sodium less than 136 mEq/L with normal serum osmolality
3. Nursing diagnoses
   a. Deficient Fluid Volume related to excessive fluid and sodium losses and inadequate intake or replacement
   b. Decreased Cardiac Output related to decreased preload
4. Collaborative management
   a. Monitor urine output, I&O, daily weight, and laboratory studies.
   b. Restore normal serum electrolyte levels.
      (1) Encourage sodium intake in diet in mild deficiency.
      (2) Administer sodium parenterally for moderate or severe deficiency.
         (a) Normal saline as prescribed
         (b) Hypertonic (3%) saline as prescribed for severe hyponatremia
            (i) Usually administered no more rapidly than 1 to 2 mL/kg/hr and no more than 400 mL per 24 hours
            (ii) Monitor closely for clinical indications of fluid overload because hypertonic saline pulls fluid into the vascular space
      (3) Potassium replacement also may be needed.
   c. Monitor for neurologic changes; institute seizure precautions.
   d. Provide frequent oral and skin care.

Hypernatremia

1. Etiology: increase in sodium and water
   a. Excess salt (sodium chloride) consumption
   b. Excess/rapid administration of normal saline or hypertonic saline solution
   c. Administration of sodium bicarbonate or sodium polystyrene sulfonate (Kayexalate)
   d. HF
   e. Renal failure
   f. Cirrhosis
   g. Steroid therapy
   h. Cushing's syndrome
   i. Primary hyperaldosteronism
   j. Saltwater near drowning, ingestion of salt water
2. Clinical presentation
   a. Subjective
      (1) Thirst
      (2) Muscle weakness and/or cramps
   b. Objective
      (1) Tachycardia
      (2) Hypertension
      (3) Low-grade fever
      (4) Edema
      (5) Dry, sticky tongue and mucous membranes
      (6) Flushed, dry skin
      (7) Muscle rigidity, twitching
      (8) Increased DTR
      (9) Central nervous system irritability: restlessness, agitation
      (10) Mental confusion, disorientation
      (11) Tremors, seizures
      (12) Oliguria
      (13) Weight gain
   c. Diagnostic
      (1) Serum sodium greater than 145 mEq/L with normal serum osmolality
3. Nursing diagnoses
   a. Risk for Excess Fluid Volume related to decreased fluid elimination and excessive fluid intake or replacement
   b. Risk for Injury related to potential seizures
4. Collaborative management

a. Monitor urine output, I&O, daily weight, and laboratory studies.
b. Treat the cause.
c. Restore normal serum electrolyte levels.
   (1) Restrict sodium.
      (a) Mild restriction: 3 to 4 g/day; commonly referred to as a "no added salt" diet
      (b) Moderate restriction: 2 g/day; consumption of only foods specifically "low sodium"
      (c) Severe restriction: 500 mg/day; low-sodium foods only with avoidance of shellfish and limitation of dairy and meat
   (2) Administer diuretics as prescribed.
d. Provide frequent oral and skin care.
e. Monitor for change in neurologic status; institute seizure precautions.

Hypokalemia

1. Etiology
   a. Poor potassium intake
      (1) Starvation
      (2) Alcoholism
      (3) Administration of potassium-deficient parenteral fluids or nutrition
      (4) Use of low-potassium dialysate
   b. Increased GI losses
      (1) GI surgery
      (2) Gastric or intestinal suction
      (3) Vomiting
      (4) Fistula
      (5) Diarrhea
      (6) Chronic malabsorption syndrome
      (7) Laxative abuse
      (8) Intestinal bypass surgery
   c. Increased renal losses
      (1) Polyuria
      (2) Renal tubular acidosis
      (3) Sodium restriction
      (4) Hypomagnesemia
      (5) Hyperaldosteronism
      (6) Licorice excess: increases aldosterone effect
      (7) Congestive heart failure
      (8) Steroid therapy or Cushing's syndrome
      (9) Cirrhosis
      (10) Stress via RAA system and release of corticosteroids
      (11) Burns (as fluid shifts back into intravascular space 48 to 72 hours after fluid resuscitation)
      (12) Drugs
         (a) Diuretics: thiazide; loop
         (b) Certain antimicrobials: aminoglycosides, amphotericin B, carbenicillin, penicillin
         (c) Corticosteroids
   d. Skin losses
      (1) Diaphoresis
   e. Extracellular to intracellular shift
      (1) Alkalosis
      (2) Insulin
      (3) Treatment of DKA
      (4) Refeeding syndrome
2. Clinical presentation
   a. Subjective
      (1) Anorexia, nausea, vomiting
      (2) Malaise, fatigue
      (3) Dizziness
      (4) Muscle cramps
   b. Objective
      (1) Orthostatic hypotension
      (2) Decreased GI motility and bowel sounds, paralytic ileus, constipation, abdominal distention
      (3) Muscle weakness, possibly flaccid paralysis
      (4) Decreased DTR
      (5) Irritability, mental confusion, drowsiness to coma
      (6) Respiratory muscle weakness causing shallow ventilation; dyspnea progressing to respiratory paralysis and respiratory arrest
      (7) Polyuria, polydipsia, inability to concentrate urine
      (8) Enhanced digitalis effect
      (9) Decreased CO, dysrhythmias, and cardiac arrest may occur
   c. Diagnostic
      (1) Serum potassium less than 3.5 mEq/L
      (2) Electrocardiogram (ECG) changes
         (a) Flat T waves and prominent U waves
         (b) Depressed ST segment
         (c) Prolonged QT and PR intervals
         (d) Dysrhythmias (e.g., premature ventricular contractions, ventricular tachycardia, or ventricular fibrillation)
3. Nursing diagnoses
   a. Decreased Cardiac Output related to dysrhythmias
   b. Ineffective Breathing Pattern related to respiratory muscle weakness
   c. Constipation related to decreased GI
4. Collaborative management
   a. Monitor urine output, I&O, daily weight, and laboratory studies.
   b. Treat the cause.
      (1) Correct alkalosis.
      (2) Correct hypomagnesemia and/or hypocalcemia; hypokalemia that is refractory to treatment frequently is accompanied by hypomagnesemia and/or hypocalcemia.
      (3) Discontinue causative drug if possible.
   c. Restore normal serum electrolyte levels.
      (1) Increase dietary potassium for mild hypokalemia; encourage use of potassium chloride salt substitute.
      (2) Administer potassium supplements orally.
         (a) Decrease gastric irritation by administering with food.
      (3) Administer potassium parenterally for severe hypokalemia.
         (a) Never administer potassium IV push.
         (b) Always use an infusion pump.

(c) Do not add to a preexisting infusion; if potassium is to be added to maintenance fluids, a new solution should be mixed to avoid uneven distribution of the potassium.

(d) Administer potassium "runs" IV usually via minibag (usual safe maximum 10 mEq/100 mL over 1 hour but may be administered at 20 mEq/hr if serum potassium is less than 2.5 mEq/L).

(i) Administer at no greater concentration than 10 mEq/100 mL if given via peripheral catheter or 20 mEq/100 mL if given via a central venous catheter.

(ii) Administer in normal saline unless contraindicated; dextrose may stimulate insulin secretion and intracellular shift of potassium.

(iii) NOTE: It takes 100 to 200 mEq of potassium to increase serum potassium by 1 mEq/L.

(iv) Monitor ECG closely when administering high concentrations of potassium.

d. Monitor for clinical indications of digitalis toxicity if patient is receiving digitalis preparation.

e. Teach patient about adequate potassium replacement if receiving diuretics; potassium-sparing diuretics may be used.

Hyperkalemia

1. Etiology

a. Increased potassium intake

(1) Excessive administration/ingestion of potassium: oral or parenteral

(2) Excessive or too rapid potassium replacement

(3) Excessive use of potassium chloride salt substitute

(4) Transfusion of banked blood; the longer the blood has been stored, the higher the extracellular potassium content

(5) Cardioplegic solution

(6) Drugs that contain potassium, such as potassium penicillin and potassium phosphate enemas

b. Decreased potassium excretion

(1) Acute and chronic renal disease

(2) Adrenal insufficiency (Addison's disease)

(3) Drugs

(a) Potassium-sparing diuretics

(b) ACE inhibitors or angiotensin receptor blockers

(c) NSAIDs

(d) Cyclosporine

c. Cellular disruption with leak of intracellular potassium

(1) Crush injuries

(2) Rhabdomyolysis

(3) Hemolysis (e.g., blood transfusion reaction or freshwater near drowning)

(4) Early burns

(5) Trauma

(6) Catabolism

(7) Lysis of tumor cells from chemotherapy

d. Intracellular to extracellular shift

(1) Acidosis

(2) Insulin deficiency

(3) Malignant hyperthermia

(4) Drugs

(a) Massive digitalis overdosage

(b) Muscle paralyzing agents (e.g., succinylcholine)

e. Pseudohyperkalemia

(1) Hemolyzed blood sample

(2) Sample drawn above an IV infusion containing potassium

(3) Traumatic venipuncture

(4) Delay in analysis of sample

2. Clinical presentation

a. Subjective

(1) Nausea, vomiting, abdominal cramping, diarrhea

(2) Numbness, paresthesia of extremities

(3) Weakness, fatigue

b. Objective

(1) Initially tachycardia progressing to bradycardia and cardiac arrest

(2) Decreased contractility, decreased CO, hypotension

(3) Abdominal distention

(4) Hyperactive bowel sounds

(5) Muscle weakness progressing to flaccid paralysis

(6) Increased DTR initially progressing to decreased to absent DTR

(7) Respiratory muscle weakness may cause hypopnea and respiratory distress

(8) Lethargy, apathy, mental confusion

(9) Oliguria

c. Diagnostic

(1) Serum potassium greater than 5 mEq/L

(a) Mild: 5 to 6 mEq/L

(b) Moderate: 6 to 7 mEq/L

(c) Severe: greater than 7 mEq/L

(2) ECG changes

(a) 5.5 to 6 mEq/L: tall, narrow, peaked T waves, shortened QT interval

(b) 6 to 7 mEq/L: wide QRS complexes, prolonged PR intervals

(c) 7 to 7.5 mEq/L: flattened to absent P waves, further widening of QRS complexes

(d) 8 or greater: fusion of QRS complexes and T waves, idioventricular rhythm, asystole

3. Nursing diagnoses

a. Decreased Cardiac Output related to decreased contractility and dysrhythmias

b. Ineffective Breathing Pattern related to respiratory muscle weakness

c. Diarrhea related to increased GI motility

4. Collaborative management
   a. Monitor urine output, I&O, daily weight, and laboratory studies.
      (1) Check BUN and creatinine levels for data about renal function.
   b. Treat the cause.
      (1) Dialysis for renal failure
      (2) Treatment of acidosis
      (3) Insulin therapy for hyperglycemia
      (4) Discontinuance of any causative drug if possible
         (a) Potassium-sparing diuretics
         (b) ACE inhibitors or angiotensin receptor blockers
         (c) NSAIDs
   c. Restore normal serum electrolyte levels.
      (1) Limit potassium intake.
         (a) Make sure that IV solution or TPN contains no potassium.
         (b) Check medications for potassium content.
      (2) Administer diuretics as prescribed: usually 40 to 80 mg furosemide (Lasix).
      (3) Initiate emergency treatment if potassium is greater than 6.5 mEq/L or dysrhythmias are present; however, patients with chronic renal failure may tolerate high levels of potassium and may not be symptomatic until 7 mEq/L or greater.
         (a) Dextrose and insulin as prescribed; this moves potassium back into the cell and the effect lasts about 4 to 6 hours; sodium polystyrene sulfonate (Kayexalate) should be given during this time
            (i) Usual dosage is 50 mL of 50% dextrose and 10 units of insulin
            (ii) Monitor for increased or decreased serum glucose
         (b) Sodium polystyrene sulfonate (Kayexalate), an exchange resin, as prescribed; exchanges sodium for potassium and moves potassium out of the body via the GI tract
            (i) Oral or by retention enema
               a) Usual dose is 15 to 50 g in 50 to 100 mL of 20% sorbitol orally
               b) 50 g in 200 mL of dextrose as retention enema
            (ii) Sorbitol, an osmotic laxative, produces a cathartic effect only when given orally and may contribute to intestinal necrosis when given by enema
         (c) Nebulized albuterol as prescribed
            (i) Usual dose is 10 to 20 mg nebulized over 15 minutes
            (ii) Adverse effect: tachycardia
         (d) Bicarbonate as prescribed to correct acidosis
            (i) Usual dose 50 mEq IV over 5 minutes
            (ii) This effect lasts 1 to 2 hours
            (iii) Adverse effects: hypernatremia, hyperosmolality
         (e) CRRT (e.g., continuous venous-venous hemodialysis) if prescribed
   d. Monitor for and prevent cardiac effects of hyperkalemia.
      (1) IV calcium as prescribed
         (a) Usual dose 5 to 10 mL of 10% calcium chloride over 2 to 5 minutes
         (b) Blocks the neuromuscular and cardiac effects
         (c) Contraindicated if patient is receiving digitalis

Hypocalcemia

1. Etiology
   a. Decreased calcium intake or absorption
      (1) Chronic insufficient dietary calcium intake
      (2) Hypoparathyroidism
      (3) Hypomagnesemia
      (4) Acute and chronic renal failure
      (5) Vitamin D deficiency or resistance
      (6) Liver disease
      (7) After gastrectomy
      (8) Chronic malabsorption syndrome
      (9) Alcoholism
      (10) Cushing's syndrome
      (11) Steroid therapy
   b. Increased calcium excretion
      (1) Diuretic therapy: loop, osmotic, potassium-sparing, carbonic anhydrase inhibitors
      (2) Chronic diarrhea
      (3) Hyperphosphatemia
      (4) Diuretic phase of acute renal failure
   c. Increased calcium binding, decreased ionized calcium
      (1) Citrated blood administration
      (2) Alkalosis
      (3) Acute pancreatitis
      (4) Drugs (e.g., aminoglycosides, cimetidine, heparin, or theophylline)
2. Clinical presentation
   a. Subjective
      (1) Abdominal cramps, biliary colic
      (2) Muscle cramps
      (3) Paresthesia of fingertips, circumoral area
   b. Objective
      (1) Chvostek's sign: facial twitching in response to tapping on the facial nerve
      (2) Trousseau's sign: carpal spasm after 3 minutes of inflation of a BP cuff to a level above systolic pressure
      (3) Muscle tremors
      (4) Increased DTR, carpopedal spasm
      (5) Irritability, confusion, psychosis
      (6) Memory loss
      (7) Laryngospasm, stridor
      (8) Tetany (characterized by cramps, twitching of the muscles, sharp flexion of the wrist and ankle joints, seizures)
      (9) Seizures
      (10) Decreased contractility, CO

(11) Oliguria, anuria if renal calculi obstructive
(12) Bruising, bleeding

c. Diagnostic
(1) Serum calcium less than 8.5 mg/dL (less than 4.5 mEq/L)
(a) If albumin is decreased, corrected total calcium can be calculated as follows: measured total calcium + 0.8 × (4 – albumin).
(b) Hypocalcemia is present if serum ionized calcium is less than 4.1 mg/dL.
(2) ECG changes
(a) Prolonged QT interval
(b) Dysrhythmias (e.g., torsades de pointes)
(3) Serum phosphate decreased

3. Nursing diagnoses
a. Risk for Ineffective Breathing Pattern related to laryngospasm
b. Risk for Decreased Cardiac Output related to altered conductivity and contractility
c. Risk for Injury related to seizures

4. Collaborative management
a. Monitor airway patency and ventilation: cricothyroidotomy may be necessary for severe laryngospasm.
b. Monitor urine output, I&O, daily weight, and laboratory studies.
c. Treat the cause.
(1) Phosphate-binding antacids as prescribed for hyperphosphatemia
(2) Calcium administration, phosphate restriction, and phosphate-binding agents for renal failure
d. Restore normal serum electrolyte levels.
(1) High-calcium, low-phosphorus diet
(2) Oral calcium with vitamin D supplements as prescribed for mild hypocalcemia
(3) Calcium gluconate or calcium chloride IV as prescribed
(a) 10 mL of calcium gluconate contains 4.5 mEq of calcium, whereas 10 mL of calcium chloride contains 13.6 mEq of calcium
(b) Slow administration: dilute in 100 mL of 5% dextrose in water and administer over 10 to 30 minutes
(c) Administration through central venous catheter if possible; if administered through a peripheral catheter, prevent extravasation that may cause necrosis and sloughing
(4) Magnesium as prescribed (hypocalcemia unresponsive to treatment may indicate concurrent hypomagnesemia)
e. Monitor for and prevent neurologic complications; institute seizure precautions.

Hypercalcemia

1. Etiology
a. Increased calcium intake
(1) Excessive intake of calcium supplements or calcium antacids
(2) Milk-alkali syndrome related to milk and antacid intake
b. Increased calcium absorption: hypophosphatemia
c. Increased mobilization of calcium from bone
(1) Hyperparathyroidism
(2) Vitamin D excess
(3) Immobility
(4) Osteolytic lesions
(5) Malignancy especially breast, lung, lymphoma, multiple myeloma
(6) Paget's disease
(7) Leukemia
(8) Granulomatous disease (e.g., sarcoidosis, tuberculosis, and histoplasmosis)
(9) Thyrotoxicosis
d. Decreased calcium excretion
(1) Thiazide diuretics
(2) Adrenal insufficiency (Addison's disease)
(3) Renal tubular acidosis
(4) Hyperparathyroidism
(5) Oliguric phase of acute renal failure
e. Increased ionized calcium: acidosis

2. Clinical presentation
a. Subjective
(1) Thirst
(2) Anorexia, nausea, vomiting, abdominal pain
(3) Malaise, fatigue, weakness
(4) Bone and/or flank pain; pathologic fractures may occur
(5) Depression
b. Objective
(1) Decreased bowel sounds, constipation, paralytic ileus
(2) Neuromuscular weakness to flaccidity; decreased DTR
(3) Agitation, confusion, lethargy, stupor, coma
(4) Subtle personality changes progressing to psychosis
(5) Renal calculi
(6) Polyuria, polydipsia
(7) Azotemia
(8) Enhanced digitalis effect
c. Diagnostic
(1) Serum calcium greater than 10.5 mg/dL (greater than 5.8 mEq/L)
(2) Serum phosphate decreased
(3) ECG changes: shortened QT interval, dysrhythmias, and/or blocks
(4) X-ray: osteoporosis

3. Nursing diagnoses
a. Decreased Cardiac Output related to dysrhythmias
b. Risk for Injury related to neurosensory changes
c. Impaired Urinary Elimination related to renal calculi
d. Constipation related to decreased bowel motility

4. Collaborative management
a. Monitor urine output, I&O, daily weight, and laboratory studies.
b. Treat the cause.
(1) Discontinuance of causative drugs
(2) Surgery, radiation, antineoplastics for malignancy
(3) Partial parathyroidectomy for hyperparathyroidism

c. Restore normal serum electrolyte levels.
   (1) Decrease calcium absorption.
      (a) Low-calcium, high-phosphorus diet
      (b) Corticosteroids
   (2) Increase calcium excretion.
      (a) Oral or parenteral fluids as prescribed; usually isotonic saline at 100 to 200 mL/hr
      (b) Any of the following as prescribed:
         (i) Loop diuretics (e.g., furosemide [Lasix])
         (ii) Calcitonin
         (iii) Phosphorus
         (iv) Etetate disodium (EDTA)
      (c) Dialysis may be used
   (3) Decrease bone resorption of calcium
      (a) Weight-bearing activities
      (b) Any of the following as prescribed:
         (i) Etidronate (Didronel)
         (ii) Pamidronate (Aredia)
         (iii) Gallium nitrate
         (iv) Corticosteroids
         (v) Plicamycin (formerly known as *mithramycin*) (Mithracin)
         (vi) Inorganic phosphate

d. Monitor for and prevent cardiac effects of hypercalcemia: administer calcium channel blockers as prescribed.

e. Prevent renal calculi while correcting hypercalcemia: agents to acidify urine may be used because acidification of urine increases solubility of calcium.

f. Monitor for clinical indications of digitalis toxicity.

Hypophosphatemia

1. Etiology
   a. Inadequate intake of phosphorus
      (1) Malnutrition
      (2) Alcoholism
      (3) Severe, prolonged vomiting
      (4) Prolonged low-phosphorus or phosphate-free IV therapy or TPN therapy
   b. Decreased GI absorption or increased intestinal loss
      (1) Excessive use of phosphate-binding gels such as aluminum hydroxide (Amphojel)
      (2) Prolonged vomiting, gastric suction, sucralfate (Carafate)
      (3) Chronic diarrhea
      (4) Chronic malabsorption syndrome
      (5) Vitamin D deficiency
   c. Increased renal excretion of phosphorus
      (1) Thiazide diuretics
      (2) Hypomagnesemia
      (3) Hypokalemia
      (4) Hyperglycemia
      (5) Hyperparathyroidism
      (6) Fanconi syndrome
   d. Extracellular to intracellular shifts
      (1) Parenteral glucose or insulin administration
      (2) Alkalosis
      (3) Large amounts of carbohydrate (refeeding syndrome)
      (4) Treatment of DKA
      (5) Beta-adrenergic drugs (e.g., albuterol [Proventil])
2. Clinical presentation
   a. Subjective
      (1) Anorexia, nausea, vomiting
      (2) Malaise, fatigue
      (3) Paresthesia
      (4) Bone pain
      (5) Chest pain
   b. Objective
      (1) Tachycardia, hypotension
      (2) Tremors
      (3) Muscle weakness
      (4) Nystagmus, anisocoria
      (5) Incoordination, ataxia
      (6) Confusion, lethargy, coma
      (7) Seizures
      (8) Memory loss
      (9) Respiratory muscle weakness and decreased respiratory excursion
      (10) Heart failure: dyspnea, crackles
      (11) Weight loss
      (12) Hemolytic anemia
      (13) Platelet dysfunction: petechiae, bleeding
      (14) Immunosuppression
   c. Diagnostic
      (1) Serum phosphate less than 3 mg/dL
      (2) Increased serum and urine calcium
      (3) ECG: dysrhythmias
      (4) X-ray: skeletal abnormalities
3. Nursing diagnoses
   a. Ineffective Breathing Pattern related to decreased respiratory muscle strength
   b. Risk for Decreased Cardiac Output related to altered conductivity and contractility
   c. Risk for Ineffective Breathing Pattern related to laryngospasm
   d. Impaired Gas Exchange related to decreased 2,3-diphosphoglyceric acid levels
   e. Risk for Injury related to seizures
4. Collaborative management
   a. Monitor urine output, I&O, daily weight, and laboratory studies.
   b. Treat the cause.
      (1) Discontinuance of phosphate binding gels
      (2) Correction of hypercalcemia if cause of hypophosphatemia
   c. Restore normal serum electrolyte levels.
      (1) High-phosphorus, low-calcium diet
      (2) Oral phosphate supplements (e.g., Neutra-Phos [sodium and potassium phosphate], Phospho-Soda [sodium phosphate], or K-Phos [potassium phosphate]) as ordered, and monitor for signs of hypocalcemia when giving supplements
      (3) Parenteral sodium phosphate or potassium phosphate IV as ordered and monitor for signs of hypocalcemia

(a) Usual dose
(i) If phosphate less than 1 mg/dL without adverse effects: usual dose is 0.6 mg/kg/hr
(ii) If phosphate less than 2 mg/dL with adverse effects: usual dose is 0.9 mg/kg/hr
(b) Use central venous catheter if possible
(c) IV phosphate is contraindicated in hypercalcemia

d. Monitor for cardiovascular, pulmonary, and neurologic effects of hypophosphatemia.

Hyperphosphatemia

1. Etiology
 a. Increased phosphorus intake
 (1) Cathartic abuse with phosphate-containing laxatives and enemas
 (2) Excessive vitamin D intake
 (3) Transfusion of stored blood
 (4) Acute elemental phosphorus poisoning
 b. Decreased phosphorus excretion
 (1) Acute or chronic renal failure
 (2) Hypoparathyroidism
 c. Intracellular to extracellular shifts
 (1) Acidosis
 (2) Malignant hyperthermia
 (3) Severe hypothermia
 d. Cellular destruction
 (1) Neoplastic disease treated with chemotherapy
 (2) Catabolism
 (3) Rhabdomyolysis
2. Clinical presentation
 a. As for hypocalcemia
 b. Diagnostic: serum phosphate greater than 4.5 mg/dL
3. Nursing diagnoses
 a. Risk for Ineffective Breathing Pattern related to laryngospasm
 b. Risk for Decreased Cardiac Output related to altered conductivity and contractility
 c. Risk for Injury related to seizures
4. Collaborative management
 a. Monitor airway patency; cricothyroidotomy may be necessary for severe laryngospasm.
 b. Monitor urine output, I&O, daily weight, and laboratory studies.
 c. Treat the cause.
 (1) Correction of hypocalcemia
 (2) Dialysis if renal failure is cause
 (3) Saline diuresis and urinary alkalinization if tumor lysis syndrome or rhabdomyolysis
 d. Restore normal serum electrolyte levels.
 (1) Low-phosphorus, high-calcium diet
 (2) Sucralfate (Carafate) or aluminum antacids to bind with phosphate in GI tract as prescribed
 (3) Glucose and insulin as prescribed to shift phosphate into the cell (transient effect only)
 e. Monitor for and prevent neurologic complications; institute seizure precautions.

Hypomagnesemia

1. Etiology
 a. Decreased magnesium intake or absorption
 (1) Protein-calorie malnutrition
 (2) Starvation
 (3) Alcoholism
 (4) Prolonged low-magnesium or magnesium-free IV therapy or TPN therapy
 b. Impaired absorption
 (1) Alcoholism
 (2) Intestinal malabsorption syndrome
 (3) Acute pancreatitis
 c. Increased magnesium loss
 (1) Drugs
 (a) Diuretics
 (b) Antimicrobials: aminoglycosides, pentamidine, amphotericin B
 (c) Ethanol
 (d) Cisplatin
 (e) Cyclosporin A
 (2) Diuretic phase of acute renal failure
 (3) Vomiting, gastric suction, fistula
 (4) Chronic diarrhea (e.g., ulcerative colitis; laxative abuse)
 (5) Hypoparathyroidism
 (6) Hyperaldosteronism
 (7) Steroids
 (8) DKA
 (9) HF
 d. Increased magnesium binding: citrated blood administration
 e. Extracellular to intracellular shift
 (1) Refeeding syndrome
 (2) Amino acid solutions
 (3) Insulin; treatment of DKA
 (4) Acute myocardial infarction
2. Clinical presentation
 a. Subjective
 (1) Anorexia, nausea, vomiting, abdominal distention
 (2) Paresthesia of fingertips, circumoral area
 (3) Muscle cramps
 (4) Syncope
 b. Objective
 (1) Tachycardia, hypotension
 (2) Chvostek's and Trousseau's signs
 (3) Tremors, increased DTR, carpopedal spasm
 (4) Ataxia, nystagmus
 (5) Laryngospasm, stridor
 (6) Tetany
 (7) Seizures
 (8) Insomnia
 (9) Confusion, psychosis
 (10) Memory loss
 (11) Decreased contractility, CO
 (12) Increased digitalis effect
 c. Diagnostic
 (1) Serum magnesium less than 1.5 mEq/L
 (a) May have concurrent hypocalcemia, hypokalemia, or hypophosphatemia

(2) ECG changes
(a) Prolonged QT interval
(b) Dysrhythmias, especially torsades de pointes
3. Nursing diagnoses
a. Risk for Ineffective Breathing Patterns related to laryngospasm
b. Risk for Decreased Cardiac Output related to altered conductivity and contractility
c. Risk for Injury related to seizures
4. Collaborative management
a. Monitor airway patency; cricothyroidotomy may be necessary for severe laryngospasm.
b. Monitor urine output, I&O, daily weight, and laboratory studies.
c. Treat the cause.
(1) Nutritional support for malnutrition
(2) Use of potassium-sparing diuretics if diuretics are needed because they spare magnesium
d. Restore normal serum electrolyte levels.
(1) High-magnesium diet
(2) Oral magnesium supplements in the form of magnesium antacids as prescribed
(3) Magnesium sulfate IV as prescribed
(a) Usually administered in 1 to 2 g over 5 to 60 minutes
(i) Usually diluted in 100 mL and administered over 1 hour
(ii) May be diluted in 10 mL and administered over 5 to 20 minutes for when life-threatening dysrhythmias (e.g., torsades de pointes) occur
(4) Calcium replacement as prescribed; most patients with hypomagnesemia are also hypocalcemic
e. Monitor for and prevent neurologic complications; institute seizure precautions.
f. Monitor for clinical indications of digitalis toxicity for patients on digitalis preparations.

Hypermagnesemia

1. Etiology
a. Increased magnesium intake
(1) Magnesium antacids
(2) Magnesium sulfate IV
(3) Magnesium-containing antacids, laxatives, enemas
b. Decreased magnesium excretion
(1) Acute or chronic renal failure
(2) Hyperparathyroidism
(3) Hypoaldosteronism
(4) Hypothyroidism
c. Intracellular to extracellular shift
(1) Untreated ketoacidosis
(2) Burns
(3) Rhabdomyolysis
d. Pseudohypermagnesemia: sample hemolysis
2. Clinical presentation
a. Subjective
(1) Weakness, fatigue
(2) Nausea, vomiting
(3) Somnolence
(4) Diplopia
b. Objective
(1) Bradycardia, hypotension
(2) Facial flushing
(3) Muscle weakness progressing to paralysis
(4) Decreased DTR: loss of patellar reflex occurs at levels greater than 8 mEq/L
(5) Respiratory muscle weakness may cause hypoventilation and dyspnea
(6) Respiratory muscle paralysis and apnea may occur with levels greater than 10 mEq/L
(7) Confusion, somnolence, lethargy, coma
(8) Cardiopulmonary arrest
c. Diagnostic
(1) Serum magnesium greater than 2.5 mEq/L
(2) ECG: prolonged PR interval, QRS complex, QT interval; bradycardias and blocks
3. Nursing diagnoses
a. Risk for Ineffective Breathing Pattern related to respiratory muscle weakness
b. Risk for Decreased Cardiac Output related to altered conductivity and contractility
c. Risk for Injury related to seizures
4. Collaborative management
a. Monitor and maintain airway and ventilation; intubation and mechanical ventilation may be necessary.
b. Monitor urine output, I&O, daily weight, and laboratory studies.
c. Treat the cause.
(1) Discontinuance of magnesium-containing antacids or laxatives, IV administered magnesium
d. Restore normal serum electrolyte levels.
(1) Low-magnesium diet
(2) Diuresis
(a) Normal saline or one-half normal saline and furosemide (1 mg/kg) as prescribed if normal renal function
(b) Monitor for hypocalcemia and hypokalemia
(3) Dialysis if renal failure is cause of hypermagnesemia
(4) Dextrose and insulin may promote movement of magnesium into the cells (transient effect only)
e. Monitor for and prevent neuromuscular, pulmonary, and cardiovascular complications.
(1) IV calcium as prescribed
(a) Usual dose 5 to 10 mL of 10% calcium chloride over 2 to 5 minutes
(b) Blocks the neuromuscular and cardiac effects
(c) Contraindicated if patient is receiving digitalis

Acute Renal Failure

Definition

Any sudden severe impairment or cessation of kidney function; characterized by accumulation of nitrogenous wastes and fluid and electrolyte imbalances

Etiology and Pathophysiology

See Figure 8-8 and Table 8-4.

Clinical Presentation

1. Subjective
   a. Flank pain may be present
   b. Uremic syndrome
      (1) Irritability
      (2) Insomnia
      (3) Inability to concentrate
      (4) Anorexia, nausea, vomiting
      (5) Metallic taste
      (6) Fatigue, weakness
      (7) Anxiety
   c. Dyspnea if pulmonary edema is present
   d. Headache
   e. Pruritus
   f. Decreased libido
   g. Weight loss or weight gain
2. Objective
   a. GU
      (1) Decrease in urine volume
         (a) Nonoliguria: dilute urine output greater than 400 mL per 24 hours
         (b) Oliguria: urine output less than 400 mL per 24 hours
         (c) Anuria: urine output less than 100 mL per 24 hours
            (i) Rare but may be seen in complete obstruction (postrenal)
      (2) Altered excretion of drugs; toxic drug levels
      (3) Bladder distention may be noted with postrenal failure
   b. Neurologic
      (1) Change in behavior
      (2) Confusion
      (3) Change in level of consciousness
      (4) Focal neurologic deficits
      (5) Tremors, twitching, increased DTR
      (6) Asterixis
      (7) Seizures
   c. GI

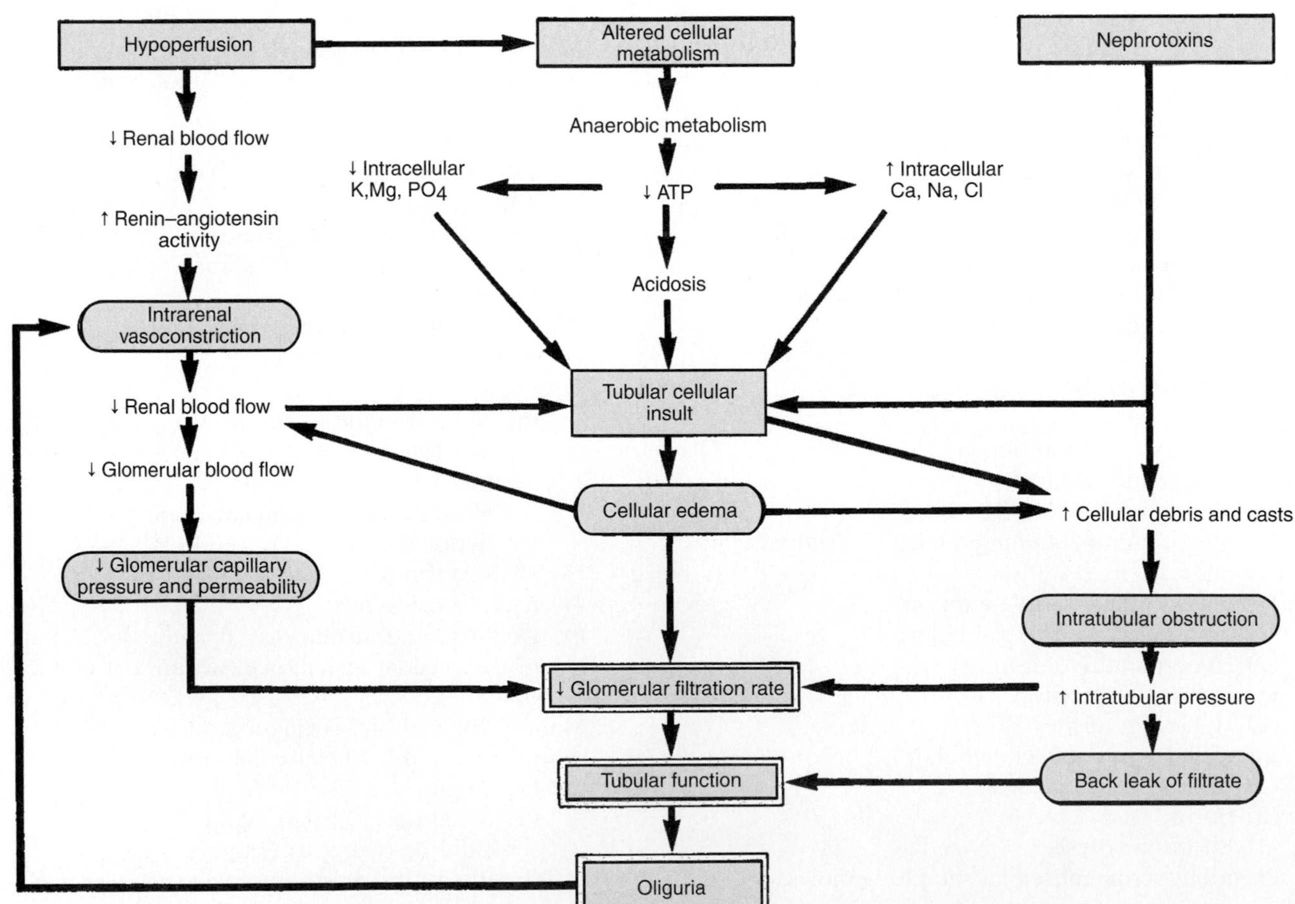

Figure 8-8 Pathophysiology of acute renal failure. *ATP*, Adenosine triphosphate. (From Kinney, M. R., Packa, D. R., & Dunbar, S. B. [1998]. *AACN's clinical reference for critical-care nursing* [4th ed.]. St. Louis: Mosby.)

Table 8-4 Etiology, Pathophysiology, Diagnostics of Acute Renal Failure

		Intrarenal: Damage to the Renal Tissue		
	Prerenal: Disrupted Blood Flow to the Kidney	Cortical	Medullary (Acute Tubular Necrosis)	Postrenal: Disrupted Urine Flow
Etiology	Decreased intravascular volume • Hemorrhage • Gastrointestinal losses: vomiting; diarrhea • Renal losses: osmotic diuresis, diuretics; diabetes insipidus • Skin losses: perspiration; burns; necrotizing fasciitis • Volume shifts: peritonitis; ileus; pancreatitis Decreased cardiac output • Myocardial infarction • Heart failure • Cardiomyopathy • Cardiac tamponade • Dysrhythmias • Pulmonary embolism Vasodilation • Sepsis • Anaphylaxis • Vasodilators Renovascular changes • Renal artery atherosclerosis or thrombosis • Abdominal aortic aneurysm	Glomerulonephritis • Acute poststreptococcal • Systemic lupus erythematosus • Goodpasture's syndrome • Bacterial endocarditis Vasculitis • Periarteritis • Hypersensitivity angioedema • Pregnancy Interstitial nephritis • Acute pyelonephritis • Allergic nephritis • Severe hypercalcemia • Uric acid nephropathy • Myeloma of the kidney • Malignant hypertension	Nephrotoxic agents • Antimicrobials • Aminoglycosides • Cephalosporins • Tetracyclines • Penicillins • Antineoplastics (e.g., cisplatin and methotrexate) • Nonsteroidal antiinflammatory drugs • Contrast dyes • Heavy metals (e.g., lead, arsenic, mercury, and uranium) • Pesticides, fungicides • Chemicals (e.g., ethylene glycol and carbon tetrachloride) • Multiple myeloma • Pigments (e.g., hemoglobin and myoglobin) Prolonged ischemic injury • Mean arterial pressure less than 60 mm Hg for 40 minutes or more • Aortic cross-clamping • Bilateral emboli to both kidneys causing renal infarction • Vasoconstriction • Vasopressors (e.g., norepinephrine [Levophed] or high-dose dopamine) Any of the causes of prerenal failure that is prolonged	Mechanical • Ureteral obstruction such as strictures, calculi, and neoplasm • Urethral obstruction such as prostatic hypertrophy • Edema Functional • Neurogenic bladder such as diabetic neuropathy and spinal cord injury • Ganglionic blocking agents
Pathophysiology	• Decreased pressure to renal artery • Decreased afferent arterial pressure • Diminished GFR • Oliguria • Usually reversible if nephrons are intact	• Renal capillary swelling • Cellular proliferation • Obstruction of glomerulus or tubular structures by edema or cellular debris • Oliguria	• Prolonged ischemia destroys tubular basement membrane • Nephrotoxic injury affects epithelial cellular layer	• Obstruction to urinary flow at or below the collecting ducts • Back pressure causes increased renal interstitial pressure • Decreased GFR • Oliguria
Diagnostics	• Oliguria • Urinary sodium less than 20 mEq/L • Increased BUN with BUN/creatinine ratio greater than 10:1 (usually 20:1)	• Urine output may be normal (nonoliguria), oliguria, or polyuria • Urine sodium greater than 20 mEq/L • BUN/creatinine increased with 10:1 ratio	• Urine output may be normal (nonoliguria), oliguria, or polyuria • Urine sodium greater than 20 mEq/L • Urine specific gravity 1.010 • BUN/creatinine increased with 10:1 ratio	• Oliguria with partial obstruction; anuria with complete obstruction • Urine sodium 20 to 40 mEq/L • BUN/creatinine increased with 10:1 ratio

Continued

Table 8-4 Etiology, Pathophysiology, Diagnostics of Acute Renal Failure—cont'd

	Prerenal: Disrupted Blood Flow to the Kidney	Intrarenal: Damage to the Renal Tissue — Cortical	Intrarenal: Damage to the Renal Tissue — Medullary (Acute Tubular Necrosis)	Postrenal: Disrupted Urine Flow
	• Urine specific gravity greater than 1.020 • Urine osmolality increased except with metabolic acidosis or diuretics • Urine pH less than 6 • No protein in urine or only minimal amount of protein in urine • Sediment in urine: hyaline casts, finely granular casts	• Urine specific gravity varies • Urine pH greater than 6 • Moderate to heavy proteinuria • Sediment in urine: RBCs, WBCs casts	• Urine specific gravity 1.010-1.015 • Urine pH greater than 6 • Minimal to moderate proteinuria • Sediment in urine: tubular epithelial cells, tubular casts, rarely RBCs	• Urine specific gravity 1.010-1.015 • Urine pH greater than 6 • Sediment in urine: RBCs, WBCs, calculi, uric acid crystals, hyaline casts • Kidney-ureter-bladder, intravenous pyelogram may obstruction and/or ureteral dilation • May have positive culture for bacteria

BUN, Blood urea nitrogen; *GFR*, glomerular filtration rate; *RBCs* red blood cells; *WBCs*, white blood cells.

(1) Bleeding gums
(2) Uremic breath
(3) Abdominal distention
(4) Malnutrition
(5) GI bleeding, melena
(6) Constipation or diarrhea
(7) May have paralytic ileus

d. Respiratory
(1) Deep, rapid breathing (Kussmaul's respirations)
(2) Pulmonary edema
(a) Bilateral crackles
(3) Hemoptysis may be seen along with acute renal failure in Goodpasture's syndrome

e. Cardiovascular
(1) Tachycardia
(2) Dysrhythmias
(3) Uremic pericarditis
(a) Pericardial friction rub
(4) Hypertension
(5) Vascular access
(a) Bruit
(b) Thrill
(c) Neurovascular assessment of limb

f. Musculoskeletal
(1) Impaired mobility
(2) Muscle weakness

g. Integument
(1) Dry skin
(2) Pruritus
(3) Edema
(4) Bruising
(5) Pallor
(6) Uremic frost (end-stage)

h. Hematologic/immunologic
(1) Increased susceptibility to infection, sepsis
(2) Petechiae, bruising, bleeding

3. Diagnostic
a. Blood
(1) Chemistry
(a) Elevated BUN, creatinine
(b) Hyperkalemia
(c) Hyperphosphatemia
(d) Hypocalcemia
(e) Hypermagnesemia
(f) Sodium level depends on water balance
(i) Normal or dilutional hyponatremia
(g) Hyperuricemia
(2) ABGs
(a) Metabolic acidosis with increased anion gap
(3) Hematology
(a) Hct, Hgb usually decreased; may be increased in prerenal failure because of dehydration
(b) Platelets: decreased
(4) Clotting profile: bleeding time may be increased
(5) For other specifics, see Table 8-4

b. Urine
(1) Varies depending on type of acute renal failure (see Table 8-4)
(2) Decreased creatinine clearance

c. Radiologic
(1) Kidney-ureter-bladder (KUB), intravenous pyelogram (IVP) may indicate cause of postrenal failure.
(2) Chest x-ray may show the following:
(a) Pericardial effusion
(b) Pleural effusion
(c) Pulmonary edema

d. Renal biopsy: most definitive diagnostic test especially for glomerulonephritis

4. Stages of acute renal failure (Table 8-5)

NOTE: Some patients (especially when acute renal failure is related to nephrotoxins) go through only three phases: onset, nonoliguric, and recovery.

Nursing Diagnoses

1. Risk for Fluid Volume Excess related to inability of kidney to eliminate fluid during the oliguric phase,

Table 8-5 **Stages of Acute Renal Failure**

	Onset	Oliguric-Anuric	Diuretic	Recovery
Definition	Time from the precipitating event to the beginning of oliguria or anuria	Time when urine output is less than 400 mL per 24 hours	Time between when urine output is greater than 400 mL per 24 hours and laboratory values stabilize	Time between when the laboratory values stabilize and they are normal
Duration	Hours to days	1-2 weeks	1-2 weeks	3-12 months
Blood urea nitrogen/ creatinine	Normal or slight increase	Increased	Begins to decrease	Almost normal
Urine output	Decreased; about 20% of normal	Less than 400 mL per 24 hours; about 5% of normal	May exceed 3 L per 24 hours; about 150%-200% of normal	Back to 100% of normal
Mortality	5%	50%-60%	25%	10%-15%
Other characteristics		• Metabolic acidosis • Water gain with dilutional hyponatremia • Hyperkalemia • Hypocalcemia • Hyperphosphatemia • Hypermagnesemia • Azotemia	• Metabolic acidosis • Sodium may be normal or decreased • Hyperkalemia continues	• Uremia, acid-base imbalances, and electrolyte imbalances gradually resolve

sodium and water retention, and failure to comply with sodium and fluid restrictions

2. Risk for Deficient Fluid Volume related to diuresis during the diuretic phase
3. Ineffective Renal Tissue Perfusion related to hypovolemia, pump failure, vasodilation, and renovascular disease
4. Risk for Injury related to uremia, electrolyte imbalance, metabolic acidosis, diminished drug metabolism, and diminished excretion
5. Risk for Infection related to suppressed immune response associated with uremia, malnutrition, and invasive devices
6. Activity Intolerance related to uremia and anemia
7. Imbalanced Nutrition: Less Than Body Requirements related to uremia, anorexia, and dietary restrictions
8. Impaired Skin Integrity related to pruritus and scratching, needle puncture sites at fistula, invasive catheters, and altered oral mucous membranes
9. Disturbed Body Image related to AV access, peritoneal access, and dependency on life-sustaining technology
10. Anxiety related to change in health status
11. Deficient Knowledge related to required lifestyle changes
12. Ineffective Individual Coping related to situational crisis, powerlessness, and change in role
13. Ineffective Family Coping related to critically ill family member

Collaborative Management

1. Treat the cause.
   a. Support renal perfusion and improve GFR through appropriate treatment.
      (1) Volume to improve preload in patients with hypovolemia as evidenced by decreased RAP and PAOP
      (2) Inotropes to improve contractility in patients with decreased contractility as evidenced by decreased right ventricular stroke work index and left ventricular stroke work index
      (3) Vasopressors to increase afterload in patients with massive vasodilation as evidenced by decreased SVR
      (4) Low-dose dopamine has shown no evidence of benefit when used in patients with acute oliguric renal failure and can predispose the patient to bowel ischemia through splanchnic vasoconstriction and is no longer recommended for the management of acute oliguric renal failure
      (5) Fenoldopam (Corlopam), a dopaminergic stimulator, may be prescribed to increase renal blood flow
      (6) Diuretic trial as prescribed if patient is not anuric
         (a) A limited trial of high-dose loop diuretics in an oliguric patient after collection of volume status is recommended because

the use of diuretics in acute renal failure has been shown to increase the risk of death (Mehta, Pascual, Soroko, & Chertow, 2002)

(b) Agents
   (i) Loop diuretics (e.g., furosemide [Lasix] or bumetanide [Bumex])
   (ii) Osmotic diuretics (e.g., mannitol [Osmitrol])
      a) Frequently used for rhabdomyolysis
      b) Contraindicated in HF and pulmonary edema

b. Administer fluids, diuretics (usually mannitol), and sodium bicarbonate for rhabdomyolysis with myoglobinuria.

c. Administer immunosuppressants and initiate plasmapheresis for immune-mediated causes of acute renal failure (e.g., Goodpasture's syndrome).

2. Maintain fluid, electrolyte, acid-base balance.
   a. Fluid
      (1) Monitor for clinical indications of fluid overload.
      (2) Maintain sodium and water restriction, and encourage the patient to remain within prescribed restrictions.
         (a) Restrict fluid intake: 24-hour restriction usually is determined by adding 500 mL (for insensible loss) to the previous day's urine output.
         (b) Space fluid allowances over the entire 24-hour period.
         (c) Treat thirst by offering ice chips (must be included as intake), wet washcloths, misting the mouth, and providing mouth care.
         (d) Restrict sodium intake (usually 1 to 2 g/day)
   b. Potassium
      (1) Monitor for clinical indications of hyperkalemia.
      (2) Maintain potassium restriction (usually 40 mEq/day); do not allow salt substitute (potassium chloride) on dietary trays.
   c. Phosphorus
      (1) Monitor for clinical indications of hyperphosphatemia.
      (2) Maintain phosphorus restrictions.
      (3) Administer phosphate-binding agents (e.g., aluminum carbonate [Basaljel] or aluminum hydroxide [Amphojel]).
         (a) These aluminum-containing phosphate-binding agents may contribute to dialysis encephalopathy because of accumulation of aluminum; calcium carbonate (Caltrate) or calcium acetate (PhosLo) may be prescribed instead.
      (4) Treat hypocalcemia with calcium administration; increasing calcium will decrease phosphorus.
   d. Magnesium
      (1) Monitor for clinical indications of hypermagnesemia.
      (2) Maintain dietary magnesium restrictions.
      (3) Do not administer magnesium-containing medications (e.g., Maalox, magnesium sulfate, or magnesium citrate).
   e. Acid-base balance
      (1) Initiate dialysis to eliminate nitrogenous wastes as prescribed for metabolic acidosis.
      (2) Administer sodium bicarbonate or Carbicarb as prescribed.
         (a) Generally used only for severe metabolic acidosis (pH less than 7.0)
         (b) Monitor for hypernatremia
         (c) Monitor for hypocalcemia caused by increased binding between albumin and calcium and decrease in ionized calcium

3. Diminish the accumulation of nitrogenous wastes.
   a. Maintain protein restriction; usually 0.6 g/kg/day initially but may be as high as 1 to 1.5 g/kg/day if patient is receving hemodialysis; 1.5 to 2 g/kg/day if patient is receiving peritoneal dialysis.
   b. Provide protein foods of high biologic value (i.e., contain all essential amino acids).
   c. Provide adequate caloric intake to prevent catabolism and use of dietary protein for energy needs: usually greater than or equal to 35 to 40 kcal/kg/day.
   d. Initiate dialysis as indicated and prescribed.
      (1) Indications for dialysis in the patient with acute renal failure generally include the following:
         (a) Volume overload (especially with pulmonary edema)
         (b) Uncontrollable hyperkalemia
         (c) Uncontrollable hyperphosphatemia
         (d) Uncontrollable acidosis
         (e) Symptomatic uremia (e.g., neurologic changes)
         (f) Pericarditis
         (g) Seizures or coma
         (h) BUN 80 to 100 mg/dL or greater, but may be initiated at BUN greater than 50 to 60 mg/dL
         (i) Serum creatinine 10 mg/dL or greater
      (2) Contraindications to dialysis
         (a) Hemodynamic instability: CRRT may be used in these situations
         (b) Inability to tolerate anticoagulation
         (c) Lack of vascular access
      (3) Maintenance of patency and prevention of infection of vascular access (if present)
         (a) Palpate shunt, fistula, AV graft for thrill; auscultate for bruit; note change bright red color in tubing in shunt; palpate pulses and check capillary refill distal to access.

(b) Do not allow venipuncture, IV cannulation, injections, BP measurements in limb with shunt, fistula, or AV graft.
(c) Monitor for constrictive clothing or dressing in limb with shunt, fistula, or AV graft.
(d) Monitor for bleeding; use pressure dressing to stop bleeding; bulldog clamps (always kept clamped to dressing) are used on shunt tubing to stop bleeding.
(e) Note any redness, induration, or purulent drainage around access; culture any purulent drainage; change dressing as for central venous catheter.
(f) Instruct patient not to disturb scabs at puncture sites at fistula or AV graft for hemodialysis.

(4) Maintenance of patency and prevention of infection of peritoneal access
(a) Note any redness, induration, or purulent drainage around access; culture any purulent drainage.
(b) Provide aseptic catheter care.
(i) Wash with antibacterial soap.
(ii) Dress with light gauze dressing.
(iii) Manipulate catheter aseptically.
(c) Culture peritoneal dialysate outflow fluid periodically or as indicated.

4. Prevent further damage to the kidney by nephrotoxic agents.
a. Note that dosages of drugs eliminated by the kidney are decreased and the interval between doses is increased.
b. Monitor peak/trough serum drug levels when appropriate (e.g., aminoglycosides).
c. Monitor urine creatinine clearance when patient is receiving nephrotoxic agents.
d. Prevent contrast dye–related nephrotoxicity.
(1) Increase oral and/or parenteral fluid intake.
(2) Administer acetylcysteine (Mucomyst) as prescribed.
(a) Acts as an oxygen free radical scavenger
(b) Usual dose is 600 mg orally every 12 hours the day before and the day of the radiologic procedure that requires contrast medium
(3) Administer fenoldopam (Corlopam) as prescribed.
(a) Acts as a dopaminergic stimulator to improve renal blood flow
(b) Usual dose is an IV infusion of 0.05 to 0.1 mcg/kg/min for 60 to 90 minutes before the injection of the contrast material and is continued for 4 hours after the injection if no adverse reactions occur
e. Monitor for changes in urine color that may indicate the presence of heavy pigments that may cause acute tubular necrosis.
(1) Myoglobinuria: tea or cola colored
(2) Hemoglobinuria: wine colored

5. Provide adequate nutrition while maintaining dietary restrictions.
a. Provide high biologic protein within protein restriction.
b. Provide enough calories to prevent catabolism of somatic protein stores.
c. Increase dietary calcium.
d. Decrease dietary sodium, potassium, and phosphorus.

6. Prevent fluid volume deficit during the diuretic phase.
a. Monitor for clinical indications of fluid volume deficit.
b. Volume may be replaced hourly during this phase by replacing the last hour's urine output during the following hour.

7. Prevent infection: initiate dialysis as prescribed when the BUN level is greater than 80 to 100 mg/dL because BUN values above this level are associated with increased risk of infection.

8. Prevent injury: initiate dialysis as prescribed when the BUN level is greater than 80 to 100 mg/dL because BUN values above this level are associated with neurologic changes

9. Monitor for and treat anemia and platelet dysfunction.
a. Monitor Hgb, Hct, and RBC count.
b. Treat anemia as prescribed.
(1) Folic acid, iron, vitamin B_{12}
(2) Recombinant erythropoietin (epoetin alfa [Epogen])
(3) Packed RBCs: only prescribed if the patient is symptomatic of anemia (e.g., dyspnea, chest pain, syncope, or hypotension)
c. Monitor for clinical indications of platelet dysfunction (e.g., petechiae, ecchymosis, or bleeding).
d. Administer desmopressin (DDAVP) as prescribed for platelet dysfunction.

10. Promote comfort.
a. Administer antipyretics as prescribed.
b. Use emollient or cornstarch baths.

11. Monitor for complications.
a. Renal: Chronic renal failure will develop in 25% to 30% of patients with acute renal failure.
b. Cardiovascular
(1) Dysrhythmias
(2) Hypertension
(3) Pericarditis, cardiac tamponade
(4) Pulmonary edema
c. Neurologic
(1) Coma
(2) Seizures
d. Metabolic
(1) Electrolyte imbalances
(a) Hyperkalemia
(b) Hyperphosphatemia
(c) Hypermagnesemia
(d) Hypocalcemia

(2) Acid-base imbalance: metabolic acidosis
e. GI
(1) Peptic ulcer disease
(2) GI hemorrhage
f. Hematologic
(1) Anemia
(2) Uremic coagulopathies
g. Infection
(1) Increased susceptibility to pneumonias
(2) Septicemias
(3) Urinary tract and wound infections
h. Miscellaneous: drug toxicity

Renal Replacement Therapy

Dialysis

1. Definition: separation of solutes by differential diffusion through a semipermeable membrane that is placed between the two solutions (Figure 8-9)
2. Purposes
   a. Eliminate excess body fluids
   b. Maintain or restore electrolyte balance
   c. Maintain or restore acid-base balance
   d. Eliminate nitrogenous wastes and toxins from the blood
3. Indications
   a. Acute or chronic renal failure
      (1) Symptomatic uremia
      (2) Uremic pericarditis

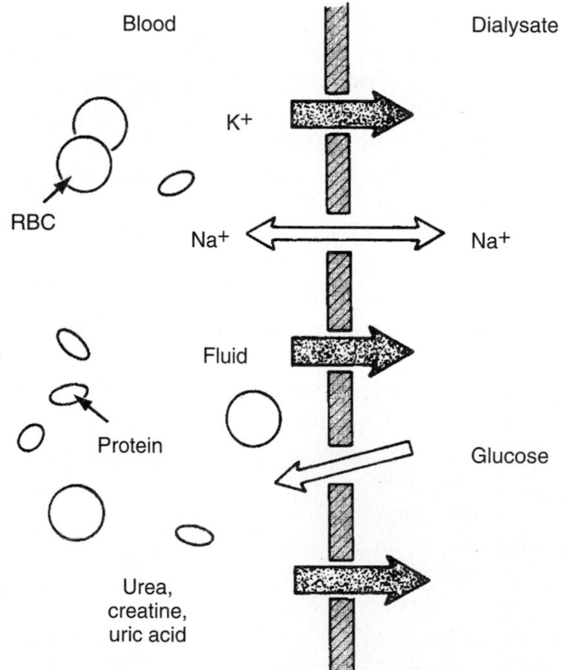

Figure 8-9 Osmosis and diffusion in dialysis. Net movement of major particles and fluid is illustrated. *RBC*, Red blood cell. (From Long, B. C., Phipps, W. J., & Cassmeyer, V. L. [1993]. *Medical-surgical nursing: A nursing process approach* [3rd ed.]. St. Louis: Mosby.)

   b. Severe water intoxication
   c. Severe electrolyte imbalance
   d. Drug intoxication (drug must be dialyzable [e.g., alcohol, salicylates, lithium, barbiturates, and some poisons])
   e. Hepatic encephalopathy/coma
4. Components
   a. Dialysate: solution of water, electrolytes (sodium, chloride, magnesium, bicarbonate), nonelectrolytes (glucose), and buffer (acetate)
      (1) Electrolyte concentration in the dialysate is adjusted to the patient's needs.
   b. Semipermeable membrane: peritoneum, extracorporeal membrane
   c. Patient's blood in contact with the membrane
5. Principles (Figure 8-10)
   a. Osmosis: A hypertonic solution is used as the dialysate to move water across the semipermeable membrane.
   b. Diffusion: The dialysate solution contains a concentration of selected solutes lower than the blood so that these solutes will move across the semipermeable membrane and into the dialysate solution.
   c. Filtration: In some forms of dialysis, there is a pressure difference between the sides of the semipermeable membrane, with the highest pressure on the forward side of the membrane to act as a hydrostatic force pushing against the membrane to provide a filtration effect.
   d. Convection (in CRRT): The transfer of solutes and solutions moving across the semipermeable membrane occurs simultaneously.
6. Variables affecting efficiency
   a. Size and number of the pores in the semipermeable membrane
   b. Surface area of the semipermeable membrane
   c. Thickness of the semipermeable membrane
   d. Size of the solute molecules
   e. Concentration of solutes in the blood
   f. Osmotic concentration
   g. Pressure gradients
   h. Temperature of the solution
   i. Rate of blood flow
7. Comparison of various types of dialysis (Table 8-6)
   a. Choice of right dialysis option
      (1) Intermittent hemodialysis: therapy of choice for most patients; use limited when patient is hemodynamically unstable
      (2) Peritoneal dialysis: suited for hemodynamically unstable patients but has low efficiency
      (3) CRRT: suitable for hemodynamically unstable patient and has a higher efficiency than peritoneal dialysis; increasingly popular for hemodynamically unstable patients with acute renal failure

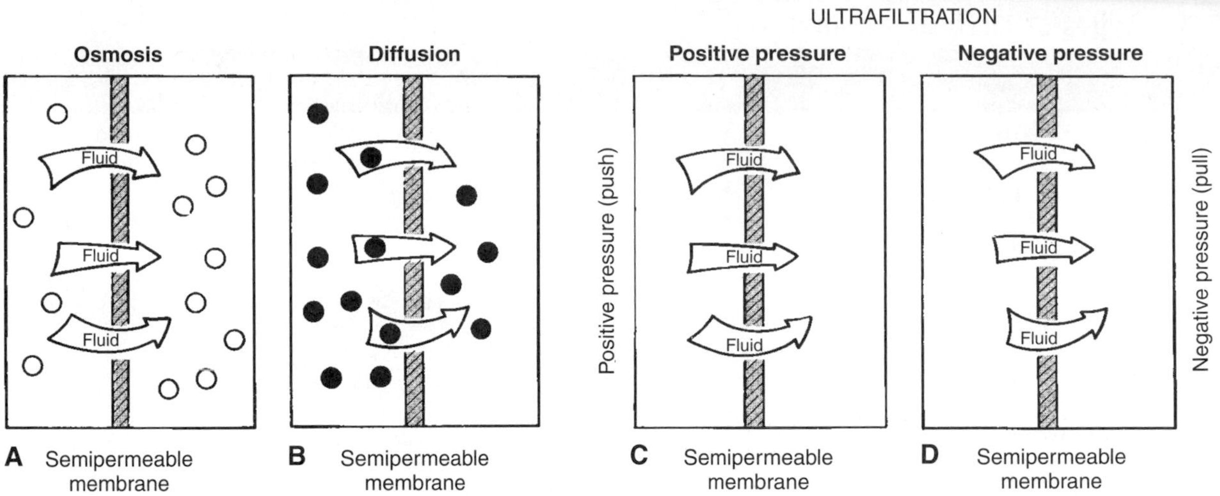

Figure 8-10 Dialysis is based on the following principles: **A,** osmosis; **B,** diffusion and ultrafiltration. Ultrafiltration occurs when positive pressure **(C)** or negative pressure **(D)** is placed on the system. Ultrafiltration is maximized by exerting positive and negative pressure on the system simultaneously. (From Long, B. C., Phipps, W. J., & Cassmeyer, V. L. [1993]. *Medical-surgical nursing: A nursing process approach* [3rd ed.]. St. Louis: Mosby.)

Table 8-6 Types of Dialysis

	Hemodialysis	Intermittent Peritoneal Dialysis	Continuous Renal Replacement Therapies (SCUF, CAVH, CVVH, CAVHD, CVVHD, CVVHDF)
Principles	• Osmosis • Diffusion • Filtration	• Osmosis • Diffusion • Filtration	• Osmosis • Diffusion • Filtration • Convection
Treatment requirements	• Membrane: extracorporeal membrane • Blood pump • Dialyzer • Dialysate • Vascular access • Anticoagulation	• Membrane: peritoneum • Dialysate: 1.5%, 2.5%, 4.25% • Access: peritoneal catheter	• Vascular access (SCUF, CAVH, and CAVHD require arterial and venous access; CVVH, CVVHD, and CVVHDF require venous access and a pump) • High-coefficient membrane hemofilter • Dialysate (usually 1.5% without potassium) • Systolic BP of at least 60 mm Hg • NOTE: Continuous venous-venous hemodialysis can be performed if a pump is added to serve as arterial pressure.
Specific indications	• Need for rapid treatment • Fluid overload unresponsive to diuretics • Electrolyte imbalance • Acute or chronic renal failure • Drug overdosage or poison intoxication with dialyzable agent • Pulmonary edema refractory to diuretics	• Fluid overload • Electrolyte imbalance • Acute or chronic renal failure • Drug overdosage or poison intoxication with dialyzable agent • Lack of availability of vascular access for hemodialysis • Inability to anticoagulate • Hemodynamic instability	• Fluid overload unresponsive to diuretics • Acute or chronic renal failure in hemodynamically unstable patient • Electrolyte imbalance • Drug overdosage or poison intoxication with dialyzable agent • Inability to tolerate hemodialysis or therapeutic anticoagulation • May also be used in heart failure, sepsis, lactic acidosis, rhabdomyolysis, multiple organ dysfunction syndrome, and hepatic failure

Continued

Table 8-6 Types of Dialysis—cont'd

	Hemodialysis	Intermittent Peritoneal Dialysis	Continuous Renal Replacement Therapies (SCUF, CAVH, CVVH, CAVHD, CVVHD, CVVHDF)
Contraindications	• Hemodynamic instability • Hypovolemia • Inadequate vascular access • Coagulopathy	• Rapid treatment required • Acute peritonitis • Recent abdominal surgery • Known abdominal adhesions • Abdominal trauma • Intraperitoneal hematoma • Recent vascular anastomosis of abdominal vessels • Respiratory distress • Sepsis • Extreme obesity • Coagulopathy	• Rapid treatment required • Systolic BP less than 60 mm Hg for CAVH and CAVHD • Lack of arterial access for SCUF, CAVH, and CAVHD • Hematocrit greater than 45% • Inability to tolerate high volumes of fluid exchange • Coagulopathy
Advantages	• Rapid and efficient; only 4-6 hours per session (usually 3 times weekly) • Very efficient; corrects biochemical disturbances quickly	• Equipment is easily and readily assembled • Fairly simple; requiring less staff and patient education • Relatively inexpensive • Minimal danger of acute electrolyte imbalance or hemorrhage • Dialysate can be individualized easily • Anticoagulation not required	• Removes solutes gradually • Decreased risk of hemodynamic instability • Provides flexibility in fluid administration • Requires only minimal heparinization • Relatively inexpensive • Fairly simple; requiring less staff education • Can be used for physiologically unstable patients
Disadvantages	• Complex procedure requiring extensive staff training • Equipment expensive • Machine availability may be limited • Requires anticoagulation • Vascular access necessary	• Relatively slow to alter biochemical imbalances, usually requiring 36 hours for therapeutic effect • May cause protein loss • May be difficult to gain and maintain peritoneal access	• Not efficient • Patient must be in bed during entire treatment • Requires anticoagulation • Vascular access necessary • Increased care requirements • Complicates dosing of certain drugs such as antibiotics and vasoactive agents
Complications	• Access complications: bleeding, clotting, infection • Acute fluid and electrolyte imbalances • Hemorrhage • Hypovolemia • Air embolus • Disequilibrium syndrome caused by too rapid a removal of waste products • Allergic reaction to membrane • Hepatitis • Dialysis encephalopathy (related to accumulation of aluminum from water used to prepare dialysate) • Infection • Dysrhythmias	• Access complications: infection, dialysate leak, bleeding, and peritonitis • Too rapid a fluid removal causing the following: ◦ Hypovolemia ◦ Hypernatremia • Hypervolemia caused by dialysate retention • Hypokalemia caused by potassium-free dialysate usage • Alkalosis caused by alkaline dialysate usage • Disequilibrium syndrome caused by too rapid a removal of waste products • Hyperglycemia caused by high glucose concentration of dialysate • Protein loss • Respiratory distress	• Hypotension • Hypothermia • Fluid, electrolyte imbalances especially fluid volume deficit if volume not adequately replaced • Acid-base imbalances • Access complications: bleeding, clotting, infection • Depletion syndrome: loss of vitamins and amino acids • Hemorrhage related to the following: ◦ Anticoagulation ◦ Disruption of filter or tubing • Infection • Air embolism

BP, Blood presssure; *CAVH*, continuous arteriovenous hemofiltration; *CAVHD*, continuous arteriovenous hemodialysis; *CVVH*, continuous venovenous hemofiltration; *CVVHD*, continuous venovenous hemodialysis; *CVVHDF*, continuous venovenous hemodiafiltration; *SCUF*, slow continuous ultrafiltration therapy.

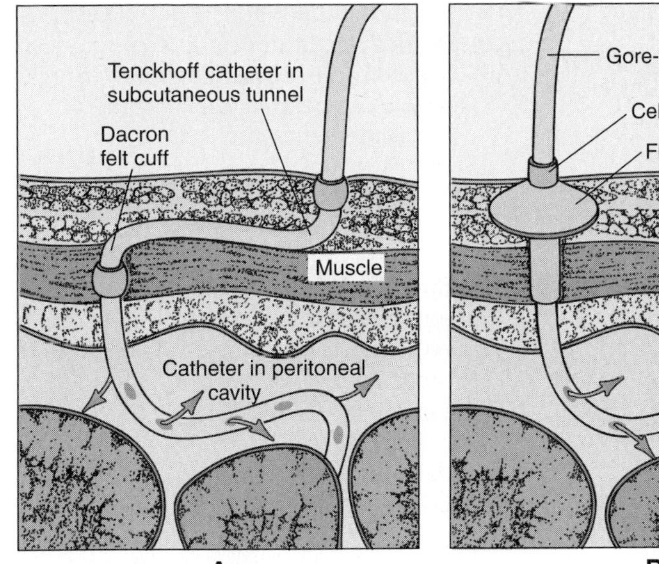

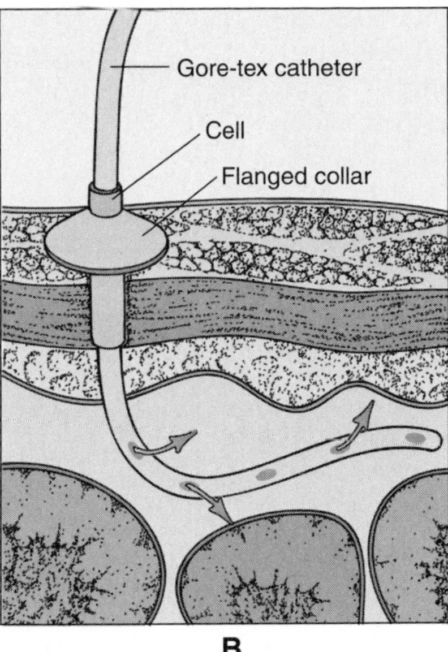

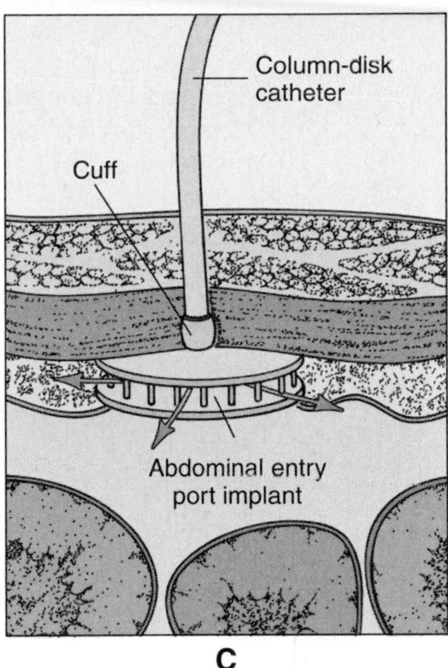

Figure 8-11 Three types of peritoneal dialysis catheters. **A,** Tenckhoff catheter has two Dacron felt cuffs that hold the catheter in place and prevent dialysate leakage and bacterial invasion. Subcutaneous tunnel also helps prevent infection. **B,** Gore-Tex catheter with Dacron cuff above flanged collar. **C,** Column-disk catheter has cuff and large abdominal entry port implant. (From Beare, P., & Myers, J. [1998]. *Adult health nursing* [3rd ed.]. St. Louis: Mosby.)

8. Collaborative management
   a. Peritoneal dialysis
      (1) Preparation
         (a) Prepare patient for insertion of peritoneal catheter (Figure 8-11)
            (i) Explain procedure to patient.
            (ii) Ask patient to void or insert urinary catheter before abdominal puncture.
         (b) Weigh patient before treatment; weigh patient daily after draining dialysate.
      (2) Procedure (Figure 8-12)
         (a) Warm dialysate to body temperature.
         (b) Add prescribed medications to dialysate: for example, heparin, potassium chloride, antibiotics, and lidocaine.
         (c) Instill between 1 and 3 L of dialysate (usually 2 L; inflow phase); this volume usually is infused at a rate of 2 L in 10 to 20 minutes.
         (d) Allow to dwell in intraperitoneal space for 20 to 30 minutes (NOTE: If this is the first exchange, do not allow dialysate to dwell; drain it immediately to ensure catheter patency and placement).
         (e) Drain and measure dialysate (outflow phase).
         (f) Assess appearance of dialysate.
            (i) Normal: clear, pale yellow or straw colored
            (ii) Cloudy: suspect infection; culture and sensitivity is indicated

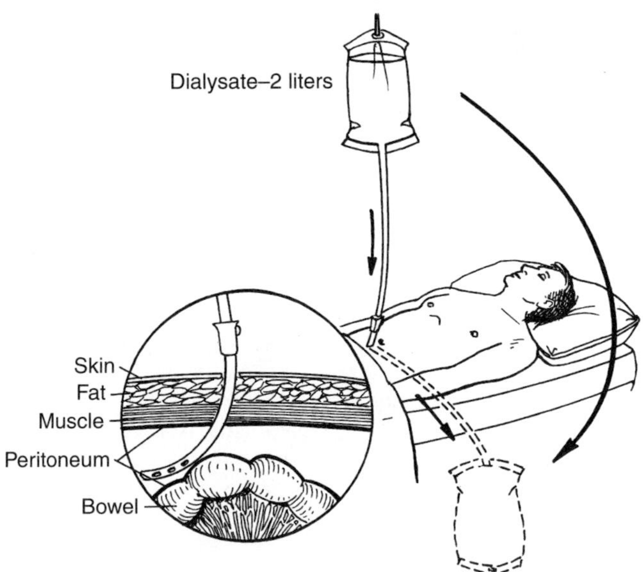

Figure 8-12 Patient receiving peritoneal dialysis. Dialysate fluid is instilled into the peritoneal cavity, is allowed to dwell for a given period, and then is drained. (From Long, B.C., Phipps. W.J., & Cassmeyer, V.L. (1993). *Medical-surgical nursing: A nursing process approach* (3rd ed.). St Louis: Mosby.)

(iii) Bloody: if occurs after the first four exchanges, suspect intraabdominal bleeding or coagulopathy
(iv) Amber: suspect bladder perforation
(v) Brownish: suspect bowel perforation
(g) If the amount drained is less than the amount instilled, do the following:
(i) Turn patient side to side.
(ii) Apply gentle pressure to the abdomen.
(3) Keep meticulous cumulative I&O records (e.g., if drain is 300 mL less than the amount instilled [+300 mL] during one exchange, but the next exchange yields a drain volume of 400 mL more than the amount instilled [–400 mL], the cumulative volume is –100 mL).
(4) Monitor patient for hypotension and respiratory distress especially during inflow phase.
(5) Monitor vital signs during outflow phase.
(6) Monitor blood glucose levels in all patients; hyperglycemia is likely to occur in diabetic patients or when 4.25% dialysate is used.
(7) Provide peritoneal catheter exit site care.
b. Hemodialysis
(1) Preparation
(a) Patient must have vascular access (Table 8-7; Figures 8-13 and 8-14).
(b) Weigh patient before hemodialysis.
(c) Do not administer drugs that may cause hypotension before hemodialysis.
(i) Antihypertensives
(ii) Antiemetics
(iii) Narcotics
(iv) Beta-blockers
(v) Calcium channel blockers
(d) Do not administer dialyzable drugs immediately before hemodialysis.
(2) Procedure (usually performed by specially trained hemodialysis nurse rather than critical care staff; Figure 8-15)
(a) Cannulate vascular access and/or connect to dialyzer.
(b) Maintain anticoagulation.
(c) Monitor blood chemistries throughout the treatment.
(d) Monitor vital signs frequently for evaluation of hemodynamic stability and tolerance.
(e) Monitor the vascular access and the hemofilter for indications of clotting.
c. Selected complications
(1) Disequilibrium syndrome
(a) Caused by toxins (e.g., urea being rapidly removed from the blood but not as rapidly removed from the cerebrospinal fluid)

Table 8-7 Forms of Vascular Accesses for Dialysis

Access	Advantages	Disadvantages	Management
Double-lumen vascular catheter (Figure 8-13) inserted into subclavian, jugular, or femoral vein	• Easy insertion • Immediate use • High flow rates are achieved • No venipuncture required for access	• Externally located • Can be dislodged easily • Prone to infection and thrombosis • Femoral catheters are associated with a higher incidence of infection	• Monitor site daily and provide site care • Restrict use of this catheter to dialysis only • Administer heparin into catheter if prescribed • A thrombolytic may be used to reestablish patency of an occluded catheter
Fistula (Figure 8-14, *A*)	• Located internally • Greater longevity • Lower clotting and infection rates than external devices • No danger of disconnection	• Requires 4 to 6 weeks to mature before use • Requires venipuncture for access • May result in ischemia to affected limb (referred to as *vascular steal syndrome*) • May thrombose	• Do not use limb for blood pressure or venipuncture • Listen for bruit, feel for thrill: indicate patency • Assess neurovascular status of affected limb frequently • Teach patient exercises to increase blood flow in fistula (e.g., squeezing a ball) • Warn patient not to wear constrictive clothing
Arteriovenous graft (Figure 8-14, *B*)	• As for fistula • May be used for patients with vessels inadequate for fistula formation • Can be used earlier than traditional fistula	• As for fistula • Infection is more serious than with traditional fistula because of risk of disintegration and hemorrhage • May cause aneurysm formation	• As for fistula • Rotating puncture sites and applying pressure on needle removal aids in prevention of aneurysm and pseudoaneurysm

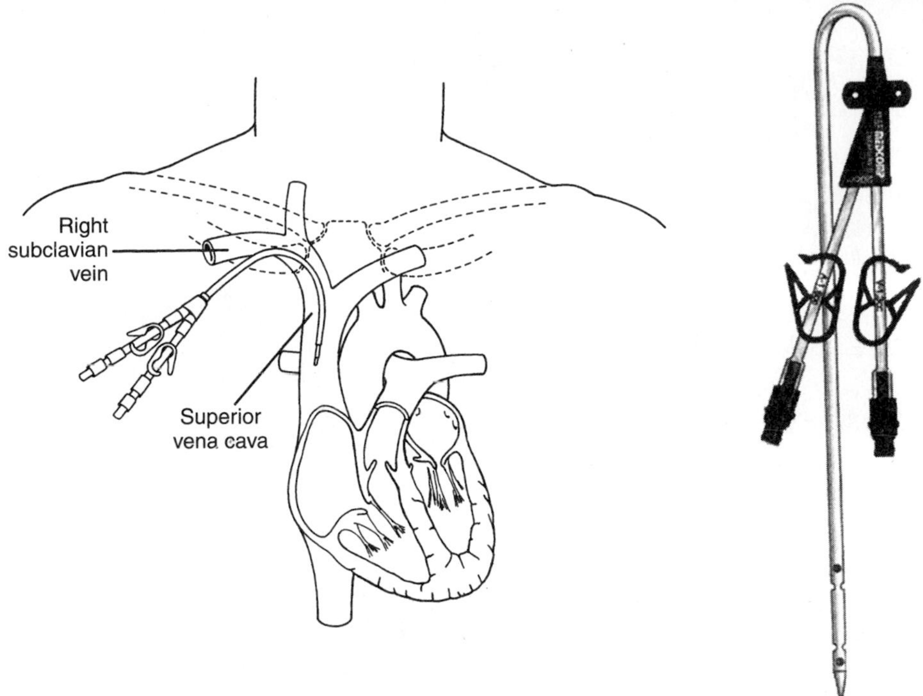

Figure 8-13 **A,** Temporary vascular access using subclavian dual-lumen venous catheter. **B,** Dual-lumen temporary catheter. (Courtesy MEDCOMP Corporation, Harleysville, PA.)

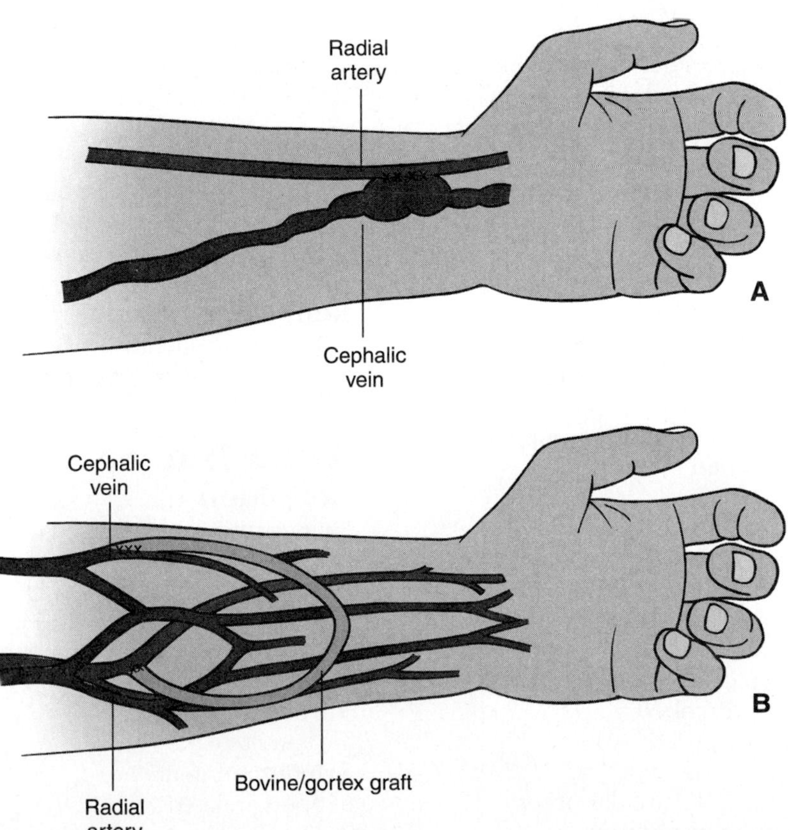

Figure 8-14 Permanent vascular accesses. **A,** AV fistula. **B,** AV graft. (From Urden, L. D., Stacy, K. M., & Lough, M. E. [2006]. *Thelan's critical care nursing: Diagnosis and management* [5th ed.]. St. Louis: Mosby.)

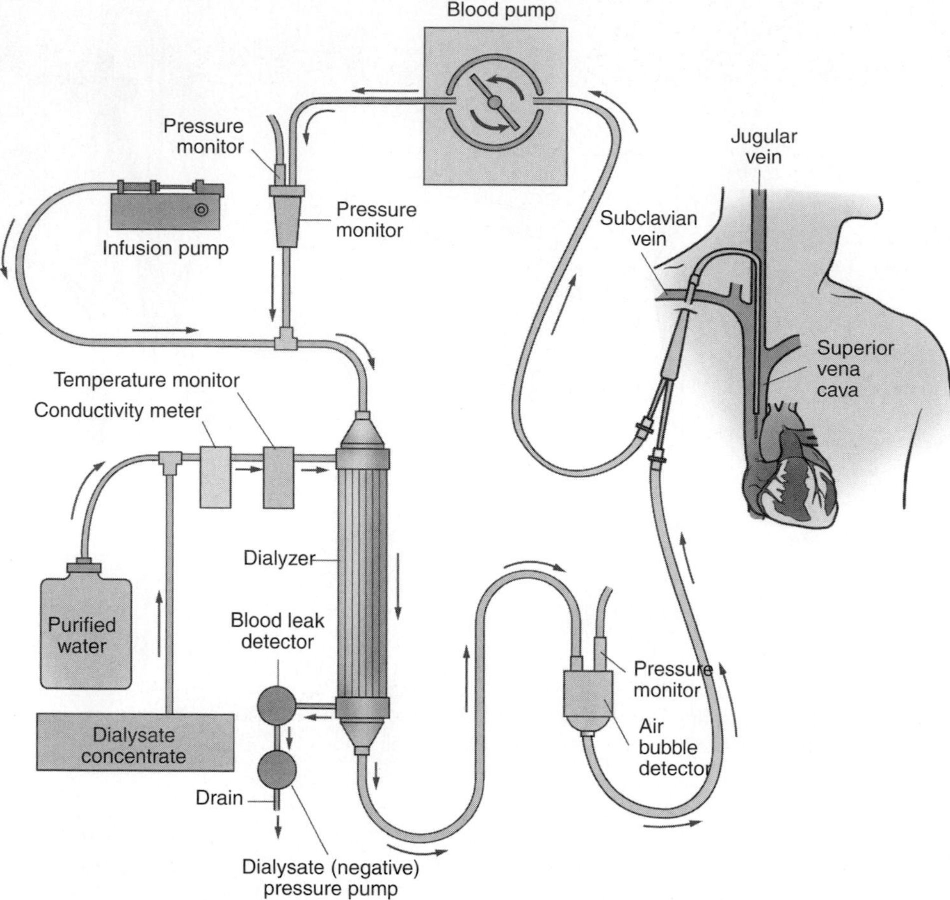

Figure 8-15 Components of a hemodialysis system. (From Urden, L. D., Stacy, K. M., & Lough, M. E. [2006]. *Thelan's critical care nursing: Diagnosis and management* [5th ed.]. St. Louis: Mosby.)

(b) The higher concentration of toxins in the brain cells may cause a shift of fluid into brain cells and cause cerebral edema
(c) Clinical indications may include nausea, vomiting, headache, hallucinations, and seizures
(d) Collaborative management
(i) Use a smaller dialyzer.
(ii) Reduce blood pump speed.
(iii) Shorten dialysis time, and dialyze more frequently.
(iv) Administer diazepam and phenytoin as prescribed for seizures.
(2) Muscle cramps
(a) Caused by rapid water removal and sodium shifts
(b) Collaborative management
(i) Administer quinine as prescribed before dialysis.
(ii) Hypertonic saline during dialysis also may be prescribed.
d. CRRT (Table 8-8 and Figure 8-16)
(1) Preparation
(a) Patient must have vascular access.
(b) Heparin is administered after baseline clotting studies are obtained.
(2) Procedure
(a) Prepare hemofilter with dialysate solution.
(b) Connect vascular access to hemofilter.
(c) Fluid replacement if calculated according to the ultrafiltration rate.
(d) Change the filter when the rate slows or if the filter ruptures or is clogged.

Renal Transplant

Renal replacement therapy for patients with chronic renal failure (see Chapter 10)

Renal Trauma

Definition

Injury to the kidney caused by blunt or penetrating impact

Etiology

1. Motor vehicle crash: The kidney is the organ most likely to be injured in a lateral impact crash.
2. Falls
3. Pedestrian injury
4. Assault
5. Industrial injury
6. Sports-related injury
7. Deceleration/acceleration injury
8. Gunshot wound
9. Stab wound

Table 8-8 **Continuous Renal Replacement Therapy**

Type	Ultrafiltration Rate	Function	Nursing Considerations
SCUF	100-300 mL/hr	• Fluid removal	• Anticoagulation may be required
CAVH or CVVH	500-800 mL/hr	• Fluid removal • Moderate solute removal by convection	• Fluid replacement required • Solute replacement may be required
CAVHD or CVVHD	500-800 mL/hr	• Fluid removal • Maximal solute removal by diffusion	• Dialysate solution is required
CVVHDF		• Maximal fluid and solute removal by convection and diffusion	• Dialysate solution required • Fluid replacement required

CAVH, Continuous arteriovenous hemofiltration; *CAVHD*, continuous arteriovenous hemodialysis; *CVVH*, continuous venovenous hemofiltration; *CVVHD*, continuous venovenous hemodialysis; *CVVHDF*, continuous venovenous hemodiafiltration; *SCUF*, slow continuous ultrafiltration.

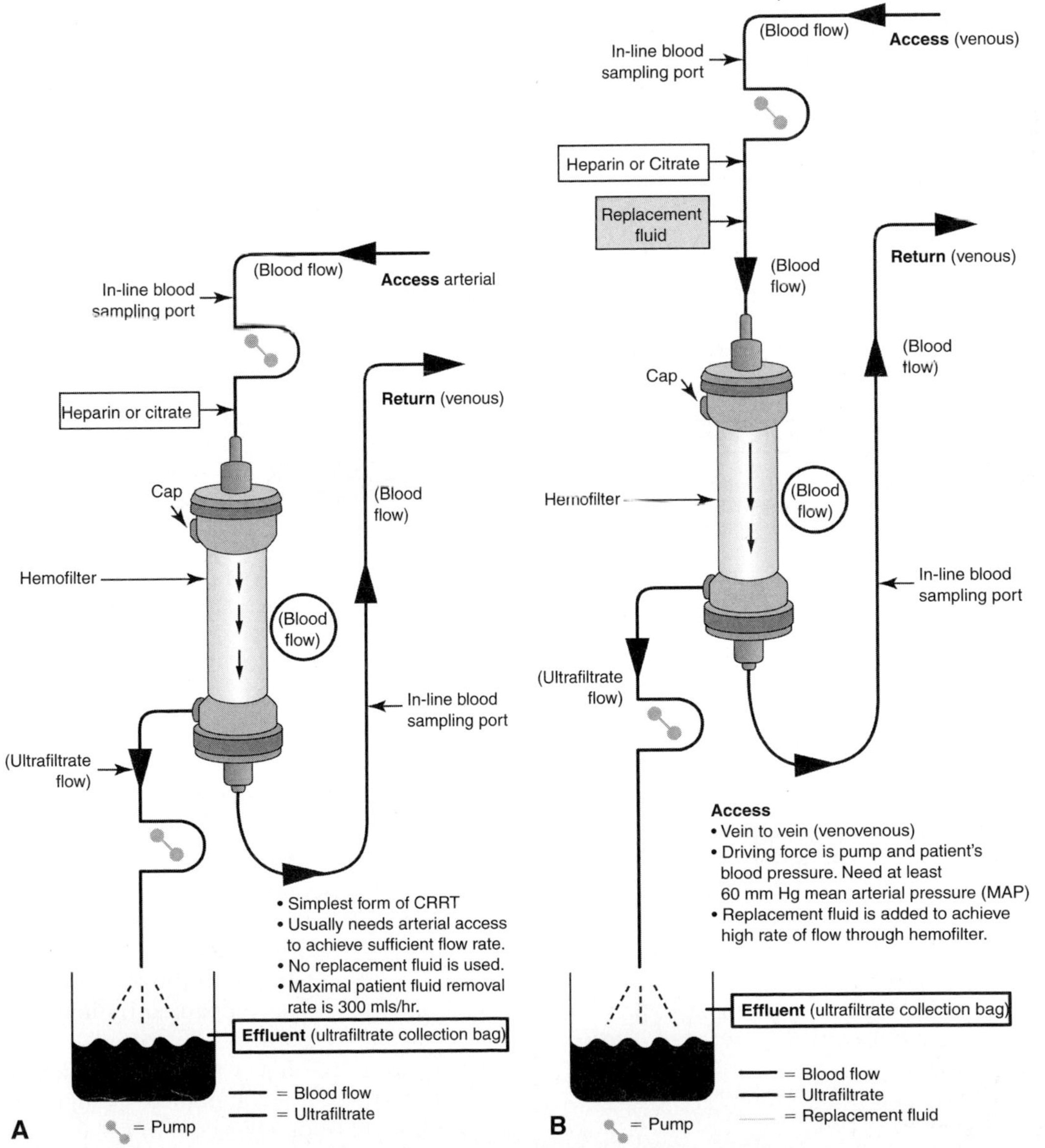

Figure 8-16 CRRT systems. **A,** Slow continuous ultrafiltration (SCUF). **B,** Continuous venovenous hemofiltration (CVVH).

Continued

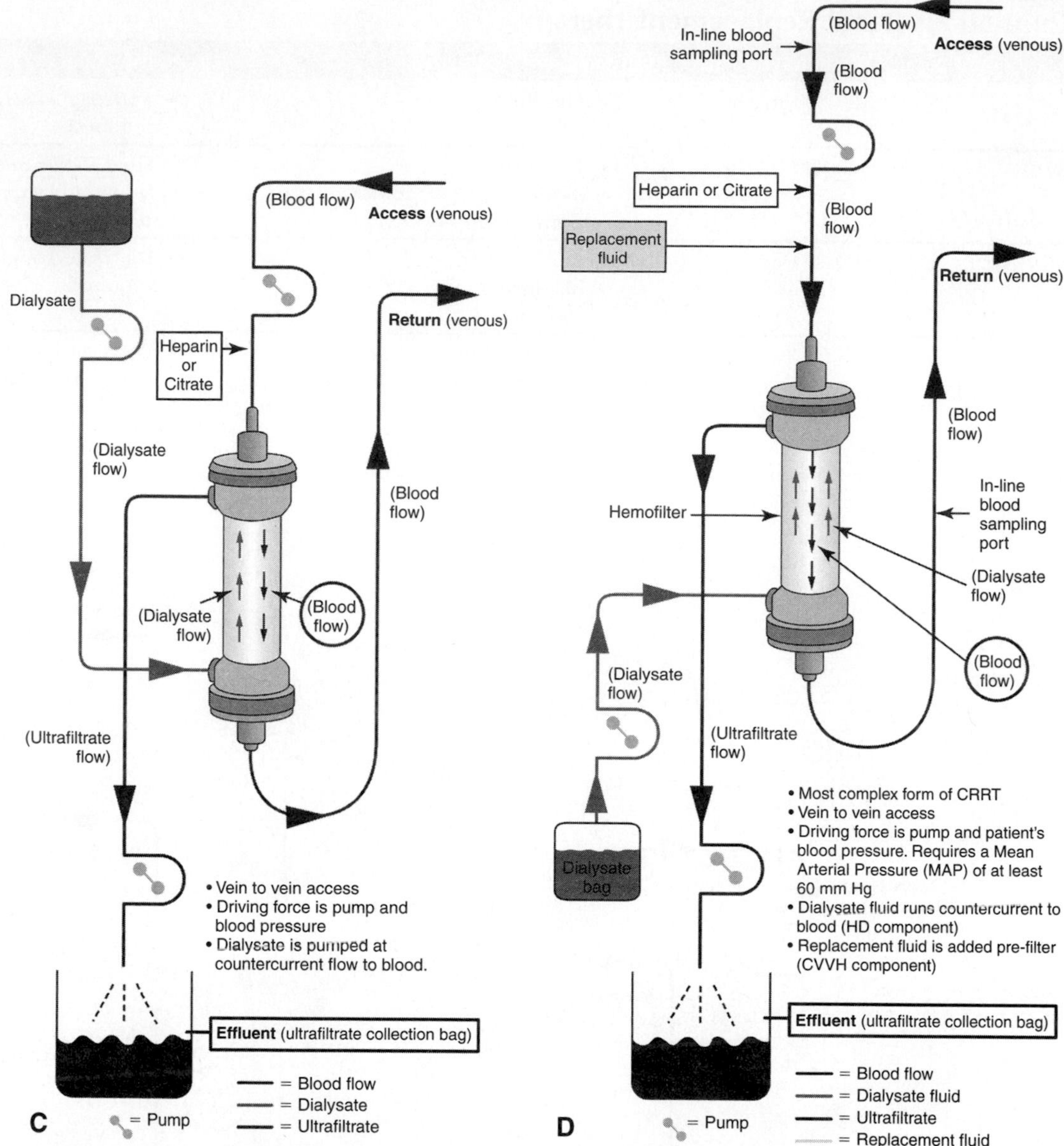

Figure 8-16, cont'd **C,** Continuous venovenous hemofiltration dialysis (CVVHD). **D,** Continuous venovenous hemodiafiltration (CVVHDF). (From Urden, L. D., Stacy, K. M., & Lough, M. E. [2006]. *Thelan's critical care nursing: Diagnosis and management* [5th ed.]. St. Louis: Mosby.)

Pathophysiology

1. Classification
   a. Mechanism of injury: The kidney is mobile and susceptible to parenchymal and vascular damage.
      (1) Blunt trauma: ~90%
         (a) Rapid deceleration
         (b) Direct impact
      (2) Penetrating trauma: ~10%
   b. Anatomic location
      (1) Cortical
      (2) Parenchyma
      (3) Pedicle: vascular
      (4) Collecting system
      (5) Anatomic issues
         (a) The right kidney is more vulnerable to injury than the left because it is lower.
         (b) Fracture of ribs 11 and 12 may cause penetration of the kidney.
         (c) Renal trauma is almost always accompanied by other system problems.
            (i) Injury to the left kidney frequently is accompanied by injury to the spleen.
            (ii) Injury to the right kidney frequently is accompanied by injury to the liver.
   c. Classification (Figure 8-17)
      (1) Class I: caused by compression of the kidney between the lower ribs and the vertebral column

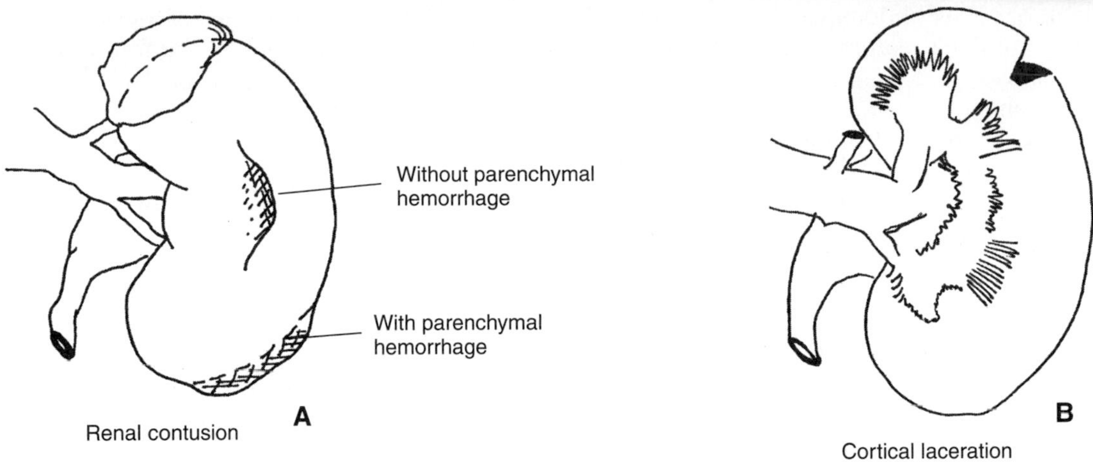

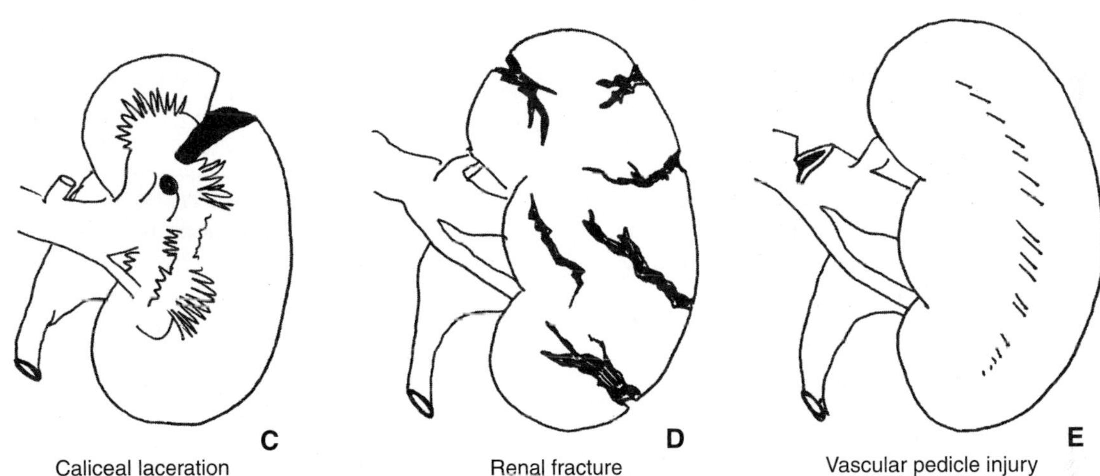

Figure 8-17 Renal trauma. **A,** Renal contusion. **B,** Cortical laceration. **C,** Caliceal laceration. **D,** Renal fracture. **E,** Vascular pedicle injury. (Drawing by Ann M. Walthall.)

(a) Contusion: hematuria but normal urologic studies
(b) Hematoma: subcapsular, nonexpanding
(c) May have minor cortical lacerations but not into the parenchyma

(2) Class II: caused by fracture of ribs 10 to 12 or the transverse process of the vertebrae
(a) Hematoma: perirenal, nonexpanding, confined to retroperitoneum
(b) Laceration: less than 1 cm parenchymal depth and without urinary extravasation

(3) Class III
(a) Laceration of more than 1 cm parenchymal depth without urinary extravasation

(4) Class IV
(a) Laceration extending through the renal cortex, medulla, and collecting system
(b) Vascular injury to the renal artery or vein with contained hemorrhage

(5) Class V
(a) Lacerations that are extensive at various sites in the renal parenchyma resulting in a completely shattered kideny
(b) Vascular injury with avulsion of the renal hilum resulting in devascularization of the kidney

d. Severity
(1) Minor: contusions, shallow cortical lacerations
(2) Major: deep cortical lacerations, caliceal laceration
(3) Critical: renal fracture, renal vascular injury

Clinical Presentation

1. Subjective
a. Information about mechanism of injury from patient, witness, or first responders
b. Pain or tenderness

(1) Flank or upper abdominal quadrant pain; persistent flank pain may indicate renal artery thrombosis
(2) CVA pain
(3) Renal colic: pain radiating from flank into groin, external genitalia, or into thigh: indicative of passage of clots

2. Objective
   a. Hematuria
      (1) Gross or microscopic
      (2) Note that 10% to 25% of significant renal injuries present without hematuria
   b. Oliguria
   c. Abrasion or hematoma over posterior aspect of eleventh or twelfth rib or in flank area
   d. Entrance/exit wound if penetrating trauma
   e. Flank swelling or mass
   f. Abdominal distention or asymmetry
   g. Abdominal bruit if renal artery thrombosis
   h. External genitalia: note any ecchymosis
   i. Urethral meatus: note any bleeding
   j. Clinical indications of retroperitoneal bleeding
      (1) Back pain
      (2) Clinical indications of hemorrhage: tachycardia, hypotension
      (3) Grey Turner's sign: ecchymosis over the flank indicative of retroperitoneal bleeding
   k. Clinical indications of extravasated urine
      (1) Midline bulging (i.e., overdistended bladder)
      (2) Lower quadrant, flank, or thigh distention (i.e., fluid collection)
      (3) Lower abdominal pain or mass (i.e., bladder rupture)
      (4) Abdominal pain, rebound tenderness (i.e., peritoneal irritation)
      (5) Hematuria (i.e., trauma to kidney or urinary tract)
      (6) Anuria (i.e., disruption of urinary tract)
   l. Presence of other injuries
      (1) Pelvic fracture
      (2) Lower rib fracture
      (3) Lumbar spine fracture
      (4) Abdominal visceral injuries
3. Diagnostic
   a. Laboratory
      (1) Serum
         (a) BUN and creatinine: may be elevated if renal damage
         (b) Hgb and Hct: may be decreased if hemorrhage
         (c) Potassium: may be elevated
      (2) Urine: may be positive for blood or protein
   b. Chest x-ray: may show fractured ribs (11 to 12) on affected side
   c. KUB: may show any of the following:
      (1) Rib fracture over kidney
      (2) Displacement of bowel
      (3) Obliteration of renal shadow
   d. Computed tomography (CT) with IV contrast
      (1) Most valuable diagnostic study for assessment of renal injury; superior to IVP
      (2) Documents extent of injury
   e. IVP may show any of the following:
      (1) Delayed excretion of dye
      (2) Renal outline enlargement
      (3) Decreased concentration of contrast media in renal parenchyma
   f. Ultrasonography: may show renal parenchymal injury
   g. Renal scan: may show renal parenchymal injury and/or defect in renal blood flow
   h. Angiogram
      (1) Indicated if the kidney cannot be visualized on CT or if extravasation of bloody urine or contrast media noted on CT
      (2) May show vascular disruption, renal infarction, hematoma

Nursing Diagnoses

1. Altered Urinary Elimination related to mechanical trauma and extravasation of urine
2. Risk for Fluid Volume Deficit related to hemorrhage
3. Risk for Infection related to bacterial contamination of urinary tract and invasive procedures
4. Pain related to trauma and surgery

Collaborative Management

1. Maintain airway, ventilation, and oxygenation.
2. Detect and control hemorrhage; replace circulating volume.
   a. Assess patient for associated injuries.
   b. Maintain patient on bed rest.
   c. Insert urinary catheter unless blood is noted at urethral meatus or resistance is met.
      (1) Prepare patient for urethrogram if resistance is met.
      (2) Assist with insertion of suprapubic catheter as indicated.
      (3) Monitor patient for hematuria.
   d. Monitor Hgb and Hct.
   e. Insert two large-gauge, short IV catheters.
      (1) Administer crystalloids or colloids as prescribed.
      (2) Type and cross-match for blood; administer blood as prescribed.
   f. Encourage oral fluid intake if injury is minor and after administration of any contrast media.
3. Administer fluid and drug therapy to maintain urine output.
   a. Administer appropriate fluid replacement.
   b. Administer fluids, diuretics, and sodium bicarbonate as prescribed for rhabdomyolysis and myoglobinuria.
4. Control pain: administer analgesics (e.g., morphine) as prescribed.
5. Prevent and/or treat infection.
   a. Maintain strict aseptic techniques.
   b. Monitor patient for clinical indications of infection (e.g., fever, chills, or pyuria).
   c. Administer antibiotics as prescribed.

6. Minimize renal damage and preserve renal function as indicated by class of injury (Table 8-9).
   a. Conservative treatment is indicated for a hemodynamically stable patient
   b. Surgery exploration, drainage, and/or partial or total nephrectomy
      (1) Indications
         (a) Excessive and persistent retroperitoneal bleeding
         (b) Pulsatile retroperitoneal hematoma
         (c) Urinary extravasation: fibrin sealant may be used
         (d) Necrotic renal parenchyma with significant amounts of nonviable tissue
         (e) Abscess
         (f) Vascular injury: embolization may be done to avoid surgery
         (g) Progressive loss of renal function
      (2) Postoperative management
         (a) Treat pain aggressively to allow for lung expansion and to prevent hypoventilation and atelectasis.
         (b) Monitor urine volume, color, and clarity.
         (c) Monitor drainage from any drainage tubes (e.g., nephrostomy tube).
         (d) Have patient ambulate after gross hematuria clears.
7. Monitor patient for complications.
   a. Hypertension
   b. Hemorrhage, shock
   c. Infection, sepsis
   d. Rhabdomyolysis
   e. Renal failure
   f. Fistula
   g. Abscess
   h. Ileus
   i. Pseudoaneurysm

Table 8-9 Management According to Renal Injury Classification

Class	Description	Management
I	Renal contusion	• Bed rest • Assessment with continuous evaluation of urine
II	Cortical laceration	• Bed rest • Assessment with continuous evaluation of urine • Antibiotics may be prescribed
III	Caliceal laceration	• Conservation ○ Bed rest ○ Blood transfusion may be necessary ○ Assessment with evaluation of urine • Aggressive: exploratory laparotomy, repair, and/or partial nephrectomy
IV	Renal fracture	• Exploratory laparotomy and nephrectomy
V	Vascular pedicle injury or renal artery thrombosis	• Emergency surgical exploration with vascular repair • Blood transfusion may be necessary

LEARNING ACTIVITIES

1. **DIRECTIONS:** Complete the following crossword puzzle related to renal anatomy and physiology.

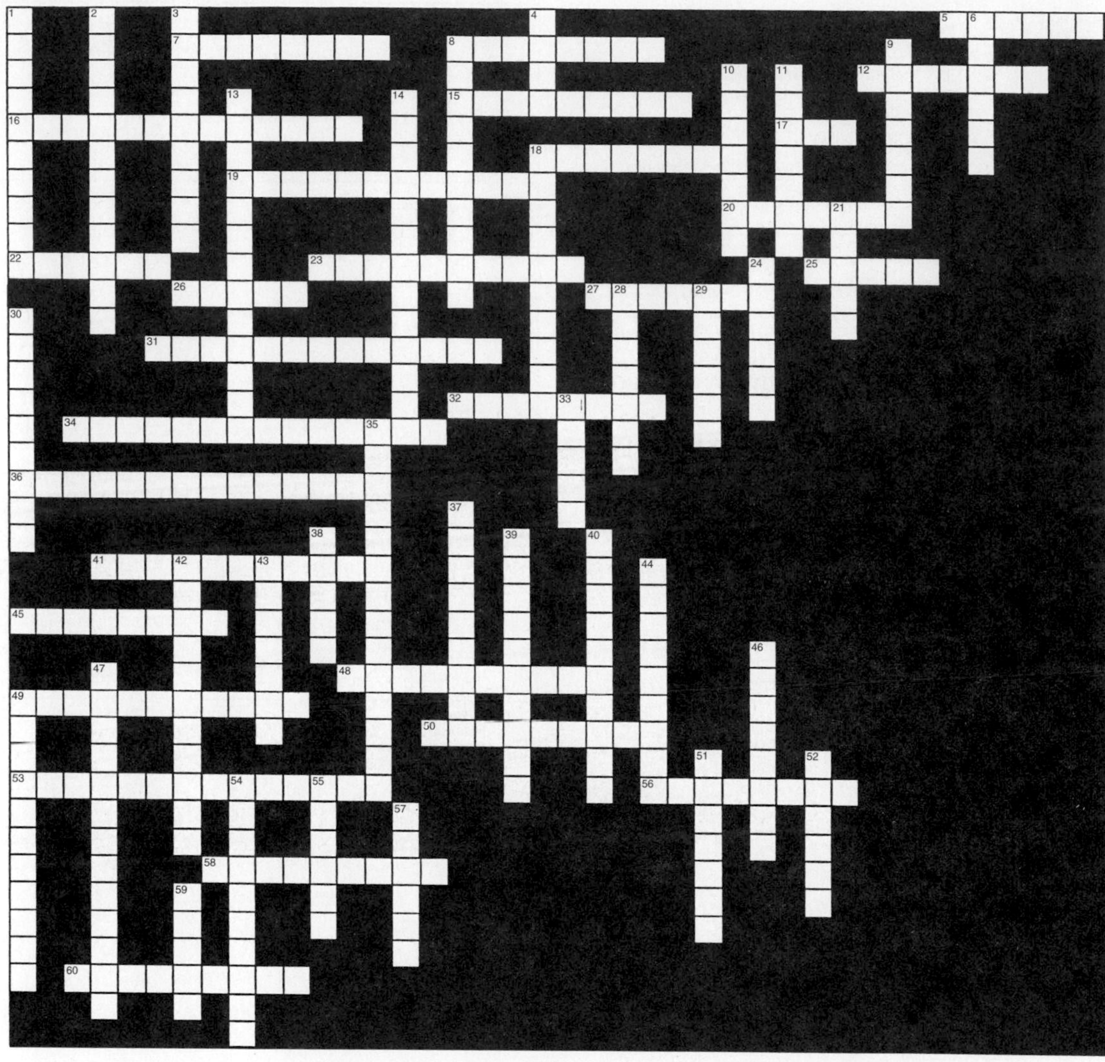

Across

5. This type of transport is against concentration gradients and requires energy
7. This arteriole leads into the glomerulus
8. The concentration of this ion determines pH
12. Microscopic functional unit of the kidney
15. The primary intracellular cation
16. Fluid outside cells
17. This hormone is produced in the hypothalamus and is released by the posterior pituitary; it causes water retention in the renal tubule
18. Indicates that the fluid has approximately the same osmolality as body fluids; example is normal saline
19. The movement of substances from the tubule back into the capillaries
20. The passageway for expulsion of urine from the bladder to the urinary meatus
22. The primary extracellular cation
23. Waste product of muscle metabolism
25. A negatively charged ion
26. Cuplike structures that drain the papillae
27. The thin layer of fibrous membrane that surrounds each kidney
31. Fluid inside cells
32. This arteriole leads out of the glomerulus
34. This type of nephron is important in the ability of the kidney to concentrate urine
36. A complex physiologic process that allows for concentration of urine
41. The kidney aids in acid-base regulation primarily by excreting and retaining this solute
45. This electrolyte works with sodium to maintain body fluid osmolality
48. This area of the kidney includes the renal cortex and medulla
49. This pressure is a pushing pressure

50. The passage of a substance from the capillary into the tubule
53. The hormone that stimulates the release of RBCs from the bone marrow
56. This type of nephron has a short loop of Henle
58. This structure consists of Bowman's capsule and the glomerulus
60. The movement of solutes from an area of high solute concentration to an area of low solute concentration

Down

1. Cluster of tightly coiled capillaries in the nephron
2. Fluid between cells
3. This electrolyte is crucial for neuromuscular transmission
4. The end product of protein metabolism
6. Site of the glomerulus and proximal and distal tubules
8. Indicates that the fluid has an osmolality more than body fluids: example, 3% saline
9. Composed of 6 to 10 pyramids
10. Vitamin D is necessary for the absorption of this mineral
11. This organ is a collapsible bag of smooth muscle
13. Another term for glomerular filtrate
14. Fluid inside vessels
18. The type of fluid loss (or gains) that cannot be measured
21. Loop diuretics such as furosemide work at the loop of _____
24. A small funnel tapering into the ureter
28. The endocrine gland that is referred to as the suprarenal gland
29. This structure collects urine from the renal pelvis and propels it to the bladder by peristaltic waves
30. The capillary network that runs parallel to the ascending and descending loop of Henle (two words)
33. The substance is secreted by the juxtaglomerular apparatus in response to low perfusion
35. The process that maintains constancy in GFR
37. An estimate of a known substance in the plasma compared with the amount in the urine
38. The human body is composed mostly of this substance
39. This electrolyte is crucial for cellular energy
40. The movement of solutes and solutions from an area of high pressure to an area of low pressure
42. The hormone of the adrenal cortex that causes retention of sodium and water and excretion of potassium
43. The movement of solution from an area of low solute concentration to an area of high solute concentration
44. Indicates that the fluid has an osmolality less than body fluids; example, one half normal saline
46. Triangular wedges of medullary tissue; composed of collecting tubules
47. This substance is made by the kidney and modulates the vasoconstrictive effects of angiotensin and norepinephrine
49. The state of internal equilibrium within the body
51. Urea is the result of the breakdown of this macronutrient
52. A positively charged ion
54. Number of osmoles per kilogram of solution; expressed as mOsm/kg
55. This structure includes proximal convoluted, loop of Henle, and distal convoluted segments
57. The inward extension of cortical tissue between the pyramids
59. Cavity filled with adipose tissue, minor and major calyces, renal pelvis, and origin of the ureter

2. DIRECTIONS: Number the structures below according to the order of their involvement in urine formation.

___ Ureters
___ Glomerulus
___ Loop of Henle
___ Proximal convoluted tubule
___ Bladder
___ Bowman's capsule
___ Collecting ducts
___ Distal convoluted tubule
___ Urethra

3. DIRECTIONS: Complete the following statements related to the movement of solutes and solutions.

Water moves by the process of __________.
Electrolytes move by the process of __________.
The sodium-potassium pump is an example of __________.
The use of a pushing pressure, such as hydrostatic pressure, is called __________.

4. A 72-year-old woman is brought to the emergency department from a long-term care facility. She recently had been started on enteral feedings. She has had a change in level of consciousness. Her sodium level is 150 mEq/L, her BUN is 80 mg/dL, and her serum glucose is 1000 mg/dL. Calculate her serum osmolality, and identify what this serum osmolality indicates. What is the most likely cause of this abnormal serum osmolality?

____

____

____

____

____

5. **Directions:** Identify the electrolyte or electrolytes that the statement describes.
   a. Serum levels of this electrolyte go up in acidosis and down in alkalosis.
   ____
   b. These three electrolytes frequently go down together.
   ____
   c. Serum levels of this electrolyte go down in hypoalbuminemia.
   ____
   d. These two electrolytes have an inverse relationship: when one goes down, the other goes up.
   ____
   e. These two electrolytes are frequently deficient in malnourished patients.
   ____
   f. Loss of either of these electrolytes causes hydrogen ions to move into the cell, resulting in metabolic alkalosis.
   ____

6. **Directions:** Identify whether these signs and symptoms are indicative of electrolyte deficit or excess.

Sign/Symptom	Excess (Hyper-)	Deficit (Hypo-)
Sodium		
Weight gain		
Abdominal cramps		
Flushed, dry skin		
Postural hypotension		
Headache		
Hypertension		
Potassium		
Flat T waves, prominent U waves		
Decreased GI motility, paralytic ileus		
Intestinal colic, diarrhea		
Muscle cramps → flaccid paralysis		
Decreased cardiac contractility		
Tall, peaked T waves; widened QRS complex		
Calcium		
Tetany		
Decreased DTR		
Neuromuscular weakness, flaccidity		
Seizures		
Bone or flank pain		
Laryngospasm		
Phosphorus		
Tetany		
Fatigue		
Chest pain		
Dyspnea		
Increased DTR		
Abdominal cramps		
Magnesium		
Decreased DTR		
Anorexia, nausea, vomiting		
Cardiopulmonary arrest		
Lethargy		
Dysrhythmias especially torsades de pointes		
Facial flushing		

7. **Directions:** Identify three major reasons for the BUN to be elevated in a patient with a normal creatinine.
   a. ______________________________
   b. ______________________________
   c. ______________________________

8. **DIRECTIONS:** Specify whether the following causes of metabolic acidosis would have a normal anion gap or an increased anion gap.

Condition	Normal Anion Gap	Increased Anion Gap
Shock		
Renal failure		
Diarrhea		
DKA		
Salicylate overdose		
Renal tubular acidosis		
Rhabdomyolysis		
Carbonic anhydrase inhibitors		
Ethylene glycol poisoning		

9. **DIRECTIONS:** Identify three electrolyte imbalances that enhance digitalis effect and increase the chance of digitalis toxicity.
   a. ______________________ c. ______________________
   b. ______________________

10. **DIRECTIONS:** Identify the fluid, electrolyte, or acid-base imbalances to which these patients would be predisposed:
    a. A patient receiving regular doses of furosemide.
       1. ______________ 4. ______________
       2. ______________ 5. ______________
       3. ______________ 6. ______________
    b. A patient with persistent vomiting.
       1. ______________ 3. ______________
       2. ______________ 4. ______________
    c. A patient with acute renal failure.
       1. ______________ 5. ______________
       2. ______________ 6. ______________
       3. ______________ 7. ______________
       4. ______________
    d. A patient with DKA (before treatment).
       1. ______________ 3. ______________
       2. ______________ 4. ______________
    e. A patient receiving multiple units of banked blood.
       1. ______________ 3. ______________
       2. ______________

11. List three indications for dialysis in a patient with acute renal failure.
    a. ______________________ c. ______________________
    b. ______________________

12. **DIRECTIONS:** Identify the following characteristics as occurring during the oliguric or diuretic phase of acute renal failure or both.

Characteristic	Oliguric Phase	Diuretic Phase	Both
Elevated BUN			
Hyperkalemia			
Hypermagnesemia			
Metabolic acidosis			
Volume deficit			
Volume excess			

13. Directions: Categorize the following causes of acute renal failure as prerenal, intrarenal, or postrenal.

Condition	Prerenal	Intrarenal	Postrenal
Acute pyelonephritis			
Aminoglycosides			
Benign prostatic hypertrophy			
Contrast dyes			
Diuretics			
Glomerulonephritis			
Goodpasture's syndrome			
Hemorrhage			
Hepatorenal syndrome			
Hypersensitivity reactions			
Intraabdominal tumor			
Malignant hypertension			
Neurogenic bladder			
Prolonged hypotension			
Renal calculi			
Rhabdomyolysis with myoglobinuria			
Septic shock			

14. Directions: List three indications of extravasation of urine into the peritoneal cavity.

a. ______________________ c. ______________________

b. ______________________

15. Directions: Complete the following crossword puzzle related to renal assessment, conditions, and treatments.

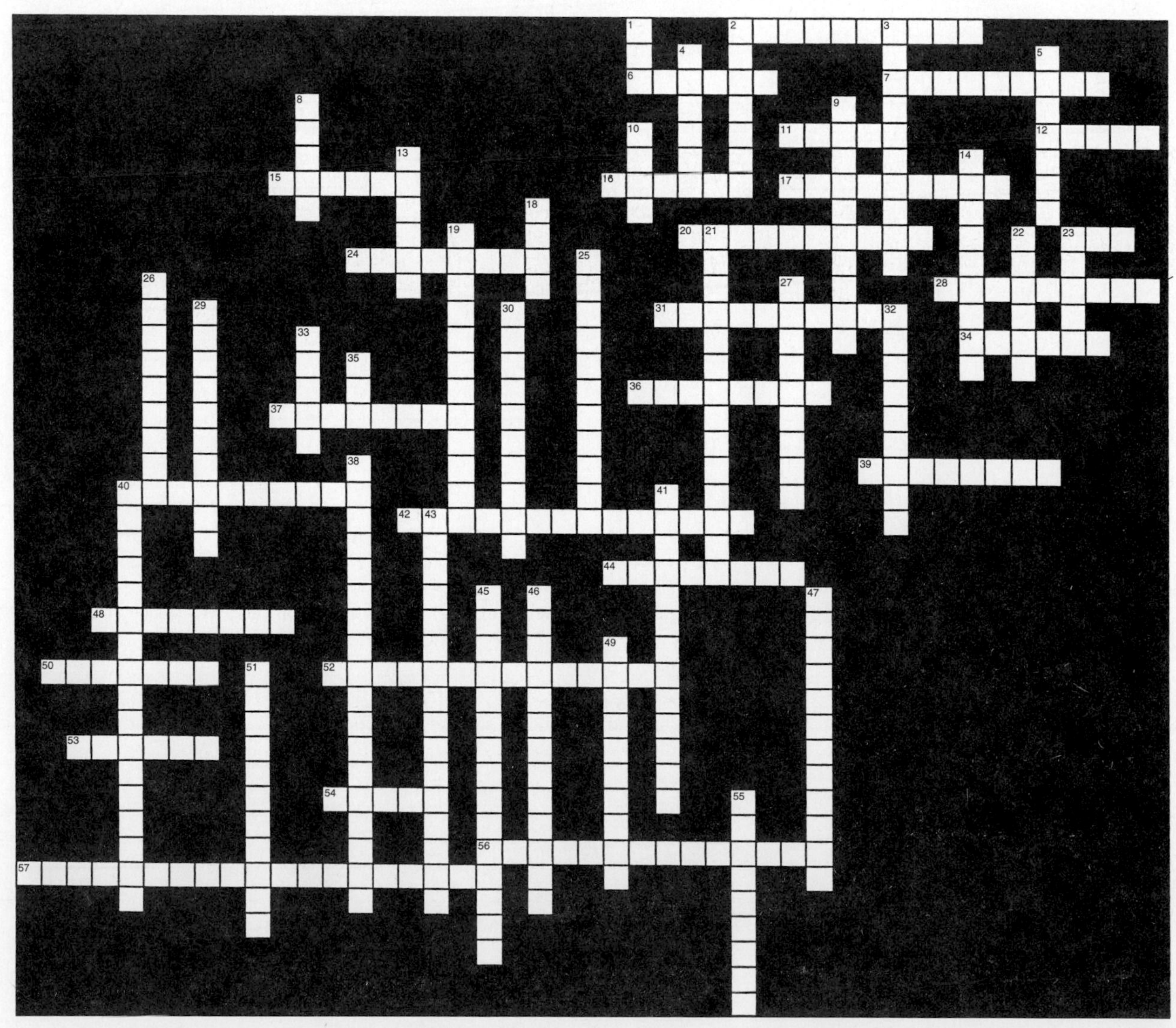

Across

2. A dopaminergic agent that increases renal flow (generic)
6. Glomerulonephritis requires a renal ____ for definitive diagnosis
7. This type of intrarenal failure is caused by nephrotoxic agents or prolonged ischemic injury
11. The amount of time that the dialysate solution remains in the peritoneal cavity in peritoneal dialysis is referred to as the _____ time
12. A common form of CRRT (abbreviation)
15. This condition occurs in renal failure and is caused by deficiency of erythropoietin
16. Increased levels of urea in the blood
17. The presence of this substance in the urine is the result of the breakdown of skeletal muscle; may cause renal failure
20. An ion exchange agent used to decrease serum potassium (brand)
23. The most common type of acute renal failure in critically ill patients (abbreviation)
24. The separation of solutes by differential diffusion through a semipermeable membrane that is placed between two solutions
28. The hand-flapping tremor seen in uremia
31. The breakdown of body protein
34. A condition characterized by cramps, convulsions, twitching of the muscles, and sharp flexion of the wrist and ankle joints
36. The renal injury that involves multiple lacerations extending into the renal collection system
37. An osmotic diuretic (generic)
39. This phase of acute renal failure is heralded by a dramatic increase in urine output
40. The categorization of acute renal failure that is caused by damage to renal tissue
42. The condition characterized by the breakdown of skeletal muscle
44. The categorization of acute renal failure that is caused by disrupted blood flow to the kidney
48. The type of intrarenal failure that is caused by infectious processes
50. The plasma protein has the most significant effect on intravascular oncotic pressure
52. Tenderness over this "angle" may indicate pyelonephritis
53. This is palpable over a fistula
54. This is audible over a fistula
56. An aldosterone antagonist (also referred to as a potassium-sparing diuretic) (generic)
57. A thiazide diuretic (generic)

Down

1. Another term for this x-ray is "flat plate of abdomen" (abbreviation)
2. A long-term vascular access consisting of an internal artery-vein anastomosis
3. This serum value goes down in overhydration and up in dehydration
4. Levels of this electrolyte are greatly affected by water balance
5. A deficiency of this electrolyte may cause paresthesia, tetany, and seizures
8. Pain in this area frequently is associated with renal conditions
9. Presence of this substance in the urine is the result of massive hemolysis; may cause renal failure
10. A renal replacement therapy that may be used in patients who cannot tolerate hemodialysis (abbreviation)
13. This type of edema frequently is associated with nephrotic syndrome
14. A solution of glucose and electrolytes used on one side of the semipermeable membrane to pull fluid and electrolytes across the semipermeable membrane in dialysis
18. Precipitation from the kidney that takes the shape of the tubule where it was formed
19. The electrolyte imbalance that occurs with crush injury, renal failure, and hemolysis
21. An oxygen free scavenger that may be used after contrast dye, especially if the patient has an elevated creatinine
22. To move the kidney down to palpable range the patient is asked to take a deep _____
23. Calculation of this gap differentiates metabolic acidosis caused by acid gain from metabolic acidosis caused by bicarbonate loss
25. The surgical procedure performed for renal fracture
26. This type of renal injury is caused by compression of the kidney between the lower ribs and the vertebral column
27. This categorization of acute renal failure is caused by disrupted renal flow; renal stone is an example of a cause of this type of renal failure
29. High levels of this electrolyte occur in renal failure; low levels occur in malnutrition
30. A loop diuretic (generic)
32. High levels of this electrolyte may cause respiratory paralysis and cardiopulmonary arrest
33. Renal patients may taste _____
35. This lab value is normally 10 times the creatinine value (abbreviation)
38. An acute inflammation of the kidney associated with beta-hemolytic streptococcal infection
40. The drugs used to prevent organ rejection in a posttransplant patient cause _____
41. The electrolyte imbalance that occurs with osteolytic lesions
43. The electrolyte imbalance primarily associated with refeeding syndrome
45. Calcium may be administered for hypocalcemia, hyperkalemia, and _____
46. A carbonic anhydrase inhibitor frequently used to treat metabolic alkalosis (abbreviation)
47. The syndrome characterized by basement membrane damage and manifested by renal failure and hemoptysis (possessive)
49. A permanent renal replacement therapy for patients with chronic renal failure
51. A cause of hypoproteinemia in renal failure
55. Significant changes in serum levels of this electrolyte causes T wave changes and dysrhythmias

LEARNING ACTIVITIES ANSWERS

1.

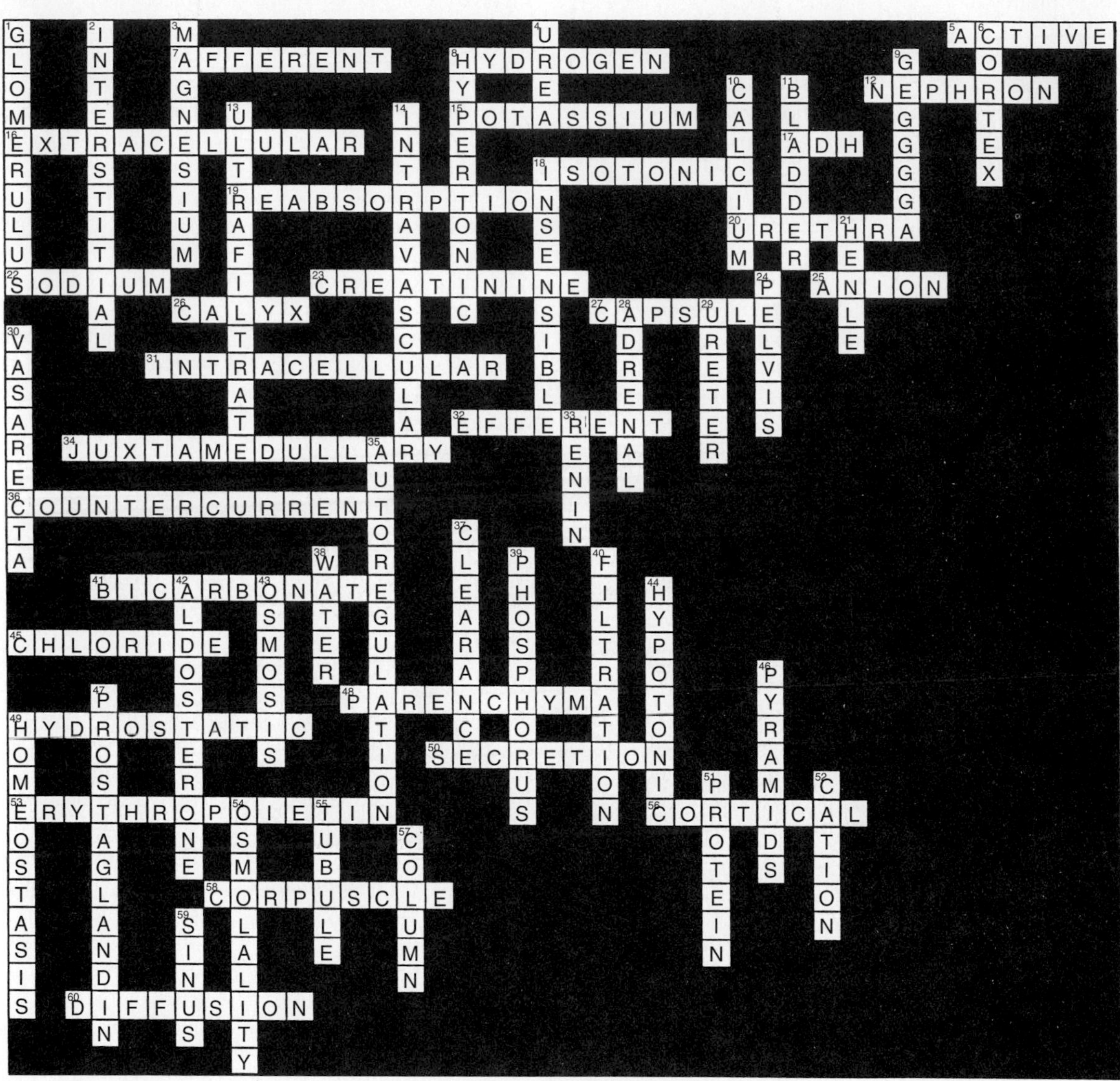

2. 7 Ureters
   1 Glomerulus
   4 Loop of Henle
   3 Proximal convoluted tubule
   8 Bladder
   2 Bowman's capsule
   6 Collecting ducts
   5 Distal convoluted tubule
   9 Urethra

3. Water moves by the process of *osmosis*.
   Electrolytes move by the process of *diffusion*.
   The sodium-potassium pump is an example of *active transport*.
   The use of a pushing pressure, such as hydrostatic pressure, is called *filtration*.

4. Serum osmolality is 433 mOsm/kg, which indicates severe dehydration. This is an example of a hyperglycemic hyperosmolar nonketotic condition caused by glucose intolerance associated with recent initiation of high-glucose enteral feedings.

5. a. Potassium
b. Potassium, calcium, magnesium
c. Calcium
d. Calcium, phosphorus
e. Magnesium, phosphorus
f. Potassium, chloride

6.

Sign/Symptom	Excess (Hyper-)	Deficit (Hypo-)
Sodium		
Weight gain	×	
Abdominal cramps		×
Flushed, dry skin	×	
Postural hypotension		×
Headache		×
Hypertension	×	
Potassium		
Flat T waves, prominent U waves		×
Decreased GI motility, paralytic ileus		×
Intestinal colic, diarrhea	×	
Muscle cramps → flaccid paralysis		×
Decreased cardiac contractility	×	
Tall, peaked T waves; widened QRS complex	×	
Calcium		
Tetany		×
Decreased DTR	×	
Neuromuscular weakness, flaccidity	×	
Seizures		×
Bone or flank pain	×	
Laryngospasm		×
Phosphorus		
Tetany	×	
Fatigue		×
Chest pain		×
Dyspnea		×
Increased DTR	×	
Abdominal cramps	×	
Magnesium		
Decreased DTR	×	
Anorexia, nausea, vomiting		×
Cardiopulmonary arrest	×	
Lethargy	×	
Dysrhythmias especially torsades de pointes		×
Facial flushing	×	

7. a. Prerenal failure caused by hypovolemia or hypoperfusion
b. Catabolism
c. GI bleeding with digestion of hemoglobin (i.e., protein)

8.

Condition	Normal Anion Gap	Increased Anion Gap
Shock		×
Renal failure		×
Diarrhea	×	
DKA		×
Salicylate overdose		×
Renal tubular acidosis	×	
Rhabdomyolysis		×
Carbonic anhydrase inhibitors	×	
Ethylene glycol poisoning		×

9. a. Hypercalcemia
b. Hypokalemia
c. Hypomagnesemia

10. a. A patient receiving regular doses of furosemide.
1. Hypovolemia
2. Hyponatremia
3. Hypokalemia
4. Hypocalcemia
5. Hypomagnesemia
6. Metabolic alkalosis (caused by hypochloremia and hypokalemia)

b. A patient with persistent vomiting.
1. Hypovolemia
2. Hyponatremia
3. Hypokalemia
4. Metabolic alkalosis (caused by hypochloremia and hypokalemia)

c. A patient with acute renal failure (oliguric phase).
1. Hypervolemia
2. Hyponatremia
3. Hyperkalemia
4. Hypocalcemia
5. Hyperphosphatemia
6. Hypermagnesemia
7. Metabolic acidosis

d. A patient with DKA (before treatment).
1. Hyperkalemia
2. Hypophosphatemia
3. Hypermagnesemia
4. Metabolic acidosis

e. A patient receiving multiple units of banked blood.
1. Hyperkalemia
2. Hypocalcemia
3. Hypomagnesemia

11. a. BUN greater than 100 mg/dL
b. Volume overload especially with pulmonary edema
c. Uncontrollable hyperkalemia
d. Uncontrollable hyperphosphatemia
e. Uncontrollable acidosis
f. Pericarditis
g. Seizures or coma
h. Symptomatic uremia

12.

Characteristic	Oliguric Phase	Diuretic Phase	Both
Elevated BUN			×
Hyperkalemia			×
Hypermagnesemia			×
Metabolic acidosis			×
Volume deficit		×	
Volume excess	×		

13.

Condition	Prerenal	Intrarenal	Postrenal
Acute pyelonephritis		×	
Aminoglycosides		×	
Benign prostatic hypertrophy			×
Contrast dyes		×	
Diuretics	×	×	
Glomerulonephritis		×	
Goodpasture's syndrome		×	
Hemorrhage	×	×*	
Hepatorenal syndrome	×	×*	
Hypersensitivity reactions		×	
Intraabdominal tumor			×
Malignant hypertension		×	
Neurogenic bladder			×
Prolonged hypotension		×	
Renal calculi			×
Rhabdomyolysis with myoglobinuria		×	
Septic shock	×	×*	

*If prolonged hypoperfusion occurs.

14. a. Midline bulging
b. Lower quadrant and flank or thigh distention
c. Lower abdominal pain or mass
d. Abdominal pain, rebound tenderness
e. Hematuria
f. Anuria

15.

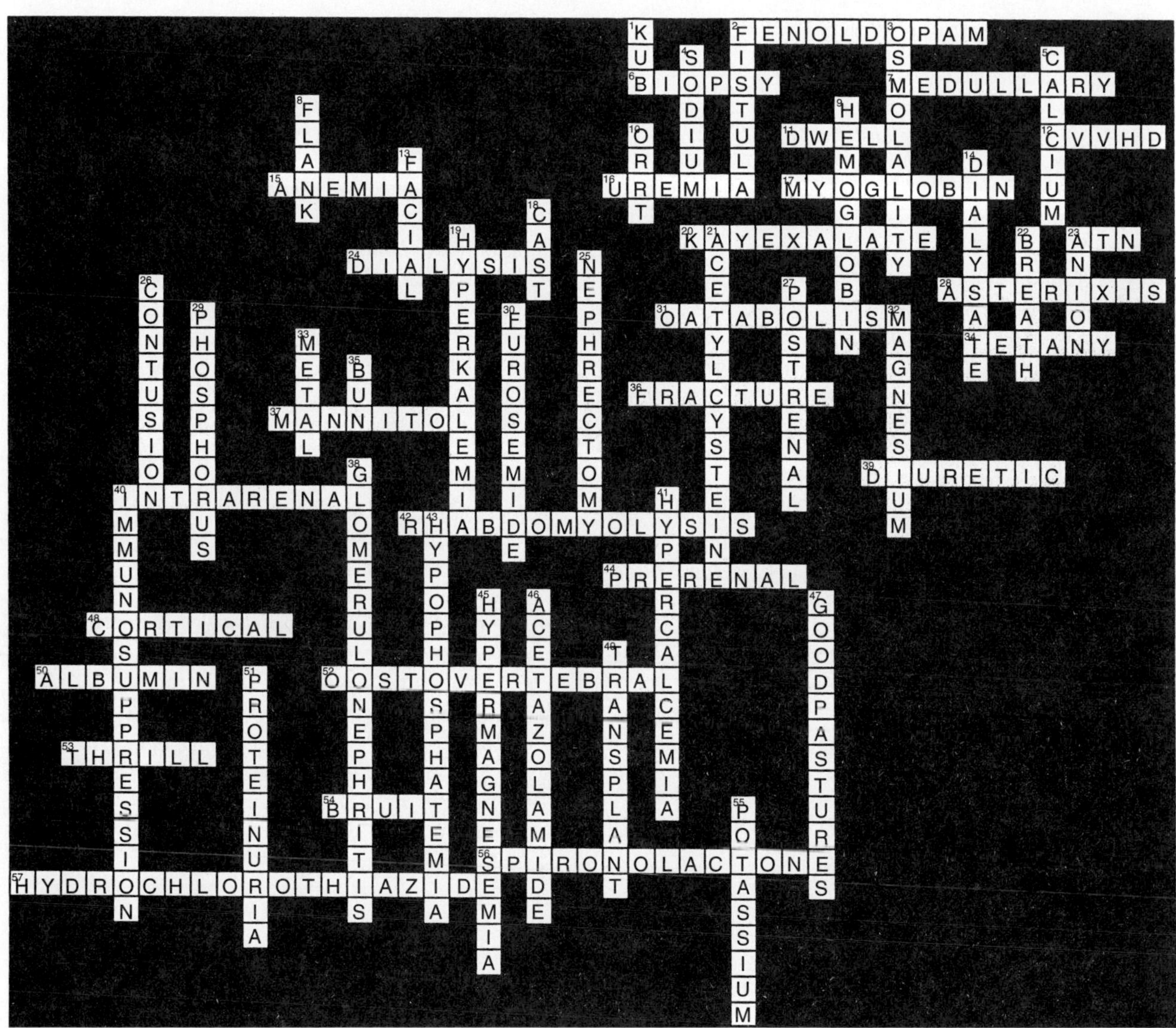

Reference

Mehta, R. L., Pascual, M. T., Soroko, S., & Chertow, G. M. (2002). Diuretics, mortality, and nonrecovery of renal function in acute renal failure. *Journal of the American Medical Association, 288*(20), 2547-2553.

Bibliography

American Heart Association. (2005). Part 10.1: Life-threatening electrolyte abnormalities. *Circulation, 112*(24 suppl.), IV121-IV125.

Bozeman, C., Carver, B., Zabari, G., Caldito, G., & Venable, D. (2004). Selective operative management of major blunt renal trauma. *Journal of Trauma, 57*(2), 305-309.

Brenner, Z. R., & Myer, S. A. (2003). Acetylcysteine and nephropathy. *American Journal of Nursing, 103*(3), 64AA-64EE.

Burger, C. M. (2004). Hyperkalemia: When serum K+ is not okay. *American Journal of Nursing, 104*(10), 66-70.

Burger, C. M. (2004). Hypokalemia: Averting crisis with early recognition and intervention. *American Journal of Nursing, 104*(11), 61-65.

Burrows-Hudson, S. (2005). Chronic kidney disease: An overview. *American Journal of Nursing, 105*(2), 40-50.

Campoy, S., & Elwell, R. (2005). Pharmacology & CKD. *American Journal of Nursing, 105*(9), 60-72.

Cassabaum, V. D., & Bourg, P. W. (2002). The ins and outs of renal trauma. *American Journal of Nursing, 102*(9 suppl.), 4-7.

Criddle, L. M. (2003). Rhabdomyolysis: Pathophysiology, recognition, and management. *Critical Care Nurse, 23*(6), 14-32.

Eckert, K. L. (2005). Penetrating and blunt abdominal trauma. *Critical Care Nursing Quarterly, 28*(1), 41-59.

Elgart, H. N. (2004). Assessment of fluids and electrolytes. *AACN Clinical Issues, 15*(4), 607-621.

Fischer, U. M., Paschalis, T., & Mehlhorn, U. (2005). Renal protection by radical scavenging in cardiac surgery patients. Retrieved January 27, 2006, from http://www.medscape.com/viewarticle/510550_print

Gutch, C. F., Stoner, M. H., & Corea, A. L. (2005). *Review of hemodialysis for nurses and dialysis personnel* (7th ed.). St. Louis, MO: Mosby.

Hammer, C., & Santucci, R. A. (2003). Effect of an institutional policy of nonoperative treatment of grades I to IV renal injuries. *Journal of Urology, 169*, 1751-1753.

Harrington, L. (2005). Potassium protocols: In search of evidence. *Clinical Nurse Specialist, 19*(3), 137-141.

Huggins, R. M., Kennedy, W. K., Melroy, M. J., & Tollerton, D. G. (2003). Cardiac arrest from succinylcholine-induced hyperkalemia. *American Journal of Health-System Pharmacy, 60*(7), 693-697.

Innerarity, S. (2000). Hypomagnesemia in acute and chronic illness. *Critical Care Nursing Quarterly, 23*(2), 1-19.

Johnson, A. L., & Criddle, L. M. (2004). Pass the salt: Indications for and implications of using hypertonic saline. *Critical Care Nurse, 24*(5), 36-48.

Kallenbach, J. Z., Gutch, C. F., Stoner, M., & Corea, A. (2005). *Review of hemodialysis for nurses and dialysis personnel* (7th ed.). St. Louis, MO: Mosby.

Kaplow, R., & Barry, R. (2002). Continuous renal replacement therapies. *American Journal of Nursing, 102*(11), 26-34.

Kinney, M., Dunbar, S., Brooks-Brunn, J. A., Molter, N., & Vitello-Cicciu, J. (1998). *AACN clinical reference for critical care nursing* (4th ed.). St. Louis, MO: Mosby.

Kruse, J. A., Fink, M. P., & Carlson, R. W. (2003). *Saunders manual of critical care*. Philadelphia: Saunders.

Kumar, S. P., & Sorrell, V. L. (2003). Renal-dose dopamine: Myth or ally in the treatment of acute renal failure? Retrieved January 27, 2006, from http://www.medscape.com/viewarticle/462075_print

Legg, V. (2005). Complications of chronic kidney disease. *American Journal of Nursing, 105*(6), 40-50.

Little, C. (2000). Renovascular hypertension. *American Journal of Nursing, 100*(2), 46.

Meister, J., & Reddy, K. (2002). Rhabdomyolysis: An overview. *American Journal of Nursing, 102*(2), 75-79.

Metnitz, P. G. H., Krenn, C. G., Steltzer, H., Lang, T., Ploder, J., Lenz, K., et al. (2002). Effect of acute renal failure requiring renal replacement therapy on outcome in critically ill patients. *Critical Care Medicine, 30*(9), 2051-2058.

Nicol, A. J., & Theunissen, D. (2002). Renal salvage in penetrating kidney injuries: A prospective analysis. *Journal of Trauma, 53*(2), 351-353.

Small, K. R., & McMullen, M. (2005). When clear becomes cloudy. *American Journal of Nursing, 105*(1), 72AA-72GG.

Sole, M. L., Klein, D. G., & Moseley, M. J. (2005). *Introduction to critical care nursing* (4th ed.). Philadelphia: Elsevier Saunders.

Thomas, N. (Ed.). (2002). *Renal nursing* (Vol. 2). Edinburgh: Bailliere Tindall.

Thompson, E. J., & King, S. L. (2003). Acetylcysteine and fenoldopam: Promising new approaches for preventing effects of contrast nephrotoxicity. *Critical Care Nurse, 23*(3), 39-46.

Urden, L. D., Stacy, K. M., & Lough, M. E. (2006). *Thelan's critical care nursing: Diagnosis and management* (5th ed.). St. Louis, MO: Mosby.

Wiegand, D. L.-M. J., & Carlson, K. K. (2005). *AACN procedure manual for critical care* (5th ed.). Philadelphia: W. B. Saunders.

Zabat, E. (2003). When your patient needs peritoneal dialysis. *Nursing 2003, 33*(8), 52-54.

The Endocrine System

CHAPTER 9

Selected Concepts in Anatomy and Physiology

Functions

The endocrine system regulates secretion of hormones that alter metabolic body functions including all of the following:

1. Chemical reactions and transport of chemicals across cell membranes
2. Growth and development
3. Metabolism
4. Fluid and electrolyte balance
5. Acid-base balance
6. Adaptation
7. Reproduction

Components

1. Glands or glandular tissue that synthesize, store, and secrete hormones
   a. An endocrine gland is ductless but highly vascular.
   b. The location of endocrine glands is depicted in Figure 9-1.
2. Hormones
   a. Definition: complex chemical substances produced in one part or organ of the body that initiate or regulate the activity of an organ or a group of cells in another part of the body
      (1) Hormones are released by endocrine glands in response to specific signals (e.g., low target gland hormone levels).
      (2) Hormones are released directly into the bloodstream to be distributed throughout the body and to the target gland or target organ to initiate a response.
   b. Types include the following:
      (1) Single amino acids (e.g., epinephrine, dopamine, and thyroid hormones)
      (2) Proteins (e.g., growth hormone and follicle-stimulating hormone)
      (3) Steroids (e.g., androgens, aldosterone, and cortisol)
   c. Endocrine glands and hormones significant in the care of critically ill patients are summarized in Table 9-1; hormones also are secreted by the following organs although these organs normally are not considered part of the endocrine system:
      (1) Gastrointestinal (GI) tract (e.g., gastrin, cholecystokinin, and somatostatin)
      (2) Heart (e.g., atrial natriuretic hormone)
      (3) Kidney (e.g., erythropoietin, renin, and calcitriol)
3. Receptor cells: located in an organ or a group of cells in another part of the body

Process of Hormone Synthesis, Secretion, Effect, and Suppression

See Figure 9-2.

Regulation of Hormones

1. The hypothalamus
   a. The hypothalamus regulates the secretion of hormones through other stimulating hormones called *releasing factors*.
   b. Releasing factors are keyed to cause the release of hormone from the target gland.
2. Neurotransmitters
   a. Sympathetic nervous system (SNS): epinephrine, norepinephrine
   b. Parasympathetic nervous system: acetylcholine
3. Feedback regulation
   a. Allows self-regulation
   b. Based on the concentration of the hormone present in the circulation
   c. Also influenced by electrolyte levels, metabolites, osmolality, fluid status, and other hormones
   d. Positive feedback: low hormone levels stimulate release of the releasing factor
   e. Negative feedback: high hormone levels inhibit the release of the releasing factor (Figure 9-3)

Endocrine Dysfunction

1. Classification
   a. Based on level of hormone activity

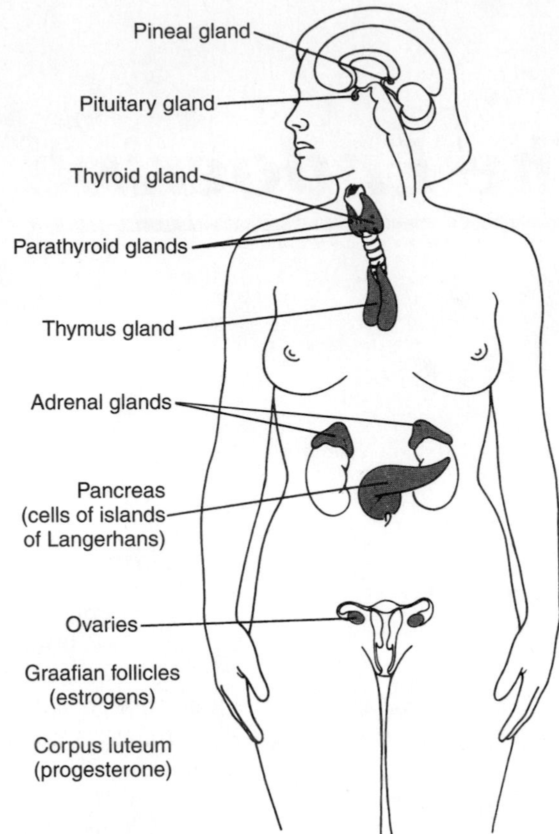

Figure 9-1 Location of endocrine glands. Testes not pictured. (From Beare, P. G., & Myer, J. L. [1994]. *Principles and practice of adult health nursing* [2nd ed.]. St. Louis: Mosby.)

(1) Hyperfunction: increased hormonal activity
(2) Hypofunction: decreased hormonal activity

b. Based on location of dysfunctional gland or response
(1) Primary disorders: disorder of the target gland (e.g., adrenal or thyroid gland)
(2) Secondary disorder: disorder of the stimulating gland (e.g., hypothalamus or pituitary gland)

c. Based on clinical course of dysfunction
(1) Acute: beginning abruptly with marked intensity
(2) Chronic: developing slowly and persisting for a long time, often for the remainder of the lifetime of the individual

2. Etiology of endocrine dysfunction
a. Dysfunction of a particular gland
b. Altered secretion of the stimulating hormones for that gland
c. Altered response to the hormone itself at the target cell

Assessment of the Endocrine System

Interview

1. Chief complaint: why is the patient seeking help and the duration of the problem; because hormones affect every body tissue, numerous symptoms may indicate endocrine dysfunction
a. General
(1) Easy fatigability, lethargy
(2) Sleep disorders
(3) Cold or heat intolerance
(4) Weight loss or gain, or rapid fluctuations in weight
(5) Increase in size of head, hands, and feet

b. Dermatologic
(1) Pruritus
(2) Hair loss
(3) Changes in hair distribution
(4) Changes in quality of hair
(5) Changes in skin color or pigmentation
(6) Striae
(7) Changes in skin moisture

c. Eyes: visual changes

d. Neck
(1) Jugular neck vein distention
(2) Enlargement or nodules

e. Cardiovascular
(1) Palpitations
(2) Syncope

f. Pulmonary: dyspnea

g. Neurologic
(1) Voice changes
(2) Tremors
(3) Nervousness

Text continued on p. 601

Table 9-1 Endocrine Glands and Hormones Significant in the Care of Critically Ill Patients

Hormone	Actions	Releasing Factors	Target	Hypersecretion	Hyposecretion
PITUITARY (HYPOPHYSIS)					
Anterior Pituitary (Adenohypophysis)					
Growth hormone (somatotropin)	• Stimulates protein anabolism • Mobilizes fatty acids • Conserves carbohydrates • Stimulates bone and cartilage growth	Growth hormone-releasing hormone from hypothalamus in response to exercise, starvation, decreased amino acid levels, stress, and hypoglycemia	All body cells capable of growth, especially muscle, bone, and cartilage cells	Giantism in children; acromegaly in adults	Dwarfism in children; possible decrease in organ weight in adults
Adrenocorticotropic hormone	• Stimulates growth and function of adrenal gland • Controls production and release of glucocorticoid hormones • Stimulates mineralocorticoid production • Stimulates androgen production	Corticotropin releasing-hormone from hypothalamus in response to hypoglycemia, decrease in cortisol levels, hypoxia, trauma, surgery, and physical and/or psychological stress	Cells of adrenal cortex	Cushing's disease	Adrenal insufficiency (chronic) and/or adrenal crisis (acute)
Thyroid-stimulating hormone (thyrotropin)	• Increases size and growth of thyroid cells • Increases synthesis of thyroid hormones • Releases stored thyroid hormones	Thyrotropin-releasing hormone from hypothalamus in response to cold temperature or a decrease in thyroid hormone levels	Cells of thyroid gland	Hyperthyroidism	Hypothyroidism
Posterior Pituitary (Neurohypophysis)					
Antidiuretic hormone (vasopressin)	• Increases water reabsorption (inhibits diuresis) by kidney tubules and collecting ducts • Vasoconstriction of arterioles • Abdominal cramping	Increase in serum osmolality; hypernatremia; hypovolemia; hypoxia; hypotension; pain; trauma; stress; nausea; pharmacologic agents	Distal renal tubules and collecting ducts; smooth muscle of arterioles and GI tract	Syndrome of inappropriate antidiuretic hormone	Diabetes insipidus

Continued

Table 9-1 Endocrine Glands and Hormones Significant in the Care of Critically Ill Patients—cont'd

Hormone	Actions	Releasing Factors	Target	Hypersecretion	Hyposecretion
THYROID GLAND					
Triiodothyronine (T_3) and thyroxine (T_4) NOTE: Triiodothyronine is more biologically active.	• Stimulate metabolic rate • Increase protein synthesis • Increase carbohydrate and fat metabolism • Increase bone growth • Increase oxygen consumption • Increase metabolism and clearance of drugs	Thyroid-stimulating hormone (TSH) from anterior pituitary; thyrotropin-releasing hormone from hypothalamus; cold temperature	Most body cells	Hyperthyroidism (chronic); thyroid storm or crisis (acute)	Hypothyroidism (chronic); myxedema coma (acute)
Thyrocalcitonin (calcitonin)	• Reduces plasma calcium levels by inhibiting bone lysis and decreasing calcium resorption by the kidney	Increase in serum calcium, magnesium, or glucagon	Bone cells and kidney cells	Not significant	Not significant
PARATHYROID GLAND					
Parathyroid hormone (parathormone)	• Increases serum calcium by accelerating bone breakdown with release of calcium into the blood, increasing calcium reabsorption from intestine, and decreasing kidney tubule reabsorption of calcium • Decreases blood phosphate levels by increasing phosphate loss in urine • Increases reabsorption of magnesium by the renal tubules	Low serum calcium; high serum magnesium or phosphate level; catecholamines; cortisol	Bone cells and cells of GI tract and kidney	Hypercalcemia and hypophosphatemia; possibly renal calculi	Hypocalcemia and bone decalcification; hyperphosphatemia

Adrenal Cortex					
Glucocorticoids such as cortisol	• Increase blood glucose by stimulating gluconeogenesis in the liver • Inhibit glucose use by the cell • Inhibit protein anabolism • Promote fatty acid mobilization • Inhibit inflammatory response	Corticotropin-releasing hormone from hypothalamus; ACTH from anterior pituitary	Most body cells	Cushing's syndrome	Addison's disease (chronic); adrenal crisis (acute)
Mineralocorticoids such as aldosterone	• Increase sodium and water reabsorption and potassium excretion	ACTH from anterior pituitary (minor effect); primary stimulus is renin-angiotensin system; decrease in serum sodium; increase in serum potassium	Distal and collecting tubules of kidney; sweat glands; salivary glands; intestines	Hyperaldosteronism	Addison's disease (chronic); adrenal crisis (acute)
Adrenal Medulla					
Catecholamines such as epinephrine and norepinephrine	• Dilate pupils • Increase heart rate and contractility • Dilation of blood vessels to heart, brain, and skeletal muscle • Constriction of blood vessels to nonessential organs such as skin, kidney, and GI tract • Bronchodilation • Increase in respiratory rate and depth • Increase in perspiration, peristalsis, and secretion in GI tract • Increase in blood sugar	Sympathetic nervous system innervation: insulin; histamine; anxiety; fear; pain; trauma; exercise; temperature extremes; hypoxia; hypotension; hypovolemia; excess thyroid hormone	Most body cells, vascular beds, and smooth muscle	Exaggeration or prolongation of normal effects; may be caused by adrenal medulla tumor called *pheochromocytoma*	May have decrease in stress response or no noticeable effect

Continued

Table 9-1 Endocrine Glands and Hormones Significant in the Care of Critically Ill Patients—cont'd

Hormone	Actions	Releasing Factors	Target	Hypersecretion	Hyposecretion
PANCREAS					
Glucagon (from alpha cells)	• Stimulates glycogenolysis and gluconeogenesis to increase blood glucose • Inhibits glycolysis • Increases lipolysis	Decrease in blood glucose; elevated blood amino acid; catecholamines; exercise; starvation	Most body cells, especially liver cells	Hyperglycemia	Hypoglycemia
Insulin (from beta cells)	• Enables glucose to move into the cell • Aids in muscle and tissue oxidation of glucose • Enhances storage of glycogen • Increases protein synthesis • Inhibits lipolysis	Increase in blood glucose; gastrin; increase in growth hormone; ACTH; glucagon	Most body cells, especially liver cells	Hypoglycemia	Hyperglycemia (diabetes mellitus)

ACTH, Adrenocorticotropic hormone; *GI*, gastrointestinal.

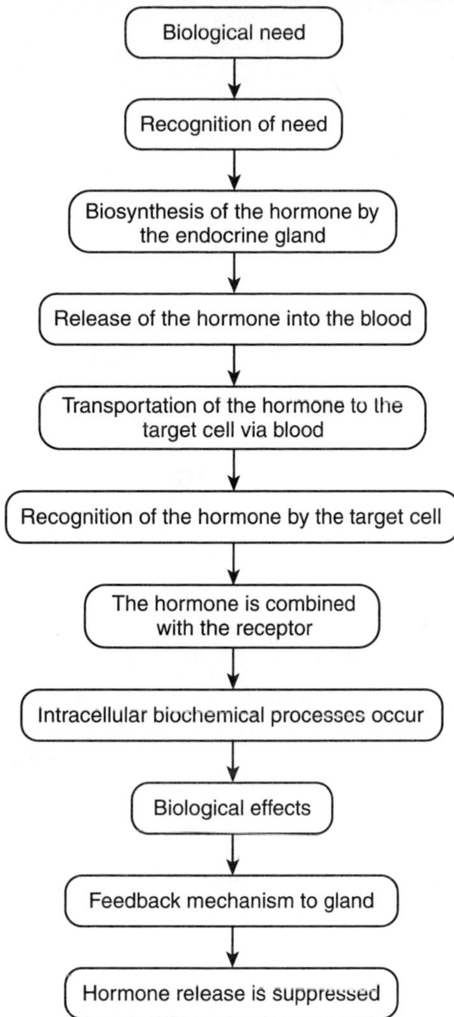

Figure 9-2 Process of hormone synthesis, secretion, effect, and suppression.

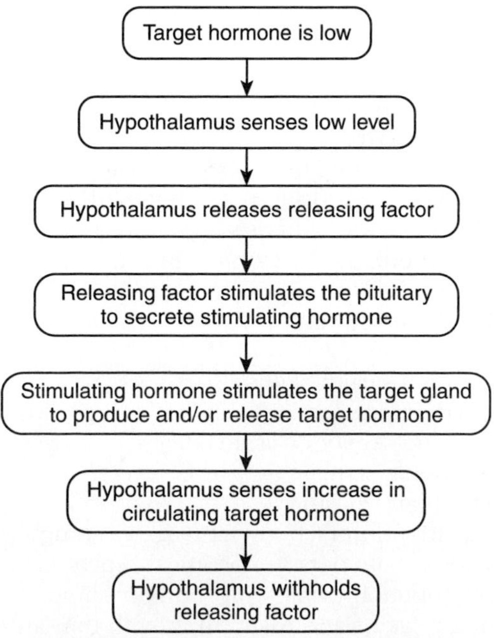

Figure 9-3 Negative feedback mechanism.

(4) Visual changes
(5) Loss of the sense of smell
(6) Headache
(7) Sensory changes
(8) Memory loss
(9) Personality changes
(10) Confusion, agitation
(11) Delusions, paranoia, depression
(12) Muscle twitching
(13) Seizures

h. GI
(1) Change in appetite
(2) Nausea, vomiting
(3) Abdominal pain
(4) Constipation or diarrhea
(5) Incontinence
(6) Polyphagia
(7) Polydipsia

i. Genitourinary (GU)
(1) Polyuria, oliguria, nocturia
(2) Incontinence
(3) Decreased libido
(4) Menstrual irregularities

j. Musculoskeletal
   (1) Muscle or joint pain or aching
   (2) Muscle weakness
   (3) Muscle cramping
   (4) Muscle wasting
   (5) Twitching
   (6) Fractures
2. History of present illness: use PQRST format (provocation, palliation, quality, quantity, region, radiation, severity, timing)
3. Past medical history: past illnesses or pathologic conditions that may result in endocrine dysfunction
   a. Trauma
   b. Ischemia or infarction
   c. Neoplasm
   d. Inflammation, infection
   e. Autoimmune conditions
   f. Acquired immunodeficiency syndrome (AIDS)
   g. Irradiation, antineoplastic drugs
   h. Surgical removal of an endocrine gland
   i. Interruption of prescribed pharmaceutical agent for treatment of a preexisting chronic endocrine dysfunction
4. Family history
   a. Diabetes mellitus (DM)
   b. Cardiovascular disease
   c. Cerebrovascular disease
   d. Cancer
5. Social history
   a. Relationship with spouse or significant other; family structure
   b. Occupation
   c. Educational level
   d. Stress level and usual coping mechanisms
   e. Recreational habits
   f. Exercise habits
   g. Dietary habits
      (1) Usual diet
      (2) Compliance with prescribed limitations
   h. Fluid intake
   i. Caffeine intake
   j. Tobacco use: recorded as pack-years (number of packs per day times the number of years patient has been smoking)
   k. Alcohol use: recorded as alcoholic beverages consumed per month, week, or day
   l. Toxin exposure
   m. Travel
6. Medication history
   a. Prescribed drug, dose, frequency, and time of last dose
   b. Nonprescribed drugs
      (1) Over-the-counter drugs, supplements
      (2) Substance abuse
   c. Patient understanding of drug actions, side effects, and sick day management
   d. Pharmacologic agents used to treat chronic endocrine dysfunction
      (1) Hormone replacement
      (2) Hormone suppressive agents
      (3) Agents that trigger release of hormone or potentiate the effect of the hormone
      (4) Vitamins or minerals necessary for body synthesis of hormones
   e. Evaluation of patient's compliance with prescribed therapy
   f. Pharmacologic agents that may alter endocrine function by stimulating or inhibiting hormone release or may interfere with hormone action at the target tissue; pharmacologic agents that may cause endocrine dysfunction are listed under Etiology for each endocrine condition

Inspection and Palpation

1. Vital signs
   a. Blood pressure (BP): lying, sitting, standing; orthostatic BP changes caused by hypovolemia may be seen in diabetes insipidus (DI) or DM
   b. Heart rate
      (1) Bradycardia frequently is seen in hypothyroidism.
      (2) Tachycardia may be associated with hyperthyroidism, infection (which may be a cause of diabetic ketoacidosis [DKA] or hyperglycemic hyperosmolar nonketotic syndrome [HHNK]), hypovolemia (which may occur in DKA, HHNK, or DI), and hypervolemia (which may occur in syndrome of inappropriate antidiuretic hormone [SIADH]).
   c. Respiratory rate
      (1) Bradypnea frequently is seen in hypothyroidism.
      (2) Tachypnea may be associated with hyperthyroidism, infection (which may be a cause of DKA or HHNK), hypovolemia (which may occur in DKA, HHNK, or DI), and hypervolemia (which may occur in SIADH).
   d. Temperature
      (1) Hypothermia may be associated with hypothyroidism.
      (2) Hyperthermia may be associated with hyperthyroidism, with extreme hyperthermia during thyroid crisis.
      (3) Hyperthermia also may indicate infection that may be a cause of DKA or HHNK.
   e. Height and weight
2. General survey
   a. Apparent health status
   b. Apparent age (consistency with chronologic age)
   c. Gross deformity or asymmetry
   d. Nutritional status
   e. Stature and posture
   f. Redistribution of body fat (e.g., Cushing's syndrome [hyperadrenocortical function] causes redistribution of fat with "buffalo hump," "moon face," and thick trunk with thin arms and legs)

g. Gynecomastia in males: may be related to hypogonadism, hyperthyroidism, or Cushing's syndrome
h. Mobility
i. Level of consciousness: changes seen in cerebral function may occur
j. Presence of Medic-Alert bracelet indicating chronic endocrine condition or steroid dependency

3. Head and neck
   a. Eyes
      (1) Eyeballs
         (a) Protruding eyeballs (exophthalmos): frequently seen in hyperthyroidism; lid lag frequently seen in patients with exophthalmos
         (b) Sunken: may be seen in hypothyroidism or dehydration
      (2) Strabismus: may be seen with hyperthyroidism
   b. Facial or periorbital edema: frequently seen in Cushing's syndrome; also may be seen in hypothyroidism
   c. Changes in visual acuity and visual fields: may be related to pituitary tumor
   d. Facial bone structure: facial changes including protruding forehead and prominent jaw seen in acromegaly
   e. Thyroid gland (the only endocrine gland that can be palpated)
      (1) Enlargement or palpable mass or nodule
      (2) Tenderness
      (3) Presence of thrill
4. Skin and appendages
   a. Skin color changes
      (1) Addison's disease causes characteristic "bronzing" of the skin.
      (2) Gray-brown pigmentation around neck and axillae may be seen in Cushing's syndrome.
      (3) Yellowish skin discoloration may be seen in hypothyroidism.
   b. Skin temperature: skin temperature changes frequently seen in thyroid conditions
   c. Skin moisture and turgor
      (1) Warm, moist, paper-thin skin may be seen in hyperthyroidism.
      (2) Dry, scaly skin may be seen in hypothyroidism.
      (3) Decreased skin turgor may be seen in dehydration, which may be seen in DI, DKA, or HHNK.
   d. Skin lesions: acne; spider angiomas
   e. Mucous membranes: note moisture
   f. Scars (especially in neck area, which may indicate prior thyroid surgery)
   g. Bruising: increased bruising may be seen in Cushing's syndrome
   h. Striae: purplish striae on abdomen may be seen in Cushing's syndrome
   i. Hair changes
      (1) Alopecia: may be seen in hyperthyroidism, hypothyroidism, and hypopituitarism
      (2) Coarse hair: frequently seen in hypothyroidism
      (3) Thin, silky hair: frequently seen in hyperthyroidism
      (4) Increased body or facial hair: may be seen in acromegaly or Cushing's disease
   j. Brittle nails: frequently seen in hypothyroidism
   k. Enlargement and protrusion of tongue: may be seen in hypothyroidism or acromegaly
5. Cardiovascular
   a. Point of maximal impulse displacement: may indicate cardiomegaly, which may be seen in hypothyroidism
   b. Heave: may be associated with heart failure (HF), which may be seen in hyperthyroidism
   c. Peripheral pulses: increased or decreased quality
6. Pulmonary
   a. Odor of breath: acetone (fruity) breath noted in DKA
   b. Respiratory rate, depth, and rhythm
7. Neurologic
   a. Level of consciousness or mental status changes: may be related to intracranial mass (e.g., pituitary tumor) or cerebral edema or dehydration (e.g., antidiuretic hormone [ADH] disorders)
   b. Pupil size, shape, and reactivity: changes may be related to intracranial mass (e.g., pituitary tumor) or cerebral edema
   c. Motor tone and strength
   d. Sensation
   e. Tremors
8. GI: abdominal mass or organ enlargement
9. GU: suprarenal mass may indicate adrenal tumor (e.g., pheochromocytoma)

Percussion

1. Neurologic: changes in deep tendon reflexes (increased or decreased) may be related to serum sodium changes seen in DI or SIADH

Auscultation

1. Head and neck: thyroid gland bruits
2. Cardiovascular: heart sound changes
   a. S_3: indicative of HF, which may be seen in patients with hyperthyroidism
   b. Systolic murmur: frequently heard in high cardiac output states (e.g., hyperthyroidism)
3. Pulmonary
   a. Crackles noted with fluid overload and pulmonary edema
   b. Stridor noted in hypocalcemia associated with hypoparathyroidism
4. GI: bowel sounds changes (hyperactive or hypoactive)

Diagnostic Studies

1. Serum
   a. Chemistry
      (1) Sodium: normal 136 to 145 mEq/L
      (2) Potassium: normal 3.5 to 5.5 mEq/L
      (3) Chloride: normal 96 to 106 mEq/L

(4) Calcium: normal 8.5 to 10.5 mg/dL
(5) Phosphorus: normal 3 to 4.5 mg/dL
(6) Magnesium: normal 1.5 to 2.2 mEq/L
(7) Glucose: normal 70 to 110 mg/dL
(8) Glycosylated hemoglobin: 4% to 7%
(9) Osmolality: normal 280 to 295 mOsm/kg
(10) Blood urea nitrogen (BUN): normal 5 to 20 mg/dL
(11) Creatinine: normal 0.7 to 1.5 mg/dL
(12) Ketones: negative

b. Hormone levels
(1) Thyroid-stimulating hormone: normal 2 to 10 milliunits/mL
(2) Triiodothyronine (T_3): normal 0.2 to 0.3 mcg/dL
(3) Thyroxine (T_4): normal 6 to 12 mcg/dL
(4) Adrenocorticotropic hormone: normal 15 to 100 pg/mL in the morning, less than 50 pg/mL in the evening
(5) Cortisol: normal 6 to 28 mcg/dL at 8 AM; 2 to 12 mcg/dL at 4 PM
(6) ADH: normal 1 to 5 pg/mL
(7) Provocation tests: these tests assess the ability of the endocrine gland to respond to stimulus
(a) Assess the reserve capacity of the endocrine gland
(b) Confirm hypofunction or hyperfunction of the endocrine gland

c. Arterial blood gases (ABGs)
(1) pH: normal 7.35 to 7.45
(2) $Paco_2$: normal 35 to 45 mm Hg
(3) Bicarbonate: normal 22 to 26 mEq/L
(4) Pao_2: normal 80 to 100 mm Hg

d. Hematology
(1) Hematocrit: normal 40% to 52% for males; 35% to 47% for females
(2) Hemoglobin: normal 13 to 18 g/dL for males; 12 to 16 g/dL for females
(3) White blood cell (WBC) count: 3500 to 11,000 cells/mm^3

2. Urine
a. Glucose: normal negative
b. Ketones: normal negative
c. Specific gravity: 1.005 to 1.03
d. Osmolality: 50 to 1200 mOsm/kg
e. 17-hydroxycorticosteroids: normal 4.5 to 10 mg per 24 hours for males; 2.5 to 10 mg per 24 hours for females
f. 17-ketosteroids: normal 8 to 15 mg per 24 hours for males; 6 to 12 mg per 24 hours for females

3. Radiologic studies
a. Skull series
b. Chest x-ray
c. Flat plate of abdomen (KUB [kidney-ureter-bladder])
d. Computed tomography scan of head or abdomen
e. Magnetic resonance imaging
f. Pancreatic scan
g. Thyroid scan
h. Thyroid ultrasound
i. Fine-needle aspiration biopsy of thyroid gland
j. Adrenal angiography
k. Brain scan

4. Other studies
a. Electrocardiogram (ECG)
b. Electroencephalogram

Diabetes Insipidus

Definition

Clinical condition characterized by impaired renal conservation of water, resulting in polyuria, low urine specific gravity, dehydration, and hypernatremia; caused by deficiency of ADH or decreased renal responsiveness to ADH

Etiology

1. Neurogenic (or central) DI: defect in synthesis or release of ADH resulting from a defect in the hypothalamus, pituitary stalk, or posterior pituitary gland
a. Primary: familiar, congenital, idiopathic
b. Secondary
(1) Intracranial tumors: especially hypothalamic or pituitary; may be primary or metastatic tumor
(2) Extracranial neoplasm: leukemia; breast cancer
(3) Central nervous system (CNS) trauma: especially basal skull fracture
(4) Craniotomy
(a) Transient: edema after craniotomy causes obstruction of stalk between hypothalamus and posterior pituitary gland
(b) Permanent: hypophysectomy requires lifelong replacement of ADH
(5) Intracerebral aneurysm, hemorrhage
(6) CNS infections (e.g., meningitis or encephalitis)
(7) Radiation
(8) Cerebral hypoxia and/or anoxic brain syndrome
(9) Granulomatous diseases (e.g., sarcoidosis or tuberculosis)
(10) Drugs that inhibit the secretion of ADH (Box 9-1)
(a) Ethanol
(b) Phenytoin (Dilantin)
(c) Chlorpromazine (Thorazine)
(d) Reserpine (Serpasil)

2. Nephrogenic DI: defect in renal tubular response to ADH; usually less severe than neurogenic DI
a. Congenital
b. Renal disease
(1) Renal insufficiency
(2) Pyelonephritis
(3) Renal transplant
(4) Polycystic kidneys
(5) Metabolic diseases affecting the kidneys
(a) Amyloidosis
(b) Sarcoidosis
(c) Multiple myeloma

BOX 9-1 Drugs Affecting the Action of Antidiuretic Hormone

Drugs That Decrease the Amount or Effect of Antidiuretic Hormone (May Cause Diabetes Insipidus)
- Alpha-adrenergic agents (e.g., norepinephrine)
- Amphotericin B
- Caffeine
- Chlorpromazine (Thorazine)
- Demeclocycline (Declomycin), a tetracycline derivative
- Ethanol
- Lithium
- Phenytoin (Dilantin)
- Reserpine (Serpasil)

Drugs That Increase the Amount or Effect of Antidiuretic Hormone (Some May Be Used to Treat Diabetes Insipidus)
- Acetaminophen
- Anticonvulsants: carbamazepine (Tegretol)
- Antihyperlipidemics: clofibrate (Atromid-S)
- Barbiturates
- Beta-adrenergic agents (e.g., isoproterenol)
- Cytotoxic agents: vincristine (Oncovin); cyclophosphamide (Cytoxan)
- General anesthetics
- Narcotics: morphine, meperidine
- Nicotine
- Oral hypoglycemics: chlorpropamide (Diabinese)
- Thiazide diuretics: hydrochlorothiazide (HydroDIURIL)
- Tricyclic antidepressants: amitriptyline (Elavil)

c. Drugs that block the effect of ADH on the renal tubules (Box 9-1)
(1) Lithium
(2) Demeclocycline (Declomycin), a tetracycline derivative
(3) Alpha-adrenergic agents (e.g., norepinephrine)
(4) Caffeine
(5) Amphotericin B
(6) Colchicine
(7) Vinblastine
d. Result of electrolyte imbalance
(1) Severe hypokalemia
(2) Hypercalcemia
3. Psychogenic DI
a. Caused by psychiatric disturbances with psychogenic polydipsia
b. Also referred to as *compulsive water drinking*
4. Dipsogenic DI: caused by an abnormality in the CNS thirst mechanism

Pathophysiology (Figure 9-4)
1. Deficiency of ADH or inadequate renal tubule response to ADH leading to inadequate antidiuresis
2. Diuresis of large volumes of hypotonic urine
3. Dehydration and hypernatremia
4. Potential shock and/or neurologic effects
5. Permanent versus temporary
a. Permanent DI follows hypophysectomy (removal of pituitary gland)
b. Temporary DI usually resolves within 3 to 5 days but may last up to 8 days

Clinical Presentation
1. History of precipitating event: usually occurs within 24 hours of precipitating event, but clinical indications may not occur for 1 to 3 days because of use of stored ADH
2. Subjective
a. Thirst, especially for cold liquids
b. Fatigue, weakness
3. Objective
a. Polyuria: 5 to 15 L per 24 hours; suspect DI if urine output is greater than 200 mL/hr for 2 hours consecutively
b. Clinical indications of dehydration and volume depletion
(1) Weight loss
(2) Poor skin turgor
(3) Dry mucous membranes
(4) Sunken eyeballs
(5) Postural hypotension, tachycardia
(6) Decrease in central venous pressure (CVP), right atrial pressure (RAP), and/or pulmonary artery occlusive pressure (PAOP)
c. Neurologic signs resulting from hyperosmolality and hypernatremia
(1) Restlessness, confusion; irritability
(2) Seizures
(3) Lethargy, coma
4. Diagnostic
a. Serum
(1) Sodium: elevated, greater than 145 mEq/L (hyperosmolar hypernatremia caused by water loss)
(2) BUN: elevated
(3) Increased serum osmolality: elevated, greater than 295 mOsm/kg
(4) Hematocrit: elevated
(5) Serum ADH level: decreased (less than 1 pg/mL)
b. Urine
(1) Specific gravity: decreased; less than 1.005
(2) Osmolality: less than serum osmolality; less than 200 mOsm/kg
c. Water deprivation test may be performed (NOTE: Because of the risks of dehydration, this test usually is not performed on a critically ill patient.)
(1) Prestudy weight, serum and urine osmolality, and urine specific gravity are measured.
(2) Fluid intake is withheld.
(3) Measurements are repeated hourly until one of the following occurs:
(a) Negative results: urine specific gravity exceeds 1.020 and urine osmolality exceeds 800 mOsm/kg
(b) Positive results: 5% of body weight is lost, or urine specific gravity does not increase after 3 hours consecutively
(4) Discontinue if hypotension, tachycardia, or lethargy occurs.

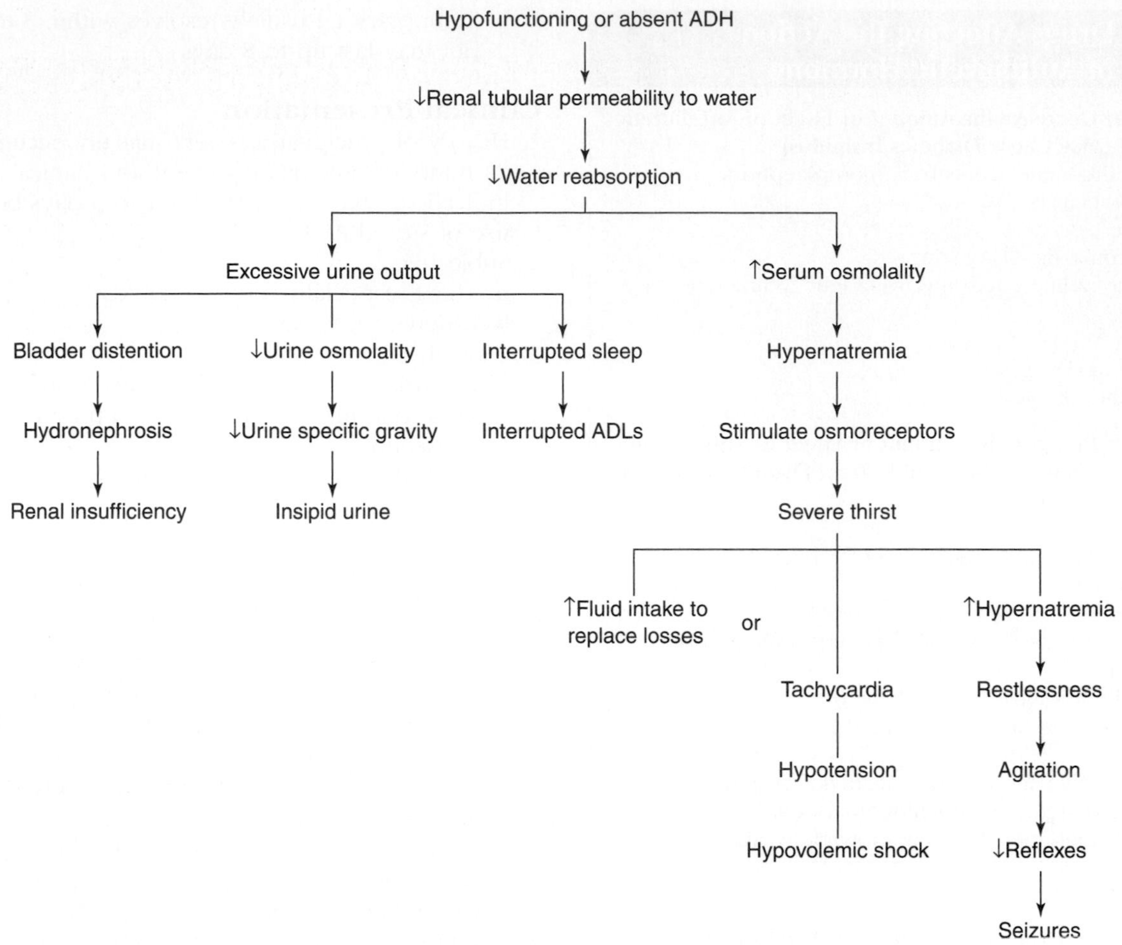

Figure 9-4 Pathophysiology of DI. *ADH*, Antidiuretic hormone; *ADL*, activities of daily living. (From Urden, L. D., Stacy, K. M., & Lough, M. E. [2006]. *Thelan's critical care nursing: Diagnosis and management* [5th ed.]. St. Louis: Mosby.)

(5) Inability to concentrate urine when fluid deprived suggests DI, and a vasopressin test should be performed.

d. Vasopressin test
   (1) Exogenous ADH (usually 5 units of aqueous vasopressin) is administered subcutaneously; urine specimens are collected every 30 minutes for 2 hours and are evaluated for quantity and osmolality.
      (a) If neurogenic DI: urine output decreases and urine osmolality increased by more than 9%
      (b) If nephrogenic DI: no response to ADH will be seen

Nursing Diagnoses

1. Deficient Fluid Volume related to diuresis caused by ADH deficiency or decreased effect of ADH on renal tubule
2. Decreased Cardiac Output related to decreased preload
3. Risk for Injury related to altered consciousness and electrolyte imbalance
4. Ineffective Individual Coping related to situational crisis, powerlessness, and change in role
5. Ineffective Family Coping related to critically ill family member
6. Deficient Knowledge related to health maintenance

Collaborative Management

1. Detect clinical indications of DI in high-risk patients.
   a. Monitor urine output hourly; measure urine specific gravity if indicated by increase in urine output.
   b. Monitor weight daily and estimate fluid loss (1 kg = 1 L).
   c. Monitor serum sodium levels.
   d. Note or calculate serum osmolality.
   e. Monitor patient for clinical indications of hypovolemia and hypoperfusion.
2. Correct fluid deficit.
   a. Type of volume replacement
      (1) Normal saline until intravascular volume is replaced (even if the patient is hypernatremic)
      (2) Hypotonic solutions such as 0.45% sodium chloride solution or 5% dextrose in water depending on degree of hyperosmolality once intravascular volume is restored
   b. Rate of volume replacement

Table 9-2 Antidiuretic Hormone Replacement

Drug	Route	Comments
SYNTHETIC ANTIDIURETIC HORMONE		
Aqueous vasopressin (Pitressin)	• IV, IM, subcutaneously: 1-10 units 2, 3, or 4 times per day • IV infusion: 2.5 units/hr	• Short duration (4-6 hours)
Vasopressin tannate (Pitressin tannate in oil)	• IM or subcutaneously: 1.25-5 units every 24-72 hours	• Never administer IV • Long duration (24 to 72 hours) • Contraindicated in patients with allergy to peanuts or peanut oil
ANTIDIURETIC HORMONE ANALOGS		
Desmopressin (DDAVP [1,deamino-8-D-arginine vasopressin])	• Nasal: 10-60 mcg every 8-24 hours (one to four sprays when 0.1 mg/mL) • IV, IM, or subcutaneously: 2-4 mcg twice per day • Oral: 100 to 300 mcg 2-3 times per day	• Relatively long duration (8-24 hours) with few side effects • May cause nasal congestion if given intranasally • Administer IV DDAVP via central vein catheter
Lysine vasopressin (Diapid)	• Nasal: 1-2 sprays per nostril 2 to 4 times per day	• Shorter duration (4-6 hours) than DDAVP

IV, Intravenous.

(1) Half of free-water deficit is replaced over the first 24 hours, with the remaining deficit being replaced over the next 48 hours.
(2) Hourly rate initially may be determined by volume of urine output and insensible losses (e.g., hourly urine output plus 50 mL/hr).
c. Close monitoring for electrolyte losses and replace accordingly
3. Treat the cause.
a. Administer exogenous ADH replacement as prescribed for neurogenic DI (Table 9-2).
(1) Side effects to monitor for: hypertension; chest pain; water intoxication; abdominal cramping
b. Assist in preoperative preparation and postoperative management after hypophysectomy if pituitary tumor is the cause; removal usually is done by transsphenoidal approach (Figure 7-40).
(1) Incision is made in the gingiva above the maxilla, and then pituitary gland is removed through the sphenoid.
(2) Antibiotic-impregnated nasal packing usually is maintained for 48 to 72 hours.
(3) Cerebrospinal fluid (CSF) leak may be seen during first 72 hours; mustache dressing is used to collect CSF.
c. Administer ADH potentiator as prescribed for nephrogenic DI (see Box 9-1).
(1) Chlorpropamide (Diabinese) is used most often.
(a) Stimulates the release of ADH from the pituitary gland and enhances its effect at the renal tubule
(b) Monitor for clinical indications of hypoglycemia
(2) Thiazide diuretics (e.g., hydrochlorothiazide) and sodium restriction also may be used.
(a) Causes mild sodium depletion, which enhances water reabsorption
(b) May be combined with indomethacin (Indocin) or amiloride (Midamor)
d. Administer pharmacologic agents as prescribed for obsessive-compulsive behavior (e.g., serotonin reuptake inhibitors, tricyclic antidepressants, or monoamine oxidase inhibitors) for psychogenic polydipsia.
4. Correct electrolyte imbalance: potassium replacement usually is required.
5. Maintain patient safety.
a. Safe environment: side rails up; call light within reach
b. Seizure precautions
c. Frequent reorientation
6. Monitor patient for complications.
a. Coma
b. Hypovolemic shock
c. Thromboembolism

Diabetic Ketoacidosis

Definitions

1. DM: a group of metabolic diseases characterized by hyperglycemia (confirmed fasting serum glucose of greater than or equal to 126 mg/dL) that results from defects in insulin secretion, insulin action, or both
a. Type 1 diabetes is characterized by beta cell destruction, usually leading to absolute insulin deficiency; previously known as *juvenile-onset, type I, insulin-dependent DM.*
b. Type 2 diabetes is a characterized by insulin resistance and a relative (rather than absolute)

insulin deficiency; previously known as *adult-onset, type II, non–insulin-dependent DM.*
2. Hyperglycemic crises
   a. DKA: hyperglycemic crisis associated with metabolic acidosis and elevated serum ketones; the most serious metabolic disturbance of type 1 DM
   b. HHNK condition: hyperglycemic crisis associated with the absence of ketone formation; most serious metabolic disturbance in type 2 DM

Etiology

1. Undiagnosed type 1 DM: 20% of patients with DKA
2. Causes in known type 1 DM
   a. Illness or infection
   b. Causes of exogenous insulin
   c. Trauma
   d. Surgery
   e. Noncompliance: too many calories
3. Causes in patients with or without diabetes
   a. Cushing's syndrome
   b. Hyperthyroidism
   c. Pancreatitis
   d. Pregnancy
   e. Drugs
      (1) Glucocorticoids (e.g., prednisone)
      (2) Thiazide diuretics (e.g., hydrochlorothiazide)
      (3) Phenytoin (Dilantin)
      (4) Sympathomimetics (e.g., epinephrine)
      (5) Diazoxide (Hyperstat)

Pathophysiology (Figure 9-5)

1. Insulin production is insufficient or the cells cannot use insulin.
2. Without insulin, glucose cannot move into the cell and it accumulates in the blood, causing hyperglycemia.
3. Hyperglycemia causes an osmotic diuresis because the hypertonic solution goes through the renal tubules and pulls more water into the tubule; this

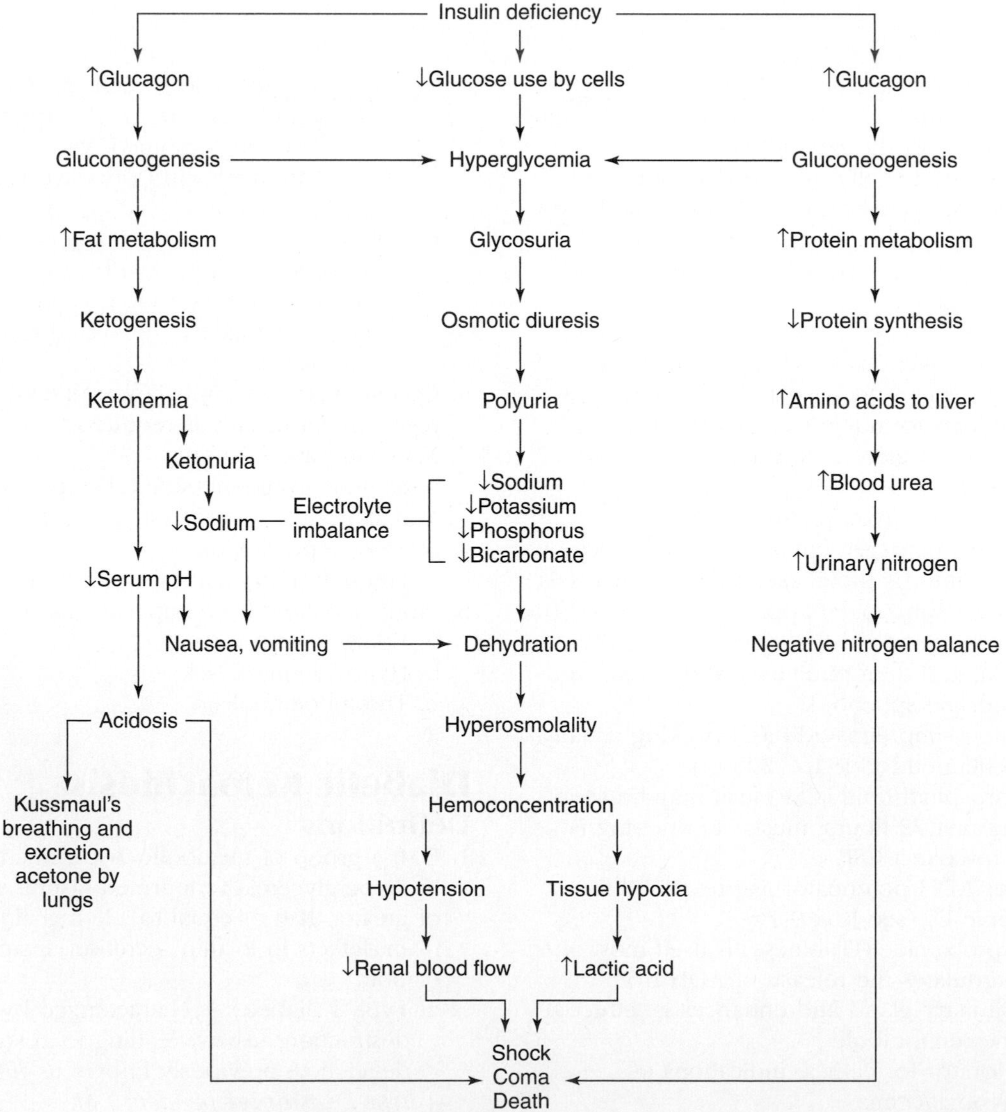

Figure 9-5 Pathophysiology of DKA. (From Urden, L. D., Stacy, K. M., & Lough, M. E. [2006]. *Thelan's critical care nursing: Diagnosis and management* [5th ed.]. St. Louis: Mosby.)

causes glycosuria, dehydration, and electrolyte imbalance.
4. Breakdown of glycogen is activated and its synthesis is inhibited; gluconeogenesis is stimulated to make new glucose from proteins and fats.
5. Impaired glucose uptake by adipose tissue causes impaired triglyceride synthesis and liberation of free fatty acids into blood.
6. Excessive fatty acids enter liver, leading to ketoacidosis.

Clinical Presentation

1. Subjective
   a. Nausea
   b. Abdominal pain
   c. Polyphagia initially; may progress to anorexia with acidosis
   d. Weakness, fatigue
   e. Polydipsia
   f. Weight loss
   g. Headache
   h. Visual disturbances
2. Objective
   a. General
      (1) Flushed, warm, dry skin
      (2) Poor skin turgor
      (3) Sunken eyeballs
      (4) Hypothermia or hyperthermia
   b. Cardiovascular
      (1) Tachycardia
      (2) Pulse may have decreased quality: 1+/3+
      (3) Orthostatic hypotension
      (4) Decreased CVP, pulmonary artery pressure, PAOP, or CO
   c. Pulmonary
      (1) Kussmaul's ventilatory pattern
      (2) Acetone (fruity) odor to breath
   d. Neurologic
      (1) Diminished deep tendon reflexes
      (2) Lethargy progressing to coma
   e. GI
      (1) Vomiting
      (2) Hypoactive bowel sounds
   f. Renal
      (1) Polyuria early
      (2) Oliguria late
3. Diagnostics
   a. Laboratory
      (1) Serum
         (a) Glucose: elevated 300 to 800 mg/dL; average 600 mg/dL
         (b) Sodium: normal, elevated, or decreased depending on hydration status
         (c) Potassium
            (i) Elevated initially
            (ii) Decreased to normal or low as pH and dehydration are corrected
            (iii) Total body potassium is low
         (d) Anion gap: elevated; greater than 15
         (e) Calcium: may be decreased
         (f) Phosphorus: normal initially but decreases with treatment with insulin and fluids
         (g) Magnesium: elevated initially and then decreased
         (h) Ketones: elevated; greater than 3 mOsm/kg
         (i) BUN elevated with BUN/creatinine ratio greater than 10:1
         (j) Serum osmolality: elevated; usually 295 to 330 mOsm/kg
         (k) Lipids: may be elevated
         (l) ABGs: metabolic acidosis frequently with some degree of respiratory compensation
            (i) pH less than 7.30
            (ii) Bicarbonate less than 15 mEq/L
            (iii) $Paco_2$ less than 35 mm Hg
         (m) Hematocrit: elevated
         (n) WBC count: elevated; unreliable indication of infection in DKA
      (2) Urine: positive for glucose and ketones
   b. ECG
      (1) May show changes associated with potassium levels
      (2) Sinus tachycardia frequently is seen

Nursing Diagnoses

1. Decreased Cardiac Output related to decreased preload and dysrhythmias caused by electrolyte imbalances
2. Deficient Fluid Volume related to osmotic diuresis, vomiting, and inadequate oral intake
3. Imbalanced Nutrition: Less Than Body Requirements related to relative deficiency of insulin
4. Ineffective Airway Clearance related to altered consciousness
5. Risk for Infection related to hyperglycemia and immunocompromise
6. Risk for Injury related to alteration in consciousness and electrolyte imbalance
7. Ineffective Individual Coping related to situational crisis, powerlessness, and change in role
8. Ineffective Family Coping related to critically ill family member
9. Deficient knowledge related to health maintenance

Collaborative Management

1. Identify and treat cause.
   a. Assess for source of infection: obtain cultures; administer antibiotics as prescribed.
   b. Assess knowledge level related to self-care; be alert to possible drug therapy errors, noncompliance with diet, and drug interactions.
2. Correct fluid volume deficit.
   a. Monitor patient for clinical and laboratory indications of dehydration, hypovolemia, and hypoperfusion.
   b. Establish intravenous (IV) access with at least one large-gauge catheter.
   c. Administer appropriate IV solution.

(1) Normal saline for the first 1 to 2 L or until the patient is hemodynamically stable; then normal (0.9%) saline if serum sodium is normal or if serum osmolality is less than 320 mOsm/kg; half-normal (0.45%) saline if patient is hypernatremic or serum osmolality is greater than 320 mOsm/kg
(2) Colloids such as albumin or plasma protein fraction may be used, especially if the patient is hypotensive
(3) Dextrose 5% is added (e.g., 5% dextrose in normal saline or 5% dextrose in one-half normal saline) when serum glucose reaches 250 to 300 mg/dL
(4) Dextrose 10% may be used if serum glucose falls to 150 mg/dL or less

d. Administer IV fluid replacement at appropriate rate.
(1) First hour: 10 to 30 mL/kg
(2) After first hour: 500 to 1000 mL/hr depending on cardiovascular status, volume deficit, and urine output
(3) Total volume deficit: usually 4 to 8 L

3. Normalize serum glucose level gradually.
a. Monitor serum glucose every hour initially.
(1) Goal of insulin therapy is to decrease serum glucose by 50 to 100 mg/dL each hour.
(2) Rapid correction of serum glucose is associated with hypoglycemia, hypokalemia, and cerebral edema.

b. Administer regular insulin IV injection as prescribed: usually 10 to 20 units (or 0.15 unit/kg) followed by infusion.

c. Initiate regular insulin IV infusion as prescribed: usually 5 to 10 units/hr (or 0.1 unit/kg/hr)
(1) Insulin is mixed in normal saline and the IV tubing is flushed with 50 mL of insulin solution to saturate binding sites on the tubing before administration.
(2) Insulin infusion usually is decreased to 3 to 5 units/hr when serum glucose is less than 250 mg/dL and usually is discontinued 1 to 2 hours after subcutaneous insulin is started.

d. Administer subcutaneous regular insulin as prescribed: usually administered by sliding scale when serum glucose is less than 250 mg/dL; pH is greater than 7.2; and bicarbonate is greater than 18 mEq/L.

4. Correct electrolyte imbalance.
a. Monitor for clinical, laboratory, and ECG indications of hyperkalemia (initially) and hypokalemia, hypophosphatemia, and hypomagnesemia (with insulin therapy).

b. Replace potassium as prescribed.
(1) Potassium levels are monitored every 1 to 2 hours initially.
(2) Usually total body potassium is severely depleted, but serum levels show normal level or hyperkalemia because of an intracellular-to-extracellular shift caused by acidosis.
(3) Potassium replacement is started when potassium level is at upper limit of normal; usually in the form of potassium chloride (KCl), but a portion may be given in form of potassium phosphate (KPO_4) depending on phosphorus levels.
(4) Refractory hypokalemia suggests hypocalcemia and/or hypomagnesemia.

c. Replace phosphorus as prescribed.
(1) Frequently low, especially with insulin therapy; replacement is indicated especially if patient is anemic; has HF, pneumonia, or any other cause of hypoxia (remember that hypophosphatemia shifts the oxyhemoglobin curve to the left and impairs tissue oxygenation); or if serum phosphate level is less than 1 mg/dL
(2) Two thirds to one half of potassium is replaced with potassium chloride and one third to one half of potassium is replaced with potassium phosphate
(3) To prevent hypocalcemia, phosphate administration should not exceed 1.5 mEq/kg per 24 hours

d. Replace magnesium as prescribed.
(1) Frequently low
(2) Usually replaced as 1 to 2 g of 10% solution if renal function adequate

5. Correct acid-base imbalance.
a. Provide adequate rehydration and insulin therapy.
b. Administer sodium bicarbonate as prescribed. NOTE: Sodium bicarbonate is only recommended today for severe acidosis (pH 7.0 or less) and should be discontinued as soon as pH is 7.20.
c. Monitor for hyperchloremic acidosis caused by sodium chloride and potassium chloride administration.

6. Ensure patient safety.
a. Prevent aspiration caused by paralytic ileus commonly seen in DKA.
(1) Keep head of bed elevated 30 degrees.
(2) Insert nasogastric tube as indicated.
b. Maintain seizure precautions.
c. Monitor serum glucose and electrolytes carefully.

7. Monitor patient for complications.
a. Cardiovascular
(1) Hypovolemic shock
(2) Dysrhythmias
(3) Thromboembolism
(4) Myocardial infarction
(5) Pulmonary edema
b. Neurologic
(1) Cerebral edema
(2) Seizures
(3) Coma
c. Pulmonary
(1) Acute respiratory distress syndrome (ARDS)
(2) Pulmonary embolism
d. Endocrine: hypoglycemia
e. Renal
(1) Acute renal failure

(2) Electrolyte imbalances: potassium; sodium; phosphorus; magnesium

f. Sepsis

8. Provide instruction and counseling regarding lifestyle modification and need for pharmacologic therapy.
   a. Nonpharmacologic therapies
      (1) Monitoring and normalization of body weight
      (2) Dietary modifications
         (a) Low saturated fat
         (b) American Diabetic Association (ADA) diet for control of serum glucose
      (3) Cessation of tobacco use
      (4) Avoidance of alcohol
      (5) Regular aerobic exercise in moderation
      (6) Complementary therapies: relaxation; imagery, biofeedback
      (7) Stress reduction
      (8) Yearly flu and pneumococcal vaccine
      (9) Recognition of symptoms of hyperglycemia and hypoglycemia and when to call the physician
      (10) Measurement of body weight
   b. Pharmacologic agents
      (1) Insulin therapy including sick day management
      (2) Control of hypertension, hyperlipidemia, and thyroid disorders

Hyperglycemic Hyperosmolar Nonketotic Syndrome

Definition

Hyperglycemic crisis associated with the absence of ketone formation; most common severe metabolic disturbance in type 2 DM

Etiology

Usually seen in patients over 50 years with glucose intolerance or type 2 DM; frequently iatrogenic

1. Noncompliance with diet or drug therapy in a patient with known type 2 DM
2. Acute illness
3. Trauma
4. Surgery
5. Infection
6. Pancreatitis
7. Burns
8. Hepatitis
9. Cushing's syndrome
10. Hyperthyroidism
11. Renal disease
    a. Peritoneal dialysis
    b. Hemodialysis
12. Hypertonic nutrition: enteral or parenteral
13. Alcohol
14. Drugs
    a. Glucocorticoids (e.g., prednisone)
    b. Thiazide diuretics (e.g., hydrochlorothiazide)
    c. Loop diuretics (e.g., furosemide [Lasix])
    d. Phenytoin (Dilantin)
    e. Diazoxide (Hyperstat)
    f. Immunosuppressive drugs
    g. Beta-blockers (e.g., propranolol [Inderal])
    h. Chlorpromazine (Thorazine)
    i. Cimetidine (Tagamet)
    j. Calcium channel blockers
    k. Mannitol
    l. Sympathomimetic drug (e.g., epinephrine)
    m. Thyroid preparations

Pathophysiology (Figure 9-6)

1. Relative insulin deficiency occurs.
2. Without insulin, glucose cannot move into the cell and accumulates in the blood, causing hyperglycemia; hyperglycemia is severe.
3. Hyperglycemia causes an osmotic diuresis as the hypertonic solution goes through the renal tubules

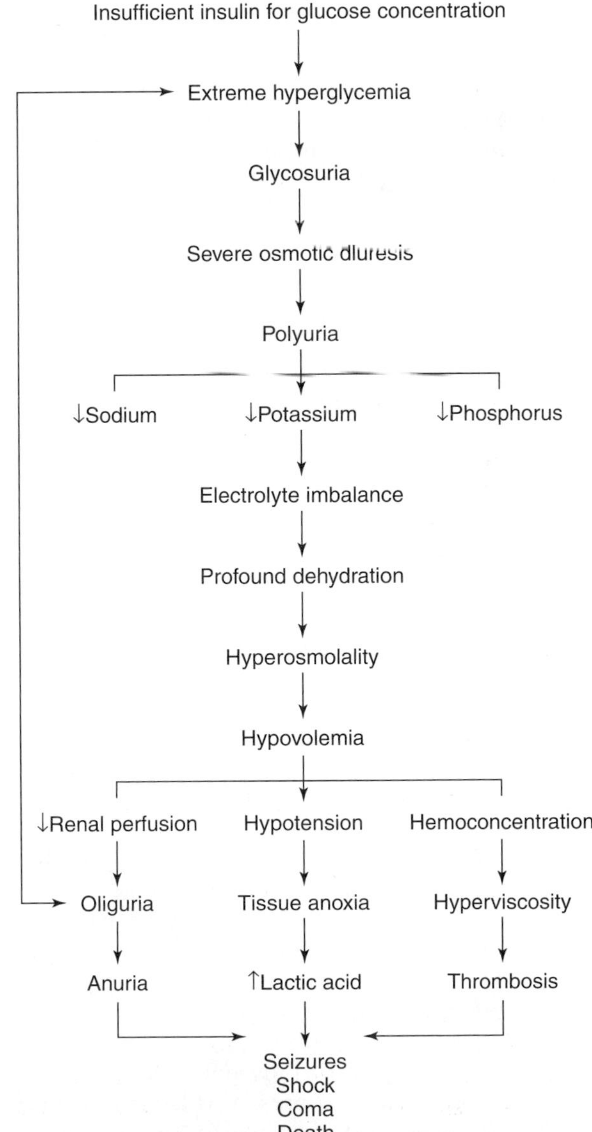

Figure 9-6 Pathophysiology of HHNK syndrome. (From Urden, L. D., Stacy, K. M., & Lough, M. E. [2006]. *Thelan's critical care nursing: Diagnosis and management* [5th ed.]. St. Louis: Mosby.)

and pulls more water into the tubule; this causes glycosuria, dehydration, and electrolyte imbalance.
4. Sufficient insulin is present to inhibit gluconeogenesis; therefore, breakdown of fat and protein with resultant ketoacidosis and muscle wasting does not occur.
5. Osmotic diuresis causes serum hyperosmolality, cellular dehydration, and decreased glomerular filtration rate.
6. Thrombosis, renal failure, and neurologic changes may result.

Clinical Presentation

1. Subjective: weakness, fatigue
2. Objective
   a. General
      (1) Weight loss
      (2) Flushed, warm, dry skin
      (3) Poor skin turgor
      (4) Polydipsia
      (5) Fever common
   b. Cardiovascular
      (1) Tachycardia
      (2) Orthostatic hypotension
      (3) Decreased CVP, RAP, PAOP, and CO/cardiac index
   c. Pulmonary: tachypnea
   d. Neurologic
      (1) Sensory deficits: paresthesia
      (2) Motor deficits: paresis, plegia
      (3) Aphasia
      (4) Decreased deep tendon reflexes
      (5) Seizures
      (6) Lethargy progressing to coma
   e. Rena
      (1) Polyuria early
      (2) Oliguria late
3. Diagnostics
   a. Serum
      (1) Glucose 600 to 2000 mg/dL; average 1100 mg/dL
      (2) Sodium: normal or elevated
      (3) Potassium: decreased
      (4) Calcium: may be decreased
      (5) Phosphorus: decreased
      (6) Magnesium: decreased
      (7) Ketones: normal or only mildly elevated
      (8) BUN and creatinine: elevated with BUN/creatinine ratio greater than 10:1
      (9) Serum osmolality: elevated; usually greater than 330 mOsm/kg; may be as high as 450 mOsm/kg
      (10) ABGs
         (a) Normal pH or only mildly acidotic
            (i) Acidosis if present is lactic acidosis related to hypoperfusion instead of ketoacidosis
      (11) Hematocrit: elevated
      (12) WBC count: elevated
   b. Urine
      (1) Glucose: positive
      (2) Ketones: negative or trace
   c. ECG
      (1) May show changes associated with potassium levels
      (2) May show sinus tachycardia

Nursing Diagnoses

1. Decreased Cardiac Output related to decreased preload and dysrhythmias caused by electrolyte imbalances
2. Deficient Fluid Volume related to osmotic diuresis
3. Imbalanced Nutrition: Less Than Body Requirements related to relative deficiency of insulin
4. Ineffective Airway Clearance related to altered consciousness
5. Risk for Infection related to hyperglycemia and immunocompromise
6. Risk for Injury related to alteration in consciousness and electrolyte imbalance
7. Ineffective Tissue Perfusion: Renal related to dehydration and thromboembolism
8. Ineffective Individual Coping related to situational crisis, powerlessness, and change in role
9. Ineffective Family Coping related to critically ill family member
10. Knowledge Deficit related to health maintenance

Collaborative Management

1. Identify and treat cause.
   a. Assess patient for source of infection: obtain cultures; administer antibiotics as prescribed.
   b. Monitor serum glucose in patients receiving enteral and parenteral nutrition, glucocorticoids, dialysis, and diuretics.
   c. Assess knowledge level related to self-care; be alert to possible drug therapy errors, noncompliance with diet, and drug interactions.
2. Correct fluid volume deficit.
   a. Monitor for clinical and laboratory indications of dehydration, hypovolemia, and hypoperfusion; hemodynamic monitoring is frequently necessary to guide fluid resuscitation because of the age and health of the patient.
   b. Establish IV access with at least one large-gauge catheter.
   c. Administer appropriate IV solution.
      (1) Normal saline usually is used for the first 1 to 2 L or until the patient is hemodynamically stable; then normal (0.9%) saline is used if serum sodium is normal or if serum osmolality is less than 320 mOsm/kg; half-normal (0.45%) saline is used if patient is hypernatremic or serum osmolality is greater than 320 mOsm/kg.
      (2) Colloids such as albumin or plasma protein fraction may be needed, especially if the patient is hypotensive.
      (3) Dextrose 5% is added (e.g., 5% dextrose in normal saline or 5% dextrose in one-half normal saline) when serum glucose reaches 250 to 300 mg/dL.

(4) Dextrose 10% may be used if serum glucose falls to 150 mg/dL or less.

d. Administer IV fluid replacement at appropriate rate.
   (1) First hour: 10 to 30 mL/kg
   (2) After first hour: 500 to 1000 mL/hour depending on cardiovascular status, volume deficit, and urine output
   (3) Total volume deficit: usually 8 to 15 L

3. Normalize serum glucose level gradually (NOTE: Even though HHNK causes higher serum glucose levels, smaller amounts of insulin are needed to normalize serum glucose).
   a. Monitor serum glucose every hour initially.
      (1) Goal of insulin therapy is to decrease serum glucose by 50 to 100 mg/dL each hour.
      (2) Rapid correction of serum glucose is associated with hypoglycemia, hypokalemia, and cerebral edema.
   b. Administer IV regular insulin injection as prescribed: usually 10 to 20 units (or 0.15 to 0.3 units/kg) followed by infusion.
   c. Initiate IV regular insulin infusion as prescribed: usually 5 to 10 units/hr (or 0.1 unit/kg/hr).
      (1) Insulin is mixed in normal saline, and the IV tubing is flushed with 50 mL of insulin solution to saturate binding sites on the IV tubing before administration.
   d. Administer subcutaneous regular insulin as prescribed.
      (1) Usually administered by sliding scale when serum glucose is less than 250 mg/dL; pH is greater than 7.2; and bicarbonate is greater than 18
      (2) IV insulin infusion usually discontinued when subcutaneous insulin is initiated; note that usually no overlap is required in HHNK

4. Correct electrolyte imbalance.
   a. Monitor patient for clinical, laboratory, and ECG indications of hyperkalemia (initially) and hypokalemia, hypophosphatemia, and hypomagnesemia (with insulin therapy).
   b. Replace potassium as prescribed.
      (1) Potassium levels are monitored every 1 to 2 hours initially.
      (2) Potassium levels usually are severely depleted; serum levels show severe hypokalemia because no intracellular-to-extracellular shift occurs because acidosis is not usually present.
      (3) Usually administered in the form of KCl, but a portion may be in form of KPO_4 depending on phosphorus levels.
      (4) Refractory hypokalemia suggests hypocalcemia and/or hypomagnesemia.
   c. Replace phosphorus as prescribed.
      (1) Frequently low especially with insulin therapy; replacement is indicated especially if patient is anemic; has HF, pneumonia, or any other cause of hypoxia (remember that hypophosphatemia shifts the oxyhemoglobin curve to the left and impairs tissue oxygenation); or if serum phosphate level is less than 1 mg/dL
      (2) Two thirds to one half of potassium is replaced with potassium chloride and one third to one half of potassium is replaced with potassium phosphate
      (3) To prevent hypocalcemia, potassium phosphate administration should not exceed 1.5 mEq/kg per 24 hours
   d. Replace magnesium as prescribed.
      (1) Frequently low
      (2) Usually replaced as 1 to 2 g of 10% solution if renal function adequate

5. Ensure patient safety.
   a. Prevent aspiration caused by paralytic ileus
      (1) Keep head of bed elevated 30 degrees.
      (2) Insert nasogastric tube as indicated.
   b. Maintain seizure precautions.
   c. Monitor serum glucose and electrolytes carefully.

6. Monitor patient for complications.
   a. Cardiovascular
      (1) Hypovolemic shock
      (2) Dysrhythmias
      (3) Thromboembolism
      (4) Myocardial infarction
      (5) Pulmonary edema
   b. Neurologic
      (1) Intracranial hypertension
      (2) Cerebral edema
      (3) Cerebral infarction
      (4) Coma
   c. Pulmonary
      (1) ARDS
      (2) Pulmonary embolism
   d. Endocrine: hypoglycemia (Figure 9-7)
   e. Renal
      (1) Acute renal failure
      (2) Electrolyte imbalances: potassium; sodium; phosphorus; magnesium
   f. Sepsis

7. Provide instruction and counseling regarding lifestyle modification and need for pharmacologic therapy.
   a. Nonpharmacologic therapies
      (1) Monitoring and normalization of body weight
      (2) Dietary modifications
         (a) Low saturated fat
         (b) ADA diet for control of serum glucose
      (3) Cessation of tobacco use
      (4) Avoidance of alcohol
      (5) Regular aerobic exercise in moderation
      (6) Complementary therapies: relaxation; imagery, biofeedback
      (7) Stress reduction
      (8) Yearly flu and pneumococcal vaccine
      (9) Recognition of symptoms of hyperglycemia and hypoglycemia and when to call the physician

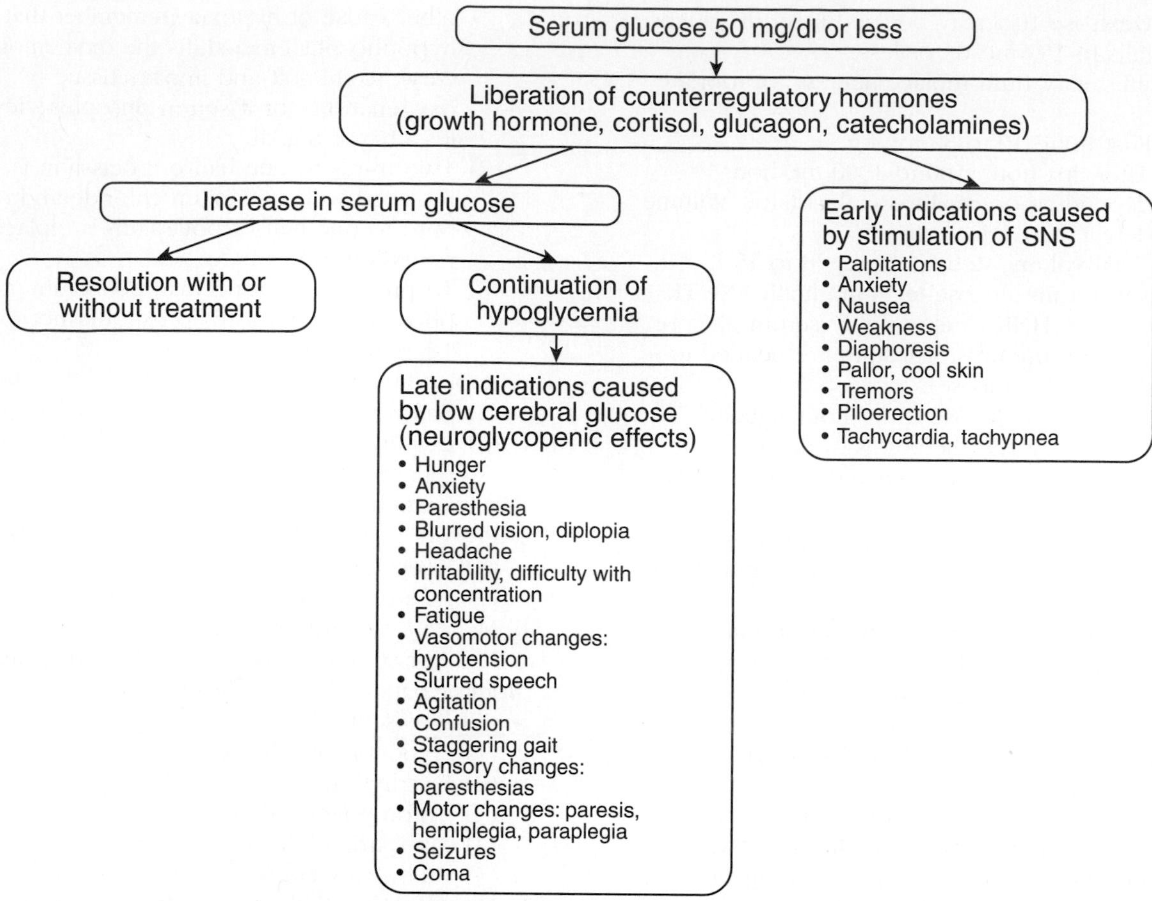

Figure 9-7 Pathophysiology of hypoglycemia. *SNS*, Sympathetic nervous system.

(10) Measurement of body weight

b. Pharmacologic agents
 (1) Insulin therapy including sick day management
 (2) Control of hypertension, hyperlipidemia, thyroid disorders

Hypoglycemia

Definition

Less than normal serum glucose level

1. Any serum glucose level of less than 70 mg/dL is hypoglycemia.
2. Symptomatic hypoglycemia generally occurs at a serum glucose level of 50 mg/dL or less, but symptoms may occur if a sudden decrease in serum glucose occurs even though the level is not less than 50 mg/dL.

Etiology

1. Insufficient nutrient intake
 a. Missed or delayed meal
 b. Nausea, vomiting
 c. Interrupted tube feedings or parenteral nutrition
2. Excessive insulin dose
 a. Poor visual acuity causing dose inaccuracy
 b. Change from pork or beef insulin to human insulin (Humulin)
 c. Injection in area of improved absorption
3. Drugs
 a. Sulfonylurea therapy
  (1) Renal insufficiency potentiates effects.
  (2) Hepatic insufficiency delays metabolism and excretion and impairs gluconeogenesis and glycogenolysis.
  (3) Potentiation occurs by salicylates, sulfonamides, phenylbutazone, alpha-glucosidase inhibitors (e.g., acarbose [Precose] and miglitol [Glyset]).
 b. Ethanol
 c. Quinidine
 d. Disopyramide
 e. Alpha-blockers
 f. Salicylates
 g. Haloperidol
 h. Trimethoprim-sulfamethoxazole
4. Inadequate production of glucose
 a. Strenuous physical exercise or stress with inadequate adjustment of food intake and/or insulin dosage
 b. Excessive alcohol intake ingested without adequate food intake
 c. Glucagon deficiency
5. After gastrectomy
6. Pancreatic islet cell necrosis: may occur with pentamidine therapy for *Pneumocystis carinii* infection; causes an acute increase in insulin release

7. Adrenal insufficiency
8. Severe liver disease
9. Pregnancy
10. Tumors
   a. Non–beta-cell tumors
      (1) Malignant: sarcoma, mesothelioma, hepatomas, lymphoma, leukemia, adrenal carcinoma
      (2) Benign: carcinoid and carcinoid-like tumors, pheochromocytoma
   b. Beta-cell tumors (i.e., insulinomas)

Pathophysiology

1. Too much insulin in relation to amount of glucose
2. Decrease in serum glucose levels to 50 mg/dL or below causes physiologic response
3. Release of counterregulatory hormones to insulin
   a. Growth hormone
   b. Cortisol
   c. Glucagon
   d. Epinephrine
      (1) SNS stimulation (NOTE: This stimulation and therefore the clinical indication may be blocked by beta-blockers.)
4. Serum glucose may increase because of glycogenolysis and gluconeogenesis triggered by the counterregulatory hormones and/or food intake
5. Serum glucose may continue to be less than normal, causing a decrease in cerebral glucose levels
   a. Neuroglycopenic effects may cause neuronal damage: the brain must have constant supply of glucose (i.e., carbohydrate) and cannot use any other substrates (e.g., protein and fat).
6. Severe neurologic injury, seizures, coma may result with severe and/or prolonged hypoglycemia

Clinical Presentation

1. Subjective
   a. Adrenergic (sympathetic) stimulation indicators
      (1) Palpitations
      (2) Anxiety
      (3) Nausea
      (4) Weakness
   b. Neuroglycopenic indicators
      (1) Hunger
      (2) Anxiety
      (3) Paresthesia
      (4) Blurred vision, diplopia
      (5) Headache
      (6) Irritability, difficulty with concentration
      (7) Fatigue
2. Objective
   a. Adrenergic (sympathetic) stimulation indicators
      (1) Diaphoresis
      (2) Pallor, cool skin
      (3) Tremors
      (4) Piloerection
      (5) Tachycardia, tachypnea
   b. Neuroglycopenic indicators
      (1) Vasomotor changes: hypotension
      (2) Slurred speech
      (3) Agitation
      (4) Confusion
      (5) Staggering gait
      (6) Sensory changes: paresthesias
      (7) Motor changes: paresis, hemiplegia, paraplegia
      (8) Seizures
      (9) Coma
   c. Nocturnal hypoglycemia
      (1) Restless sleep
      (2) Nightmares
      (3) Early morning headache
3. Diagnostic
   a. Serum glucose: 50 mg/dL or less
      (1) 20 to 40 mg/dL is associated with seizures
      (2) Less than 20 mg/dL is associated with coma
   b. ECG: sinus tachycardia is seen
   c. BUN, creatinine, liver function studies indicated
   d. Drug screen for possible drug cause may be indicated

Nursing Diagnoses

1. Risk for Injury related to alteration in consciousness and seizures
2. Risk for Decreased Adaptive Capacity: Intracranial related to neuroglycopenic effects

Collaborative Management

1. Restore normal serum glucose level.
   a. Measure serum glucose level immediately when clinical indications of hypoglycemia occur.
   b. Administer 10 to 15 g (40 to 60 calories) of carbohydrates for conscious patients; for examples, see Box 9-2.
      (1) Glucose tablets or gel is *required* if the patient has been receiving an alpha-glucosidase inhibitor (e.g., acarbose [Precose] or miglitol [Glyset]) because these agents block the conversion of carbohydrates to glucose.
   c. Administer glucose parenterally if patient is unconscious.

BOX 9-2 Foods Providing 10 to 15 g of Carbohydrates for Relief of Hypoglycemia

4 oz of apple or orange juice
4 oz of cola or other carbonated beverage
8 oz of skim or 1% milk
4 cubes or 2 packets sugar
2 oz of corn syrup, honey, or grape jelly
6 Life Savers or jelly beans
10 gumdrops
2 tablespoons raisins
½ cup regular gelatin dessert
2 to 3 squares of graham crackers
1 small (2-oz) serving of cake decorating icing
3 (5-g) glucose tablets
25 mL of 50% dextrose in water if patient is unable to take calories orally

Table 9-3 Characteristics of Insulin Preparations

Insulin	Onset	Peak	Duration
Human regular (IV)	Immediate	15-30 minutes	1-2 hours
Human lispro (subcutaneously)	15 minutes	½-1½ hours	3-5 hours
Human regular (subcutaneously)	½-1 hour	2-3 hours	5-7 hours
Human NPH (subcutaneously)	2-4 hours	4-10 hours	14-18 hours
Human Lente (subcutaneously)	3-4 hours	4-12 hours	16-20 hours
Human Ultralente (subcutaneously)	6-10 hours	14-24 hours	20-36 hours

(1) Injection of 50% dextrose in water: usually 50 mL (25 g) over 3 to 5 minutes
(a) Thiamine 100 mg IV recommended before dextrose administration especially in alcoholics to prevent Wernicke's encephalopathy
(b) Infusion of 10% dextrose in water or 5% dextrose in water to follow as prescribed
(2) Glucagon 0.5 to 1 mg intramuscularly may be given to unconscious patients if unable to gain IV access
d. Provide longer-acting carbohydrate source (milk, cheese, crackers) or regularly scheduled meal to avoid recurrence.
e. Reassess serum glucose 15 minutes after treatment and every 15 minutes until serum glucose is within normal range: an additional 50 mL of 50% dextrose in water may be required for refractory hypoglycemia.

2. Prevent injury.
a. Maintain airway if patient is unconscious.
b. Monitor closely for seizures; maintain seizure precautions.

3. Identify and treat cause of hypoglycemia.
a. Assess serum glucose by laboratory or bedside glucose monitoring device as indicated.
b. Anticipate times when the patient is most likely to exhibit hypoglycemia.
(1) Be aware of peak times for administered insulin therapy (Table 9-3).
(2) Be aware of missed or late meals or snacks that predispose the patient to hypoglycemia.
(3) Be aware of excessive exertion that may predispose the patient to hypoglycemia.
(4) Note any drugs that the patient is receiving that may potentiate insulin.
(5) Be aware (and make patient and family aware) that beta-blockers block the SNS (early) symptoms of hypoglycemia; serum glucose testing should be done more frequently in patients taking beta-blockers.
c. Assess knowledge level related to self-care; be alert to possible drug therapy errors, noncompliance with diet, and drug interactions.
d. Assist with additional diagnostic studies if hypoglycemia is experienced by a patient who is not a known diabetic.
e. Consider Somogyi phenomenon (insulin-induced posthypoglycemic hyperglycemia) as cause of early morning hyperglycemia.
(1) The result of counterregulatory hormone secretion in response to hypoglycemia
(2) Results in early morning hyperglycemia after nighttime hypoglycemia; needs to be differentiated from dawn phenomenon (hyperglycemia caused by nocturnal elevations in growth hormone)
(3) Best documented by 3 AM serum glucose
(4) Treated by a decrease in insulin dose and/or bedtime snack

4. Monitor for complications.
a. Myocardial ischemia or infarction
b. Seizures
c. Coma
d. Irreversible neurologic damage

5. Provide instruction and counseling regarding lifestyle modification and need for pharmacologic therapy.
a. Importance of not skipping meals
b. Recognition of symptoms of hyperglycemia and hypoglycemia and when to call the physician
c. Insulin and/or oral hypoglycemic agents including sick day management
d. Control of hypertension, hyperlipidemia, and thyroid disorders

LEARNING ACTIVITIES

1. **DIRECTIONS:** Complete the following crossword puzzle.

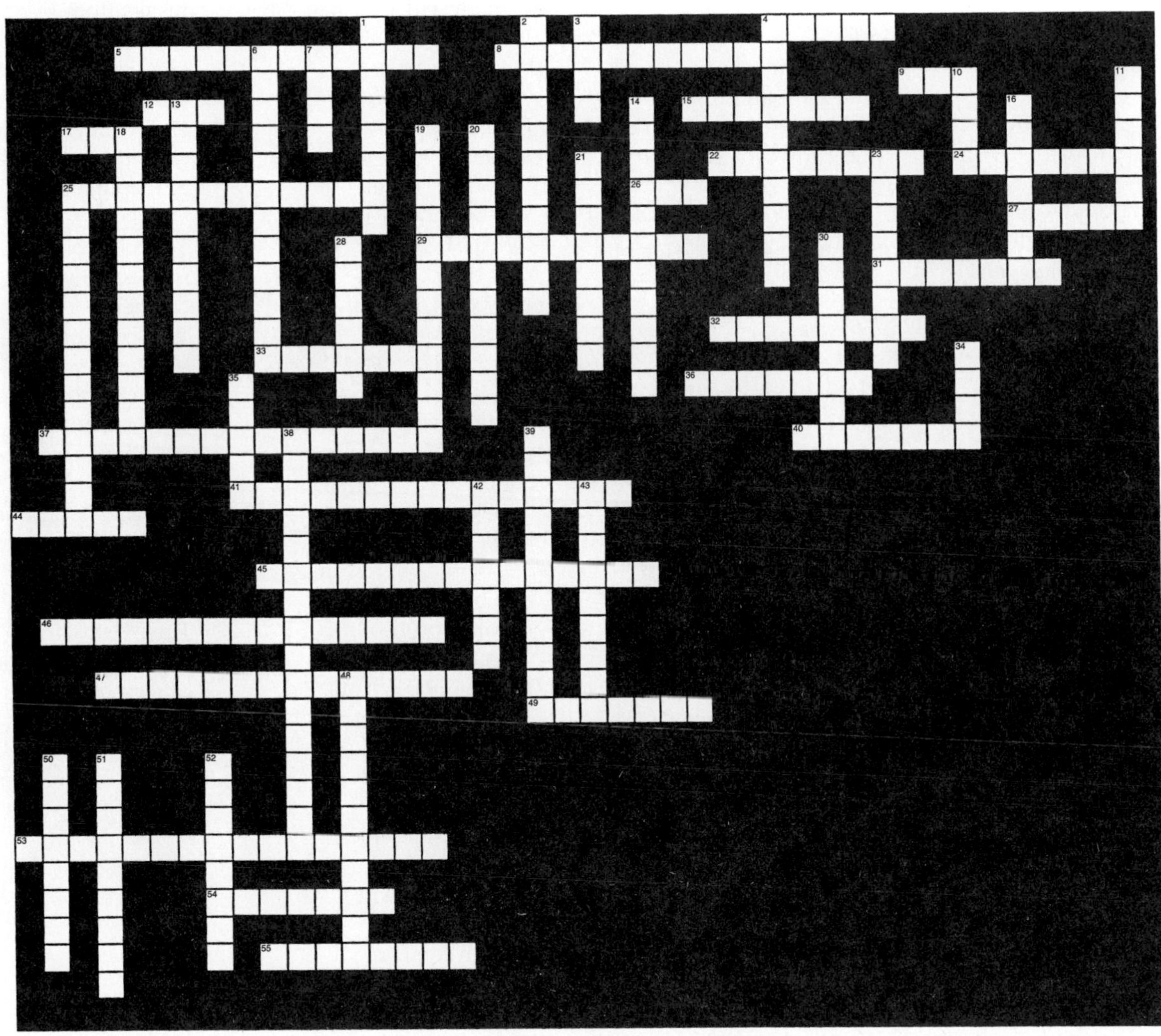

Across

4. DKA causes an increase in this "gap"
5. The treatment for hypoglycemia in a conscious patient is 10 to 15 g of ____
8. This type of DI is caused by decreased responsiveness of the renal tubule to ADH
9. This hyperglycemic crisis occurs in type 1 DM (abbreviation)
12. The initial symptoms of hypoglycemia are caused by stimulation of the ___ (abbreviation)
15. This occurs in DKA but not in HHNK syndrome
17. This hormone is produced by the hypothalamus and is stored in and released by the posterior pituitary gland (abbreviation)
22. This type of regulation controls the release or retention of hormones
24. Insulin manufactured using recombinant DNA technology (trade)
25. This electrolyte imbalance is noted in DKA caused by acidosis
26. This hormone is produced by the anterior pituitary gland and stimulates the thyroid gland (abbreviation)
27. _____'s disease is the most common cause of thyrotoxicosis
29. This electrolyte imbalance is noted as the acidosis is corrected
31. This hormone enables glucose to move into the cell
32. This hormone triggers glycogenolysis and gluconeogenesis
33. This endocrine gland is located on top of the kidney

36. This endocrine gland is located in the neck and produces hormones that control metabolic rate
37. Another term for the posterior pituitary gland
40. This area of the adrenal gland produces epinephrine and norepinephrine
41. Another term for the anterior pituitary gland
44. This form of vasopressin replacement is used nasally in patients with permanent DI (abbreviation)
45. A complication in HHNK syndrome caused by the severe dehydration
46. These hypoglycemic effects are caused by low brain glucose
47. This oral hypoglycemic agent protentiates the action of ADH on the renal tubules; may be used for nephrogenic DI (generic)
49. _____'s syndrome is caused by an excess of hormones from the adrenal cotex
53. This electrolyte imbalance occurs with insulin therapy in DKA because glucose moves into the cell and increased amounts of adenosine triphosphate are produced
54. _____'s disease is caused by a deficiency of hormones from the adrenal gland
55. Severe hypothyroidism may cause _____ coma, which results in hypothermia, hypotension, bradycardia, and coma

Down

1. This organ produces glucagon and insulin
2. This type of drug blocks the early symptoms of hypoglycemia
3. This hyperglycemic crisis occurs in type 2 DM or in patients with glucose intolerance (abbreviation)
4. This disorder is caused by excessive secretion of growth hormone in an adult
6. A serum glucose less than 50 mg/dL
7. This hyperglycemic effect is caused by nocturnal elevations of growth hormone
10. This hormone is produced by the anterior pituitary gland and causes the production and release of hormones from the adrenal cortex (abbreviation)
11. The color of the skin in a patient with Addison's disease
13. This type of DI results from a deficiency in the secretion of ADH from the posterior pituitary gland
14. This drug used for *Pneumocystis carinii* pneumonia may cause hypoglycemia (generic)
16. Hyperglycemia caused by release of counterregulatory hormones released in response to hypoglycemia
18. In DI and HHNK syndrome the serum becomes _____
19. Protruding eyeballs seen in hyperthyroidism
20. This is another name for ADH
21. This type of diabetes is caused by insulin deficiency
23. This hormone is considered a stress hormone and is produced by the adrenal cortex
25. This is most likely the result of insulin deficiency but also may be caused by stress, steroids, or insulin resistance
28. The hormones from this area of the adrenal gland can be remembered as sugar (cortisol), salt (aldosterone), and sex (androgen)
30. This is given with glucose for hypoglycemia in patients with substance abuse to prevent Wernicke's encephalopathy
34. These cells produce insulin
35. These cells produce glucagon
38. This benign tumor of the adrenal medulla causes labile hypertension
39. This type of DI results from excessive water consumption
42. This type of endocrine disorder is caused by a problem in the target gland
43. This type of diabetes is caused by ADH deficiency
48. This hormone is secreted by the adrenal cortex and causes the retention of sodium and water
50. The change in urine output that occurs in DI, DKA, and HHNK syndrome
51. This type of endocrine disorder is caused by a problem with the stimulating gland
52. _____'s respirations are seen in DKA caused by metabolic acidosis

2. **Directions:** Identify whether these factors increase or decrease the release or action of ADH.

Lithium	
Alcohol	
Chlorpropamide (Diabinese)	
Positive pressure ventilation	
Chlorpromazine (Thorazine)	
Phenytoin (Dilantin)	
Hydrochlorothiazide (HydroDIURIL)	
Anesthetic agents	
Demeclocycline (Declomycin)	
Beta stimulants	
Morphine sulfate	

3. **Directions:** Identify whether these factors are increased or decreased in DI.

	Diabetes Insipidus
Serum ADH	
Urine output	
Urine specific gravity	
Urine osmolality	
Serum osmolality	
Serum sodium	
RAP/PAOP	

4. **Directions:** A 45 year-old man was admitted to the surgical intensive care unit yesterday after a craniotomy. Today his urine output has increased dramatically over the last couple of hours. His urine output has been 600 mL over the last 2 hours, and the urine is dilute with a specific gravity of 1.004. Calculate his serum osmolality, and identify the likely cause of the following laboratory values:

Serum sodium	158 mEq/L
Serum potassium	3.8 mEq/L
Serum glucose	110 mg/dL
BUN	32 mg/dL
Serum creatinine	1 mg/dL
Hematocrit	45%
Urine osmolality	195 mOsm/kg

___

___

___

5. **Directions:** Complete this table.

	Diabetic Ketoacidosis	Hyperglycemic Hyperosmolar Nonketotic Syndrome
Age		
Type of DM		
Average serum glucose		
Presence of ketosis		
pH		
Anion gap		
Respiratory pattern		
Breath odor		
Serum osmolality		
Serum sodium		
Serum potassium		
BUN		
Average fluid deficit		

6. **Directions:** Identify the following clinical indications as DKA, HHNK, or both.

Serum glucose greater than 300 mg/dL	
Kussmaul's respirations	
pH less than 7.3	
Positive serum and urine ketones	
Abdominal pain	
Dehydration	
Lethargy → coma	
Serum glucose greater than 1000 mg/dL	

7. **DIRECTIONS:** Identify the following clinical indications as DKA, hypoglycemia, or both.

Headache	
Serum glucose greater than 300 mg/dL	
Abdominal pain	
Cold, clammy skin	
Nervousness, tremors	
Polyuria	
Lethargy → coma	
Seizures	
Glycosuria	
Tachycardia	
Agitation, difficulty with concentration	
Weakness, fatigue	
Fruity breath	
Serum glucose less than 50 mg/dL	

8. **DIRECTIONS:** Match the following endocrine conditions with appropriate pharmacologic therapy. More than one therapy may be listed for each condition.

___ 1. Neurogenic DI
___ 2. Nephrogenic DI
___ 3. DKA
___ 4. HHNK
___ 5. Hypoglycemia

a. 50% dextrose
b. Chlorpropamide (Diabinese)
c. Parenteral fluids
d. Insulin
e. Thiazide diuretics
f. Vasopressin
g. Potassium
h. Glucagon

LEARNING ACTIVITIES ANSWERS

1.

1 PANCREAS
2 BETABLOCKER
3 HHNK
4 ANION
4 ACROMEGALY
5 CARBOHYDRATE
6 HYPOGLYCEMIA
7 DAWN
8 NEPHROGENIC
9 DKA
10 ACTH
11 BRONZE
12 SNS
13 NEUROGENIC
14 PENTAMIDINE
15 KETOSIS
16 SOMOGY
17 ADH
18 HYPEROSMOLA
19 EXOPHTHALMO
20 VASOPRESSIN
21 MELLITUS
22 FEEDBACK
23 CORTISOL
24 HUMULIN
25 HYPERKALEMIA
25 HYPERGLYCEMI
26 TSH
27 GRAVE
28 CORTEX
29 HYPOKALEMIA
30 THIAMIN
31 INSULIN
32 GLUCAGON
33 ADRENAL
34 BETA
35 ALPHA
36 THYROID
37 NEUROHYPOPHYSIS
38 PHEOCHROMOCYTOMA
39 PSYCHOGENIC
40 MEDULLA
41 ADENOHYPOPHYSIS
42 PRIMARY
43 INSIPIDUS
44 DDAVP
45 THROMBOEMBOLISM
46 NEUROGLYCOPENIC
47 CHLORPROPAMIDE
48 ALDOSTERON
49 CUSHING
50 POYYURIA
51 SECONDARY
52 KUSSMAUL
53 HYPOPHOSPHATEMIA
54 ADDISON
55 MYXEDEMA

2.

Lithium	Decrease
Alcohol	Decrease
Chlorpropamide (Diabinese)	Increase
Positive pressure ventilation	Increase
Chlorpromazine (Thorazine)	Decrease
Phenytoin (Dilantin)	Decrease
Hydrochlorothiazide (HydroDIURIL)	Increase
Anesthetic agents	Increase
Demeclocycline (Declomycin)	Decrease
Beta stimulants	Increase
Morphine sulfate	Increase

3.

	Diabetes Insipidus
Serum ADH	↓ if neurogenic Normal if nephrogenic
Urine output	↑
Urine specific gravity	↓
Urine osmolality	↓
Serum osmolality	↑
Serum sodium	↑ (concentration effect)
RAP/PAOP	↓

4. To calculate the serum osmolality: (Serum sodium [158]) × 2 + (BUN [32] ÷ 2.6]) + (Serum glucose [110] ÷ 18) = Serum osmolality of 334.4 mOsm/kg. The most likely cause of the increase in urine output and the laboratory findings is DI.

5.

	Diabetic Ketoacidosis	Hyperglycemic Hyperosmolar Nonketotic Syndrome
Age	Young	Old
Type of DM	1 (IDDM)	2 (NIDDM) or none
Average serum glucose	600 mg/dL	1100 mg/dL
Presence of ketosis	Positive	Negative
pH	May be very acidotic	Normal or minimally acidotic
Anion gap	Increased	Normal
Respiratory pattern	Kussmaul's (rapid and deep)	Normal or tachypneic (rapid and shallow)
Breath odor	Acetone (fruity)	Normal
Serum osmolality	295-330 mOsm/kg	330-450 mOsm/kg
Serum sodium	Decreased, normal, or increased	Normal or increased
Serum potassium	Increased initially; drops with rehydration and correction of acidosis	Decreased
BUN	Mildly increased	Severely increased
Average fluid deficit	4-8 L	8-15 L

6.

Serum glucose greater than 300 mg/dL	Both
Kussmaul's respirations	DKA
pH less than 7.30	DKA
Positive serum and urine ketones	DKA
Abdominal pain	DKA
Dehydration	Both
Lethargy → coma	Both
Serum glucose greater than 1000 mg/dL	HHNK

7.

Headache	Hypoglycemia
Serum glucose greater than 300 mg/dL	DKA
Abdominal pain	DKA
Cold, clammy skin	Hypoglycemia
Nervousness, tremors	Hypoglycemia
Polyuria	DKA
Lethargy → coma	DKA
Seizures	Hypoglycemia
Glycosuria	DKA
Tachycardia	Both
Agitation, difficulty with concentration	Hypoglycemia
Weakness, fatigue	DKA
Fruity breath	DKA
Serum glucose less than 50 mg/dL	Hypoglycemia

8.

c, f — 1. Neurogenic DI
b, e — 2. Nephrogenic DI
c, d, g — 3. DKA
c, d, g — 4. HHNK syndrome
a, h — 5. Hypoglycemia

Bibliography

Bardsley, J. K., & Want, L. L. (2004). Overview of diabetes. *Critical Care Nursing Quarterly, 27*(2), 106-112.

DiNardo, M. M., Korytkowski, M. T., & Siminerio, L. S. (2004). The importance of normoglycemia in critically ill patients. *Critical Care Nursing Quarterly, 27*(2), 126-134.

Guthrie, R. A., & Guthrie, D. W. (2004). Pathophysiology of diabetes mellitus. *Critical Care Nursing Quarterly, 27*(2), 113-125.

Kinney, M., Dunbar, S., Brooks-Brunn, J. A., Molter, N., & Vitello-Cicciu, J. (1998). *AACN clinical reference for critical care nursing* (4th ed.). St. Louis, MO: Mosby.

Kruse, J. A., Fink, M. P., & Carlson, R. W. (2003). *Saunders manual of critical care*. Philadelphia: Saunders.

Langdon, C. D., & Shriver, R. L. (2004). Clinical issues in the care of the critically ill diabetic patients. *Critical Care Nursing Quarterly, 27*(2), 162-171.

Mayes, J., Dennis, V., & Hoogwerf, B. (2000). Pancreas transplantation in type 1 diabetes: Hope vs reality. *Cleveland Clinic Journal of Medicine, 67*(4), 281-286.

Parrillo, J. E., & Dellinger, R. P. (2002). *Critical care medicine: Principles of diagnosis and management in the adult* (2nd ed.). St. Louis, MO: Mosby.

Robinson, L. E., & van Soeren, M. H. (2004). Insulin resistance and hyperglycemia in critical illness. *AACN Clinical Issues, 15*(1), 45-62.

Sole, M. L., Klein, D. G., & Moseley, M. J. (2005). *Introduction to critical care nursing* (4th ed.). Philadelphia: Elsevier Saunders.

Tkacs, N. (2002). Hypoglycemia unawareness. *American Journal of Nursing, 102*(2), 34-41.

Urden, L. D., Stacy, K. M., & Lough, M. E. (2006). *Thelan's critical care nursing: Diagnosis and management* (5th ed.). St. Louis, MO: Mosby.

Wiegand, D. L.-M. J., & Carlson, K. K. (2005). *AACN procedure manual for critical care* (5th ed.). Philadelphia: W. B. Saunders.

The Hematologic and Immunologic Systems

CHAPTER 10

Selected Concepts in Anatomy and Physiology

Purposes of the Hematologic and Immunologic Systems

1. Hematologic
   a. Provides the medium for transportation of oxygen, carbon dioxide, and nutrients to the tissues
   b. Maintains hemostasis
   c. Maintains internal environment, including participation in regulation of temperature and acid-base balance
2. Immunologic
   a. Protects the internal milieu of the body against invading organisms and the development, growth, and dissemination of abnormal cells
   b. Maintains homeostasis by removing damaged cells from the circulation

Bone Marrow

1. Adults have 30 to 50 mL of bone marrow per kilogram of body mass.
2. Most functioning bone marrow in adults is located in flat bones (vertebrae, skull, pelvic and shoulder girdles, clavicle, ribs, sternum) and proximal epiphysis of long bones.
3. The functions of the bone marrow include the following:
   a. Production of the following:
      (1) Erythrocytes (red blood cells [RBCs])
      (2) Leukocytes (white blood cells [WBCs]) including granulocytes, agranulocytes, and lymphocytes
      (3) Thrombocytes (platelets)
   b. Recognition and removal of senescent cells
   c. Participation in cellular and humoral immunity

Spleen

1. White pulp: primarily concerned with humoral immunity; performs the following functions:
   a. Production of lymphocytes
   b. Stimulation of B cell activity to produce immunoglobulins; therefore, splenectomized patients have a greatly increased risk of sepsis
2. Red pulp: contains reticuloendothelial tissue; performs the following functions
   a. Storage and release of RBCs into the circulation
      (1) Caused by contraction of smooth muscle in the capsule surrounding the spleen and in invaginations of the capsule, called *trabeculae*
      (2) When stimulated by the sympathetic nervous system (SNS), as much as 100 mL of concentrated RBCs can be released into the circulation, raising the hematocrit by 1% to 2%
   b. Filtering and destruction (by the process of phagocytosis) of damaged or old erythrocytes (referred to as *culling*)
      (1) Removes particles from intact RBCs without destroying them (referred to as *pitting*)
      (2) Catabolizes hemoglobin released from RBCs that have been destroyed by the spleen; iron returned to the bone marrow for reuse
   c. Filtering and trapping foreign material, including bacteria and viruses
   d. Storage and release of platelets; destruction of damaged or senescent platelets

Liver

Performs the following functions:

1. Filtering of blood as it comes from the gastrointestinal (GI) tract
   a. Removal of foreign material including microorganisms, damaged or old RBCs, and other degradation products by the Kupffer cells lining the sinusoidal beds of the liver
   b. Destruction of RBCs produces bilirubin, which the liver converts to bile, which is necessary for fat digestion
2. Elimination of immune complexes (e.g., antigen-antibody complexes) from the blood
3. Detoxification of toxic substances that enter the blood
4. Manufacture of some clotting factors and antithrombin

5. Storage of blood (e.g., in heart failure, the liver becomes engorged with blood)

Lymphatic System

1. Lymph: pale yellow fluid that transports lymphocytes
   a. Composition
      (1) Contains lymphocytes, granulocytes, enzymes, and antibodies
      (2) Deficient in platelets and fibrinogen, so it coagulates slowly
   b. Function: returns proteins and fat from GI tract, certain hormones, and excess interstitial fluid to the blood
2. Lymph circulation
   a. Lymphatic capillaries are somewhat larger than blood capillaries and are irregular in diameter.
   b. Lymphatic vessels are formed by lymphatic capillaries.
   c. Lymph ducts drain into subclavian veins.
      (1) The right lymphatic duct collects lymph from right side of head, neck, thorax, right arm, right lung, right side of heart, and right upper surface of diaphragm.
      (2) The thoracic duct collects lymph from all other parts of the body.
   d. Lymph nodes are small, bean-shaped organs located along lymph vessels
      (1) Spongy and multichanneled on inside
      (2) Sites of B and T cell lymphocyte production and distribution
      (3) Functions
         (a) Lymph nodes filter out and allow WBCs to phagocytose bacteria and foreign material carried by lymph.
         (b) Granulocytes, macrophages, and lymphocytes pass through the lymph node to return to the blood.
      (4) Enlargement of lymph nodes
         (a) This occurs with infection or malignancy.
         (b) Enlargement of superficial nodes can be palpated; enlarged deep nodes can be visualized only on x-ray.
   e. Additional lymphoid tissue synthesizes immunoglobulin A (IgA) and immunoglobulin E (IgE) and is located in the submucosa of the respiratory, intestinal, or genitourinary (GU) tracts.
      (1) Mucosal-associated lymphoid tissues: clusters of T and B lymphocytes and phagocytes dispersed in the mucosal linings of the respiratory, GI, and GU tracts
      (2) Gut-associated lymphoid tissue: Peyer's patches in the intestinal tract
3. Thymus
   a. Location: anterosuperior mediastinum below the thyroid gland; each lobe packed with lymphocytes
   b. Function
      (1) Site of maturation and distribution of T lymphocytes
      (2) Secretes a hormone, thymosin, which is thought to stimulate immune function

Blood

1. Plasma composes 55% of total blood volume.
   a. Composed of serum and plasma proteins including albumin, serum globulins, fibrinogen, prothrombin, and plasminogen
   b. Hematocrit expresses the percentage of RBCs in the total blood volume
2. All blood cells originate from pluripotential stem cells.
   a. Erythroid stem cells (pronormoblasts) develop into reticulocytes and finally into erythrocytes.
   b. Myeloid stem cells (myeloblasts or monoblasts) develop into granulocytes and monocytes.
   c. Lymphoid stem cells (lymphoblasts) develop into B and T lymphocytes.
   d. Thrombocytic stem cells (megakaryoblasts) develop into thrombocytes.
3. Erythrocytes also are referred to as *red blood cells*.
   a. Structure
      (1) Erythrocytes are nonnucleated, round, biconcave cells.
      (2) The inner part of the RBC (referred to as *stoma*) is the location of hemoglobin attachment and contains the antigens that determine ABO and Rh blood type.
   b. Function of RBCs
      (1) Transportation of oxygen from lungs to tissues
      (2) Participation in maintenance of acid-base balance
      (3) Highly permeable to hydrogen, chloride, and bicarbonate ions and water
   c. Types of RBCs
      (1) Reticulocytes: immature RBCs
         (a) Useful in assessing erythrocyte production; elevated reticulocyte count means that production of new RBCs is greater than usual such as may occur in acute hemorrhage
         (b) Maturation to erythrocyte takes 1 to 4 days
      (2) Erythrocytes: mature RBCs
         (a) Life span is approximately 120 days
         (b) The spleen acts as RBC reservoir; contains 1% to 2% of circulating RBCs
   d. Erythropoiesis
      (1) Regulation
         (a) Determined by relationship of cellular oxygen requirement and general metabolic activity
         (b) Bone marrow stimulated to make more RBCs by the hormone erythropoietin; erythropoietin secreted by the kidney in response to hypoxemia
      (2) Nutritional requirements for RBC and hemoglobin production
         (a) Iron
         (b) Vitamin B_{12}
         (c) Folic acid

(3) Process
(a) Stem cell
(b) Erythroblast (has a nucleus)
(c) Expulsion of nucleus
(d) Erythrocyte
(4) Hemoglobin synthesis
(a) Synthesis takes place in bone marrow.
(b) Hemoglobin consists of four globin chains and four heme groups per hemoglobin molecule; each hemoglobin molecule has two different types of globin (e.g., normal adult hemoglobin [referred to as *hemoglobin A*]) and has two alpha chains and two beta chains.

e. Destruction (hemolysis) of erythrocytes
(1) Destruction of old and immature RBCs occurs in the liver and spleen.
(2) Destruction of immature RBCs occurs primarily because they are misshapen or damaged.
(3) Presenescent RBCs are removed from the circulation by the spleen, liver, or bone marrow for any of the following reasons:
(a) RBC membrane abnormalities
(b) Hemoglobin abnormalities
(c) Abnormal metabolic functions
(d) Physical trauma to the RBC
(e) Antibodies
(f) Infectious agents and toxins
(4) Hemoglobin and iron are returned to the bone marrow for reuse.
(5) Erythrocyte destruction increases bilirubin production; bilirubin is transported to the liver attached to albumin.
(a) Indirect bilirubin is unconjugated; this is before the liver has converted it to be water soluble; indirect bilirubin becomes elevated in hemolytic states that overwhelm the ability of the liver to conjugate or in liver disease where the liver is unable to adequately conjugate
(b) Direct bilirubin is conjugated: this is after the liver has converted it to a water-soluble substance that will be excreted into the bile; direct bilirubin becomes elevated in biliary obstruction.

4. Leukocytes: phagocytic and immunologic systems
a. Cytokines: protein hormones synthesized by the various leukocytes (Table 10-1)
(1) Act as chemical mediators of immunity and inflammation
(2) Important in regulation of normal immune and inflammatory responses
(3) Are causative factors in systemic inflammatory response syndrome (SIRS) (see Chapter 11)
(4) Types of cytokines
(a) Monokines are synthesized by mononuclear phagocytes.
(b) Lymphokines are synthesized by lymphocytes.

b. Granulocytes: active phagocytes
(1) Neutrophils (also known as *polymorphonuclear leukocytes*); largest component of circulating WBC mass (40% to 80%)
(a) Function
(i) Neutrophils leave the blood vessel, migrate through the tissues, and search for microorganisms or damaged or old body cells; they then engulf, kill, and digest these cells through the process of phagocytosis (Table 10-2 and Figure 10-1 describe some selected cellular processes of leukocytes, including phagocytosis).
a) Neutrophils are the most actively phagocytic of granulocytes.
b) After phagocytosis, the neutrophil dies.
c) Pus is the end product of neutrophil death.
d) Neutrophils exhibit a burst of oxygen consumption during phagocytosis known as a *respiratory burst;* this produces superoxide, hydrogen peroxide, and hydroxyl radicals; these oxygen-derived radicals normally function in destruction of microorganisms but may be injurious to normal body tissue.
(ii) Neutrophils contain cytoplasmic granules that include lysosomal enzymes, which aid in killing the microorganism.
(b) Life span after maturation: half-life is 4 to 10 hours
(c) Maturity
(i) Bands are immature neutrophils.
a) Phagocytic
b) Increase in bands seen in acute infection; frequently referred to as a *shift to the left*
(ii) Segmented neutrophils (referred to as *segs*) are mature neutrophils.
a) Phagocytic
b) Increase in segmented neutrophils seen in liver disease and pernicious anemia; frequently referred to as a *shift to the right*
(d) Recruitment
(i) Movement into the tissues is stimulated by microorganisms or antigen-antibody reactions.
(ii) The bone marrow speeds maturation and release when more neutrophils are needed for phagocytosis.
(e) Destruction: lost from the blood via the GI tract, pulmonary or oral secretions, and urine and into the tissues

Table 10-1 Cytokines

Factor	Action
Chemotactic factors	• Attract macrophages and granulocytes to area of antigen
Granulocyte-macrophage colony-stimulating factor	• Enhances production of neutrophils in the bone marrow
Interferon	• Inhibition of viruses • Activates NK cells
Interleukin-1 (IL-1)	• Augments the immune response • Mediates the inflammatory response • Activates T cells • Activates phagocytes • Promotes prostaglandin production • Induces fever
Interleukin-2 (IL-2)	• Induces T cells to proliferate • Enhances activity of NK cells and cytotoxic T cells
Interleukin-3 (IL-3)	• Regulates growth and differentiation of leukocytes in the bone marrow
Interleukin-4 (IL-4)	• Enhances antibody production through B cell activation
Interleukin-5 (IL-5)	• Promotes growth and differentiation of B lymphocytes into immunoglobulin A–secreting cells
Interleukin-6 (IL-6)	• Promotes the differentiation of B lymphocytes to plasma cells • Promotes hematopoiesis • Enhances the inflammatory process
Interleukin-7 (IL-7)	• Induces growth of immature T and B cells
Interleukin-8 (IL-8)	• Stimulates chemotaxis • Activates T lymphocytes and neutrophils
Interleukin-9 (IL-9)	• Induces growth of T cells and mast cells
Interleukin-10 (IL-10)	• Inhibits proliferation of helper T cells • Decreases production of some other cytokines (an antiinflammatory effect)
Lymphotoxin	• Cytotoxic: directly destroys the antigen
Macrophage activation factor	• Enhances functioning of macrophages
Migration inhibition factor	• Prevents migration of macrophages to area of antigen
Transfer factor	• Changes nonsensitized T lymphocytes to sensitized T lymphocytes
Transforming growth factor	• Stimulates fibroblasts for wound healing • Inhibits the immune response
Tumor necrosis factor (TNF) (also called *cachectin*)	• Cytotoxic to tumor cells • Induces fever • In high concentrations (e.g., septic shock) causes endothelial cell damage and increases vascular permeability

NK, Natural killer.

Table 10-2 Definitions of Selected Leukocyte Activities

Opsonization	The process by which opsonins render bacteria more susceptible to phagocytosis by leukocytes; an opsonin is an antibody or complement split product that when attached to foreign material, microorganism, or antigen, enhances phagocytosis of the substances by leukocytes and other macrophages
Chemotaxis (Figure 10-1)	The movement toward (positive) or away from (negative) a chemical stimulus; movement of neutrophils and monocytes toward an invading microorganism
Margination (Figure 10-1)	The process of the WBC sticking to the wall of the capillary
Diapedesis (Figure 10-1)	The passage of WBCs through the walls of the vessels that contain them without damage to the vessels
Phagocytosis	The process by which certain cells engulf and destroy microorganisms and cellular debris; involves invagination, engulfment, internalization and formation of phagocyte vacuole, digestion of phagocytosed material by lysosomes and oxygen-derived radicals, and release of digested microbial products
Lysis	The destruction or dissolution of a cell through the action of a specific agent

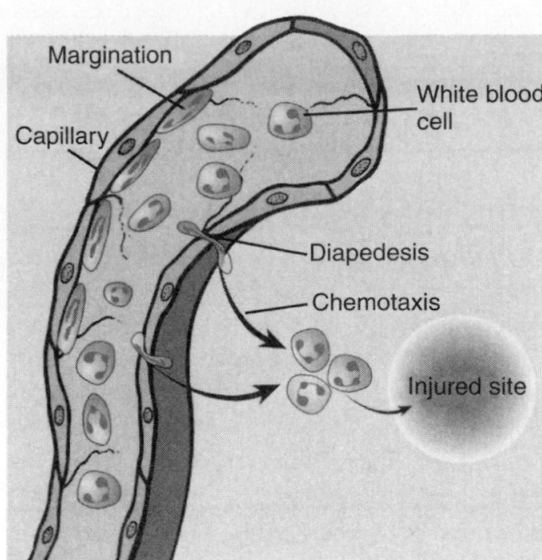

Figure 10-1 Illustration of margination, diapedesis, and chemotaxis. (From Lewis, S. M., Heitkemper, M. M., & Dirksen, S. R. [2004]. *Medical-surgical nursing: Assessment and management of clinical problems* [6th ed.]. St. Louis: Mosby.)

(2) Eosinophils: compose 0% to 5% of WBC mass
(a) Functions
(i) Ingest immune complexes (antigen-antibody complexes) and inactive mediators of allergic response
(ii) Some phagocytic activity
(iii) Probably most important during parasitic infections and allergic reactions; especially important in helminth infections because these parasitic worms are too large to be phagocytized and eosinophils secrete chemicals that destroy the surface of the helminth
(b) Life span after maturation: half-life in circulation approximately 30 minutes; in tissues 12 days
(c) Tissue eosinophils are present in large numbers on mucosal surfaces of the respiratory and GI systems and the skin because these locations are common entry points for foreign material
(3) Basophils: compose 0% to 2% of WBC mass
(a) Function
(i) Like mast cells, basophils contain heparin and histamine, which are released as the basophils degranulate during acute local or systemic allergic reactions; mast cells stay in the tissue, whereas basophils stay in the circulatory system; if a basophil leaves the circulatory system to stay in the tissue, it becomes a mast cell.
(ii) Basophils do not participate in phagocytic activity.
(b) Life span after maturation: unknown

c. Agranulocytes
(1) Mononuclear phagocytes
(a) Monocytes: compose 3% to 8% of WBC mass
(i) Function
a) Some phagocytic activity
b) Differentiate into macrophages as they migrate into the tissues
(ii) Life span after maturation: circulating half-life is 8 to 10 hours
(b) Macrophages (not measured in WBC count because of their location)
(i) Function
a) Greater phagocytic ability than polymorphonuclear neutrophils or monocytes; especially involved in removal of damaged or senescent cells, cellular debris, and mutant or cancer cells
b) Produce the cytokine interleukin-1 (IL-1), which increases proliferation of T cells, stimulates the growth and development of B lymphocytes, causes fever, and stimulates the release of prostaglandin
c) Produces the cytokine interferon-alpha, which is important in the bodily defense against viruses and tumors
d) Also produce interleukin-6 (IL-6), interleukin-8 (IL-8), and tumor necrosis factor (TNF)
(ii) Fixed or mobile
a) Fixed (or tissue) macrophages: stay in one organ and phagocytize live and dead debris
i) Lung: alveolar macrophages
ii) Brain: microglia
iii) Liver: Kupffer cells
iv) Bone: osteoclast
v) Peritoneum: peritoneal macrophages
vi) Kidney: mesangial cells
b) Mobile macrophages: found primarily at sites of inflammation and in peritoneal, pleural, and synovial spaces; migrate through the circulatory system as monocytes
(iii) Life span: months or years
(2) Lymphocytes: compose 10% to 40% of WBC mass
(a) T cells: compose 70% to 80% of lymphocytes
(i) Develop in the bone marrow; mature and differentiate in the thymus
(ii) Function: cellular immunity

(iii) Types of T cells
a) Helper T cells (also referred to as *CD4 T lymphocytes, T4 lymphocytes*, or T_H) detect foreign cells and produce lymphokines to stimulate the production or activation of other cells to fight infection; lymphokines are soluble proteins that function as chemical communicators to transmit instructions to macrophages, lymphocytes, and tissue cells.
b) Cytotoxic T cells (also referred to as *killer cells* or T_c) emit chemicals that dissolve the membrane of a foreign cell to kill the cell before the invader can use it as a base for multiplication.
c) Suppressor T cells (also referred to as *CD8 T lymphocytes, T8 lymphocytes*, or T_S) modulate the overall immune system by signaling B cells and T cells to slow down or stop their activity.
d) Memory T cells circulate in blood and lymph after the initial infection to allow ready response to subsequent invasion by the same organism.
e) Helper T cells typically carry the CD4 surface molecule and suppressor, and cytotoxic T cells typically carry the CD8 surface molecule; normally there are twice as many CD4 cells as CD8 cells.

(b) B cells: compose 10% to 20% of lymphocytes
(i) Develop and matures in the bone marrow (bursa)
(ii) Function: production of immunoglobulins (humoral immunity)
a) Once activated, B cells become plasma cells.
i) Recognize specific foreign material
ii) Develop specific immunoglobulins to that antigen
b) Memory B cells circulate in blood and lymph after the initial infection to allow ready response to subsequent invasion by the same organism.

(c) Natural killer (NK) cells (also referred to as *null cells*) compose approximately 10% of lymphocytes.
(i) Large granular cytotoxic lymphocytes that are not T cells or B cells (no surface marker exist on these lymphocytes)
(ii) Function
a) Kill nonspecifically and do not need prior exposure for activation
b) Involved in surveillance against tumors, some parasites, and viruses

Inflammation

1. Sequential physiologic response the body makes to injuries, immunologic processes, or foreign substances in the body; may be acute or chronic
a. Occurs at sites of tissue damage irrespective of cause
b. May be local only or can become systemic; systemic response now is referred to as *systemic inflammatory response syndrome* (discussion of systemic inflammatory response syndrome and multiple organ dysfunction syndrome (MODS) is in Chapter 11)
2. Process
a. Stage I: vascular stage
(1) Phases
(a) Phase 1: immediate but temporary vasoconstriction caused by trauma to vascular smooth muscle
(b) Phase 2
(i) Warmth, redness, swelling, pain, and loss of function are the five classic symptoms of the inflammatory response.
(ii) Injured tissues and cells secrete chemical mediators (Table 10-3); predominant effect is vasodilation and increase in capillary permeability causing warmth, redness, and swelling.
a) Healing is enhanced by the increase in mobilization of nutrients to the area.
b) Tissue injury is decreased by diluting toxins or microorganisms that enter the area.
c) Pain is caused by tissue stretching and histamine and prostaglandin release.
d) Loss of function is caused by tissue swelling and pain.
(2) The major leukocyte in this stage of inflammation is the tissue macrophage
(a) Response is immediate because the tissue macrophage is already in the tissue.
(b) Granulocyte colony-stimulating factor is secreted by the macrophage to stimulate the bone marrow to speed up the maturation and release of leukocytes.
(c) Cytokines secreted by the macrophage attract neutrophils to the area of injury or invasion.
b. Stage II: cellular stage; major leukocyte in this stage of inflammation is the neutrophil, which attacks and destroys foreign material and removes necrotic tissue

Table 10-3 Chemical Mediators of the Inflammatory Process

Chemical Mediator	Actions
Bradykinin	• Causes vasodilation • Increases capillary permeability • Enhances chemotaxis • Causes pain • Converts plasminogen to plasmin • Produces smooth muscle contraction (e.g., bronchospasm)
Collagenase	• Degrades clots
Complement cascade	• Triggers neutrophil aggregation • Increases capillary permeability • Activates mast cells and basophils
Elastase	• Degrades clots
Endorphin	• Causes vasodilation • Produces analgesia
Fibrinolysin	• Digests fibrin
Histamine	• Causes vasodilation • Increases capillary permeability • Increases heart rate and contractility • Produces bronchospasm • Increases secretion of mucus and gastric acid • Inhibits T cells
Interleukin-1 (IL-1)	• Stimulates protein catabolism • Causes fever • Activates lymphocytes • Stimulates fibroblasts
Interleukin-2 (IL-2)	• Activates B lymphocytes to make antibodies • Activates macrophages
Leukotriene	• Causes vasoconstriction • Increases capillary permeability • Produces smooth muscle contraction (e.g., bronchospasm)
Lipase	• Degrades fat
Plasminogen	• Degrades clots when activated to plasmin
Prostacyclin	• Causes vasodilation • Inhibits platelet aggregation • Increases capillary permeability
Prostaglandin (PGD_2, PGF_{2a})	• Vasoconstriction • Bronchoconstriction
Prostaglandin (PGE_2, PGI_2)	• Causes vasodilation • Produces smooth muscle relaxation (e.g., bronchodilation) • Promotes platelet aggregation • Increases capillary permeability • Activates lysosomal enzymes • Potentiates leukotrienes • Causes pain
Serotonin	• Causes vasodilation • Increases capillary permeability • Causes pulmonary vasoconstriction • Produces smooth muscle contraction (e.g., bronchospasm)
Thromboxane	• Causes vasoconstriction and endothelial damage • Causes pulmonary vasoconstriction • Acts as a potent platelet aggregator
Tumor necrosis factor (TNF)	• Causes necrosis of bacteria or tissue • Stimulates muscle catabolism • Induces fever

c. Stage III: tissue repair and replacement
   (1) Initiated at the time of injury
   (2) Regeneration: replacement of lost cells with the same type of cells
   (3) Repair: replacement of lost cells with connective tissue cells to form scar tissue; some loss of function occurs with the degree of loss depending on the percentage of previously functional tissue replaced by scar tissue

Immunity

1. Definition: the protection of the body against pathogenic organisms or other foreign material; dependent on ability to recognize self from nonself
   a. Self is determined genetically; it is anything synthesized by a person's own particular DNA code
   b. Nonself describes anything that is different in its chromosome structure and evokes a response from the immune system; antigens are chemical substances (almost always protein) that are viewed by the body as foreign (nonself)
2. Lines of defense
   a. First: skin and mucous membranes, acid secretions and enzymes, and natural immunoglobulins
   b. Second: macrophages and neutrophils
   c. Third: cellular and humoral immunity
3. Innate immunity: inherent immune mechanisms; present at birth; do not require prior exposure to antigen for activation
   a. Anatomic: skin and mucous membranes
   b. Chemical
      (1) Acid secretions in stomach, vagina, and mouth
      (2) Digestive enzymes in the GI tract
      (3) Tears, perspiration
      (4) Lysosomes
      (5) Natural immunoglobulins
      (6) Cytokines
      (7) Pyrogen (produced by granulocytes to cause an increase in body temperature)
   c. Cellular
      (1) Normal bacterial flora: GI tract, vagina, and respiratory tract
      (2) Tissue macrophages
      (3) Leukocytes and mobile macrophages
      (4) Inflammatory process

4. Acquired immunity: immunity developed by the body through the creation of antibodies and formation of T and B memory cells in response to exposure to foreign material (antigen)
   a. Types
      (1) Passive acquired immunity: produced by the injection of antibodies or sensitized lymphocytes
      (2) Active acquired immunity: produced by natural exposure to an antigen (e.g., infection)
   b. Cell-mediated immunity
      (1) Particularly effective against viruses, parasites, some fungi, and bacteria harbored inside of cells; responsible for delayed hypersensitivity, transplant rejection, and malignancy surveillance and, possibly, destruction
      (2) Primarily mediated by T cells
      (3) Induced and regulated primarily through the production and activity of cytokines (Table 10-1)
      (4) Process
         (a) The macrophage is the first cell to detect most antigens.
         (b) The macrophage processes the antigen and "presents" it to T and B cells.
         (c) T cells recognize the antigen when it is on the macrophage cell membrane.
         (d) The antigen binds with an antigen receptor on the surface of the T cell, sensitizing the T cell.
         (e) Sensitized T cells secrete lymphokines (Table 10-1), which regulate and coordinate the immune response to combat foreign cells, protect the body against mutant or cancer cells, and destroy foreign tissue; IL-8 is secreted by the macrophage and stimulates T cell division.
         (f) T cells are programmed to recognize the body's own tissue (self) from nonself (antigenic); autoimmune diseases are caused when the immune system cannot recognize self and the body is damaged by the immune system.
         (g) NK cells also contribute to cellular immunity, especially in relation to cancer cell surveillance.
   c. Humoral-mediated immunity
      (1) Primarily effective against bacteria and viruses
      (2) Primarily mediated by B cells
      (3) Process (Figure 10-2)
         (a) Once activated, B cells become plasma cells and recognize specific foreign cells or antigen.
         (b) Plasma cells make antibodies (also called *immunoglobulins*; Table 10-4).
            (i) Immunoglobulins (antibodies) are serum proteins that bind to specific antigens; they begin the process that causes lysis or phagocytosis of an offending antigen.

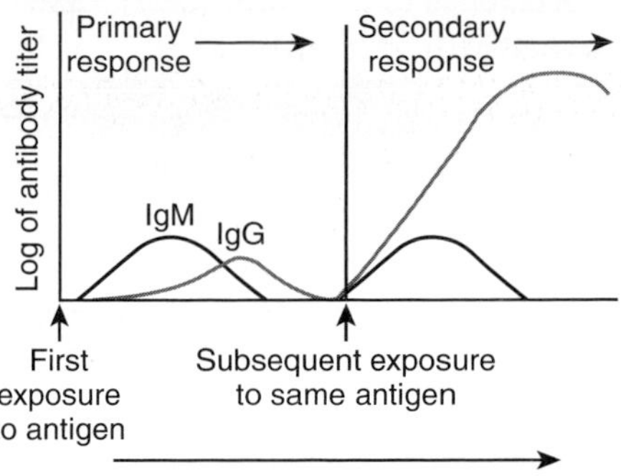

Figure 10-2 Primary and secondary immune responses. The introduction of antigen induces a response dominated by two classes of immunoglobulins: immunoglobulin M and immunoglobulin G. Immunoglobulin M predominates in the primary response, with some immunoglobulin G appearing later. After the immune system of the host is primed, another challenge with the same antigen induces the secondary response, in which some immunoglobulin M and large amounts of immunoglobulin G are produced. (From McCance, K. L., & Huether, S. E. [2006]. *Pathophysiology: The biologic basis for disease in adults and children* [5th ed.]. St. Louis: Mosby.)

            (ii) One end of the immunoglobulin molecule has a constant fragment with a fixed sequence of amino acids that is constant within the category of the immunoglobulin (e.g., IgG or IgM).
            (iii) The other end of the immunoglobulin has an antigen binding fragment with an amino acid sequence specific to the antigen for which it was formed.
         (c) The first exposure to an antigen is followed by a latent phase in which no antibody levels are detected.
         (d) Primary response follows as serum antibody levels rise rapidly; maximal antibody response takes 3 to 5 days.
         (e) Levels of immunoglobulin plateau and finally decline.
         (f) Subsequent exposure to the antigen results in more rapid production of antibodies to that antigen and higher concentrations of the antibody; this is the basis for immunizations.
         (g) Inflammation occurs because antigen-antibody complexes (referred to as *immune complexes*) attract WBCs.
      (4) Immune complexes activate the complement cascade (Figure 10-3).
         (a) Complement is a group of blood proteins: there are more than 20 of these proteins, but 11 are considered the primary complement elements.
            (i) These are labeled C1 to C9, with C1 having three subunits (C1q, C1r, C1s).
            (ii) C1 is synthesized primarily by the intestinal epithelium.

Table 10-4 Immunoglobulins

Immunoglobulin	Actions	Comments
IgG	• Coats microorganisms (primarily bacteria and viruses) to enhance phagocytosis • Activates complement system	• Most abundant immunoglobulin (75%-80% of total) • Present in intravascular and extravascular spaces • Crosses the placental barrier and provides natural immunity
IgA	• Protects epithelial surfaces against antigen adhesion and invasion • Protects against entry via the respiratory tract and genitourinary and gastrointestinal tracts • Activates complement system	• Present in many body secretions (e.g., saliva, tears, sweat, mucus, and breast milk) • 10%-15% of total
IgM	• Kills bacteria in bloodstream • Activates complement system	• First responder to bacterial or viral invasion • Present mostly in intravascular space • 5%-10% of total immunoglobulin
IgD	• Not well understood • May activate B cells	• 1% of total immunoglobulins
IgE	• Attaches to mast cells and basophils and causes them to release their contents (e.g., histamine) in response to contact with specific antigens	• Present in serum, interstitial space, exocrine secretions, and on basophils and mast cells • Very small (0.002) percentage of total immunoglobulins

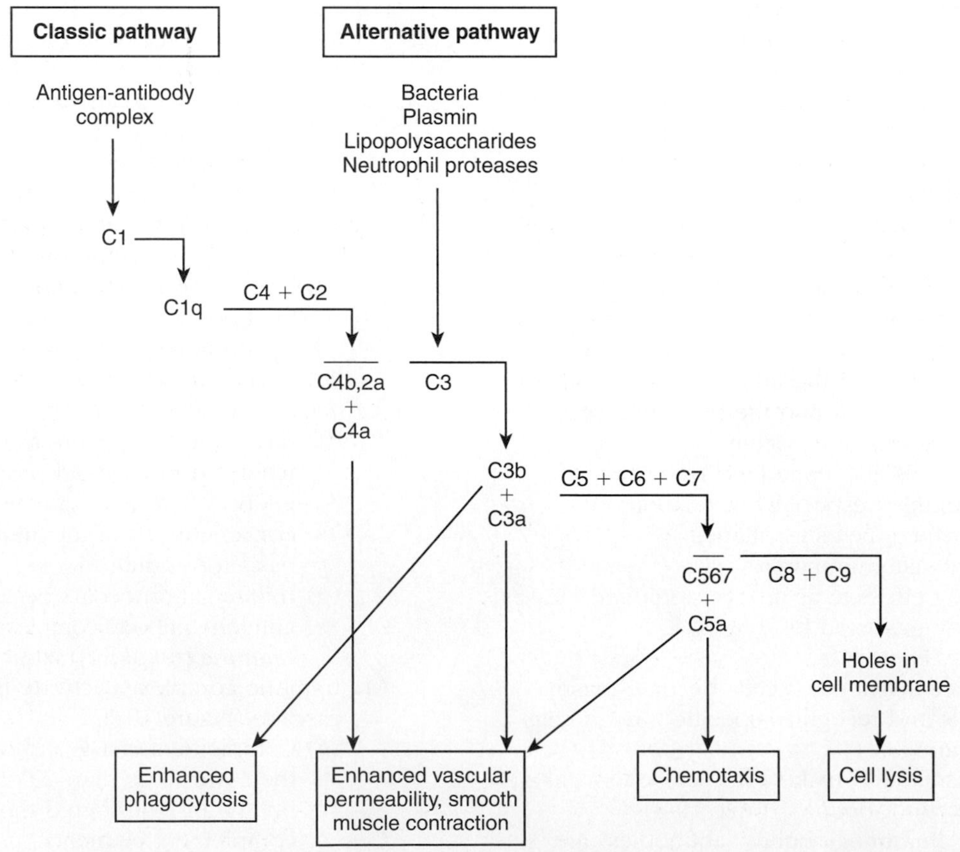

Figure 10-3 The complement cascade. (From Lewis, S. M., Heitkemper, M. M., & Dirksen, S. R. [2004]. *Medical-surgical nursing: Assessment and management of clinical problems* [6th ed.]. St. Louis: Mosby.)

(iii) C2 and C4 are produced by macrophages.
(iv) C3, C6, and C9 are synthesized by the liver.
(v) C5 and C8 are synthesized by the spleen.
(b) When activated, complements function as mediators to enhance various aspects of inflammatory response; they also do the following:
(i) Attract and stimulate polymorphonuclear neutrophils
(ii) Kill microorganisms by punching holes in their cell membranes, allowing intracellular fluid to leak out; mononuclear phagocytes and monocytes then clear the debris from the bloodstream
(iii) Agglutinate the bacteria
(iv) Activate basophils and mast cells
(c) They may be activated with or without previous exposure to the antigen.
(i) Anaphylactoid reaction: no previous exposure to the antigen; no true antigen-antibody interaction
(ii) Anaphylactic reaction: previous exposure to the antigen; involves antigen-antibody interaction
(iii) A more detailed description of anaphylactoid and anaphylactic reactions is in Chapter 11

d. Hypersensitivity (allergic) reactions
(1) Type I: immediate hypersensitivity reactions ranging from mild reaction with localized response to a severe systemic reaction referred to as *anaphylaxis*
(a) Reaction occurs within minutes (usually 5 to 20 minutes) of exposure to even a minute amount of the antigen
(b) Caused by IgE specific to the antigen; the antigen binds to one end of IgE; IgE is bound to a mast cell or basophil; when the antigen is attached, the mast cell or basophil degranulates and histamine is released; slow-reacting substance of anaphylaxis (SRS-A) and eosinophil chemotactic factor of anaphylaxis are also released; eosinophils are recruited to the site
(c) Example: anaphylactic reaction to a penicillin, insect venom, foods, or pollen
(2) Type II: cytotoxic hypersensitivity
(a) Reaction is usually within minutes to days
(b) Caused by the combination of IgG, IgM, or IgA antibody and antigenic receptors on membranes of cells; complement cascade is activated; NK cells are involved in destruction of the immune complex and the cell to which it is attached, and macrophages may phagocytize the immune complexes
(c) Example: mismatched blood transfusion reaction
(3) Type III: immune complex–mediated reaction
(a) Reaction is usually within hours
(b) Caused by large quantities of antigen-antibody (IgG, IgM, or IgA) complexes that cannot be cleared quickly and efficiently by the reticuloendothelial system; complement cascade is activated; neutrophils are activated at the site of deposition; inflammatory process is stimulated and mediators are released
(c) Example: environmental antigens (e.g., pollen and some drugs)
(4) Type IV: delayed or cell-mediated hypersensitivity
(a) Reaction is within 1 day or more
(b) Cause is poorly understood but is presumed to be cells that require time to migrate to the site; probably caused by previously sensitized lymphocytes and lymphokines that activate the inflammatory response at the site
(c) Examples: skin testing for tuberculosis and contact dermatitis

Hemostasis

1. Definition: the termination of bleeding by a complex process that involves integrated interactions among blood vessels, platelets, clotting factors, and the fibrinolytic system
2. Hemostatic mechanisms
a. Vascular response
(1) Disruption of vascular integrity causes an SNS response resulting in vasospasm and blood vessel constriction in the injured vessel.
(2) Thromboxane A_2, endothelin, the alpha-adrenergic system, and serotonin are thought to mediate this response.
b. Platelets aggregation (thrombocytes)
(1) Thrombocytes (platelets)
(a) Produced in bone marrow
(b) Life span is 9 to 12 days
(c) Thrombopoiesis
(i) Thrombopoietin (a hormone like erythropoietin for RBCs) is postulated to stimulate the production and release of thrombocytes.
(ii) Iron is needed for thrombopoiesis.
(d) Thrombocytes stored in and destroyed by the spleen
(2) Process
(a) Endothelial damage exposes the basement membrane of the subendothelial collagen.

(b) Damaged tissues release chemicals (e.g., thromboplastin) to activate platelets.
(c) Activated platelets swell and develop hairlike projections.
(d) Swelling increases the surface area of the platelet for platelet adhesion and makes platelet more likely to aggregate.
(e) Granules and components necessary for the clotting process are released from the platelets; adenosine diphosphate released by degranulation of the platelet enhances adhesiveness and aggregation.
  (i) Adhesiveness: stickiness that aids in ability to stick to vessel walls
  (ii) Aggregation: process of platelets adhering or clumping together to form the "platelet plug"
(f) Activated platelets become adhesive and aggregate.
(g) Platelet aggregation becomes large enough to form a platelet plug (sometimes referred to as a *white clot*) that seals the damaged blood vessel.
(h) During aggregation of the platelets, platelet factor III, an important contributor in the intrinsic pathway, is released.
(i) Platelets contain factor XIII (fibrin stabilizing factor) essential in the formation of a stable fibrin clot.

(3) Platelet function is affected by qualitative and quantitative factors
  (a) Qualitative changes
    (i) Drugs that decrease the ability of the platelets to aggregate
      a) Alcohol
      b) Aspirin (ASA)
      c) Ticlopidine (Ticlid)
      d) Clopidogrel (Plavix)
      e) Glycoprotein IIb/IIIa platelet receptor blockers (e.g., abciximab [ReoPro], eptifibatide [Integrilin], and tirofiban [Aggrastat])
      f) Nonsteroidal antiinflammatory drugs (NSAIDs) (e.g., phenylbutazone [Butazolidin] and ibuprofen [Motrin])
      g) Quinidine
      h) Dextran 40 (low-molecular-weight dextran)
      i) Heparin
  (b) Quantitative changes
    (i) Thrombocytopenia
      a) Significance
        i) Platelet counts greater than 50,000/mm^3: surgery generally can be tolerated
        ii) Platelet counts 20,000-30,000/mm^3: spontaneous bleeding may occur
        iii) Platelet counts less than 10,000/mm^3: spontaneous intracranial hemorrhages likely
      b) Etiology
        i) Decreased production (e.g., bone marrow depression or vitamin B_{12} or folic acid deficiency)
        ii) Increased destruction (e.g., idiopathic thrombocytopenic purpura, disseminated intravascular coagulation [DIC], or sepsis)
        iii) Hypersplenism (e.g., portal hypertension)
        iv) Heparin-induced thrombocytopenia and thrombosis (HITT): also called *heparin-associated thrombocytopenia and thrombosis* (HATT) or *white clot syndrome;* immune-mediated response caused by heparin
        v) Dilutional thrombocytopenia: caused by large volumes of fluids that do not contain platelets
    (ii) Thrombocytosis
      a) Significance: may cause excessive thrombosis or bleeding, depending on the quality of the platelets
      b) Etiology
        i) Malignancy
        ii) Polycythemia vera
        iii) Leukemia
        iv) Postsplenectomy
        v) Rheumatoid arthritis
        vi) Trauma

c. Coagulation
  (1) Depends on presence of clotting factors and functioning of the pathways
  (2) Blood coagulation factors (Table 10-5)
    (a) Consist of proteins, lipoproteins, and calcium, which is critical in the intrinsic, extrinsic, and common pathways
    (b) Circulate as inactive; activated in a cascade fashion

NOTE: The letter "a" after the factor indicates an activated factor.

  (3) Clotting pathways (Figure 10-4)
    (a) Pathways are cascades in which one action depends on a preceding action or interaction.
    (b) A fibrin clot may be produced through activation of the intrinsic or extrinsic pathway.
      (i) Intrinsic pathway
        a) Initiated by damage to RBCs or platelets
        b) Time from activation through intrinsic pathway and common pathway to a clot: 2 to 6 minutes
        c) Tested by partial thromboplastin time (PTT)

Table 10-5 Blood Coagulation Factors

Factor	Name(s)	Comments
I	Fibrinogen	• Synthesized in liver • Precursor to fibrin (Ia)
Ia	Fibrin	• Activated fibrinogen (I) becomes fibrin (Ia)
II	Prothrombin	• Synthesized in liver • Vitamin K dependent • Precursor to thrombin (IIa)
IIa	Thrombin	• Activated prothrombin becomes thrombin
III	Tissue thromboplastin Tissue factor	• First factor of extrinsic pathway
IV	Calcium	• Acts as an enzyme cofactor for most of the activation steps in intrinsic, extrinsic, and common pathways
V	Proaccelerin Labile factor Accelerator globulin	• Synthesized in liver • Combines with Xa and phospholipid to accelerate conversion of prothrombin (II) to thrombin (IIa)
VI	There is no designated factor VI	
VII	Proconvertin Stable factor	• Synthesized in liver • Vitamin K dependent • Part of extrinsic pathway • Complexes with tissue thromboplastin (III) to activate X
VIII	Antihemophiliac factor A	• Part of intrinsic pathway • Complexes with IXa and platelet phospholipid to activate X
IX	Plasma thromboplastin component Christmas factor Antihemophiliac factor B	• Synthesized in liver • Vitamin K dependent • Associated with factors VIII, XI, and XII in the intrinsic pathway
X	Stuart-Prower factor	• Synthesized in liver • Vitamin K dependent • Part of intrinsic and extrinsic pathways • Complexes with V and phospholipid to accelerate prothrombin (II) conversion
XI	Plasma thromboplastin antecedent	• May be synthesized in liver • May be vitamin K dependent • Part of intrinsic pathway • Associated with factors VIII, IX, and XII in the intrinsic pathway
XII	Hageman factor Contact factor	• First factor in intrinsic factor • Indirectly activates plasmin and complement cascades
XIII	Fibrin-stabilizing factor Fibrinase Laki-Lorand factor	• May be synthesized in liver • Activated by thrombin (IIa) • Produces a stronger, insoluble clot; stabilizes clot formation

(ii) Extrinsic pathway
- a) Initiated by injured tissue
- b) Time from activation through extrinsic pathway and common pathway to a clot: as short as 15 to 20 seconds
- c) Tested by prothrombin time (PT)

(c) Common pathway
- (i) Platelet factor III and tissue thromboplastin combine to become a prothrombin activator.
- (ii) Prothrombin is converted to thrombin.
- (iii) Fibrinogen is converted to fibrin.
- (iv) Fibrin clot is formed.
- (v) Pathway is tested by PTT, PT, and thrombin time.

d. Anticoagulant mechanisms in normal system
- (1) Fibrinolytic system (Figure 10-5)
  - (a) Activated clotting factors are cleared by the reticuloendothelial system.
  - (b) Clot-lysing activities maintain blood in fluid state.
    - (i) Process of clot breakdown takes approximately 7 to 10 days.

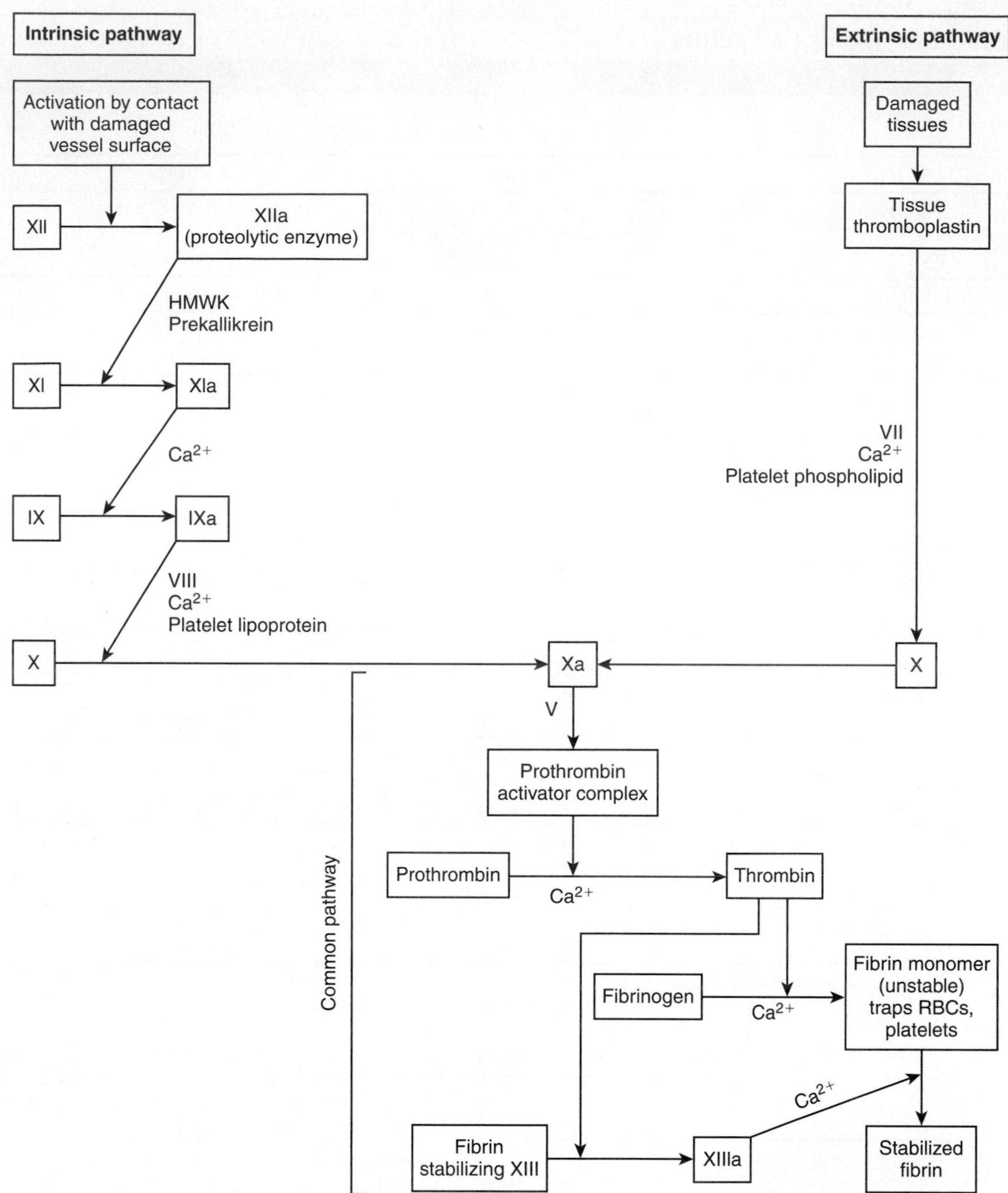

Figure 10-4 The clotting pathways: intrinsic, extrinsic, and common. *HMWK*, High-molecular-weight kininogen; *RBC*, red blood cell. (From Lewis, S. M., Heitkemper, M. M., & Dirksen, S. R. [2004]. *Medical-surgical nursing: Assessment and management of clinical problems* [6th ed.]. St. Louis: Mosby.)

(ii) Blood (intrinsic pathway) or tissue (extrinsic pathway) plasminogen activators activate plasminogen to plasmin; therefore, once a clot is developed, steps are initiated to eliminate it.

(iii) Plasmin works to lyse fibrin clots producing fibrin split products (FSPs) (also referred to as *fibrin degradation products*) increased amounts of FSPs increase potential for patient to bleed.

(iv) Fibrinolytic agents speed up this process by directly providing tissue plasminogen activator (e.g., alteplase [Activase] or reteplase [Retavase]) or tenecteplase (TNKase) or by triggering the process by adding a complex to cause the activation of the fibrinolytic system (streptokinase [Streptase]) (discussion of these agents and implications is located under Myocardial Infarction in Chapter 3 and in Chapter 13).

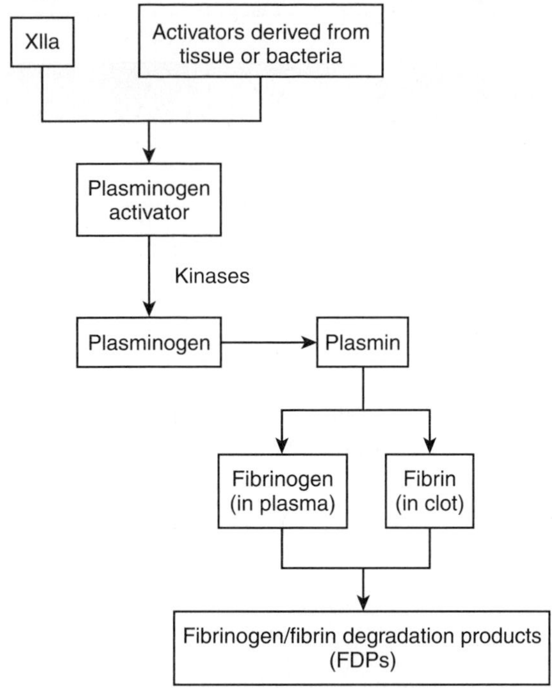

Figure 10-5 The fibrinolytic process. (From Lewis, S. M., Heitkemper, M. M., & Dirksen, S. R. [2004]. *Medical-surgical nursing: Assessment and management of clinical problems* [6th ed.]. St. Louis: Mosby.)

(c) Controls of fibrinolysis
(i) Plasminogen activator inhibitor type 1 inactivates tissue plasminogen activator
(ii) Alpha$_2$-antiplasmin is an inhibitor of plasmin
(2) Antithrombin system
(a) Defends against excessive clotting
(b) Release of antithrombin III from mast cells
(c) Neutralizes the clotting capability of thrombin

Blood Groups

1. Three systems describe the most important antigens on RBCs, tissues, and other cells.
a. ABO system (Table 10-6)
(1) This system is concerned with antigens on the RBC, which are designated A and B; the presence of these antigens is genetically controlled.
(2) Blood type is named for the antigen that is present on the RBC.
(3) Antibodies are present in the plasma for the antigen or antigens that are not present (e.g., B antibodies are found in group A blood because B antigens are absent).
(4) Agglutination that occurs in mismatched blood is the basis for typing and crossmatching.
(a) Blood typing detects the major antigens: A, B, Rh.
(b) Crossmatching detects the presence of major or minor RBC antigens.
b. Rh system (Table 10-7)
(1) This system is concerned with a series of six common types of Rh antigens, each called an *Rh factor*.
(2) Each person has one of each of three pairs, so they have three of these Rh factors designated c, C, d, D, e, and E.
(3) Only C, D, and E are antigenic enough to cause significant development of anti-Rh antibodies (and therefore potentially to cause blood transfusion reaction if nonmatched blood is administered).
(4) If C, D, or E antigens are present, the person is Rh+; if none of these three antigens are present, the person is Rh–; most (85%) of Americans are Rh+.
(5) Rh antibodies do not develop spontaneously; they only occur after exposure to Rh antigen (e.g., second exposure to non–Rh-matched blood or Rh– mothers pregnant with the second Rh+ fetus if anti-Rh globin [RhoGAM] was not given); delayed transfusion reactions can occur even after the first exposure to Rh+ blood and can cause a mild transfusion reaction.
c. Other red cell antigens
(1) Cold agglutinins
(a) These are antibodies that cause erythrocytes to coagulate when blood plasma temperature is below normal body temperature.
(b) Banked blood must be warmed to normal body temperature (37°C) before given to a patient who has cold agglutinins.
(2) Coombs' test: used to determine presence of hemolyzing antibodies
(a) Direct: detects antibodies attached to red cells
(b) Indirect: detects antibodies in serum
d. Uncrossmatched type O negative packed RBCs may be used safely in an exsanguinating patient.
(1) Whole blood is avoided to decrease the risk of reaction caused by anti-A and anti-B antibodies in type O plasma.
(2) Blood antigen-antibody complexes may complicate later crossmatching and may cause future blood transfusion reaction to own blood type unless it is O negative.
(3) Type-specific blood may be preferable, and type matching takes only 5 to 15 minutes.
e. Human leukocyte antigen (HLA)
(1) Concerned with a group of antigenic substances found on many cell types (including WBCs and platelets but not on erythrocytes)
(2) Detected serologically by cytotoxicity assays; HLA-A, HLA-B, and HLA-C are found on all nucleated cells, but HLA-D and HLA-DR antigens are located only on B lymphocytes, monocytes, epidermal cells, and endothelial cells
(3) Important in organ and tissue transplantation histocompatibility

Table 10-6 ABO Blood Groups

Patient's ABO Group	Percentage of Population	Antigen on Red Blood Cell	Antibodies in Plasma	Compatible Red Blood Cells	Compatible Plasma
O	47%	None	Anti-A; anti-B	O	O, A, B, AB
A	41%	A	Anti-B	O, A	A, AB
B	9%	B	Anti-A	O, B	B, AB
AB	3%	A and B	None	O, A, B, AB	AB

Table 10-7 Rh Compatibility

Patient's Rh Type	Red Blood Cell Rh Type for Transfusion	Plasma Rh Type for Transfusion
Positive	Positive or negative	Positive or negative
Negative	Negative	Positive or negative

Assessment of the Hematologic and Immunologic Systems

Interview

1. Chief complaint: why the patient is seeking help and duration of the problem
   a. Symptoms that may be related to hematologic or immunologic conditions
      (1) General
         (a) Fatigue
         (b) Weakness
         (c) Chills
         (d) Fever
         (e) Weight loss
         (f) Night sweats
         (g) Apathy
         (h) Lethargy
         (i) Malaise
         (j) Abnormal bleeding, bruising, or swelling
         (k) Chronic or recurrent infections
         (l) Poor wound healing
         (m) Enlarged and/or tender lymph nodes
      (2) Specific
         (a) Skin
            (i) Dry, coarse skin
            (ii) Bruising or bleeding
               a) Prolonged bleeding
               b) Petechiae
               c) Bruising easily
            (iii) Color changes
               a) Jaundice
               b) Pallor
               c) Cyanosis
            (iv) Rash
            (v) Pruritus
            (vi) Lesions
            (vii) Wounds: poor healing
            (viii) Inflammation
         (b) Eyes
            (i) Visual disturbances (e.g., blurring or diplopia)
            (ii) Blindness related to retinal hemorrhage
            (iii) Conjunctival pallor or inflammation
         (c) Ears
            (i) Vertigo
            (ii) Tinnitus
         (d) Nasopharynx and mouth
            (i) Epistaxis
            (ii) Dysphagia
            (iii) Gingival bleeding
            (iv) Painful lesions on mouth and lips
            (v) Sore tongue
            (vi) Sore throat
            (vii) Persistent hoarseness
         (e) Neck: nuchal rigidity
         (f) Lymph nodes
            (i) Swelling
            (ii) Tenderness
         (g) Cardiovascular
            (i) Chest pain
            (ii) Sternal tenderness
            (iii) Palpitations
            (iv) Known murmurs
         (h) Pulmonary
            (i) Exertional dyspnea
            (ii) Cough
            (iii) Sputum
            (iv) Orthopnea
            (v) Respiratory tract infections including *Pneumocystis* pneumonia in immunodeficient patients
            (vi) Hemoptysis
         (i) GI
            (i) Anorexia
            (ii) Abdominal pain and cramping
            (iii) Abdominal fullness
            (iv) Eructation
            (v) Bloody or black stools
            (vi) Vomiting of blood or coffee-ground material
            (vii) Ulcers
            (viii) Change in bowel habits
               a) Diarrhea
               b) Constipation
            (ix) Rectal pain or bleeding
         (j) GU
            (i) Hematuria

(ii) Pyuria
(iii) Menorrhagia
(iv) Amenorrhea
(v) Incontinence, dysuria, hesitancy, frequency
(vi) Urinary retention
(vii) Pelvic or flank pain
(k) Neurologic
(i) Change in level of consciousness (LOC)
(ii) Confusion
(iii) Irritability
(iv) Memory loss
(v) Headache
(vi) Ataxia
(vii) Sensory changes: paresthesia, anesthesia
(viii) Syncope, vertigo
(l) Back and extremities
(i) Pain and/or tenderness in joints, back, shoulder, or bone
(ii) Joint stiffness or swelling
(iii) Muscle weakness

2. Medical history
a. Surgical history
(1) Splenectomy
(2) Tumor removal
(3) Thymectomy
(4) Breast implants
(5) Organ or tissue transplant
(6) Prosthetic heart valves
(7) Tonsillectomy
(8) Surgical excision of duodenum
(9) Total or partial gastrectomy
(10) Response to dental extractions (e.g., excessive bleeding)
b. Medical problems
(1) Recurrent infections
(2) Problems with wound healing
(3) Anemia
(4) Asthma
(5) Mononucleosis
(6) Malignancy, especially leukemia, lymphoma, multiple myeloma
(7) Autoimmune disease (e.g., lupus erythematosus)
(8) Radiation therapy
(9) Malabsorption syndrome
(10) Liver disease
(11) Renal failure
(12) Spleen disorders
(13) Diabetes mellitus
(14) Sexually transmitted disease
(15) Human immunodeficiency virus (HIV)/acquired immunodeficiency syndrome (AIDS)
(16) Prolonged or excessive bleeding (e.g., after dental procedures, injury, or surgery)
(17) Deep vein thrombosis or pulmonary embolus
(18) Vitamin K deficiency
c. Allergies
(1) Known allergies and type of reaction
(a) Inhalants
(b) Contactants
(c) Injectables
(d) Ingestibles
(2) Transfusion with blood or blood products
d. Immunizations: types, dates, any adverse reactions

3. Family history
a. Congenital immune deficiency
b. Congenital bleeding disorder (e.g., hemophilia)
c. Congenital RBC dyscrasias (e.g., sickle cell disease)
d. Congenital anemia (e.g., thalassemia)
e. Asthma
f. Allergies
g. Anemia
h. Jaundice
i. Malignancies
j. Autoimmune disease (e.g., systemic lupus erythematosus [SLE] or rheumatoid arthritis)

4. Social history
a. Relationship with spouse or significant other; family structure
b. Occupation
(1) Occupational exposure to radiation
(2) Occupational exposure to chemicals (e.g., lead, benzene, ethylene oxide, insecticides, or vinyl chloride)
(3) Military service; exposure to toxins
c. Educational level
d. Stress level and usual coping mechanisms; lifestyle changes
e. Recreational habits
f. Exercise habits
g. Dietary habits; dietary deficiency: iron, folic acid, vitamin B_{12}
h. Caffeine intake
i. Tobacco use: record as pack-years (number of packs per day times the number of years the patient has been smoking)
j. Alcohol use: record as alcoholic beverages consumed per month, week, or day
k. Recent foreign travel
l. Sexuality
(1) Safe sex practices
(2) Sexual preference: heterosexual; homosexual; bisexual
(3) Multiple sexual partners
(4) Sexual activity with prostitutes, homosexuals, or bisexuals

5. Medication history
a. Agents used to treat existing hematologic conditions
(1) Drugs used for erythropoiesis: iron, vitamin B_{12}, pyridoxine, folic acid, recombinant human erythropoietin
(2) Drugs used for bleeding or clotting disorders: cryoprecipitate, anticoagulants
(3) Antineoplastic agents
(4) Antiviral agents

(5) Drugs to augment the immune system (e.g., interferon, interleukin-2, and colony-stimulating factors)

b. Agents that may exert a negative effect on hematologic/immunologic system
   (1) Allergy medication
   (2) Analgesics
      (a) Acetaminophen: may decrease platelets; may cause hemolytic anemia
      (b) Antiinflammatory agents
         (i) Antigout drugs (e.g., colchicine): may cause aplastic anemia
         (ii) Aspirin: inhibits platelet aggregation; decreases macrophage activity
         (iii) Corticosteroids (e.g., prednisone): suppresses the immune/inflammatory process
         (iv) NSAIDs (e.g., phenylbutazone [Butazolidin] or ibuprofen [Motrin]): inhibit platelet aggregation; depress bone marrow and may cause aplastic anemia; lyse T, B, and NK cells; inhibit interferon production; inhibit IL-1 and IL-2 production
      (c) Narcotics
         (i) Heroin: may decrease platelets
         (ii) Morphine sulfate: may decrease platelets
   (3) Antibiotics
      (a) Oral antibiotics: may kill vitamin K–producing bacteria in the GI tract
      (b) All antibiotics may cause opportunistic infections by altering normal flora in GI tract, mouth, and vagina; *Clostridium difficile* is an organism frequently seen in critical care units that causes severe diarrhea
      (c) Tetracyclines: inhibit chemotaxis; inhibit activation of the lymphocytes
      (d) Sulfonamides: inhibit chemotaxis; inhibit activation of the lymphocytes; may cause aplastic anemia; may decrease platelets
      (e) Chloramphenicol: depresses WBC production; may cause aplastic anemia
      (f) Penicillin: may decrease platelets
      (g) Rifampicin: may decrease platelets
   (4) Anticonvulsants
      (a) Phenytoin (Dilantin): inhibits the effects of corticosteroids; may cause lymph node hyperplasia; may cause anemia or thrombocytopenia
      (b) Phenobarbital: may cause aplastic anemia
   (5) Antidysrhythmic drugs
      (a) Procainamide: may cause hemolytic anemia, thrombocytopenia; decreases production of WBCs
      (b) Quinidine: may cause hemolytic anemia or thrombocytopenia
      (c) Propranolol: inhibits platelet aggregation
   (6) Antifungals
      (a) Amphotericin B: may cause anemia or thrombocytopenia
   (7) Antihypertensives
      (a) Captopril (Capoten): may cause pancytopenia
      (b) Methyldopa (Aldomet): may cause thrombocytopenia, anemia
   (8) Antituberculin drugs (e.g., *p*-aminosalicylic acid or isoniazid [INH])
   (9) Diuretics
      (a) Chlorothiazide (Diuril): may cause anemia or thrombocytopenia
      (b) Furosemide (Lasix): may cause anemia or thrombocytopenia
   (10) Heparin: may decrease platelets
   (11) Histamine receptor antagonists (e.g., ranitidine): may decrease platelets
   (12) Immunosuppressives
   (13) Oral contraceptives and diethylstilbestrol
   (14) Oral hypoglycemic agents (e.g., chlorpropamide): may cause anemia or thrombocytopenia
   (15) Sympathomimetics (e.g., epinephrine): decrease chemotaxis; decrease WBC production and response to antigens; alter antibody production
   (16) Anesthetic agents (e.g., halothane, nitrous oxide, or cyclopropane): decrease phagocytosis and inhibit T cell function

c. Nonprescribed drug use
   (1) Over-the-counter drugs
   (2) Vitamins, minerals, herbs
   (3) Substance abuse: injectable drug use especially if needles are shared
      (a) Intravenous (IV) drug use
      (b) Intramuscular steroid use
      (c) Intradermal "poppers"

Physical Examination

1. Vital signs
   a. Weight: weight loss
   b. Heart rate: tachycardia frequently seen with blood loss or infection
   c. Blood pressure: hypotension seen with blood loss
   d. Temperature: hyperthermia frequently seen with infection but less likely seen in elderly patients
2. Inspection
   a. Skin and appendages
      (1) Color
         (a) Pallor or flushing of mucous membranes and palmar creases
         (b) Pallor of conjunctivae
         (c) Cyanosis
         (d) Jaundice
         (e) Brownish skin discoloration
         (f) Areas of hyperpigmentation
         (g) Signs of inflammation
      (2) Bleeding
         (a) Petechiae

(b) Ecchymosis
(c) Purpura
(d) Mucous membrane bleeding
(e) Gingival bleeding
(f) Retinal hemorrhages
(g) Hemorrhage from orifices
(3) Moisture
(a) Dry, rough skin (xeroderma)
(b) Moisture-related skin breakdown may occur at skin folds (e.g., axillae, groin, and perineal areas); fungal infections are common in these areas
(4) Lesions and wounds
(a) Rash
(b) Excoriated skin
(c) Leg ulcers
(d) IV catheter insertion sites
(e) Chest tube insertion site
(f) Surgical or traumatic wounds
(g) Orthopedic devices
(h) Drains
(5) Pitting edema of extremities
(6) Hair: alopecia
(7) Nail and nailbed
(a) Pallor of nailbeds
(b) Spoon nails
(c) Clubbing
b. Mouth
(1) Dryness of the mouth (xerostomia)
(2) Gingival and mucosal ulceration
(3) Swollen, reddened, bleeding gums
(4) Smooth tongue texture
(5) White coating on tongue (candidiasis, also called *thrush*)
(6) White, irregular lesions on lateral surfaces of tongue (oral hairy leukoplakia frequently seen in HIV-positive patients)
(7) Purplish lesions on tongue
(8) Beefy, red tongue
c. GI: nasogastric tube
d. Neuromuscular
(1) Decreased LOC
(2) Pupil changes
(3) Decreased sensation
(4) Muscle weakness
3. Palpation
a. Enlargement or tenderness of superficial lymph nodes
b. Tenderness during sternal or rib palpation
c. Tenderness during abdominal palpation
d. Hepatomegaly
e. Splenomegaly
4. Percussion
a. Decreased deep tendon reflexes
b. Diaphragmatic excursion
c. Hepatomegaly
d. Splenomegaly
5. Auscultation
a. Cardiovascular
(1) Dysrhythmia
(2) S_3
(3) S_4
(4) Murmur
(5) Rub
(6) Bruits over carotid arteries and aorta
b. Pulmonary
(1) Crackles
(2) Pleural rub
c. Abdomen
(1) Bowel sounds
(2) Peritoneal friction rub

Diagnostic Studies

1. Blood
a. Hematology
(1) RBCs: normal 4.4 to 5.9 × 10^6 cells/mL for males; 3.8 to 5.2 × 10^6 cells/mL for females
(a) Quantity
(i) Elevated in dehydration, chronic hypoxemia, or high altitudes; may increase temporarily after a cold shower or with intense emotions
(ii) Decreased in hemorrhage, anemias, leukemias, or hypothyroidism
(b) Quality
(i) Microcytic: RBCs too small
(ii) Macrocytic: RBCs too large
(iii) Hypochromic: hemoglobin concentration too low
(iv) Hyperchromic: hemoglobin concentration too high
(2) Reticulocyte count: normal 0.5% to 1.5% of RBC count
(a) Young RBCs
(b) Assesses the responsiveness and potential of the bone marrow to respond to bleeding or hemolysis
(3) Erythrocyte sedimentation rate: normal 1 to 13 mm/hr for males, 1 to 20 mm/hr for females
(a) Nonspecific test; measures the amount of RBCs that settle in 1 hour
(b) Elevated in inflammatory processes (e.g., rheumatoid arthritis, malignancy, rheumatic fever, hemolytic anemia, thyroid disorders, autoimmune disorders, and nephrotic syndrome)
(c) Decreased in polycythemia vera, hypofibrinogenemia, sickle cell anemia, and heart failure
(4) Hemoglobin: normal 13 to 18 g/dL for males; 12 to 16 g/dL for females
(a) Elevated in polycythemia, which may occur in chronic hypoxia or high altitudes
(b) Decreased in anemia and hemorrhage
(5) Hematocrit: normal 40% to 52% for males; 35% to 47% for females
(a) Elevated in dehydration or polycythemia
(b) Decreased with anemia, leukemia, or normal hemoglobin and water overload

(6) Red cell indexes
  (a) Mean corpuscular volume (an average of size): normal 80 to 100 fL
  (b) Mean corpuscular hemoglobin (an average of weight of hemoglobin in an RBC): normal 26.6 to 34 pg
  (c) Mean corpuscular hemoglobin concentration: normal 31.4 to 36.3 g/dL
(7) Peripheral smear: evaluation of blood cell size, shape, and composition
(8) WBC count: 3500 to 11,000 cells/mm^3
  (a) Elevated in infection; trauma; surgery; acute leukemia; stress
  (b) Decreased in bone marrow depression (e.g., aplastic anemia, agranulocytosis, chronic leukemia, sepsis, and autoimmune disorders)
(9) Differential
  (a) Neutrophils: normal 40% to 80%
    (i) Elevated in infection, inflammatory processes, malignancy, trauma, hemorrhage, burns, tissue necrosis (e.g., myocardial infarction), and ketoacidosis
    (ii) Decreased in overwhelming infection, bone marrow depression, vitamin B_{12} or folic acid deficiency, and hypersplenism
  (b) Eosinophils: normal 0% to 5%
    (i) Elevated in the following:
      a) Allergic conditions
        i) Asthma
        ii) Eczema
      b) Leukemia
      c) Autoimmune disorders
      d) Parasitic infection especially helminthic infections
    (ii) Decreased in the following:
      a) Adrenocortical stimulation
      b) Stress
      c) Cushing's syndrome
      d) SLE
  (c) Basophils: 0% to 2%
    (i) Elevated in allergic conditions, inflammatory processes, graft rejection, acute leukemia, and recent splenectomy
    (ii) Decreased in hyperthyroidism and long-term corticosteroid therapy
  (d) Monocytes: 3% to 8%
    (i) Elevated in chronic inflammatory conditions, anemia, malignancy, mononucleosis, and acute HIV infection
    (ii) Decreased in immunodeficiency disorders
  (e) Lymphocytes: 10% to 40%
    (i) Elevated in chronic lymphocytic leukemia; chronic infections: bacterial and viral; multiple myeloma; mononucleosis; Cushing's syndrome

Table 10-8 Lymphocyte Assays

Lymphocyte Type	Percentage or Ratio of Lymphocytes
Total T cells	70%-80%
CD4 (helper T cells)	29%-60%
CD8 (suppressor T cells)	18%-42%
CD4/CD8 (helper/suppressor ratio)	0.8:2.9
Total B cells	10%-20%

    (ii) Decreased in immunodeficiency disorders (e.g., AIDS, SLE, leukemia, antineoplastic drug use, steroid use, and sepsis)
    (iii) Lymphocyte assays (Table 10-8)
      a) T cells
      b) B cells
      c) NK cells
  (f) Changes in differential
    (i) Shift to the left: increased percentage of bands; seen in infection
    (ii) Shift to the right: increased percentage of segmented neutrophils; seen in pernicious anemia or hepatic disease
    (iii) Regenerative shift: elevated WBC with increased percentage of bands; indicative of stimulation of bone marrow
    (iv) Degenerative shift: decreased WBC with increased percentage of bands; indicative of bone marrow depression
(10) Platelets: normal 150,000 to 400,000/mm^3; decreased in SLE, HIV infection, idiopathic thrombocytopenic purpura, and DIC
  (a) 50,000 to 100,000/mm^3: prolonged bleeding times, increased risk of bleeding after severe trauma or surgery
  (b) Fewer than 50,000/mm^3: increased risk of bleeding after minor trauma
  (c) Fewer than 20,000/mm^3: risk of spontaneous bleeding, including intracranial bleeding

b. Clotting profile
(1) PT: normal 12 to 15 seconds; assesses extrinsic coagulation pathway and the common pathway
(2) International normalized ratio: therapeutic ratio is usually 2 to 3 but may be higher depending on indications for anticoagulant therapy
  (a) Mathematical calculation that accounts for the differences in sensitivity between reagents; therefore, it standardizes PT values

(3) aPTT: normal 25 to 38 seconds; assesses intrinsic coagulation pathway and the common pathway
(4) Activated clotting time (ACT): therapeutic activated clotting time during procedures that require anticoagulation (e.g., percutaneous coronary intervention) is usually 300 to 350 seconds
  (a) Bedside test used to monitor heparin-induced anticoagulation
  (b) Sheath removal generally is delayed until activated clotting time is less than 150 seconds
(5) Thrombin time: normal 10 to 15 seconds; assesses time for thrombin to convert fibrinogen to a fibrin clot
(6) Bleeding time: normal 1 to 4 minutes; assesses platelet function
(7) Lee White clotting time: normal 6 to 12 minutes; nonspecific test for clotting abnormalities
(8) Fibrinogen: normal 200 to 400 mg/dL
  (a) Elevated in hypercoagulable states and inflammatory conditions
  (b) Decreased in hypocoagulable states with propensity to bleed
(9) FSPs (also referred to as *fibrin degradation products*: normal 0-10 mcg/dL; elevated in excessive fibrinolysis (e.g., DIC)
(10) D dimer: normal less than 250 ng/mL; elevated in DIC
(11) Specific factor assays: measure amounts of each factor in the blood

c. Serum proteins
(1) Total protein: normal 6 to 8 g/dL
(2) Albumin: normal 3.5 to 4.5 g/dL
(3) C-reactive protein: normal less than 0.8 mg/dL; nonspecific test for evaluating severity and course of inflammatory conditions
(4) Serum protein electrophoresis: immunoglobulin analysis (Table 10-9)
(5) Complement assay
  (a) Components
    (i) Total complement: normal 41 to 90 hemolytic units
    (ii) C1 esterase inhibitor: normal 16 to 33 mg/dL
    (iii) C3: normal 88 to 252 mg/dL in men; 88 to 206 mg/dL in women
    (iv) C4: normal 12 to 72 mg/dL in men; 13 to 75 mg/dL in women
  (b) Decreased total complement levels occurs in the following:
    (i) SLE
    (ii) Acute poststreptococcal glomerulonephritis
    (iii) Acute serum sickness
    (iv) Cirrhosis of the liver
    (v) Multiple myeloma
    (vi) Severe immunodeficiency
    (vii) Rapidly rejecting allografts

Table 10-9 Immunoglobulin Analysis

Immunoglobulin	Increased	Decreased
IgG	• Infection • Hepatitis A • Glomerulonephritis • Rheumatoid arthritis • SLE • AIDS • IgG myeloma	• Agammaglobulinemia • Chronic lymphocytic leukemia
IgM	• Hepatitis A and B • Chronic infections • SLE • Rheumatoid arthritis • Sjögren syndrome • AIDS	• Hypogammaglobulinemia • Chronic lymphocytic leukemia • IgG myeloma • IgA myeloma • Agammaglobulinemia
IgA	• SLE • Rheumatoid arthritis • IgA myeloma	• IgA deficiency • Acute and chronic lymphocytic leukemia • Agammaglobulinemia • IgG myeloma • Chronic infections
IgE	• Allergic rhinitis • Allergic asthma • Parasitic infection	• IgA deficiency • Intrinsic asthma
IgD	• Eczema • Skin disorders	• Unknown

AIDS, Acquired immunodeficiency syndrome; *SLE*, systemic lupus erythematosus.

(c) Elevated total complement levels occur in the following:
(i) Obstructive jaundice
(ii) Thyroiditis
(iii) Acute rheumatic fever
(iv) Rheumatoid arthritis
(v) Acute myocardial infarction
(vi) Ulcerative colitis
(vii) Diabetes mellitus

d. Chemistry
(1) Calcium: normal 8.5 to 10.5 mg/dL
(2) Bilirubin: normal total bilirubin 0.3 to 1.3 mg/dL
(a) Indirect (before being conjugated by liver): 0.1 to 1 mg/dL
(b) Direct (after being conjugated by liver): 0.1 to 0.3 mg/dL
(3) Iron: normal 50 to 150 mcg/dL
(4) Total iron-binding capacity: normal 250 to 410 mcg/dL

e. Type and crossmatch
(1) Blood typing: determined by agglutination studies
(2) Rh factor determination
(3) Coombs' test: detects immune antibodies important in crossmatching
(a) Direct: normal negative; measures antibodies (IgG) attached to RBCs
(b) Indirect: normal negative; measures antibodies (IgG) in the serum

f. HLA: evaluates tissue compatibility
(1) Tissue
(a) Complement-dependent cytotoxic assay
(b) Mixed lymphocyte culture
(2) Crossmatching

g. Immune profile
(1) CD4 cell count: normal 800 cells/mm^3; varies with age
(a) Measured helper T cells
(b) Decreased in HIV infection and AIDS; assists in staging HIV infection
(2) T4/T8 (CD4/CD8) ratio
(a) Helper cells: suppressor/cytotoxic cells ratio: normal 1.8
(b) Normally more CD4 cells than CD8 cells
(c) Reverse ratio in HIV infection or AIDS

h. HIV antibody screening: normal negative
(1) Detects antibodies to HIV; present with exposure to HIV, but absence does not mean that the patient has not been exposed because time is required for development of antibodies
(2) Does not indicate immunity
(3) Types of tests
(a) Enzyme-linked immunosorbent assay (ELISA): screening test subject to error; up to 10% false-positive results
(b) Western blot: more specific than ELISA

i. HIV virus screening (e.g., polymerase chain reaction: normal negative)

j. HIV viral load testing
(1) May range from imperceptible (less than 25 to 5000 copies of HIV per milliliter) to 1 million or more copies per milliliter; consider that the higher the viral load, the more rapid the damage from HIV
(2) Used to evaluate the effectiveness of antiretroviral therapy

2. Culture and sensitivity: various body secretions (e.g., blood, urine, or wound secretions)
a. Gram stain: identification of gram-positive or gram-negative bacteria
b. Culture: identification of microorganism
c. Sensitivity
(1) Minimum inhibitory concentration: the smallest concentration of antibiotic that effectively inhibits bacterial growth; reported as antibiotic concentration per milliliter of solution necessary for growth inhibition
(2) This is compared with the achievable blood level of the antibiotic
(a) If this level is less than the minimum inhibitory concentration, the bacterium is considered resistant to that antibiotic.
(b) If this level is greater than the minimum inhibitory concentration, the bacterium is considered sensitive to that antibiotic.
(3) Other factors such as known adverse effects of the antibiotic also are considered

3. Urine
a. RBCs: normal 0 to 2 per low-power field; RBCs in the urine may indicate trauma (e.g., renal calculi) or bleeding disorder (e.g., DIC)
b. WBCs: normal 0 to 4 per low-power field; WBCs in the catheterized urine specimen indicate urinary tract infection
c. Bilirubin: normal none; urobilinogen indicates biliary obstruction or liver disease

4. Stool
a. Blood: may be grossly bloody or guaiac positive in bleeding disorders
b. Culture and/or toxins: may show opportunistic infections (e.g., *Clostridium difficile* in immunodeficient patients)

5. Radiologic and radioisotope studies
a. Chest x-ray
b. Flat plate of abdomen
c. Lymphangiography: visualizes the lymph system after injection of dye; assists in node assessment
d. Isotopic lymphangiography: uses technetium 99m and is less invasive than radiographic lymphangiography
e. Scans: liver, spleen, or bone
f. Computed tomography scan of abdomen for evaluation of liver, spleen, and lymph nodes

6. Biopsy
a. Bone marrow
b. Lymph node
(1) Open: direct visualization; performed in operating room
(2) Closed or needle: performed at bedside

c. Synovial
d. Biopsy of transplanted organs to look for indications of rejection
7. Anergy panel testing
a. Administration of antigen for observation of a delayed inflammatory skin reaction
(1) Tuberculosis, mumps, *Candida*, and trichophytin are used most frequently.
(2) Mumps antigen is contraindicated in patients allergic to chicken or eggs.
b. Normal response: a negative response to tuberculosis (unless the patient previously has been exposed to tuberculosis) and a positive reaction to several of the other antigens within 24 to 72 hours
c. Abnormal responses
(1) Anergy: failure to respond to any of the injections
(2) Immunodeficiency: induration of less than 5 mm in diameter

Anemia

Definition

Decrease in the quantity or quality of circulating RBCs caused by the following:

1. Decrease in RBC or hemoglobin production
2. Excessive loss of RBCs
3. Excessive lysis of RBCs earlier than the 120-day life expectancy of the RBC

Etiology

1. Iron deficiency anemia
a. Inadequate intake of iron-rich foods
b. Absorption deficiency
c. Ingestion or occupational exposure to lead
2. Pernicious anemia: deficiency of intrinsic factor necessary for absorption of vitamin B_{12}
a. Hereditary, affecting primarily persons of northern European descent but also may affect persons of African and Hispanic descent
b. Autoimmune disorder
c. GI disorders
(1) Gastritis
(2) Gastric resection
(3) Crohn's disease
(4) Bowel resection
(5) Pancreatic insufficiency
d. Medications such as proton pump inhibitors and antineoplastics
3. Folic acid deficiency anemia
a. Inadequate intake of folic acid–rich foods
b. Anorexia nervosa
c. Elderly
4. Acute blood loss anemia
a. GI: esophageal varices, gastric ulcers, lower GI bleed
b. GU: renal trauma, menorrhagia
c. Trauma: bleeding may be overt or occult
d. Coagulopathies
5. Anemia of chronic illness
a. Renal failure
b. Cancer
6. Aplastic anemia: failure of the bone marrow to produce blood cells; some degree of pancytopenia is present
a. Congenital
b. Acquired
(1) Idiopathic
(2) Chemicals
(a) Benzene
(b) Benzene-containing chemicals
(i) Kerosene
(ii) Carbon tetrachloride
(iii) Toluene
(3) Drugs
(a) Antineoplastics
(b) Antiarthritics
(c) Antibiotics
(d) Anticonvulsants
(e) Antidysrhythmic drugs
(f) Antihypertensives
(g) Antithyroid agents
(h) Diuretics
(i) NSAIDs
(j) Oral hypoglycemic agents
(k) Platelet aggregation inhibitors
(l) Psychotropics
(4) Radiation
(5) Viruses
(6) Pregnancy
7. Sickle cell anemia: hereditary, affecting primarily persons of African descent but also may affect persons of Hispanic, Mediterranean, or Middle Eastern descent

Pathophysiology

1. General
a. Reduced oxygen-carrying capacity of the blood
b. Tissue ischemia
c. Anaerobic metabolism
d. Local acidosis
e. Cellular edema
2. Specific to pernicious anemia
a. Inherited autoimmune disorder that produces parietal cell antibodies, or excessive drinking or smoking or gastric resection
b. Defective gastric secretion of the glycoprotein intrinsic factor
c. Ineffective erythropoiesis
3. Specific to aplastic anemia: stem cell defect or injury or destruction of hematopoietic cells
4. Specific to sickle cell anemia
a. Hereditary disorder causes presence of hemoglobin S, an abnormal form of hemoglobin A.
b. Crystallization of the abnormal hemoglobin is promoted by deoxygenation, dehydration, acidosis, temperature changes.
c. RBCs become crescent or sickle shaped after they release oxygen.

d. These misshapen RBCs get stuck in the blood vessels, causing occlusion, tissue injury, and pain.
e. Vascular occlusion may cause myocardial infarction, ischemic stroke, splenic or hepatic infarction, blindness, and bone necrosis.
f. Chronic hemolysis occurs because sickled RBCs are destroyed within 15 days.
g. Immunocompromise occurs because spleen function is compromised.

Clinical Presentation

1. Subjective
   a. Weakness, fatigue
   b. Anorexia, indigestion, epigastric pain, oral pain related to glossitis
   c. Exertional dyspnea
   d. Palpitations
   e. Chest pain
   f. Paresthesia
2. Objective
   a. Pallor
   b. Tachycardia
   c. Tachypnea
   d. Glossitis
   e. Brittle or fine hair
   f. Diarrhea or constipation
   g. Flow murmur (i.e., systolic murmur associated with the turbulence of increased flow of blood through the heart)
   h. Impaired proprioception progressing to ataxia
3. Diagnostic
   a. RBC quantity: less than 4.4 to 5.9 × 10^6 cells/mL for males or 3.8 to 5.2 × 10^6 cells/mL for females
   b. RBC quality
      (1) Microcytic, hypochromic
      (2) Normocytic, normochromic
      (3) Macrocytic, normochromic
4. Specifics depending on type of anemia
   a. Specifically iron deficiency anemia
      (1) Microcytic, hypochromic RBCs
   b. Specific to pernicious anemia
      (1) Neurologic changes such as paresthesias and numbness progressing to loss of balance and dementia
      (2) Decreased RBC, hemoglobin, and hematocrit
      (3) Macrocytic, normocytic RBCs
      (4) Increased mean corpuscular volume, normal mean corpuscular hemoglobin
      (5) Increased serum bilirubin
      (6) Decreased fasting serum vitamin B_{12}
      (7) Normal serum folate (to rule out folate deficiency)
      (8) Schilling test: abnormal; indicates impaired vitamin B_{12} absorption
   c. Specific to folic acid deficiency anemia: macrocytic, normocytic RBCs
   d. Specific to acute blood loss anemia: normocytic, normochromic
   e. Specific to anemia of chronic illness: normocytic, normochromic or macrocytic, normocytic
   f. Specific to aplastic anemia: normocytic, normochromic
   g. Specific to sickle cell crisis
      (1) Chest pain
      (2) Fever
      (3) Jaundice with chronic hemolysis
      (4) Complete blood count
         (a) Severe reduction in RBC count, hemoglobin, and hematocrit
         (b) Reticulocyte count: decreased
         (c) Presence of nucleated RBCs and sickled RBCs
      (5) Chest x-ray: pulmonary infiltrates

Nursing Diagnoses

1. Deficient Fluid Volume related to inadequate circulating blood volume
2. Ineffective Tissue Perfusion related to inadequate hemoglobin
3. Decreased Cardiac Output related to decreased or increased preload
4. Risk for Excess Fluid Volume related to too rapid an administration of blood
5. Risk for Injury related to transfusion reaction and blood-transmitted disease

Collaborative Practice

1. Improve oxygen-carrying capacity.
   a. Oxygen to increase Sao_2 by pulse oximetry (Spo_2) to at least 95% unless contraindicated
   b. IV administration of fluids to ensure adequate intravascular volume
   c. Blood and blood products as prescribed (Table 10-10)
      (1) Administer blood and blood products safely.
         (a) Insert or ensure patency of IV catheter; do not use a catheter (or lumen) smaller than 20 gauge.
         (b) Ensure that the type and crossmatch has been done and that blood or blood component is available.
         (c) Assess vital signs: notify physician if temperature is 37.8°C (100°F) or higher.
         (d) Request blood or blood component from blood bank when ready to administer it within 20 to 30 minutes; if you cannot begin the transfusion within 30 minutes after receiving it, return it to the blood bank.
         (e) Check all of the following before administration of blood or blood component:
            (i) Physician prescription for blood or blood product
            (ii) Consent form signed by the patient (according to hospital policy)

Table 10-10 Blood and Blood Products

Product	Contents	Compatibility Required	Uses	Volume/Unit	Comments
Whole blood	RBCs, WBCs, platelets, plasma, and clotting factors	ABO, Rh specific NOTE: In emergency situations, type-specific blood or O-negative blood may be used.	Restores blood volume and oxygen-carrying capacity	Approximately 500 mL	• Must be fresh (less than 4 hours old) to preserve platelet function • Administer over 2-4 hours • Best for hemorrhagic shock
Packed RBCs	RBCs and 20% plasma	ABO, Rh specific preferred; ABO, Rh compatible required	Restores oxygen-carrying capacity	Approximately 250 mL	• Increases hemoglobin by 1 g/dL/unit and hematocrit by 2%-3% per unit; this change takes at least 6-12 hours • Administer over 2-4 hours
Washed RBCs	RBCs and 20% plasma with fewer WBCs and platelets than packed RBCs	ABO, Rh specific preferred; ABO, Rh compatible required	Restores oxygen-carrying capacity in patients previously sensitized by transfusions	Approximately 250 mL	• As for packed RBCs • Must be administered within 24 hours of washing
Leukocyte-poor RBCs	RBCs, plasma but no leukocytes	ABO, Rh specific preferred; ABO, Rh compatible required	Restores oxygen-carrying capacity in patients susceptible to febrile reactions	Approximately 250 mL	• As for packed RBCs
Platelets	Platelets, WBCs, plasma	ABO, Rh specific or compatible	Corrects low platelet levels to aid in clotting	Approximately 50 mL	• Administer 1 unit over 10 minutes • Will increase platelet count by 5000-10,000/mm^3 • Agitate often as platelets tend to settle
Fresh frozen plasma	Water, plasma proteins, clotting factors	Rh compatibility required; ABO compatibility preferred	Expands blood volume Restores clotting factor deficiencies Contains no Platelets	Approximately 250 mL	• Takes 20 minutes to thaw • Must be given within 6 hours of thawing • Administer 1 unit over 1-2 hours or more rapidly if for hemorrhage
Granulocytes	WBCs, small amount of plasma	ABO, Rh compatible; human leukocyte antigen compatible if possible	Restores granulocytes in life-threatening granulocytopenia	Approximately 300 mL	• Administer rapidly • Chills and fever may occur; steroids and antihistamines may be given; meperidine may be used for shivering • Administer over 2-6 hours
Cryoprecipitate	Factors VIII and XIII, fibrinogen, fibronectin	ABO specific or compatible	Replaces clotting factors	Approximately 10 mL; usually 10 bags pooled	• Administer rapidly immediately after thawing • May administer 30 units at one time

Continued

Table 10-10 Blood and Blood Products—cont'd

Product	Contents	Compatibility Required	Uses	Volume/Unit	Comments
Albumin	Albumin from plasma	No compatibility required	Provides volume expansion (no clotting factors)	5%: 200 or 500 mL 25%: 50 mL or 100 mL	• Administer 1 mL/min or more rapidly if patient is in shock • Chemically processed, so no risk of hepatitis
Plasma protein fraction	Albumin and globulin in saline solution	No compatibility required	Provides volume expansion (no clotting factors)	5%: 200-500 mL	• Administer 10 mL/min • Chemically processed, so no risk of hepatitis

RBCs, Red blood cells; *WBCs,* white blood cells.

(iii) Confirm the following with another registered nurse:
a) Patient's name and hospital number on patient identification bracelet
b) Type of blood component
c) Patient's blood group and Rh type
d) Donor's blood group and Rh type
e) Unit number of blood or blood component
f) Expiration date of the blood or blood component

(f) Sign the transfusion record along with the registered nurse who confirmed the required information.

(g) Prime the blood administration set with normal (0.9%) saline, allowing the normal saline to cover the filter; use only normal saline; do not use dextrose-containing solutions or lactated Ringer's solution.

(h) Warm the blood if indicated.
(i) Blood may be warmed to avoid hypothermia in the patient receiving four or more units over 6 hours or in the patient who has tested positive for cold agglutinins.
(ii) Warm the blood to between 32° and 37°C using a blood-warming device in these situations.

(i) Clamp off the saline, and start the blood or blood component.

(j) Adjust rate to administer slowly 25 to 50 mL within the first 15 minutes.

(k) Monitor for transfusion reaction (Table 10-11 and Box 10-1).

Table 10-11 Types of Transfusion Reactions

Type of Reaction	Etiology	Clinical Indications	Timing	Treatment
Febrile (nonhemolytic; the most common type of transfusion reaction)	Antigen-antibody reaction to white blood cells, platelets, or plasma proteins in the blood product	• Fever (rise in temperature greater than 1°C) • Chills • Headache • Nausea, vomiting • Flushing • Anxiety • Muscle pain	Immediately or up to 6 hours after transfusion	• Stop transfusion • Keep vein open with saline • Notify physician and blood bank • Send blood specimens to blood bank • Administer antipyretics as indicated • Steroids may be prescribed • Washed or leukocyte-poor blood should be considered for future transfusions
Mild allergic (type I hypersensitivity reaction)	Allergic reaction to plasma-soluble antigen in blood product	• Flushing • Itching • Urticaria • Hives	During transfusion or up to 1 hour after transfusion	• If febrile, stop transfusion • If afebrile, slow transfusion to keep-vein-open rate until advised by physician • Notify physician and blood bank • Monitor vital signs • Administer antihistamines as prescribed

Table 10-11 Types of Transfusion Reactions—cont'd

Type of Reaction	Etiology	Clinical Indications	Timing	Treatment
Anaphylaxis (type I hypersensitivity reaction)	Allergic reaction in patients with IgA deficiency sensitized to IgA through previous transfusion or pregnancy	• Anxiety • Urticaria • Facial edema • Dysphagia • Abdominal cramps, diarrhea • Urinary incontinence • Dyspnea • Stridor • Wheezing • Cyanosis • Chest pain or pulmonary edema may occur • Shock may occur • Cardiopulmonary arrest may occur	Immediately; after transfusion of only a few milliliters of blood	• Stop transfusion • Keep vein open with saline • Notify physician and blood bank • Administer oxygen • Administer antihistamines, steroids, and/or aqueous epinephrine as prescribed • Emergency airway and/or cardiopulmonary resuscitation may be necessary • Washed or leukocyte-poor blood or blood from IgA–deficient donor should be considered for future transfusions
Acute hemolytic (type II hypersensitivity reaction)	ABO group incompatibility; antibodies in recipient's plasma attach to antigens in transfused RBCs, causing RBC destruction	• Burning sensation along vein • Lumbar pain • Chills • Fever • Flushing • Nausea, vomiting • Tachycardia, tachypnea • Hypotension (may be only sign in unconscious patient) • May even have the following: ◦ Dyspnea ◦ Chest pain ◦ Hemoglobinemia ◦ Hemoglobinuria ◦ Anuria ◦ Disseminated intravascular coagulation • Shock may occur • Cardiopulmonary arrest may occur	Usually within 15 minutes after initiation of transfusion but may occur anytime during transfusion; may be delayed if Rh incompatibility	• Stop transfusion • Keep vein open with saline • Notify physician and blood bank • Send blood unit and blood sample from the patient to the blood bank immediately • Monitor vital signs and urine output • Administer fluids for shock as prescribed • Diuretics (usually mannitol) may be prescribed, especially if hemoglobinuria occurs • Monitor for acute renal failure and shock • Request new crossmatch
Delayed hemolytic	Alloimmune response causes slow hemolysis	• Fever • Mild jaundice • Purpura • Anemia	Days to weeks after completion of transfusion	• Monitor urine output and hemoglobin and hematocrit levels
Noncardiac pulmonary edema	Donor antibodies react with recipient human leukocyte antigen	• Fever, chills • Dyspnea • Cough • Crackles • Hypoxemia • Shock	During transfusion or shortly after the transfusion	• Stop transfusion • Administer oxygen • Intubation and mechanical ventilation may be necessary • Steroids may be prescribed
Circulatory overload	Fluid administered faster than the cardiovascular system can accommodate	• Tachycardia • Hypertension • Headache • Jugular venous distention	During transfusion or shortly after the transfusion	• Administer RBCs no more rapidly than 4 mL/kg/hr unless severe hemorrhage is occurring • Slow or stop transfusion

Continued

Table 10-11 Types of Transfusion Reactions—cont'd

Type of Reaction	Etiology	Clinical Indications	Timing	Treatment
		• Increased RAP, PAP, PAOP • Dyspnea • Cough • Crackles		• Continue intravenous administration of saline slowly if transfusion is discontinued • Position patient upright with legs over the side of bed • Administer oxygen as indicated • Administer diuretics or venous vasodilators as indicated
Sepsis	Transfusion of contaminated blood components (blood should be infused within 4 hours)	• Chills • Fever • Vomiting • Abdominal pain • Diarrhea (may be bloody) • Hypotension • Shock	During or after transfusion	• Stop the transfusion • Obtain cultures of patient's blood and send with remaining blood to blood bank • Administer antibiotics as prescribed • Administer fluids or steroids as prescribed • Vasopressors may be needed
Graft-versus-host disease	Occurs in immunodeficient patients who receive lymphocytes; involves donor's lymphocytes mounting an attack against the recipient's tissues	• Fever • Rash • Stomatitis • Hepatitis • Severe diarrhea • Bone marrow suppression • Infection • Lymphadenopathy • Hepatosplenomegaly	Days to weeks after transfusion	• Steroids as prescribed • Methotrexate or azathioprine (Imuran) may be prescribed

PAOP, Pulmonary artery occlusive pressure; *PAP,* pulmonary artery pressure; *RAP,* right arterial pressure; *RBCs,* red blood cells.

BOX 10-1 Clinical Indications of Blood Transfusion Reaction in an Unconscious or Sedated Patient

Bleeding
Fever
Hypotension
Oliguria or anuria
Tachycardia or bradycardia
Visible signs of hemoglobin in urine

(i) Ask the patient to notify the nurse if he or she develops chills, low back pain, shortness of breath, nausea, sweating, itching, hives, or anxiety.
(ii) Assess patient for clinical indications of transfusion reaction (Table 10-12).
(iii) Take appropriate action for transfusion reactions (Table 10-12 and Box 10-2) if they occur.
(iv) Monitor vital signs every 15 minutes for the first hour and then every 30 minutes until transfusion is complete or according to hospital policy.
(v) Adjust rate to infuse blood within 4 hours of initiating the infusion; fresh frozen plasma, platelet, and granulocytes are administered rapidly; if the blood slows, do the following:
a) Ensure that the roller clamp is open.
b) Increase the height of the blood bag.
c) Gently squeeze the bag several times to agitate the blood cells.
d) Gently squeeze the tubing and flashbulb.
e) Remove dressing and check site.
f) Close the blood and open the saline to allow 50 to 100 mL to irrigate the line, and then restart the blood.
(vi) Flush administration set tubing with saline after transfusion is complete.
(vii) Disconnect the empty blood bag from the administration set, and dispose of these according to hospital policy.

(2) Monitor patient for adverse effects (Table 10-12) and complications.

d. Transfusion-related infections and complications
(1) Hepatitis
(a) Hepatitis B transmission has been reduced by mandatory testing of all donor blood for hepatitis B surface antigen.

Table **10-12 Potential Adverse Effects of Blood Transfusion**

Complications	Clinical Indications	Prevention/Treatment
Citrate intoxication and hypocalcemia caused by binding of citrate with calcium	• Paresthesia of fingertips and circumoral area • Chvostek's sign • Trousseau's sign • Muscle cramps, tremors • Increased deep tendon reflexes, carpopedal spasm • Abdominal cramps, biliary colic • Confusion, psychosis • Memory loss • Laryngospasm, stridor • Tetany (characterized by cramps, twitching of the muscles, sharp flexion of the wrist and ankle joints, and seizures) • Electrocardiogram changes ◦ Prolonged QT interval ◦ Dysrhythmias	• Monitor calcium in patients receiving multiple transfusions and/or patients with hepatic or renal disease • Administer 500 mg to 1 g of calcium every three to five units of blood as prescribed
Hyperkalemia caused by hemolysis of stored blood and liberation of potassium (NOTE: The older the blood, the higher the potassium content in the blood.)	• Tachycardia progressing to bradycardia and cardiac arrest • Nausea, vomiting, intestinal colic, diarrhea • Muscle weakness progressing to flaccid paralysis • Numbness, tingling of extremities • Increased deep tendon reflexes • Fatigue • Lethargy, apathy, mental confusion • Respiratory muscle weakness may cause hypopnea, dyspnea • Respiratory distress • Oliguria • Decreased contractility, cardiac output • Electrocardiogram changes ◦ Tall, peaked T waves ◦ Wide QRS complex ◦ Prolonged PR interval ◦ Flattened to absent P wave ◦ Bradycardia ◦ Dysrhythmias	• Monitor potassium closely in patients receiving stored blood (especially patients with renal insufficiency) • Dextrose and insulin may be prescribed acutely for patients with cardiac effects of hyperkalemia
Loss of 2,3-diphosphoglycerate (2,3-DPG) (2,3-DPG is a by-product of glucose metabolism on the hemoglobin molecule; banked [refrigerated] blood is low in 2,3-DPG; 2,3-DPG encourages unloading between hemoglobin and oxygen)	• Clinical indications of hypoxia (e.g., tachycardia, dysrhythmias, cyanosis, restlessness, and confusion)	• Especially a problem if massive amounts of banked blood are administered • Give fresh whole blood when possible for patients in need of multiple transfusions
Ammonia intoxication Occurs in older blood; especially a problem for patients with hepatic disease	• Decreased cardiac output: hypotension • Confusion • Altered level of consciousness • Elevated serum ammonia	• Avoid use of older blood, especially for massive transfusion • Monitor for ammonia intoxication in patients with hepatic disease
Dilutional coagulopathy	• Prolonged prothrombin time and partial thromboplastin time • Bleeding from needle site and wound	• Administer 2 units of fresh frozen plasma and/or platelets for every 10 units of packed red blood cells as prescribed
Hypothermia	• Decrease in body temperature • Decrease in tissue delivery of oxygen caused by shift of the oxyhemoglobin dissociation curve to the left, resulting in increased affinity between hemoglobin and oxygen	• Warm blood to 35° to 37°C if large quantities of blood are being administered

BOX 10-2 Nursing Actions for Suspected Transfusion Reaction

1. Stop transfusion.
2. Maintain intravenous access with normal saline and new administration set.
3. Reassure the patient; stay at the bedside.
4. Notify physician and blood bank.
5. Recheck blood numbers and type.
6. Treat symptoms appropriately.
7. Return unused portion of blood in blood bag and administration set to the blood bank.
8. Collect and send blood and urine samples to the laboratory; send another urine specimen 24 hours after transfusion reaction.
9. Document the transfusion reaction and treatment administered.

(b) Non-A, non-B hepatitis (also referred to as *type C hepatitis*) accounts for 90% of transfusion-related hepatitis.

(2) HIV
  (a) HIV transmission through blood transfusion has been reduced greatly by screening for HIV antibody, which started in 1985, and by careful history taking of potential donors for risk factors for HIV

(3) Cytomegalovirus (CMV)
  (a) CMV is usually not a problem for immunocompetent patients but may be life-threatening in immunodeficient patients.
  (b) Clinical indications of CMV infection include mild fever, mild splenomegaly, and atypical serum lymphocytes.
  (c) CMV-negative blood products are indicated for immunodeficient patients.

(4) Creutzfeldt-Jakob disease (i.e., "mad cow disease")
  (a) No confirmed cases, but concern continues

(5) Transfusion-related acute lung injury or acute respiratory distress syndrome (ARDS)

(6) Systemic inflammatory response syndrome

2. Specific to iron deficiency anemia
   a. Treatment of cause.
      (1) Identify any source of slow, chronic blood loss.
         (a) GI bleeding
         (b) Menorrhagia
         (c) Pregnancy
         (d) Zinc deficiency
      (2) Encourage dietary consumption of iron-rich foods.
   b. Administer multivitamins with iron or iron supplements orally or parenterally.
      (1) Instruct the patient to take oral iron supplements with meals to decrease the GI side effects.
      (2) Inject parenteral iron deep intramuscularly using Z-track method.
   c. Assist with chelation to remove lead from the blood if caused by lead ingestion or exposure.
3. Specific to pernicious anemia
   a. Eliminate cause (e.g., discontinue offending drug).
   b. Administer vitamin B_{12} as prescribed.
      (1) Usual dose is 1000 units intramuscularly daily for 1 week, then weekly for 1 month, and then monthly for life.
      (2) Inform patient that pain or burning at the injection site may occur.
4. Specific to folic acid deficiency anemia
   a. Encourage dietary consumption of foods rich in folic acid
   b. Administer folic acid orally as prescribed
5. Specific to acute blood loss anemia
   a. Assist with treatment of cause (e.g., compress compressible vessels and prepare patient for surgery).
   b. Administer isotonic IV fluids as prescribed.
   c. Administer blood and/or blood products as prescribed.
   d. Use other approaches to reduce the need for blood component transfusions.
      (1) Thromboelastography
         (a) Allows for assessment of hemostatic function through point of care testing
         (b) Administration of the specifically needed products
      (2) Limitation of diagnostic blood loss
      (3) Erythropoietin (epoetin alpha [Epogen])
      (4) Readministration of cell-saver blood
      (5) Autotransfusion if appropriate
         (a) Advantages
            (i) Readily available
            (ii) Less costly than banked blood
            (iii) No chance of transfusion reaction
            (iv) Near-normal half-life for RBCs
            (v) Near-normal clotting factors, pH, and electrolytes
         (b) Risks of autotransfusion
            (i) Sepsis: blood should be administered within 6 hours of collection
            (ii) Coagulopathy, RBC damage
            (iii) Citrate toxicity, calcium deficiency
      (6) Autologous transfusion if blood loss was anticipated and blood donation was made before loss (e.g., surgery)
6. Specific to anemia of chronic illness: administer RBC colony-stimulating factor (e.g., erythropoietin [Epogen])
7. Specific to aplastic anemia
   a. Administer immunosuppressive agents as prescribed.
      (1) Antithymocyte globulin
      (2) Cyclosporine
      (3) Corticosteroids
      (4) Cyclophosphamide

b. Prepare patient for allogeneic hematopoietic stem cell transplantation.
   (1) Pretransplantation workup
   (2) Monitoring for complications
      (a) GI: nausea, vomiting, mucositis, hepatoxicity
      (b) Hematologic: anemia, thrombocytopenia, neutropenia,
      (c) Immunologic: infection, sepsis
      (d) Neurologic: neurotoxicity
      (e) Cardiovascular: cardiomyopathy
      (f) Pulmonary: pulmonary toxicity, pulmonary infections
      (g) Renal: renal insufficiency or failure, urosepsis
      (h) Graft failure (i.e., lack of stem cell differentiation or proliferation after initial indications of donor cell engraftment)
      (i) Acute graft-versus-host disease
   (3) Immunosuppressive therapy
8. Specific to sickle cell anemia
   a. Encourage patient to prevent stress, dehydration, and extreme changes in temperature and altitude.
   b. Increase dietary folic acid ingestion, or administer folic acid supplements.
   c. Assist with management of sickle cell crisis.
      (1) Oxygen to maintain Sao_2 by pulse oximetry at least 95%.
      (2) IV fluids
         (a) Usually 5% dextrose in one-half normal saline; the hypotonic solution allows rehydration of RBCs
         (b) Usually 150 to 200 mL/hr initially
      (3) Analgesics
         (a) Opiates, usually morphine 510 mg every 2 to 4 hours
         (b) NSAID
      (4) Antibiotics if cause of crisis was infection
      (5) Drugs to improve blood flow and reduce sickling
         (a) Nitric oxide as prescribed
            (i) Vasodilates
            (ii) Slows and reverses sickling
         (b) Oral administration of clotrimazole and hydroxyurea as prescribed
            (i) Maintains RBC hydration and reduces sickling by preventing potassium loss
            (ii) Decreases severity of anemia
            (iii) Decreases hemolysis
         (c) Poloxamer 188 (RheothRx) or purified poloxamer 188 (Flocor)
            (i) Coats RBCs and allows them to move more freely to improve blood flow
      (6) Extracorporeal membrane oxygenation may be considered
      (7) Bone marrow transplantation may be considered
   d. Monitor for complications.
      (1) Acute sequestration crisis
         (a) Clinical indications: abdominal pain, weakness, fatigue, dyspnea, vomiting, pallor, enlarging spleen, decreased hemoglobin and hematocrit, shock
         (b) Collaborative management: blood transfusion, emergency splenectomy
      (2) Aplastic crisis
         (a) Clinical indications: weakness, pallor, dyspnea, syncope, decreased hemoglobin, hematocrit, RBCs
         (b) Collaborative management: blood transfusion
      (3) Acute chest syndrome: may involve fat embolism and/or pulmonary infection
         (a) Clinical indicators: chest pain, fever, tachypnea, hypoxia, cough, changes in LOC, seizures
         (b) Collaborative management: hydration, oxygen, analgesics, antibiotics, blood transfusions
      (4) Infection
         (a) Clinical indications: fever, leukocytosis, and indications specific to site
         (b) Collaborative management: antibiotics
      (5) Multiple organ dysfunction syndrome
         (a) Clinical indications: organ failure, pain, change in LOC
         (b) Collaborative management: supportive therapies, blood transfusion

Disseminated Intravascular Coagulation

Definition

1. A syndrome characterized by thrombus formation and hemorrhage resulting from overstimulation of the normal coagulation process with resultant decrease in clotting factors and platelets
2. DIC may be acute or chronic, but this discussion is limited to acute DIC

Etiology

Always secondary

1. Vascular disorders
   a. Shock
   b. Vasculitis
   c. Giant hemangioma
   d. Dissecting aneurysm
2. Infection and sepsis
   a. Bacterial
      (1) Gram negative (e.g., *Escherichia coli* or meningococci)
      (2) Gram positive (e.g., *Staphylococcus* or *Streptococcus*)
   b. Viral (e.g., influenza or herpes)
   c. Rickettsial (e.g., Rocky Mountain spotted fever)
   d. Protozoal (e.g., malaria)
   e. Fungal (e.g., *Aspergillus*)

3. Hematologic/immunologic
   a. Hemolytic blood transfusion reaction
   b. Massive blood transfusion
   c. Prolonged cardiopulmonary bypass
   d. Sickle cell crisis
   e. Thalassemia major
   f. Polycythemia vera
   g. Anaphylaxis
   h. SLE
   i. Transplant rejection
4. Trauma
   a. Multiple trauma
   b. Burns
   c. Acute anoxia
   d. Heat stroke
   e. Crush injury
   f. Head injury
   g. Surgery
5. Neoplastic disorders
   a. Adenocarcinoma
      (1) Pancreatic cancer
      (2) Breast cancer
      (3) Prostate cancer
      (4) Ovarian cancer
      (5) Lung cancer
      (6) Colon cancer
      (7) Stomach cancer
   b. Cancer of the urinary tract
   c. Sarcoma
   d. Leukemia
   e. Pheochromocytoma
6. Obstetric complications
   a. Abruptio placentae
   b. Retained dead fetus
   c. Retained placenta
   d. Septic abortion
   e. Hydatidiform mole
   f. Amniotic fluid embolism
   g. Acute fatty liver of pregnancy
   h. Toxemia
7. Embolism
   a. Pulmonary embolism
   b. Fat embolism
   c. Amniotic fluid embolism
8. GI and accessory organs
   a. Necrotizing enterocolitis
   b. Pancreatitis
   c. Obstructive jaundice
   d. Hepatitis
   e. Cirrhosis
   f. Acute hepatic failure
9. Pulmonary
   a. ARDS
   b. Pulmonary embolism
10. Toxins
    a. Snake bites
    b. Aspirin poisoning
    c. Impure IV drugs
11. Prosthetic devices
    a. LeVeen or Denver shunt
    b. Intraaortic balloon pump

Pathophysiology

Figure 10-6 summarizes pathophysiology and relates therapy to the pathophysiology.

1. The paradox of DIC: bleeding after clotting
2. Triggered by the following:
   a. Intrinsic coagulation system activation: damage to vascular endothelium
   b. Extrinsic coagulation system activation: release of tissue thromboplastin
   c. Red cell or platelet injury
3. Clotting causes ischemia and tissue and organ necrosis; this leads to multiple organ dysfunction syndrome
   a. Tissue damage releases thromboplastin into circulation.
   b. Thromboplastin converts prothrombin into thrombin.
   c. Abundant intravascular thrombin is produced that converts fibrinogen to a fibrin clot and enhances platelet aggregation.
   d. Excessive blood coagulation creates microvascular thrombi (referred to as *microclots*) in the microcirculation, causing ischemia.
4. Bleeding causes loss of hemoglobin and oxygen-carrying capacity; this leads to hypoxia and ischemia
   a. Excessive aggregation of platelets causes a thrombocytopenia, and excessive blood coagulation causes depletion of clotting factors (this is why DIC frequently is referred to as a *consumptive coagulopathy*).
   b. A stable clot, therefore, cannot be formed at injury sites, predisposing the patient to hemorrhage.
5. Fibrinolysis causes the destruction of once stable clots and more bleeding
   a. Activation of plasminogen to plasmin causes lysis of preexisting clots and surface bleeding.
   b. Naturally occurring antithrombins, which inhibit thrombin, are inactivated by plasmin.
   c. Fibrinolysis causes production of FSPs, also referred to as *FDPs*.
   d. FSPs normally are cleared by the reticuloendothelial system, but overproduction overwhelms the system.
   e. FSPs act as an anticoagulant, perpetuating bleeding.
      (1) FSPs coat the platelets and interfere with platelet function.
      (2) FSPs interfere with thrombin and disrupt coagulation.
      (3) FSPs attach to fibrinogen, which interferes with the polymerization process necessary to form a stable clot.

Clinical Presentation

1. Subjective
   a. History of predisposing factor
   b. Symptoms related to ischemia
      (1) Chest pain

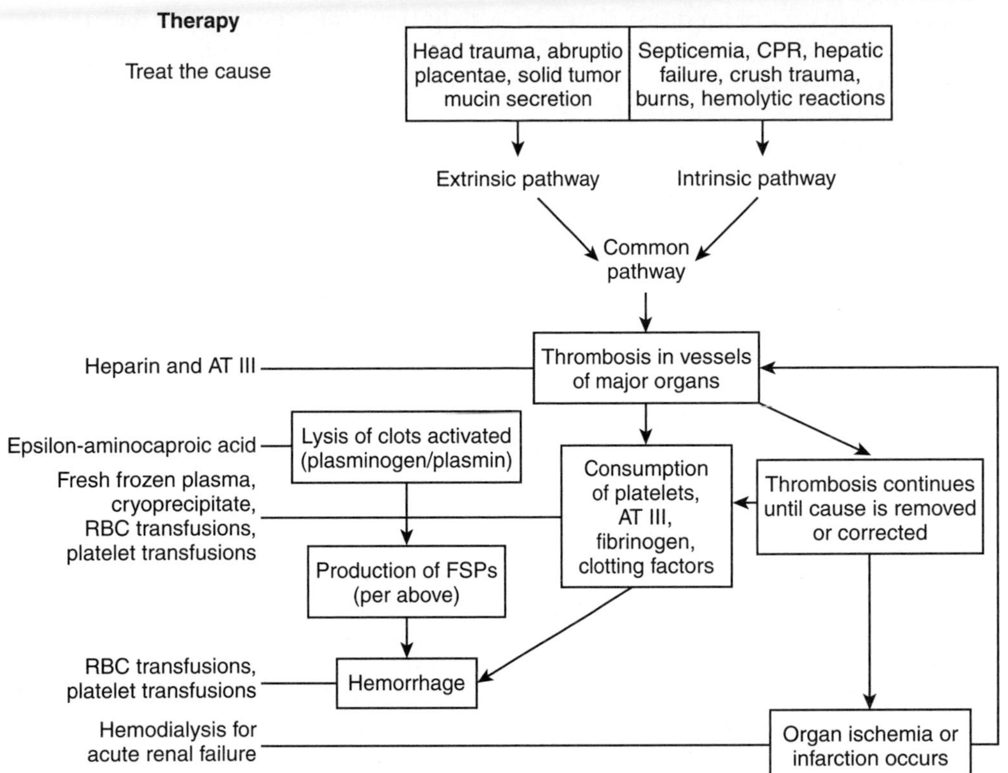

Figure 10-6 Pathophysiology and intended sites of action for therapies in DIC. *AT III*, Antithrombin III; *CPR*, cardiopulmonary resuscitation; *FSPs*, fibrin split products; *RBC*, red blood cell. (From Lewis, S. M., Heitkemper, M. M., & Dirksen, S. R. [2004]. *Medical-surgical nursing: Assessment and management of clinical problems* [6th ed.]. St. Louis: Mosby.)

(2) Dyspnea
(3) Abdominal pain

2. Objective
   a. Clinical indications of decreased perfusion (subjective included)
      (1) Brain: change in LOC; focal neurologic signs; seizures
      (2) Heart: chest pain; ST segment elevation or depression; clinical indications of hypoperfusion
      (3) Lung: dyspnea; chest pain; clinical indications of hypoxemia
      (4) Kidney: decreased urine output; proteinuria; electrolyte imbalance
      (5) GI tract: abdominal pain; diarrhea (may be bloody)
      (6) Skin: acral cyanosis of toes, fingers, lips, nose, ears; mottling; coldness; necrosis
   b. Clinical indications of platelet dysfunction
      (1) Petechiae: frequently the first indication of DIC
      (2) Ecchymoses
      (3) Purpura
   c. Clinical indications of hemorrhage
      (1) Tachycardia
         (a) Initially postural only, then profound tachycardia
      (2) Hypotension
         (a) Initially narrowed pulse pressure
         (b) Then postural hypotension
         (c) Then profound hypotension
      (3) Tachypnea
      (4) Overt bleeding in a patient with no previous bleeding history
         (a) Mucosal surfaces: gingival bleeding; epistaxis
         (b) GU: hematuria
         (c) GI: hematemesis, hematochezia, melena, guaiac-positive stool
         (d) Pulmonary: hemoptysis
         (e) Gynecologic: vaginal bleeding
         (f) Skin: prolonged oozing from puncture points, IV sites, and wounds (referred to as *surface bleeding*), bruising
      (5) Occult bleeding
         (a) Swollen joints and joint pain may indicate bleeding into the joint.
         (b) Abdominal distention and rebound tenderness may indicate intraperitoneal bleeding.
         (c) Back pain, leg numbness, and hypotension may indicate retroperitoneal bleeding.
         (d) Headache, change in LOC, and pupillary changes may indicate intracerebral hemorrhage.

(e) Visual changes (e.g., blurred vision or loss of visual fields) may indicate retinal hemorrhage.
(f) Alterations in hemodynamic parameters occur: right atrial pressure, pulmonary artery wedge pressure, cardiac output/cardiac index may be decreased.

3. Diagnostic: All that bleeds is not DIC; diagnostic studies are definitive.
   a. Serum
      (1) Platelet count: decreased (less than 150,000/mm^3)
      (2) PT: prolonged (usually greater than 40 seconds)
      (3) aPTT: prolonged (usually greater than 70 seconds)
      (4) Thrombin time: prolonged (greater than 15 seconds)
      (5) Fibrinogen level: decreased by 50% or more or less than 200 mg/dL
         (a) Because fibrinogen is elevated in pregnancy, sepsis, and neoplastic conditions, a decrease of 50% is a more accurate indicator of DIC than an absolute value in these patients.
      (6) Thrombin-antithrombin III complex: decreased (usually less than 70% activity)
         (a) Evaluates the activation of the coagulation system that occurs when thrombin is generated
         (b) Decreased antithrombin III indicates accelerated coagulation
      (7) FSPs (also referred to as *FDPs*): elevated (usually greater than 40 mcg/mL)
         (a) Measures the results of fibrin and fibrinogen degradation
      (8) D dimer (end product of fibrin degradation): elevated (greater than 250 ng/mL)
         (a) Specific to the results of fibrin degradation
         (b) More specific for DIC than FSPs, but less sensitive
      (9) Protamine sulfate test: strongly positive
         (a) Protamine sulfate is added to plasma to see whether fibrin strands are formed
         (b) A positive test reflects the formation of excessive amounts of thrombin
      (10) Clotting factor analysis: shows a decrease in factors I, V, and VIII and fibrinogen
      (11) Peripheral smear: shows presence of schistocytes, helmet cells, and red cell fragments
      (12) Hemoglobin and hematocrit: may be decreased if blood loss is significant
      (13) Arterial blood gases (ABGs): respiratory alkalosis initially progressing to metabolic acidosis because of lactic acidosis
   b. Urine: may be positive for blood
   c. Stool: may be positive for blood
   d. Sputum: may be positive for blood

Nursing Diagnosis

1. Ineffective Peripheral, Cardiopulmonary, Cerebral, and Renal Tissue Perfusion related to microclots and/or hemorrhage
2. Risk for Deficient Fluid Volume related to hemorrhage
3. Decreased Cardiac Output related to decreased preload
4. Impaired Gas Exchange related to microclots in pulmonary circulation and shunting
5. Risk for Injury related to altered clotting and prescribed therapies
6. Pain related to ischemia and necrosis
7. Anxiety related to acute change in health status
8. Ineffective Individual Coping related to situational crisis, powerlessness, and change in role
9. Interrupted Family Processes related to critically ill family member

Collaborative Management

1. Identify and closely assess high-risk groups for clinical indications of DIC.
   a. Monitor patient closely for thrombosis or bleeding.
      (1) Note petechiae, ecchymosis, and acrocyanosis.
      (2) Test nasogastric aspirate or vomitus, stools, and urine for blood.
      (3) Monitor oral secretions, pulmonary secretions, and gums for bleeding.
      (4) Monitor peripheral pulses and capillary refill.
   b. Monitor laboratory studies for diagnostic indications of DIC.
   c. Monitor patient closely for clinical indications of hypoperfusion or intracranial hemorrhage.
   d. Monitor hemodynamic parameters as indicated; insert indwelling urinary catheter to monitor hourly urine output.
2. Control underlying causative factors.
   a. Surgery
      (1) Surgical débridement
      (2) Abscess drainage
      (3) Evacuation of the uterus
      (4) Removal of tumor
   b. Antimicrobials for infection
   c. Antineoplastics for malignancy
3. Maintain airway, ventilation, and oxygenation.
   a. Administer oxygen to maintain PaO_2 of 80 mm Hg and SaO_2 by pulse oximetry of 95%.
   b. Assist with intubation and mechanical ventilation as necessary.
   c. Suction only as necessary and with low suction to avoid trauma to the tracheobronchial mucosa.

4. Correct hypovolemia, hypotension, hypoxia, and acidosis.
   a. Insert or ensure patency of peripheral IV catheter.
   b. Administer normal saline to replace volume until type and crossmatch is completed and blood is available.
   c. Administer volume replacement, inotropes, and/or vasopressors as prescribed to maintain mean arterial pressure (MAP) greater than 60 mm Hg.
5. Stop the microclotting to maintain perfusion and protect vital organ function.
   a. Administer heparin IV (usually 5 to 15 units/kg/hr) as prescribed; desirable aPTT is 1.5 to 2 times the control.
      (1) Used primarily for patients with thrombosis who continue to bleed despite other rigorous treatment; often effective with underlying malignancy, acute promyelocytic leukemia, and purpura fulminans (may be seen in sepsis)
      (2) Prevents further thrombosis in the microvasculature and prevents platelet aggregation; works with antithrombin III to neutralize circulating thrombin
      (3) Continues to be controversial because it may potentiate or prolong bleeding, but it is thrombosis of small vessels that has the greatest effect on morbidity and mortality in DIC, not hemorrhage
      (4) Contraindicated in central nervous system (CNS) or GI hemorrhage, DIC associated with hepatic failure, hemorrhagic obstetric causes (e.g., abruptio placentae), and recent surgical procedures
   b. Administer antithrombin III as prescribed: antithrombin III inhibits the action of thrombin; it may be administered if antithrombin levels are low.
   c. Assist with plasmapheresis (may be used in severe cases).
   d. NOTE: Table 10-13 describes rationale and controversies regarding selected treatments.
6. Stop the bleeding by supporting coagulation.
   a. Administer blood products as prescribed to replace missing clotting factors.
      (1) Fresh frozen plasma (contains all clotting factors): used for bleeding patients with greatly prolonged PT and aPTT
      (2) Cryoprecipitate (contains factors VIII and XIII and fibrinogen): maintain fibrinogen levels above 125 mg/dL
      (3) Platelets: maintain platelet count greater than 50,000/mm^3
         (a) Desmopressin acetate may be prescribed to improve platelet function when platelet dysfunction is due to dextran, NSAIDs, or aspirin; monitor for fluid overload, hyponatremia, and tachycardia.
      (4) Packed RBCs: may be needed if blood loss is significant
      (5) May potentiate or prolong the clotting (fuel to the fire theory), so heparin may be given first
   b. Administer hemostatic cofactors as prescribed.
      (1) Vitamin K: needed for liver production of several clotting factors
      (2) Folic acid: folic acid deficiency may cause thrombocytopenia
   c. Administer an antifibrinolytic agent (epsilon-aminocaproic acid [Amicar] or tranexamic acid [Cyclokapron]) as prescribed for primary fibrinolysis.
      (1) Should be avoided in all other situations because it may enhance deposition of fibrin in the microcirculation and macrocirculation and lead to fatal DIC

Table 10-13 Treatments for Disseminated Intravascular Coagulation

Treatment	Rationale	Controversy
Heparin	• Prevents further microclots and prevents platelet aggregation • Works with antithrombin III to neutralize circulating thrombin	• May perpetuate bleeding
Antithrombin III	• Works with heparin to neutralize circulating thrombin	• May perpetuate bleeding
Clotting factors • Fresh frozen plasma • Cryoprecipitate • Platelets	• Reestablishes normal hemostatic potential	• "Fuel to the fire" theory attests that until the clotting process is stopped, clotting factors just increase the thrombosis and microclotting
Epsilon-aminocaproic acid (Amicar)	• Blocks the fibrinolytic system so that stable clots are not degraded • Decreases amount of fibrin split products that act as anticoagulant	• Clearance of microclots from occluded vessels may be delayed • Indicated only in primary fibrinolysis

(2) Requires concurrent heparin therapy in DIC
d. Apply thrombin-soaked gauze, pressure dressings, and/or ice packs to control bleeding sites.
e. Maintain normal body temperature because hypothermia contributes to coagulopathy.
7. Treat ischemic pain.
a. Administer analgesics as prescribed.
b. Apply cold compresses for pain caused by bleeding into joints and tissues.
8. Maintain skin integrity and minimize tissue trauma.
a. Provide meticulous skin care.
(1) Turn patient gently and frequently to assess skin.
(2) Keep the skin moist with lubricating lotions.
(3) Use specialized beds as needed.
b. Provide careful mouth care; use alcohol-free mouthwash and swabs.
c. Provide careful perianal care; avoid use of rectal thermometers and suppositories.
d. Alternate activity with rest; mobilize patient and have him or her ambulate progressively.
e. Use an electric rather than straight-edged razor.
f. Avoid tape if possible; use adhesive remover to remove tape.
g. Apply local pressure to any break in skin integrity.
(1) Avoid intramuscular and subcutaneous infections.
(2) Use an arterial line or heparin lock for blood sampling.
(a) If venous puncture is necessary, apply pressure for 3 to 5 minutes after venous puncture.
(b) If arterial puncture is necessary, apply pressure for 10 to 15 minutes after arterial puncture.
h. Reduce frequency of taking blood pressure by cuff sphygmomanometer: an arterial line is ideal for pressure monitoring and obtaining blood specimens.
i. Do not give aspirin or NSAIDs because of their effect on platelet aggregation.
j. Teach patient to avoid Valsalva maneuver.
k. Do not disturb any clot.
9. Provide psychological support and reassurance: reassure patient that treatment is being provided to stop the bleeding (hemorrhage causes extreme anxiety).
10. Monitor patient for complications.
a. Intracerebral hemorrhage (a major cause of death)
b. Hemorrhagic shock
c. ARDS
d. GI dysfunction
e. Renal failure
f. Infection, sepsis

Immunodeficiency

Definition

A state of decreased responsiveness or unresponsiveness of the immune system, causing an impaired ability to defend the body against antigens

Etiology

1. Congenital immunodeficiency
2. Acquired immunodeficiency
a. Acute and/or overwhelming infections
(1) Bacterial
(2) Viral
b. Physical agents, chemicals, drugs
(1) Radiation
(2) Antibiotics
(3) Antineoplastic agents
(4) Steroids
(5) Antacids, histamine$_2$ receptor antagonists
(6) Immunosuppressive agents (e.g., for posttransplant patients)
(7) Anesthetic agents
(8) Alcohol
c. Surgery
d. Stress
(1) Physiologic
(2) Psychological, including noise
e. Bone marrow depression
f. After splenectomy
g. Cancer, especially leukemia, lymphoma, multiple myeloma
h. Chronic diseases (e.g., diabetes mellitus, inflammatory bowel disease, hepatic cirrhosis and/or failure, chronic renal failure, and psychiatric illness)
i. Malnutrition
(1) Protein-calorie malnutrition
(2) Zinc deficiency
j. Alcohol or drug abuse
k. Anaphylaxis
l. HIV infection or AIDS
m. Aging (immunosenescence)
n. CNS depression

Pathophysiology

1. In addition to previously mentioned etiologic factors, critically ill patients are likely to have the following:
a. Invasive catheters, nasogastric tubes, endotracheal tubes, chest tubes, indwelling urinary bladder catheter, trauma, burns, surgery, skin lesions that alter skin barrier or mucous membranes
b. Stress that promotes catabolism, impairs healing, and causes immunodeficiency
c. Sleep deprivation that alters the immune function by reducing interleukin-1, reducing cellular immunity
d. Multiple infections that may overwhelm the immune system and bone marrow, causing a consumptive leukopenia

e. Impaired consciousness, artificial airways, and/or feeding tubes, which cause impaired gag, swallowing, and cough reflexes
f. Increased gastric pH caused by antacids, histamine$_2$-receptor antagonists, and proton pump inhibitors, which allows proliferation of bacteria in the stomach that may migrate or be aspirated into the tracheobronchial tree and lungs
g. Malnutrition caused by preexisting disease or inadequate nutritional replacement
h. Altered perfusion of the intestinal tract that results in impaired integrity of the intestinal wall and translocation of microorganisms or their toxins from intestinal lumen into the blood
i. Prolonged hospitalization that increases risk of exposure to microorganisms in the hospital environment from contaminated objects, other patients, or hospital personnel

2. These factors reduce resistance to infection because of a decrease in number or effectiveness of leukocytes and lymphocytes and suppression of the immune system in the patient
3. Infection
   a. Chain of infection includes the following components:
      (1) Source of infection
      (2) Mechanism of spread
         (a) Understaffing has been linked to increased risk of nosocomial infection because routine nursing interventions such as turning, suction, and compliance with aseptic standards may decline
         (b) Unit design also may affect risk of nosocomial infection because hand washing needs to be convenient; the use of alcohol-based cleansers at multiple convenient locations is helpful
         (c) Avoidance of artificial nails and/or polish
         (d) Avoidance of rings with stones
         (e) Careful placement of patients with infections to avoid cross-contamination
      (3) Susceptible host
   b. Nosocomial infection
      (1) 80% of nosocomial infections are within one of the following categories:
         (a) Urinary tract infection
         (b) Surgical site infection
         (c) Pneumonia
         (d) Intravascular catheter–related bloodstream infection
      (2) 70% of nosocomial infections are caused by the following microorganisms:
         (a) Gram-positive microorganisms
            (i) *Staphylococcus aureus*
            (ii) Coagulase-negative staphylococci
            (iii) Enterococci
         (b) Gram-negative microorganisms
            (i) *Escherichia coli*
            (ii) *Pseudomonas aeruginosa*
            (iii) *Enterobacter*
            (iv) *Klebsiella pneumoniae*
   c. Drug-resistance infections
      (1) Underlying principles of antimicrobial resistance (Levy, 1998)
         (a) Given sufficient time and antimicrobial use, resistance will occur.
         (b) Resistance is progressive, from low to high levels.
         (c) Organisms resistant to one antimicrobial are likely to become resistant to others.
         (d) Resistance is slow to decline, if it declines at all.
         (e) Use of antimicrobials by one person affects others in the immediate and extended environment.
      (2) Factors that contribute to microbial resistance include the following:
         (a) Increased use and misuse of antimicrobials
         (b) Increase in the number of susceptible hosts
         (c) Increase in use of invasive procedures and devices
         (d) Lack of diligence with infection control practices
      (3) Examples
         (a) Methicillin-resistant *Staphylococcus aureus* (MRSA)
         (b) Vancomycin-resistant enterococci
         (c) Vancomycin-resistant intermediate *S. aureus*
         (d) Vancomycin resistant *S. aureus*
         (e) Penicillin-resistant *Streptococcus pneumoniae*
         (f) Extended-spectrum beta-lactamase–producing microorganisms
   d. Opportunistic infection
      (1) Etiology
         (a) Immunocompromise
         (b) Suppression of normal flora
            (i) Candidiasis
               a) Oral (i.e., thrush)
               b) Systemic
            (ii) *Clostridium difficile*
               a) Causes diarrhea
               b) Treated with metronidazole (Flagyl) or vancomycin

Clinical Presentation

1. Subjective
   a. History of precipitating condition
   b. Increased susceptibility to infection
      (1) Immunodeficiency is suspected when an individual experiences chronic, recurrent infections that do not respond to therapy or do respond but recur.
2. Objective
   a. Fever: greater than 101°F, or 38.3°C
      (1) Fever may be the only sign of infection in patients with leukopenia.

(2) Not all patients can develop a fever because the immune system (cytokines) is responsible for fever, so in immune-deficient patients, temperature may be normal or below normal even in the presence of infection.

b. Skin rash
c. Poor wound healing
d. Redness, swelling, induration at IV site, wounds, incisions
e. Recurrent abscess
f. Osteomyelitis
g. Hepatosplenomegaly
h. Presence of opportunistic infections (e.g., *Pneumocystis* pneumonia or oral candidiasis)
i. Presence of opportunistic malignancy (e.g., Kaposi sarcoma)
j. Chronic diarrhea
k. Clinical indications of sepsis or septic shock may be seen

3. Diagnostic
   a. Serum
      (1) WBC: total WBC may be decreased, or one component of the differential may be decreased
      (2) T cell count: may be decreased or T cell count may be normal, but T cell function may be impaired
      (3) Albumin and total proteins: may be decreased if protein malnutrition is a causative factor
   b. Cultures: may show causative organism(s)
   c. Anergy profile: delayed or absent response to skin tests
   d. Antibody titers: may be abnormal

Nursing Diagnosis

1. Risk for Infection related to immune system impairment
2. Impaired Skin Integrity related to invasive procedures and devices, edema, malnutrition, immunosuppression
3. Imbalanced Nutrition related to anorexia and hypermetabolism
4. Ineffective Individual Coping related to situational crisis, powerlessness, and change in role
5. Interrupted Family Processes related to critically ill family member
6. Deficient Knowledge related to health maintenance

Collaborative Management

1. Prevent and monitor for clinical indications of infection.
   a. Place patient in private room; limit number of visitors.
   b. Avoid contact with visitors or hospital staff who have any of the following:
      (1) Fever
      (2) Upper respiratory infection
      (3) Diarrhea
      (4) Open skin lesions
      (5) Exposure to contagious disease
   c. Maintain appropriate isolation or precautionary measures.
   d. Minimize potential of cross-contamination; do not assign this patient and a patient with an infection to the same nurse.
   e. Institute and emphasize good hand washing.
      (1) The wearing of gloves does not eliminate the need to wash hands because microorganisms can permeate gloves and because applying gloves over dirty hands may transfer microorganisms to the outside of the glove and, therefore, to the patient.
      (2) Wash hands at the following times:
         (a) Before and after patient contact
         (b) Before and after invasive procedures
         (c) After contact with soiled items
         (d) After toileting
         (e) Before and after using gloves
         (f) Before handling food
      (3) Technique
         (a) Use alcohol-based cleansers when the hands are not obviously soiled.
         (b) Hand washing with soap and water is recommended when the hands are soiled and at least every 5 times of using gloves.
            (i) Wet hands under running water.
            (ii) Apply 5 mL of soap and distribute thoroughly over both hands.
            (iii) Using friction, wash all surfaces of the hands and fingers for at least 15 seconds, including under nails.
            (iv) Rinse and dry thoroughly.
            (v) Turn off faucets with a paper towel if there is not an automatic shutoff or foot controls.
   f. Ensure proper cleaning, storage, disinfection, and sterilization of medical equipment as appropriate.
   g. Provide only food that is cooked, pasteurized, or sterilized; avoid unpeeled fruit.
   h. Provide sterile water for drinking as indicated.
   i. Minimize introduction of organisms.
      (1) Avoid cut flowers, potted plants, and standing water.
      (2) Damp dust with disinfectant solution at least every 24 hours.
   j. Culture common sources of contamination (e.g., ventilator tubing).
   k. Avoid intrusive procedures and invasive devices if possible.
   l. Teach patient and encourage necessary personal hygiene techniques.
   m. Assess oral mucosa daily and maintain oral hygiene.
   n. Decrease stress, noise, bright lights, and other stressors.
   o. Do not administer live vaccines.
   p. Encourage a high-protein, high-calorie diet.

q. Administer a granulocyte colony-stimulating factor (filgrastim [Neupogen]) and a granulocyte-macrophage colony-stimulating factor (sargramostim [Leukine or Prokine]) as prescribed.
  (1) These drugs stimulate proliferation and differentiation of hematopoietic cells, specifically neutrophils or neutrophils and monocytes
  (2) Indicated to decrease incidence of infection in patients with nonmyeloid malignancy receiving bone marrow suppressive antineoplastic agents and for ganciclovir-induced neutropenia in AIDS patients

2. Provide appropriate nutritional support.
  a. Enteral nutrition is preferred over parenteral nutrition because it helps to prevent translocation of gram-negative bacteria from the GI tract and helps to prevent stress ulcers.
  b. Nutritional support containing glutamine and arginine also may be helpful in prevention of sepsis.
3. Prevent breaks in skin integrity.
4. Maintain activity, but provide for adequate rest.
5. Assist in patient and family adjustment: provide appropriate reassurance that measures are being taken to stop the bleeding.
6. Monitor for complications.
  a. Poor wound healing
  b. Opportunistic infections
  c. Secondary infections
  d. Sepsis
  e. Septic shock

Acquired Immunodeficiency Syndrome

Definition

A syndrome of immunodeficiency caused by HIV

Etiology

1. Exposure to the causative agent: HIV, a CD4 cell retrovirus
2. High-risk groups
  a. Participants of high-risk sexual behavior; unprotected sex
    (1) Anal: highest risk during unprotected intercourse
    (2) Vaginal
    (3) Oral
  b. Sex partners (heterosexual or homosexual) of infected persons
  c. Injectable drug users who share needles
    (1) IV drug users
    (2) Intramuscular steroid users (e.g., athletes)
    (3) Users of "skin poppers"
  d. Recipients of blood products, especially before 1985; hemophiliacs significantly affected
  e. Newborns or breast-fed infants of infected mothers

Pathophysiology

1. Infection with HIV
  a. A Lentivirus, a subgroup of retroviruses
    (1) Known for the following:
      (a) Latency
      (b) Persistent viremia
      (c) Infection of the nervous system
      (d) Weak host immune responses
    (2) Two types of HIV that cause AIDS: HIV-1 and HIV-2
      (a) There are various subtypes of HIV-1; more than half of all new HIV infections worldwide are caused by subtype C.
      (b) There are no known subtypes of HIV-2.
  b. HIV primarily infects CD4 T lymphocytes and monocytes
    (1) CD4 is an antigen on the surface of T helper cells that acts as the primary receptor for HIV.
  c. HIV binds to CD4 cells and becomes internalized.
  d. HIV replicates itself by generating a DNA copy by reverse transcriptase
  e. Viral DNA becomes incorporated into the host DNA, enabling further replication
  f. Destruction of CD4 cells, CD4 progenitor cells in bone marrow, thymus, and peripheral lymphoid organs, and CD4 cells within the nervous system (e.g., microglia)
  g. Destruction of T4 cells and imbalance between T4 and T8 cells caused by HIV using the T4 cell DNA for reproduction
  h. Failure of T cell production and eventual immune suppression
  i. Decrease in cell-mediated immunity because T cells lack ability to destroy foreign organisms that enter the body
  j. General decline in the immune system
  k. Presence of opportunistic infections and malignancies
2. Transmission of HIV
  a. Unprotected sexual contact with an infected partner
  b. Exposure to infected blood or blood products or other body fluids with high concentration of HIV (e.g., cerebrospinal fluid of an infected person)
  c. From mother to child during pregnancy, birth, breast-feeding
3. Clinical course from exposure to HIV to AIDS
  a. Window period from exposure to seroconversion: approximately 6 weeks to 6 months; may take a year or longer in some persons; therefore repeated testing necessary after suspected exposure
    (1) Acute primary infection: lasts 1 to 2 weeks
  b. Asymptomatic phase from seroconversion to symptoms: period is 6 months to 10 years; average 2 to 5 years
  c. HIV-related disease with persistent generalized lymphadenopathy: 1 to 5 years
  d. AIDS: 1 to 3 years

Clinical Presentation

1. Subjective
   a. High-risk group or activity by history
   b. Acute retroviral syndrome: about 70% of patients with primary HIV infection develop a mononucleosis-like syndrome within 2 to 6 weeks after the initial infection
      (1) Fever
      (2) Fatigue
      (3) Headache
      (4) Nausea, vomiting, diarrhea
      (5) Weight loss
      (6) Neurologic symptoms
      (7) Sore throat
      (8) Muscle and joint discomfort
      (9) Night sweats
   c. Fatigue, lethargy, weakness
   d. Anorexia, nausea, vomiting, dysphagia, diarrhea, abdominal pain
   e. Headache, visual changes
   f. Skin dryness, itching
   g. Night sweats, chills
   h. Joint pain
   i. Bruising, bleeding
   j. Dyspnea, cough
   k. Recurrent infections: upper respiratory infection; shingles
   l. Depression, personality change
2. Objective
   a. Acute retroviral syndrome
      (1) Lymphadenopathy
      (2) Pharyngitis; exudates may be present
      (3) Oral ulcers
      (4) Maculopapular rash
      (5) Oral candidiasis (i.e., thrush)
      (6) Hepatomegaly
      (7) Genital ulcers
   b. Fever: recurrent
   c. Rash
   d. Weight loss: rapid, unplanned (may be referred to as *HIV wasting*)
   e. White spots or sores in mouth
   f. Decrease in visual acuity
   g. Generalized lymphadenopathy
   h. CMV retinitis; cotton-wool spots noted on funduscopic exam
   i. Splenomegaly, hepatomegaly
   j. Genital or anal warts
3. AIDS-defining illnesses
   a. Opportunistic infection: infections in the patient with HIV tend to be severe, to be disseminated, and to recur.
      (1) Candidiasis: esophagus; trachea; bronchi; lungs
      (2) Coccidioidomycosis: disseminated or extrapulmonary
      (3) Cryptococcosis: extrapulmonary
      (4) Cryptosporidia diarrhea for over 1 month
      (5) CMV disease or retinitis
      (6) Encephalopathy: HIV-related
      (7) Herpes simplex: skin ulcers for over 1 month; pneumonia; bronchitis; esophagitis
      (8) Histoplasmosis: disseminated or extrapulmonary
      (9) Isosporiasis: chronic diarrhea for more than 1 month
      (10) *Mycobacterium avium-intracellulare* or *M. kansasii:* disseminated or extrapulmonary
      (11) *M. tuberculosis:* pulmonary or extrapulmonary
      (12) *Mycobacterium:* other species disseminated or extrapulmonary
      (13) *Pneumocystis carinii* pneumonia: most common reason for admission to the critical care unit
      (14) Pneumonia: recurrent
      (15) Progressive multifocal leukoencephalopathy
      (16) *Salmonella* septicemia: recurrent
      (17) Toxoplasmic encephalitis
   b. Malignancy: Malignancy in the patient with HIV tends to be more aggressive and responds more poorly to therapy.
      (1) Cervical cancer: invasive
      (2) Kaposi sarcoma: in patients less than 60 years of age
      (3) Lymphoma
         (a) Burkitt's
         (b) Immunoblastic
         (c) Primary lymphoma of the brain
   c. Wasting syndrome caused by HIV
4. Diagnostic
   a. Acute retroviral syndrome: leukopenia, elevated liver enzymes
   b. Serum
      (1) Tests for the antibody to HIV
         (a) ELISA: screening test with high sensitivity, and so used to rule out HIV
         (b) Western blot: high specificity, and so used to rule in HIV
      (2) Test for the antigen (i.e., virus): nucleic acid detection
         (a) Cell culture
         (b) Polymerase chain reaction (PCR)
         (c) Viral load testing: important in detection of resistance to antivirals
         (d) Viral resistance testing: indicates resistance mutations of the virus
            (i) HIV genotype
            (ii) Phenotypic testing
      (3) Tests for immunocompetence
         (a) CD4 lymphocyte cell count
            (i) Normal: ~1000 cells/mm^3
            (ii) AIDS: CD4 less than 200 cells/mm^3
         (b) CD4 below 14%
         (c) Ratio of CD4 to CD8+ cells: less than 1
      (4) Immune substances
         (a) Acid-labile alpha interferon
         (b) HLA DR5
         (c) Immunoglobulins: may be elevated in number but decreased in function
      (5) Hemoglobin and hematocrit: may be decreased
      (6) WBCs: may be decreased

(7) Platelets: may be decreased
(8) Total protein, albumin, transferrin: decreased in protein malnutrition

c. Skin tests: may be decreased or absent delayed hypersensitivity reactions to common antigens (e.g., *Candida*, mumps, and purified protein derivative)
d. Chest x-ray: may reveal pneumonia
e. Bronchoscopy with lavage and/or biopsy: may be performed for diagnosis of *Pneumocystis carinii* pneumonia (also called *PCP*), Kaposi sarcoma, and tuberculosis

Nursing Diagnoses

1. Risk for Infection related to immunodeficiency
2. Impaired Tissue Integrity related to infection
3. Impaired Gas Exchange related to *Pneumocystis carinii* pneumonia
4. Imbalanced Nutrition: Less Than Body Requirements related to HIV and adverse drug effects
5. Diarrhea related to adverse drug effects and HIV
6. Anticipatory Grieving related to diagnosis of disease with no known cure
7. Anxiety related to acute change in health status
8. Ineffective Individual Coping related to situational crisis, powerlessness, and change in role
9. Interrupted Family Processes related to critically ill family member
10. Deficient Knowledge related to health maintenance

Collaborative Management

1. Minimize further immune system damage.
   a. Administer highly active antiretroviral therapy (HAART) as prescribed (included in Table 10-14).
      (1) Types of antiretrovirals

Table 10-14 Selected Antivirals and Antiinfectives for Human Immunodeficiency Virus/Acquired Immunodeficiency Syndrome

Drug	Also Called	Indication	Adverse Effects
Abacavir (Ziagen)	1592/ABC	HIV: NRTI antiretroviral	• Systemic hypersensitivity reaction • Nausea, vomiting • Fever • Malaise
Acyclovir (Zovirax)		Viral infections • Herpes simplex 1 and 2 • Varicella zoster	• Anorexia, nausea, vomiting, abdominal pain, diarrhea (oral administration) • Rash • Headache • Bone marrow depression (IV administration) • Nephrotoxicity (IV administration)
Amphotericin B (Fungizone)		Disseminated fungal infections	• Chills, fever • Anorexia, nausea, vomiting, diarrhea • Headache • Muscle and joint pain • Hypotension • Electrolyte imbalance ◦ Hypokalemia ◦ Hypomagnesemia • Bone marrow depression ◦ Leukopenia ◦ Thrombocytopenia ◦ Anemia • Hepatotoxicity • Nephrotoxicity • Seizures
Amprenavir (Agenerase)		HIV; protease inhibitor antiretroviral	• Nausea, vomiting • Rash • Increased liver enzymes • Fat redistribution • Hyperglycemia
Atazanavir (Reyataz)		HIV; protease inhibitor antiretroviral	• Headache • Rash • Nausea, abdominal discomfort, diarrhea • Elevated bilirubin • Elevated liver enzymes • Peripheral neuropathy • Atrioventricular conduction abnormalities

Continued

Table 10-14 Selected Antivirals and Antiinfectives for Human Immunodeficiency Virus/Acquired Immunodeficiency Syndrome—cont'd

Drug	Also Called	Indication	Adverse Effects
Dapsone		*Pneumocystis carinii* pneumonia prophylaxis	• Nausea, vomiting • Headache • Peripheral neuropathy • Anemia • Methemoglobinemia • Leukopenia • Hepatotoxicity • Nephrotoxicity • Visual changes
Delavirdine (Rescriptor)	DLV	HIV: NNRTI antiretroviral	• Nausea • Fever • Rash

Didanosine (Videx)	ddI	HIV: NRTI antiretroviral Indicated for patients who cannot tolerate zidovudine (Retrovir) or who have become resistant to Retrovir	• Anorexia, nausea, vomiting, abdominal pain, diarrhea
			• Dry mouth
			• Headache
			• Peripheral neuropathy
			• Seizures
			• Pancreatitis
			• Elevated liver enzymes; hepatotoxicity
			• Bone marrow depression
			  ◦ Leukopenia
			  ◦ Thrombocytopenia
			  ◦ Anemia

Efavirenz (Sustiva)	DMP 266	HIV: NNRTI antiretroviral	• Dizziness • Rash • Hepatitis • Confusion • Insomnia
Enfuvirtide (Fuzeon)		HIV; fusion inhibitor	• Skin reactions at injection site (administered subcutaneously) • Headache • Pain • Peripheral neuropathy • Dizziness • Insomnia
Fluconazole (Diflucan)		Fungal infections	• Nausea, vomiting, abdominal pain, diarrhea • Headache • Rash • Elevated liver enzymes
Foscarnet (Foscavir)		Pulmonary CMV	• Anorexia, nausea, vomiting, diarrhea • Dysrhythmias • Elevated liver enzymes • Nephrotoxicity • Electrolyte imbalance • Bone marrow depression • Bronchospasm • Myalgia • Seizures

Ganciclovir (Cytovene)		CMV	• Chills, fever
			• Anorexia, nausea, vomiting, diarrhea
			• Rash
			• Bone marrow depression
			  ◦ Leukopenia
			  ◦ Thrombocytopenia
			  ◦ Anemia
			• Elevated liver enzymes
			• Disorientation, confusion

Table 10-14 Selected Antivirals and Antiinfectives for Human Immunodeficiency Virus/Acquired Immunodeficiency Syndrome—cont'd

Drug	Also Called	Indication	Adverse Effects
Indinavir (Crixivan)	IND	HIV: protease inhibitor antiretroviral	• Diarrhea, abdominal pain, nausea, vomiting, anorexia • Headache • Renal stones • Hyperbilirubinemia • Elevated liver enzymes • Elevated cholesterol and triglycerides • Hyperglycemia • Fat redistribution
Lamivudine (Epivir)	3TC	HIV: NRTI antiretroviral	• Nausea, vomiting, anorexia, abdominal pain, diarrhea, dyspepsia • Headache • Pancreatitis • Photophobia • Rash • Renal stones • Myalgia, arthralgia • Bone marrow depression ◦ Leukopenia ◦ Thrombocytopenia ◦ Anemia
Lopinavir and ritonavir (Kaletra)		HIV; protease inhibitor antiretroviral	• Nausea, vomiting • Elevated cholesterol and triglycerides • Elevated liver enzymes • Rash • Headache
Nelfinavir (Viracept)	NFV	HIV: protease inhibitor antiretroviral	• Diarrhea • Elevated liver enzymes • Elevated cholesterol and triglycerides • Hyperglycemia • Fat redistribution
Nevirapine (Viramune)	NVP	HIV: NNRTI antiretroviral	• Nausea • Rash; Stevens-Johnson syndrome • Fever
Pentamidine (Pentam)		*Pneumocystis carinii* pneumonia	• Nausea, vomiting • Metallic taste • Chills, facial flushing • Hypertension • Rash • Hypotension • Dysrhythmias • Hyperglycemia • Hyperkalemia • Nephrotoxicity • Elevated liver enzymes • Pancreatitis • Leukopenia • Thrombocytopenia
Ritonavir (Norvir)	RTV	HIV: protease inhibitor antiretroviral	• Anorexia, nausea, vomiting, abdominal pain, diarrhea • Buccal mucosa ulceration • Dry mouth; bitter taste • Headache • Paresthesia • Rash • Elevated cholesterol and triglycerides • Hyperglycemia • Fat redistribution

Continued

Table 10-14 Selected Antivirals and Antiinfectives for Human Immunodeficiency Virus/Acquired Immunodeficiency Syndrome—cont'd

Drug	Also Called	Indication	Adverse Effects
Saquinavir (originally Invirase, now Fortovase)	SQV	HIV: protease inhibitor antiretroviral	• Anorexia, nausea, vomiting, abdominal pain, diarrhea • Elevated cholesterol and triglycerides • Fat redistribution • Dry mouth • Headache • Somnolence • Rash
Stavudine (Zerit)	d4T	HIV: NRTI antiretroviral Advanced HIV infection not responsive to other antiretrovirals	• Nausea, vomiting, anorexia, diarrhea, dyspepsia, stomatitis, pancreatitis • Hepatotoxicity • Bone marrow depression: anemia • Peripheral neuropathy • Myalgia, arthralgia • Photosensitivity • Rash
Tenofivir (Viread)		HIV; NtRTI	• Nausea, vomiting, diarrhea, flatulence • Hepatomegaly • Lactic acidosis

Trimethoprim-Sulfamethoxazole (TMP-SMZ)	TMP-SMX	*Pneumocystis carinii* pneumonia
		Isospora belli infection
		Salmonella infection
		Shigella infection
			• Rash
			• Fever
			• Nausea, vomiting
			• Peripheral neuritis
			• Bone marrow depression
			  ◦ Leukopenia
			  ◦ Thrombocytopenia
			• Headache
			• Elevated liver enzymes

Zalcitabine (Hivid)	ddC	HIV: NRTI antiretroviral combination treatment with zidovudine CD4 count of 300 cells/mm^3 or less in patients who have demonstrated clinical or immune system deterioration	• Anorexia, nausea, vomiting, abdominal pain, diarrhea, stomatitis
			• Rash, pruritus
			• Headache
			• Elevated liver enzymes
			• Bone marrow depression
			  ◦ Leukopenia
			  ◦ Thrombocytopenia
			• Peripheral neuropathy
			• Pancreatitis
			• Nephrotoxicity

Zidovudine (Retrovir)	AZT	HIV: NRTI antiretroviral
		CD4 count of 500/mm^3 or lower even if asymptomatic
			• Bone marrow depression
			  ◦ Anemia
			  ◦ Leukopenia
			  ◦ Thrombocytopenia
			• Nausea, vomiting, abdominal pain, diarrhea
			• Taste changes
			• Rash, acne
			• Headache
			• Fatigue, malaise
			• Myalgia
			• Insomnia

Zidovudine and lamivudine (Combivir)		HIV: both of these drugs are NRTI antiretrovirals	• Bone marrow depression
			  ◦ Anemia
			  ◦ Leukopenia
			  ◦ Thrombocytopenia

Zidovudine, lamivudine, and abacavir (Trizivir)		HIV: all of these drugs are NRTI antiretrovirals	• Bone marrow depression
			  ◦ Anemia
			  ◦ Leukopenia
			  ◦ Thrombocytopenia

HIV, Human immunodeficiency virus; *IV*, intravenous; *NNRTI*, nonnucleoside reverse transcriptase inhibitor; *NRTI*, nucleoside reverse transcriptase inhibitor; *NtRTI*, nucleotide reverse transcriptase inhibitor.

(a) Analog nucleoside reverse transcriptase inhibitors (NRTI)
(i) First class of antiretroviral agents introduced
(ii) Prevent the viral enzyme reverse transcriptase from synthesizing DNA from viral RNA
(iii) Examples include zidovudine (Retrovir), didanosine (Videx), zalcitabine (Hivid), lamivudine (Epivir), and stavudine (Zerit)
(b) Nonnucleoside reverse transcriptase inhibitors (NNRTI)
(i) Interfere directly with reverse transcriptase
(ii) Resistance is common, so generally reserved for use in three-drug combinations
(iii) Examples include nevirapine, delavirdine, and efavirenz
(c) Protease inhibitors
(i) Prevents viral protein from being broken down into usable segments by the enzyme protease
(ii) Generally given in combination with two or more antiretroviral agents because of concern about HIV resistance
(iii) Combinations of two protease inhibitors are being used because of enhancement of effectiveness
(iv) Examples include ritonavir (Norvir), saquinavir (Invirase), indinavir (Crixivan), and nelfinavir (Viracept)
(d) Nucleotide reverse transcriptase inhibitor (NtRTI)
(i) Prevents HIV from reproducing in uninfected cells
(ii) Example: tenofovir (Viread)
(e) Fusion inhibitor
(i) Prevents the entry of HIV into the cell by preventing fusion of the virus coat and the cell membrane
(ii) Only approved for advanced HIV disease
(iii) Example: enfuvirtide (Fuzeon)
(2) Multiple drug therapy is preferred because of the rapid development of resistance with monotherapy
(a) Recommendation is to use three or more drugs, using agents from two or more classes
(i) Different mechanisms of action
(ii) Nonoverlapping toxicity
(b) Common combinations include the following:
(i) Two nucleoside analogs + one or two protease inhibitors
(ii) Two nucleoside analogs + one nonnucleoside reverse transcriptase inhibitor
(3) HIV viral load testing along with CD4 cell count are used to monitor the therapeutic effect of drugs
(4) Complications of highly active antiretroviral therapy
(a) Lipodystrophy: redistribution of body fat
(b) Alteration in blood lipid levels along with altered blood glucose metabolism
(i) Hypertriglyceridemia may cause acute pancreatitis.
(c) Anemia
(d) Virologic failure with resultant increase in viral load
(5) Discuss the importance of taking all the prescribed doses of the drugs
b. Encourage adequate rest and nutrition.
c. Encourage avoidance of alcohol and nonprescribed drugs.
2. Prevent infection.
a. Use good hand-washing techniques.
b. Place patient in private room if possible to prevent transmission of infection to the patient.
c. Decrease number of visitors, and do not permit visitors with infections (e.g., upper respiratory infection).
3. Identify and treat opportunistic infections and malignancy (Table 10-15).
a. Monitor for complications of HIV and of drug therapy.
b. Treat fever with antipyretics, tepid sponge baths, and fluid replacement.
c. Monitor for and treat *Pneumocystic carinii* pneumonia and acute respiratory failure.
(1) Early symptoms include nonproductive cough, dyspnea, fever, chills, and chest pain.
(2) Assist with symptom management.
(a) Positioning
(b) Cool air by fan
(c) Pursed lip breathing
(d) Relaxation techniques: guided imagery, music, massage, meditation, prayer
(e) Oxygen
(f) Opiates
(g) Anxiolytics
(h) Bronchodilators (e.g., beta-2 stimulants)
(3) Diagnostic studies include chest x-ray (findings similar to ARDS), sputum culture that frequently requires inducement with saline lavage, and/or bronchoscopy with bronchial lavage or brushing.
(4) Collaborative management includes the following:
(a) Administer trimethoprim-sulfamethoxazole (TMP-SMX) orally or IV or pentamidine (Pentam) by inhalation or IV.
(i) Trimethoprim-sulfamethoxazole administered IV requires dilution in a large volume of fluid and may cause fluid overload.

Table 10-15 Opportunistic Infections and Malignancies Seen in Acquired Immunodeficiency Syndrome and Treatment

Infection or Malignancy	Treatment
BACTERIAL INFECTIONS	
Mycobacterium tuberculosis	• Isoniazid (INH) • Ethambutol (Myambutol) • Rifampin (Rifadin) • Pyrazinamide • Streptomycin • Para-aminosalicylic acid
Mycobacterium avium-intracellulare	• Clarithromycin • Azithromycin (Zithromax) • Ethambutol (Myambutol) • Isoniazid (INH) • Rifampin (Rifadin) • Streptomycin • Amikacin (Amikin) • Ciprofloxacin (Cipro) • Clofazimine (Lamprene) • Rifabutin (Mycobutin) • Cycloserine (Seromycin)
Salmonella	• Chloramphenicol (Chloromycetin) • Ampicillin • Amoxicillin • Trimethoprim-sulfamethoxazole (TMP-SMX) • Ceftriaxone (Rocephin) • Ciprofloxacin (Cipro)
Shigella	• Trimethoprim-sulfamethoxazole (TMP-SMX) • Ciprofloxacin (Cipro) • Ampicillin • Nalidixic acid (NegGram) • Furazolidone
Treponema pallidum (syphilis)	• Penicillin
Neisseria gonorrhoeae	• Ceftriaxone sodium (Rocephin) • Cefixime (Suprax) • Ciprofloxacin (Cipro) • Ofloxacin (Floxin)
PROTOZOAL INFECTIONS	
Pneumocystis carinii	• Trimethoprim-sulfamethoxazole (TMP-SMX) • Pentamidine (Pentam) • Dapsone-trimethoprim
Cryptosporidium enteritidis	• Amphotericin B (Fungizone) • Spiramycin (Rovamycin)
Toxoplasma gondii	• Pyrimethamine (Daraprim) • Sulfadiazine • Pyrimethamine-sulfadoxine (Fansidar) • Clindamycin (Cleocin)
Isospora belli	• Trimethoprim-sulfamethoxazole (TMP-SMX)
VIRAL INFECTIONS	
Herpes (1 and 2)	• Acyclovir (Zovirax) • Foscarnet • Vidarabine (Vira-A)
Cytomegalovirus	• Ganciclovir (Cytovene) • Foscarnet (Foscavir) Retinitis
Varicella zoster	• Acyclovir (Zovirax) • Foscarnet • Vidarabine (Vira-A)
Hepatitis A, B, or non-A/non-B	• Interferon alfa-2b for B and non-A/non-B
FUNGAL INFECTIONS	
Candida albicans	• Nystatin rinses (for oral candidiasis) • Clotrimazole (Mycelex) • Amphotericin B (Fungizone) • Fluconazole (Diflucan) • Ketoconazole (Nizoral) • Itraconazole (Sporanox)
Cryptococcus neoformans	• Amphotericin B (Fungizone) • Fluconazole (Diflucan) • Ketoconazole (Nizoral) • Itraconazole (Sporanox)
Histoplasma capsulatum	• Amphotericin B (Fungizone) • Fluconazole (Diflucan) • Ketoconazole (Nizoral) • Itraconazole (Sporanox)
Coccidioides immitis	• Amphotericin B (Fungizone) • Fluconazole (Diflucan) • Itraconazole (Sporanox) • Ketoconazole (Nizoral)
MALIGNANCIES	
Kaposi sarcoma	• Radiation • Surgical excision • Cryotherapy • Chemotherapy • Interferon alfa-2a • Doxorubicin (Adriamycin) • Bleomycin (Blenoxane) • Vinblastine (Velban) • Vincristine (Oncovin) • Methotrexate (Folex) • Cyclophosphamide (Cytoxan)
Central nervous system lymphoma	• Radiation
Hodgkin's lymphoma	• Radiation • Chemotherapy
Non-Hodgkin's lymphoma	• Radiation • Steroids • Chemotherapy

(ii) Pentamidine administration by inhalation may cause bronchospasm.
(iii) Pentamidine administered IV may cause hypotension.
(b) Administer oxygen for hypoxemia.
(c) Initiate mechanical ventilation as prescribed for respiratory acidosis and fatigue.
(d) Bronchodilators may be necessary for bronchospasm.
(e) Provide appropriate rest periods.
(f) Encourage fluid intake to liquefy secretions.
(g) Encourage sustained inspiration and incentive spirometry; encourage the patient to cough; suction secretions only if necessary.
(h) Provide frequent oral and nasal care to prevent candidiasis.

4. Provide appropriate nutritional support.
a. Monitor nutritional status and electrolyte balance.
b. Monitor for and treat HIV wasting indicated by unexplained weight loss of more than 10% of body weight.
(1) Provide diet that is high in protein and calories.
(a) Discourage ingestion of "empty calorie" foods.
(b) Administer multivitamins as ordered.
(2) Provide small, frequent meals with snacks as desired.
(3) Provide the patient's favorite foods.
c. Identify causes for anorexia and provide symptomatic relief.
(1) Possible causes of anorexia in the patient with HIV include adverse medication effects, altered taste, dysphagia, nausea, vomiting, weakness, and lethargy.
(2) Avoid providing fatty, spicy, or overly sweet foods.
(3) Avoid metallic utensils and foods from metal cans.
(4) Administer antiemetics as prescribed.
(5) Administer megestrol (Megace), dronabinol (Marinol), and oxandrolone (Oxandrin) as prescribed.
d. Provide symptomatic relief for stomatitis.
(1) Provide a mixture of viscous lidocaine, diphenhydramine (Benadryl) elixir, and a magnesium or aluminum salt product such as Mylanta or sucralfate (Carafate) suspension before meals to reduce mouth pain in the patient while eating.
(2) Provide meticulous mouth care.
(3) Administer nystatin (Mycostatin) as prescribed for oral candidiasis.
e. Provide symptomatic relief of diarrhea.
(1) Replace fluids and electrolytes.
(a) High-potassium foods
(b) Electrolyte-containing fluids (e.g., Gatorade) may be helpful
(2) Provide diet low in fat and lactose and high in soluble fiber (e.g., oatmeal and fruit).
(3) Avoid extreme temperature in foods.
(4) Avoid caffeine.
(5) Administer antidiarrheal drugs as prescribed; acidophilus or Lactaid also may be helpful.
f. Provide symptomatic relief of dysphagia.
(1) Provide soft, bland, nutrient-dense foods and supplements; gelatin, yogurt, and pudding are easy to swallow.
(2) Provide small, frequent meals.
g. Administer enteral or parenteral nutritional support as prescribed.
(1) Assist with placement of an enteral feeding tube or vascular access.
(2) Use medium chain triglycerides (e.g., Lipisorb or Peptamen) or elemental formulae (e.g., Vivonex TEN) as prescribed.

5. Prevent transmission of HIV.
a. Consider all body secretions as potentially infectious.
b. Use protective barriers when exposure to blood or body fluids is likely.
(1) Wear gloves when hands will come in contact with blood, body fluids, nonintact skin, or items or surfaces soiled with blood or body fluids.
(2) Wear gown, mask, and goggles whenever there is a chance of spattering of body fluids, especially blood.
(3) Wear masks whenever there is an airborne infection (e.g., tuberculosis).
(4) Use mouthpieces and manual resuscitation bags for resuscitation.
c. Wash hands immediately after removing gloves and anytime hands are contaminated with blood or other infectious substances.
d. Use caution with sharp instruments (e.g., needles and scalpels), and dispose of these objects safely.
(1) Do not recap needles.
(2) Place all sharps in puncture-resistant container.
e. Double-bag and label linens as infectious.
f. Decontaminate surfaces exposed to body fluids with 1:10 dilution of bleach solution.
g. Ensure that reusable equipment is washed and autoclaved.
h. Teach patient and significant others about transmission of HIV.
(1) HIV is not transmitted by casual contact.
(2) Saliva has not been shown to be a transmission medium, so eating utensils do not need to be disposable and simply should be washed after use.
(3) HIV is transmitted via venereal fluids, blood, and breast milk and perinatally.
(a) Toothbrushes, razors, needles, or other items that may be contaminated with blood should not be shared.

(b) Sexual transmission should be prevented though the use of condoms with nonoxynol-9, which has been shown to kill HIV and prevent other sexually transmitted diseases.
(i) Remember: this practice is considered safer than not using a condom, but is not safe.
(c) HIV-positive women should not breast-feed infants; use of antiretrovirals perinatally has been shown to decrease transmission of the virus to the unborn child.
(d) HIV-positive persons should not donate blood or expose anyone else to their blood.
(e) HIV-positive persons should inform their dentist and other health care professionals of their HIV status.
(f) Injectable drug users should discard needles and syringes safely or should clean syringes and needles with a 1:10 dilution of bleach solution; syringes and needles should not be shared.

6. Provide compassionate emotional support and health counseling.
   a. Be nonjudgmental, and use scientific knowledge instead of prejudice in health counseling.
   b. Assess the following:
      (1) The patient's level of knowledge about HIV and AIDS
      (2) The patient's past experiences with others with HIV and AIDS
      (3) The patient's perception of HIV and AIDS in light of their cultural and religious beliefs
   c. Teach patient how to prevent transmission of HIV to others.
   d. Teach significant others what they can do to help and support the patient and to protect themselves from HIV.
   e. Teach clinical indications of infection and what to do if they occur.
   f. Spend time listening to the patient's fears and concerns; allow the patient to express fear and grief.
7. Monitor patient for complications.
   a. Acute respiratory failure
   b. Septic shock
   c. Meningitis
   d. CNS lymphoma
   e. HIV encephalopathy
   f. Coagulopathy
      (1) DIC
      (2) Thrombocytopenic purpura
   g. CMV retinitis
   h. Heart failure
   i. Pulmonary embolism
   j. GI bleeding
   k. Adrenal crisis

Organ Transplantation

Donor

1. Sources of organ donors
   a. Deceased donors (previously referred to as *cadaver donor*)
      (1) Patient has been declared brain dead.
         (a) Irreversible cessation of all functions of the entire brain, including the brainstem
            (i) Recognizable cause of coma (e.g., severe head trauma, intracranial hemorrhage, anoxic encephalopathy following cardiac arrest, drowning, or asphyxiation)
            (ii) Potentially reversible causes of coma (sedative drugs including alcohol, neuromuscular blocking agents, hypothermia, or metabolic or endocrine disturbance) excluded or eradicated
            (iii) No spontaneous ventilation when tested for a sufficient time; usually 3 to 5 minutes of $Paco_2$ of greater than 60 mm Hg; apnea testing is performed by doing the following:
               a) Disconnect the mechanical ventilator.
               b) Deliver 100% oxygen.
               c) Monitor for ventilatory effort.
               d) Measure ABGs after 8 minutes to confirm $Paco_2$ greater than 60 mm Hg.
               e) Reconnect the ventilator.
            (iv) No brainstem reflexes
               a) No pupillary light reflex
               b) No corneal reflex
               c) No oculocephalic reflex (doll's eyes)
               d) No oculovestibular reflex (caloric)
               e) No gag reflex
            (v) No motor response to central pain stimulation
            (vi) Electroencephalogram: no electrical activity during a period of at least 30 minutes
            (vii) Cerebral angiography: no intracerebral filling in circle of Willis or at carotid bifurcation
            (viii) Cerebral blood flow scan: no uptake of radionuclide in brain parenchyma, indicating no cerebral blood flow
   b. Deceased after cardiac death donors; previously referred to as a *non–heart-beating donor*
      (1) Irreversible cessation of circulatory and respiratory function
      (2) Constitutes only approximately 1% of cadaveric organ donors each year, but use is increasing

(3) Kidney retrieval is most likely because the kidneys generally can withstand more anoxic damage than other organs; liver retrieval is also possible
(4) Two types of those deceased after cardiac death
(a) Uncontrolled recovery: organs are removed after a sudden cardiopulmonary arrest
(b) Controlled recovery: life-sustaining treatment is discontinued while interventions to maintain viability of organs are maintained; organs are retrieved after cardiopulmonary function ceases

c. Living donors
(1) May be used for kidney, part of liver, lung, or pancreas
(2) Types
(a) Living, related donor: family member who donates to another related family member
(b) Living, unrelated donor
(i) Person not related by blood (e.g., husband, wife, in-law, or friend)
(ii) Stranger-to-stranger

2. General organ donor criteria
a. Organ function acceptable to transplant program
b. No prolonged hypotension or cardiopulmonary arrest
c. No active sepsis or cancer (exception primary brain tumor)
d. Consent from next of kin or signed organ donation card
e. Exclusions (NOTE: Recipients may be given a choice of accepting "risky" organs, and they may accept if they feel it is their only hope for survival.)
(1) General
(a) Untreated bacterial, fungal, or viral infection or sepsis
(b) Malignancy other than primary brain tumor or minor skin lesions
(c) Communicable disease (e.g., HIV)
(i) Hepatitis B donor may be matched to hepatitis B recipient, hepatitis C donor to hepatitis C recipient
(2) Heart
(a) History of cardiac disease
(b) Suboptimal cardiac function after intervention
(3) Lungs
(a) Positive sputum Gram stain
(b) Pulmonary edema
(c) Pulmonary contusion
(d) Aspiration
(e) Previous thoracic surgery on donor side
(4) Pancreas
(a) History of diabetes mellitus
(5) Kidneys
(a) Biopsy may be performed if donor history of hypertension or diabetes mellitus
(b) Congenital kidney

3. Preoperative assessment of donor to evaluate current status of organ to be transplanted
a. General for all donors
(1) Blood urea nitrogen, creatinine
(2) Electrolytes
(3) Complete blood count with platelet count
(4) Serum glucose
(5) ABGs
(6) Blood type
(7) Urinalysis
(8) Weight
(9) Psychological and emotional status if living donor
(10) Potential sources of postoperative infection
b. Heart
(1) Age: males less than 40 years old and females less than 45 years old; older donors may be accepted by an older recipient as long as no evidence of coronary artery disease or cardiac abnormalities
(2) Electrocardiagram
(3) Echocardiogram
(4) Cardiac enzymes and isoenzymes, troponin
(5) Chest x-ray
(6) Cardiac catheterization may be indicated
c. Lung
(1) ABGs
(2) Gram stain and culture of sputum
(3) Chest x-ray
(4) Pulmonary function studies
d. Liver
(1) Liver function studies: aspartate transaminase, alanine transaminase, alkaline phosphatase, gamma-glutamyl transpeptidase, lactate dehydrogenase
(2) Bilirubin: indirect and direct
(3) Hemoglobin, hematocrit
(4) PT, aPTT
(5) Total protein, albumin
(6) Type and crossmatch
e. Pancreas
(1) Serum amylase
(2) Urine culture
f. Kidney
(1) Urine culture

4. Tissue histocompatibility to evaluate donor and recipient
a. ABO compatibility: detects surface antigens on RBCs and other tissues
b. Minor red cell antigen testing: detects surface antigens on RBCs
c. Microlymphocytotoxicity testing: detects Class I HLA and match between donor and recipients
d. Mixed leukocyte culture or mixed lymphocyte culture: detects Class II HLA (NOTE: This test takes too long to be used for cadaver organs; it is used for living kidney donors.)

e. White cell crossmatch: detects presence of preformed circulating cytotoxic antibodies in recipient to antigens on the lymphocytes of the donor
f. Mixed lymphocyte crossmatch: detects presence of preformed circulating cytotoxic antibodies in recipient to antigens on the lymphocytes of the donor

5. Collaborative management of the donor before transplant
   a. Recognize the patient as a potential organ donor according to donor criteria, and follow hospital protocol for notification of the local organ procurement organization.
   b. Collaborate with the physician and organ procurement coordinator in obtaining consent for organ donation from closest family member; if family is not available, look for signed organ donor card.
      (1) Offer the patient's family the option of organ donation as soon as brain death has been declared.
      (2) Ensure that the person who approaches the family is an expert regarding organ donation and has the time to spend with the family.
      (3) Approach the family in a private, quiet location.
      (4) Allow time for the family to accept the death.
      (5) Use the word *dead* not *nearly dead*, *almost dead*, or *for all practical purposes dead;* avoid the term *brain dead* because families then tend to believe that there is something worse than brain dead; brain death is permanent and irreversible, and when the brain is dead, the person is dead.
      (6) Use *recover*, *retrieve*, or *remove* organs; avoid the word *harvest*.
      (7) Avoid the term *life support* or indicate that the patient is being "kept alive," because it implies that the patient is not truly dead; use *mechanical ventilation*.
      (8) Use the patient's name and do not refer to the patient as the "donor."
      (9) Believe in the benefit to the family of the donor and to the recipient.
      (10) Ensure confidentiality of the donor family and transplant recipients.
   c. Obtain necessary measurements and laboratory data.
      (1) Height and weight
      (2) Serology screening for hepatitis antigen and antibody; HIV, syphilis, and CMV
      (3) Blood type and crossmatch
      (4) Tissue typing
      (5) Diagnostic studies to evaluate organ status
   d. Maintain airway, oxygenation, and ventilation.
      (1) Ensure a patent airway.
      (2) Elevate head of the bed to 30 degrees until hypotension results.
      (3) Administer oxygen to maintain $Pa{O_2}$ of at least 80 mm Hg and arterial oxygen saturation greater than 95%.
      (4) Use mechanical ventilation to maintain $Pa{CO_2}$ at 35 to 45 mm Hg.
      (5) Use sequential compression devices to prevent deep venous thrombosis.
      (6) Maintain orogastric suction to low intermittent suction to aid in prevention of aspiration.
      (7) Administer beta-2 stimulants as prescribed for bronchospasm.
   e. Maintain adequate organ perfusion and tissue oxygenation.
      (1) Monitor vital signs, urine output, and hemodynamic parameters.
      (2) Administer IV fluids, inotropes, and/or vasopressors as prescribed to maintain systolic blood pressure of 100 mm Hg, mean arterial pressure of greater than 70 mm Hg, and urine output greater than 100 mL/hr.
      (3) Administer proton pump inhibitor as prescribed to aid in prevention of stress ulcer.
   f. Maintain adequate hydration and electrolyte balance.
      (1) Monitor serum osmolality and electrolytes.
      (2) Replace fluids and electrolytes as prescribed.
         (a) Careful monitoring is required; though it is important to perfuse organs, the lungs are susceptible to adverse effects of overhydration.
      (3) Control diabetes insipidus with administration of aqueous vasopressin as prescribed.
      (4) Monitor serum glucose every 2 hours by finger stick, and administer insulin as required.
   g. Maintain normal body temperature.
      (1) Use warm blankets, radiant heat lamps, warm inspired air by the ventilator, and/or warm IV fluids as indicated for hypothermia.
      (2) Use antipyretics and tepid sponge baths as indicated for hyperthermia; aspirin is preferred as an antipyretic because of the potential adverse liver effects of acetaminophen.
   h. Prevent infection.
      (1) Monitor patient for clinical indications of infection.
      (2) Avoid intrusive procedures if possible.
      (3) Use strict aseptic technique in IV, airway, and tube management.
      (4) Administer antibiotics as prescribed.
   i. Transport the patient to the operating room when the organ procurement organization has found recipients for all of the organs that will be donated.

Recipient

1. General organ recipient criteria
   a. End-stage organ disease
   b. Positive psychosocial assessment factors
   c. Absence of the following:
      (1) Infection or transmittable disease
      (2) Malignancy
      (3) Substance abuse
      (4) Other organ system failure
2. Preoperative assessment of recipient
   a. General for all donors
      (1) Blood urea nitrogen, creatinine

(2) Electrolytes
(3) Complete blood count with platelet count
(4) Serum glucose
(5) ABGs
(6) Blood type
(7) Urinalysis
(8) Weight
(9) Tissue histocompatibility to evaluate donor and recipient (described under Donor)

b. Heart
(1) Electrocardiogram
(2) Echocardiogram
(3) Stress test: exercise if capable or pharmacologic
(4) Cardiac enzymes and isoenzymes; troponin
(5) Chest x-ray
(6) Cardiac catheterization
(7) Pulmonary function studies
(8) Carotid Doppler ultrasonography studies

c. Lung
(1) ABGs
(2) Gram stain and culture of sputum
(3) Chest x-ray
(4) Pulmonary function studies

d. Liver
(1) Liver function studies: aspartate transaminase (AST), alanine aminotransferase (ALT), alkaline phosphatase (ALP), gamma-glutamyl transpeptidase (GGTP), lactate dehydrogenase (LDH)
(2) Bilirubin: indirect and direct
(3) Hemoglobin, hematocrit
(4) PT, aPTT
(5) Total protein, albumin
(6) Type and crossmatch

e. Pancreas
(1) Serum amylase
(2) Urine culture

f. Kidney
(1) Urine culture

3. Nursing Diagnoses for the recipient after transplant
   a. Risk for Infection related to immunosuppression
   b. Excess or Deficient Fluid Volume related to heart failure, overhydration, hemorrhage, and third spacing
   c. Impaired Gas Exchange related to heart failure and lung transplant
   d. Pain related to surgical procedure
   e. Ineffective Individual Coping related to situational crisis, powerlessness, and change in role
   f. Interrupted Family Processes related to critically ill family member
   g. Deficient Knowledge related to health maintenance
4. Collaborative management of the recipient after transplant
   a. Relieve pain and anxiety.
      (1) Administer narcotics (e.g., morphine) for pain relief.
         (a) Not given after liver transplant until patient is awake and LOC can be assessed because of the risk of intracerebral hemorrhage
      (2) Administer anxiolytics (e.g., diazepam) as needed.
      (3) Allow patient the opportunity to discuss feelings and concerns regarding the surgery and chances of success.
   b. Protect patient from infection.
      (1) Monitor patient for clinical indications of infection; CMV is one common serious infection in immunodeficient patients.
         (a) Clinical indications: fever; malaise; leukopenia, thrombocytopenia, or anemia; abnormal liver function studies; pneumonitis; hepatic or splenic enlargement; impaired graft function
         (b) Diagnosis by CMV antigen
      (2) Administer antimicrobials and antivirals as prescribed.
   c. Prevent and detect acute rejection of transplant (Figure 10-7 illustrates the pathophysiology of rejection; Table 10-16 summarizes forms of rejection).
      (1) Administer antirejection agents (Table 10-17); corticosteroids and azathioprine (Imuran) or cyclosporine (Neoral) or tacrolimus (Prograf) usually are used for maintenance; other agents may be substituted or added for acute rejection.

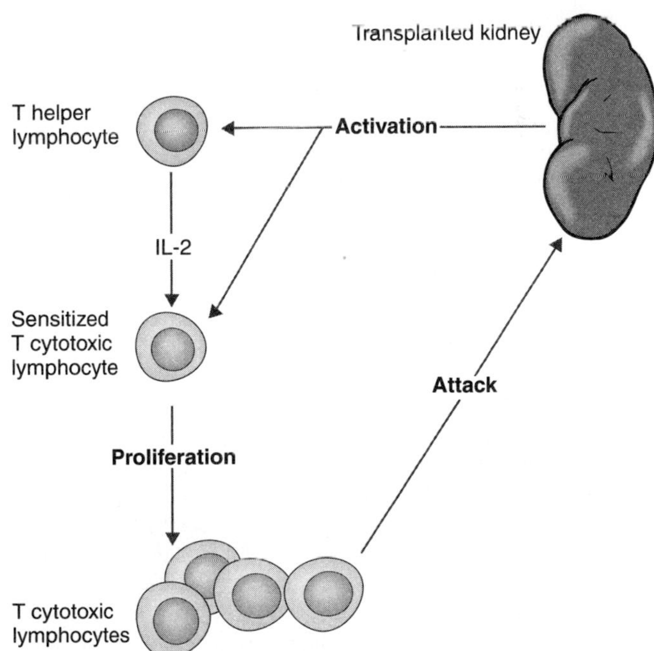

Figure 10-7 Mechanism of action of T cytotoxic lymphocyte activation and attack of renal transplanted tissue. The transplanted kidney is recognized as foreign and activates the immune system. T helper cells are activated to produce interleukin-2, and T cytotoxic lymphocytes are sensitized. After these T cytotoxic cells proliferate, they attack the transplanted kidney. (From Lewis, S. M., Heitkemper, M. M., & Dirksen, S. R. [2004]. *Medical-surgical nursing: Assessment and management of clinical problems* [6th ed.]. St. Louis: Mosby.)

Table 10-16 Forms of Rejection

Form	Time Frame	Mechanism	Treatment
Hyperacute	Minutes to hours	Humoral response involving preexisting antibodies; results in infarction occurring before the end of the transplantation procedure or within a few hours after the surgical procedure	• Immediate graft failure occurs, so removal is required
Accelerated	Within 3 days	Cellular response; results in organ failure	• High-dose steroids • Response to treatment: poor
Acute	1 week to 1 year	Cellular response to antigens on the cells of the transplanted graft	• High-dose steroids • Response to treatment: good
Chronic	1 to 5 years	Humoral-mediated and cell-mediated responses; result in chronic inflammation with diffuse scarring of the organ, stenosis of the vasculature, and ischemia and necrosis of the organ tissue	• Rescue agents such as rabbit antithymocyte globulin • Response to treatment: poor since progressive process

Table 10-17 Antirejection Agents

Drug	Effects	Adverse Effects
Steroids Inhibit production of T cell lymphokines		
• Prednisone (Deltasone, Orasone)	• Inhibits inflammation by inhibiting production of prostaglandin • Impairs the sensitivity of the T cells to an antigen • Prevents proliferation of sensitized T cells • Impairs the production of interleukins • Decreases macrophage mobility • Used for maintenance therapy and to treat acute rejection	• Cushingoid appearance • Gastrointestinal irritation and/or hemorrhage • Sodium and water retention • Hypertension • Hyperglycemia • Mood swings • Protein catabolism • Delayed healing • Development of cataracts • Development of neoplasms • Aseptic bone necrosis • Decreased resistance to infection
Calcineurin Inhibitors Inhibit calcineurin activity, thereby interfering with the function of interleukin-2		
• Cyclosporine (Neoral, Gengraf)	• Interferes with the production and activity of cytotoxic and helper T cells • Interferes with the secretion of interleukins by helper T cells and the ability of cytotoxic T cells to respond to interleukins • Interferes with the ability of macrophages to secrete interleukin • Associated with less risk of infection than corticosteroids because more cellular immunity specific • Used as a maintenance immunosuppressive agent	• Nausea • Gingival hyperplasia • Headache • Leg cramps • Hirsutism • Hypertension • Nephrotoxicity • Hepatotoxicity • Electrolyte imbalance: hyperkalemia; hypomagnesemia • Tremors, seizures • Lymphocytopenia • Development of neoplasms: lymphomas • Increased susceptibility to infection, especially viral or fungal infections

Table 10-17 Antirejection Agents—cont'd

Drug	Effects	Adverse Effects
• Tacrolimus (Prograf) ◦ Formerly referred to as *FK 506*	• Blocks production of IL-2 and other lymphokines that help activate T lymphocytes • Associated with fewer adverse effects than cyclosporine; not as nephrotoxic and does not cause hypertension • Used as a maintenance immunosuppressive agent	• Anorexia, nausea, vomiting, abdominal pain, diarrhea • Headache • Circumoral numbness and tingling, tremors, seizures • Insomnia, nightmares • Flushing • Chest pain • Anemia • Edema • Elevated liver enzymes • Nephrotoxicity • Electrolyte imbalance: hyperkalemia, hypomagnesemia • Hypertension • Rash if given with cyclosporine; cyclosporine must be discontinued 24 hours before FK 506 initiated • Decreased resistance to infection
ANTIMETABOLITES Interfere with DNA and RNA synthesis, thereby resulting in the inhibition of the proliferation of T and B lymphocytes • Azathioprine (Imuran)	• Interferes with the purine synthesis necessary for the production of antibodies • Prevents synthesis of DNA/RNA in leukocytes • Prevents activation and rapid proliferation of T cells responding to an antigen • Used as a maintenance immunosuppressive agent	• Nausea, vomiting • Stomatitis • Pancreatitis • Hepatotoxicity • Bone marrow depression: leukopenia, anemia, thrombocytopenia • Alopecia • Coagulopathy • Development of neoplasms • Decreased resistance to infection
• Mycophenolate mofetil (CellCept)	• Inhibits the proliferative responses of T and B lymphocytes • Blocks antibody formation • Blocks the generation of cytotoxic T cell production • Preferable to azathioprine because it does not cause global bone marrow depression • Used as a maintenance immunosuppressive agent	• Nausea, vomiting, diarrhea • Dyspnea • Hypertension • Thrombocytopenia • Leukopenia • Hematuria • Electrolyte imbalance: hypokalemia
MONOCLONAL ANTIBODIES Interfere with antigen recognition; used for induction therapy and treatment of refractory chronic rejection • Daclizumab (Zenapax)	• Blocks interleukin-2 receptor sites • Used for induction therapy and acute rejection	• Nausea, vomiting, diarrhea • Chills • Tremors • Dyspnea, wheezing • Nephrotoxicity • Pulmonary edema
• Muromonab-CD3 (Orthoclone OKT3)	• Removes T cells with the T3 surface antigen from the circulation • Alters T cell function so that they are unable to recognize antigens • Used for induction therapy (5 to 7 days and then stopped)	• Fever, chills • Nausea, vomiting, diarrhea • Malaise • Headache • Dyspnea • Chest pain

Continued

Table 10-17 Antirejection Agents—cont'd

Drug	Effects	Adverse Effects
		• Wheezing • Tremors • Fluid retention • Thrombocytopenia • Leukopenia • Muscle and bone pain • Allergic reactions; pretreat initial doses with diphenhydramine and acetaminophen • Increased incidence of malignancy • Increased susceptibility to infections especially viral infections (e.g., cytomegalovirus and herpes)
• Sirolimus (Rapamycin, Rapamune)	• Blocks activation of T and B cell lymphocytes by cytokines • Used as a maintenance immunosuppressive agent	• Thrombocytopenia • Leukopenia • Elevated serum lipid levels • May delay wound healing
POLYCLONAL ANTIBODIES Interfere with the interaction of antibodies with antigens to decrease T lymphocytes • Rabbit antithymocyte globulin (Thymoglobulin)	• Reduces number of circulating T cells • Reduces the proliferative function of the T cell • Used for induction therapy 5 to 7 days for lung transplants • Used for acute rejection in other transplants	• Allergic reactions • Thrombocytopenia • Anaphylaxis • Increased incidence of malignancy • Decreased resistance to infection especially viral infections (e.g., cytomegalovirus and herpes)

(2) Monitor for clinical indications of acute rejection.
  (a) General: fever; tachycardia; flulike symptoms
  (b) Organ specific: usually pain around the transplanted organ (with exception of the heart because of denervation) and failure of the transplanted organ; organ biopsy is definitive for rejection
    (i) Heart
      a) Clinical indications of heart failure: S_3, dyspnea, crackles, peripheral edema, jugular venous distention, fatigue, elevated RAP and PAOP
      b) Dysrhythmias
      c) Decreased cardiac output/cardiac index with resultant clinical indicators of hypoperfusion (e.g., hypotension, restlessness, cool skin, decreased bowel sounds, and decreased urine output)
    (ii) Lung
      a) Malaise
      b) Dyspnea, pleuritic chest pain
      c) Nonproductive cough
      d) Oxygen desaturation with activity; progressive hypoxemia
      e) Breath sound changes: diminished breath sounds; crackles
      f) Abnormal pulmonary function studies (e.g., decreased forced expiratory volumes and vital capacity)
      g) Pulmonary infiltrates on chest x-ray
    (iii) Liver
      a) Itching, jaundice
      b) Back pain or abdominal pain
      c) Elevated bilirubin, liver enzymes, and ammonia (late)
      d) Hepatomegaly
    (iv) Pancreas
      a) Elevated serum glucose
      b) Abdominal pain
      c) Decrease in urine amylase (in patient with exocrine urinary diversion)
    (v) Kidney
      a) Hypertension
      b) Swollen, tender kidneys; remember that transplanted kidneys are placed in the pelvis; therefore, pelvic rather than flank pain occurs (Figure 10-8)
      c) Decreased urine volume
      d) Elevated BUN and creatinine

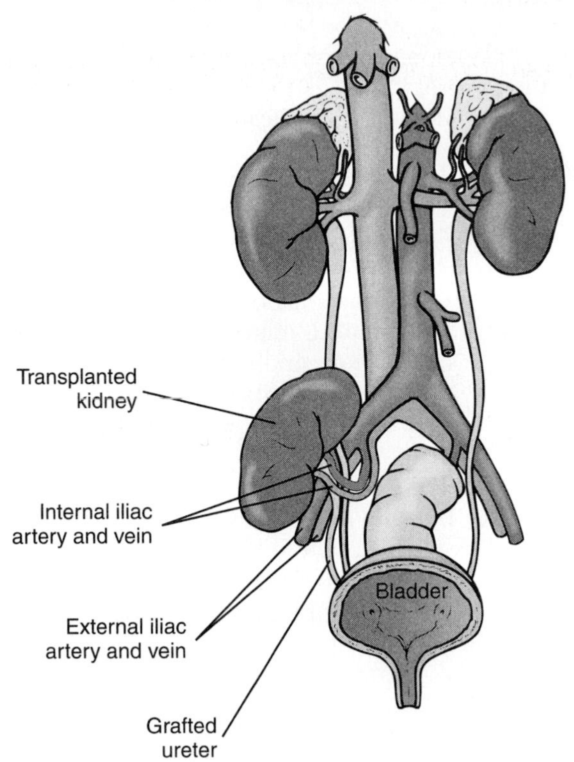

Figure 10-8 Location of transplanted kidney. (From Lewis, S. M., Heitkemper, M. M., & Dirksen, S. R. [2004]. *Medical-surgical nursing: Assessment and management of clinical problems* [6th ed.]. St. Louis: Mosby.)

e) Electrolyte imbalances, particularly hyperkalemia
f) Weight gain and peripheral edema

(3) Teach patient about immunosuppressive drugs.
(a) Explain that they are the main defense against transplant rejection.
(b) Discuss the side effects of the prescribed medications.
(c) Stress that medications cannot be withdrawn suddenly.
(d) Teach the patient to notify the physician immediately of any indications of infection.
(e) Advise the patient to inform health care providers that they are receiving immunosuppressive drugs; they should not receive vaccination with live, attenuated organisms.
(f) Instruct patient regarding pets.
(i) No birds
(ii) Approval for other pets

d. Participate in collaborative management specific to types of transplant.
(1) Heart
(a) Monitor for and treat clinical indications of hypoperfusion.
(i) Hemodynamic monitoring is indicated.
(ii) Inotropes frequently are required initially.
a) Isoproterenol (Isuprel): increases heart rate and contractility, and decreases pulmonary vascular resistance
b) Dopamine or dobutamine: increases contractility
c) Temporary pacing: may be required to increase heart rate
(b) Monitor for and treat clinical indications of hypervolemia or hypovolemia: fluids, diuretics, or vasodilators may be required.
(c) Monitor for and treat coagulopathy.
(i) Protamine is given to reverse the heparin used while patient is on cardiopulmonary bypass.
(ii) Clotting factors, in the form of fresh frozen plasma, may be necessary.
(iii) Blood administration may be necessary.
(d) Monitor for and treat dysrhythmias.
(i) Note that two P waves are common after heterotopic heart transplant (less than 5% of heart transplants).
(ii) Note that transplanted hearts are denervated and do not respond to atropine and have little response to digoxin.
(iii) Epinephrine or isoproterenol and/or pacemaker may be used for bradycardia; denervated heart does not respond to atropine and has a minimal response to digoxin.
(e) Monitor for and treat cardiac tamponade.
(2) Lung
(a) Maintain airway, ventilation, and oxygenation.
(i) Monitor ABGs closely.
(ii) Administer oxygen to maintain Sao_2 of at least 90%; mechanical ventilation may be necessary initially.
(iii) Ensure bronchial hygiene: turn; deep breathe; incentive spirometry; coughing; humidification.
a) Thick secretions are expected.
b) Denervated lung eliminates cough reflex.
(b) Monitor for and treat hypervolemia or hypovolemia.
(i) Monitor hemodynamic parameters, chest tube drainage, and wound drainage.
(ii) Administer diuretics and/or venous vasodilators and use PEEP as prescribed to prevent or treat pulmonary edema.
(iii) Replace intravascular fluid volume cautiously.
(c) Monitor for and treat dysrhythmias.
(d) Monitor for and treat coagulopathy.

(i) Protamine is given to reverse the heparin used if the patient was put on cardiopulmonary bypass.
(ii) Blood that is CMV-negative may be administered.

(e) Monitor for clinical indications of anastomotic leak (e.g., subcutaneous emphysema and pneumothorax).

(3) Liver
(a) Monitor for indications of biliary obstruction (e.g., decreased T tube drainage and jaundice).
(b) Monitor for intraabdominal bleeding (e.g., increase in abdominal girth, bleeding into Jackson-Pratt drains, and melena).
(c) Monitor for indications of coagulopathy (e.g., prolonged PT, aPTT, and abnormal bleeding); administer fresh frozen plasma and platelets as prescribed.
(i) If coagulopathy does not correct within 24 hours, a nonfunctioning graft is probable.
(d) Monitor for electrolyte imbalance, especially hypokalemia and hypocalcemia; replace electrolytes as prescribed.
(e) Monitor for hypoglycemia.
(f) Monitor for renal impairment.

(4) Pancreas
(a) Monitor for indications of hypoglycemia or hyperglycemia.
(i) Maintain insulin drip as prescribed.
(ii) Administration of 10% dextrose in water may be required.
(b) Monitor for clinical indications of peritoneal irritation: abdominal pain; abdominal distention; absent bowel sounds; rebound tenderness.
(c) Monitor for metabolic acidosis if exocrine drainage through bladder: sodium bicarbonate may be required.

(5) Renal
(a) Maintain patency of vascular access.
(b) Monitor renal function.
(i) Monitor hourly urine output.
(ii) Monitor blood urea nitrogen and creatinine.
(c) Monitor for clinical indications of extravasation of urine (e.g., abdominal pain, rebound tenderness, diminished bowel sounds, and abdominal distention).

LEARNING ACTIVITIES

1. Complete the following crossword puzzle.

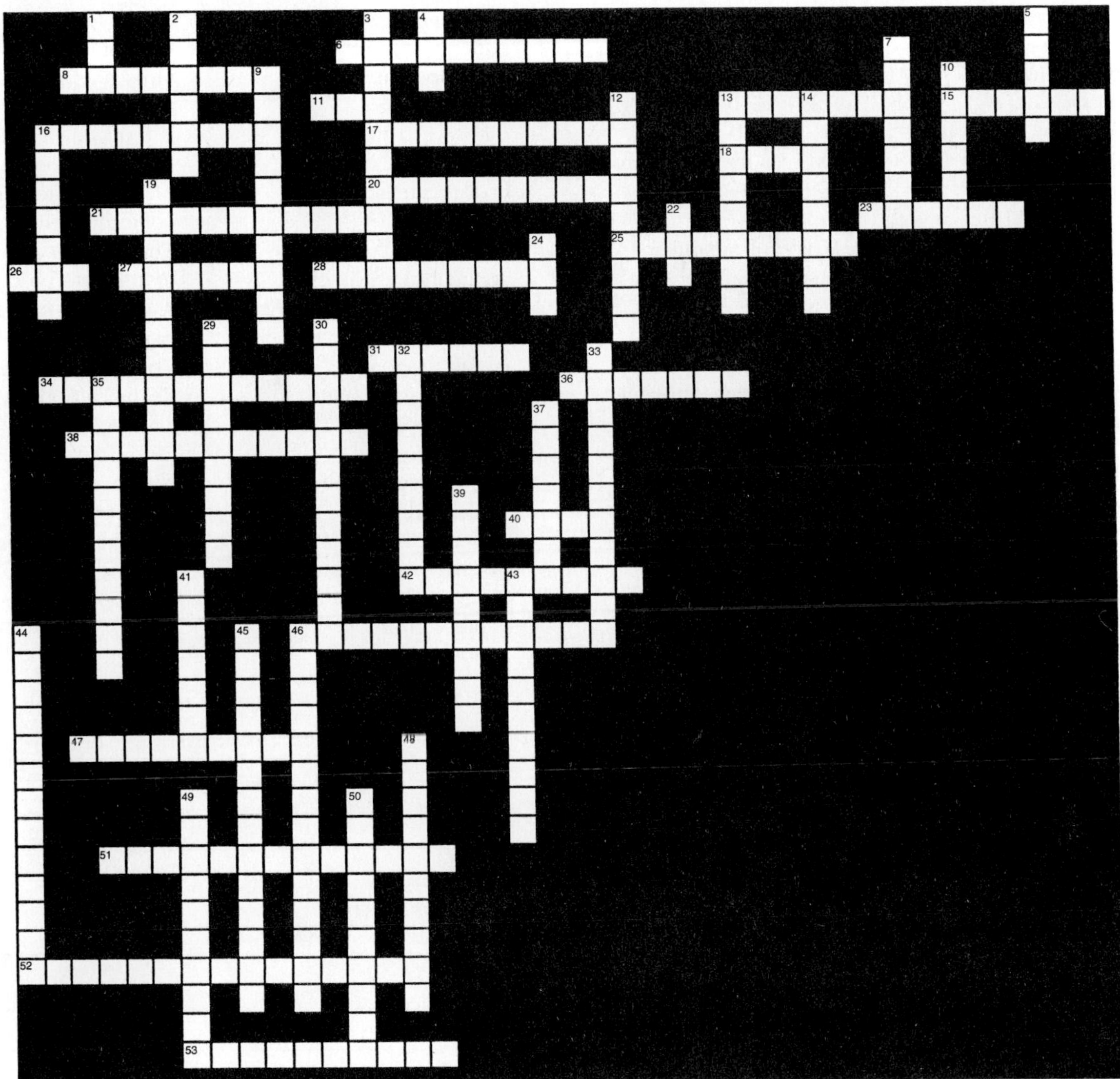

Across

6. The type of granulocyte that is significant in allergic reactions
8. The granulocyte that releases heparin and histamine
11. The end result of fibrinolysis (abbreviation)
13. This electrolyte may decrease with administration of banked blood
15. This type of T cell is decreased in AIDS
16. This electrolyte may increase with administration of banked blood
17. A cytokine synthesized by lymphocytes is called a _____
18. An increase in the number of bands causes a shift to the ____
20. This agranulocyte is the major phagocyte of the leukocytes
21. This mediator causes vasoconstriction, pulmonary vasoconstriction, and platelet aggregation
23. The liquid portion of blood
25. The type of reaction that occurs with mismatched blood transfusion
26. The virus that causes AIDS (abbreviation)
27. Immunodeficient condition characterized by lack of or diminished reaction to an antigen
28. The clotting pathway that is initiated by endothelial injury
31. The site of B cell distribution
34. An immature erythrocyte
36. A fungal infection frequently seen in patients with immunocompromise; oral infection with this organism is referred to as thrush
38. A mature RBC
40. One of the first antibiotic-resistant bacterial strains (abbreviation)

42. The clotting pathway that is initiated by tissue injury
46. The sequential physiologic response of the body to injury or invasion
47. This mediator is the endogenous opiate of the body
51. The process by which stem cells develop and differentiate into different types of blood cells
52. This blood product is administered to replace factor VIII in patients with hemophilia
53. This type of T cell serves to modulate the immune response; increased in AIDS

Down

1. A drug frequently administered to decrease platelet aggregation (abbreviation)
2. _____ sarcoma is a malignancy frequently seen in patients with AIDS
3. A cascading system that can result in direct killing of invading organism
4. The consumptive coagulopathy seen in critical illness (abbreviation)
5. The yellowish fluid that transports lymphocytes
7. This type of immunity is mediated by B cells; involves the development of antigen-specific antibodies
9. A type of agranular leukocyte; B cells and T cells are examples
10. The site of T cell distribution
12. The first sign of platelet dysfunction
13. This type of immunity is mediated by the T cell
14. Chemical mediators of immunity and inflammation
16. Activated plasminogen; the active agent in the fibrinolytic process
19. A leukocyte that releases granules when it ruptures
22. The virus that is a serious problem for immunocompromised patients (abbreviation)
24. This type of pneumonia is frequently seen in patients with severe immunocompromise such as AIDS (abbreviation)
29. The product of erythrocyte destruction
30. Heparin and _____ maintain the fluidity of the blood
32. This type of cell can engulf and digest microorganisms and cellular debris
33. The adherence of phagocytes to the vessel wall
35. A synonym for platelet
37. Parenterally administered anticoagulant acts as an indirect thrombin inhibitor (generic)
39. This mediator is released by the basophil cell in allergic reactions; causes vasodilation and increased capillary permeability
41. These cells are fixed macrophages in the liver
43. A cytokine that inhibits viruses and activates NK cells
44. A term for infections that are more likely when the immune system is compromised
45. The process of erythrocyte production
46. A synonym for antibody; made by B cells
48. This blood protein becomes fibrin when activated
49. The movement of neutrophils and phagocytes through pores of small blood vessels
50. The movement of neutrophils and monocytes toward an antigen

2. List the five major clinical indications of inflammation.

a. ____________________

b. ____________________

c. ____________________

d. ____________________

e. ____________________

3. Identify which type of hypersensitivity reaction the following situations demonstrate.

Example	Type
Skin testing for tuberculosis	
Inhalation allergies	
Anaphylaxis to penicillin	
Hemolytic blood transfusion reaction	

4. Complete the following table.

	Platelet Plug	Intrinsic Pathway	Extrinsic Pathway	Common Pathway	Fibrinolytic System
Activation					
Laboratory test					

5. Match the type of anemia to the possible cause.

a. Esophageal varices
b. Radiation or drugs
c. Hereditary
d. Malignancy
e. Lead poisoning
f. Crohn's disease
g. Anorexia nervosa

___ 1. Iron deficiency anemia
___ 2. Pernicious anemia
___ 3. Folic acid deficiency anemia
___ 4. Sickle cell anemia
___ 5. Aplastic anemia
___ 6. Acute blood loss anemia
___ 7. Anemia of chronic illness

6. Identify the appropriate actions to take for suspected transfusion reaction.

a. ______________________________
b. ______________________________
c. ______________________________
d. ______________________________
e. ______________________________
f. ______________________________
g. ______________________________
h. ______________________________
i. ______________________________

7. Briefly describe the three major phases of DIC.

1. ______________________________
2. ______________________________
3. ______________________________

8. Identify the direction of change of the following laboratory values in DIC.

Platelets	
PT	
Partial thromboplastin time	
FSPs	
Factors V and VIII	
Fibrinogen	

9. Discuss the controversy of the following therapies in the treatment of DIC.

a. Heparin	
b. Clotting factors	

10. List five factors encountered in the critical care unit that affect the patient's immune response and may cause immunodeficiency.

1. ______________________________
2. ______________________________
3. ______________________________
4. ______________________________
5. ______________________________

11. Identify three major adverse effects of the following antiretroviral agents.

Zidovudine (Retrovir)	1. 2. 3.
Didanosine (Videx)	1. 2. 3.
Zalcitabine (Hivid)	1. 2. 3.

12. Identify general and organ-specific indications of rejection after organ transplantation.

General: ______________________________

Heart: ______________________________

Lung: ______________________________

Liver: ______________________________

Pancreas: ______________________________

Kidney: ______________________________

13. Identify three major adverse effects of the following immunosuppressive agents.

Agent	Adverse effects
Azathioprine (Imuran)	1. 2. 3.
Cyclosporine (Neoral)	1. 2. 3.
Muromonab-CD3 (Orthoclone OKT3)	1. 2. 3.
Prednisone	1. 2. 3.

LEARNING ACTIVITIES ANSWERS

1.

2. a. Warmth
   b. Redness
   c. Swelling
   d. Pain
   e. Loss of function

3.

Example	Type
Skin testing for tuberculosis	IV
Inhalation allergies	III
Anaphylaxis to penicillin	I
Hemolytic blood transfusion reaction	II

4.

	Platelet Plug	Intrinsic Pathway	Extrinsic Pathway	Common Pathway	Fibrinolytic System
Activation	Intimal defect	Hageman factor (XII)	Tissue thromboplastin (III)	Stuart-Prower factor (X)	Tissue plasminogen activator
Laboratory test	Bleeding time	PTT	PT	PTT, thrombin time	FSPs

5.

e 1. Iron deficiency anemia
f 2. Pernicious anemia
g 3. Folic acid deficiency anemia
c 4. Sickle cell anemia
b 5. Aplastic anemia
a 6. Acute blood loss anemia
d 7. Anemia of chronic illness

6. a. Stop transfusion.
b. Maintain IV access with normal saline and new administration set.
c. Reassure the patient; stay at the bedside.
d. Notify physician and blood bank.
e. Recheck blood numbers and type.
f. Treat symptoms appropriately.
g. Return unused portion of blood in blood bag and administration set to the blood bank.
h. Collect and send blood and urine samples to the laboratory; send another urine specimen 24 hours after transfusion reaction.
i. Document the transfusion reaction and treatment administered.

7. 1. Clotting (caused by activation of the clotting cascade)
2. Bleeding (caused by consumption of clotting factors)
3. More bleeding (caused by activation of the fibrinolytic system)

8.

Platelets	↓
PT	↑
PTT	↑
FSPs	↑
Factors V and VIII	↓
Fibrinogen	↓

9.

a. Heparin	May perpetuate bleeding
b. Clotting factors	May perpetuate clotting

10. Any five of the factors listed below.
Anesthetic agents
Antacids
Histamine$_2$ receptor antagonists
Immunosuppressive agents
Invasive procedures
Malnutrition
Massive antibiotic therapy
Steroids
Stress

11.

Zidovudine (Retrovir)	1. Bone marrow depression 2. GI symptoms 3. Headache Or any adverse effects listed in Table 10-14
Didanosine (Videx)	1. Peripheral neuropathy 2. Pancreatitis 3. GI symptoms Or any adverse effects listed in Table 10-14
Zalcitabine (Hivid)	1. Peripheral neuropathy 2. Bone marrow depression 3. GI symptoms Or any adverse effects listed in Table 10-14

12.

General: Flulike symptoms, fever, tachycardia
Heart: Heart failure, dysrhythmias, decreased cardiac index with clinical indications of hypoperfusion
Lung: Hypoxemia especially with exertion, pulmonary infiltrates, pleuritic chest pain
Liver: Itching, jaundice, back or abdominal pain, elevated bilirubin and liver enzymes, hepatomegaly
Pancreas: Abdominal pain, hyperglycemia, decrease in urine amylase
Kidney: Hypertension; swollen, tender kidneys; decrease in urine output; elevated blood urea nitrogen; creatinine

13. Increased susceptibility to infection applies to all of these agents.

Azathioprine (Imuran)	1. Bone marrow depression 2. Hepatotoxicity 3. Pancreatitis Or any adverse effects listed in Table 10-17
Cyclosporine (Neoral)	1. Nephrotoxicity 2. Hepatotoxicity 3. Hypertension Or any adverse effects listed in Table 10-17
Muromonab-CD3 (Orthoclone OKT3)	1. Leukopenia 2. Thrombocytopenia 3. Allergic reactions Or any adverse effects listed in Table 10-17
Prednisone	1. Sodium and water retention 2. Hypertension 3. Hyperglycemia Or any adverse effects listed in Table 10-17

Reference

Levy, S. B. (1998). Multidrug resistance: A sign of the times. *New England Journal of Medicine, 338*, 1376-1378.

Bibliography

Angerio, A. D. (2003). Sickle cell crisis and endothelin antagonists. *Critical Care Nursing Quarterly, 27*(3), 225-229.

Caiola, E. (2000). Heparin-induced thrombocytopenia: How to manage it, how to avoid it. *Cleveland Clinic Journal of Medicine, 67*(9), 621.

Coe, P. (2000). Managing pulmonary hypertension in heart transplantation: Meeting the challenge. *Critical Care Nurse, 20*(2), 22-30.

Coyne, P. J., Lyne, M. E., & Watson, A. C. (2002). Symptom management in people with AIDS. *American Journal of Nursing, 102*(9), 48-57.

Day, S. W., & Wynn, L. W. (2000). Sickle cell pain and hydroxyurea. *American Journal of Nursing, 100*(11), 34-39.

Exley, M., White, N., & Martin, J. H. (2002). Why families say no to organ donation. *Critical Care Nurse, 22*(6), 44-51.

Gando, S., Iba, T., Yutaka, E., Ohtomo, Y., Okamoto, K., Koseki, K., et al. (2006). A multicenter, prospective validation of disseminated intravascular coagulation diagnostic criteria for critically ill patients: Comparing current criteria. *Critical Care Medicine, 34*(3), 625-631.

George, E. L., Hoffman, L. A., Boujoukos, A., & Zullo, T. G. (2002). Effect of positioning of oxygenation in single-lung transplant recipients. *American Journal of Critical Care, 11*(1), 66-75.

Gilcreast, D. M., Avella, P., Camarillo, E., & Mullane, G. (2001). Treating severe anemia in a trauma patient who is a Jehovah's Witness. *Critical Care Nurse, 21*(2), 69-82.

Holcomb, S. S. (2001). Anemias: Road signs to the real problems. *Dimensions of Critical Care Nursing, 20*(3), 2-11.

Kruse, J. A., Fink, M. P., & Carlson, R. W. (2003). *Saunders manual of critical care*. Philadelphia: Saunders.

Lanuza, D., & McCabe, M. A. (2001). Care before and after lung transplant and quality of life research. *AACN Clinical Issues, 12*(2), 186-201.

Lapointe, L. A., & Von Rueden, K. T. (2002). Coagulapathies in trauma patients. *AACN Clinical Issues, 13*(2), 192-203.

Lewis, S. M., Heitkemper, M. M., & Dirksen, S. R. (2004). *Medical-surgical nursing: Assessment and management of clinical problems* (6th ed.). St. Louis, MO: Mosby.

Maxson, J. H. (2000). Management of disseminated intravascular coagulation. *Critical Care Nursing Clinics of North America, 12*(3), 341-352.

McCance, K. L., & Huether, S. E. (2006). *Pathophysiology: The biologic basis for disease in adults and children* (5th ed.). St. Louis, MO: Mosby.

Myer, S. A., & Oliva, J. (2002). Severe aplastic anemia and allogenic hematopoietic stem cell transplantation. *AACN Clinical Issues, 13*(2), 169-191.

Navuluri, R. (2001). Understanding hemostasis. *American Journal of Nursing, 101*(9), 24B-24C.

Rankin, J. A. (2004). Biological mediators of acute inflammation. *AACN Clinical Issues, 15*(1), 3-17.

Rempher, K. J., & Little, J. (2004). Assessment of red blood cell and coagulation laboratory data. *AACN Clinical Issues, 15*(4), 622-637.

Ress, B. (2001). Caring for patients with HIV disease in the new millennium. *Critical Care Nurse, 21*(1), 69-76.

Ress, B. (2003). HIV disease and aging: The hidden epidemic. *Critical Care Nurse, 23*(5), 38-44.

Ricards, M., Thursky, K., & Buising, K. (2003). Epidemiology, prevalence, and sites of infection in intensive care units. *Seminars in Respiratory Critical Care Medicine, 24*(1), 3-22.

Richard, N. M., & Giuliano, K. K. (2002). Transfusion practices in critical care. *American Journal of Nursing, 102*(5 suppl.), 16-22.

Sole, M. L., Klein, D. G., & Moseley, M. J. (2005). *Introduction to critical care nursing* (4th ed.). Philadelphia: Elsevier Saunders.

Taylor, R. W., Manganaro, L., O'Brien, J., Trottier, S. J., Parkar, N., & Veremakis, C. (2002). Impact of allogenic packed red blood cell transfusion on nosocomial infection rates in the critically ill patient. *Critical Care Medicine, 30*(10), 2249-2254.

Tokarczyk, T. R. (2003). Cardiac transplantation as a treatment option for the heart failure patient. *Critical Care Nursing Quarterly, 26*(1), 61-68.

Trzcianowska, H., & Mortensen, E. (2001). HIV and AIDS: Separating fact from fiction. *American Journal of Nursing, 101*(6), 53-60.

Ungvarski, P. J. (2001). The past 20 years of AIDS. *American Journal of Nursing, 101*(6), 26.

Urden, L. D., Stacy, K. M., & Lough, M. E. (2005). *Thelan's critical care nursing: Diagnosis and management* (5th ed.). St. Louis, MO: Mosby.

Vernon, S., & Pfeifer, G. M. (2003). Blood management strategies for critical care patients. *Critical Care Nurse, 23*(6), 34-41.

Multisystem

CHAPTER 11

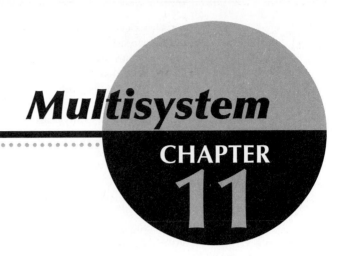

NOTE: The CCRN blueprint includes Cardiogenic Shock and Hypovolemic in Cardiovascular, Anaphylactic Shock in Hematology/Immunology, and Neurogenic Shock in Neurologic, but it is logical to discuss the similarities of all shock states together and then discuss their differences.

Shock

Definitions

1. Shock: the condition of insufficient perfusion of cells and vital organs, causing tissue hypoxia; perfusion is inadequate to sustain life and results in cellular, metabolic, and hemodynamic derangements
2. Systemic inflammatory response syndrome (SIRS): the systemic response to a variety of insults that begin as local inflammation; consider the vasodilation and increased capillary permeability of local inflammation as a normal healing process and the more global vasodilation and increased capillary permeability of SIRS as life-threatening
3. Multiple organ dysfunction syndrome (MODS): failure of more than one organ in an acutely ill patient with SIRS to such an extent that homeostasis cannot be maintained without intervention

Classification by Etiology

1. Hypovolemic: caused by inadequate intravascular volume
2. Cardiogenic: caused by impaired ability of the heart to pump blood effectively
3. Distributive: caused by massive vasodilation and a resultant relative hypovolemia
   a. Septic: resulting from massive vasodilation caused by release of mediators of the inflammatory process in response to overwhelming infection
   b. Anaphylactic: resulting from massive vasodilation caused by release of histamine in response to a severe allergic reaction
   c. Neurogenic: resulting from massive vasodilation caused by suppression of the sympathetic nervous system (SNS)

Pathophysiology

1. Stages of shock
   a. Initial stage: subclinical hypoperfusion caused by inadequate delivery and/or inadequate extraction of oxygen
      (1) Shock is initiated by decreased tissue oxygenation caused by any of the following:
         (a) Decrease in circulating blood volume (hypovolemic)
         (b) Decrease in ability of the heart to pump blood (cardiogenic)
         (c) Decrease in vascular tone (distributive; may also be referred to as *vasogenic*)
      (2) Cardiac output and index are decreased, but there are no *clinical* indications of hypoperfusion; this decrease in cardiac output and cardiac index would be detected by invasive hemodynamic monitoring
   b. Compensatory stage: attempts of the neuroendocrine systems to compensate and restore tissue perfusion to vital organs
      (1) SNS stimulation
         (a) Baroreceptor reflex: Decrease in blood pressure stimulates the baroreceptors, which then stimulate the vasomotor center in the medulla to activate the SNS
         (b) SNS: Epinephrine and norepinephrine released from adrenal medulla cause the following physiologic responses:
            (i) Cardiac effects
               a) Positive chronotropic (i.e., increase in heart rate)
               b) Positive inotropic (i.e., increase in contractility)
               c) Positive dromotropic (i.e., increase in conductivity)
            (ii) Vascular effects
               a) Arterial vasoconstriction
                  i) Systemic response increases systemic vascular resistance (SVR) and blood pressure.
                  ii) Constriction of afferent and efferent arterioles of kidneys decreases glomerular filtration rate (GFR) and urine output.

b) Venous vasoconstriction
   i) Widespread reflex venoconstriction increases venous return to the heart, which increases preload.
   ii) Increased venous return and preload increase myocardial contractility by increasing myofibril stretch (Starling's Law of the Heart).
(iii) Redistribution of blood flow from nonessential (e.g., skin, bowel, and kidney) to essential (e.g., heart and brain) organs
(c) Central nervous system (CNS) ischemic response
   (i) Low oxygen levels stimulate chemoreceptors to increase rate and depth of ventilation.
   (ii) Hyperventilation causes respiratory alkalosis and cerebral vasoconstriction and, potentially, cerebral ischemia.
   (iii) Also, a CNS ischemic response occurs when mean arterial pressure (MAP) falls to less than 50 mm Hg.
   (iv) CNS ischemia causes powerful stimulation of the SNS.
(2) Hormonal compensation
   (a) Hypoperfusion of the kidney causes the activation of renin-angiotensin-aldosterone system (Figure 2-22 in Chapter 2).
      (i) Vasoconstriction of arteries and arterioles caused by angiotensin II
      (ii) Increase in reabsorption of sodium and water by the renal tubule caused by aldosterone
   (b) Hypothalamic stimulation causes release of antidiuretic hormone (ADH) from posterior pituitary gland and adrenocorticotopic hormone (ACTH) from anterior pituitary gland.
      (i) ADH: vasoconstriction and retention of water at renal tubules
      (ii) ACTH stimulates the adrenal cortex to release the following:
         a) Glucocorticoids: stimulate glycogenolysis and gluconeogenesis to mobilize glucose for cellular energy
         b) Aldosterone: stimulates the reabsorption of sodium and water at the renal tubules

c. Progressive stage: the inability of the compensatory mechanisms to maintain tissue perfusion
   (1) Myocardial depression
      (a) Coronary artery perfusion pressure is dramatically reduced by decrease in MAP to less than 60 mm Hg, which causes myocardial ischemia.
      (b) Myocardial depressant factor (MDF) is released by the ischemic pancreas.
   (2) Vasomotor center depression caused by severe cerebral ischemia
      (a) Increases capillary permeability
      (b) Decreases circulating volume
      (c) Results in decreased flow to vital organs
   (3) Deterioration of microcirculation
      (a) Spasm of the precapillary sphincter and venules occurs.
      (b) Continuing ischemia and local acidosis causes dilation of the precapillary sphincters, whereas the venules are more resistant to the effects of acidosis and remain constricted.
      (c) Blood enters capillaries and pools.
      (d) Stagnant blood increases capillary hydrostatic pressure and increases tissue edema.
   (4) Thrombosis of small vessels
      (a) Microcirculation is sluggish.
      (b) Microclots develop, which lead to organ ischemia, anoxia, and consumption of clotting factors, potentially leading to disseminated intravascular coagulation (DIC).
   (5) Cellular deterioration
      (a) Reduced delivery of oxygen to tissues
      (b) Change from aerobic to anaerobic metabolism
         (i) Metabolic acidosis occurs because lactic acid is produced as a by-product of anaerobic metabolism and accumulates in the blood.
         (ii) Depletion of cellular adenosine triphosphate (ATP) reserves occurs because aerobic metabolism results in 18 times more ATP than the same amount of glucose metabolized anaerobically.
      (c) Failure of sodium-potassium pump, an active transport system that requires ATP
      (d) Organelle edema
         (i) Lysosomes may rupture, releasing active enzymes into the cell.
         (ii) Mitochondria can no longer use glucose and oxygen to make ATP, worsening the ATP deficiency.
      (e) Cellular destruction
         (i) Cellular edema is caused by failure of sodium-potassium pump.
         (ii) Apoptosis (i.e., preprogrammed cellular suicide) is activated by injury.
      (f) Organ failure
   (6) Massive ischemia of tissues leading to the release of mediators of the inflammatory process and SIRS (see next section on SIRS)

(7) Effects of shock on specific organs and organ systems
  (a) Heart
    (i) Dysrhythmias occur because of the failure of the sodium-potassium pump resulting from decreased ATP, hypoxemia, ischemia, and acidosis.
    (ii) Cardiac failure may occur because of ischemia, acidosis, and myocardial depressant factor.
  (b) Lung
    (i) Endothelial damage in the capillary bed and precapillary arterioles along with damage to the type II pneumocytes may cause acute lung injury or acute respiratory distress syndrome (ARDS).
    (ii) Hypoxemia causes hypoxemic vasoconstriction of pulmonary circulation and pulmonary hypertension.
    (iii) Ventilation-perfusion mismatch occurs because of disturbances in ventilation and perfusion.
    (iv) Pulmonary edema may result from disruption of the alveolar-capillary membrane, ARDS, heart failure, or from overaggressive fluid resuscitation.
  (c) Brain
    (i) Loss of autoregulation and brain ischemia occurs when cerebral perfusion pressure is less than 50 mm Hg.
    (ii) SNS dysfunction, depression of cardiac and respiratory centers, and impaired thermoregulation occur.
    (iii) Cerebral infarction may occur.
  (d) Kidney
    (i) Renal vasoconstriction and hypoperfusion of the kidney decreases GFR.
    (ii) Prolonged ischemia causes acute tubular necrosis and renal failure.
    (iii) Metabolic acids accumulate in the blood, worsening the metabolic acidosis caused by lactic acid production during anaerobic metabolism.
  (e) Liver
    (i) Hypoperfusion damages the reticuloendothelial cells, which causes recirculation of bacteria and cellular debris and predisposes the patient to bacteremia and sepsis.
    (ii) Damage to the hepatocytes causes the liver to be unable to detoxify drugs, toxins, or hormones or to conjugate bilirubin.
    (iii) Hepatic dysfunction causes a decreased ability to mobilize carbohydrate, protein, and fat stores, which results in hypoglycemia.
  (f) Pancreas
    (i) Pancreatic enzymes are released by the ischemic and damaged pancreas.
    (ii) Pancreatic ischemia causes the release of MDF, which results in depression of cardiac contractility.
    (iii) Hyperglycemia occurs as the result of endogenous and/or exogenous corticosteroids and insulin resistance. Hyperglycemia results in the following:
      a) Dehydration and electrolyte imbalances related to osmotic diuresis
      b) Impairment of leukocyte function, causing decreased phagocytosis and increased risk of infection
      c) Depression of immune response
      d) Impairment in gastric motility
      e) Shifts in the substrate availability from glucose to free fatty acids or lactate
      f) Negative nitrogen balance and decreased wound healing
  (g) Gastrointestinal
    (i) Ischemia and increased gastric acid production caused by glucocorticoids increase risk of stress ulcer.
    (ii) Prolonged vasoconstriction and ischemia lead to the inability of the intestinal walls to act as intact barriers to prevent the migration of bacteria out of the gastrointestinal tract; this may allow translocation of bacteria from the gastrointestinal tract into the lymphatic and vascular beds, increasing the risk for sepsis.
  (h) Hematologic/immunologic
    (i) Hypoxia and release of inflammatory cytokines impair blood flow and result in microvascular thrombosis.
    (ii) Sluggish blood flow, massive tissue trauma, and consumption of clotting factors may cause DIC.
    (iii) The bone marrow mobilizes the release of white blood cells.
      a) Causes leukocytosis early in shock
      b) Causes leukopenia as depletion of white blood cells in blood and in bone marrow occurs
    (iv) Massive tissue injury caused by widespread ischemia stimulates a SIRS with massive release of mediators of the inflammatory process.

2. Refractory stage is irreversible and refractory to conventional therapy.
   a. Clinical indications of profound hypoperfusion and profound hypotension unresponsive to potent vasopressors

b. Clinical indications of MODS (i.e., failure of two or more body systems)
    (1) ARDS
    (2) DIC
    (3) Hepatic dysfunction or failure
    (4) Acute tubular necrosis (ATN) or renal failure
    (5) Myocardial ischemia, infarction, or failure
    (6) Cerebral ischemia or infarction
c. Death from ineffective tissue perfusion caused by failure of the circulation to meet the oxygen needs of the cell

Clinical Presentation (Table 11-1)

1. Initial stage: no clinical indications; expert nurse may detect that "something is different"
2. Compensatory stage: SNS stimulation
    a. Subjective
        (1) Anxiety, fear, feeling of impending doom
        (2) Thirst
    b. Objective
        (1) Tachycardia
        (2) Blood pressure changes
            (a) Systolic blood pressure (BP) increases or stays the same while diastolic BP increases, resulting in a decrease in pulse pressure.
                (i) Because diastolic BP is a reflection of arterial elasticity, the vasoconstriction caused by the SNS causes an elevation in diastolic BP and a narrowing of the pulse pressure earlier than a decrease in systolic BP or MAP.
            (b) Orthostatic effects occur, with the BP decreasing when the patient is repositioned from lying to sitting.
        (3) Tachypnea
        (4) Skin: cool, pale, clammy
        (5) Gastrointestinal (GI): decreased bowel sounds
        (6) Renal: oliguria (i.e., less than 0.5 mL/kg/hr)
        (7) CNS: irritability, restlessness, confusion
            (a) Because the CNS is sensitive to changes in oxygen and glucose, neurologic signs and symptoms occur early.
3. Progressive stage: hypoperfusion
    a. Subjective
        (1) Anorexia, nausea
        (2) Chest pain; palpitations may occur
        (3) Dyspnea may occur
    b. Objective
        (1) Tachycardia, dysrhythmias
        (2) Hypotension
        (3) Hypothermia (except early septic)
        (4) Tachypnea
        (5) Skin
            (a) Bluish, mottled appearance
            (b) Peripheral cyanosis
        (6) GI: vomiting, absent bowel sound
        (7) Renal: anuria (i.e., negligible or less than 100 mL per 24 hours)
        (8) CNS: lethargy, coma
4. Refractory stage: profound hypoperfusion and evidence of MODS
    a. ARDS: clinical indications of respiratory distress; crackles; decreased PaO_2, SaO_2; decreased pulmonary compliance; diffuse pulmonary infiltrates on chest x-ray
    b. DIC: bleeding in a patient without a history of bleeding; petechiae; blood in sputum, vomitus, nasogastric aspirate, urine, stool; elevated prothrombin time (PT), partial thromboplastin time (PTT), decreased platelets, elevated (FSP), positive D-dimer

Table 11-1 Clinical Presentation of the Stages of Shock

	Initial: Subclinical Hypoperfusion	Compensatory: Sympathetic Nervous System	Progressive: Hypoperfusion	Refractory: Profound Hypoperfusion
Cardiac index	2.2-2.5 L/min/m^2	2-2.2 L/min/m^2	Less than 2 L/min/m^2	Less than 1.8 L/min/m^2
Clinical indications	• No clinical indications of hypoperfusion, but "something is different" • Detected by invasive hemodynamic monitoring	• Tachycardia • Narrowed pulse pressure • Tachypnea • Cool skin • Oliguria • Diminished bowel sounds • Restlessness → confusion	• Dysrhythmias • Hypotension • Tachypnea • Cold, clammy skin • Anuria • Absent bowel sounds • Lethargy → coma	• Life-threatening dysrhythmias • Hypotension despite potent vasopressors • MODS ∘ ARDS ∘ DIC ∘ Hepatic dysfunction/failure ∘ ATN ∘ Mesenteric ischemia/infarction ∘ Myocardial ischemia/infarction/failure ∘ Cerebral ischemia/infarction

ARDS, Acute respiratory distress syndrome; *ATN,* acute tubular necrosis; *DIC,* disseminated intravascular coagulation; *MODS,* multiple organ dysfunction syndrome.

c. Hepatic dysfunction or failure: jaundice; elevated bilirubin; elevated aspartate transaminase (AST), alanine transaminase (ALT), and lactate dehydrogenase (LDH); hypoglycemia
d. GI: paralytic ileus; gastrointestinal bleeding
e. ATN/renal failure: oliguria or anuria; elevated blood urea nitrogen (BUN) and creatinine; decreased urine creatinine clearance
f. Myocardial ischemia, infarction, or failure: chest pain; electrocardiogram (ECG) indicators of myocardial infarction (MI); positive creatine kinase (myocardial bound) (CK-MB) and troponin; clinical indicator of left ventricular and/or right ventricular failure
g. Cerebral ischemia or infarction: change in level of consciousness; change in Glasgow Coma Scale score of 1 or more; focal signs (e.g., hemiparesis or hemiplegia; aphasia)

5. Hemodynamic parameters (Table 11-2)
   a. Decreased oxygen delivery to the tissues (DO_2): common to all forms of shock except early septic shock, in which DO_2 is increased but extraction and use are impaired (For more information regarding DO_2, consult the hemodynamic monitoring section of Chapter 2.)
      (1) $DO_2 = CO \times (Hgb \times 1.34 \times Sao_2) \times 10$ where *CO* is cardiac output and *Hgb* is hemoglobin saturation
      (2) Normal: approximately 1000 mL/min ($600\ mL/min/m^2$)
   b. Gastric tonometry may be used to assess tissue perfusion (For more information on gastric tonometry, consult the Hemodynamic Monitoring section of Chapter 2.)
6. Diagnostic
   a. Serum
      (1) Sodium: increased early; increased or decreased late
      (2) Potassium: decreased early; increased late
      (3) Chloride: decreased early; increased late
      (4) Bicarbonate: normal early; decreased late
      (5) Carbon dioxide (CO_2): normal early; decreased late
      (6) Glucose: increased early; decreased late
      (7) BUN: increased
      (8) Creatinine: increased
      (9) Total protein, albumin: decreased
      (10) Bilirubin: increased late
      (11) Amylase, lipase: increased late
      (12) Ammonia: increased late
      (13) CK: increased
      (14) Liver enzymes (AST, ALT, LDH): increased
      (15) Lactate: increased (should be done on arterial blood)
         (a) Correlates with the degree of hypoperfusion
         (b) Above 2 mmol/L is associated with increased mortality
      (16) Hemoglobin, hematocrit: decreased if caused by hemorrhage
      (17) Hematocrit: increased if caused hypovolemia other than hemorrhage
      (18) White blood cell (WBC): increased early, decreased late
      (19) PT, PTT: may be prolonged
      (20) Platelets: may be decreased
      (21) Arterial blood gases: respiratory alkalosis progressing to metabolic acidosis; Pao_2 and Sao_2 may be decreased
      (22) Blood cultures: may identify organism if septic shock
   b. Urine
      (1) Urine creatinine clearance: decreased
      (2) Urine specific gravity: increased early, decreased late
      (3) Urine osmolality: increased early, decreased late
      (4) Urine sodium: decreased
      (5) Presence of heavy pigments
         (a) Myoglobinuria occurs with muscle tissue destruction (e.g., crush injuries, muscle ischemia/necrosis, electrical burns, and seizures).
         (b) Hemoglobinuria occurs with mismatched blood transfusion reaction and freshwater near-drowning.
   c. Other diagnostic studies may be done to evaluate the reason for shock.

Table 11-2 Hemodynamic Alterations in Shock

	Hypovolemic	Cardiogenic	Early Septic	Late Septic	Anaphylactic	Neurogenic
Heart rate	High	High	High	High	High	Normal or low
Blood pressure	Normal → low	Normal → low	Normal → low	Low	Normal → low	Normal → low
CO/CI	Low	Low	High	Low	Normal → low	Normal → low
RAP/PAOP	Low	High	Low	Variable	Low	Low
SVR/SVRI	High	High	Low	Variable	Low	Low
Svo_2	Low	Low	High	Low	Low	Low

CO/CI, Cardiac output/cardiac index; *RAP/PAOP,* right atrial pressure/pulmonary artery occlusive pressure; *SVR/SVRI,* systemic vascular resistance/systemic vascular resistance index; *Svo_2,* venous oxygen saturation.

Nursing Diagnoses

1. Ineffective Tissue Perfusion related to decreased effective blood volume, decreased cardiac output, and decreased vascular tone
   a. Ineffective Cerebral Tissue Perfusion related to hypoxia and cerebral hypoperfusion
   b. Ineffective Peripheral Tissue Perfusion related to hypovolemia, fluid shifts, and decreased blood flow secondary to IABP catheter position and vasopressors
2. Decreased Cardiac Output related to inadequate volume, inadequate cardiac contractility, inadequate vascular tone, dysrhythmias, and ineffective timing of IABP
3. Deficient Fluid Volume related to blood or fluid loss
4. Ineffective Airway Clearance related to altered consciousness, tracheobronchial obstruction caused by laryngeal edema, laryngeal spasm, bronchospasm, increased secretions, and artificial airways
5. Impaired Gas Exchange related to alveolar-capillary membrane changes resulting from increased capillary permeability associated with histamine, ventilation/perfusion mismatch, and intrapulmonary shunt
6. Ineffective Breathing Pattern related to immobility and analgesics
7. Imbalanced Nutrition: Less Than Body Requirements related to hypermetabolism, paralytic ileus, and decreased absorption
8. Impaired Urinary Elimination related to hypoperfusion and excretion of pigments (e.g., myoglobin and hemoglobin)
9. Risk for Infection related to invasive procedures and immunocompromise
10. Pain related to invasive procedures
11. Risk for Injury related to intubation, invasive procedures, and hemorrhage resulting from clotting abnormalities
12. Risk for Electrolyte Imbalance related to fluid shifts and potential hemolysis
13. Interrupted Family Processes related to sudden critical illness
14. Anxiety related to sudden critical illness, fear of the unknown, fear of death, change in role relationships, and change in self-concept

Collaborative Management

1. Maximize oxygen delivery to the tissues (Hgb, SaO_2, CO/CI).
   a. Maintain optimal hemoglobin and vascular volume: monitor and use CVP or PAOP when available.
      (1) Insert two intravenous catheters immediately, especially in cases of hemorrhage; these catheters should be short and large gauge.
      (2) Volume replacement for hypovolemic and vasogenic shock; may be necessary even in cardiogenic shock to achieve optimal PAOP.
         (a) Types of fluids used for fluid resuscitation (Box 11-1)
            (i) Crystalloids: solutions with dextrose or electrolytes; safe, effective, inexpensive, and usually the initial fluid type (Table 11-3)
            (ii) Colloids: large molecule (protein or starch) solutions; considered when the patient's response to initial efforts are insufficient
               a) Not only stay in the vascular space better than crystalloids but contribute to intravascular colloidal oncotic pressure to pull more fluid into the vascular space
               b) May be used in hypovolemic shock (except early burns) or neurogenic shock; because septic and anaphylactic shock are associated with increased capillary permeability, avoid colloids at least initially
               c) Examples
                  i) Albumin: plasma protein component; costly
                  ii) Dextran: contains polymers of high-molecular-weight polysaccharides; may cause coagulopathy by decreasing platelet aggregation; may cause allergic reactions; may cause

BOX 11-1 Types of Fluids Used for Fluid Resuscitation

Crystalloids
- Isotonic: NS; LR (D_5NS, D_5LR)
- Hypotonic: ½NS (D_5 ½ NS, D_5W)
- Hypertonic: 3% saline; D_{10}W; TPN

Colloids
- Albumin
- Dextran 70/75
- Hetastarch (Hespan)

Blood and Blood Products
- Whole blood
- Packed RBCs
- Fresh frozen plasma

NS, normal (0.9%) saline; *LR,* lactated Ringer's solution; *D_5NS,* 5% dextrose in normal saline; *D_5LR,* 5% dextrose in lactated Ringer's solution; *½ NS,* 0.45% saline; *D_5 ½ NS,* 5% dextrose in 0.45% saline; *D_5W,* 5% dextrose in water; *D_{10}W,* 10% dextrose in water; *TPN,* total parenteral nutrition (usually 25% dextrose); *RBCs,* red blood cells.

NOTE: Dextrose solutions are in parentheses because even though 5% dextrose adds to osmolality in the bottle or bag, this small amount of dextrose is metabolized so quickly when in the body that it should not be considered in the osmolality of the solution. So, consider D_5NS as NS, D_5 ½ NS as ½ NS, and D_5W as water. This last example is why D_5W is avoided except in extreme hyperosmolar conditions. In significant volumes, D_5W will dilute electrolytes, particularly sodium, and potentially cause neurologic changes including seizures.

Table 11-3 Crystalloids

	Isotonic	Hypotonic	Hypertonic
Osmolarity	250 to 350 mOsm/L (which is similar to blood osmolarity of 280-295 mOsm/kg)	Less than 250 mOsm/L	Greater than 350 mOsm/L
Uses	• Tend to stay in the vascular space better than other crystalloids • Require replacement with 3 mL for every 1 mL lost because they do equilibrate across fluid compartments	• Tend to leave the vascular space and replace the interstitial space better than the vascular space	• Pull fluid from the interstitial space into the intravascular space • Expand intravascular volume over isotonic crystalloid without the adverse effects of colloids • Monitor closely for clinical indications of fluid overload when these solutions are administered
Examples	*0.9% saline* • Composition ◦ 154 mEq sodium ◦ 154 mEq chloride ◦ Water • Osmolarity is 289 mOsm/L • pH is 5.7 • Large volumes may cause metabolic (hyperchloremic) acidosis *Lactated Ringer's solution* • Composition ◦ 130 mEq/L sodium ◦ 109 mEq/L chloride ◦ 4 mEq/L potassium ◦ 3 mEq/L calcium ◦ 28 mEq/L lactate ◦ Water • Osmolarity is 273 mOsm/L • pH 6.7 • Lactate is added as a buffer to make the solution less acidic (than without the lactate) • Lactate is converted to bicarbonate by the liver, so large volumes may cause metabolic alkalosis; this solution should be avoided in patients who have liver disease	*Half normal (0.45%) saline* • Composition ◦ 77 mEq sodium ◦ 77 mEq chloride ◦ Water *D_5W (5% dextrose in water)* • Composition ◦ 50 g dextrose ◦ Water • Note that though D_5W is isotonic in the bottle, the body quickly metabolizes the dextrose and free water is left; avoid this solution except in extremely hyperosmolar patients (e.g., HHNK, DI)	*Hypertonic (3% saline)* • 513 mEq sodium • 513 mEq chloride *$D_{10}W$ (10% dextrose in water)* • Composition ◦ 100 g dextrose per liter ◦ Water *$D_{50}W$ (50% dextrose in water)* • Composition ◦ 25 g dextrose per 50 mL ampule ◦ Water *Parenteral nutrition solution* • Central ◦ 250 g dextrose per liter ◦ Protein, electrolytes, vitamins vary ◦ Water • Peripheral ◦ 100 g dextrose per liter ◦ Protein, electrolytes, vitamins vary ◦ Water

HHNK, Hyperglycemic hyperosmolar nonketotic syndrome; *DI,* diabetes insipidus.

acute tubular necrosis (ATN) and renal failure, but this is rare

iii) Hetastarch: contains polymers of hydroxyethyl starch; may cause coagulopathy by decreasing platelet aggregation; may elevate serum amylase levels, but they return to normal at 5 to 7 days after hetastarch administration

(iii) Blood and blood products: used only to achieve a specific physiologic goal, such as to increase oxygen delivery or clotting capability

a) Contain plasma proteins present to add to intravascular colloidal oncotic pressure; only solution that increases the CaO_2 (content of oxygen in arterial blood) because 97% of all oxygen is carried on the hemoglobin molecule

b) Indicated when the patient has lost blood and there are clinical indications of hypoperfusion

c) Hematocrit of 30% to 32% probably is a reasonable goal because no significant increase in oxygen delivery is achieved and blood flow may become sluggish with a greater hematocrit

d) Major disadvantages of blood and blood products: cost and risk of blood transfusion reaction or blood-transmitted disease

e) For more information on blood and blood products and administration of blood, see Chapter 10

(b) Selection of solution for replacement
   (i) Colloids should not be used in situations with increased capillary permeability.
   (ii) In other situations, there is no difference in effectiveness (Alderson, Schierhout, Roberts, & Bunn, 2004), and colloids are considerably more costly.
   (iii) Blood should be used when the patient has lost blood and shows clinical indications of hypoperfusion.

(c) Volume
   (i) Typical fluid challenge is 250 to 500 mL of normal saline over 5 minutes (Figure 11-1).
   (ii) Monitor BP, CVP, and PAOP as available.
   (iii) Monitor for clinical indicators of fluid overload (e.g., dyspnea, jugular venous distention, S_3, systolic flow murmur, and crackles).

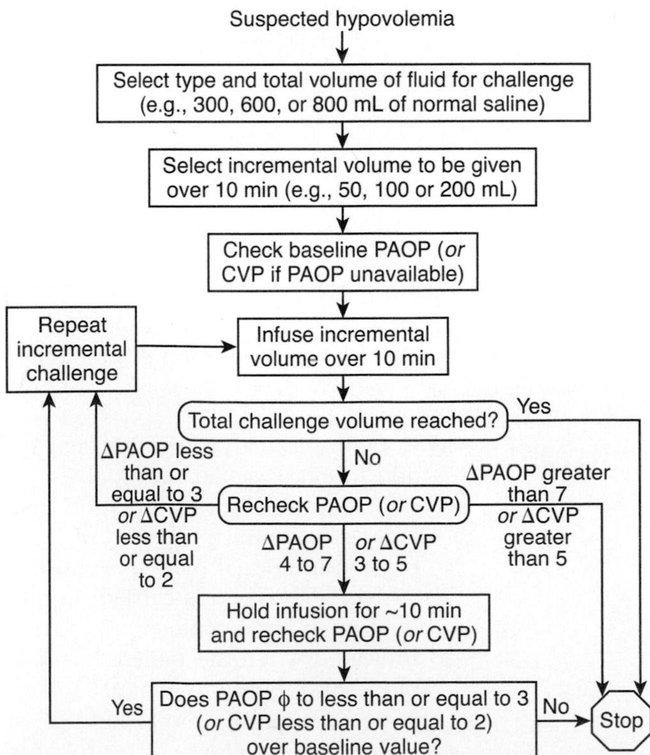

Figure 11-1 Fluid challenge algorithm. (From Kruse, J. A., Fink, M. P., & Carlson, R. W. [2003]. *Saunders manual of critical care*. Philadelphia: Saunders.)

(3) Type and crossmatch blood immediately if patient is hemorrhaging; type specific blood or O negative may be given in severe hemorrhage but may make future crossmatching more difficult.

(4) Take care during fluid resuscitation to prevent hypothermia; fluids may need to be warmed if the patient's body temperature is low (35°C [95°F] or less) at the initiation of fluid resuscitation or if multiple units of blood or multiple liters of IV fluids are needed.

(5) Administer venous vasodilators and/or diuretics as prescribed to decrease the preload (PAOP) in cardiogenic shock.

b. Maintain optimal cardiac contractility and cardiac output.
   (1) Monitor ECG, MAP, right atrial pressure (RAP), pulmonary artery pressure (PAP), PAOP, cardiac output/cardiac index (CO/CI), left ventricular stroke work index (LVSWI), right ventricular stroke work index (RVSWI), and neurologic status.
   (2) Administer inotropes (e.g., dobutamine) as prescribed.
   (3) Administer diuretics (e.g., furosemide) as prescribed.
   (4) Administer vasoactive agents.
      (a) Administer arterial vasodilators (e.g., nitroprusside [NTP]) to decrease afterload (SVR) and/or venous vasodilators (e.g., nitroglycerin [NTG]) to decrease preload (PAOP) as prescribed; these agents typically are needed in cardiogenic shock.
      (b) Administer vasopressors (e.g., norepinephrine [Levophed] or dopamine [Intropin]) as prescribed and in the lowest doses necessary to achieve desired effects.
         (i) Vasopressors are generally contraindicated in patients with cardiogenic shock because they increase afterload (SVR) and myocardial oxygen consumption.
         (ii) Vasopressors sometimes are used in an effort to maintain MAP greater than 60 mm Hg to maintain perfusion pressure, but by constricting the vessels they actually may decrease blood flow to organs, even through the MAP is higher.
   (5) Correct metabolic acidosis because it affects cardiac contractility.
      (a) Improve oxygenation and perfusion by improving hemoglobin, Sa_{O_2}, and CO.
      (b) Administer sodium bicarbonate as prescribed; it is indicated only if pH is 7.0 or less.
   (6) Avoid overheating the patient, which may cause vasodilation and a decrease in preload.

c. Maintain optimal oxygen saturation.
   (1) Monitor Spo_2, Svo_2, and arterial blood gases.
   (2) Ensure adequate airway; endotracheal intubation frequently is necessary.
   (3) Administer oxygen at 5 to 6 L/min initially.
      (a) Higher concentrations may be necessary depending on Spo_2 and arterial blood gas values.
      (b) Continuous positive airway pressure (CPAP) or positive end-expiratory pressure (PEEP) may be required for refractory hypoxemia.
   (4) Initiate mechanical ventilation as prescribed for respiratory muscle fatigue, respiratory acidosis, and/or refractory hypoxemia.
   (5) Monitor patient closely for changes in Spo_2, arterial blood gases, pulmonary vascular resistance, chest x-rays, and lung compliance indicative of ARDS.
   (6) Assist with extracorporeal membrane oxygenation (ECMO) as required.

2. Minimize oxygen consumption of the tissues.
   a. Maintain patient comfort.
      (1) Maintain patient on bed rest, and provide adequate rest periods.
      (2) Administer analgesics and anxiolytics as required, but be cautious to avoid cumulative effect.
   b. Control body temperature.
      (1) Treat hyperthermia with cooling blankets as necessary: set at 1°C below patient's temperature to avoid drift and resultant shivering.
      (2) Avoid overheating, which may increase myocardial oxygen consumption.
   c. Monitor work of breathing; initiate mechanical ventilation as prescribed for respiratory fatigue.
   d. Treat pain and anxiety.
      (1) Administer analgesics and/or anxiolytics as prescribed and indicated.
   e. Provide patient and family support.
      (1) Keep patient and family informed.
      (2) Encourage the patient and family to discuss fear and concerns.
3. Prevent injury caused by decreased perfusion.
   a. Limit sedatives and other CNS depressants.
   b. Administer drugs only by IV route because peripheral perfusion and drug absorption is impaired; a central venous catheter with multiple-lumen catheter is preferred.
4. Maintain or improve nutritional status.
   a. Provide enteral feedings unless absolutely contraindicated (e.g., paralytic ileus or structural obstruction).
      (1) Use of the GI tract is important to prevent bacterial translocation.
      (2) Glutamine, arginine, and omega-3 fatty acids may be important in the prevention and treatment of sepsis, septic shock, SIRS, and MODS.
   b. Provide parenteral feeding if enteral feedings are contraindicated or if parenteral supplementation of enteral feedings is needed to meet calorie and protein requirements.
   c. Monitor serum potassium, magnesium, and phosphate closely; replace or restrict as indicated.
   d. Add trace elements and vitamins as prescribed.
5. Maintain renal perfusion and GFR.
   a. Insert Foley catheter to monitor hourly urine output.
   b. Monitor BUN, creatinine, urine creatinine clearance, and urine sodium.
   c. Replace volume as indicated by CVP or PAOP.
   d. Monitor closely for change in color of urine, which may indicate myoglobinuria or hemoglobinuria.
6. Maintain glycemic control.
   a. Recognize that hyperglycemia is related to stress and insulin resistance and occurs in patients without diagnosis of diabetes mellitus.
   b. Maintain serum glucose less than 150 mg/dL, preferably between 70 and 110 mg/dL.
      (1) Measure serum glucose by point-of-care testing every hour until serum glucose is less than 150 mg/dL, and then measure every 4 hours.
         (a) Fingerstick measurements may be inaccurate in edematous, vasoconstricted, or poorly perfused patients; place an arterial or venous catheter for sampling.
      (2) Administer insulin by infusion (usually 1 unit/mL), and adjust rate according to serum glucose level.
      (3) Administer 10% dextrose in water for hypoglycemia.
7. Monitor patient for complications.
   a. Dysrhythmias: close monitoring and appropriate antidysrhythmic agents depending on rhythm
   b. GI ulceration: stress ulcer prophylaxis with H_2 receptor antagonists or proton pump inhibitors
   c. Deep venous thrombosis: prophylaxis with low-molecular-weight heparin subcutaneously
   d. Mesenteric ischemia, infarction: monitoring for abdominal pain, bloody diarrhea; surgery required if intestinal perforation occurs
8. Monitor for indications of organ failure and MODS
   a. Acute respiratory failure (ARDS)
   b. DIC
   c. Hepatic failure
   d. Acute tubular necrosis (ATN)
   e. MI
   f. Cerebral infarction
9. Provide emotional support to the patient and family.
   a. Inform the patient regarding what is going to occur and why.
   b. Provide the family with accurate information; maintain hope, but do not give false reassurance.

Hypovolemic Shock

Definition

Caused by inadequate intravascular volume

Etiology

1. External losses
   a. Blood
      (1) Gastrointestinal (e.g., esophageal varices, peptic ulcer, or hemorrhoids)
      (2) Genitourinary (e.g., antepartal or postpartum bleeding or hematuria)
      (3) Amputations
      (4) Major blood vessel disruption (also may be occult)
      (5) Coagulopathy
         (a) Congenital coagulopathy (e.g., hemophilia)
         (b) Acquired coagulopathy (e.g., DIC or excessive anticoagulation)
   b. Fluid
      (1) Gastrointestinal (e.g., vomiting, diarrhea, or nasogastric suction)
      (2) Renal
         (a) Diabetic ketoacidosis (DKA)
         (b) Hyperglycemic hyperosmolar nonketotic syndrome (HHNK)
         (c) Diabetes insipidus
         (d) Hypoaldosteronism (Addison's disease)
         (e) Diuretics
         (f) Osmotic dyes
      (3) Cutaneous
         (a) Burns
         (b) Exudative wounds
         (c) Excessive perspiration (e.g., heat exhaustion)
2. Internal sequestration
   a. Blood
      (1) Hemoperitoneum or retroperitoneal (e.g., hemorrhagic pancreatitis, ruptured spleen, or lacerated liver)
      (2) Thoracic trauma with hemothorax or hemomediastinum
      (3) Dissecting aortic aneurysm
      (4) Pelvic or long bone fractures
   b. Fluid
      (1) Ascites: peritonitis; pancreatitis; cirrhosis; intraabdominal malignancies (e.g., liver or ovarian)
      (2) Pleural effusion
      (3) Intestinal obstruction

Pathophysiology

See Figure 11-2.

Clinical Presentation

Same as for shock and including the following:
1. Subjective: history of precipitating factor
2. Objective
   a. Flat neck veins
   b. Abdominal girth may be increased if intraabdominal bleeding

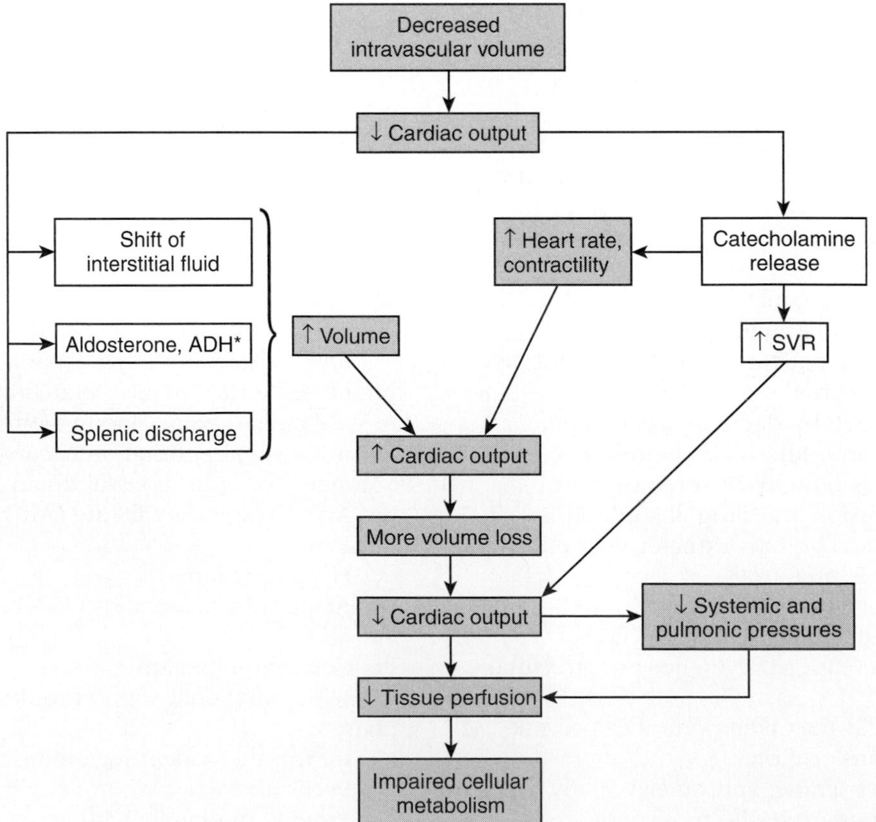

Figure 11-2 Pathophysiology of hypovolemic shock. (From McCance, K. L., & Huether, S. E. [2006]. *Pathophysiology: The biologic basis for disease in adults and children* [5th ed.]. St. Louis: Mosby.)

(1) Measure at same location on abdomen and mark with pen.
(2) One inch increase in abdominal girth is equal to an increase in intraabdominal volume of 500 to 1000 mL.

c. Daily weight
(1) Use same scale, same time of day, same clothing, and linens.
(2) 1 kg is equal to 1 L (1000 mL).

d. Intake and output: 1 L is equal to 1 kg
(1) Consider insensible losses.
(2) Weigh dressings and convert to volume using 1 kg equal to 1000 mL.
(3) Include all drainage tubes outputs.

e. Parameters used for evaluation of severity of hemorrhagic shock (Table 11-4)

3. Hemodynamics: Table 11-2
4. Diagnostic
   a. Hematocrit
      (1) Elevated if resulting from dehydration
      (2) Decreased if resulting from blood loss
   b. Diagnostic peritoneal lavage to detect intraabdominal bleeding
   c. Computed tomography of chest or abdomen to detect source of bleeding

Nursing Diagnoses

1. Ineffective Tissue Perfusion related to decreased effective blood volume
2. Decreased Cardiac Output related to decreased preload
3. Deficient Fluid Volume related to blood or fluid loss or sequestration
4. Ineffective Airway Clearance related to altered consciousness
5. Impaired Gas Exchange related to ventilation/perfusion mismatch or intrapulmonary shunt
6. Ineffective Breathing Patterns related to immobility and analgesics
7. Imbalanced Nutrition: Less Than Body Requirements related to protein loss, increased metabolic requirements, and decreased absorption
8. Impaired Urinary Elimination related to hypoperfusion and excretion of pigments (e.g., myoglobin and hemoglobin)
9. Risk for Infection related to invasive procedures and immunocompromise
10. Pain related to invasive procedures
11. Risk for Injury related to intubation, invasive procedures, and hemorrhage resulting from clotting abnormalities
12. Risk for Electrolyte Imbalance related to fluid shifts and potential hemolysis
13. Interrupted Family Processes related to sudden critical illness
14. Anxiety related to sudden critical illness, fear of the unknown, fear of death, change in role relationships, and change in self-concept

Collaborative Management

Same as for shock and including the following:

1. Identify high-risk patient, and monitor patient for clinical indications of hypoperfusion.
2. Treat the cause.
   a. Compress any compressible vessels.
   b. Surgery may be necessary to control bleeding.
   c. Administer antidiarrheals for diarrhea, insulin for hyperglycemia, and other necessary treatments specific to the cause.
3. Administer appropriate volume replacement.
   a. Two large-gauge intravenous catheters
   b. Normal saline at rapid rate initially
   c. Monitoring for fluid overload
4. Use autotransfusion if appropriate; autotransfusion is used primarily in chest trauma (or chest surgery) to decrease the risk of transfusion-transmitted disease (for more detailed discussion, see Chest Surgery and Chest Tubes in Chapter 5).

Table 11-4 Severity of Hemorrhagic Shock

	Class			
Indicators	**I**	**II**	**III**	**IV**
Blood loss (percent of blood volume)	Less than 15%	15-30%	30-40%	Greater than 40%
Blood loss (mL)	Less than 750 mL	750-1500 mL	1500-2000 mL	Greater than 2000 mL
Heart rate per minute	Less than 100	Greater than 100	Greater than 120	140 or greater
Blood pressure	Normal	Normal	Decreased	Decreased
Pulse pressure	Widened or normal	Narrowed	Narrowed	Narrowed
Capillary refill	Normal	Delayed	Delayed	Delayed or absent
Ventilatory rate per minute	14-20	20-30	30-40	Greater than 35
Urine output (mL/hr)	30 or greater	20-30	Less than 20	Negligible
Skin appearance	Cool, pink	Cool, pale	Cold, moist, pale	Cold, clammy, cyanotic
Neurologic status	Slightly anxious	Mildly anxious	Anxious, confused	Confused, lethargy

Modified from American College of Surgeons, Advanced Trauma Life Support program for physicians, Chicago, 1993.

Cardiogenic Shock

Definition

Shock caused by impaired ability of the heart to pump blood effectively

Etiology

1. Decreased contractility
   a. Coronary artery disease
      (1) Acute MI
         (a) Loss of 40% of left ventricular myocardium
            (i) Large anterior MI
            (ii) MI with history of previous MI
         (b) MI with preexisting left ventricular dysfunction
      (2) Myocardial ischemia with preexisting left ventricular dysfunction
   b. Myocardial contusion
   c. Cardiomyopathy
   d. Myocarditis
   e. Severe heart failure (HF)
   f. Ventricular aneurysm
   g. Overdosage of myocardial depressant drugs (e.g., beta-blockers, calcium channel blockers, or barbiturates)
   h. Stunned myocardium: transient cardiogenic shock
      (1) Cardiac surgery: related to hypothermia, cardioplegic arrest, surgical incisions
      (2) Reperfusion injury
      (3) After CPR
      (4) Hypoxemia
      (5) Acidosis
      (6) Hypoglycemia
      (7) Electrolyte imbalance
   i. Acute rejection of cardiac transplant
2. Impaired filling
   a. Dysrhythmias
   b. Cardiac tamponade
   c. Noncompliant ventricle (e.g., left ventricular hypertrophy or right ventricular hypertrophy)
3. Impaired emptying (may be referred to as *obstructive*)
   a. Valvular dysfunction
      (1) Chronic: stenosis or regurgitation
      (2) Acute: papillary muscle rupture
   b. Ventricular septal rupture
   c. Intracardiac tumor
   d. Massive pulmonary embolism
   e. Tension pneumothorax
   f. Dissecting thoracic aortic aneurysm

Pathophysiology

See Figure 11-3.

Clinical Presentation

Same as for shock and including the following:

1. Subjective
   a. History of precipitating factor
   b. Chest pain
   c. Dyspnea

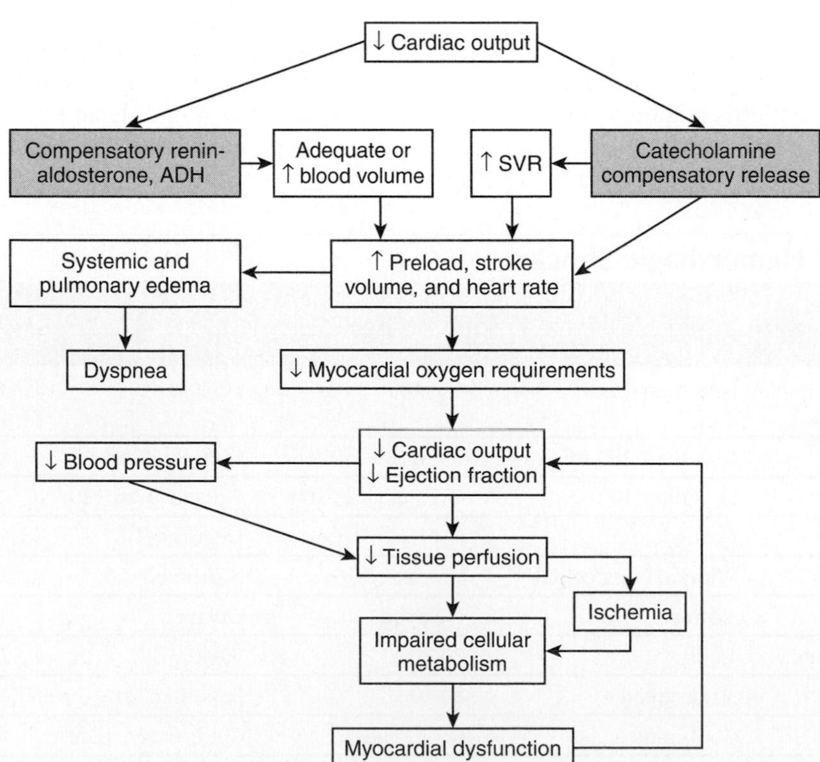

Figure 11-3 Pathophysiology of cardiogenic shock. (From McCance, K. L., & Huether, S. E. [2006]. *Pathophysiology: The biologic basis for disease in adults and children* [5th ed.]. St. Louis: Mosby.)

d. Thirst
e. Anxiety, fear, feeling of impending doom

2. Objectives
   a. Clinical indicators of left ventricular failure (LVF)
      (1) Tachycardia
      (2) Dysrhythmias
      (3) Pulsus alternans
      (4) Tachypnea
      (5) Heart sound changes: S_3
      (6) Breath sound changes: crackles
   b. Clinical indicators of right ventricular failure (RVF)
      (1) Jugular venous distention
      (2) Peripheral edema
      (3) Hepatosplenomegaly
3. Hemodynamics: Table 11-2; defining characteristics of cardiogenic shock
   a. CO/CI: less than 2 L/min/m^2
   b. RAP, PAP, and PAOP increased; PAOP usually greater than 18 mm Hg
   c. SVR and SVRI increased; SVR usually greater than 2000 dynes/sec/cm^{-5}
4. Diagnostic
   a. Serum
      (1) Enzymes and troponin: elevated if acute MI
      (2) Electrolytes: note any abnormality
      (3) Arterial blood gases: may reveal significant hypoxemia in pulmonary edema, respiratory acidosis as patient fatigues and acute respiratory failure occurs, and eventually metabolic acidosis with tissue hypoxia occurs, causing lactic acidosis
   b. ECG
      (1) May reveal acute (i.e., ST segment elevation and pathologic Q waves) or old (pathologic Q waves without ST segment elevation) MI
      (2) May reveal ventricular aneurysm (i.e., persistent ST segment elevation in anterior leads)
      (3) May reveal dysrhythmias
   c. Chest x-ray: may show pulmonary vascular congestion
   d. Cardiac catheterization
      (1) May reveal cause of cardiogenic shock
      (2) May reveal abnormal intracardiac pressures
   e. Echocardiography: may reveal cause of cardiogenic shock
      (1) Ventricular wall motion abnormality
         (a) Regional wall motional abnormality: myocardial in myocardial ischemia or infarction
         (b) Global wall motion abnormality in cardiomyopathy or myocarditis
      (2) Valvular abnormality (e.g., ruptured ventricular septum, ruptured papillary muscle with acute mitral regurgitation)
      (3) Cardiac tamponade

Nursing Diagnoses

1. Ineffective Tissue Perfusion related to decreased cardiac output
   a. Ineffective Cardiopulmonary Tissue Perfusion related to decreased coronary artery perfusion pressure and myocardial ischemia
   b. Ineffective Cerebral Tissue Perfusion related to cerebral hypoperfusion
   c. Ineffective Peripheral Tissue Perfusion related to hypovolemia, fluid shifts, decreased blood flow resulting from IABP catheter position and vasopressors
2. Decreased Cardiac Output related to inadequate volume, inadequate cardiac contractility, inadequate vascular tone, dysrhythmias, and ineffective timing of IABP
3. Ineffective Airway Clearance related to altered consciousness
4. Impaired Gas Exchange related to pulmonary edema, ventilation/perfusion mismatch, and intrapulmonary shunt
5. Ineffective Breathing Patterns related to immobility and analgesics
6. Imbalanced Nutrition: Less Than Body Requirements related to increased metabolic requirements and decreased absorption
7. Impaired Urinary Elimination related to hypoperfusion and excretion of pigments (e.g., myoglobin and hemoglobin)
8. Risk for Infection related to invasive procedures and immunocompromise
9. Pain related to invasive procedures
10. Risk for Injury related to intubation, invasive procedures, and hemorrhage resulting from clotting abnormalities
11. Risk for Electrolyte Imbalance related to fluid shifts and potential hemolysis
12. Interrupted Family Processes related to sudden critical illness
13. Anxiety related to sudden critical illness, fear of the unknown, fear of death, change in role relationships, and change in self-concept

Collaborative Management

Same as for shock and including the following:

1. Identify high-risk patient and monitor for clinical indications of hypoperfusion; use invasive hemodynamic monitoring if appropriate for early detection of changes in cardiac index.
2. Prevent and treat the cause.
   a. Early reperfusion for acute MI
   b. Pericardiocentesis for cardiac tamponade
   c. Fibrinolytics and anticoagulants for pulmonary embolus
   d. Surgery for removal of intracardiac tumors, valve replacement, and septal repair
   e. Emergency decompression followed by chest tube insertion for tension pneumothorax
3. Improve oxygenation.
   a. Oxygen by nasal cannula to achieve an SaO_2 of at least 95%; non-rebreathing face mask may be

required to achieve this $Sa{O_2}$, but the mask may increase dyspnea.
   b. Mask CPAP may be helpful to improve oxygenation, especially for patients with significant pulmonary edema, but it is likely to increase dyspnea.
   c. Intubation and mechanical ventilation may be required to decrease the work of breathing as well and improve ventilation and oxygenation.
4. Improve myocardial perfusion.
   a. Administer nitrates for ischemia while being careful not to decrease blood pressure and coronary artery perfusion pressure; because one nitroglycerin tablet sublingually is 400 mcg, titratable intravenously administered nitroglycerin is preferred.
   b. Make prompt evaluation for emergency reperfusion options if acute MI occurs.
      (1) Primary percutaneous coronary intervention (PCI): preferred if facilities available
      (2) Fibrinolytics may be used
      (3) Coronary artery bypass graft (CABG)
5. Optimize cardiac output and improve tissue perfusion.
   a. Inotropes (e.g., dobutamine) to increase *contractility*
   b. Diuretics (e.g., furosemide) or venous vasodilators (e.g., nitroglycerin [NTG]) to decrease *preload* (PAOP)
   c. Arterial vasodilators (e.g., nitroprusside) to decrease *afterload* if no contraindications
      (1) Nitroprusside is contraindicated in acute myocardial ischemia because of the risk of coronary artery steal with shunting of blood from ischemic areas to nonischemic areas.
      (2) Use caution with all arterial vasodilators in acute myocardial ischemia because they are likely to decrease aortic root pressure and coronary artery perfusion pressure.
      (3) Careful titration of all vasodilators is required to maintain the MAP greater than the 60 mm Hg required to perfuse vital organs; afterload reduction may need to be achieved nonpharmacologically through the use of an IABP.
   d. Antidysrhythmics as required to control *heart rate*
      (1) Anxiolytics (e.g., lorazepam [Ativan]) may be helpful to decrease heart rate by decreasing anxiety.
      (2) Beta-blockers are contraindicated during cardiogenic shock states because they decrease contractility.
   e. Mechanical supports (e.g., IABP; Figures 3-19 and 3-20 and Table 3-14) or ventricular assist devices (Table 3-19)
      (1) IABP is especially helpful in patients who have very high afterload that is refractory to arterial vasodilators or who are too hypotensive to use arterial vasodilators to reduce afterload.
      (2) IABP or ventricular assist devices also may serve as a bridge to transplantation if the patient is a candidate for cardiac transplantation.
6. Registration of the patient for cardiac transplantation if appropriate.

Anaphylactic Shock

Definition

Results from massive vasodilation caused by release of histamine in response to a severe allergic reaction

Etiology

1. Foods, especially the following:
   a. Fish
   b. Shellfish
   c. Eggs
   d. Milk and milk products
   e. Wheat
   f. Strawberries
   g. Legumes (e.g., peanuts and soybeans)
   h. Nuts (e.g., walnuts and pecans)
   i. Chocolate
   j. Food additives
      (1) Artificial coloring
      (2) Preservatives: sulfites, monosodium glutamate (MSG)
2. Drugs
   a. Angiotensin-converting enzyme (ACE) inhibitors (e.g., captopril or enalapril)
   b. Acetylcysteine (Mucomyst)
   c. Allergic extracts in hyposensitization therapy
   d. Anesthetics
      (1) Local anesthetics: lidocaine, cocaine
      (2) General anesthetics: thiopental, etomidate, ketamine
   e. Animal serums: antitoxins, antivenoms
   f. Antibiotics
      (1) Beta-lactam antibiotics
         (a) Penicillin
         (b) Cephalosporins
      (2) Tetracycline
      (3) Macrolides
   g. Barbiturates
   h. Blood and blood products: blood transfusion incompatibilities, gamma globulin, albumin
   i. Dextran
   j. Enzymes
      (1) Pancreatic
      (2) Papaya enzyme
         (a) Chymopapain (used in chemical diskectomy)
         (b) Meat tenderizer
   k. Insulin: pork or beef
   l. Iodine-containing contrast media (e.g., diatrizoate [Renografin])
   m. Narcotics: morphine, meperidine, codeine
   n. Neuromuscular blocker
   o. Nonsteroidal antiinflammatory drugs: aspirin, ibuprofen, indomethacin
   p. Protamine sulfate
   q. Thiazide diuretics (e.g., hydrochlorothiazide)

3. Venoms
   a. Snakes
   b. Hymenoptera: wasps, hornets, bees, yellow jackets, fire ants
   c. Spiders
   d. Jellyfish
   e. Stingrays
   f. Deer flies
   g. Scorpions
4. Other chemicals or biologics
   a. Materials (e.g., latex)
   b. Hand lotions
   c. Soap
   d. Perfume
   e. Iodine-containing solutions (e.g., povidone-iodine [Betadine])
   f. Animal dander

Pathophysiology (Figure 11-4)

1. Anaphylactic reaction requires previous exposure to the antigen.
   a. With first exposure to the antigen, specific immunoglobulin E (IgE) antibody is formed.
   b. The antibody binds to the mass cells and basophils.
   c. Repeat exposure triggers a response by the IgE antibodies.
   d. Mast cells are triggered to degranulate.
   e. Bioactive mediators are released.
2. Anaphylactoid reaction is clinically indistinguishable from anaphylactic reaction but does not require previous exposure to the antigen.
   a. Non-IgE mediated
   b. Direct activation and degranulation of mast cells thought to be triggered by the complement system

Clinical Presentation

Same as for shock and including the following:

1. Subjective
   a. History of precipitating factor
   b. Anxiety, vague uneasiness
   c. Warmth
   d. Nausea, abdominal cramping, abdominal pain
   e. Chest tightness, palpitations
   f. Dyspnea
   g. Dizziness, vertigo
   h. Pruritus
   i. Feeling of a lump in throat
2. Objective
   a. Cutaneous
      (1) An identifiable site of allergen exposure, bite, sting, or envenomation may be evident as localized redness, swelling, and pruritus
      (2) May be generalized
         (a) Angioedema (edema of membranous tissues): swelling of eyes, lips, tongue, hands, feet, and genitalia
         (b) Flushing

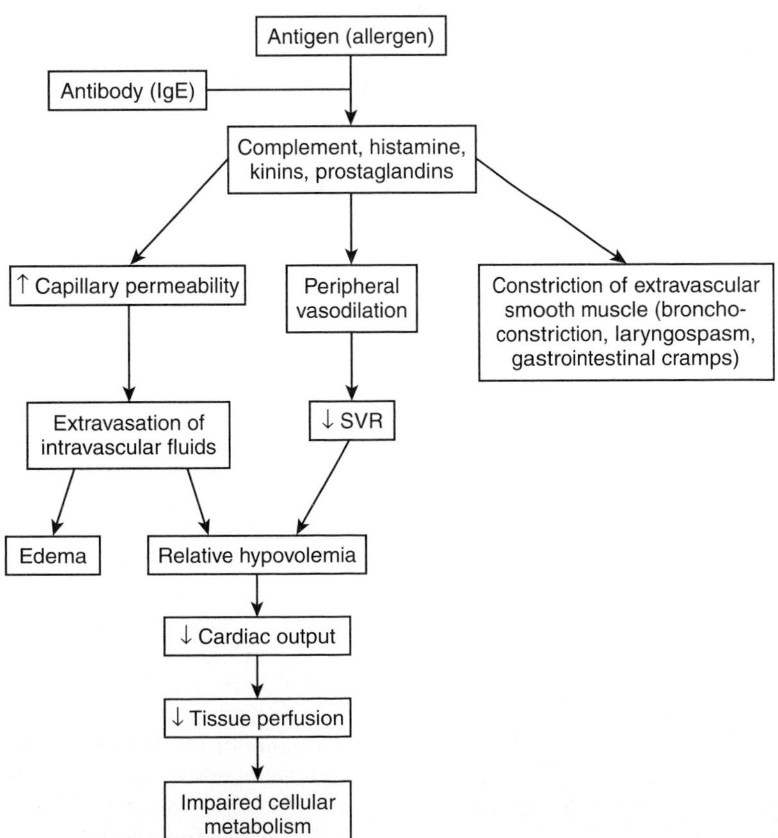

Figure 11-4 Pathophysiology of anaphylactic shock. (From McCance, K. L., & Huether, S. E. [2006]. *Pathophysiology: The biologic basis for disease in adults and children* [5th ed.]. St. Louis: Mosby.)

(c) Warm to hot skin
(d) Urticaria
(e) Conjunctival injection, tearing
(f) Watery rhinorrhea, sneezing
(g) Erythema more in upper extremities

b. Cardiovascular
(1) Tachycardia
(2) Hypotension
(3) Dysrhythmias
(4) ST segment and T wave changes consistent with ischemia
(5) Shock
(6) Cardiac arrest may occur

c. Pulmonary
(1) Hoarseness
(2) Cough
(3) Prolonged expiration
(4) Breath sound changes: stridor; wheezing; crackles; rhonchi
(5) Respiratory arrest may occur

d. Neurologic
(1) Restlessness
(2) Headache
(3) Paresthesia
(4) Change in level of consciousness
(5) Seizures

e. Genitourinary
(1) Urinary incontinence
(2) Urine output: may be decreased
(3) Vaginal bleeding

f. Gastrointestinal
(1) Dysphagia
(2) Vomiting
(3) Hyperactive bowel sounds
(4) Diarrhea

3. Hemodynamics: Table 11-2
4. Diagnostic
a. Serum
(1) IgE levels may be used to confirm allergic origin
(2) Eosinophils elevated
(3) Arterial blood gases: initially respiratory alkalosis with hypoxemia, eventually respiratory and metabolic acidosis as hypoventilation and tissue hypoxia occur

Nursing Diagnoses

1. Ineffective Airway Clearance related to altered consciousness, tracheobronchial obstruction caused by laryngeal edema, laryngeal spasm, bronchospasm, increased secretions, and artificial airways
2. Ineffective Tissue Perfusion related to decreased vascular tone
   a. Ineffective Cerebral Tissue Perfusion related to hypoxia and cerebral hypoperfusion
   b. Ineffective Peripheral Tissue Perfusion related to hypovolemia, fluid shifts, and vasopressors
3. Decreased Cardiac Output related to inadequate vascular tone and dysrhythmias
4. Impaired Gas Exchange related to alveolar-capillary membrane changes resulting from increased capillary permeability associated with histamine, ARDS, ventilation/perfusion mismatch, and intrapulmonary shunt
5. Imbalanced Nutrition: Less Than Body Requirements related to increased metabolic requirements and decreased absorption
6. Impaired Urinary Elimination related to hypoperfusion
7. Impaired Skin Integrity caused by urticaria and angioedema
8. Risk for Infection related to invasive procedures and immunocompromise
9. Pain related to invasive procedures
10. Risk for Injury related to intubation, invasive procedures, and hemorrhage resulting from clotting abnormalities
11. Risk for Electrolyte Imbalance related to fluid shifts and potential hemolysis
12. Interrupted Family Processes related to sudden critical illness
13. Anxiety related to sudden critical illness, fear of the unknown, fear of death, change in role relationships, and change in self-concept

Collaborative Management

Same as for shock and including the following:

1. Identify high-risk patient, and monitor patient for clinical indications of allergic reaction and hypoperfusion.
2. Provide CPR as required.
3. Maintain airway, oxygenation, and ventilation.
   a. Airway
      (1) Assess airway for clinical indications of angioedema (i.e., edema of uvula, respiratory distress, stridor, and hypoxemia).
      (2) If angioedema is present, assist with endotracheal tube insertion early to prevent complete airway obstruction; cricothyrotomy may be necessary because of laryngeal edema.
   b. Oxygen at 5 to 6 L initially; adjust to maintain Spo_2 at 95% unless contraindicated; 100% oxygen by non-rebreathing mask may be required, but the mask may increase the sensation of dyspnea
   c. Mechanical ventilation as prescribed
4. Remove the offending agent or slow absorption of antigen.
   a. Removal of stinger if anaphylaxis is due to a sting and the stinger can be removed easily without squeezing
   b. Ice if anaphylaxis is due to sting or bite
   c. Discontinuance of infusion of dye, drug, or blood
   d. Dermal decontamination with soap and water if skin exposure to allergen
   e. Gastric lavage not recommended to remove an ingested antigen
5. Modify or block the effects of biochemical mediators.
   a. Sympathomimetic agents
      (1) Epinephrine
         (a) Intravenous
            (i) IV injection: 0.1 mg (100 mcg) over 5 to 10 minutes initially

if clinical indications of cardiovascular compromise are present: stop injection if dysrhythmias or chest pain occur
    (ii) IV infusion: 1 to 4 mcg/min if inadequate response to IV injection
  (b) Intramuscular injection: 0.3 to 0.5 mg every 5 to 10 minutes for patients with less severe symptoms; thigh injection preferred over upper arm
 (2) Glucagon 1 mg IV every 5 minutes for patients taking beta-blockers with hypotension refractory to epinephrine and fluids
  (a) Glucagon can stimulate an increase in heart rate and contractility even with beta-blockade.
  (b) Monitor patient for nausea, vomiting, hypokalemia, and hyperglycemia.

b. Crystalloids: 1 to 2 L of normal saline
c. Antihistamines as prescribed to block histamine receptors
 (1) Diphenhydramine (Benadryl) 25 to 50 mg IV, IM, or PO
 (2) Ranitidine (Zantac) 50 mg IV or cimetidine (Tagamet) 150 mg IV
d. Steroids as prescribed to stabilize mast cells, decrease capillary permeability, and prevent delayed reaction
 (1) Methylprednisolone sodium succinate (Solu-Medrol): 125 mg IV or hydrocortisone sodium succinate (Solu-Cortef) 100 to 200 to 500 mg IV
 (2) Prednisone 40 to 60 mg PO daily
e. Bronchodilators as prescribed to reverse the bronchoconstriction caused by histamine, slow-reacting substance of anaphylaxis (SRS-A), and bradykinin
 (1) Albuterol, intermittent or continuous nebulizer for wheezing refractory to epinephrine
 (2) Ipratropium bromide (Atrovent) or magnesium also may be used

6. Maintain MAP and tissue perfusion: fluids, inotropes, and/or vasopressors may be necessary.

Neurogenic Shock

Definition

Shock resulting from massive vasodilation caused by suppression of the SNS

Etiology

1. Cervical spinal cord injury
2. Head injury
3. Insulin shock
4. General anesthesia
5. Spinal anesthesia
6. Epidural block
7. Drugs
   a. Barbiturates
   b. Phenothiazines
   c. Sympathetic blocking agents (e.g., antihypertensives)
8. Exposure to unpleasant circumstances (e.g., fright or pain)

Pathophysiology

See Figure 11-5.

Clinical Presentation

1. Subjective: history of precipitating factor
2. Objective
   a. Bradycardia
   b. Hypotension
   c. Hypothermia
   d. Skin warm, dry, flushed
   e. Definite neurologic deficit
3. Hemodynamics: Table 11-2

Nursing Diagnoses

1. Ineffective Tissue Perfusion related to decreased vascular tone
   a. Ineffective Cerebral Tissue Perfusion related to hypoxia and cerebral hypoperfusion
   b. Ineffective Peripheral Tissue Perfusion related to hypovolemia, fluid shifts, and vasopressors
2. Decreased Cardiac Output related to inadequate vascular tone and dysrhythmias
3. Ineffective Airway Clearance related to altered consciousness and artificial airways
4. Impaired Gas Exchange related to alveolar-capillary membrane changes resulting from increased capillary permeability associated with ARDS, ventilation/perfusion mismatch, and intrapulmonary shunt
5. Ineffective Breathing Patterns related to immobility and analgesics

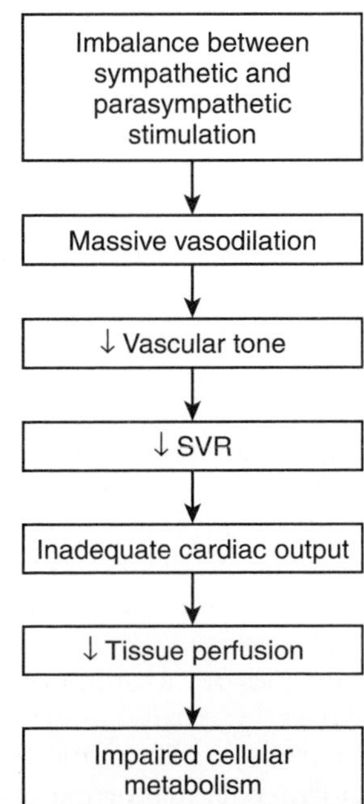

Figure 11-5 Pathophysiology of neurogenic shock. (From McCance, K. L., & Huether, S. E. [2006]. *Pathophysiology: The biologic basis for disease in adults and children* [5th ed.]. St. Louis: Mosby.)

6. Hypothermia related to impaired thermoregulation
7. Imbalanced Nutrition: Less Than Body Requirements related to increased metabolic requirements, paralytic ileus, and decreased absorption
8. Impaired Urinary Elimination related to hypoperfusion and excretion of pigments (e.g., myoglobin and hemoglobin)
9. Risk for Infection related to invasive procedures and immunocompromise
10. Pain related to invasive procedures
11. Risk for Injury related to intubation, invasive procedures, and hemorrhage resulting from clotting abnormalities
12. Risk for Electrolyte Imbalance related to fluid shifts and potential hemolysis
13. Interrupted Family Processes related to sudden critical illness
14. Anxiety related to sudden critical illness, fear of the unknown, fear of death, change in role relationships, and change in self-concept

Collaborative Management

Same as for shock and including the following:

1. Identify high-risk patient, and monitor patient for clinical indications of hypoperfusion.
2. Prevent and treat the cause.
   a. Suspected spinal cord injury
      (1) Early immobilization of the spine with suspected spinal injury
      (2) Elevate the head of the bed to 30 degrees to decrease spinal cord edema
   b. Anesthesia: reverse anesthesia, rewarm
   c. Insulin shock
      (1) Monitor patient for clinical indications of hypoglycemia, and measure serum glucose as required.
      (2) Administer 10 to 15 g of carbohydrates (see Box 9-2 in Chapter 9) if the patient is conscious or 50 mL of 50% dextrose in water ($D_{50}W$) if patient is unconscious.
3. Maintain MAP and tissue perfusion.
   a. Maintain MAP at greater than 70 mm Hg.
      (1) Fluids
         (a) Crystalloids: Hypertonic saline may be used.
         (b) Colloids: Although albumin traditionally has been advocated, recent studies and a meta-analysis show no benefit to the use of colloids, including in patients with neurologic problems (Alderson et al., 2004).
         (c) Monitor patient closely for pulmonary or cerebral edema.
      (2) Inotropes and/or vasopressors may be necessary
   b. Maintain heart rate at 60 to 100 beats/min: atropine and/or pacemaker may be necessary.
4. Prevent venous stasis and deep venous thrombosis: administer anticoagulants (e.g., mini-heparin) as prescribed.

Septic Shock

Definitions

1. Infection: an inflammatory response to microorganisms
2. Bacteremia: the presence of viable bacteria in the blood
3. Sepsis: SIRS caused by infection
4. Severe sepsis: sepsis with associated organ dysfunction
5. Septic shock: shock resulting from massive vasodilation caused by release of mediators of the inflammatory process in response to overwhelming infection; sepsis with hypotension despite adequate fluid resuscitation along with the presence of perfusion abnormalities

Etiology

1. Factors that cause immunosuppression
   a. Extremes of age
   b. Malnutrition
   c. Alcoholism or drug abuse
   d. Debilitation
   e. Malignancy
   f. Acquired immunodeficiency syndrome (AIDS)
   g. History of splenectomy
   h. Chronic health problems (diabetes mellitus, liver disease, heart disease [e.g., coronary artery disease or heart failure], renal failure)
   i. Bone marrow suppression
   j. Immunosuppressive therapies (e.g., immunosuppressive drugs, antineoplastic drugs, antibiotic therapy, or corticosteroids)
2. Factors that cause bacteremia and septicemia
   a. Invasive procedures and devices
   b. Pulmonary procedures
   c. Diagnostic procedures
   d. Surgical procedures or wounds
   e. Traumatic wounds or burns
   f. Genitourinary infection
   g. Untreated GI disease (cholelithiasis, intestinal obstruction, appendicitis, diverticulitis)
   h. Peritonitis
   i. Food poisoning
   j. Prolonged hospitalization
   k. Translocation of GI bacteria: nothing-by-mouth (NPO) status, decreased peristalsis, and GI ischemia contribute to proliferation of gastrointestinal bacterial and translocation of these bacterial into blood or lymph
3. Microorganisms
   a. Gram-negative bacteria (*most likely)
      (1) *Escherichia coli**
      (2) *Klebsiella*
      (3) *Enterobacter**
      (4) *Pseudomonas aeruginosa**
      (5) *Proteus mirabilis*
      (6) *Enterococcus*
      (7) *Serratia marcescens*
      (8) *Bacteroides* organisms
      (9) *Haemophilus influenzae*

b. Gram-positive organisms
   (1) *Staphylococcus aureus*
   (2) *Staphylococcus epidermidis*
   (3) *Streptococcus pneumoniae*
   (4) *Clostridium* organisms
c. Less likely
   (1) Viruses
   (2) Fungi
   (3) Rickettsieae
   (4) *Spirochaeta*
   (5) Protozoa
   (6) Parasites

Pathophysiology (Figure 11-6)

1. Triad of inflammation, hypercoagulability, and impaired fibrinolysis (Figure 11-7)
2. Activated protein C levels have been shown to correlate positively with survival, hence the use of recombinant activated protein C

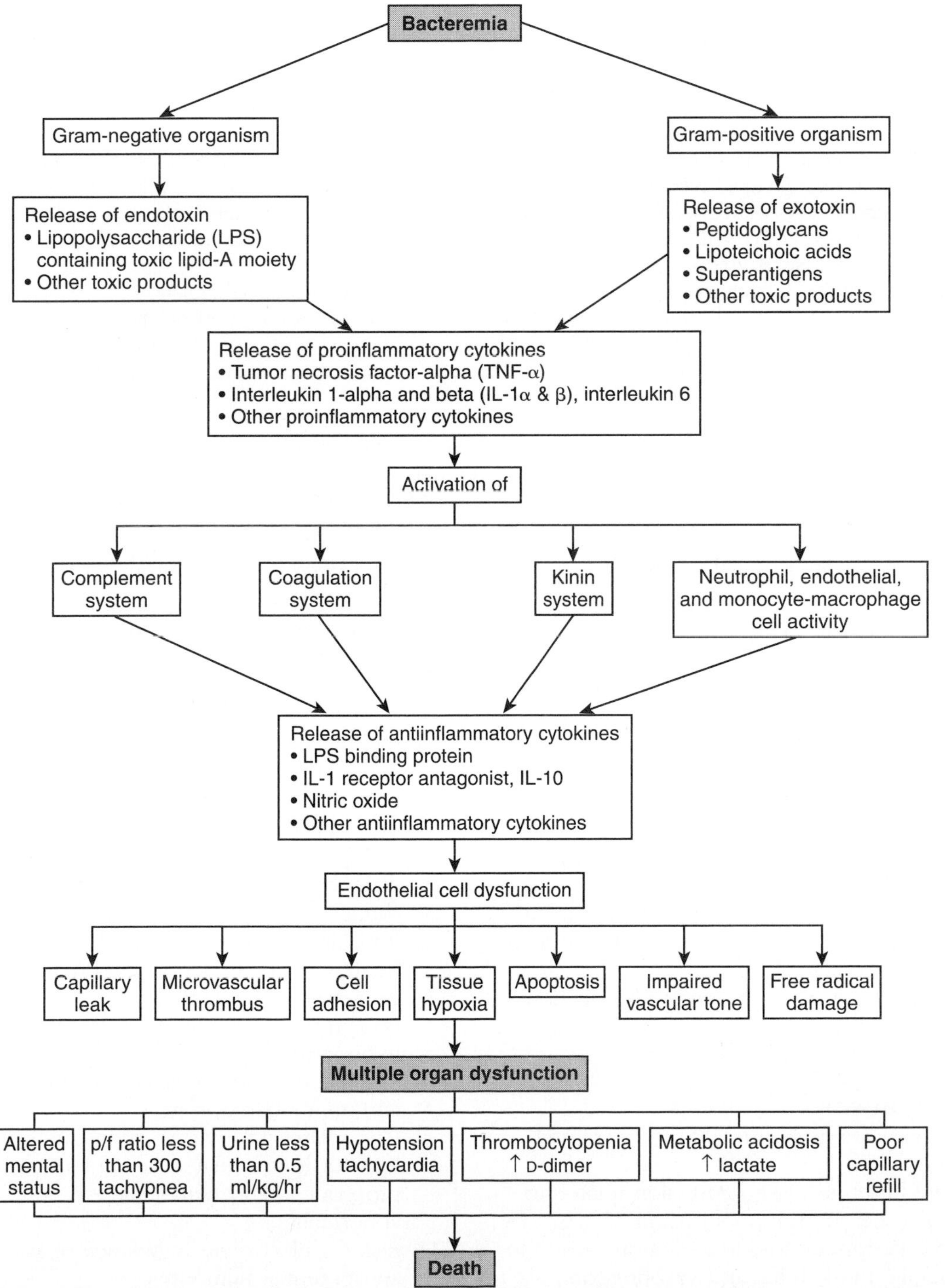

Figure 11-6 Pathophysiology of septic shock. *p/f,* (Pa_{O_2})/(Fi_{O_2}) = oxygen ratio. (From McCance, K. L., & Huether, S. E. [2006]. *Pathophysiology: The biologic basis for disease in adults and children* [5th ed.]. St. Louis: Mosby.)

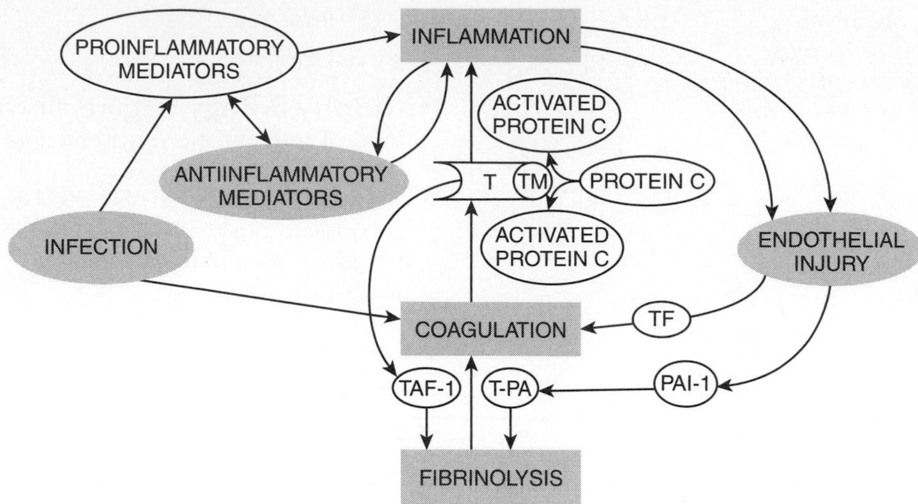

Figure 11-7 Severe sepsis is associated with three integrated components:

- Infection with the systemic activation of inflammation. During progression of sepsis, a wide variety of proinflammatory cytokines is released. Endotoxin induces rapid increases in the levels of tumor necrosis factor (TNF), interleukin-1 (IL-1), and interleukin-6 (IL-6) in experimental models of sepsis. These proinflammatory cytokines are linked to the development of the clinical signs of sepsis. Release of proinflammatory cytokines is associated with endothelial injury and vascular bed–specific changes in the thrombogenicity of the endothelium. These can include increased tissue factor (TF) expression in a subset of endothelial cells and release of plasminogen activator inhibitor-1 (PAI-1).
- Activation of coagulation. Inflammatory changes trigger the extrinsic pathway of coagulation. Activation of coagulation in patients with sepsis is not always disseminated intravascular coagulation. Instead, in most patients, activation of coagulation is a subclinical activation of the hemostatic system as indicated by changes in commonly measured hemostatic parameters. Experimentally, there are increases in thrombin-antithrombin (TAT) complexes. Clinical laboratory findings include significant increases in D-dimer, a marker of coagulation and associated fibrinolysis.
- Impairment of fibrinolysis. In patients with sepsis, plasminogen levels fall rapidly while antiplasmin levels remain normal. This decreases the normal fibrinolytic response. Fibrinolysis is impaired further by release of PAI-1 and the generation of increased amounts of thrombin-activatable fibrinolysis inhibitor (TAFI). Although the plasminogen/antiplasmin ratio and PAI-1 levels remain abnormal in nonsurviving patients, they tend to normalize in survivors. (Courtesy Eli Lilly.)

Clinical Presentation (Table 11-5)

1. Severe sepsis
   a. Known or suspected infection
   b. Two or more clinical indications of SIRS
      (1) Heart rate greater than 90 beats/min (sinus rhythm)
      (2) Hyperthermia (temperature above 38°C, or 100.4°F) or hypothermia (temperature below 36°C, or 96.8°F) (Note that hypothermia is more common in elderly patients.)
      (3) Respiratory rate above 20 breaths/min or $Paco_2$ below 32 mm Hg
      (4) White blood cell count greater than 12,000 cells/mm^3, less than 4000 cells/mm^3, or more than 10% bands
      (5) Evidence of at least one organ dysfunction (Figure 11-8)
2. Hemodynamics: Table 11-2

Nursing Diagnoses

1. Ineffective Tissue Perfusion related to decreased vascular tone
   a. Ineffective Cerebral Tissue Perfusion related to hypoxia and cerebral hypoperfusion
   b. Ineffective Peripheral Tissue Perfusion related to hypovolemia, fluid shifts, and vasopressors
   c. Ineffective Renal Tissue Perfusion related to hypovolemia, fluid shifts, and vasopressors
2. Decreased Cardiac Output related to inadequate volume, inadequate cardiac contractility, inadequate vascular tone, dysrhythmias, and ineffective timing of IABP
3. Deficient Fluid Volume related to increased vascular capacitance
4. Ineffective Airway Clearance related to altered consciousness and artificial airways
5. Impaired Gas Exchange related to alveolar-capillary membrane changes resulting from increased capillary permeability associated with ventilation/perfusion mismatch and intrapulmonary shunt
6. Imbalanced Nutrition: Less Than Body Requirements related to hypermetabolism and decreased absorption
7. Impaired Urinary Elimination related to hypoperfusion
8. Risk for Infection related to invasive procedures and immunocompromise
9. Pain related to invasive procedures
10. Risk for Injury related to intubation, invasive procedures, and hemorrhage resulting from clotting abnormalities
11. Risk for Electrolyte Imbalance related to fluid shifts and potential hemolysis
12. Interrupted Family Processes related to sudden critical illness

Table 11-5 Stages of Septic Shock

Early (Hyperdynamic; Looks Like Infection)	Late (Hypodynamic; Looks Like Shock)
Objective	
• Tachycardia	• Tachycardia
• Pulses bounding	• Pulses weak and thready
• Blood pressure: normal or low	• Hypotension
• Wide pulse pressure	• Narrow pulse pressure
• Skin warm, flushed	• Skin cool, pale
• Hyperpnea	• Bradypnea or tachypnea
• Change in mental status (e.g., irritability and confusion)	• Decreased level of consciousness (e.g., lethargy or coma)
• Oliguria	• Anuria
• Hyperthermia	• Hypothermia
Hemodynamic	
• CO/CI increased	• CO/CI decreased
• RAP/PAP/PAOP decreased	• RAP/PAP/PAOP variable
• SVR/SVRI decreased	• SVR/SVRI variable
• Svo_2 increased	• Svo_2 decreased
Diagnostic	
• ABGs: respiratory alkalosis with hypoxemia	• ABGs: metabolic acidosis with hypoxemia
• PT and PTT increased	• PT and PTT increased
• Platelets decreased	• Platelets decreased
• WBC increased	• WBC decreased
• Glucose increased	• Glucose decreased
	• BUN, creatinine increased
	• Serum arterial lactate increased
	• Amylase, lipase increased
	• AST, ALT, LDH increased

CO, Cardiac output; *CI,* cardiac index; *RAP,* right atrial pressure; *PAP,* pulmonary artery pressure; *PAOP,* pulmonary artery occlusive pressure; *SVR,* systemic vascular resistance; *SVRI,* systemic vascular resistance index; *Svo_2,* oxygen saturation of venous blood; *ABGs,* arterial blood gases; *PT,* prothrombin time; *PTT,* partial thromboplastin time; *WBC,* white blood cell; *BUN,* blood urea nitrogen; *AST,* aspartate aminotransferase; *ALT,* alanine aminotransferase; *LDH,* lactic dehydrogenase.

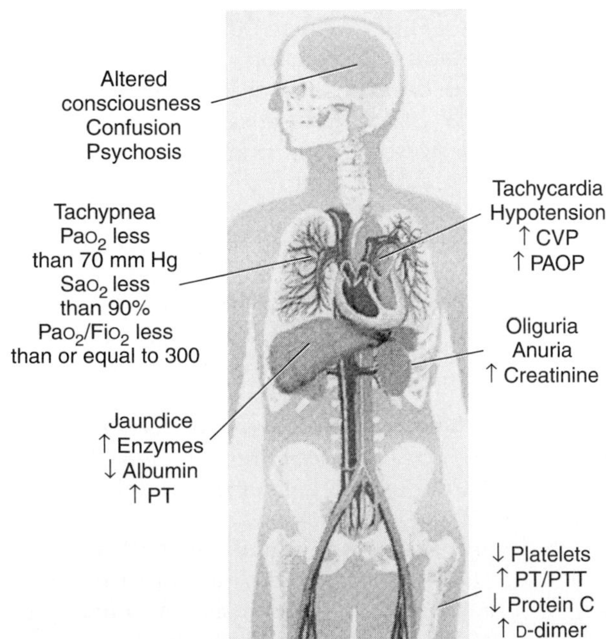

Figure 11-8 Acute organ dysfunction as a marker of severe sepsis. (Courtesy Eli Lilly.)

13. Anxiety related to sudden critical illness, fear of the unknown, fear of death, change in role relationships, and change in self-concept

Collaborative Management

Same as for shock and including the following:

1. Identify high-risk patient, and monitor for clinical indications of infection and sepsis; note any of the following:
   a. Hyperthermia
   b. Increase in respiratory rate
   c. Elevated glucose caused by insulin resistance
   d. Poor gastric motility and retention of enteral feedings
   e. Elevated serum lactate despite clinical picture of increased cardiac output
2. Prevent infection and sepsis.
   a. Use good hand-washing techniques and prevent cross-contamination.
   b. Avoid intrusive procedures if possible.
   c. Participate in early identification of focus of infection.
      (1) Monitor color, characteristics of sputum, urine, stools, and wounds.
      (2) Culture secretions and wounds as indicated.

d. Prepare patient for surgery as indicated for any of the following:
   (1) Removal of all necrotic tissue
   (2) Drainage of abscess
   (3) Early débridement of burn eschar
   (4) Prompt stabilization of fractures to minimize soft tissue damage, inflammation, and infection
e. Perform meticulous oral and airway care; silent aspiration of oral, nasopharyngeal, and sinus secretions around the endotracheal tube cuff occurs and is a cause of nosocomial pneumonia.
f. Perform meticulous intravenous, intraarterial, pulmonary arterial, and urinary catheter care according to Centers for Disease Control and Prevention (CDC) guidelines or hospital policy.
g. Perform meticulous wound care as indicated by type and appearance of wound.
h. Avoid NPO status to prevent translocation of enteric bacteria into the lymphatics and vascular bed.
   (1) Enteral feedings should be given if at all possible.
   (2) Selective gut decontamination (gut sterilization) with a nonabsorbable aminoglycoside (e.g., neomycin) has been advocated for use in patients that must have NPO (e.g., functional or structural obstruction of the GI tract).
      (a) Controversial
      (b) Parenteral nutrition would be provided for nutritional support
i. Administer prophylactic antibiotic therapy as prescribed.
   (1) Controversial today as more and more microorganisms become resistant to available antibiotic therapy
   (2) Many physicians prefer to have clinical indications of infection before prescribing antibiotic therapy
j. Prevent ventilator-associated pneumonia as described in Chapter 5.

3. Restore tissue perfusion and normalize cellular metabolism.
   a. Provide early goal-directed therapy during first 6 hours after severe sepsis or septic shock are recognized (Loma Linda University Medical Center Department of Emergency Medicine et al. for STOP Sepsis Working Group, 2006; Figure 11-9)
      (1) Indications
         (a) Two or more indications of SIRS
         (b) Suspected or confirmed infection
         (c) MAP less than 65 mm Hg after 20 mL/kg fluid bolus *or* serum lactate of at least 4 mmol/L
      (2) Goals include the following:
         (a) CVP of 8 to 12 mm Hg
         (b) MAP of 65 mm Hg or greater
         (c) Central venous oxygen saturation ($Scvo_2$) or Svo_2 of 70% or greater
         (d) Urine output greater than 0.5 mL/kg/hr
      (3) Initial treatment includes the following:
         (a) Intubation and mechanical ventilation when required for respiratory distress; use the following setting to avoid ventilator-induced lung injury (VILI):
            (i) Tidal volume at 6 mL/kg
            (ii) Peak inspiratory plateau pressure of no more than 30 cm H_2O
         (b) Antimicrobial agents following blood cultures
            (i) Cultures
               a) One blood draw should be percutaneous.
               b) One blood draw should be through each vascular access that has been in place more than 48 hours.
               c) Other cultures from other sites (e.g., CSF, pulmonary secretions, urine, and wound) may be indicated.
            (ii) Antimicrobials
               a) Initiated within 1 hour of recognition of severe sepsis
               b) One or more antimicrobials active against the likely pathogens
               c) Reassessed after 48 to 72 hours
         (c) Preload correction
            (i) If CVP less than 8 mm Hg: crystalloid fluid boluses until CVP is 8 to 12 mm Hg
               a) Colloids are not indicated and may be harmful.
               b) Hypertonic crystalloids also are not recommended at this time.
            (ii) If CVP greater than 15 mm Hg and MAP greater than 110 mm Hg: nitroglycerin until CVP less than 12 or MAP less than 90 mm Hg
         (d) Afterload correction
            (i) If MAP is less than 65 mm Hg after 20 mL/kg of crystalloids, administer vasopressors as necessary to maintain a MAP of at least 65 mm Hg.
               a) The preferred agent is still debatable; norepinephrine (2 to 20 mcg/min) frequently is advocated as the initial agent; dopamine (5 to 20 mcg/kg/min) also may be used.
                  i) Low-dose dopamine (previously thought to provide renal protection) is not advocated.
               b) Phenylephrine is preferred if heart rate is greater than 120 beats/min.
               c) Vasopressin
                  i) Very low doses (0.01 to 0.04 units/min) of vasopressin have been shown to improve MAP in septic shock.
                  ii) Terlipressin, a longer-acting synthetic analog of vasopressin,

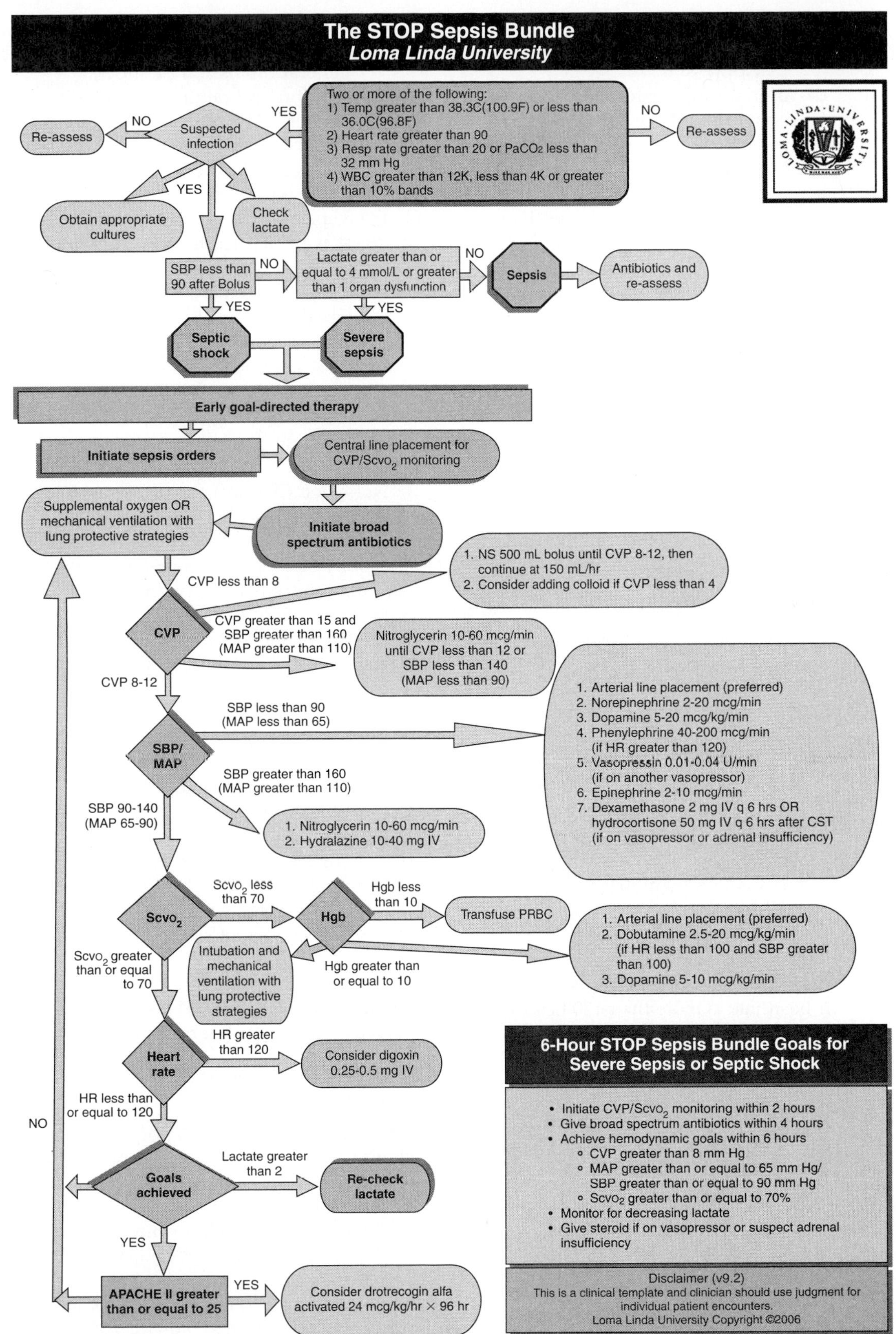

Figure 11-9 Early goal-directed therapy for sepsis. *APACHE*, Acute Physiology and Chronic Health Evaluation. (From STOP Sepsis Working Group of Loma Linda University Medical Center, Loma Linda, Calif.)

has a longer half-life and similar hemodynamic effects to vasopressin.
d) Arterial catheter for continuous monitoring of blood pressure is indicated.
(ii) Corticosteroids should be considered if patient is vasopressor dependent.
a) Cosyntropin stimulation test is recommended: baseline cortisol level, ACTH 250 mcg IV, remeasurement of cortisol at 30 minutes and 60 minutes; change in cortisol of less than 9 mcg/dL suggests adrenal insufficiency
b) Hydrocortisone 50 mg IV every 6 hours along with fludrocortisone 50 mcg PO daily is recommended for adrenal insufficiency in severe sepsis
(iii) If MAP is greater than 110 mm Hg, nitroglycerin or hydralazine may be used.
(e) Optimize oxygen delivery.
(i) If $Scvo_2$ is less than 70% after appropriate therapies (see earlier discussions) and hemoglobin is less than 10 g/dL, administration of red blood cells is indicated.
a) Platelets are indicated if platelet counts are less than 5000/mm^3 or when less than 30,000 mm^3 if there is significant risk for bleeding.
(ii) If $Scvo_2$ is less than 70% after appropriate therapies (see earlier discussions) and hemoglobin in greater than 10 g/dL, administration of dobutamine or dopamine is indicated.
(iii) If heart rate is more than 120 beats/min, digoxin administration may be considered.

b. Decrease inflammation and antithrombotic aspects of sepsis.
(1) Activated protein C (drotrecogin alfa [Xigris]) for patients with severe sepsis who have a high risk of death (i.e., severe sepsis with evidence of organ dysfunction) (For more specifics, see Chapter 13.)
(a) Actions
(i) Antiinflammatory
(ii) Anticoagulant
(iii) Profibrinolytic
(b) Dose: 24 mcg/kg/hr for a total infusion duration of 96 hours
(c) Contraindications: The primary contraindication is bleeding or increased risk of bleeding, especially intracranial or intraspinal bleeding.
(d) Adverse effect: bleeding
(2) Corticosteroids as prescribed
(3) Control of serum glucose as described in the general discussion of shock

4. Treat infection and neutralize toxins.
   a. Administer antimicrobials as prescribed.
   b. Prepare the patient for surgery as requested.
      (1) Drainage of abscess
      (2) Débridement of wound
      (3) Repair of intestinal perforation
   c. Assist with plasmapheresis or continuous venovenous hemodialysis (CVVHD) to remove bacterial by-products.
5. Modify mediators (controversial because these mediators are important to the inflammatory process, but excess amounts may need to be modified or blocked).
   a. Antihistamines (e.g., diphenhydramine [Benadryl] or ranitidine [Zantac]) to modify and/or block histamine
   b. Naloxone (Narcan) to modify and/or block endorphins
   c. Ibuprofen (Motrin) and indomethacin (Indocin) to modify and/or block prostaglandins
   d. Corticosteroids (e.g., hydrocortisone sodium succinate [Solu-Cortef]) may modify several mediators and stabilize the cell membrane
   e. Angiotensin-converting enzyme inhibitors (e.g., captopril [Capoten]) to modify and/or block angiotensin II
   f. Anticoagulants (e.g., heparin) to modify the clotting cascade by blocking the conversion of prothrombin to thrombin
6. Control hyperthermia.
   a. Monitor core body temperature.
   b. Administer antipyretics as indicated.
   c. Use cooling blankets and tepid soaks.
7. Monitor patient for complications of shock and clinical indications of organ failure.

Systemic Inflammatory Response Syndrome and Multiple Organ Dysfunction Syndrome

Definitions

1. SIRS (Figure 11-10): "Widespread inflammation (or clinical response to that inflammation) that can occur in patients with patients with such diverse disorders as infection, pancreatitis, ischemia, multiple trauma, shock, or immunologically-mediated organ injury" (Bone, Sprung, & Sibbald, 1992)
2. MODS (Figure 11-11): "Presence of altered organ function in an acutely ill patient such that homeostasis cannot be maintained without intervention" (Bone, Sprung, & Sibbald, 1992)
   a. "Primary multiple organ dysfunction syndrome occurs when there is a direct injury to the organ that [then] becomes dysfunctional" (Bone, Sprung, & Sibbald, 1992)

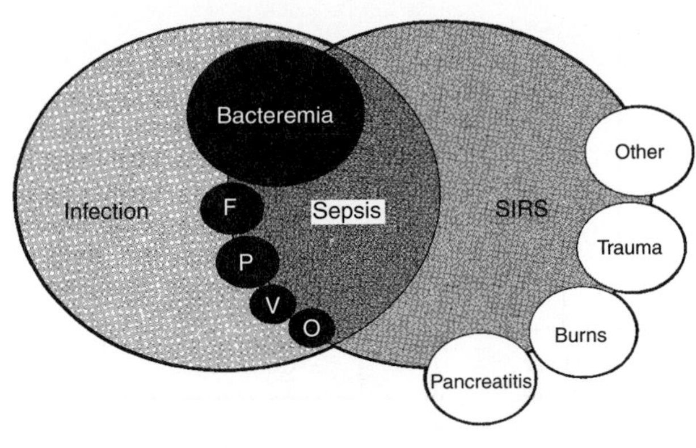

Figure 11-10 Interrelationships among systemic inflammatory response syndrome *(SIRS),* sepsis, and infection. (From American College of Chest Physicians/Society of Critical Care Medicine Consensus Conference Committee. [1992]. *Critical Care Medicine,* 20[6], 865.)

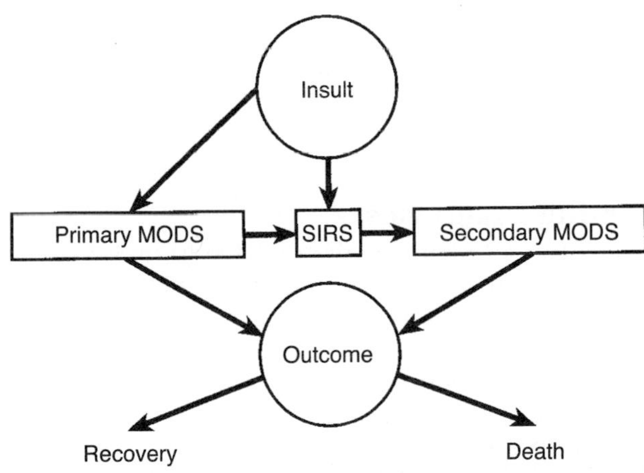

Figure 11-11 Relationship of systemic inflammatory response syndrome and multiple organ dysfunction syndrome. (From American College of Chest Physicians/Society of Critical Care Medicine Consensus Conference Committee. [1992]. *Critical Care Medicine,* 20[6], 866.)

b. "Secondary multiple organ dysfunction syndrome occurs as a consequence of trauma or infection in one part of the system that results in the systemic inflammatory response and dysfunction of organs elsewhere" (Bone, Sprung, & Sibbald, 1992)

Etiology

1. Mechanical tissue damage: trauma, burns, crush injuries, surgical procedures
2. Abscesses: intraabdominal, intracranial
3. Ischemic/necrotic tissue: prolonged shock, MI, pancreatitis, DIC
4. Microbial invasion: immunosuppressed states, surgery/trauma, community exposure, nosocomial exposure
5. Endotoxin release: gram-negative sepsis, translocation of bacteria from gut (sepsis is the most common single etiologic factor, but 40% to 50% of MODS patients do not have positive blood cultures)
6. Global perfusion deficits: shock, cardiopulmonary arrest
7. Regional perfusion deficits: vascular injury, vascular repair procedures, thromboembolic events

Pathophysiology

1. May be triggered by infection or noninfective processes such as injury, ischemia, and necrosis
2. Cascade of inflammation (Figure 11-12): although the inflammatory process is necessary and helpful when localized, it may be destructive when generalized or systemic
3. Mediators (Table 11-6): mediators and other chemicals cause systemic effects
4. CNS, autonomic nervous system, endocrine system, hematologic system, and immunologic system respond as if there is an infection
5. MODS may occur because of hypoperfusion and generalized inflammatory process (Figure 11-13)

Clinical Presentation

1. SIRS
   a. Criteria—two or more of the following (Bone, 1991):
      (1) Tachycardia (more than 90 beats/min)
      (2) Hyperpnea (respiratory rate above 20 breaths/min or $Paco_2$ less than 32 mm Hg)
      (3) Hyperthermia (temperature above 38°C, or 100.4°F) or hypothermia (temperature below 36°C, or 96.8°F); hypothermia is more common in elderly patients
      (4) WBC count greater than 12,000 cells/mm^3 or less than 4000 cells/mm^3 or more than 10% bands
   b. System assessment (Table 11-7)
2. MODS: dysfunction of more than one of the following organs
   a. Pulmonary (ARDS): absence of pulmonary embolism or bilateral pneumonia with the following
      (1) Predisposing factor such as sepsis
      (2) Unexplained hypoxemia
      (3) Bilateral pulmonary infiltrates consistent with pulmonary edema
      (4) Pao_2/Fio_2 ratio less than 300
      (5) PAOP less than 18 mm Hg (to rule out cardiac pulmonary edema)
   b. Hematologic (DIC): absence of liver failure, major hematoma, or anticoagulation therapy with the following
      (1) FSP greater than 1:40 or D-dimer greater than 2 mg/L
      (2) Thrombocytopenia or a 25% drop from a previous value

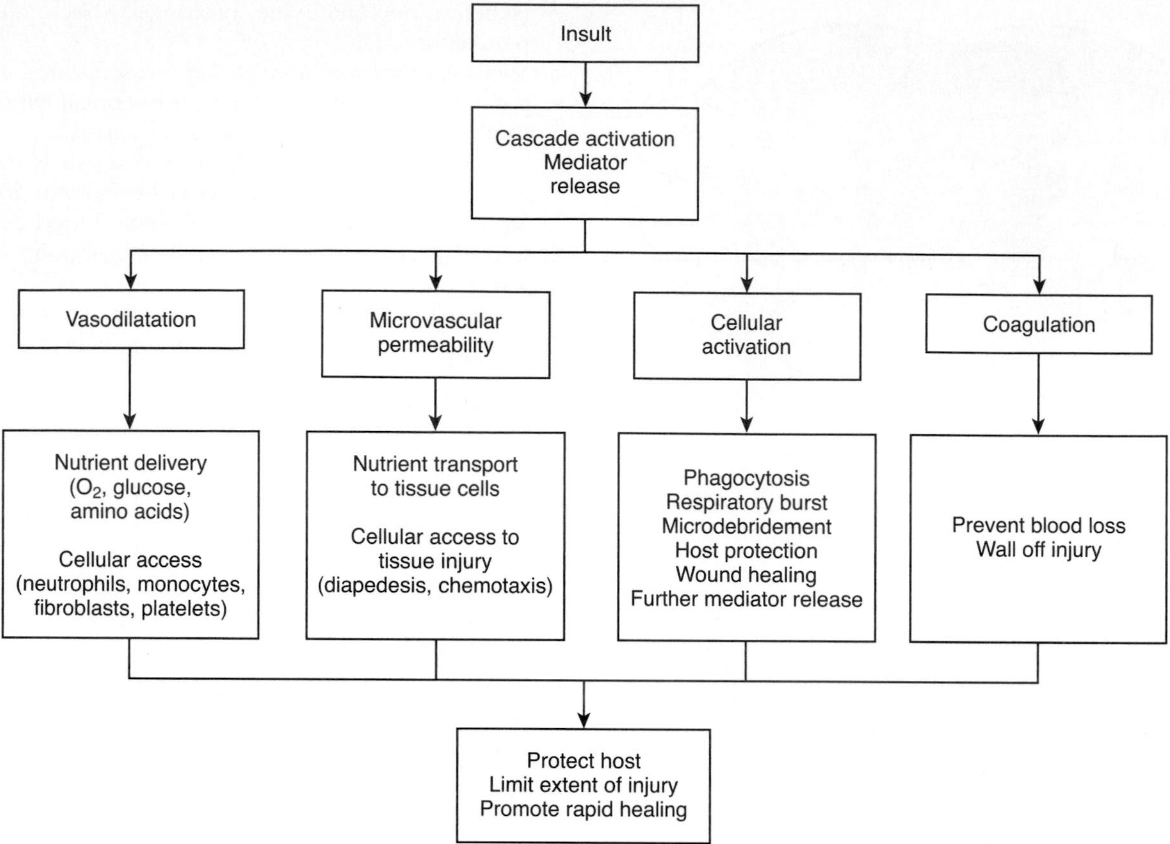

Figure 11-12 Cascade of inflammation. (From Huddleston Secor, V. [1996]. *Multiple organ dysfunction and failure* [2nd ed.]. St. Louis: Mosby.)

(3) PTT prolonged
(4) International normalized ratio (INR) greater than 1.2
(5) May have clinical evidence of bleeding

c. Renal: absence of diuretic within 2 hours of urine analysis with the following:
(1) Urine output less than 0.5 mL/kg/min
(2) Serum creatinine abnormal and urinary sodium is greater than 40 mmol/L
(3) If previous renal insufficiency, an increase in creatinine by 2 mg/dL not caused by myoglobinuria

d. Hepatobiliary: absence of preexisting liver disease with the following:
(1) Serum bilirubin greater than 2 mg/dL for 2 days
(2) Alkaline phosphatase, ALT, AST, gamma-glutamyl transferase (GGT) more than twice laboratory normal

e. CNS: absence of sedation or paralyzing agents that would alter the patient's ability to respond with decrease in Glasgow Coma Scale score by one point

f. Metabolic: serum lactate level increased

g. Degrees of organ dysfunction are described in Table 11-8

Nursing Diagnoses

1. Ineffective Tissue Perfusion related to massive vasodilation and increased capillary permeability
   a. Ineffective Cerebral Tissue Perfusion related to hypoxia and cerebral hypoperfusion
   b. Ineffective Peripheral Tissue Perfusion related to relative hypovolemia, fluid shifts, and vasopressors
   c. Ineffective Renal Tissue Perfusion related to relative hypovolemia, fluid shifts, and vasopressors
2. Decreased Cardiac Output related to inadequate volume, inadequate cardiac contractility, inadequate vascular tone, and dysrhythmias
3. Deficient Fluid Volume related to increased vascular capacitance
4. Ineffective Airway Clearance related to altered consciousness, increased secretions, and artificial airways
5. Impaired Gas Exchange related to alveolar-capillary membrane changes resulting from increased capillary permeability associated with ventilation/perfusion mismatch and intrapulmonary shunt
6. Imbalanced Nutrition: Less Than Body Requirements related to hypermetabolism, paralytic ileus, and decreased absorption

Table 11-6 Mediators

Effect	Chemical Mediators and Triggers
Selective vasoconstriction	• Angiotensin II • ADH • Catecholamines: epinephrine; norepinephrine • Leukotrienes • Thromboxane • Prostaglandins (PGD_2, PGF_{2a}) • Platelet-activating factor • Oxygen-free radicals
Peripheral vasodilation	• Histamine • Prostaglandins (PGE_2, PGI_2) • Prostacyclin • Kinins • Serotonin • Endorphins
Increased capillary permeability	• Leukotrienes • Histamine • Prostaglandins (PGE_2, PGI_2) • Prostacyclin • Kinins
Coagulation	• Neutrophils • Platelets • Complement • Hageman factor • Vasoconstriction
Endothelial damage	• Acidosis • Complement • Endotoxin • Histamine • Hypoxia • Oxygen-free radicals • Platelet-activating factor • Polymorphonuclear cell aggregation • Tumor necrosis factor • Interleukin-1
Depressed myocardial contractility	• Complement • Endorphins • Histamine • Impaired adrenergic response • Lactic acid • Myocardial depressant factor
Enhanced polymorphonuclear activity	• Cellular debris • Complement • Elastase • Kinins • Interleukin-1 • Leukotrienes • Platelet-activating factor • Platelet aggregation • Prostaglandins • TNF
Tissue breakdown	• Interleukin-1 • Cachectin (TNF) • Collagenase • Elastase

ADH, antidiuretic hormone; *TNF,* tumor necrosis factor.

7. Impaired Urinary Elimination related to hypoperfusion and excretion of pigments (e.g., myoglobin and hemoglobin)
8. Risk for Infection related to invasive procedures and immunocompromise
9. Pain related to invasive procedures
10. High Risk for Injury related to intubation, invasive procedures, and hemorrhage resulting from clotting abnormalities
11. Risk for Electrolyte Imbalance related to fluid shifts and potential hemolysis
12. Anxiety related to sudden critical illness, fear of the unknown, fear of death, change in role relationships, and change in self-concept
13. Interrupted Family Processes related to sudden critical illness

Collaborative Management

1. Prevent and treat infection (see Septic Shock).
2. Maximize oxygen delivery to the tissues (see Shock).
   a. Maintain cardiac index within normal limits (NOTE: Current research has not shown that increasing the CI to 4.5 L/min/m^2 or greater is effective in reducing mortality.)
      (1) Administer fluids: crystalloids are used because capillary permeability is increased.
      (2) Administer inotropes (e.g., dobutamine) as prescribed.
      (3) Administer vasopressors (e.g., dopamine or norepinephrine) as prescribed when SVR is very low.
   b. Maintain hematocrit at approximately 30% to 32%.
      (1) Administer blood and blood products as prescribed.
      (2) Correct coagulopathies; administer fresh frozen plasma, platelets, and vitamin K as prescribed.
   c. Maintain Sao_2 at greater than 95%.
      (1) Ensure adequate airway.
      (2) Administer oxygen as needed.
      (3) Initiate mechanical ventilation as needed; positive end-expiratory pressure also may be necessary.
   d. Monitor Svo_2.
      (1) Decreased SvO_2 to less than 60% indicates that oxygen delivery is impaired or oxygen consumption is increased.
         (a) Assess Sao_2.
         (b) Assess cardiac output/cardiac index.
         (c) Assess hemoglobin.
         (d) Assess patient for causes of increased consumption (e.g., shivering, fever, and seizures).
      (2) Increased Svo_2 to greater than 80% indicates that oxygen extraction is impaired.
3. Minimize oxygen consumption of the tissues (see Shock).
4. Maintain or improve nutritional status (see Shock).

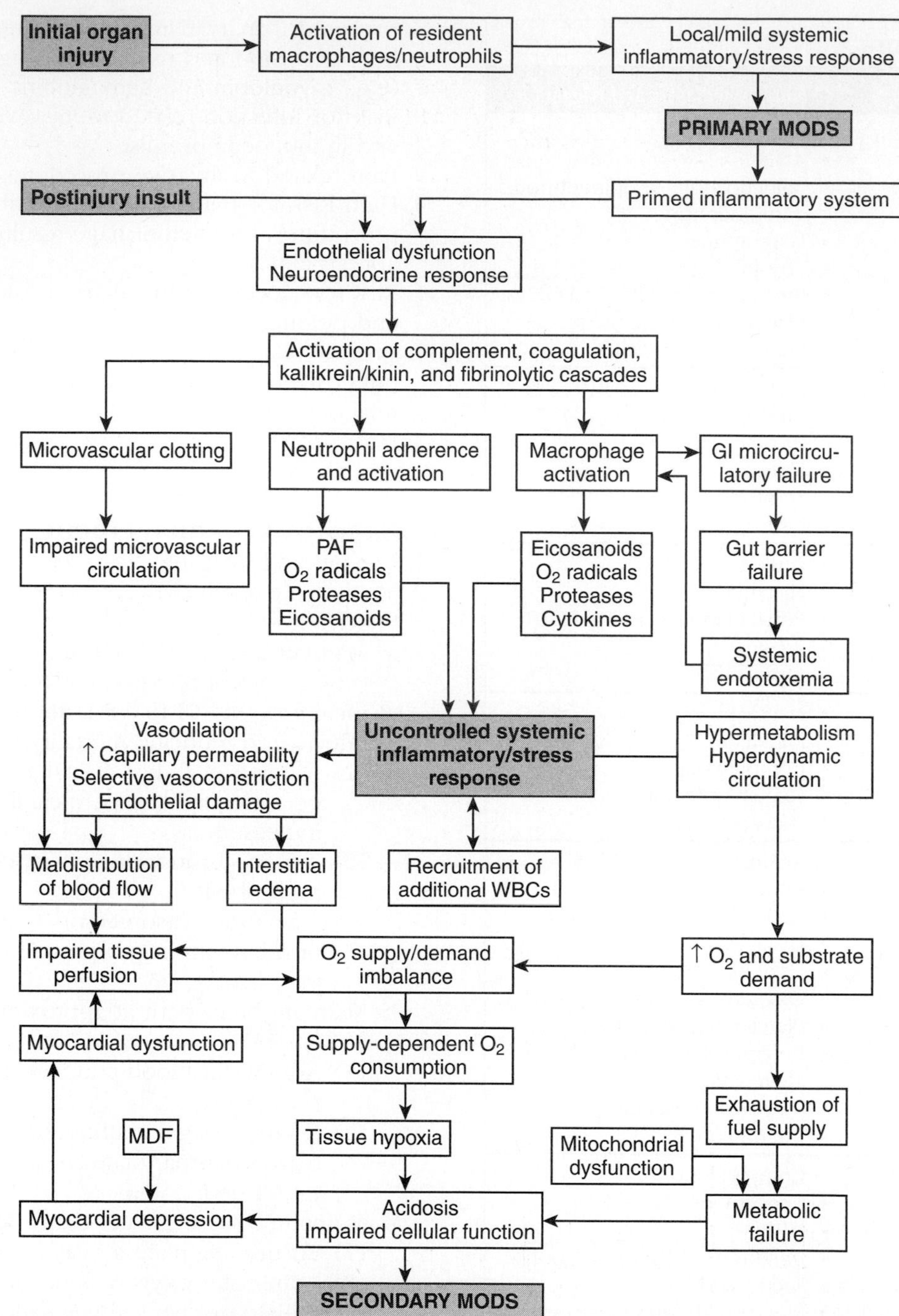

Figure 11-13 Pathophysiology of multiple organ dysfunction syndrome. *MODS,* Multiple organ dysfunction syndrome; *GI,* gastrointestinal; *PAF,* platelet-activating factor; *WBCs,* white blood cells; *MDF,* myocardial depressant factor. (From McCance, K. L., & Huether, S. E. [2006]. *Pathophysiology: The biologic basis for disease in adults and children* [5th ed.]. St. Louis: Mosby.)

5. Use experimental therapies as prescribed; these may be available only for compassionate use.
   a. Modify cytokine response.
      (1) Antioxidants: allopurinol (Zyloprim); mannitol; vitamins C and E; superoxide dismutase (SOD)
      (2) Antiprostaglandin: ibuprofen (Motrin)
      (3) Antihistamines: diphenhydramine (Benadryl) and ranitidine (Zantac)
      (4) Opiate receptor blockers: naloxone (Narcan)
      (5) Corticosteroids: block neutrophils, lysosomes, arachidonic acid and complement cascades, interleukins, and inflammation
   b. Use ECMO: blood is removed from body, taken through a bubble oxygenator, and then returned to the body in an oxygenated state.
6. Monitor patient for complications.
   a. Shock (if not caused by shock)
   b. Organ failure
   c. Death

Table 11-7 Systems Assessment with Potential Inflammatory/Immune Impact and Complications

System	Risk Factors	Impact on Inflammatory/Immune Response	Assessment	Potential Complications
Central nervous	• Invasive drains • ICP monitoring • Surgical incision • Cranial nerve involvement • Spinal cord injury	• Increased microbial access • Inflammatory/immune response activation • Impaired natural defenses	• LOC, GCS • CCP • Inflammation at wound • Respiratory depression • Skin breakdown	• CNS infection • Aspiration • Corneal abrasions • Skin breakdown
Pulmonary	• Artificial airway • Mechanical ventilation • Barotrauma • High FiO_2 levels	• Bypass of natural airway defenses • Increased microbial access • Activation of alveolar macrophages with toxic mediator release • Altered surfactant production	• Dyspnea • Use of accessory muscles • Thick, discolored sputum • Wheezes, crackles, rhonchi • Decreased compliance • Increased ventilation/ perfusion mismatching • Increased intrapulmonary shunt infiltrates on chest x-ray • Respiratory acidosis ($\downarrow$ pH, $\uparrow$ $PaCO_2$) • Hypoxemia ($\downarrow$ PaO_2, $\downarrow$ SaO_2, SpO_2) • Hypoxia ($\downarrow$ SvO_2, $\uparrow$ lactate)	• Aspiration • Atelectasis • Pneumonia • Acute respiratory distress syndrome • Oxygen toxicity
Central venous	• Invasive monitoring • Poor perfusion	• Increased microbial access • Tissue ischemia $\rightarrow$ inflammatory/immune response activation with third spacing and edema • Cellular activation and mediator release	• Changes in HR, BP, CO/CI, PAP, PAOP, CVP/RAP, SVR • Cold, pale skin • Inflammation at access sites • Diminished pulses • Narrowed pulse pressure • Urine output • Dysrhythmias • Myocardial ischemia or infarction • Positive cardiac isoenzymes, troponin • $\uparrow$ Lactate	• Reperfusion injury • Cellulitis • Bacteremia/ sepsis • Endothelial damage and clotting abnormalities
Gastrointestinal	• Nasogastric tube • Antacid therapy • H_2-blocker therapy • Stress ulceration • Antibiotics • Ileus	• Gastric pH $\rightarrow$ bacterial colonization • IIR activation • Inhibition of normal flora-protective function • Inability to clear bacterial load	• Bowel sounds • Upper or lower gastrointestinal bleeding • Abdominal distention • Diarrhea • Constipation, impaction • Ileus • Stress ulceration/erosion • Guaiac-positive stool • Enteric organisms on blood culture • Jaundice • Ascites • Drug clearance • Abnormal bleeding • Liver enzymes • Hypoglycemia • Ammonia • Plasma proteins • Clotting factors • Hepatomegaly/ splenomegaly	• Colonization of esophagus and tracheobronchial tree • Pneumonia • Overgrowth of pathogenic organisms in the GI tract (e.g., *Clostridium difficile*) • Translocation of bacteria to the lymph and blood

Continued

Table 11-7 Systems Assessment with Potential Inflammatory/Immune Impact and Complications—cont'd

System	Risk Factors	Impact on Inflammatory/Immune Response	Assessment	Potential Complications
Genitourinary	• Bladder catheter • Antibiotics • Hyperglycemia	• Increased microbial access • Altered normal flora in vagina • Promotion of yeast growth	• Changes in urine output • Malodorous urine or vaginal discharge • Peripheral edema • CVP/RAP, PAP, PAOP • BUN and creatinine • Metabolic acidosis (↓ pH, ↓ HCO_3)	• Urinary tract infection • Septicemia • *Candida* infections

Modified from Huddleston Secor, V. (1996). *Multiple organ dysfunction and failure* (2nd ed.). St. Louis: Mosby.
ICP, Intracranial pressure; *LOC,* level of consciousness; *GCS,* Glasgow Coma Scale; *CCP,* cerebral perfusion pressure; *CNS,* Central nervous system; *Fio*$_2$, fraction of inspired oxygen; *Sao*$_2$, arterial oxygen saturation; *Spo*$_2$, oxygen saturation by pulse oximetry; *Svo*$_2$, venous oxygen saturation; *HR,* heart rate; *BP,* blood pressure; *CO/CI,* cardiac output/cardiac index; *PAP,* pulmonary artery pressure; *PAOP,* pulmonary artery occlusive pressure; *CVP/RAP,* central venous pressure/right atrial pressure; *SVR,* systemic vascular resistance; *GI,* gastrointestinal; *BUN,* blood urea nitrogen; *HCO*$_3$, bicarbonate; *IIR,* inflammatory/immune response.

Table 11-8 Definitions of Degrees of Organ Dysfunction

			Organ Dysfunction			
Organ System	Parameter	Normal	Mild	Moderate	Severe	Extreme
Central venous	Systolic blood pressure (mm Hg)	Greater than 90	Less than 90, but fluid responsive	Less than 90, not fluid responsive	Less than 90, not fluid responsive	Less than 90, not fluid responsive
	Arterial pH	Greater than or equal to 7.3	Greater than or equal to 7.3	Greater than or equal to 7.3	Less than 7.3	Less than 7.2
Pulmonary	Pao_2/Fio_2 (mm Hg)	Greater than 400	301-400	201-300	101-200	Less than 100
Central nervous	Glasgow Coma Scale score	15	13-14	10-12	7-9	Greater than or equal to 6
Hematologic (coagulation)	Platelet count (1000/mL)	Greater than 120	81-102	51-80	21-50	Greater than or equal to 20
Renal	Creatinine (mg/dL)	Less than 1.5	1.5-1.9	2-3.4	3.5-4.9	Greater than or equal to 5
Hepatic	Bilirubin (mg/dL)	Less than 1.2	1.2-3.5	3.6-7	7.1-14	Greater than 14

Bone, R. (1997). Managing sepsis: what treatments can we use today? *Journal of Critical Illness, 12*(1), 15.
Fio$_2$, Fraction of inspired oxygen.

Drug Intoxication and Poisoning

Definition

Drug ingestion in amounts greater than recommended or the ingestion or absorption of a substance toxic to the human body

Etiology

1. Accidental or intentional overdosage of prescribed medication
   a. Intentional overdosage often involves more than one agent; frequently includes alcohol and/or illegal drugs.
   b. Intentional overdosage may be a suicide attempt or an attention-seeking behavior (i.e., suicide gesture).
   c. Accidental overdosage may be due to knowledge deficit regarding drug dosing or confusion.
2. Accidental overdosage of illegal drugs
   a. Overdosage frequently caused by changes in drug purity.
   b. Patient may be mentally ill and have tendency to be violent.
3. Ingestion/absorption of poison or toxin

Pathophysiology

Dependent on the following:

1. Drug ingested
   a. Fatal drug intoxications are most likely caused by analgesics, antidepressants, carbon monoxide, and cardiovascular drugs.
2. Amount of drug(s) or toxin ingested or absorbed

3. Time from ingestion to treatment
4. Preexisting condition of patient: cardiovascular, hepatic, or renal disease may increase drug effect by impairing biotransformation and excretion

Clinical Presentation (Table 11-9)

1. Subjective: For drug-specific symptoms, see Table 11-9.
   a. History of drug ingestion or exposure to toxin
      (1) Ask the patient why the overdosage occurred; listen carefully.
      (2) Patients are often inaccurate in relating drug ingestion and may minimize or exaggerate the amount of the drug; verify information with family, friends, police officers, and paramedics.
      (3) Identify the following:
         (a) Drug or toxin
         (b) Route
         (c) Dose
         (d) Length of time elapsed since exposure to drug or toxin
         (e) Reason for exposure (e.g., dose confusion, suicide attempt, or inadvertent exposure to toxin)
         (f) Previous exposure to drug or toxin
         (g) Source
            (i) Prescription
            (ii) Over-the-counter
            (iii) Street

Text continued on p. 725

Table 11-9 Drugs and Toxins

Drug or Toxin	Clinical Presentation of Intoxication	Specific Collaborative Management
Acetaminophen	Stage 1: first 24 hours • May be asymptomatic • Anorexia, nausea, vomiting • Diaphoresis • Malaise • Pallor Stage 2: 24 to 48 hours • Nausea, fatigue, malaise • Signs of hepatotoxicity may occur: liver enzymes elevated, bilirubin may be elevated, right upper quadrant pain • Gradual return to normal may occur Stage 3: 72 to 96 hours • Anorexia, nausea, vomiting • Hepatic failure ○ More likely if ethanol consumption, malnutrition, short-term fasting ○ Jaundice, elevated bilirubin ○ Hepatosplenomegaly ○ Prolonged prothrombin time (PT), gastrointestinal (GI) bleeding ○ Hypoglycemia ○ Metabolic acidosis ○ Hepatic encephalopathy: confusion → coma • Acute tubular necrosis and renal failure may develop • Dysrhythmias and shock may occur • Death may result from severe metabolic disturbances, cerebral edema, and coagulopathy Stage 4: 4 days to 2 weeks • Gradual return of liver function in patients who recover	• Gastric lavage only if within 1 hour of ingestion • Activated charcoal (single dose) if patient arrives within 4-6 hours after ingestion (though activated charcoal does adsorb *N*-acetylcysteine and reduces its peak serum levels, the loading dose of *N*-acetylcysteine does not need to be increased) • *N*-acetylcysteine (Mucomyst) 140 mg/kg initially, then 70 mg/kg every 4 hours for 17 doses to total of 1330 mg/kg ○ If given PO, dilute in juice or carbonated beverage; if given via nasogastric or duodenal tube, dilute 3:1 with juice or carbonated beverage – May cause anorexia, nausea, vomiting, diarrhea; repeat dose if vomiting occurs within 1 hour ○ Intravenous preparation (Acetadote) recently has been approved; 20-hour protocol • Treat vomiting with metoclopramide (Reglan); ondansetron (Zofran) or droperidol (Inapsine) for refractory vomiting • Monitor for bleeding; vitamin K may be prescribed especially if hepatic failure occurs • Dextrose (e.g., $D_{50}W$) may be needed for hypoglycemia • Antidysrhythmics may be needed • Registration for hepatic transplantation if indicated
Barbiturates • Pentobarbital (Nembutal) • Phenobarbital (Luminal) • Secobarbital (Seconal)	• Bradycardia, cardiac dysrhythmias • Hypotension • Hypothermia • Respiratory depression → respiratory arrest • Headache • Nystagmus, dysconjugate eye movements • Dysarthria • Ataxia	• Gastric lavage only if within 1 hour of ingestion • Multiple doses of activated charcoal with cathartic added to first dose • Phenobarbital: sodium bicarbonate to alkalinize the urine and increase rate of barbiturate excretion; maintain urine pH greater than 7.50

Continued

Table 11-9 Drugs and Toxins—cont'd

Drug or Toxin	Clinical Presentation of Intoxication	Specific Collaborative Management
	• Depressed deep tendon reflexes • Confusion, stupor, coma • Hemorrhagic blisters • Gastric irritation (chloral hydrate) • Pulmonary edema (meprobamate) • Hypertonicity, hyperreflexia, myoclonus, seizures (methaqualone)	○ Monitor potassium, calcium, and magnesium levels • Anticonvulsants (e.g., diazepam, phenytoin, or phenobarbital) for seizures • Hemodialysis or hemoperfusion may be required
Benzodiazepines • Diazepam (Valium) • Flurazepam (Dalmane) • Lorazepam (Ativan) • Midazolam (Versed) • Oxazepam (Serax)	• Hypotension • Respiratory depression • Diminished or absent bowel sounds • Decreased deep tendon reflexes (DTR) • Confusion, drowsiness, stupor, coma	• Gastric lavage only if within 1 hour of ingestion • Activated charcoal (single dose) • Flumazenil (Romazicon), a benzodiazepine receptor antagonist may be prescribed ○ Contraindicated if patient has coingested tricyclic antidepressants; use cautiously if patient has history of long-term use of benzodiazepines ○ Monitor for seizures, agitation, flushing, nausea and vomiting as side effects of flumazenil • Intubation and mechanical ventilation may be necessary
Beta-blockers	• Sinus bradycardia, arrest, block • Junctional escape rhythm • Atrioventricular nodal block • Bundle branch block (usually right) • Hypotension • Heart failure • Cardiogenic shock • Cardiac arrest • Decreased level of consciousness (LOC) • Seizures • Respiratory depression, apnea • Bronchospasm • Hyperglycemia or hypoglycemia	• Gastric lavage only if within 1 hour of ingestion • Multiple doses of activated charcoal with cathartic added to first dose • Bowel irrigation if sustained-release preparations ingested • Atropine, epinephrine, dopamine, or isoproterenol for bradycardia and hypotension; temporary pacing may be required • Glucagon 3-5 mg IV, IM, or subcutaneously, followed by infusion of 1-5 mg/hr $D_{50}W$ for hypoglycemia • Anticonvulsants (e.g., diazepam or phenobarbital) for seizures; phenytoin is contraindicated
Calcium channel blockers	• Sinus bradycardia, arrest, block • Sinoatrial blocks (diltiazem) • Atrioventricular blocks (verapamil) • Hypotension • Heart failure • Confusion, agitation, dizziness, lethargy, slurred speech • Seizures • Nausea, vomiting • Paralytic ileus • Hyperglycemia	• Gastric lavage only if within 1 hour of ingestion • Activated charcoal; multiple dose with cathartic added to first dose if massive ingestion or ingestion of sustained-release preparations • Bowel irrigation if sustained-release preparations ingested • Calcium chloride 5 mL (500 mg) to 10 mL (1 g) of 10% solution • Atropine, epinephrine, dopamine, or isoproterenol for bradycardia and hypotension; temporary pacing may be required • Glucagon 3-5 mg IV, IM, or subcutaneously, followed by infusion of 1-5 mg/hr • Anticonvulsants (e.g., diazepam, phenytoin, or phenobarbital) for seizures
Cannabinoids • Hashish • Marijuana	• Euphoria • Slowed thinking and reaction time • Confusion • Impaired balance and coordination	• Supportive care
Carbon monoxide (CO) • NOTE: The affinity between CO and hemoglobin (Hgb) is approximately 200 times the affinity between oxygen and Hgb	• Dysrhythmias • Impaired hearing or vision • Pallor; cherry red skin may be seen • Elevated carboxyhemoglobin (HbCO) levels; normal 0%-3% for nonsmoker and 3%-8% for smoker • 10%-20%: mild headache, flushing, dyspnea or angina on vigorous exertion, nausea, dizziness	• Removal from contaminated area • Oxygenation ○ 100% oxygen via mask initially; CPAP by mask may be used ○ Intubation and mechanical ventilation until HbCO less than 5%; PEEP may be used

Table 11-9 **Drugs and Toxins—cont'd**

Drug or Toxin	Clinical Presentation of Intoxication	Specific Collaborative Management
	• 20%-30%: throbbing headache, nausea, vomiting, weakness, dyspnea on moderate exertion, ST segment depression • 30%-40%: severe headache, visual disturbances, syncope, vomiting • 40%-50%: tachypnea, tachycardia, chest pain, worsening syncope • 50%-60%: chest pain, respiratory failure, shock, seizures, coma • 60%-70%: respiratory failure, shock, coma, death	◦ Hyperbaric oxygen (at 3 atomspheres) as soon as available if: – Carboxyhemoglobin (COHb) greater than 25% – COHb greater than 15% if history of cardiovascular disease, acute ECG changes, or CNS symptoms • Fluids, diuretics, urine alkalinization to treat myoglobinuria if present • Anticonvulsants (e.g., diazepam, phenytoin, or phenobarbital) for seizures
Caustic poisoning • Acids (e.g., battery acid, drain cleaners, or hydrochloric acid) • Alkalis (e.g., drain cleaners, refrigerants, fertilizers, or photographic developers)	• Burning sensation in the oral cavity, pharynx, esophageal area • Dysphagia • Respiratory distress: dyspnea, stridor, tachypnea, hoarseness • Soapy-white mucous membrane *Acid* • Oral ulcerations and/or blisters • May have signs of gastric perforation (e.g., abdominal pain, distention, absent bowel sounds, and rebound tenderness) • May have signs of shock *Alkali* • May have signs of esophageal perforation (e.g., chest pain or subcutaneous emphysema)	• Diluent: flush mouth with copious volumes of water; drink water or milk (approximately 250 mL) • Do not induce vomiting or perform gastric lavage • Esophagogastroscopy to assess damage • Corticosteroids may be prescribed for alkali poisoning
Cocaine including "crack" cocaine	• Tachycardia, dysrhythmias, conduction defects • Hypertension or hypotension • Tachypnea or hyperpnea • Cocaine-induced myocardial infarction (MI) • Pallor or cyanosis • Euphoria, hyperexcitability, anxiety • Headache • Hyperthermia, diaphoresis • Nausea, vomiting, abdominal pain • Dilated but reactive pupils • Confusion, delirium, hallucinations • Seizures • Coma • Respiratory arrest	• Swabbing of inside of nose to remove any residual drug if cocaine was snorted • Bowel irrigation for "body packers" • Anxiolytics (e.g., lorazepam or diazepam) • Anticonvulsants (e.g., benzodiazepine, phenytoin, or phenobarbital) for seizures • Antidysrhythmics, usually lidocaine; calcium channel blockers also may be used (they also may help with coronary artery spasm) • Antihypertensives: vasodilators (e.g., nitroprusside [Nipride]) • Vasopressors (e.g., norepinephrine) for hypotension • Hypothermia blanket, ice packs, ice-water sponge baths for hyperthermia ◦ Dantrolene (Dantrium) may be prescribed for malignant hyperthermia • Fluids, diuretics, urine alkalinization to treat myoglobinuria if present
Cyanide	• Anxiety, restlessness, hyperventilation initially • Bradycardia followed by tachycardia • Hypertension followed by hypotension • Dysrhythmias • Bitter almond odor to breath • Cherry-red mucous membranes • Nausea • Dyspnea • Headache • Dizziness • Pupil dilation • Confusion	• 100% oxygen initially by mask ◦ Hyperbaric oxygen may be needed ◦ Intubation and mechanical ventilation are frequently necessary • Supportive care if only anxiety, restlessness, hyperventilation • Discontinuance of causative agent (e.g., nitroprusside) • Antidotes for more serious symptoms ◦ Amyl nitrite by inhalation ◦ Sodium nitrite IV ◦ Sodium thiosulfate IV

Continued

Table 11-9 Drugs and Toxins—cont'd

Drug or Toxin	Clinical Presentation of Intoxication	Specific Collaborative Management
	• Stupor, seizures, coma, death • Elevated cyanide level ○ 0.5 mcg/mL or less: asymptomatic ○ 0.5 to 1 mcg/mL: tachycardia, flushing ○ 1 to 2.5 mcg/mL: agitation or decreased LOC ○ 2.5 to 3 mcg/mL: coma ○ More than 3 mcg/mL: potentially fatal	• Gastric lavage only if within 1 hour of ingestion • Activated charcoal if cyanide was ingested • Flushing of eyes and/or skin with water if dermal contamination; removal and isolation of clothing • Fluids, vasopressors for blood pressure support • Anticonvulsants (e.g., diazepam, phenytoin, or phenobarbital) for seizures • Antidysrhythmics (e.g., lidocaine) for ventricular dysrhythmia, atropine for bradydysrhythmias • Sodium bicarbonate for severe metabolic acidosis • Vitamin B_{12} may be prescribed
Digitalis preparations	• Anorexia • Nausea • Vomiting • Headache • Restlessness • Visual changes • Sinus bradycardia, block, or arrest • Paroxysmal atrial tachycardia with atrioventricular block • Junctional tachycardia • Atrioventricular (AV) blocks: first, second type I, third • Premature ventricular contractions (PVCs): bigeminy, trigeminy, quadrigeminy • Ventricular tachycardia: especially bidirectional • Ventricular fibrillation	• Gastric lavage only if within 1 hour of ingestion • Multiple doses of activated charcoal with cathartic added to first dose • Cholestyramine • Bowel irrigation for large ingestions • Correction of hypoxia and electrolyte imbalance (especially potassium) • Treatment of dysrhythmias: ○ For symptomatic bradydysrhythmias and blocks – Atropine – External pacemaker ○ For symptomatic tachydysrhythmias – Lidocaine – Phenytoin – Magnesium if hypomagnesemia or hyperkalemia present – Cardioversion at lowest effective voltage and only if life-threatening dysrhythmias exist – Defibrillation for ventricular fibrillation – Verapamil if supraventricular tachycardia (SVT) • Digoxin immune FAB (Digibind) if greater than 10 mg ingested (adult), serum digoxin greater than 10 ng/mL, or serum potassium greater than 5 mEq/L • Monitor closely for exacerbation of condition for which digitalis was being used (i.e., increase in heart rate and heart failure)
Dissociative anesthetics • Ketamine • Phencyclidine (PCP)	• Tachycardia • Hypertensive crisis initially; may cause hypotension later • Hyperthermia • Agitation, hyperactivity • Nystagmus • Blank stare • Hypoglycemia • Violent, psychotic behavior • Ataxia • Seizures • Myoglobinuria, renal failure • Lethargy, coma • Cardiac arrest	• Quiet environment • Gastric lavage only if within 1 hour of ingestion • Activated charcoal • Gastric suction • Benzodiazepines (e.g., diazepam) for anxiety and agitation • Antidysrhythmics if required • Antihypertensives: vasodilators (e.g., nitroprusside [Nipride]) • Hypothermia blanket, ice packs, ice-water sponge baths for hyperthermia ○ Dantrolene (dantrium) may be prescribed for malignant hyperthermia • Anticonvulsants (e.g., diazepam, phenytoin, or phenobarbital) for seizures • Haloperidol (Haldol) for acute psychotic reactions • Fluids and diuretics for myoglobinuria; sodium bicarbonate is contraindicated because urinary alkalinization interferes with urinary elimination of PCP

Table 11-9 Drugs and Toxins—cont'd

Drug or Toxin	Clinical Presentation of Intoxication	Specific Collaborative Management
Ethanol	Increased ethanol concentration (mg/dL) • Less than 25: sense of warmth and well-being, talkativeness, self-confidence, mild incoordination • 25-50: euphoria, decreased judgment and control • 50-100: decreased sensorium, worsened coordination, ataxia, decreased reflexes and reaction time • 100-250: nausea, vomiting, ataxia, diplopia, slurred speech, visual impairment, nystagmus, emotional lability, confusion, stupor • 250-400: stupor or coma, incontinence, respiratory depression • Greater than 400: respiratory paralysis, loss of protective reflexes, hypothermia, death • NOTE: A wide variability exists between these signs/symptoms and blood ethanol levels; these signs/symptoms are for a non–alcohol-dependent person Also: • Alcohol odor to breath • Hypoglycemia • Seizures • Metabolic acidosis	• Gastric lavage if within 1 hour of ingestion • Fluid and electrolyte replacement (potassium, magnesium, and calcium may be needed) • Anticonvulsants (e.g., diazepam, phenytoin, or phenobarbital) for seizures • Monitor blood glucose and administer glucose for hypoglycemia and multivitamins including thiamine and folic acid ○ NOTE: Thiamine is necessary for the brain to use glucose; thiamine deficiency in alcoholic patients may cause Wernicke's encephalopathy. • Hemodialysis may be necessary
Ethylene glycol	First 12 hours after ingestion • Appears "drunk" without the odor of ethanol on breath • Nausea, vomiting, hematemesis • Focal seizures, coma • Nystagmus, depressed reflexes, tetany • Metabolic acidosis with increased anion gap 12-24 hours after ingestion • Tachycardia • Mild hypertension • Pulmonary edema • Heart failure 24-72 hours after ingestion • Flank pain, costovertebral tenderness • Acute renal failure	• Gastric lavage only if within 1 hour of ingestion • 10% ethanol in D_5W IV to maintain serum ethanol level at 100-200 mg/dL • Fomepizole (Antizol) IV may be used instead of ethanol • Fluid and electrolyte replacement (particularly calcium, but potassium and magnesium may also be needed) • Sodium bicarbonate for severe metabolic acidosis • Glucose for hypoglycemia and multivitamins including thiamine, folic acid, and pyridoxine ○ NOTE: Thiamine is necessary for the brain to use glucose; thiamine deficiency in alcoholic patients may cause Wernicke's encephalopathy. • Anticonvulsants (e.g., diazepam, phenytoin, or phenobarbital) for seizures • Hemodialysis may be needed
Hallucinogens (e.g., D-lysergic acid diethylamide [LSD])	• Tachycardia, hypertension • Hyperthermia • Anorexia, nausea • Headaches • Dizziness • Agitation, anxiety • Impaired judgment • Distortion and intensification of sensory perception • Toxic psychosis • Dilated pupils • Rambling speech • Polyuria	• Reassurance • Quiet environment with soft lighting • If ingested orally: activated charcoal may be used • Benzodiazepines (e.g., diazepam or lorazepam) for anxiety and agitation • Anticonvulsants (e.g., phenytoin or phenobarbital) for seizures • Restraints only if necessary to protect patient

Continued

Table 11-9 **Drugs and Toxins—cont'd**

Drug or Toxin	Clinical Presentation of Intoxication	Specific Collaborative Management
Inhalants • Gases such as butane, propane, aerosol propellants, and nitrous oxide • Nitrites and nitrates such as amyl nitrite, butyl nitrite, and cyclohexyl nitrate • Solvents such as paint thinner, gasoline, and glue	• Mental status changes • Depression • Muscle weakness • Memory impairment • CNS damage • Sudden death	• Oxygen • Supportive care
Isopropanol (i.e., rubbing alcohol)	• Gastrointestinal distress (e.g., nausea, vomiting, and abdominal pain) • Headache • CNS depression, areflexia, ataxia • Respiratory depression • Hypothermia; hypotension	• Gastric lavage only if within 1 hour of ingestion • Gastric suction • Hemodialysis may be needed • Fluids and vasopressors for hypoperfusion
Lithium	Mild • Vomiting, diarrhea • Lethargy, weakness • Polyuria, polydipsia • Nystagmus • Fine tremors Severe • Hypotension • Severe thirst • Tinnitus • Hyperreflexia • Coarse tremors • Ataxia • Seizures • Confusion • Coma • Dilute urine, renal failure • Heart failure	• Gastric lavage only if within 1 hour of ingestion • Hydration with normal saline • Anticonvulsants (e.g., phenytoin or phenobarbital) for seizures • Bowel irrigation • Hemodialysis may be necessary • Treatment of nephrogenic diabetes insipidus with amiloride (Midamor)
Methanol	• Nausea and vomiting • Hyperpnea, dyspnea • Visual disturbances ranging from blurring to blindness • Speech difficulty • Headache • CNS depression • Motor dysfunction with rigidity, spasticity, and hypokinesis • Metabolic acidosis with anion gap	• Gastric lavage only if within 1 hour of ingestion • 10% ethanol in D_5W IV to maintain serum ethanol level at 100-200 mg/dL • Sodium bicarbonate for severe metabolic acidosis • Hemodialysis if visual impairment, base deficit greater than 15, renal insufficiency, or blood methanol concentration greater than 30 mmol/L

Methemoglobinemia (caused by nitrites, nitrates, sulfa drugs, local anesthetics such as benzocaine, and others)	• Tachycardia
	• Fatigue
	• Nausea
	• Dizziness
	• Cyanosis in the presence of a normal Pao_2; failure of cyanosis to resolve with oxygen therapy
	• Dark red or brown blood
	• Elevated methemoglobin levels
	  ◦ 15% to 30%: nausea, headache, dizziness, fatigue, headache, cyanosis
		• Oxygen
		• Removal of cause
		  ◦ Stop nitroglycerin, nitroprusside, sulfa drugs, anesthetic agents, or other causative agent
		  ◦ Gastric lavage only if within 1 hour of ingestion
		  ◦ Multiple doses of activated charcoal with cathartic added to first dose if agent ingested
		• Methylene blue
		  ◦ If stupor, coma, angina, or respiratory depression or if level greater than 30%

Table 11-9 Drugs and Toxins—cont'd

Drug or Toxin	Clinical Presentation of Intoxication	Specific Collaborative Management
	◦ 30% to 50%: tachycardia, tachypnea, dyspnea, weakness, marked cyanosis ◦ 50% to 70%: dysrhythmias, respiratory depression, seizures, coma ◦ Greater than 70%: potentially fatal	◦ Administered at 1 to 2 mg/kg over 5 minutes; repeated at 1 mg/kg if patient still symptomatic after 30-60 minutes; total dose should not exceed 7 mg/kg • Ascorbic acid may be administered in large doses
Opioids and opiates • Cocaine • Fentanyl • Heroin • Methadone • Morphine • Opium	• Bradycardia • Hypotension • Decreased level of consciousness • Respiratory depression → respiratory arrest • Hypothermia • Miosis • Diminished bowel sounds • Needle tracks, abscesses • Seizures • Pulmonary edema (especially with heroin)	• Gastric lavage only if within 1 hour of ingestion • Activated charcoal • Bowel irrigation for "body packers" • Naloxone (Narcan) 0.4-2 mg IV, IM, or transtracheally, or nalmefene (Revex) 0.5 mg IV ◦ Duration of action of naloxone is 1-2 hours, whereas nalmefene has a duration of action of 4-8 hours (heroin and morphine 4-6 hours, meperidine 2-4 hours) • Anticonvulsants (e.g., diazepam, phenytoin, or phenobarbital) for seizures • Intubation and mechanical ventilation may be required; PEEP may be needed for pulmonary edema
Organophosphate and carbamate (cholinesterase inhibitors)	• Bradycardia • Nausea, vomiting, diarrhea • Abdominal pain and cramping • Increased oral secretions • Dyspnea • Slurred speech • Constricted pupils • Visual changes • Unsteady gait • Urinary incontinence • Poor motor control • Twitching • Change in level of consciousness • Seizures	• Gastric lavage only if within 1 hour of ingestion • Activated charcoal if ingested • Washing of skin with soap and water and then ethanol if dermal contamination; removal and isolation of clothing • Atropine 1-2 mg IV or IM; repeated as required • Pralidoxime chloride (Protopam) 1-2 g IV over 15-30 minutes followed by infusion of 10-20 mg/kg may be used for organophosphates • Anticonvulsants (e.g., diazepam, phenytoin, or phenobarbital) for seizures
Petroleum distillates	• Flushed skin • Hyperthermia • Vomiting • Diarrhea • Abdominal pain • Tachypnea • Dyspnea • Cyanosis • Coughing • Breath sound changes: crackles; rhonchi; diminished breath sounds • Staggering gait • Confusion • CNS depression or excitation	• Washing of skin with soap and water if dermal contamination; removal and isolation of clothing • Oxygen • Positioning on left side • Bronchodilators may be required • Antiemetics
Salicylates	Initial • Hyperthermia • Burning sensation in mouth or throat • Change in level of consciousness • Petechiae Later • Hyperventilation (respiratory alkalosis) • Nausea, vomiting, epigastric pain, GI bleeding	• Gastric lavage only if within 1 hour of ingestion • Multiple doses of activated charcoal with cathartic added to first dose • Bowel irrigation if enteric-coated salicylates ingested • Fluids with dextrose (e.g., $D_5\frac{1}{2}NS$) to maintain urine output at 2 mL/kg/hr • Hypothermia blanket, ice packs, ice-water sponge baths for hyperthermia

Continued

Table 11-9 Drugs and Toxins—cont'd

Drug or Toxin	Clinical Presentation of Intoxication	Specific Collaborative Management
	• Thirst • Tinnitus • Diaphoresis Late • Hearing loss • Motor weakness • Vasodilation and hypotension • Oliguria, renal failure • Pulmonary edema, respiratory depression → respiratory arrest • Metabolic acidosis • Prolonged PT, bleeding time • Hypokalemia, hypocalcemia	○ Dantrolene (Dantrium) may be prescribed for malignant hyperthermia • Sodium bicarbonate to alkalinize the urine and increase rate of salicylate excretion; maintain urine pH greater than 7.50 ○ Monitor potassium, calcium, and magnesium levels • Hemodialysis may be necessary • Monitoring for bleeding; vitamin K may be needed • Monitoring and correction of potassium, calcium levels • Anticonvulsants (e.g., diazepam, phenytoin, or phenobarbital) for seizures • H_2 receptor blocker or proton pump inhibitor for gastric ulcer prophylaxis
Stimulants • Amphetamines (e.g., biphetamine or dextroamphetamine [Dexedrine]) • Methylenedioxymethamphetamine (MDMA) (i.e., Ecstasy) • Methylphenidate (i.e., meth) • Methylphenidate (Ritalin) • Gamma-hydroxybutyrate (GHB) (i.e., liquid Ecstasy, liquid X)	• Tachycardia • Hypertension or hypotension • Tachypnea • Dysrhythmias • Hyperthermia, diaphoresis • Dilated but reactive pupils • Dry mouth • Urinary retention • Headache • Paranoid-type psychotic behavior • Hallucinations • Hyperactivity, anxiety • Hyperactive deep tendon reflexes, tremor, seizures • Confusion, stupor, coma	• Calm, quiet environment ○ Avoid overstimulation of patient ○ Do not speak loudly or move quickly ○ Do not approach from behind ○ Avoid touching the patient unless you are sure it is safe • Gastric lavage only if within 1 hour of ingestion • Activated charcoal (single dose) • Diazepam (Valium) or lorazepam (Ativan) for agitation • Phentolamine (Regitine) for hypertension • Anticonvulsants (e.g., diazepam, phenytoin, or phenobarbital) for seizures • Antidysrhythmics (e.g., lidocaine) for ventricular dysrhythmias • Haloperidol (Haldol) for acute psychotic reactions • Hypothermia blanket, ice packs, ice-water sponge baths for hyperthermia ○ Dantrolene (Dantrium) may be prescribed for malignant hyperthermia
Tricyclic antidepressants • Amitriptyline (Elavil) Desipramine (Norpramin) • Doxepin (Sinequan) • Imipramine (Tofranil) • Nortriptyline (Aventyl) • Trimipramine (Surmontil)	Anticholinergic • Tachycardia, palpitations • Dysrhythmias • Hyperthermia • Headache • Restlessness • Mydriasis • Dry mouth • Nausea, vomiting • Dysphagia • Decreased bowel sounds • Urinary retention • Decreased deep tendon reflexes • Restlessness, euphoria • Hallucinations • Seizures • Coma Anti–alpha-adrenergic • Hypotension • QT interval prolongation and quinidine-like dysrhythmias (including torsades de pointes) • AV and bundle branch blocks • Clinical indications of heart failure	• Gastric lavage only if within 1 hour of ingestion • Activated charcoal if agent ingested • Sodium bicarbonate to alkalinize the urine and increase rate of tricyclic antidepressant (TCA) excretion; maintain urine pH greater than 7.50 ○ Monitor potassium, calcium, and magnesium levels • Hyperventilation may be used to produce alkalosis • Physostigmine (Antilirium) may be prescribed • Cardioversion, defibrillation, pacemaker as needed for dysrhythmias; avoid quinidine, lidocaine, digitalis; phenytoin or beta-blockers may be used to shorten QRS complex duration; overdrive pacing for torsades de pointes • Anticonvulsants (e.g., diazepam, phenytoin, or phenobarbital) for seizures • Fluids and vasopressors for hypotension • Bethanechol (Urecholine) for urinary retention

b. May have history of depression or psychiatric illness
c. May have history of previous drug overdosage/toxin ingestion
d. May have history of chemical dependency
e. May have history of complicated drug regimen with or without confusion
f. Note any history of cardiovascular, renal, or hepatic disease

2. Objective: Focus assessment on the following (for drug-specific signs, see Table 11-9).
   a. Vital signs
   b. Mental status
   c. Seizures
   d. Pupils
   e. Ventilation
   f. Skin and mucous membranes
   g. Peristalsis
   h. Odors
   i. Urine color
   j. Also note the following:
      (1) Needle marks
      (2) Evidence of self-injury (e.g., cutting on forearms)
   k. Physiologic grading of the severity of poisoning (Table 11-10)
3. Diagnostic
   a. Toxicology
      (1) Rapid drug screens (qualitative)
         (a) Serum
            (i) Acetaminophen
            (ii) Ethanol
            (iii) Salicylates
            (iv) Tricyclic antidepressants
         (b) Urine
            (i) Amphetamines
            (ii) Barbiturates
            (iii) Benzodiazepines
            (iv) Cannabinoids
            (v) Cocaine
            (vi) Methadol
            (vii) Opiates
            (viii) Phencyclidine
            (ix) Propoxyphene
      (2) Quantitative drug levels may be required to determine appropriate treatment
         (a) Carbamazepine
         (b) Carbon monoxide
         (c) Digoxin
         (d) Ethylene glycol
         (e) Lithium
         (f) Methanol
         (g) Methemoglobin
         (h) Phenytoin
         (i) Theophylline
   b. Arterial blood gas
      (1) Respiratory acidosis caused by hypoventilation when drugs or toxin depress ventilation
      (2) Metabolic acidosis
         (a) With increased anion gap (for more information on anion gap, see Chapter 8)
            (i) Paraldehyde, ethylene glycol, methanol, toluene, salicylates
            (ii) Agents that cause hypoxia and resultant increase in serum lactate
         (b) With decreased anion gap: lithium, bromide, iodide
   c. ECG: dysrhythmias frequently seen, depending on the drug or toxin
   d. Flat plate of abdomen (i.e., kidney, ureter, bladder [KUB]): to assess for presence of radiopaque agents
   e. Computed tomography (CT) scan: may be done to rule out pathologic condition
   f. Lumbar puncture: may be done to rule out pathologic condition

Nursing Diagnoses

1. Ineffective Airway Clearance related to drug effects on respiratory center and artificial airway
2. Ineffective Breathing Patterns related to drug effects on respiratory center
3. Decreased Cardiac Output related to dysrhythmias, diuresis, vasodilation, and negative inotropic effects

Table 11-10 Physiologic Grading of the Severity of Poisoning

	Signs and Symptoms	
Severity	**Stimulant Poisoning**	**Depressant Poisoning**
Grade 1	Agitation, anxiety, diaphoresis, hyperreflexia, mydriasis, tremors	Ataxia, confusion, lethargy, weakness, verbal, able to follow commands
Grade 2	Confusion, fever, hyperactivity, hypertension, tachycardia, tachypnea	Mild coma (nonverbal but responsive to pain), brainstem and deep tendon reflexes intact
Grade 3	Delirium, hallucinations, hyperpyrexia, tachydysrhythmias	Moderate coma (respiratory depression, unresponsive to pain), some but not all reflexes absent
Grade 4	Coma, cardiovascular collapse, seizures	Deep coma (apnea, cardiovascular depression), all reflexes absent

Irwin, R. S., & Rippe, J. M. (2003). *Irwin and Rippe's intensive care medicine* (Vol. 5). Philadelphia: Lippincott Williams & Wilkins.

4. Ineffective Cerebral Tissue Perfusion related to hypoxia, cerebral hypoperfusion, and intracranial hypertension
5. Risk for Injury related to seizures, intubation, aspiration, invasive procedures, and hemorrhage
6. Risk for Electrolyte Imbalance related to fluid shifts and potential hemolysis
7. Interrupted Family Processes related to sudden critical illness

Collaborative Management

1. Maintain airway, oxygenation, and ventilation.
   a. Administer oxygen, dextrose, thiamine, and naloxone (Narcan) (sometimes referred to as a *coma cocktail*) for altered mental status with no known cause.
      (1) Administer oxygen to reverse hypoxemia as a cause of loss of consciousness.
         (a) Goal is to achieve a SaO_2 of 95% unless contraindicated; if patient has a history of chronic obstructive pulmonary disease, goal is to achieve a SaO_2 of 90%
         (b) Contraindicated if the herbicide paraquat is ingested because it is likely to increase alveolar injury caused by oxygen free radicals
      (2) Administer dextrose to reverse possible hypoglycemia as the cause of loss of consciousness.
         (a) Usual dose is 50 to 100 mL 50% dextrose IV.
      (3) Administer thiamine to prevent Wernicke's encephalopathy especially if there is a history of alcoholism or chronic drug abuse.
         (a) Usual dose is 50 to 100 mg thiamine IV or IM
         (b) Also helpful in ethylene glycol intoxication because thiamine may prevent formation of toxic metabolites
      (4) Administer naloxone (Narcan) to reverse possible opiate intoxication as a cause of loss of consciousness.
         (a) Dose is usually 1 to 2 mg naloxone IV, IM, or transtracheally; dose of up to 10 mg may be required.
         (b) Goal is to reverse the CNS and respiratory depression, not to obtain full consciousness.
         (c) Sudden narcotic withdrawal occurs in patients with opiate intoxication, so exercise caution to prevent the patient from injuring himself or herself or health care providers.
   b. Maintain head tilt–chin lift position to maintain open airway; use jaw thrust technique if cervical spine injury may exist.
   c. Use an oropharyngeal or nasopharyngeal airway to keep the tongue away from the hypopharynx.
      (1) Choose appropriate airway: oropharyngeal airways should not be used in conscious patients because of their propensity to cause vomiting by stimulating the gag reflex.
      (2) Place patient in a left side-lying position.
      (3) Have suction equipment available.
   d. Assist with endotracheal intubation if gag and cough reflexes are depressed or if gastric lavage is initiated in lethargic patient.
   e. Monitor breath sounds and chest x-ray for aspiration and pulmonary edema.
   f. Administer oxygen therapy; adjust flow rate or oxygen concentration to keep SpO_2 at approximately 95% unless contraindicated; in patients with chronic hypercapnia, adjust flow rate or oxygen concentration to keep SpO_2 at approximately 90%.
   g. Assist with initiation of mechanical ventilation for acute respiratory failure or respiratory failure and respiratory acidosis.
2. Maintain cardiovascular function.
   a. Monitor electrocardiogram rhythm for conduction changes or dysrhythmias, especially if tricyclic antidepressant overdosage.
   b. Administer antidysrhythmic agents as prescribed.
   c. Assist with treatment of hypotension if required.
      (1) Insertion of intravenous catheter
      (2) Treatment of hypovolemia by infusion of isotonic crystalloids
      (3) Administration of vasopressors for vasodilation
         (a) Alpha stimulants for tricyclic antidepressants
         (b) Alpha and beta stimulants for beta-blocker or calcium channel blocker intoxication
         (c) Calcium may be administered for calcium channel blocker intoxication
   d. Assist with treatment of hypertension if required.
      (1) Sedation with benzodiazepine as prescribed
      (2) Alpha-blocker and beta-blocker (e.g., labetalol [Normodyne]) as prescribed for hypertension with tachycardia
      (3) Peripheral vasodilator if hypertension with normal heart rate or bradycardia
   e. Apply blankets and radiant heat lamps if needed for hypothermia.
3. Prevent further absorption of drug or toxin depending on the route of absorption.
   a. Eye: immediate irrigation of the eyes with large quantities of isotonic saline
   b. Skin
      (1) Protect yourself with gloves, gown, and goggles.
      (2) Remove and discard clothing.
      (3) Rinse with water until skin pH is normal if toxin is a strong acid or alkaline.
      (4) Wash body with soap and water.
   c. Ingestion
      (1) Induced emesis using ipecac: may be used in prehospital environment in alert patients with active gag reflex but is unlikely to be effective in removing poisons from the stomach and increases risk of aspiration

(2) Gastric lavage: especially helpful if patient arrives within 60 minutes of ingestion of drug or toxin
   (a) Assist with endotracheal intubation before gastric lavage in patients who have decreased level of consciousness and a diminished gag reflex.
   (b) Consider contraindications.
      (i) Ingestion of hydrocarbons or corrosives
         a) Use dilution: give water or milk (usually approximately 250 mL).
      (ii) Airway cannot be protected
      (iii) Seizures
   (c) Use large-bore (32 to 40 French) orogastric tube (Ewald).
      (i) Viscous lidocaine on tube may decrease gag reflex.
      (ii) Confirm placement by aspirating gastric contents.
   (d) Place patient in a left side-lying, head-down position; have suction equipment available.
   (e) Use approximately 5 to 10 L of warm tap water; inject 150 to 200 mL at a time and aspirate completely before injecting any more lavage fluid.
   (f) Monitor for potential complications (e.g., esophageal or gastric perforation, aspiration pneumonitis, laryngospasm, epistaxis, hypothermia, or hyponatremia).
   (g) Do not remove tube until after activated charcoal has been given.
(3) Adsorbent therapy
   (a) Administer activated charcoal as prescribed, usually 0.5 to 1 g/kg.
      (i) Indicated if patient presents within 1 hour of ingestion of a potentially toxic amount of drug or toxin that does bind to charcoal
      (ii) Contraindications
         a) More than an hour after ingestion of the drug or toxin
            i) May be used if more than 1 hour since ingestion if a significant overdosage of a drug slows gastric emptying and if the airway is protected
         b) Substances not bound to charcoal, including the following:
            i) Metal salts: iron, lithium, potassium
            ii) Alcohols: ethanol, ethylene glycol, glycol, methanol
            iii) Hydrocarbons, solvents, corrosives, acids, alkalis
            iv) Pesticides
            v) Cyanide
         c) Airway cannot be protected
         d) Oral antidote is given
      (iii) Multiple doses as prescribed
         a) Usually administered as 0.5 g/kg of body mass every 2 to 6 hours until serum drug level is normal
         b) Indicated for life-threatening overdosage of the following agents:
            i) Carbamazepine (Tegretol)
            ii) Dapsone
            iii) Theophylline
            iv) Phenobarbital
            v) Quinine
      (iv) Cathartics: necessity and safety now questioned, so likely to be prescribed only with multiple doses of activated charcoal
         a) Administer sorbitol with first dose of activated charcoal as prescribed
         b) Repeated doses may cause intractable diarrhea
(4) Bowel irrigation
   (a) Administer nonabsorbable, osmotically active solution (e.g., polyethylene glycol lavage electrolyte solution [GoLYTELY, Colyte]) as prescribed orally or by nasogastric tube, usually at a rate of 1 to 2 L/hr for 4 to 6 hours or until the patient is having clear stools
   (b) Indications
      (i) Large ingestions of drugs or toxins not adsorbed to activated charcoal
      (ii) Large ingestions of sustained-release or enteric-coated drugs
      (iii) "Body packers" and "body stuffers"; surgical intervention also may be required in these situations
         a) "Body packers" swallow condoms or balloons filled with a drug to smuggle it
         b) "Body stuffers" swallow drugs to prevent detection by police; these drugs are not specially prepared to prevent absorption in the gastrointestinal tract, so they present great risk of overdosage
      (iv) Formed concretions of drugs in the gastrointestinal tract
   (c) Contraindicated if the patient has significant gastrointestinal pathologic condition or dysfunction
   (d) Monitor patient for vomiting
(5) Assist with gastroscopy if indicated: may be necessary to remove coalesced mass of pills

4. Facilitate removal of drug.
   a. Forced diuresis: intravenously administered fluids and osmotic or loop diuretics were used to cause a forced osmotic diuresis in ethanol, methanol, and ethylene glycol intoxication in the past but are no longer recommended

b. Urine alkalization
   (1) Intravenous sodium bicarbonate is used.
   (2) Treatment is indicated for salicylates, tricyclic antidepressants, phenobarbital, and chlorpropamide.
   (3) Goal is urine pH of 7.5 to 8.5.
   (4) Monitoring of potassium is required.

c. Acidification of the urine previously was used for overdose of phencyclidine (PCP) and amphetamines but currently is avoided because of the incidence of rhabdomyolysis and resultant myoglobinuria that may cause acute renal failure

d. Hemodialysis or hemoperfusion as prescribed
   (1) Indications for hemodialysis include the following:
      (a) Heavy metals
      (b) Salicylate intoxication with severe acid-base imbalance or seizures unresponsive to treatment
      (c) Severe poisoning of a dialyzable drug (Box 11-2)
      (d) Ingestion of an agent known to produce delayed toxicity
      (e) Drug-induced renal or hepatic toxicity
   (2) Hemoperfusion is more effective for drugs that are bound to plasma proteins, but it is not effective in correcting acid-base imbalances.
      (a) May be used for the following:
         (i) *Amanita* (mushroom) poisoning
         (ii) Carbamazepine
         (iii) Colchicine
         (iv) Phenobarbital
         (v) Theophylline
   (3) Hemodialysis and hemoperfusion require double-venous vascular catheter.

e. Appropriate antidote if available and prescribed (listed where applicable in Table 11-9)

5. Maintain renal function.
   a. Administer intravenous fluids to maintain urine output at 0.5 to 1 mL/kg/hr.

BOX 11-2 Selected Dialyzable Drugs/Toxins

Acetaminophen
Alcohols: ethanol; ethylene glycol; methanol
Amphetamines
Antibiotics (most)
Barbiturates
Electrolytes: potassium; calcium; magnesium
Lithium
Phenobarbital
Salicylates
Theophylline

   b. Monitor patient for myoglobinuria; administer fluids and diuretics as prescribed.
6. Monitor patient's hepatic function: liver function studies; coagulation studies.
7. Monitor patient for complications.
   a. Acute respiratory failure (type II) caused by respiratory depression
   b. Aspiration pneumonitis
   c. Dysrhythmias
   d. Hypotension
   e. Heart failure
   f. Nephrotoxicity, acute renal failure
   g. Hepatotoxicity, acute hepatic failure
   h. Gastrointestinal ileus, bleeding, or perforation
   i. Seizures
   j. Coma, neurologic injury
   k. Hyperthermia or hypothermia
   l. Fluid and electrolyte imbalance
   m. Acid-base imbalance
   n. Repeat overdosage
8. Ensure appropriate psychologic counseling.
   a. Allow patient to express feelings; maintain a noncondemning approach.
   b. Monitor environment for safety hazards; maintain suicide precautions if indicated.
   c. Refer the patient to a substance abuse program if appropriate.
   d. Request psychiatric consultation for destructive behavior if appropriate.

LEARNING ACTIVITIES

1. **DIRECTIONS:** Complete the following crossword puzzle related to shock, systemic inflammatory response syndrome, and multiple organ dysfunction syndrome.

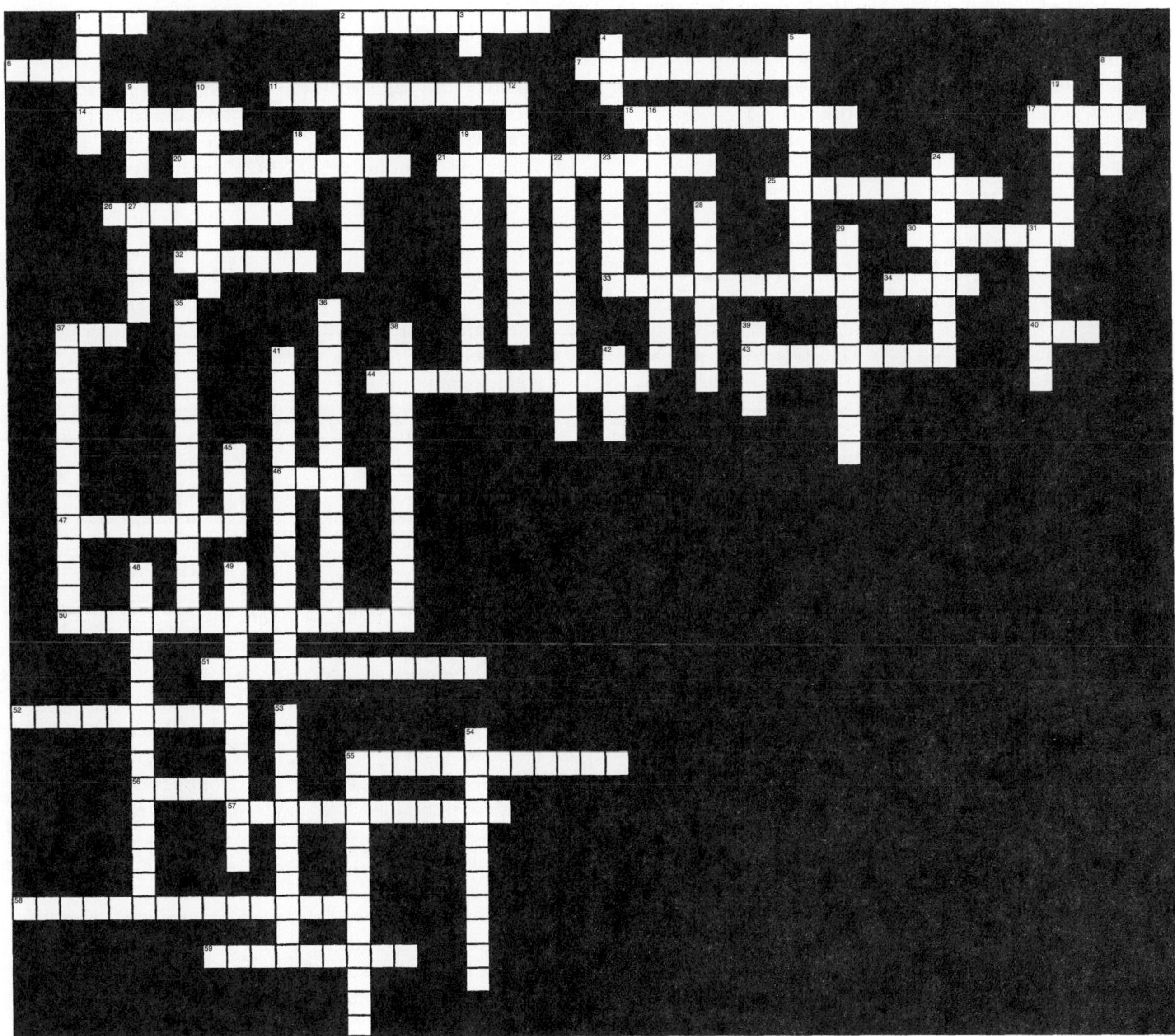

Across

1. The hemodynamic parameter that is increased in hypovolemic and cardiogenic shock (abbreviation)
2. The mediator seen in anaphylactic shock that causes vasodilation and increased capillary permeability
6. This hemodynamic parameter differentiates hypovolemic from cardiogenic shock and cardiac from noncardiac pulmonary edema (abbreviation)
7. The term for the edema of the mucous membranes seen in anaphylactic shock
11. This stage of septic shock also is referred to as late or cold septic shock
14. This stage of shock is associated with a decrease in tissue oxygenation but no clinical indications of hypoperfusion
15. The stage of shock associated with irreversible organ damage
17. This type of intravenous infusion is required for hemorrhage to the point of hypoperfusion
20. The drug most commonly associated with anaphylactic shock (generic)

21. This type of intravenous fluid contains solutes and may be categorized as hypotonic, isotonic, or hypertonic
25. The type of shock caused by suppression of the SNS
26. This drug may be used in anaphylactic shock if the patient is taking beta-blockers (generic)
30. A colloid solution that contains large starch molecules; affects platelet aggregation (trade)
32. This type of shock is associated with mediator released in response to overwhelming infection
33. This type of shock is caused by the inability of the heart to pump effectively
34. This anterior pituitary hormone stimulates the release of aldosterone and glucocorticoids (abbreviation)
37. The type of acute renal failure seen in MODS (abbreviation)
40. Cellular energy (abbreviation)
43. An oral antiprostaglandin (generic)
44. The stage of shock dominated by neuroendocrine responses to hypoperfusion
46. A mechanical therapy used in cardiogenic shock to increase coronary artery perfusion pressure and decrease afterload (abbreviation)
47. This type of intravenous fluid is used to increase intravascular colloidal oncotic pressure (plural)
50. This recombinant drug is used in severe sepsis (generic; two words)
51. This stage of shock is associated with fever, increased CO/CI, and decreased SVR
52. The inotropic agent used most often in cardiogenic shock (generic)
55. This type of drug may be used to decrease preload or afterload in cardiogenic shock (plural)
56. This physiologic response to infection increases oxygen consumption
57. Third spacing is the shift of fluid from the intravascular space to the _____ space, pleural space, pericardial space, and/or peritoneal space
58. H_1 receptor antagonist (generic)
59. Lactated Ringer's solution may cause metabolic _____

Down

1. Infection with SIRS
2. Type of shock caused by loss of intravascular volume
3. The most common cause of cardiogenic shock (abbreviation)
4. The branch of the autonomic nervous system responsible for the early compensatory response to hypoperfusion in shock (abbreviation)
5. This vasopressor is likely to improve BP more effectively than other vasopressors when significant acidosis occurs (generic)
8. The condition of insufficient perfusion of cells and vital organs
9. A systemic response of the immune system to microorganism, tissue trauma, toxins, and burns (abbreviation)
10. This device may be required in neurogenic shock
12. VO_2 is oxygen _____
13. The plasma protein with the greatest effect on plasma oncotic pressure
16. The first-line drug for anaphylactic shock (generic)
18. The type of coagulopathy seen in MODS (abbreviation)
19. The stage of shock when compensatory mechanisms are no longer effective in maintaining tissue perfusion
22. This type of shock is caused by antigen-antibody response, IgE, and the release of histamine and other mediators
23. Anaerobic metabolism cause production of this acid
24. An inflammatory response to microorganisms
27. Hypoglycemia is a early sign of dysfunction of this organ
28. DO_2 is oxygen _____
29. The presence of viable bacteria in the blood
31. Hetastarch may cause transient elevation of this serum level
35. This drug is indicated in septic shock when the patient is vasopressor dependent or steroid depleted (generic)
36. A consequence of hemolytic blood transfusion reaction; may cause renal failure
37. An anaphylactic-like reaction that does not require previous exposure; not mediated by IgE, probably triggered by the complement system
38. The consequence of muscle destruction; may cause renal failure
39. Low tidal volumes and peak inspiratory pressures are advocated to prevent __________ (abbreviation)
41. The vasopressor that usually is considered first-line for septic shock (generic)
42. The type of acute respiratory failure seen in MODS (abbreviation)
45. The frequently fatal result of SIRS; previously referred to as multisystem organ failure (abbreviation)
48. A method of returning the patient's hemorrhaged blood to his intravascular volume; greatest risks are infection and coagulopathy
49. This vasopressor is the preferred agent in a patient with septic shock and tachycardia (generic)
53. A complication of administering large volumes of fluid and blood intravenously; shifts the oxyhemoglobin dissociation curve to the left
54. An alkaline buffer used for severe metabolic acidosis
55. This group of drugs may be used in vasogenic shock to restore normal vascular tone (plural)

2. **Directions:** Identify which type of shock the following pathologic conditions or procedures may cause.

Condition	Hypovolemic	Cardiogenic	Septic	Anaphylactic	Neurogenic
Ascites					
Bee sting					
Blood transfusion reaction					
Burns					
Chemotherapy					
Diarrhea					
Esophageal varices					
Head injury					
Insulin shock					
Invasive procedures					
Intravenous pyelography dye					
Malnutrition					
Myocardial infarction					
Pulmonary embolism					
Ruptured gallbladder					
Ruptured papillary muscle					
Spinal anesthesia					
Spinal cord injury					
Trauma					

3. **Directions:** Match the pathophysiologic condition with the type of shock.

___ 1. Cardiogenic
___ 2. Septic
___ 3. Anaphylactic
___ 4. Neurogenic
___ 5. Hypovolemic

a. Vasodilation resulting from stimulation of the inflammatory and immune systems by microorganisms
b. Inability of the heart to pump effectively
c. Inadequate amount of circulating volume
d. Vasodilation resulting from the release of histamine from mast cells caused by major allergic reaction
e. Vasodilation resulting from suppression or loss of the SNS

4. **Directions:** Identify the following signs/symptoms of shock as occurring during the compensatory, progressive, and/or refractory stages of shock.

Sign/Symptom	Compensatory	Progressive	Refractory
Anuria			
Cool, pale skin			
Decreased bowel sounds			
Dysrhythmias			
Hypotension			
Mottling of extremities			
Narrow pulse pressure			
Nausea			
Neurologic changes: coma, focal signs			
Neurologic changes: irritability, confusion			
Neurologic changes: lethargy, coma			
Oliguria			
Profound hypotension despite vasopressors			
Profound hypoxemia, increased pulmonary vascular resistance, decreased lung compliance (ARDS)			
Tachycardia			
Thirst			
Uncontrollable bleeding (DIC)			

ARDS, Acute respiratory distress syndrome; *DIC,* disseminated intravascular coagulation.

5. **Directions:** Complete this table by putting ↑, ↓, or *normal* in the empty cells.

Type of Shock	CO/CI	RAP/PAP/PAOP	SVR	Svo_2
Anaphylactic				
Cardiogenic				
Hypovolemic				
Neurologic				
Early septic				
Late septic				

CO, Cardiac output; *CI,* cardiac index; *RAP,* right atrial pressure; *PAP,* pulmonary artery pressure; *PAOP,* pulmonary artery occlusive pressure; *SVR,* systemic vascular resistance; Svo_2, venous oxygen saturation.

6. **Directions:** List two fluids in each category.

Crystalloids		
Isotonic		
Hypotonic		
Hypertonic		
Colloids		
Blood or blood products		

7. **Directions:** Identify the three factors that affect oxygen delivery.
a. ____________________
b. ____________________
c. ____________________

8. **Directions:** Match the following therapies with the type of shock for which they may be used. You may list more than one therapy for each form of shock, and the therapies may be used more than once.

___ 1. Anaphylactic
___ 2. Cardiogenic
___ 3. Hypovolemic
___ 4. Neurogenic
___ 5. Septic

a. Intravenous fluids
b. Corticosteroids
c. Blood
d. Vasopressors
e. Inotropes
f. Intraaortic balloon pump (IABP)
g. Pacemaker
h. Epinephrine
i. Antihistamines
j. Antimicrobials
k. Treat the cause
l. Oxygen
m. Vasodilators

9. **Directions:** Match the sign/symptom of dysfunction with the organ that is dysfunctional.

___ 1. Brain
___ 2. Heart
___ 3. Blood
___ 4. Kidneys
___ 5. Liver
___ 6. Lungs

a. Decreased Pao_2/Fio_2 ratio
b. Oliguria
c. Hypoglycemia
d. Decrease in Glasgow Coma Scale score
e. Prolonged PT, PTT, decreased platelets
f. Increased PAOP

10. **Directions:** Complete the following table that describes the four physiologic alterations that are likely to be seen in systemic inflammatory response syndrome. The criteria for systemic inflammatory response syndrome are two of these four parameters.

Heart rate	Greater than ____			
Respiratory rate	Greater than ____	OR	$Paco_2$	Less than ____
Temperature	Greater than ____	OR	Less than ____	
WBC	Greater than ____	OR	Less than ____	

11. DIRECTIONS: Identify the two interventions used for most (but not all) overdosages to decrease absorption of the drug.

a. ___

b. ___

12. DIRECTIONS: Match the following antidotes to the appropriate drug or toxin.

___ 1. Acetaminophen		a. Glucagon
___ 2. Benzodiazepines (eg., diazepam)		b. 100% oxygen, hyperbaric oxygenation if possible
___ 3. Beta-blocker		c. Digoxin immune FAB (Digibind)
___ 4. Calcium channel blockers		d. Fomepizole (Antizol)
___ 5. Carbon monoxide		e. Ethanol
___ 6. Cyanide		f. Methylene blue
___ 7. Digoxin		g. Calcium
___ 8. Ethylene glycol		h. Amyl nitrate
___ 9. Methanol		i. Atropine
___ 10. Methemoglobinemia		j. Acetylcysteine (Mucomyst)
___ 11. Opiates (e.g., morphine sulfate)		k. Flumazenil (Romazicon)
___ 12. Organophosphates		l. Naloxone (Narcan)

13. DIRECTIONS: Complete the following crossword puzzle related to drug overdosage or toxin exposure.

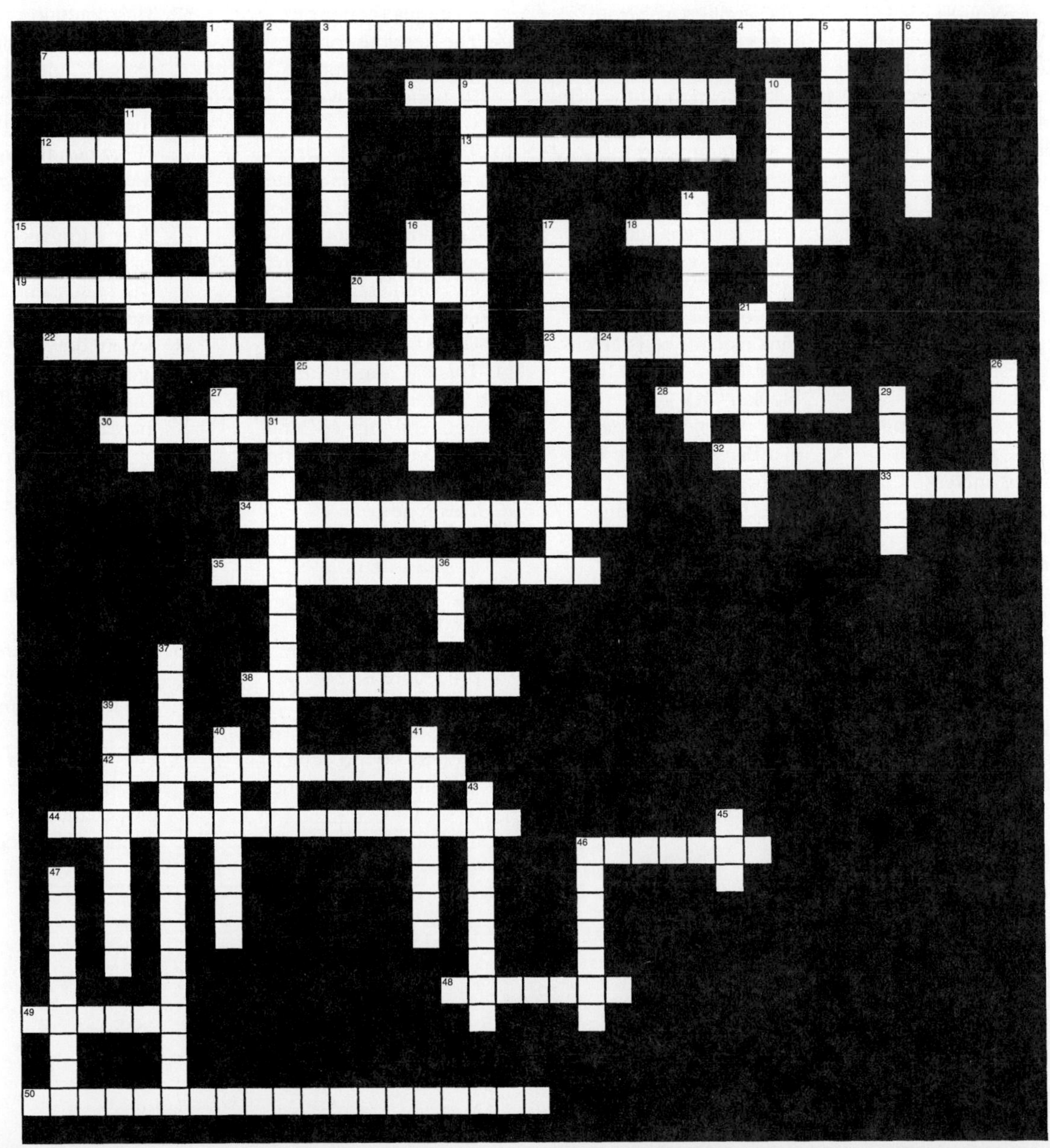

Across

3. Dilution is used rather than gastric lavage if this type of chemical is ingested
4. This drug may be used intravenously in methanol or ethylene glycol intoxication
7. A new antidote used for ethylene glycol intoxication (trade)
8. A blood cleansing procedure that may be used to remove some drugs or toxins from the blood
12. This type of consultation should always be requested for patients with drug overdose (OD)
13. This type of blood test is done to determine what drugs have been ingested
15. This drug can stimulate the beta-receptors even in the presence of beta-blockade; used for beta-blocker overdose
18. This B vitamin must be given with dextrose to malnourished patients to prevent Wernicke's encephalopathy
19. This osmotic laxative is added to first dose of activated charcoal if multiple doses are going to be used
20. This "gap" is increased in alcohol intoxication
22. The antidote for acetaminophen (trade)
23. This device may be required for the bradycardia seen in beta-blocker or calcium channel blocker overdose
25. This type of overdose causes metabolic acidosis and respiratory alkalosis
28. Drug overdose in an attempt to get attention is referred to as a suicide _____
30. This antiemetic frequently is used for acetaminophen overdose (generic)
32. This drug may cause necrosis and perforation of the nasal septum (generic)
33. This quality of the urine may be helpful to identify the drug consumed
34. The affinity between hemoglobin and this substance is much greater than the affinity between hemoglobin and oxygen (two words)
35. This drug may bind with digoxin in the gut (generic)
38. The greatest risk with ingestion of petroleum distillates
42. Alkalinization of the urine with sodium bicarbonate is recommended for overdose of this barbiturate (generic)
44. Term for hemoglobin saturated with carbon monoxide rather than oxygen
46. This electrolyte is given for calcium channel blocker OD
48. This type of behavior is a danger to staff; may occur with rapid reversion of sedating drugs and dissociative agents
49. The procedure to flush the drug or toxin from the stomach; indicated if patient arrives within 1 hour of ingestion for most substances
50. This procedure is used to assess injury after ingestion of caustic agents

Down

1. This antidote for benzodiazepines should not be given if the patient has coingested tricyclic antidepressants
2. This drug is used for malignant hyperthermia that occurs in some drug overdosages (generic)
3. The adsorbent agent used in most drug overdosages
5. This drug used for the bradycardia seen in beta-blocker or calcium channel blocker OD (generic)
6. Toxicity of this drug causes nystagmus, tremors, ataxia, seizures, and nephrogenic diabetes insipidus (generic)
9. The antidote for methemoglobinemia (generic and two words)
10. This antidote is given if digoxin level is greater than 10 ng/mL (trade)
11. The drug most often involved in intentional and unintentional drug OD in the United States
14. This calcium channel blocker is used most frequently for cocaine-induced coronary artery spasm (generic)
16. This type of antidepressant may cause torsades de pointes, especially at toxic levels
17. This blood cleansing procedure is more effective than hemodialysis for plasma protein–bound drugs
21. A coma cocktail consists of oxygen, _____, thiamine, and naloxone
24. A toxin that may cause a bitter almond odor to the breath
26. This organ is most likely to be injured by acetaminophen overdose
27. This dissociative agent is associated with violent behavior (abbreviation)
29. Induced vomiting, previously stimulated by this drug, is no longer recommended, especially in the hospital setting (trade)
31. Insecticides are frequently this type; they have a cholinergic effect
36. Carbon monoxide poisoning causes the skin to be very _____
37. This condition that may be caused by nitrites, nitrates, sulfa drugs, and local anesthetics
39. High pressure; this type of oxygen therapy is used in carbon monoxide poisoning
40. Bowel irrigation with this solution is used for OD of sustained-release drugs (trade)
41. An antidote for opiates (generic)
43. This serum level is increased in stage 2 or 3 of acetaminophen overdose
45. This radiologic procedure may be used to identify the presence of radiopaque agents (abbreviation)
46. The forearms are the most common site for this form of self-injury
47. The category of toxins that include aerosol propellants, paint thinner, and glue

LEARNING ACTIVITIES ANSWERS

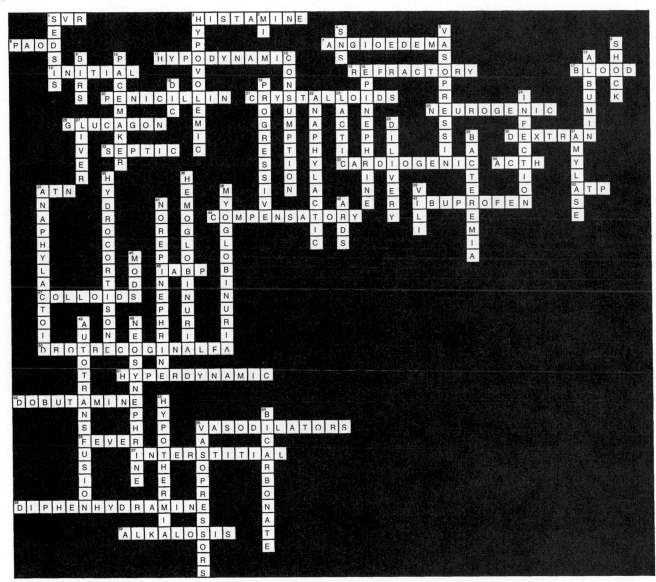

1.

2.

Condition	Hypovolemic	Cardiogenic	Septic	Anaphylactic	Neurogenic
Ascites	✓				
Bee sting				✓	
Blood transfusion reaction				✓	
Burns	✓		✓		
Chemotherapy			✓	✓	
Diarrhea	✓				
Esophageal varices	✓				
Head injury					✓
Insulin shock					✓
Invasive procedures			✓		
Intravenous pyelography dye	✓			✓	
Malnutrition			✓		
Myocardial infarction		✓			
Pulmonary embolism		✓			
Ruptured gallbladder			✓		
Ruptured papillary muscle		✓			
Spinal anesthesia					✓
Spinal cord injury					✓
Trauma	✓		✓		

3.

b 1. Cardiogenic
a 2. Septic
d 3. Anaphylactic
e 4. Neurogenic
c 5. Hypovolemic

4.

Sign/Symptom	Compensatory	Progressive	Refractory
Anuria		✓	✓
Cool, pale skin	✓		
Decreased bowel sounds	✓	✓	✓
Dysrhythmias		✓	✓
Hypotension		✓	✓
Mottling of extremities		✓	✓
Narrow pulse pressure	✓		
Nausea		✓	
Neurologic changes: coma, focal signs			✓
Neurologic changes: irritability, confusion	✓		
Neurologic changes: lethargy, coma		✓	✓
Oliguria	✓		
Profound hypotension despite vasopressors			✓
Profound hypoxemia, increased pulmonary vascular resistance, decreased lung compliance (ARDS)			✓
Tachycardia	✓	✓	
Thirst	✓		
Uncontrollable bleeding (DIC)			✓

ARDS, Acute respiratory distress syndrome; *DIC,* disseminated intravascular coagulation.

5.

Type of Shock	CO/CI	RAP/PAP/PAOP	SVR	SvO_2
Hypovolemic	↓	↓	↑	↓
Cardiogenic	↓	↑	↑	↓
Early septic	↑	↓	↓	↑
Late septic	↓	Variable	Variable	↓
Anaphylactic	↓	↓	↓	↓
Neurologic	↓	↓	↓	↓

CO, Cardiac output; *CI,* cardiac index; *RAP,* right atrial pressure; *PAP,* pulmonary artery pressure; *PAOP,* pulmonary artery occlusive pressure; *SVR,* systemic vascular resistance; *Svo_2,* venous oxygen saturation.

6.

Crystalloids		
Isotonic	Normal (0.9%) saline	Lactated Ringer's solution
Hypotonic	Half-normal (0.45%) saline	5% dextrose in water
Hypertonic	3% saline	10% dextrose in water or TPN solution
Colloids	Albumin	Dextran 70 or hetastarch
Blood or blood products	Whole blood	Red blood cells

7.

a. Arterial oxygen saturation (Sao_2) b. Hemoglobin c. Cardiac output

8.

a, b, d, h, i, k, l
e, f, k, l, m, and possibly c and g
a, k, l, and possibly c
a, d, g, k, l
a, b, d, j, k, l, and possibly c and e

1. Anaphylactic
2. Cardiogenic
3. Hypovolemic
4. Neurogenic
5. Septic

9.

d 1. Brain
f 2. Heart
e 3. Blood
b 4. Kidneys
c 5. Liver
d 6. Lungs

10.

Heart rate	Greater than 90 beats/min			
Respiratory rate	Greater than 20 breaths/min	**OR**	$Paco_2$	Less than 32 mm Hg
Temperature	Greater than 38°C (100.4°F)	**OR**	Less than 36°C (96.8°F)	
WBC	Greater than 12,000 cells/mm^3	**OR**	Less than 4000 cells/mm^3	

11.

a. Gastric lavage b. Activated charcoal

12.

j 1. Acetaminophen
k 2. Benzodiazepines (e.g., diazepam)
a 3. Beta-blocker
g 4. Calcium channel blockers
b 5. Carbon monoxide
h 6. Cyanide
c 7. Digoxin
d or e 8. Ethylene glycol
e 9. Methanol
f 10. Methemoglobinemia
l 11. Opiates (e.g., morphine sulfate)
i 12. Organophosphates

13.

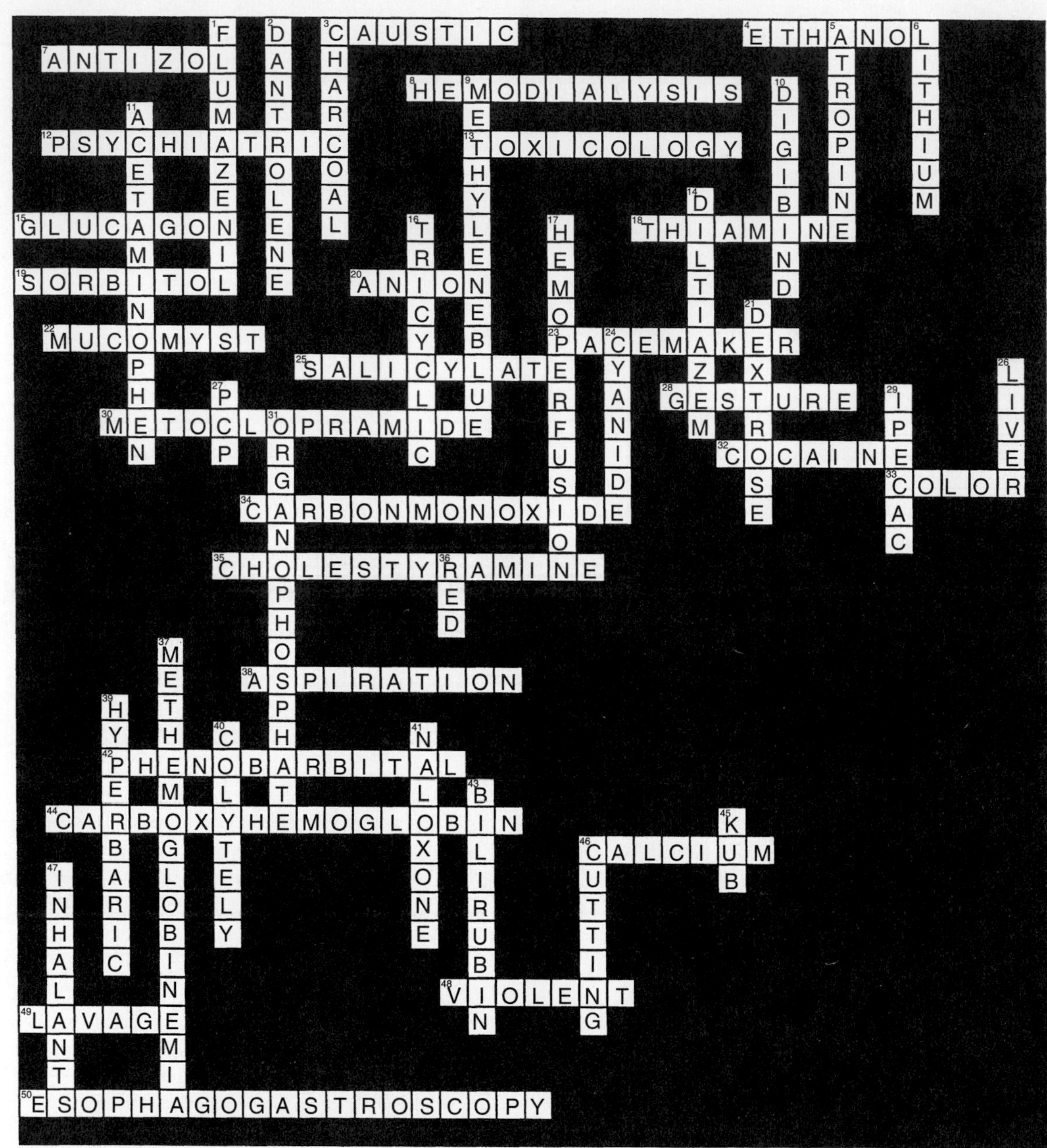

References

Alderson, P., Schierhout, G., Roberts, I., & Bunn, F. (2004). Colloids versus crystalloids for fluid resuscitation in critically ill patients. Cochrane Database System Reviews, 4:CD000567. Retrieved May 31, 2005, from http://www.medscape.com/viewarticle/485370_print

Bone, R., Sprung, C., & Sibbald, W. (1992). Definitions for sepsis and organ failure. *Critical Care Medicine, 20*(6), 724.

STOP Sepsis Working Group. (2006). *The STOP Sepsis Bundle Toolkit*. Retrieved April 24, 2006, from http://www.llu.edu/llumc/emergency/patientcare/documents/patientcare-sepsis.pdf?PHPSESSID=0ec53300a00d8305710882972d9e9706

Bibliography

American Heart Association. (2005). Part 10.2: Toxicology in ECC. *Circulation, 112*(24 suppl.), IV126-IV132.

American Heart Association. (2005). Part 10.4: Hypothermia. *Circulation, 112*(24 suppl.), IV136-IV138.

American Heart Association. (2005). Part 10.6: Anaphylaxis. *Circulation, 112*(24 suppl.), IV143-IV145.

Barclay, L. (2003). Selective decontamination of GI tract improved ICU outcome [Electronic Version]. *Medscape Medical News*. Retrieved October 15, 2003, from http://www.medscape.com/viewarticle/462056_print

Bartlett, D. (2004). The coma cocktail: Indications, contraindications, adverse effects, proper dose, and proper route. *Journal of Emergency Nursing, 30*(6), 572-574.

Berg, R. A. (2004). A long-acting vasopressin analog for septic shock: Brilliant idea or dangerous folly? *Pediatric Critical Care Medicine, 5*(2), 188-189.

Bernard, G. R., Vincent, J. L., Laterre, P. F., LaRosa, S. P., Dhainaut, J. F., Lopez-Rodriguez, A., et al. (2001). Efficacy and safety of recombinant human activated protein C for severe sepsis. *New England Journal of Medicine, 344*(10), 699-709.

Blank-Reid, C. (2004). Abdominal trauma: Dealing with the damage. *Nursing 2004, 34*(9), 36-42.

Boylston, M., & Beer, D. (2002). Methemoglobinemia: A case study. *Critical Care Nurse, 22*(4), 50-55.

Bridges, E. J., & Dukes, S. (2005). Cardiovascular aspects of septic shock: Pathophysiology, monitoring, and treatment. *Critical Care Medicine, 25*(2), 14-42.

Bromet, D. S., & Klein, L. W. (2004). Cardiogenic shock: Art and science. *Critical Care Medicine, 32*(1), 293-294.

Brown, T. (2001). Hibernating myocardium. *American Journal of Critical Care, 10*(2), 84-93.

Calandra, T., & Cohen, J. (2005). The International Sepsis Forum Consensus Conference on Definitions of Infection in the Intensive Care Unit. *Critical Care Medicine, 33*(7), 1538-1548.

Cunneen, J., & Cartwright, M. (2004). The puzzle of sepsis: Fitting the pieces of the inflammatory response with treatment. *AACN Clinical Issues, 15*(1), 18-44.

De Jong, M. J., & Fausett, M. B. (2003). Anaphylactoid syndrome of pregnancy: A devastating complication requiring intensive care. *Critical Care Nurse, 23*(6), 42-48.

Deitch, E. A., Vincent, J. L., & Windsor, A. (Eds.). (2002). *Sepsis and multiple organ dysfunction: A multidisciplinary approach.* London: W. B. Saunders.

Dellinger, R. P., Carlet, J. M., Masur, H., Gerlach, H., Calandra, T., Cohen, J., et al. (2004). Surviving Sepsis Campaign guidelines for management of severe sepsis and septic shock. *Critical Care Medicine, 32*(3), 858-873.

Dettenmeier, P., Swindell, B., Stroud, M., Arkins, N., & Howard, A. (2003). Role of activated protein C in the pathophysiology of severe sepsis. *American Journal of Critical Care, 12*(6), 518-526.

DiNardo, M. M., Korytkowski, M. T., & Siminerio, L. S. (2004). The importance of normoglycemia in critically ill patients. *Critical Care Nursing Quarterly, 27*(2), 126-134.

Ely, E. W., Kleinpell, R. M., & Goyette, R. E. (2003). Advances in the understanding of clinical manifestations and therapy of severe sepsis: An update for critical care nurses. *American Journal of Critical Care, 12*(2), 120-135.

Flynn, M. B., & Bonini, S. (1999). Blunt chest trauma: Case report. *Critical Care Nurse, 19*(5), 68-79.

Fritsch, D. E., & Steinmann, R. A. (2000). Managing trauma with abdominal compartment syndrome. *Critical Care Nurse, 20*(6), 48-58.

Gropper, M. A. (2004). Evidence-based management of critically ill patients: Analysis and implementation. *Anesthesia and Analgesia, 99,* 566-572.

Hamm, J. (2000). Acute acetaminophen overdose in adolescents and adults. *Critical Care Nurse, 20*(3), 69-74.

Hasdai, D., Topol, E. J., Califf, R. M., Berger, P. B., Holmes, J., & David, R. (2000). Cardiogenic shock complicating acute coronary syndromes. *Lancet, 356,* 749-756.

Haynes, J. (2000). Acquired methemoglobinemia following benzocaine anesthesia of the pharynx. *American Journal of Critical Care, 9*(3), 199-201.

Hess, D., & Deboer, S. (2002). Ectasy. *American Journal of Nursing, 102*(4), 45-47.

Honderick, T., Williams, D., Seaberg, D., & Wears, R. (2003). A prospective, randomized, controlled trial of benzodiazepines and nitroglycerine or nitroglycerine alone in the treatment of cocaine-associated acute coronary syndromes. *American Journal of Emergency Medicine, 21*(1), 39-42.

Irwin, R. S., & Rippe, J. M. (2003). *Irwin and Rippe's intensive care medicine* (Vol. 5). Philadelphia: Lippincott Williams & Wilkins.

Jones, A. L., & Dargan, P. I. (2001). *Churchill's pocketbook of toxicology.* Edinburgh: Churchill Livingstone.

Kinasewitz, G. T., Yan, S. B., Basson, B., Comp, P., Russell, J. A., Cariou, A., et al. (2004). Universal changes in biomarkers of coagulation and inflammation occur in patients with severe sepsis, regardless of causative microorganism [Electronic Version]. *Critical Care 8,* R82-R90. Retrieved March 30, 2004, from http://www.medscape.com/viewarticle/470755_print.

Kleinpell, R. M. (2003). Advances in treating patients with severe sepsis: Role of drotrecogin alfa (activated). *Critical Care Nurse, 23*(3), 16-29.

Kleinpell, R. M. (2003). The role of the critical care nurse in the assessment and management of the patient with severe sepsis. *Critical Care Nursing Clinics of North America, 15*(1), 27-34.

Kortgen, A., Niederprum, P., & Bauer, M. (2006). Implementation of an evidence-based "standard operating procedure" and outcome in septic shock. *Critical Care Medicine, 34*(3), 943-949.

Kruse, J. A., Fink, M. P., & Carlson, R. W. (2003). *Saunders manual of critical care.* Philadelphia: Saunders.

Kumar, A., & Mann, H. J. (2004). Appraisal of four novel approaches to the prevention and treatment of sepsis. *American Journal of Health-System Pharmacy, 61*(8), 765-774.

Lewis-Abney, K. (2000). Overdoses of tricyclic antidepressants: Grandchildren and grandparents. *Critical Care Nurse, 20*(5), 69-77.

Linden, C. H., Rippe, J. M., & Irwin, R. S. (2006). *Manual of overdoses and poisoning.* Philadelphia: Lippincott Williams & Wilkins.

Lobert, S. (2000). Ethanol, isopropanol, methanol, and ethylene glycol poisoning. *Critical Care Nurse, 20*(6), 41-47.

Luiking, Y. C., Poeze, M., Dejong, C. H., Ramsey, G., & Deutz, N. (2004). Sepsis: An arginine deficiency state? *Critical Care Medicine, 32*(10), 2135-2145.

Martin, G. S. (2001). Fluid replacement in critical care: A new look at an old issue. Retrieved May 31, 2005, from http://www.medscape.com/viewarticle/416592.

Martin, G. S. (2003). Hypertonic saline in the treatment of sepsis [Electronic Version]. *Medscape Critical Care, 4,* 1. Retrieved September 10, 2003, from http://www.medscape.com/viewarticle/460245_print

Martin, G. S. (2003). The use of inotropic agents in septic shock [Electronic Version]. *Medscape Critical Care, 4,* 1. Retrieved April 10, 2003, from http://www.medscape.com/viewarticle/451456_print

Martin, T., & Lobert, S. (2003). Chemical warfare: Toxicity of nerve agents. *Critical Care Nurse, 23*(5), 15-22.

McKinley, M. G. (2005). Alcohol withdrawal syndrome: Overlooked and mismanaged? *Critical Care Nurse, 25*(3), 40-49.

Melum, M. F. (2001). Organophosphate toxicity. *American Journal of Nursing, 101*(5), 57-58.

Micek, S. T., Shah, R. A., & Kollef, M. H. (2003). Management of severe sepsis: Integration of multiple pharmacologic interventions. *Pharmacotherapy, 23*(11), 1486-1496.

Milonovich, L. M., Headrick, C. L., Seikaly, M., & Morriss, F. C. (2001). Charcoal hemoperfusion via a continuous venovenous hemofiltration circuit to treat carbamazepine overdose. *Critical Care Nurse, 21*(6), 25-28.

Mower-Wade, D. M., Bartley, M. K., & Chiari-Allwein, J. L. (2001). How to respond to shock. *Dimensions of Critical Care Nursing, 20*(2), 22-27.

Murray, T. A., & Patterson, L. A. (2002). Prone positioning of trauma patients with acute respiratory distress syndrome and open abdominal incisions. *Critical Care Nurse, 22*(3), 52-56.

O'Hollaren, M. T. (2002). Anaphylaxis: New clues to clinical patterns and optimum treatment [Electronic Version]. *Medscape Allergy & Clinical Immunology, 2,* 1-5. Retrieved August 23, 2002, from http://www.medscape.com/viewarticle/439721_print.

O'Hollaren, M. T. (2002). Anaphylaxis: New clues to clinical patterns and optimum treatment. *Medscape Allergy and Clinical Immunology* Retrieved August 23, 2002, from http://www.medscape.com/viewarticle/439721_print

Ostrow, L., Hupp, E., & Topjian, D. (1994). The effect of Trendelenburg and modified Trendelenburg positions on cardiac output, blood pressure, and oxygenation: A preliminary study. *American Journal of Critical Care, 3*(5), 382.

Peck, P. (2004). Low-dose steroids are beneficial in sepsis [Electronic Version]. *Medscape Medical News.* Retrieved March 13, 2004, from http://www.medscape.com/viewarticle/470471_print

Peck, P. (2005). STOP sepsis bundle significantly reduces sepsis mortality [Electronic Version]. *Medscape Medical News.* Retrieved January 25, 2005, from http://www.medscape.com/viewarticle/497764_print

Piano, M. R. (2005). The cardiovascular effects of alcohol: The good and the bad. *American Journal of Nursing, 105*(7), 87-91.

Pooler, C., & Barkman, A. (2002). Myocardial injury: Contrasting infarction and contusion. *Critical Care Nurse, 22*(1), 15-26.

Powers, J., & Jacobi, J. (2003). Treatment of severe sepsis. *Clinical Nurse Specialist, 17*(3), 128-130.

Rankin, J. A. (2004). Biological mediators of acute inflammation. *AACN Clinical Issues, 15*(1), 3-17.

Rice, T. W., & Wheeler, A. P. (2003). Severe sepsis [Electronic Version]. *Infectious Medicine, 20,* 184-193. Retrieved November 19, 2005, from http://www.medscape.com/viewarticle/452425_print

Robinson, L. E., & van Soeren, M. H. (2004). Insulin resistance and hyperglycemia in critical illness. *AACN Clinical Issues, 15*(1), 45-62.

Rosenthal, L. D. (2006). Carbon monoxide poisoning: Immediate diagnosis and treatment are crucial to avoid complications. *American Journal of Nursing, 106*(3), 40-47.

Sachse, D. (2000). Delirium tremens. *American Journal of Nursing, 100*(5), 41-42.

Schulman, C., & Hare, K. (2003). New thoughts of sepsis: The unifier of critical care. *Dimensions of Critical Care Nursing, 22*(1), 20-30.

Sharma, S., & Kumar, A. (2003). Septic shock, multiple organ failure, and acute respiratory distress syndrome [Electronic Version]. *Curr Opin Pulm Med 9,* 199-209. Retrieved November 29, 2005, from http://www.medscape.com/viewarticle/452476_print

Smith-Alnimer, M., & Watford, M. F. (2004). Alcohol withdrawal and delirium tremens. *American Journal of Nursing, 104*(5), 72A-72G.

Sommers, M. S. (2002). "Nurse, I only had a couple of beers": Validity of self-reported drinking before serious vehicular injury. *American Journal of Critical Care, 11*(2), 106-114.

Stanchina, M. L., & Levy, M. M. (2004). Vasoactive drug use in septic shock. *Seminars in Respiratory Critical Care Medicine, 25*(6), 673-681.

Stanley, K. M., Amabile, C. M., Simpson, K. N., Couillard, D., Norcross, E. D., & Worrall, C. L. (2003). Impact of an alcohol withdrawal syndrome practice guideline on surgical patient outcomes. *Pharmacotherapy, 23*(7), 843-854.

Tazbir, J. (2004). Sepsis and the role of activated protein C. *Critical Care Nurse, 24*(6), 40-45.

Urden, L. D., Stacy, K. M., & Lough, M. E. (2005). *Thelan's critical care nursing: Diagnosis and management* (5th ed.). St. Louis, MO: Mosby.

Walker, J., & Criddle, L. M. (2003). Pathophysiology and management of abdominal compartment syndrome. *American Journal of Critical Care, 12*(4), 367-373.

Professional Caring and Ethical Practice

CHAPTER 12

Critical Care Nursing: General Concepts

Nursing

1. What do nurses do?
   a. "Nursing places its focus not only on a particular health problem, but on the whole patient and his or her response to treatment. Care of the patient and a firm base of scientific knowledge are indispensable elements" (American Nurses Association [ANA], 2006)
   b. "They [nurses] save lives, prevent complications, prevent suffering, and save money" (Gordon, 2006)
2. The nursing process (ANA, 2006)
   a. Assessment: collecting and analyzing physical, psychological, and sociocultural data about a patient
   b. Diagnosis: making a judgment on the cause, condition, and path of the illness
   c. Planning: creating a care plan that sets specific treatment goals
   d. Implementation: supervising or carrying out the actual treatment plan
   e. Evaluation: continuous assessment of the plan

Critical Care Nursing

1. Definition: "the specialty within nursing that deals with human responses to life-threatening health problems" (American Association of Critical-Care Nurses [AACN], 2006)
2. *Standards for Acute and Critical Care Nursing Practice* are available at *www.aacn.org*

The Critically Ill Patient

"Those patients who are at high risk for actual or potential life-threatening health problems. The more critically ill the patient the more likely he/she is to be highly vulnerable, unstable and complex, thereby requiring intense and vigilant nursing care" (AACN, 2005b)

The Critical Care Environment

"Critical care nurses work wherever critically ill patients are found—intensive care units, pediatric ICUs, neonatal ICUs, cardiac care units, cardiac catheter labs, telemetry units, progressive care units, emergency departments and recovery rooms. Increasingly, critical care nurses work in home healthcare, managed care organizations, nursing schools, outpatient surgery centers and clinics" (AACN, 2005b)

Clinical Judgment

Description

"Clinical judgment is clinical reasoning, which includes clinical decision making, critical thinking, and a global grasp of the situation, coupled with the nursing skills acquired through a process of formal and informal experiential knowledge and evidence-based guidelines" (AACN Certification Corporation, 2005).

Decision Making

1. Involves a number of steps by which information is assimilated, integrated, weighed, and valued to arrive at the selection of a course of action from among a number of possible alternatives
2. Consists of six steps
   a. Define the problem, the issue, or the situation.
   b. Gather data.
   c. Analyze the data to refine the problem statement and identify possible solutions.
   d. Identify possible solutions or actions.
   e. Analyze the possible consequences of each solution or action.
   f. Select the best possible solution or action for implementation.
   g. Implement the solution or action.
   h. Evaluate the results.

Critical Thinking, Clinical Judgment, and Clinical Reasoning

1. Definitions
   a. Critical thinking: "a disciplined process that requires validation of data, including any

assumptions that may influence your thoughts, and then careful reflection on the entire process while evaluating the effectiveness of what you have determined is the necessary action to take" (Jackson, Ignatavicius, & Case, 2006)
   b. Clinical judgment: "the development of opinions in the clinical practice setting, based on experience and knowledge, to guide the decisions you will make regarding the care of the patient" (Jackson et al., 2006)
   c. Clinical reasoning: use of "clinically specific data regarding specific populations or disease processes and making evaluations regarding their meaning" (Jackson et al., 2006)
2. Relationship between clinical judgment, clinical reasoning, and critical thinking (Figure 12-1)
3. Nine key questions of clinical judgment (Alfaro-LeFevre, 2003)
   a. What outcomes are expected in this person, family, or group when the plan of care is terminated?
   b. What problems or issues must be addressed to achieve these outcomes?
   c. What are the circumstances?
   d. What knowledge is required?
   e. How much room is there for error?
   f. How much time do I have?
   g. What resources can help me?
   h. Whose perspectives must be considered?
   i. What is influencing my thinking?
4. Strategies enhancing critical thinking (Alfaro-LeFevre, 1995)
   a. Anticipate the questions others might ask.
   b. Ask "why?"
   c. Ask "what else?"
   d. Ask "what if?"
   e. Paraphrase in your own words.
   f. Compare and contrast.
   g. Organize and reorganize information.
   h. Look for flaws in your thinking.
   i. Ask someone else to look for flaws in your thinking.
   j. Develop good habits of inquiry.
   k. Revisit information.
   l. Replace the phases "I don't know" or "I'm not sure" with "I need to find out."
   m. Turn errors into learning opportunities.
   n. Share your mistakes—they are valuable.

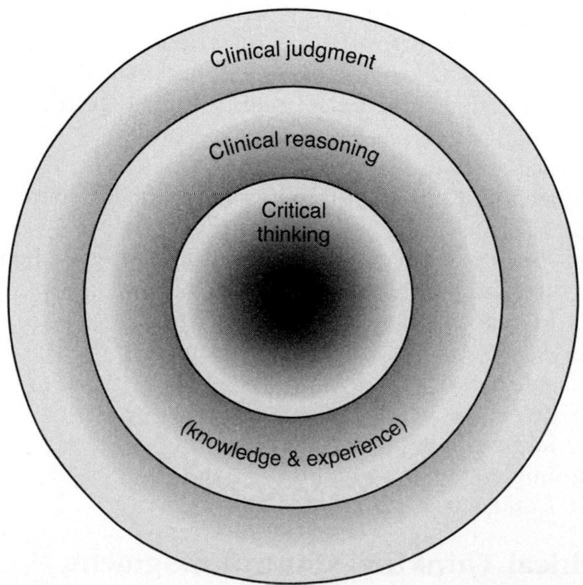

Figure 12-1 Relationship between clinical judgment, clinical reasoning, and critical thinking. (From Jackson, M., Ignatavicius, D. D., & Case, B. [2006]. *Conversations in critical thinking and clinical judgment.* Boston: Jones and Bartlett.)

Clinical Knowledge and Skills (Refer to Chapters 2 through 11)

Advocacy/Moral Agency

Description

"Advocacy is working on another's behalf and representing the concerns of the patient, family, and community; moral agency is serving as a moral agent in identifying and helping to resolve ethical and clinical concerns within the clinical setting" (AACN Certification Corporation, 2005).

Definitions and Concepts Related to Ethical Decision Making

1. Advocacy refers to respecting and supporting the basic values, rights, and beliefs of the critically ill patient (AACN, 2005c)
   a. The nurse should do the following (AACN, 2005c):
      (1) Respect and support the right of the patient or the patient's designated surrogate to autonomous, informed decision making.
      (2) Intervene when the best interest of the patient is in question.
      (3) Help the patient obtain necessary care.
      (4) Respect the values, beliefs, and rights of the patient.
      (5) Provide education and support to help the patient or the patient's designated surrogate make decisions.
      (6) Represent the patient in accordance with the patient's choices.
      (7) Support the decisions of the patient or the patient's designated surrogate or transfer care to an equally qualified critical care nurse.
      (8) Intercede for patients who cannot speak for themselves in situations that require immediate action.
      (9) Monitor and safeguard the quality of care the patient receives.
      (10) Act as liaison between the patient, the patient's family, and health care professionals.
2. Moral agency: ability to serve as a moral agent in identifying and resolving ethical and clinical concerns (Curley, 1998)

3. Ethics: systems of valued behaviors and beliefs that govern proper conduct to ensure the protection of an individual's rights; involves judgments that help to differentiate right from wrong or indicate how things ought to be
4. Values: personal beliefs about the truth and the worth of thoughts, objects, and behavior
5. Accountability: answerability or responsibility
   a. Personal accountability: to oneself and to the patient
   b. Public accountability: to employer and to society
6. Ethical principles
   a. Autonomy: an individual's obligation to respect a person's right of self-determination, independence, and freedom
      (1) The nurse must be willing to respect the patient's right to make decisions about his or her own care, even if the nurse does not agree with those decisions.
      (2) Limitations to autonomy include the following:
         (a) When the rights of one person interfere with another individual's rights, health, or well-being
         (b) When there is a high probability that a person may injure himself or others
   b. Beneficence: an individual's obligation to do good and not harm
      (1) Conflicts that may occur include the following decisions:
         (a) What is best for another person
         (b) Who should make the decision
         (c) Long-term or short-term benefit (a temporary harm eventually may produce a greater good)
   c. Nonmaleficence: an individual's obligation to do no harm, intentionally or unintentionally
      (1) It includes protecting mentally incompetent persons, unresponsive persons, children, and any other persons who cannot protect themselves.
      (2) This principle is not absolute; an example of a conflict related to nonmaleficence is when surgical trauma causes a ultimate cure or improvement in the patient's condition.
   d. Veracity: an individual's obligation to tell the truth and not intentionally to deceive or mislead the patient
      (1) This principle is not absolute; an example of a conflict related to veracity is when telling the patient the truth may cause harm.
   e. Justice: an individual's obligation to be fair to all persons
      (1) Individuals have the right to be treated fairly and equally regardless of race, sex, marital status, medical diagnosis, social standing, economic level, or religious belief; this also includes equal access to health care for all.
   f. Paternalism: an individual's obligation to assist an person to make a decision when that person does not have sufficient data or expertise
      (1) Undesirable when the entire decision if taken away from the patient
   g. Fidelity: an individual's obligation to be faithful or loyal to agreements and responsibilities that the individual has accepted
      (1) Fidelity is one of the key elements of accountability.
      (2) A conflict may occur between fidelity to patients and fidelity to employer, government, and society.
   h. Confidentiality: an individual's responsibility to respect privileged information
      (1) Access to patient data is limited to those individuals with a "need to know."
      (2) Others wishing access to patient data must have the patient's permission.
      (3) Information about the patient (status and simply his or her presence in the institution) is limited to those persons whom the patient has identified.
      (4) The patient does have the right to access his or her medical record; if this occurs while the patient is still hospitalized, a nurse should be available to explain entries about which the patient has questions.
      (5) The computerized patient record introduces new challenges to ensuring the confidentiality of patient data.
         (a) Never give out your password.
         (b) Never leave a computer terminal unattended on which you have signed in; log off when leaving the terminal.
         (c) Do not allow anyone to view the screen while you are viewing patient data.
         (d) Do not view things that you do not "need to know."

Ethical Approaches: Vary in the Basis for Ethical Decisions

1. Deontology: Actions are right or wrong based on a set of morals or rules.
   a. Emphasizes duty or obligation to another person
   b. Only acceptable ethical theory for decision making in health care
2. Teleology: Actions are right or wrong based on the action's consequences and usefulness; it looks at outcome; the end justifies the means.
3. Utilitarianism: The morally right thing to do is whatever produces the greatest good for the greatest number; it is derived from teleology.
4. Egoism: Actions are right or wrong based on self-interest and self-preservation.
5. Paternalism: Beneficence should take precedence over autonomy.
6. Social contract theory: People give up some rights to a government to receive social order. Right to the greatest degree of liberty possible.
7. Natural law: Actions are morally or ethically right when they are in accord with human nature.

Moral Distress

Moral distress is when one knows the right thing to do but cannot pursue the right action; obstacles may be internal or external.

1. The Four As to Rise Above Moral Distress (AACN, 2004)
   a. Ask: Determine whether the nurse is experiencing moral distress.
      (1) Expressions of anger, resentment, or frustration
      (2) Statements such as "why are we doing this?"
      (3) Physical symptoms such as change in weight, sleep patterns, or depression
   b. Affirm.
      (1) Affirm the distress.
      (2) Affirm professional obligations as described in the ANA Code of Ethics for Nurses.
   c. Assess.
      (1) Identify sources and severity of moral distress.
      (2) Identify barriers, risks, and strengths.
   d. Act: based on self-exploration regarding obligations, responsibilities, and risks.

Ethical Dilemmas

Ethical dilemmas are situations that require a choice between two or more equally undesirable alternatives.

1. Characteristics of an ethical dilemma (Curtin, 1982)
   a. The problem cannot be solved using only empirical data.
   b. The problem is so perplexing that it is difficult to decide what facts and data should be used to make the decision.
   c. There are far-reaching effects to the decision.
2. Conflicts related to rights of the individual: autonomy versus paternalism
   a. Informed consent
   b. Technology versus quality of life
   c. Resuscitate versus do not resuscitate
   d. Behavior control
      (1) Behavior control may be misused to suppress personal freedom (e.g., use of restraints or sedating drugs).
      (2) Individual's right to freedom may conflict with society's obligation to maintain social order.
3. Conflicts related to resource allocations: justice versus utilitarianism
   a. Triage decisions
   b. Quality of life decisions
   c. Inability to pay and/or lack of health insurance
   d. Organ transplantation decisions
      (1) Living donors: rights of donor, recipient, families, society
      (2) Choice of one recipient over another: potential for elitism
      (3) Use of health care resources: tremendous cost of organ transplantation
      (4) Designation of death: when can an organ or organs be removed
4. Conflicts related to the role of the nurse: veracity versus fidelity
   a. Withholding therapy
   b. Right to die
      (1) Positive euthanasia (also referred to as *active euthanasia* or *mercy killing*): life support systems are withdrawn or a medication, treatment, or procedure is used to cause death (e.g., assisted suicide)
      (2) Negative euthanasia (also referred to as *passive euthanasia*): no extraordinary or heroic life support measures are used to save a person's life (e.g., do-not-resuscitate orders)
5. Conflicts related to personal values: professional integrity versus personal ethical and moral beliefs
   a. Nurse participation in treatments or therapies against the nurse's ethical or moral beliefs (e.g., abortion)
   b. Nurse providing care for patients whose practices are against nurse's ethical or moral beliefs (e.g., domestic violence)

Factors Affecting Ethical Issues and Ethical Decision Making

See Figure 12-2.

Ethical Decision Making Process

1. Collect, analyze, and interpret the data.
2. State the dilemma as clearly as possible.
3. Identify the ethical principles involved in the dilemma.
4. Consider whether this dilemma can be resolved or influenced by the nurse.
5. Examine all possible solutions to the dilemma.
6. Evaluate the likely outcome of each solution and the advantages and consequences of each solution.
7. Choose the solution with the outcome most consistent with personal values and ethical principles.
8. Carry out the decision.
9. Evaluation the impact of the action.

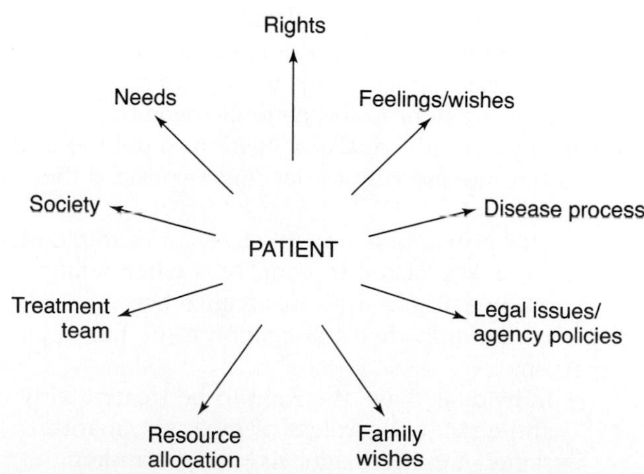

Figure 12-2 Factors affecting ethical issues and ethical decision making in nursing. (From Kinney, M., Dunbar, S., Brooks-Brunn, J. A., Molter, N., & Vitello-Cicciu, J. [1998]. *AACN clinical reference for critical care nursing* [4th ed.]. St. Louis: Mosby.)

Ethical Codes

Ethical codes are guidelines that outline the nurse's responsibility to the patient, to the employer, and to society.

1. ANA Ethical Code for Nurses (Box 12-1)

Rights

1. Ethical rights (moral rights)
   a. Based on moral or ethical principle
   b. Backed by general opinion of society or culture
   c. Often privileges are allotted to certain individuals or groups of individuals
2. Legal rights: life, liberty, property, individual freedoms, due process
   a. Based on a legal entitlement to some good or benefit
   b. Guaranteed by laws, and if violated, can be upheld in the legal system
3. Entitlements: statutory rights for a defined group (e.g., Medicare)
4. The American Hospital Association Patient's Bill of Rights has been replaced by a patient information brochure titled *The Patient Care Partnership,* which identifies the following expectations during a hospital stay (American Hospital Association, 2003):
   a. High-quality hospital care
   b. A clean and safe environment
   c. Involvement in your care
   d. Protection of your privacy
   e. Help with your bill and filing insurance claims

BOX 12-1 American Nurses Association Code of Ethics for Nurses

1. The nurse, in all professional relationships, practices with compassion and respect for the inherent dignity, worth, and uniqueness of every individual, unrestricted by considerations of social or economic status, personal attributes, or the nature of health problems.
2. The nurse's primary commitment is to the patient, whether an individual, family, group, or community.
3. The nurse promotes, advocates for, and strives to protect the health, safety, and rights of the patient.
4. The nurse is responsible and accountable for individual nursing practice and determines the appropriate delegation of tasks consistent with the nurse's obligation to provide optimum patient care.
5. The nurse owes the same duties to self as to others, including the responsibility to preserve integrity and safety, to maintain competence, and to continue personal and professional growth.
6. The nurse participates in establishing, maintaining, and improving health care environments and conditions of employment conducive to the provision of quality health care and consistent with the values of the profession through individual and collective action.
7. The nurse participates in the advancement of the profession through contributions to practice, education, administration, and knowledge development.
8. The nurse collaborates with other health professionals and the public in promoting community, national, and international efforts to meet health needs.
9. The profession of nursing, as represented by associations and their members, is responsible for articulating nursing values, for maintaining the integrity of the profession and its practice, and for shaping social policy.

From American Nurses Association. (2001). *Code of ethics for nurses with interpretative statements.* Washington, DC: American Nurses Publishing.

Legal Issues

1. Sources of law
   a. A constitution establishes the basis of a governing system.
   b. Statutes are laws that govern.
      (1) Made, voted on, and passed by legislative bodies
      (2) Nurse practice acts are statutes:
         (a) Define and limit the practice of nursing
         (b) May vary state to state, but all must be consistent with federal provisions and statutes
   c. Administrative agencies (e.g., state boards of nursing) create rules and regulations that enforce statutory laws.
   d. Court decisions are made when the courts interpret legal issues that are in dispute.
   e. Common law consists of board and comprehensive principles based on justice, reason, and common sense rather than rules and regulations.
2. Types of court cases
   a. Criminal: charges filed by the state or federal attorney general for crimes committed against an individual or society
      (1) Burden of proof is on the filing agency; the defendant is presumed innocent and must be proved guilty beyond a reasonable doubt.
      (2) Consequences if found guilty are imprisonment or even death.
      (3) An example would be a nurse who intentionally administered drugs that caused a patient's death.
   b. Civil: one individual sues another
      (1) Burden of proof to be found guilty is a preponderance of the evidence.
      (2) Consequences are monetary.
      (3) An example would be a nurse sued for wrongful death because the nurse failed to do something that would have prevented the death.
      (4) Intentional torts
         (a) Definition: A tort is a legal wrong committed against a person or property, independent of a contract, that renders the person who commits it liable for damages in a civil action; an intentional tort is a direct invasion of someone's legal rights.
         (b) Examples include assault, battery, false imprisonment, invasion of privacy, defamation, and slander.

c. Administrative: charges filed by a state or federal governmental agency (e.g., state board of nursing)
   (1) Burden of proof to be found guilty is a preponderance of the evidence.
   (2) Consequences may be monetary, disciplinary, or loss of privileges (e.g., professional license).
   (3) An example would be failure to obtain a new license at the predetermined time.

3. Malpractice (i.e., professional negligence)
   a. Definition: the omission to do something that a reasonable and prudent professional would do or as doing something that a reasonable and prudent professional would not do; an unintentional tort
      (1) Reasonable and prudent: average judgment, foresight, intelligence, and skill that would be expected of a person with similar training and experience
   b. Elements that must be present for a professional to be held liable for malpractice
      (1) Duty: the nurse had a duty to provide care and follow an acceptable standard of care
      (2) Breach: there was a breach of duty (i.e., the nurse failed to adhere to the standard of care)
      (3) Causation: the failure to meet the standard of care must have caused injury to the patient
      (4) Damages: the patient must have suffered injuries as a result of the nurse's breach of duty
   c. Avoidance of malpractice claims (Marquis & Huston, 2006)
      (1) Practice within the scope of the Nursing Practice Act of your state.
      (2) Follow the policies and procedures of your institution.
      (3) Model your practice after established practice standards.
      (4) Make patients' rights and welfare the priority.
      (5) Make rational decisions based on the biologic, psychological, and social sciences and be aware of laws and legal doctrines.
      (6) Practice within your area of competence.
      (7) Continue to update and upgrade your technical skills and seek specialty certification.
      (8) Purchase professional liability insurance and know the limits of your policy.
      (9) Document thoroughly in the patient's record and incident reports.
         (a) Document
            (i) Patient status with factual observations along with time, date, and signature (may be electronic signature)
            (ii) Any deviations from standard practice and reasons for such deviations
            (iii) Notification of physician for changes in status and the physician's response
         (b) Common problems made in documentation
            (i) Omissions without explanation
            (ii) Vague and ambiguous language
            (iii) Unapproved abbreviations
            (iv) Error correction
            (v) Spelling and grammar errors
            (vi) Illegibility
   d. Remember that patients are health care consumers and that they want good service; try to exceed your patient's expectations

4. Consent
   a. Blanket consent: The person gives permission for routine and customary care; this type of consent is required before admission.
   b. Informed consent: The person gives consent for a specific procedure after being informed and understanding the following:
      (1) Explanation of the treatment/procedure
      (2) Expected results/benefits
      (3) Risks involved
      (4) Alternatives including absence of treatment
      (5) Name of person performing the treatment/procedure
      (6) Disclosure that the patient may withdraw consent at any time
   c. Implied consent: Patient is unable to sign, but treatment is needed immediately and the treatment is in the patient's best interest.
   d. Express consent: Though the person who will perform the procedure is responsible for obtaining the consent, the nurse may be asked to have the patient sign a consent form.
      (1) The patient signed the form.
      (2) The patient knows what he or she is consenting to by signing the consent form; the nurse has an ethical responsibility to notify the person who will perform the procedure if the nurse believes that the patient does not understand the procedure.

5. Incident reports
   a. These are internal documents completed for any unusual occurrence, including errors.
   b. These reports should include facts about the incident and care given to the patient such as diagnostic studies, medications, and consults.
   c. Avoid statements of guilt or blame in the incident report and do not allude to the incident report in the patient's chart.
   d. A national trend is to disclose fully all errors to the patient, and some studies have found fewer lawsuits when the patient was informed of the error.

6. Terms related to end-of-life care
   a. Advance directive: a legal document that expresses what the patient prefers related to end-of-life issues
      (1) Must be developed by a competent adult (i.e., 18 years of age or older)
      (2) Must be witnessed by two persons

(3) May be revoked verbally, in writing, or by destruction of the document at any time
(4) Becomes effective when the person is certified by two physicians to be terminally ill or to have an irreversible condition with loss of decision-making capability
(5) Does not contraindicate the use of treatments for pain or suffering

b. Living will: an advance directive that expresses what the patient wants done if the patient becomes terminally ill and is not able to make health care decisions

c. Durable power of attorney for health care: an advance directive that designates someone to make health care decisions for the patient if the patient is unable to make the decisions

Caring Practices

Description

Caring practices are the nursing activities that are responsive to the uniqueness of the patient and family and that create a compassionate and therapeutic environment, with the aim of promoting comfort and preventing suffering (AACN Certification Corporation, 2005).

The Critically Ill Patient

1. Psychosocial characteristics of the healthy adult (Erikson, 1968)
   a. Young adulthood (18 to 40 years of age)
      (1) Intimacy versus self-isolation or self-absorption
      (2) Developmental tasks
         (a) Accepts self
         (b) Establishes independence
         (c) Establishes a vocation to make worthwhile contributions
         (d) Learns to appraise and express love responsibly
         (e) Establishes intimate bond with another
         (f) Establishes and manages residence
         (g) Finds congenial social group
         (h) Decides on option of a family
         (i) Formulates philosophy of life
         (j) Establishes role in community
   b. Middle adulthood (40 to 60 years of age)
      (1) Generativity versus self-absorption and stagnation
      (2) Developmental tasks
         (a) Develops new satisfaction as a mate
         (b) Supportive to mate
         (c) Develops sense of unity with mate
         (d) Assists offspring to become happy, responsible adults
         (e) Takes pride in accomplishments of self and mate
         (f) Balances work with other roles; assists aging parents
         (g) Achieves social and civic responsibility
         (h) Maintains active organizational membership
         (i) Accepts physical changes of middle age
         (j) Makes an art of friendship
         (k) Balances leisure with service pursuits
         (l) Develops more depth of personal philosophy by reevaluating values and examining assets
   c. Older adulthood (60 years of age to death)
      (1) Integrity versus despair
      (2) Developmental tasks
         (a) Continued self-development
         (b) Adapting to family responsibilities
         (c) Maintaining self-worth, pride, and usefulness
         (d) Dealing with loss of spouse, friends, upcoming end to life
2. Basic human needs
   a. Basic needs may be the same, but the manner in which they are fulfilled depends on personal abilities, environment, and life experience.
   b. Maslow's hierarchy of needs (Maslow, 1968) is progressive; primary needs must be met before dealing with higher level needs (Table 12-1).
3. Human needs of the critically ill patient (Figure 12-3)

Psychosocial Responses to the Critical Illness and Critical Care Environment

1. Stress
   a. Definition: mental, emotional, or physical tension or strain
   b. Two types: distress (to noxious stimuli) and eustress (to nonthreatening stimuli)
   c. Admission to a critical care unit is frightening and anxiety producing
   d. Sensory deprivation and sensory overload are stress factors within a critical care unit
   c. Interventions to decrease or eliminate stress
      (1) Maintaining a calm, restful environment
      (2) Providing for as much independence of the patient as possible
      (3) Providing contact with reality and outside world
      (4) Encourage use of coping mechanisms (Table 12-2)

Table 12-1 Maslow's Hierarchy of Needs

Level	Needs
Physiologic	Oxygen, food, water, sleep
Safety and security	Protection; freedom from anxiety
Love and belonging	Freedom from loneliness and alienation
Esteem and recognition	Freedom from sense of worthlessness, inferiority, and helplessness
Self-actualization	Aesthetic needs, self-fulfillment, creativity, spirituality

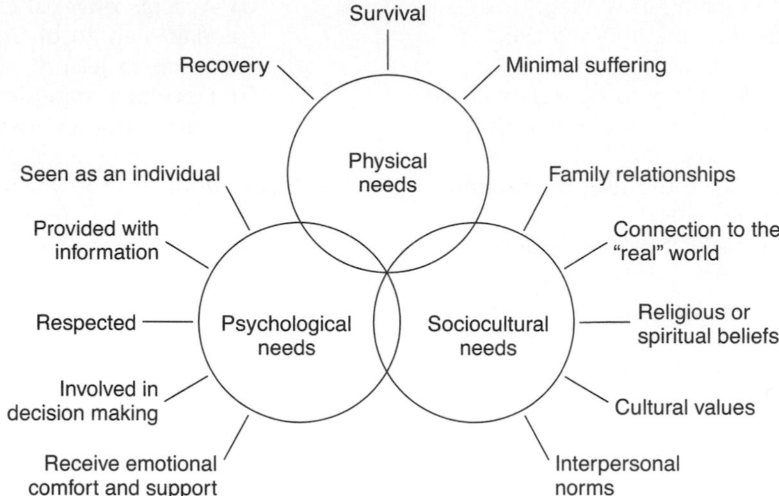

Figure 12-3 Human needs of the critically ill patient. (From Kinney, M., Dunbar, S., Brooks-Brunn, J. A., Molter, N., & Vitello-Cicciu, J. [1998]. *AACN clinical reference for critical care nursing* [4th ed.]. St. Louis: Mosby.)

2. Crisis
   a. Definition: an acute state of stress in which the person feels overwhelmed by stressors
      (1) Involves an attempt to regain equilibrium
      (2) Self-limited and allows for growth
   b. May be maturational, adventitious, or situational in focus
      (1) Maturational: arises as a result of growth and development and involves changes in self-concept and roles
      (2) Adventitious: follows accidental and uncommon events leading to major environmental changes (e.g., natural disasters)
      (3) Situational: follows an external event or experience and its associated losses and changes
   c. Stages
      (1) Shock and disbelief
      (2) Disorganization: may be demanding, irrational, angry
      (3) Reorganization: difficulty making decisions, forced to confront critical questions
      (4) Resolution

Table 12-2 Coping Mechanisms to Stress

Type	Example
Action	Taking walks, cleaning house, gardening, singing
Cognitive	Problem solving, reading about an issue
Spiritual	Prayer
Interpersonal	Talking with support person
Emotional	Use of psychological defense mechanisms (see Table 12-3)

Table 12-3 Psychological Defense Mechanisms

Defense Mechanism	Description
Suppression	Conscious, deliberate forgetting of unacceptable or painful thoughts, impulses, feelings, or acts
Repression	Unconscious, involuntary forgetting of unacceptable or painful thoughts, impulses, feelings, or acts
Denial	Treating obvious reality factors as though they do not exist because they are consciously intolerable
Rationalization	Attempting to justify feelings, behavior, and motives that otherwise would be intolerable by offering a socially acceptable, intellectual, and apparently logical explanation for an act or decision
Compensation	Making extra effort to achieve in one area to offset real or imagined deficiencies in another area
Sublimation	Directing energy from unacceptable drives into socially acceptable behavior
Projection	Unconsciously attributing one's own unacceptable qualities and emotions to others
Regression	Going back to an earlier level of emotional development and organization
Withdrawal	Separating oneself from interpersonal relationships in order to avoid emotional expression or responsiveness

d. Interventions to assist the patient in crisis
   (1) Listen to the patient's perception of the situation
   (2) Encourage the patient to express his or her feelings about the situation
   (3) Assist the patient to gain an understanding of the situation by discussing losses and positive outcomes
   (4) Assist the patient in developing a viable solution

3. Fear/anxiety
   a. Definition: fear is an unpleasant feeling specific to a known threat; anxiety is an unpleasant feeling to an unknown threat.
   b. Anxiety can produce psychological and physiologic symptoms; manifestations may include restlessness, irritability, increase in questions, insomnia, tachycardia, and tremors.
   c. Interventions to decrease feelings of fear and anxiety
      (1) Communicate honestly and empathetically.
      (2) Refer patient to psychologist, psychiatric liaison nurse, or chaplain if appropriate.
      (3) Identify adaptive and maladaptive coping mechanisms being used.
      (4) Encourage expression of fears and concerns.
      (5) Reduce sensory overload.
      (6) Teach relaxation and imagery techniques.
      (7) Encourage the patient to ask questions.
      (8) Encourage the patient to participate in his or her care.
      (9) Explore the patient's desire for spiritual or psychological counseling.
4. Loneliness
   a. Definition: discomfort caused by separation from significant relationships, places, events, and objects
   b. Manifestations may include crying and withdrawal
   c. Interventions to decrease loneliness
      (1) Encourage participation in decision making and self-care.
      (2) Encourage discussion of fears and to ask questions.
      (3) Encourage the patient to talk about his or her life, family, work, or pet.
      (4) Ask the family to bring in familiar and loved objects.
5. Powerlessness
   a. Definition: a perceived lack of control over the outcome of a specific situation or problem and the patient's perception that any action he or she takes will not affect the outcome
   b. May be manifested by apathy, withdrawal, resignation, fatalism, lack of decision making, aggression, or anger
   c. Interventions to decrease feelings of powerlessness
      (1) Recognize the potential for feelings of powerlessness; particularly at risk are individuals who are usually in a position of power or control in their daily life.
      (2) Support the patient's sense of control by offering alternatives related to activity times, treatment times, diet, routine hygiene, diversionary activities, and visitation.
      (3) Assist the patient in identifying activities that he or she can perform independently.
      (4) Keep the patient informed about his or her treatment.
      (5) Encourage the patient's involvement in decision making related to treatment.
      (6) Increase the patient's control as his or her condition improves.
6. Sensory overload
   a. Definition: increased frequency and intensity of stimulation of the senses with nonmeaningful stimuli
   b. Contributing factors: constant noise and lights, alarms, chatter of unfamiliar voices
   c. Intervention: eliminate or limit nonmeaningful sensory stimulation
7. Sensory deprivation
   a. Definition: decreased frequency, intensity, or variety of stimulation of the senses with meaningful stimuli
   b. Contributing factors: absence of windows, clocks, calendars; constant noise, lights, technical language, lack of familiar faces; deprivation of familiar touches, sounds, smells, and tastes of the usual environment
   c. Interventions
      (1) Encourage family visitation.
      (2) Encourage the family to bring familiar objects to the hospital.
      (3) Place calendar and clock where the patient can see them.
8. Anger
   a. Definition: feeling of great displeasure, hostility, exasperation
   b. May be manifested by clenching of teeth or muscles, avoidance of eye contact, sarcasm, insulting comments, screaming, argumentativeness, demanding behavior
   c. Interventions to decrease feelings of anger
      (1) Assist in identifying the cause of anger.
      (2) Give the patient permission to be angry.
      (3) Assist the patient in identifying appropriate ways to express the anger.
9. Depression
   a. Definition: feeling of sadness, hopelessness
   b. May be manifested by loss of interest in people, dissatisfaction, difficulty making decisions, crying; may say that he or she is a failure, that he or she is being punished, or that he or she is considering hurting himself or herself
   c. Interventions to decrease feelings of depression
      (1) Provide information necessary to identify patient's needs and realistically to visualize the future.
      (2) Inspire hope and facilitate coping.

10. Denial
    a. Definition: refusal to acknowledge the truth; allows the patient to come to grips with reality a little at a time
    b. Denial may be manifested by shrugging off symptoms; refusing to discuss the illness; appearing cheerful; and verbalizing the illness while ignoring restrictions
    c. Interventions
        (1) Allow the patient to express his or her feelings.
        (2) Do not confront the patient with the truth.
11. ICU (intensive care unit) syndrome
    a. Definition: confusion or psychosis associated with the critical care environment
    b. Also known as ICU psychosis, postcardiotomy delirium, postoperative psychosis, intensive care delirium, acute confusion, and impaired psychological response
    c. Usually occurs after 48 hours in the critical care unit; usually clears within 48 hours after transfer from the critical care unit
    d. Contributing factors include sleep deprivation, sensory deprivation, sensory overload, age, severe illness, history of mental illness or psychological problems, noise, isolation, immobilization, cardiopulmonary bypass, prolonged surgery, electrolyte imbalance, hypothermia, endocrine disorders, and medication
    e. May be manifested by altered consciousness, deceased attention span, disorientation, memory loss, labile emotions, perceptual distortions, hallucinations, paranoia, and combativeness
    f. Interventions to decrease incidence or severity of ICU syndrome
        (1) Reduce the sleep deprivation, sensory deprivation, and sensory overload.
        (2) Provide continuity of nursing staff to lessen the number of adjustments required by the patient.
        (3) Reorient the patient frequently.
        (4) Plan uninterrupted sleep time; do not awaken the patient unless truly necessary.
            (a) In a recent study by Tamburri, DiBrienza, Zozula, and Redeker (2004), the mean number of care interactions per night was 42.6, and patients had 2 to 3 hours of uninterrupted sleep on only 6% of the nights observed.
        (5) Decrease noise level on alarms and decrease extraneous conversation and other noise; earplugs also may be used.
            (a) The Environmental Protection Agency (1974) recommends that daytime noise levels in a hospital not exceed 45 dB and that nighttime levels not exceed 35 dB.
        (6) Adjust lighting to simulate night and day, and maintain sleep-wake cycles while allowing for short naps throughout the day.
        (7) Place a clock and calendar in the room.
        (8) Encourage the family to visit and reorient the patient.
        (9) Encourage placement of personal belongings at bedside.
12. Near-death experience (NDE)
    a. Definition: a vivid series of events reported by some individuals after periods of clinical death
    b. Manifestations include the following events (Sommers, 1994):
        (1) Time interval without feeling
        (2) Separation of mind and body
        (3) Propulsion through space or a long, dark tunnel
        (4) Interaction with a bright light
        (5) Meeting an escort (often a decreased family member or friend) who accompanies them to a warm, peaceful, bright area
        (6) Experiencing a life review
        (7) The choice of whether to go back or being told to go back
        (8) Return to the body
    c. Interventions
        (1) Be alert for indications that the patient has had a near-death experience, especially in patients who have experienced cardiac arrest, electrophysiologic studies, or any life-threatening crisis; the patient may do any of the following:
            (a) Say, "I had the strangest dream," or something similar
            (b) Be angry, withdrawn, or unusually calm
        (2) Provide the patient with an opportunity to discuss the experience, such as, "Did anything happen when you were very sick yesterday that you want to talk about?"
        (3) Explore your own feelings about near-death experience.
        (4) Listen to the patient and avoid judgment.
        (5) Reassure the patient who has a near-death experience that he or she is not "crazy" and that many persons have had this experience.
        (6) Refer the patient to books to read or a support group if available.
13. Death and dying
    a. Definition: dying is a psychophysiologic process that ultimately terminates in death for the individual and grieving for significant others.
    b. Stages of death and dying (Kübler-Ross, 1969; Table 12-4)
    c. Interventions to assist the patient deal with death and dying
        (1) Develop a personal philosophy of death in order to deal effectively with dying patients and living families.
        (2) Do not eliminate hope.
            (a) Hope is the expectation that a desire will be fulfilled.
            (b) Hope aids in the tolerance of pain and suffering throughout the dying process.

Table 12-4 Stages of Death and Dying

Stage	The Patient May Say the Following:
Shock and disbelief	"I can't be dying; you're wrong"; "No, not me"
Denial	"Most people with this disease die, but not me"
Anger	"Why me? What have I done to deserve this"
Bargaining	"If I do this …; let me live till …"
Depression	"What's the use?"
Acceptance	"I'm ready to die"

From Kübler-Ross, E. (1969). *On death and dying*. New York: Macmillan.

(3) Encourage the patient and family to discuss their fears and concerns; listen attentively.
(4) Provide your presence and your compassion.
(5) Provide comfort measures and analgesia.

d. Interventions to assist the family
(1) Allow the family to be with the patient.
(2) Encourage the family to participate in the care of the patient.
(3) Reassure the family of the patient's analgesia and comfort.
(4) Provide information about the patient's status frequently, especially the patient's imminent death.
(5) Encourage ventilation of anxiety, fears, and concerns.
(6) Ensure a private, comfortable area for the family.
(7) Refer the family to other sources of support, such as the chaplain, social worker, or support group.

14. Transfer anxiety
a. Definition: anxiety caused by anticipation of transfer or transfer from one nursing unit to another; frequently most significant when moving from a more closely monitored unit such as a critical care unit to a unit with lower nurse-to-patient ratios
b. Represents the need to start over in developing trust and security with a new environment and staff
c. Interventions to decrease transfer anxiety
(1) Provide opportunities for the patient and family to voice their concerns and fears.
(2) Demonstrate trust in the competence of the receiving nurse and unit.
(3) Emphasize that the transfer is an indication of patient progress.

Pain Management

1. Definition of pain: anything the patient says it is and occurs whenever he or she says it does (McCaffery, 1968)
a. Acute pain: pain that follows injury and ends when healing occurs; example is surgical pain
b. Chronic pain: pain that lasts longer than the normal healing period; example is low back pain
c. Neuropathic pain: chronic pain caused by nerve damage; example is diabetic neuropathy

2. Assessment
a. Self-report
(1) Pain scales
(a) Numeric (0-to-10) pain scale
(b) Wong-Baker faces scale
(c) Verbal graphic rating scale
(d) Behavioral pain scale
(2) Guidelines for teaching your patient to use a pain rating scale (McCaffery, 2002)
(a) Explain the purpose of the scale.
(b) Explain the increments of the scale.
(c) Explain what is meant by "pain."
(d) Ask the patient to give an example of pain to practice using the scale.
(e) Ask the patient to practice using the scale to rate the pain.
(f) Assist the patient to set a comfort goal.
b. Verbal cues: moaning, crying
c. Nonverbal cues: rubbing, splinting, guarding
d. Facial expressions: grimacing, frowning

3. Pharmacologic management
a. Pharmacologic agents
(1) Opioids (e.g., morphine, fentanyl, or hydromorphone)
(2) Nonsteroidal antiinflammatory agents (e.g., ibuprofen or ketorolac)
(3) Local anesthetics (e.g., lidocaine or bupivacaine)
b. Drug delivery methods used in critical care areas
(1) Analgesia
(a) Oral agents, especially sustained-release agents
(b) Intravenous
(i) Continuous infusion
(ii) Intermittent injection
(iii) Patient-controlled: usually consists of a continuous infusion with patient-controlled injection for breakthough pain
(c) Epidural
(i) Continuous infusion
(ii) Patient-controlled: usually consists of a continuous infusion with patient-controlled injection for breakthough pain
(2) Regional anesthesia
(a) Transdermal
(b) Peripheral nerve catheter: delivers local anesthetic directly to the nerve sheath
(c) Intrapleural: delivers local anesthetic directly to the parietal pleura

4. Nonpharmacologic
a. Application of heat or cold
b. Relaxation techniques
c. Distraction (e.g., music, television, reading, needlepoint, coloring, drawing, writing, and visitors)
d. Other complementary therapies are outlined next

Complementary Therapies

Complementary therapies are used with conventional therapies; most are intended in cause relaxation, decrease anxiety, and augment pain management.

1. Progressive muscle relaxation (PMR)
   a. Involves progressive tensing and relaxing of successive muscle groups
   b. Helps the patient eventually to sense muscle tension without having to progress through the tensing and relaxing of successive muscle groups
   c. Decreases stress and anxiety
   d. Frequently accompanied by diaphragmatic breathing
2. Breathing
   a. Involves instruction, practice, and encouragement in the use of breathing techniques, such as diaphragmatic breathing or pursed lip breathing
   b. Decreases stress and anxiety; may improve effectiveness of ventilation especially in dyspneic patients
3. Meditation
   a. Involves intentional concentration and repetition of a word, phrase, or muscular activity
   b. Encourage use of a word or phrase that holds a special meaning for the patient
   c. Decreases stress and anxiety
4. Comeditation
   a. Involves concentrating on certain sounds, images, or words
      (1) An assistant utters the words, which is frequently a script written by the patient
      (2) Efforts are made to synchronize the word with the rhythm of the patient's exhalations
   b. Decreases stress and anxiety
5. Guided imagery
   a. Involves focusing and directing the imagination through the use of specific words and suggestions
   b. Identifies the patient's concept of a relaxing location or situation and verbally guides the patient's thoughts there
   c. Decreases stress and anxiety, decreases fear and anxiety, and enhances the immune system
6. Massage
   a. Involves a technique of controlled touch to manipulate soft tissue
   b. Effects depend on type and speed of movements; pressure exerted by the hands, fingers, or thumbs; and the area of the body being massaged
   c. Decreases stress and anxiety, reduces muscle tension and spasm, reduces edema, and causes release of endorphin to augment pain relief
   d. Aromatherapy and music may enhance the effectiveness
7. Hypnosis
   a. Involves suggestion to enable a person to experience the imaginary as real, allowing deep relaxation
   b. Decreases stress and anxiety
8. Biofeedback
   a. Involves use of conscious mental effort to control involuntary body function, such as blood pressure, heart rate, and respiratory rate
      (1) A biofeedback instrument is used initially to alert the patient to the cues that signal a developing symptom (e.g., tension in neck and shoulders); audible tones are given.
      (2) Relaxation techniques are taught to decrease muscle tension.
   b. Decreases stress and anxiety and causes muscle relaxation
9. Therapeutic (or healing) touch
   a. Involves the transfer of energy from the practitioner's hands to the patient, without actually touching, to potentiate the healing process of one who is ill or injured
   b. Consists of the following steps: centering, assessment, unruffling, modulating, and evaluation
   c. Used to help restore the balance of the energy field and to provide additional energy to be used for healing
10. Purposeful touch
   a. Involves hand holding; stroking or patting a patient's arm, hand, or face; placing one's hand on the patient's shoulder; placing one's arm around the patient's shoulder; or hugging
   b. Also may be referred to as *affective touch, comforting touch,* or *empathetic touch*
   c. Reduces stress and communicates encouragement, support, or affection
11. Music therapy
   a. Involves use of music to soothe and relax
   b. Identify the patient's music preferences; any simple, repetitive, low-pitched music is appropriate for relaxation
   c. The most soothing music has a 3/4 beat; chants, folk songs, and lullabies are relaxing
   d. Causes endorphin release, distraction from pain or anxiety, and relaxation and improves quantity and quality of sleep
12. Aromatherapy
   a. Involves the use of essential oils extracted from flowers, leaves, stalks, fruits, and roots for therapeutic purposes
   b. May be used in massage, baths, compresses, or inhalation
   c. Effects vary depending on the essential oil used; may alter mood, reduce anxiety, cause relaxation, cause decongestion, reduce inflammation, increase circulation, relieve pain
13. Pet therapy
   a. Involves visitation by the patient's own pet or a list of pet visitation animals (usually dogs)
   b. Decreases stress and anxiety; may decrease heart rate and blood pressure
   c. Adhere to specific guidelines to ensure the safety and security of the patient, family, and staff

14. Humor
    a. Humor involves using word and images to elicit laughter.
    b. Humor decreases stress and anxiety, enhances the patient's ability to cope and his or her feelings of well-being, decreases tension in a difficult situation, causes endorphin release, augments the immune system, and causes muscle relaxation.
    c. Conduct a humor assessment to determine the patient's receptiveness to humor and which type of humor is appropriate or inappropriate.
    d. Timing of humor is crucial; humor may be inappropriate during a crisis or laughing may cause pain.
    e. Some forms of humor are inappropriate, such as humor that demeans (e.g., racial or ethnic jokes) or sexually oriented humor (e.g. "dirty" jokes).
15. Acupuncture
    a. Involves the insertion of needles into specific points in the body for therapeutic purposes; may also involve use of heat (moxibustion), pressure (acupressure), or electromagnetic energy to stimulate acupuncture points
    b. Causes endorphin release and decrease in pain

The Family of the Critically Ill Adult

1. Assessment
    a. Availability of family
    b. Structure and communication patterns within the family
        (1) Role of patient within family
        (2) Primary decision maker
        (3) Family spokesperson
        (4) Conflicts within the family
    c. Perceptions and understanding
        (1) Knowledge of patient condition
        (2) Past experience with critical care
        (3) Past experience with similar health situations (e.g., myocardial infarction or cancer)
        (4) Need for information about the patient
        (5) Expectations of outcome
    d. Coping patterns
        (1) Previous responses to crises
        (2) Usual coping mechanism
    e. Family resources and needs related to resources
        (1) Transportation
        (2) Lodging
        (3) Finances
        (4) Spirituality
    f. Family health maintenance needs
        (1) Dietary
        (2) Hygiene
        (3) Rest/sleep
        (4) Medications
2. Stressors
    a. Observation of a loved one in a life-threatening situation
    b. Overwhelming technology in the critical care environment
    c. Separation from the family member
3. Most important needs of families (Leske, 1991)
    a. To have questions answered honestly
    b. To be assured that the best care possible is being given to the patient
    c. To know the prognosis
    d. To feel there is hope
    e. To know specific facts about the patient's progress
    f. To be called at home about changes in the patient's condition
    g. To know how the patient is being treated medically
    h. To feel that hospital personnel care about the patient
    i. To receive information about the patient daily
    j. To have understandable explanations
    k. To know exactly what is being done for the patient
    l. To know why things were done for the patient
    m. To see the patient frequently
    n. To talk to the doctor every day
    o. To be told about transfer plans
4. Responses
    a. Fear of death, pain, discomfort of their loved one
    b. Anxiety
    c. Financial concerns
    d. Fear of temporary or permanent changes in the roles of the patient and other family members
    e. Severe dysfunction: argumentativeness, aggression, intoxication, guilt, blame, or verbal or physical abuse toward health care workers
5. Interventions
    a. Provide information about the status of the patient; on request, at designated times including during visiting hours, and at the time of any significant change in condition.
    b. Be available during family visitation to answer questions and provide explanations.
    c. Encourage family members to make notes regarding information that the physician or nurse have given or questions that they would like to ask during the next interaction with the nurse or physician.
    d. Encourage the designation of one family member to phone or be phoned who will then communicate to the other family members.
    e. Provide a brochure describing the unit, usual activities, visitation policies, and other useful information.
    f. Introduce yourself and ask names and relationships of family members.
    g. Identify family members by name if possible.
    h. Use touch therapeutically as indicated and allowed by the family members.
    i. Individualize visiting times based on the needs and response of the patient and the family.
        (1) Previous cited concerns about open visiting hours have not been supported through research (Berwick & Kotagal, 2004)

(a) Physiologic stress for the patient
(b) Barriers to the provision of care
(c) Exhaustion of family and friends
(2) In a study by Gonzalez, Carroll, Elliott, Fitzgerald, and Vallent (2004), family members preferred visits of 35 to 55 minutes, 3 to 4 times day, with usually no more than three visitors; patients were satisfied if the visiting guidelines were flexible to meet their needs and the needs of their family members.

j. Explain to the family if visitation is interrupted or postponed by a procedure or crisis.
k. Warn the family and explain the reason for a patient's unusual behavior (e.g., confusion).
l. Encourage the family to touch the patient, hold the patient's hand, and express their feelings.
m. Involve the family in decision making.
n. Encourage family participation in care if they desire.
o. Respect the cultural beliefs and rituals of the family; accommodate these beliefs and rituals if at all possible.
p. Encourage the family members to take care of their own basic needs (eat, sleep, bathe).
q. Provide a comfortable area for visitors close to the unit with bathroom facilities and a telephone; have private area available for family meetings and family-physician discussion.
r. Encourage participation in a support group if available.
s. Be empathetic; empathy is a "special emotion that comes as the result of a close identification and connection with another person" (Dracup & Bryan-Brown, 1999).

6. Family or significant other presence for invasive procedures and resuscitation interventions
   a. Benefits
      (1) Less anxiety about what is happening to the patient
      (2) More likely to believe that everything possible was being done
      (3) Greater ability to provide emotional support to the patient
      (4) Studies have shown that almost all family members would be present again if a similar event were to occur and patients reported feeling comfort and support because the family member(s) were present
   b. Commonly cited concerns that have *not* been demonstrated in research studies on the subjects
      (1) Disruption in the delivery of emergency care
      (2) Adverse psychological effects on the family
   c. Role of family facilitator is recommended (Mangurten et al., 2005)
      (1) Prepares the family and explains that patient care is the priority
      (2) Provides the family with personal protective equipment if appropriate
      (3) Escorts the family members (maximum of two) to the beside and remains with the family to provide comfort measures; facilitates seeing, touching, and talking to the patient; and provides opportunities for asking questions
      (4) Escorts the family member from the room if that person becomes ill, disruptive, or overwhelmed
      (5) Provides debriefing, comfort, and answers to questions after the procedure or resuscitation
7. Guidelines for giving bad news
   a. Present information clearly; ask if there are any questions.
   b. Avoid euphemisms such as "passed" because they may be misunderstood; also avoid platitudes such as "he's better off now."
   c. Be silent if you do not know what to say; offer your presence.
   d. Offer to call the family's pastor, priest, rabbi, or other religious leader; honor the family's cultural and religious beliefs.
   e. Monitor the family for any physical complaints because stress may cause exacerbation of any preexisting condition.
   f. Provide privacy for saying good-bye and assist as the family packs the dead person's belongings; explain what to expect so that they will not be surprised.
   g. If the patient is a candidate to be an organ donor (see Chapter 11), work with the organ donation coordinator to discuss donation and organ procurement with the family.
8. Guidelines for giving bad news by phone
   a. Ask for the closest family member by name.
   b. Introduce yourself: name, title, hospital.
   c. Inform the closest family member of the incident that caused the patient to be brought to the hospital or of a change in the patient's status if the patient has been in the hospital.
   d. Ask if that family member can come to the hospital; suggest that the person come to the hospital with another family member or friend if possible.
   e. Avoid telling the family by phone that the patient has died, but tell the truth if they ask; if the family lives a long distance from the hospital, they need to be informed of the death by phone, preferably by the physician, but it may be the responsibility of the nurse in some situations.
   f. If the patient is a candidate to be an organ donor (see Chapter 11), work with the organ donation coordinator to discuss donation and organ procurement with the family.

Collaboration

Description

"Collaboration is working with others in a way that promotes and encourages each person's contributions toward achieving optimal and realistic patient goals;

collaboration involves intra- and interdisciplinary work with all colleagues" (AACN Certification Corporation, 2005).

Definitions

1. Collaboration: working together
   a. Attributes of an effective team (McGregor as cited in Yoder-Wise, 2003)
      (1) Working environment: informal, comfortable, relaxed
      (2) Discussion: focused, shared by almost everyone
      (3) Objectives: well understood and accepted
      (4) Listening: respectful, facilitation of participation
      (5) Ability to handle conflict: comfortable with disagreement, open discussion of conflicts
      (6) Decision making: usually reached by consensus, general agreement necessary for action; dissenters free to voice opinions
      (7) Criticism: frequent, frank, constructive
      (8) Leadership: shared; changes from time to time
      (9) Assignments: clearly stated, accepted by all despite disagreements
      (10) Feelings: freely expressed, open for discussion
      (11) Self-regulation: frequent and ongoing, focused on solutions
   b. Basic rules to create synergy (Jackson as cited in Yoder-Wise, 2003)
      (1) Establish a clear purpose.
      (2) Listen actively.
      (3) Be compassionate.
      (4) Tell the truth.
      (5) Be flexible.
      (6) Commit to resolution.
2. Collaborative practice: when members of the medical and nursing professions, together with members of other related health care disciplines, work together to ensure quality patient and family care; includes the following critical aspects:
   a. Sharing in planning, decision making, problem solving, goal setting, and responsibility
   b. Communicating openly and respectfully
   c. Coordinating
   d. Cooperating
   e. Recognizing and accepting of separate and interrelated spheres of practice
3. Consultation: process of seeking, giving, and receiving help; may be formal (written) or informal (verbal)

Essential Elements of Collaboration

1. Communication
2. Trust
3. Respect
4. Understanding and acceptance of team members' roles
5. Competence
6. Shared responsibility and accountability
7. Shared goal setting
8. Flexibility
9. Administrative support

Components of Collaborative Practice

1. Unit co-directors: a physician and a nurse
2. Collaborative practice committee
3. Primary nurse and primary physician
4. Autonomy for clinical decision making
5. Integrated patient records
6. Multidisciplinary review of care

Blocks to Collaboration

1. Nurses and physicians
   a. Authoritative (sometimes aggressive) physicians
   b. Nonassertive (sometimes submissive) nurses
   c. Team members satisfied with traditional hierarchy
2. Misunderstanding or lack of understanding regarding the role and practice of professional nursing
   a. Nurses have their own license; they do not practice under the license of the physician.
   b. Physicians cannot discipline or fire nurses employed by the hospital.
   c. Nursing is not medicine; these are two separate and interrelated professions; if an umbrella term is needed, let it be "health care" not "medicine."
   d. Nurses are nurses because they chose to be; it was not because they were not or are not intelligent enough to be physicians.
   e. Nurses have independent functions and dependent functions; they can perform these independent functions without a physician's order (prescription is a much better word than order).
   f. Nursing research has established a unique body of scientific knowledge.
   g. Nurses control nursing practice.
3. Ineffective or lack of communication between the professions
4. Lack of administrative support
5. Systems issues

Strategies for Improving Collaboration

1. Evaluate current interdisciplinary relationships in your institution and on your unit.
   a. Are team members sought out for communication about the patient?
   b. Is communication peer to peer?
   c. Is there recognition of each team member's role in enhancing patient outcomes?
   d. Are team members willing to accept responsibility and accountability for patient outcomes?
   e. What are the steps taken when conflicts arise between team members?
2. Establish a multidisciplinary critical care committee cochaired by a nurse and a physician.
   a. Disciplines have equal representation and decision making.
   b. The committee should deal with issues related to practice, communication, and improving effectiveness or efficiency.

3. Establish multidisciplinary professional activities such as the following:
   a. Rounds
   b. Patient records
   c. Orientation
   d. Education programs
   e. Task forces for problem resolution
   f. Research
4. Establish a professional nursing environment.
   a. Assurance of competency
   b. Knowledge of and ability to articulate the unique role of nursing
   c. Encouragement of professional development of nursing staff

Communication

1. Types of communication
   a. Spoken
   b. Symbolic gestures
   c. Written words
   d. Visual images
   e. Multimedia
2. Rules for good communication
   a. Be clear in your mind as to what you want to communicate.
   b. Deliver the message as succinctly as possible.
   c. Ensure that the message has been understood clearly and correctly; ask for feedback.
3. Pitfalls (Yoder-Wise, 2003)
   a. Advice giving
   b. Making others wrong
   c. Defensiveness
   d. Judging the other person
   e. Patronizing
   f. Giving false reassurance
   g. Asking why questions
   h. Blaming others

Conflict Resolution

1. Types of conflict
   a. Intrapersonal: within a person
   b. Intragroup: between two or more groups
   c. Interpersonal: between two or more persons
2. The conflict process
   a. Frustration
   b. Conceptualization
   c. Action
   d. Outcomes
3. Common strategies
   a. Avoiding: Parties involved in the conflict do not acknowledge it or try to resolve it.
   b. Cooperating: One party sacrifices and allows the other party to win.
   c. Smoothing: Another person smooths the parties involved in the conflict.
   d. Competing/coercing: One party pursues what it wants at the expense of the other party.
   e. Negotiating/compromising: Each party gives up something it wants.
   f. Collaborating: All parties set aside their original goals and work together to establish a common goal.
4. Guidelines for dealing with interpersonal conflict
   a. Communicate with the angry person.
   b. Identify common goals (e.g., quality patient care).
   c. Discuss only one issue at a time; do not bring up old issues and anger.
   d. Discuss facts, not opinions, judgments, or what others are saying; do not make personal attacks.
   e. Communicate with the person involved; do not jump to a higher organizational level.

Delegation

1. Definition: "Achieving performance of care outcomes for which you are accountable and responsible by sharing activities with other individuals who have the appropriate authority to accomplish the work" (Yoder-Wise, 2003).
   a. Direct delegation: The delegation is the result of the registered nurse actively deciding what to delegate.
   b. Indirect delegation: The decision to delegate is the result of organizational protocols that designate specific tasks as appropriate for another to perform.
2. Process
   a. Identify desired outcome.
   b. Identify necessary skills and competencies.
   c. Select the individual or team most capable to accomplish the desired outcome.
   d. Communicate clearly the desired outcome but do not dictate how to get there.
   e. Empower the delegate to complete the task.
   f. Set deadlines and monitor progress along the way.
   g. Provide guidance through the process.
   h. Evaluate performance and reward accomplishment.
3. The five rights of delegation
   a. The right task
   b. The right circumstances
   c. The right person
   d. The right direction
   e. The right supervision
4. Delegation to unlicensed assistive personnel
   a. Recognize what may not be delegated (ANA, 1995)
      (1) Initial and subsequent nursing assessments requiring the professional judgment of a registered nurse
      (2) Determination of nursing diagnoses, care goals, care plans, and progress
      (3) Interventions that require the knowledge and skill of a registered nurse
   b. Be aware of the job description, skills, and knowledge of the individual
   c. Never delegate any task that requires the skill or knowledge of a registered nurse

Systems Thinking

Description

"Systems thinking is the body of knowledge and tools that allows the nurse to appreciate the care environment from a perspective that recognizes the holistic interrelationship that exists within and across health care systems" (AACN Certification Corporation, 2005).

System

A system is "a collection of interdependent elements that interact to achieve a common purpose" (Nolan, 1998).

1. Nursing is one aspect of patient care; nurses must work together, with other members of the health care team, and understand the organizational structure of the institution.
2. The AACN (2005a) is committed to fostering work and care environments that are "safe, healing, humane and respectful of the rights, responsibilities, needs, and contributions of all people—including patients, their families and nurses"; the standards for establishing and sustaining health work environments are as follows:
   a. Nurses must be as proficient in communication skills as they are in clinical skills.
   b. Nurses must be relentless in pursuing and fostering true collaboration.
   c. Nurses must be valued and committed partners in making policy, directing and evaluating clinical care, and leading organizational operations.
   d. Staffing must ensure the effective match between patient needs and nurse competencies.
   e. Nurses must be recognized and must recognize others for the value each brings to the work of the organization.
   f. Nurse leaders must fully embrace the imperative of a healthy work environment, authentically live it, and engage others in its achievement.

Types of Organizational Structure

1. Bureaucracy: formal, centralized, hierarchical
   a. Rules, policies, and procedures ensure consistency and promote efficiency and productivity.
   b. Communication and decisions flow from top to bottom with limited employee autonomy.
2. Matrix: focus on product and function
   a. Hybrid of bureaucratic and flat structures
   b. Sometimes referred to as *product line management*
3. Flat: less formal and hierarchical than bureaucratic organizations
   a. Fewer rules and policies than bureaucratic organizations
   b. Provides authority to make decisions at the point of interaction with the client
4. Self-governance: organizational structure that allows the staff to govern themselves
   a. Sometimes referred to as *professional practice models*
   b. Authority, responsibility, and accountability belongs to the nurse delivering care

Patient Care Delivery Systems: Method Nurses Use to Provide Care to Patients

See Table 12-5.

Delivery of Care Models

1. Patient-centered care
   a. Goal: provide patients a "seamless" health care experience and decrease fragmentation of care; focus is meeting the needs of the patient

Table 12-5 Patient Care Delivery Systems

	Functional Nursing	Team Nursing	Primary Nursing	Total Patient Care
Description	Task oriented; nurses perform tasks (e.g., charge, medicine, and treatments) as assigned	Group oriented; team leader (registered nurse [RN]) with team members deliver care to a group of patients	Patient oriented; nurse is responsible for all aspects of care for assigned patients; accountable for care delivered during entire hospitalization	As for Primary Nursing except that the nurse is accountable for care delivered during the entire shift
Advantages	• Cost-effective • Each person becomes efficient at specific tasks	• Cost-effective • Increased staff satisfaction	• Increased staff satisfaction, though nurses may be dissatisfied with the number of nonnursing tasks that do not require their degree of skill and knowledge • Improved quality of care • Improved continuity of care in primary nursing	
Disadvantages	• Fragmented nursing care • Diminished continuity of care • Diminished staff satisfaction	• Diminished continuity of care • Team leader must have leadership skills, especially effective delegation skills	• Cost-effectiveness questionable since an RN is expensive and is performing tasks that do not require the skill and knowledge of an RN; use of unlicensed assistive personnel to perform nonnursing tasks increases cost-effectiveness • Restricted opportunity for evening and night shift nurses to be assigned as "primary nurse"	

b. Key components
   (1) Care for each patient coordinated by an registered nurse or case manager
   (2) Cross-training of staff to provide up to 90% of patient services
   (3) Assignment of ancillary personnel to patient care units
   (4) Team approach between licensed and unlicensed members
   (5) Location of services closer to the patient
c. Benefits
   (1) To hospital
      (a) Reduction in management layers
      (b) Emphasis on shared governance and self-directed work teams
   (2) To patient
      (a) Interaction with a decreased number of health care providers
      (b) Improved coordination of care to enhance quality of care and increase patient satisfaction
   (3) To society: reduction of health care costs

2. Family-centered care
   a. Definition: "a philosophical approach to care that recognizes the needs of patient's family members as well as the important role that family members play during a patient's illness" (Henneman & Cardin, 2002)
   b. Goal: allow the patient and family members to maintain their normal roles as much as possible, including communication between the interdisciplinary team and patient and family members
   c. Considers the nurse, patient, and family as partners in the care of the patient and the impact of the patient's illness on the family unit
3. Cooperative care
   a. Similar to that of home health care: the patient and the family are in charge
   b. Goal: early self-management by providing patients with a wellness-oriented hospital environment
   c. Hospital environment viewed as an extension of the home rather than as an interruption
   d. An integrated, multidisciplinary health care team focusing on therapeutic care and education allows response to patient's need in a timely manner
   e. Patients have the right and responsibility to participate in their own health care as full partners to maximize their ability for self-management on discharge
   f. Inclusion of the patient's family and support system as care partners during the hospital stay leads to more humanistic hospital care and enhances the potential for improved treatment compliance and self-management after discharge
4. Holistic care
   a. Designed for the chronically ill patient with complex medical conditions that require frequent acute care admissions; addresses the physical, mental, emotional, and spiritual health of the patient and family—mind, body, and spirit
   b. Goal: maximize wellness, minimize complications, and provide an inner peace
   c. Includes common holistic therapies such as relaxation therapy, humor, massage, music, art, recreation, imagery, and pet therapy to reduce physiologic and psychological stress
   d. Characteristics of the holistic team include the following:
      (1) Excellent psychosocial and physical assessment skills
      (2) Informed, flexible practitioners
      (3) Ability to manage without the security of routines
      (4) Mature and refined interpersonal skills and self-awareness
      (5) Knowledge of family theory and the impact of illness on family functioning
5. Transitional care (also known as *subacute care*)
   a. Developed to provide the need for a more cost-effective approach to the treatment of patients with complex medical conditions and rehabilitation needs
   b. Goal: to achieve desired outcomes in a low-cost, humane setting
   c. Severity of the patient's condition requires the following:
      (1) Frequent on-site visits from the physician
      (2) Professional nursing care
      (3) Significant ancillary services
      (4) Outcomes-focused, interdisciplinary approach using a professional team
      (5) Complex medical and/or rehabilitation care
6. Case management
   a. Definition: a strategy to coordinate care, maintain quality, and contain costs (Cohen & Cesta, 2001); though a designated case manager provides comprehensive care for patients with complex health problems, all nurses have case management responsibilities
   b. Tools
      (1) Critical paths: a grid that outlines critical events expected to happen each day of the patient's hospitalization based on the Diagnosis-Related Group classification
      (2) Care Multidisciplinary Action Plan (MAP): a combination of a nursing care plan and critical path

Change Process

1. Change is one constant in health care organizations
2. Types of change
   a. Unplanned: reactive process to change that was not planned
   b. Planned: active process with predetermined goals; intentional, thought-out, mutual goal setting, and equal power distribution; there are many models of planned change (Table 12-6)
3. The change agent: the person who works to bring about the change
   a. Key qualities of effective change agents
      (1) Excellent communication skills

Table 12-6 Selected Models for Planned Change

Author	Steps in the Planned Change Process
Lewin (1951)	• Status quo (diagnose the problem) • Unfreezing (develop the solutions) • Disequilibrium (overcome resistance) • Moving (implement change) • Refreezing (reestablish balance) • Equilibrium
Lippitt, Watson, & Westley (1958) Seven Phases of Planned Change	• Aware of the need for change • Development of a relationship between the client system and change agent • Definition of the change problem • Establishment of change goals and exploration of options for achievement • Implementation of the plan for change • Acceptance and stabilization of the change • Redefinition of the relationships of the change entities
Havelock (1973) Six Phases of Planned Change	• Building a relationship • Diagnosing the problem • Acquiring relevant resources • Choosing the solution • Gaining acceptance • Stabilizing the innovation and generating self-renewal
Rogers (1995) Diffusion of Innovation Model	• Knowledge • Persuasion • Decision • Implementation • Confirmation
Prochaska, Prochaska, & Levesque (2001) and Prochaska (2000) Transtheoretical Model	• Precontemplation: the individual is not thinking of change • Contemplation: the individual is thinking of but not committed to change in the near future • Preparation: the individual intends to change in the near future • Action: the individual actively attempts to change • Maintenance: the individual sustains the change over time
Kotter & Cohen (2002)	• Establish a sense of urgency • Form a powerful guiding coalition • Create a vision • Communicate the vision • Empower others to act on the vision • Plan for and create short-term wins • Consolidate improvements and produce still more change • Institutionalize new approaches
Berwick (2003) From Description to Prescription	• Find sound innovations • Find and support innovators • Invest in early adopters • Make early adopter activity observable • Trust and enable reinvention • Create slack for change • Lead by change

(2) Observational skills to monitor change
(3) Knowledge of group dynamics
(4) Perceptive nature about political issues
(5) Supportive attitude toward change participants
(6) Ability to establish trusting relationships

b. Tips for leading change
(1) Involve all stakeholders in the process of planning for the change.
(2) Share the vision and create goals.
(3) Select a change model; different models will work better for different change processes.
(4) Identify champions among each of the major groups of stakeholders.
(5) Identify facilitators and barriers and adjust your plan accordingly.
(6) Create a detailed plan but be flexible.

Response to Diversity

Description

"Response to diversity is the sensitivity to recognize, appreciate, and incorporate differences into the provision of care" (AACN Certification Corporation, 2005).

Cultural Diversity

1. Definitions
   a. Diversity: those differences that make each person unique; includes national origin, religion, age, gender, sexual orientation, race, ethnicity, education, socioeconomic status, and abilities/disabilities
   b. Culture: the learned, shared and transmitted values, beliefs, and practices of a particular group that guide thinking, actions, behaviors, interactions with others, emotional reactions to daily living, and one's worldview; subculture: a recognizable segment of a larger cultural group that shares some characteristics of the larger group but with unique features of its own
   c. Cultural sensitivity: a learned skill in which a person has an awareness of and appreciation for another's cultural uniqueness; also referred to as *ethnosensitivity*
   d. Cultural competence: "a set of congruent behaviors, attitudes, and policies that come together in a system, agency, or among professionals that enables effective work in cross-cultural situations" (Health Resources and Services Administration, 2001)
   e. Culturally congruent nursing care: use of cognitively based nursing techniques that incorporate an individual's cultural values, beliefs, and life ways; these techniques facilitate, assist, support, and/or enable an individual toward health and well-being or to face illness or death in culturally meaningful ways
   f. Race: a group of persons related by common descent of heredity who have similar physical characteristics such as skin color, facial form, and eye shape

g. Ethnic group: subset of culture; a smaller group that identifies itself as distinct because of shared characteristics, such as culture, language, traditions, appearance, and social heritage
h. Nationality: a people from a place with specified political and geographic boundaries
i. Customs: patterns and practices within a cultural group that encompass collective learned behaviors (includes diet and health behaviors)
j. Rituals: culturally prescribed codes of behavior (may guide practices and decisions including health and wellness)
k. Values: personal standards of what is good or useful in relationship to oneself and to others
l. Norms: commonly shared customs and standards of behavior that are acceptable within a given group of individuals
m. Cultural paradigms: abstract explanation used by a cultural group to account for major life events
n. Enculturation: the process by which culture is transmitted from one generation to the next by means of social learning
o. Acculturation: the process by which an individual or group takes on the behaviors and practices of the dominant culture; factors that influence the degree and pace of an individual's acculturation include length of time in the new culture, age, economic/educational status, and discriminatory practices of the dominant culture
p. Ethnocentrism: the belief that one's own ethnic group, way of life, beliefs, and values are superior to others
q. Cultural imposition: the practice of imposing one's cultural beliefs upon others with the belief that those beliefs are best or superior
r. Cultural relativism: the attitude that the differences in ways of doing things hold equal validity
s. Cultural pain: the discomfort, suffering experienced by an individual or group resulting from the insensitivity of others who have different beliefs and/or cultural norms

2. Significance
   a. Of the developed countries in the world, the United States experiences the greatest increase in population and diversity of inhabitants; immigration accounts for at least one third of the increase.
      (1) The percentage of whites of European origin (the dominant culture in the United States) will continue to decline, creating a more multicultural power base.
   b. Nurses must be aware that issues of culture, race, gender, and socioeconomics strongly influence health status and use of the health care system.
      (1) Culturally inappropriate care and inattention to cultural differences in care may affect health outcomes negatively.
      (2) Individuals from different cultures and illegal immigrants often delay seeking medical attention because of language, cost, and cultural barriers; these delays often result in more serious conditions.
   c. Health care reform is resulting in cultural competence guidelines and enforcement by state agencies.
3. Aspects of cultural sensitivity
   a. Acknowledgment that cultural diversity exists
   b. Avoidance of stereotypes with appreciation of the uniqueness of each patient, with culture as one aspect that enhances the patient's uniqueness
   c. Respect of the unfamiliar
   d. Appreciation that cultural values are ingrained and difficult to change
   e. Modification of care to include consistency with the patient's culture
   f. Examination of personal cultural beliefs and values
   g. Realization that the patient's health practices may be different from yours but that each cultural group has health practices that attempt to improve health and temper illness
   h. Recognition that all persons within a cultural group do not respond to illness the same; there is diversity within cultures
4. Cultural assessment
   a. Assess degree of acculturation (how well language of the dominant culture is spoken, language spoken in the home, length of time in country, and food preferences).
   b. Encourage the patient to discuss cultural beliefs and practices; definitions of health/illness and origin of illnesses may differ within cultures.
   c. Make efforts to respect and understand different communication styles.
   d. Honor time and value orientation.
   e. Provide privacy according to individual's needs; be aware that in many cultures, it is important for family members to be present during assessments.
   f. Identify the decision maker within families; it may be someone other than the patient.
   g. Recognize that patients' reactions to pain are culturally driven.
   h. Be aware of biologic variations among cultures such as body structure, skin/hair color, population-specific diseases, and psychological coping characteristics.
   i. Recognize that dietary/religious practices and cultural taboos have important implications related to nursing care.
   j. Identify hobbies.
   k. Note cultural practices and modify care as necessary.
5. Cultural phenomena affecting nursing care (Figure 12-4 and Table 12-7)
6. Cultural aspects of pain
   a. Pain is not purely a neurophysiologic response; cultural, social, and psychological denominators influence pain.

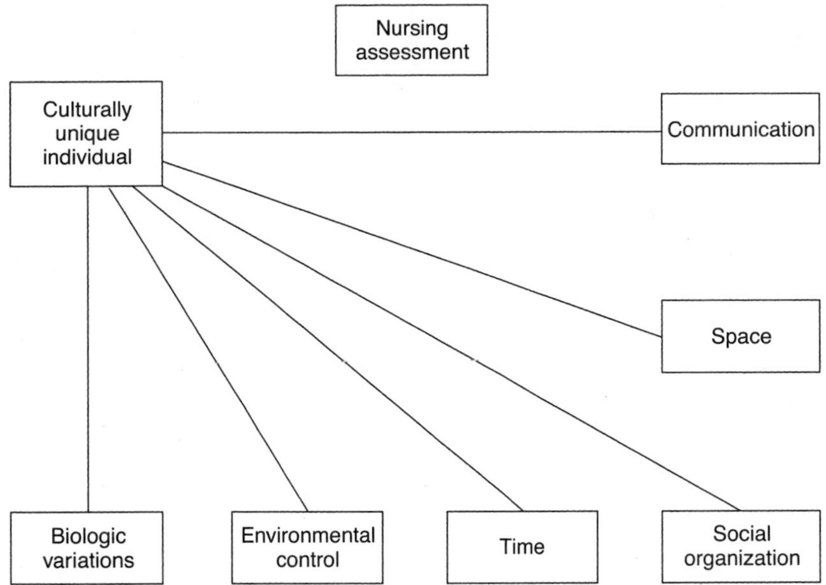

Figure 12-4 Application of cultural phenomena to nursing care and nursing practice. (From Davidhizer, R., & Giger, J. [1999]. *Transcultural nursing assessment and intervention* [3rd ed.]. St. Louis: Mosby.)

b. Pain intensity, expression, tolerance, and expected responses from caretakers are influenced by culture.
c. A patient's attitude and beliefs about pain are determined by culture.
d. Each culture has its own language of distress.
  (1) Facial expressions
  (2) Sounds
  (3) Changes in activity
  (4) Words to describe feelings
e. Nurses must always remember that regardless of the patient's cultural background, pain is what the patient says it is and it occurs when the patient says it does.
  (1) All pain should be considered "real" and treated compassionately.
  (2) Be aware that patients that do not verbally express the presence of pain may not be pain free.

7. Drug polymorphism
  a. Age, drug, gender, body size, and body composition affect individual response to drugs.
  b. Factors that influence drug polymorphism vary among ethnic groups and can be categorized as environmental, genetic, and cultural; these do not include all the aspects that affect patient's response to drugs but raise awareness regarding possible differences in response.
  c. Drug metabolism is genetically determined.
  d. Race may affect response; also called *genetic polymorphism*.
  e. Environmental factors include diet, alcohol, smoking, malnutrition, vitamin deficiencies, stress, fever, and physiologic rhythms; each of these can affect drug absorption.
  f. Cultural factors include values, beliefs, compliance, family influence, and prior drug experience; patients may be taking herbal or homeopathic remedies that can alter response to drug absorption.
  g. Nurses must become familiar with drugs that affect patients of different ethnicity; one example of this is that angiotensin-converting enzyme inhibitors (e.g., captopril) are ineffective or minimally effective in blacks (the new angiotensin II blocker valsartan [Diovan] or a calcium channel blocker or beta-blocker are more likely to be used for hypertension in blacks)
8. Cultural behaviors relevant to nursing care (Table 12-8)
  a. Respect and embrace diversity among patient and health care team members.
  b. Have a cultural reference available on your unit.
  c. Have a list of employees who speak another language and are willing to assist with translation and how to contact them.
9. Problems in providing culturally congruent health care; all of the following issues can lead to poor health outcomes:
  a. Stereotyping, prejudice, ignoring blind spots, and labeling
  b. Personal biases and bigotry
  c. Cultural differences, patients being labeled by nurses as "the difficult patient and/or family"
  d. Lack of interpreters and educational materials in patient's language
  e. Lack of diversity among nursing staff
  f. Lack of time (with culturally congruent care, listening to stories is important)
  g. Lack of flexibility with teaching methods

Table 12-7 Cultural Phenomena Affecting Nursing Care

Nations of Origin	Communication	Space	Time Orientation	Social Organization	Environmental Control	Biological Variation
Asian • China • Hawaii • Philippines • Korea • Japan • Southeast Asia (Laos, Cambodia, Vietnam)	• National language preference • Dialects, written characters • Use of silence • Nonverbal and contextual cuing	• Noncontact people	• Present	• Family: hierarchical structure, loyalty • Devotion to tradition • Many religions, including Taoism, Buddhism, Islam, and Christianity • Community social organizations	• Traditional health and illness beliefs • Use of traditional medicines • Traditional practitioners: Chinese doctors and herbalists	• Liver cancer • Stomach cancer • Coccidioidomycosis • Hypertension • Lactose intolerance
African • West Coast (as slaves) • Many African countries • West Indian Islands • Dominican Republic • Haiti • Jamaica	• National languages • Dialect: pidgin, Creole, Spanish, and French	• Close personal space	• Present over future	• Family: many female, single parent • Large, extended family networks • Strong church affiliation within community • Community social organizations	• Traditional health and illness beliefs • Folk medicine tradition • Traditional healer: root-worker	• Sickle cell anemia • Hypertension • Cancer of the esophagus • Stomach cancer • Coccidioidomycosis • Lactose intolerance
Europe • Germany • England • Italy • Ireland • Other European countries	• National languages • Many learn English immediately	• Noncontact people • Aloof • Distant • Southern countries: closer contact and touch	• Future over present	• Nuclear families • Extended families • Judeo-Christian religions • Community social organizations	• Primary reliance on modern health care system • Traditional health and illness beliefs • Some remaining folk medicine traditions	• Breast cancer • Heart disease • Diabetes mellitus • Thalassemia
Native American • 500 Native American tribes • Aleuts • Eskimos	• Tribal languages • Use of silence and body language	• Space very important and has no boundaries	• Present	• Extremely family oriented • Biological and extended families • Children taught to respect traditions • Community social organizations	• Traditional health and illness beliefs • Folk medicine tradition • Traditional healer: medicine man	• Accidents • Heart disease • Cirrhosis of the liver • Diabetes mellitus
Hispanic countries • Spain • Cuba • Mexico • Central and South America	• Spanish or Portuguese primary language	• Tactile relationships • Touch • Handshakes • Embracing • Value physical presence	• Present	• Nuclear family • Extended families • *Compadrazza:* godparents • Community social organizations	• Traditional health and illness beliefs • Folk medicine tradition • Traditional healers: *curandero, espiritisco, portera, señoro*	• Diabetes mellitus • Parasites • Coccidioidomycosis • Lactose intolerance

Compiled by Rachel Spector, RN, PhD, from Davidhizer R, Giger J: *Transcultural nursing assessment and intervention,* ed 3, St Louis, 1999, Mosby.

Table 12-8 Cultural Behaviors Relavent to Nursing Care

Cultural Group	Cultural Variations (Common Belief/Practice)	Nursing Implications
African Americans	• Dialect and slang terms require careful communication to prevent error (e.g., "bad" may mean "good").	• Question the client's meaning or intent.
Mexican Americans	• Eye behavior is important. An individual who looks at and admires a child without touching the child has given the child the "evil eye."	• Always touch the child you are examining or admiring.
Native Americans	• Eye contact is considered a sign of disrespect and is thus avoided.	• Recognize that the client may be attentive and interested even though eye contact is avoided.
Appalachians	• Eye contact is considered impolite or a sign of hostility. Verbal patter may be confusing.	• Avoid excessive eye contact. • Clarify statements.
American Eskimos	• Body language is important. The individual seldom disagrees publicly with others. Client may nod yes to be polite, even if not in agreement.	• Monitor own body language closely, as well as client's to detect meaning.
Jewish Americans	• Orthodox Jews consider excess touching, particularly from members of the opposite sex, offensive.	• Establish whether client is an Orthodox Jew and avoid excessive touch.
Chinese Americans	• Individual may nod head to indicate yes or shake head to indicate no. • Excessive eye contact indicates rudeness. • Excessive touch is offensive.	• Ask questions carefully and clarify responses. • Avoid excessive eye contact and touch.
Filipino Americans	• Offending people is to be avoided at all cost. • Nonverbal behavior is important.	• Monitor nonverbal behaviors of self and client, being sensitive to physical and emotional discomfort or concerns of the client.
Haitian Americans	• Touch is used in conversation. • Direct eye contact is used to gain attention and respect during communication.	• Use direct eye contact when communicating.
East Indian Hindu Americans	• Women avoid eye contact as a sign of respect.	• Be aware that men may view eye contact by women as offensive. Avoid eye contact.
Vietnamese Americans	• Avoidance of eye contact is a sign of respect. • The head is considered sacred; it is not polite to pat the head. • An upturned palm is offensive in communication.	• Limit eye contact. • Touch the head only when mandated and explain clearly before proceeding to do so. • Avoid hand gesturing.

From Davidhizer R, Giger.J: *Transcultural nursing assessment and intervention,* ed 3. St Louis, 1999, Mosby.

Religious Diversity

1. Definitions
   a. Spirituality: a basic human phenomenon that helps create meaning in the world
      (1) Encompasses a person's ideology, view of the world, and meaning of life
      (2) It gives an individual a sense of inner peace and harmony
   b. Spiritual distress: disruption in the life principle that pervades a person's entire being and that integrates and transcends one's biologic and psychosocial nature
   c. Religion: a specific unified system of an expression of the belief in and reverence for a supernatural power accepted as the creator and governor of the universe
   d. Religious symbols: symbols used in the expression of faith (e.g., rosary, prayer cloth, prayer rug, medicine bundles, red ribbon, charms, and "the garment")
   e. Meditation: a devotional exercise of contemplation
   f. Prayer: an intimate conversation between an individual and God or other Higher Being
   g. Hope: to wish for something with expectation of its fulfillment
   h. Faith: confident belief in the truth of a person, idea, or thing (e.g., God); belief is not based on logical proof or material evidence
2. Significance
   a. Exclusion of the important role of spirituality for patients and families can affect recovery and health.
   b. Care of the whole person enhances healing and health.

c. Spiritual beliefs of providers may be an important consideration for many patients when selecting a health care provider.
3. Causes of spiritual distress
   a. Separation from religious and cultural ties
   b. Challenged belief and value systems
   c. Sense of meaninglessness or purposelessness
   d. Remoteness from God
   e. Disrupted spiritual trust
   f. Moral or ethical nature of therapy
   g. Sense of guilt and shame
   h. Intense suffering
   i. Unresolved feelings about death
   j. Anger toward God
4. Aspects of spiritual sensitivity include the following:
   a. Perform self-exploration of your own values and beliefs.
   b. Acknowledge that you may not agree with every aspect of the patient's spiritual beliefs and practices; be nonjudgmental and respect the patient's right to worship the Supreme Being of the patient's choice.
   c. Develop good listening skills; encourage the patient to discuss spiritual concerns.
   d. Know your limits; if you are uncomfortable discussing spiritual needs with the patient or praying with the patient, contact the patient's personal spiritual advisor or consult hospital chaplain service as requested by the patient and/or family.
   e. Schedule physical care to allow religious rituals and practices.
   f. Respect the patient's rights and privacy.
   g. Increase your knowledge regarding different faiths (Table 12-9 identifies selected faiths and nursing implications).
5. Perform spiritual needs assessment.
   a. Assess the patient's spiritual or religious beliefs, values, and practices.

Table 12-9 Religious Beliefs of Selected Religions and Appropriate Nursing Interventions

Religion	Belief	Interventions
Catholicism	• God does not cause suffering but allows it for furthering human growth. • Baptism is necessary for salvation.	• Inform patient that Holy Communion is available. • Have Catholic priest/deacon available to perform Anointing of the Sick. • If patient is close to death and a Catholic religious representative is not available, any Christian may perform the baptism and then notify the priest immediately. • Make all efforts to leave religious symbols (e.g., rosary) in place.
Christian Scientist	• Sin, sickness, and death can be overcome by a full understanding of the divine principle of Jesus' teaching and healing. • Disease and illness are a delusion of the nonspiritual mind and can be overcome by prayer.	• Be aware that medical care may be refused. • Person may use the services of physicians for the purpose of setting bones, treating malignancies, and delivering babies. • Pain medications may be accepted for severe pain only. • There is no clergy or priesthood.
Hinduism	• Illness may result from misuse of the body or sins from a previous lifetime. • Meditation and prayer must be done at specific times throughout the day. • Females cannot be left in the presence of an unfamiliar male.	• Plan care around religious practices. • Provide same-sex caregivers. • Provide vegetarian meals as requested. • May refuse medication by capsule because many capsules are made from beef. • Allow the family to wash the family member's body following death if desired; do not remove any sacred threads that are placed on the body.
Islam (Muslim)	• Adherents submit to Allah's will in matters of health. • Prayer and washing are required 5 times a day. • The left hand is considered unclean; food will not be handled with the left hand.	• Provide privacy and plan care to accommodate prayer times. • Educate the patient regarding pain-reduction techniques. • Provide diet with dietary restrictions as requested. • Pork and some other foods are prohibited. • Person may refuse to take capsules because many are made from pork. • Follow patient and family wishes regarding therapies; prolonging life by life support machinery is many times seen as unacceptable. • Allow family to stay with relative during process of dying. • Allow family to wash body after death. • Turn deceased person's face toward the right.

Table 12-9 Religious Beliefs of Selected Religions and Appropriate Nursing Interventions—cont'd

Religion	Belief	Interventions
Jehovah's Witnesses	• Opposed to transfusions of blood obtained from a blood bank and some blood products (the source of the soul is believed to be in the blood). • Opposed to eating foods to which blood has been added. • Do not celebrate national holidays (including Christmas) and birthdays, and do not salute flags; it is believed that violators will spend an eternity in nothingness.	• Assess the patient's religious beliefs and practices before administering blood or blood products. • Most Witnesses carry cards indicating types of acceptable transfusions. • "Mature minors," according to Jehovah's Witnesses' standards, may refuse blood transfusions. • Be aware that the patient may refuse surgical or medical interventions that will require blood transfusion. • Consider the use of volume expanders such as saline, lactated Ringer's solution, or hetastarch (Hespan). • Implement blood-conservation strategies, especially in children. • Consult a hematologist and/or medical centers familiar with bloodless medicine and surgery management, if needed. • Respect patient and family decisions to refuse blood products. • Avoid foods to which blood has been added (e.g., certain sausages and lunch meats). • Avoid attempts to involve the patient in preparations for celebrations of national holidays.
Judaism	• Sabbath begins at sundown on Friday and ends at sundown on Saturday. • There is hope for recovery until death is imminent. • May not eat non-kosher foods. • Orthodox Jews: work of any kind is prohibited on the Sabbath, including driving or using the telephone. • Orthodox Jews: prayer required 3 times a day. • A person must stay with a critically ill or dying family member until death so that the soul will not feel alone.	• Provide kosher diet as requested. • Provide privacy and plan care considering prayer times. • Allow a relative to stay with the dying patient. ◦ Notify rabbi/rebbe according to family's wishes. ◦ Caregivers should leave the body untouched for approximately one half hour after death to allow the soul to depart. ◦ After death, by Judaic law, the body cannot be left alone. ◦ Autopsies generally are not allowed unless required by law. • Assist and respect practices of the Sabbath. • Do not shave body hair of Hasidic Jews. • Hasidic/Orthodox: provide same-sex caregivers.
Seventh-Day Adventist	• Sabbath is recognized as dusk on Friday to dusk on Saturday. • The body is a temple of God and should be kept healthy.	• Provide diet with dietary restrictions as requested. • The church encourages a vegetarian diet. • Be aware that patient may avoid seafood, meat, caffeine, alcohol, drugs, and tobacco. • Protein and iodine deficiency may occur. • Be aware that the patient may refuse procedures (medical or surgical) that occur on the Sabbath.

b. Listen for verbal cues regarding spirituality (e.g., referring to God/spiritualist, talking about church, prayer, or synagogue).
c. Note the presence of religious symbols (e.g., crucifix, Star of David, Bible, Torah, Qur'an or other spiritual books, prayer cloth) in room during interview.
d. Listen for expressions of spiritual distress (expressed hopelessness or guilt, crying, sleep disturbances, disrupted spiritual trust, loss of meaning and purpose in life).
e. Be alert to comments related to spiritual concerns or conflicts (e.g., "why me God?" "I'm being punished for my sins").
f. Determine whether there are religious or spiritual practices (such as communion) in which the patient wishes to participate during hospitalization.
g. Identify specific religious concerns such as dietary needs and refusal of blood.

6. Provide care sensitive to the patient's spiritual/religious needs.
   a. Convey a caring, nonjudgmental attitude.
   b. Inform the patient and family of the availability of spiritual/religious services (e.g., pastoral care, chapel, religious services, religious books, communion, baptism, and last rites).
   c. Inform the patient and family of policies related to clergy visitation.
   d. Provide privacy and opportunities for religious practices, such as prayer and meditation.
   e. Prepare the patient for desired religious rituals.

f. Join in prayer or reading of scripture if comfortable.
   (1) If you are comfortable praying with the patient and family, the following suggestions may be helpful:
      (a) Trust God or other Higher Power to enable you to know what to do and what to say.
      (b) Really listen to the patient so that you know what the patient's and family's greatest concerns are.
      (c) Explore the spiritual needs of the patient; ask the patient what he or she would like for God or other Higher Power to do.
      (d) Keep prayers realistic (e.g., comfort versus miraculous healing).
      (e) Be sensitive and respectful.
      (f) Hold the patient's hand or stroke the arm, if culturally appropriate.
   (2) If you are not comfortable praying with or providing other spiritual support for the patient and family, call patient's own spiritual advisor or a representative of pastoral care to pray with or comfort the patient and family.
g. Notify a chaplain or the patient's own spiritual advisor of the patient's spiritual distress (with the patient's permission).
h. Provide honest information to aid in informed decision making when spiritual beliefs and therapeutic regimens are in conflict.

7. Problems in providing spirituality sensitive health care
   a. Avoiding or minimizing the role of spirituality in patient healing
   b. Treating religious beliefs as mental illness
   c. Failure to involve patient and family in decision making
   d. Giving information that can lead to false hope
   e. Not allowing the patient an opportunity to work through grief

Generational Diversity

1. Each generation has a peer personality that lends itself to a collective mind-set (Johnson & Romanello, 2005) (Table 12-10).
2. Avoid overgeneralizing; not everyone in each age group fits the description (or every aspect of the description) of the age group.

Clinical Inquiry or Innovator/Evaluator

Description

"Clinical inquiry is the ongoing process of questioning and evaluating practice, providing informed practice, and innovating through research and experiential learning" (AACN Certification Corporation, 2005).

Table 12-10 Characteristics of Today's Generations

Generation	Born Between	Characteristics
Silent Generation (sometimes called the Veteran Generation) ~10% of today's workforce	1925 and 1942	• Tend to be practical, hard working, thrifty, and disciplined • Possess traditional values • Appreciate conformity, consistency, and uniformity at work and value the system over the individual • Tend to work at large corporations that offer security and reward longevity • Prefer direct orders • Prefer assignments that are structured and task oriented
Baby Boomers: ~45% of today's workforce	1943 and 1960	• Tend to be optimistic, rebellious, and questioning of the status quo • Equate work with self-worth • Are driven and dedicated; willing to work overtime • May be resistant to technology • Prefer facilitation • Prefer assignments that require flexibility, independent thinking, and creativity
Generation X: ~30% of today's workforce	1961 and 1981	• Tend to be skeptical, cynical, and resourceful • Balance work and leisure time; less likely to work overtime • Are more independent; do not belong to any group • Are comfortable with technology • Embrace diversity • Adapt well to change • Attempt to attain several goals at once • Prefer coaching with feedback and credit for accomplishments • Prefer assignments that allow self-direction

Table 12-10 Characteristics of Today's Generations—cont'd

Generation	Born Between	Characteristics
Millennials (sometimes called Nexters or Generation Y) 15% of today's workforce	1982 and 2002	• Tend to be optimistic, assertive, self-confident, friendly • Accept authority and prefer to be led • Are cooperative team players; prefer to work in groups and teams • Have difficulty focusing on one task; prefer to multitask • Are technology savvy • Prefer collegiality and mentoring • Prefer assignments that challenge and stretch their capabilities

Evidence-Based Practice

1. Definition: the integration of the following:
   a. Best evidence
   b. Clinician expertise
   c. Patient values
   d. Circumstances
2. Five-step process for ensuring that clinical decisions are based on best evidence (Sackett, Straus, Richardson, Rosenberg, & Haynes, 2000)
   a. Converting information into clear questions
      (1) PICO format frequently used (Melnyk & Fineout-Overholt, 2002)
         (a) *P:* problem or population
         (b) *I:* intervention
         (c) *C:* comparison intervention
         (d) *O:* outcome
      (2) Remember: the best questions come from clinicians
   b. Seeking evidence to answer those questions
      (1) Published research reports
         (a) Use search engines such as CINAHL, PubMed/MEDLINE, and Google scholar.
         (b) Scour the bibliographies of the articles that you found helpful.
      (2) Unpublished research reports
         (a) Consult known researchers regarding the issue.
         (b) This is important because research studies with statistically insignificant results are frequently not published; either the researcher chooses not to publish or the report is rejected for publication (i.e., publication bias).
   c. Evaluating (critically appraising) the evidence for its validity (truthfulness) and usefulness
      (1) Grading the evidence
         (a) Quality: the aggregate of quality ratings for individual studies, predicated on the extent to which bias was minimized (i.e., level of evidence)
            (i) Study designs
               a) Traditional hierarchy of evidence is based on study designs; note that all grading systems include all of these as valid evidence, especially manufacturer's recommendations and expert opinion, because they are more likely to be biased.
                  i) Randomized controlled trials (double-blinded)
                  ii) Nonblinded randomized clinical trials
                  iii) Nonrandomized clinical trials
                  iv) Prospective cohort studies
                  v) Case control studies
                  vi) Case reports
                  vii) Expert opinion (including consensus groups)
                  viii) Manufacturer's recommendations
               b) Randomized controlled trials are considered the gold standard, but many nursing questions are not answered using quantitative techniques.
            (ii) Sample size
            (iii) Control of extraneous variables
         (b) Quantity: the magnitude of effect, numbers of studies, and sample size or power (i.e., strength of evidence)
         (c) Consistency: the extent to which similar findings are reported using similar and different study designs
         (d) Relevance: the similarity of the study question to the clinical question and the extent to which the findings from the study can be applied in other clinical settings to different patients
   d. Integrating findings with clinical expertise, patient values, and circumstances, and if appropriate, applying these findings
   e. Evaluating performance and the outcomes of the clinical practice

The Cycle of Knowledge Transformation Using the ACE Star Model (Stevens, 2005)

See Figure 12-5.

1. Knowledge discovery: research
   a. Primary goal of nursing research: develop a specialized, scientifically based body of nursing

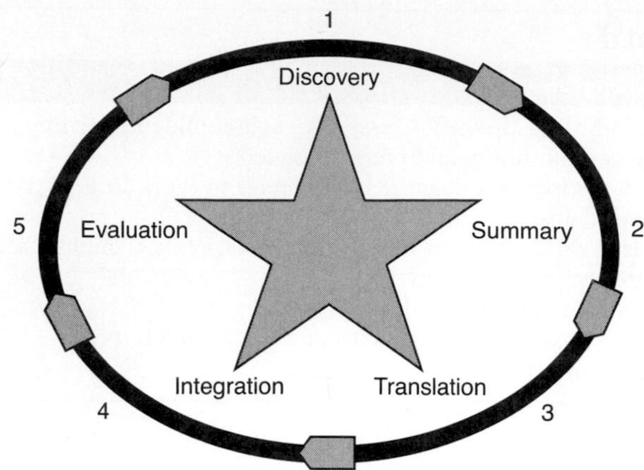

Figure 12-5 ACE Star Model of Knowledge Transformation (From Stevens, K. R. [2005]. *ACE Star Model of Knowledge Transformation*. Retrieved August 6, 2006, from http://www.acestar.uthscsa.edu/Learn_model.htm)

knowledge to facilitate improvement in patient care

b. Definitions
   (1) Scientific method: systematic approach to solving problems that controls variables and biases
   (2) Basic research: research to advance knowledge; helps in understanding relationships among phenomena
   (3) Applied research: research to solve a particular problem; helps in making decisions or evaluating techniques
   (4) Variable: a measurable concept that varies among the subjects in a research study
      (a) Independent variable: the variable that is being observed, introduced, or manipulated in a research study; may be referred to as the *treatment variable*
      (b) Dependent variable: the variable that is being observed for a change after the intervention
      (c) Extraneous variables: variables that are not being studied but may or may not be relevant to the results of the study; these variables can affect the dependent variable and interfere with research results
   (5) Hypothesis: statement that predicts a relationship among two or more variables; may be simple, complex, directional, nondirectional, or null

c. Research types
   (1) Quantitative research: deductive process that tests hypotheses and examines cause and effect relationships to examine specific phenomena; emphasizes facts and data to validate or extend existing knowledge
      (a) Experimental: uses randomization and a control group to test the effects of an intervention
      (b) Quasi-experimental: involves manipulation of variables but lacks a comparison group or randomization
      (c) Nonexperimental
         (i) Descriptive: describes situations, experiences and phenomena as they exist
         (ii) Ex post facto (correlational): describes relationships between variables
   (2) Qualitative research: inductive process used to understand phenomena in a defined contest; emphasizes development of new insights, theory, and knowledge
      (a) Relies less on numbers and measurements and more on nursing strategies, interpersonal communication techniques, intuition, and collaboration between nurse and patient to discover underlying relationships
      (b) Includes case studies, open-ended questions, field studies, and participant observation

d. Steps in the research process
   (1) Formulate the research problem.
   (2) Review related literature.
   (3) Formulate the hypothesis.
   (4) Select the research design.
   (5) Identify the population to be studied.
   (6) Specify methods of data collection.
   (7) Design the study.
   (8) Conduct the study.
   (9) Analyze the data.
   (10) Interpret the results.
   (11) Communicate the findings.
   (12) Use the findings to improve patient care.

e. Ethical responsibilities related to nursing research studies
   (1) Protect the rights of research subjects.
   (2) Ensure that the potential benefits of the study outweigh any potential risk to the subjects.
   (3) Submit the proposed study for review by the investigational review committee.
   (4) Obtain informed consent from each subject.

f. Nursing responsibilities related to research
   (1) Identify problem areas and research questions for investigation.
   (2) Assist in collection of data as requested.
   (3) Read and interpret reports of nursing research.
   (4) Assess the quality of nursing research studies and applicability to practice.
   (5) Apply research findings to change clinical practice and improve patient care.
   (6) Share research findings with peers.
   (7) Design and conduct nursing research.

2. Evidence synthesis: systematic reviews
   a. Definition: a summary of all evidence related to a specific research question using a rigorous method
      (1) Quantitative systematic reviews are conducted using meta-analysis statistical techniques

(2) Qualitative systematic reviews are a descriptive summary of the review of existing studies

b. Advantage to using systematic reviews (Stevens, 2005)
   (1) Preappraised so in more usable form
      (a) For clinicians making clinical decisions
      (b) For policy makers making policy decisions
      (c) For administrations making economic decisions
      (d) For researchers making decisions about future research designs
   (2) Shortens time between research and clinical implementation
   (3) Provides a distillation of large quantities of information into a manageable form with an answer

c. Finding systematic reviews
   (1) Agency for Healthcare Research and Quality: *www.ahrq.gov*
   (2) The Cochrane Collaboration: *www.cochrane.org*
   (3) The Campbell Collaboration: *www.campbellcollaboration.org*
   (4) The Joanna Briggs Institute: *www.joannabriggs.edu.au*

3. Translation into practice recommendations: clinical practice guidelines (CPGs)
   a. Definition: a "systemically developed statement designed to assist clinician and patient decisions about appropriate health care for specific clinical circumstances" (Sackett et al., 2000)
      (1) *Evidence-based* CPGs: explicitly articulate the link between the clinical recommendation and the strength of supporting evidence (Stevens, 2005)
   b. Advantage of CPG: "can help to overcome the barriers to research use because they eliminate the need to search for journal and articles, overcome nurses' limited skills in critical analysis, and minimize the impact of research jargon and unfamiliar terminology because most guidelines are published as clinical application documents" (Ciliska, Pinelli, DiCenso, & Cullum, 2001)
      (1) CPGs may be incorporated into standards of care, care MAPS, policies and procedures, and protocols.
   c. Topic of a clinical guideline
      (1) A condition (e.g., myocardial infarction)
      (2) A symptom (e.g., chest pain)
      (3) A clinical procedure (e.g., percutaneous coronary intervention)
   d. Clinical guidelines: purpose
      (1) Encourage treatment that offers individual patients maximum likelihood of benefit and minimum harm and is acceptable in terms of cost
      (2) Reduce inappropriate variations in practice
         (a) Common reasons for variations
            (i) Variations in clinical decision making
            (ii) Differing approaches to problem solving
            (iii) Varied routines and standards
            (iv) Availability of resources
            (v) Lack of consensus related to appropriate treatment for given conditions
      (3) Promote the delivery of evidence-based health care
      (4) Provide ready evaluation criteria by which health care professionals can be made accountable for clinical performance
      (5) May reduce the cost of health care
   e. Finding CPGs
      (1) Governmental agencies
         (a) National Guideline Clearinghouse: *www.guidelines.gov*
         (b) Scottish Intercollegiate Guideline Network: *www.sign.ac.uk/guidelines/index.html*
      (2) Professional associations
         (a) Sigma Theta Tau International: *www.stti.org*
         (b) AACN: *www.aacn.org*
         (c) Registered Nurses' Association of Ontario: *www.rnao.org/bestpractices/index.asp*
      (3) EBP centers:
         (a) *www.joannabriggs.edu.au*
   f. Tool for evaluation of guidelines: Appraisal of Guidelines for Research and Evaluation (AGREE) Instrument: *www.agreecollaboration.org*
   g. Toolkit for implementation of a guideline: Registered Nurses' Association of Ontario Toolkit for Implementation of CPG: *www.rnao.org/Storage/12/668_BPG_Toolkit.pdf*

4. Implementation into practice
   a. Select an EBP change model (e.g., Iowa model, Stetler model, or Rosswurm-Larrabee model).
   b. Consider organizational barriers to EBP.
   c. Use organizational strategies to facilitate EBP.
      (1) Foster an environment that values inquiry and critical thinking.
         (a) Encouragement of formal education
         (b) Provision of time to read research and evaluate applicability to setting
         (c) Provision of access to the Internet, electronic journals, library, and photocopying
         (d) Provision of opportunities to attend conferences, continuing education, and in-service education including education regarding critical appraisal of research
         (e) Addition of scholarship to the nurse's role so that dissemination through local, regional, and national presentations and publication is encouraged and expected
         (f) Establishment of nursing leadership to spearhead EBP activities, such as a nurse researcher, clinical nurse specialist, or nurse practitioner

(g) Encouragement of the questioning of the status quo and nursing rituals
(h) Development of collaborative teams across disciplines; "EBP is a multi-disciplinary practice" (Gray, 1997)
(2) Communicate the expectation of EBP.
(a) Incorporation of EBP activities in job descriptions, performance appraisals, merit raises, and career ladder promotions.
(b) Leaders asking, "Why are you doing that?" "Why are you doing that in that way?" and "What is the evidence?"
(3) Increase nurse autonomy over practice.
(a) Decentralization of administration
(b) Establishment of shared governance with appropriate nursing department council and committee structures
(c) Establishment of unit-level EBP committees
(4) Eliminate the gap between theory and practice.
(a) Establishment of more joint appointments between academic and practice settings
(b) Appointment of a nurse researcher on staff
(c) Use of expert consultants as necessary
(d) Provision of support for EBP committees and research activities
(e) Development of research presentations (e.g., Nursing Research Grand Rounds)
(f) Establishment of journal clubs
(g) Publication of a monthly research newsletter
(5) Use resources appropriately.
(a) Commitment of expertise, money, and time to EBP activities, including having adequate staffing
(b) Use of systematic reviews and implementation of CPGs

5. Evaluation of the impact of EBP
   a. Patient health outcomes
   b. Patient satisfaction
   c. Staff satisfaction
   d. Cost-benefit analysis

Quality Management and Quality Improvement

1. Goals
   a. Quality management emphasizes achievement of optimal patient outcomes along with the involvement of employees in the process of monitoring quality, identifying problems, and devising solutions.
   b. Quality improvement emphasizes progressive improvement through innovation.
2. Areas of focus (Yoder-Wise, 2003)
   a. Customer rather than provider
   b. Prevention rather than detection
   c. Process rather than individual
3. Principles (Yoder-Wise, 2003)
   a. Quality management is most effective within a flat, democratic organizational structure.
   b. Managers and workers must be committed to quality improvement.
   c. Emphasis is on improving systems and processes rather than assigning blame.
   d. Customers define quality.
   e. Quality improvement focuses on outcomes.
   f. Decisions must be based on data.
4. Quality improvement process
   a. Identify the needs.
   b. Assemble a multidisciplinary team.
   c. Collect data to measure current status.
      (1) Structure evaluation: examine the components of services, such as the setting and environment, that affect quality of care
      (2) Process evaluation: examine activities and behaviors of the health care provider (e.g., nurse)
      (3) Outcome evaluation: measure changes in patients
         (a) The five *D*s
            (i) Death
            (ii) Disease
            (iii) Disability
            (iv) Discomfort
            (v) Dissatisfaction
         (b) Other indicators that are more positive and broader in scope (e.g., functional status and quality of life).
         (c) Clinical indicators should reflect desired outcomes and represent high-quality care delivery.
   d. Establish outcomes.
      (1) Comparison of observed practice with expectations
         (a) Retrospective review: examination of completed health care delivery by reviewing charts, conducting conferences or interviews, and reviewing questionnaires
         (b) Concurrent review: evaluation of a patient's health status (outcome audit) or management (process) while ongoing by chart reviews, interviews, and observation of the patient
      (2) Benchmarks
         (a) Reference points or standards against which performance or achievements can be compared
         (b) Sources of standards
            (i) Internal policies and procedures
            (ii) State Nursing Practice Acts
            (iii) Accrediting bodies (e.g., Joint Commission on Accreditation of Healthcare Organizations)
            (iv) Professional associations (e.g., ANA)

(v) Governmental agencies (Agency for Healthcare Research and Quality)
(vi) Other hospitals

(3) Nursing Minimum Data Set: collection of essential nursing information for comparisons across patient populations
(a) Nursing care
(i) Nursing diagnosis
(ii) Nursing intervention
(iii) Nursing outcome
(iv) Intensity of nursing care
(b) Demographics
(i) Personal identification
(ii) Date of birth
(iii) Sex
(iv) Race and ethnicity
(v) Residency
(c) Service
(i) Unique facility or service agency number
(ii) Unique health record number of the patient
(iii) Unique number of a principal registered nurse provider
(iv) Episode, admission, or encounter date
(v) Discharge or termination
(vi) Disposition of patient or client
(vii) Expected payer for most of the bill

(4) National Database of Nursing Quality Indicators
(a) Developed by the ANA to promote and facilitate the standardization of information submitted by hospitals across the United States on nursing quality and patient outcomes
(b) Nurse-sensitive indicators: those indicators that capture care or its outcomes most affected by nursing care (ANA, 1999)
(i) Mix of registered nurses, licensed practical nurses, and unlicensed staff caring for patients in acute care settings
(ii) Total nursing care hours provided per patient day
(iii) Pressure ulcers
(iv) Patient falls
(v) Patient satisfaction with pain management
(vi) Patient satisfaction with educational information
(vii) Patient satisfaction with overall care
(viii) Patient satisfaction with nursing care
(ix) Nosocomial infection rate
(x) Nurse staff satisfaction

e. Select and implement a plan to reconcile discrepancies between observations and expectations
f. Evaluate the implementation of the plan and the achievement of outcomes

5. Rapid cycle change for improvement
a. The Model for Improvement (Figure 12-6) is advocated by the Institute for Healthcare Improvement for accelerating improvement.
b. The model has two parts (Institute for Healthcare Improvement, nd):
(1) Three fundamental questions, which can be addressed in any order:
(a) What are we trying to accomplish?
(b) How will we know that the change is an improvement?
(c) What changes can we make that will result in improvement?
(2) The plan-do-study-act (PDSA) is a cycle to test and implement changes in real work settings.
c. Selection of members for the process improvement team is critical to a successful improvement effort (Institute for Healthcare Improvement, nd).

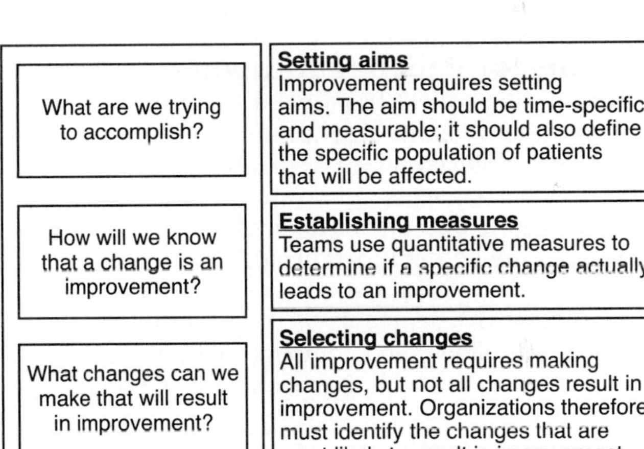

What are we trying to accomplish?
How will we know that a change is an improvement?
What changes can we make that will result in improvement?
Setting aims
Improvement requires setting aims. The aim should be time-specific and measurable; it should also define the specific population of patients that will be affected.
Establishing measures
Teams use quantitative measures to determine if a specific change actually leads to an improvement.
Selecting changes
All improvement requires making changes, but not all changes result in improvement. Organizations therefore must identify the changes that are most likely to result in improvement.

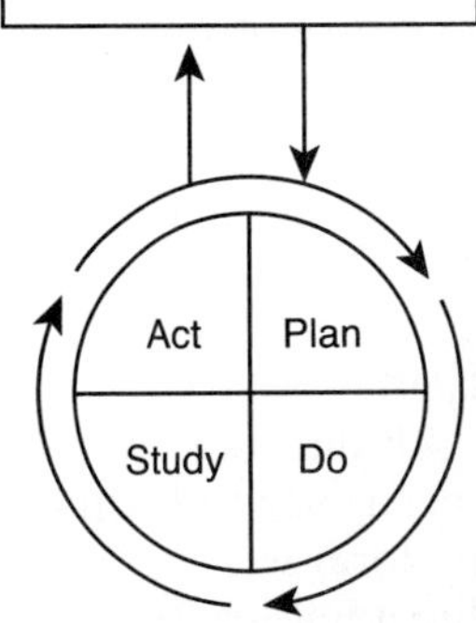

Testing changes
The Plan-Do-Study-Act (PDSA) cycle is shorthand for testing a change in the real work setting—by planning it, trying it, observing the results, and acting on what is learned. This is the scientific method used for action-oriented learning.

Implementing changes
After testing a change on a small scale, learning from each test, and refining the change through several PDSA cycles, the team can implement the change on a broader scale—for example, for an entire pilot population or on an entire unit.

Spreading changes
After successful implementation of a change or package of changes for a pilot population or an entire unit, the team can spread the changes to other parts of the organization or in other organizations.

Figure 12-6 Model for improvement (From Langley, G. L., Nolan, K. M., Nolan, T. W., Norman, C. L., & Provost, L. P. [1996]. *The improvement guide: A practical approach to enhancing organizational performance.* San Francisco: Jossey-Bass.)

Facilitator of Learning of Patient/Family Educator

Description

One who has the ability to facilitate patient and family learning (AACN Certification Corporation, 2005).

Definitions

1. Teaching: the process of facilitating learning; an interaction designed to help a person learn to do something that he or she currently is unable to do; a two-way interaction
2. Learning: the process by which a person becomes capable of doing something he or she could not do before, including a wide range of behavior from motor skills to intellectual skills; an emotional experience that can be negative or positive, traumatic or pleasant
3. Patient education: the process of teaching patients and their families about the illness, treatment, and other health-related matters, including how to adhere to the regimen and helping them change their behavior

Reasons for Patient Education

1. Because the patient has a need and a right to know those things that are relevant to his or her condition, disease, or situation
2. To produce changes in knowledge, skills, attitudes, appreciation, and understanding
3. To promote and improve health
4. To encourage the patient to assume responsibility for disease management
5. To prevent illness and complications
6. To aid in coping with illness and adaptation to change
7. To promote compliance with the therapeutic regimen
8. To reduce anxiety (including family stress and anxiety)
9. To reduce number of physician's office and/or emergency department visits and number and length of hospitalizations

Principles of Adult Education

1. Qualities of the adult learner: a self-directed independent person who becomes ready to learn when the need to know or to perform is experienced; characteristics of the adult learner include the following:
   a. Goal oriented
   b. Less flexible
   c. Requires longer time in the performance of learning tasks
   d. Impatient in the pursuit of objectives
   e. Finds little use for isolated facts
   f. Strives for recognition and success
   g. Has multiple responsibilities, all of which draw upon his or her time
   h. Experienced in the "school of life"
   i. Requires a more constant and ideal learning environment
   j. Usually comes to the teaching program on a voluntary basis
   k. Wishes to be involved in mutual planning of learning experiences
   l. Likes to participate in diagnosing needs for learning, formulating learning objectives, and evaluating learning
   m. Expects a climate of mutual respect, trust, and collaboration that supports learning
2. Educational concepts useful with adults
   a. Pacing
      (1) Allow adults to set their own pace, if possible.
      (2) Tasks or methods involving significant time pressure are likely to be difficult for adults.
   b. Arousal anxiety
      (1) Some degree of arousal is necessary for learning; however, older adults may become anxious in a learning situation.
      (2) Allow individuals an opportunity to become familiar with the situation.
      (3) Minimize the role of competition and evaluation.
   c. Fatigue
      (1) Some tasks may produce considerable mental or physical fatigue, a problem that is likely particularly to affect older adults.
      (2) Shorten the instruction sessions or provide frequent rest breaks.
   d. Difficulty: arrange materials from the simple to the complex in order to build individual's confidence and skills
   e. Errors: structure the tasks so errors are avoided and do not have to be unlearned
   f. Practice: provide an opportunity for practice on similar but different tasks; such practice helps to develop generalizable skills
   g. Feedback: provide information on the adequacy of previous responses
   h. Cues
      (1) Materials should be presented to compensate for the potential sensory problems of older adults.
      (2) Direct attention toward the relevant aspects of the task.
      (3) Reduce the level of irrelevant information to a minimum.
   i. Organization
      (1) Learning and remembering often require that information be grouped or related in some way.
      (2) Instruct individuals in the use of various mnemonic techniques (mental images, verbal associations) that may be useful to elaborate or organize the material.
   j. Relevance/experience
      (1) Individuals learn and remember what is important to them.
      (2) Attempt to make the task relevant to individual's concerns.

(3) Performance is likely to be facilitated to the extent that the individuals are able to integrate the new information with known information.

Barriers to Teaching/Learning

1. Nurse factors: lack of time; lack of knowledge; consideration of teaching as a lower priority than physical care
2. Physician interference
3. Patient factors
   a. Physiologic instability
   b. Psychological factors (e.g., anxiety or pain)
   c. Poor language or reading skills
   d. Sensory deficits: vision, hearing
   e. Poor manual dexterity for psychomotor skills
   f. Attitudes and beliefs that conflict with teaching

Teaching/Learning Process

1. Assessment
   a. Readiness to learn
      (1) Desire to know (e.g., asking questions)
      (2) Absence of acute distress (e.g., pain and dyspnea)
      (3) Adequate energy
   b. Sensory deficits (e.g., use of eyeglasses and hearing aid)
   c. Educational level and reading ability
   d. Learning style
      (1) Environment
         (a) Formal or informal
         (b) Tolerance to distraction
      (2) Alone or in a group
      (3) Preferred learning mode
         (a) Reading: print materials
         (b) Seeing: pictorial materials
         (c) Listening: auditory
         (d) Manipulating: tactile, kinesthetic
2. Plan
   a. Identify objectives; parts of the objective should include the following:
      (1) What should the learner be able to do? (behavior)
         (a) Cognitive
         (b) Affective
         (c) Psychomotor
      (2) How well should he or she be able to do it? (the criteria)
      (3) Under what conditions should he or she be able to do it? (the condition)
   b. Identify content to teach.
      (1) Language and terminology
      (2) Health care system: personnel, organization and structure, routines and procedures, norms and expectations, immediate environment
      (3) Basic anatomy and physiology of affected body system
      (4) Diagnosis, disease process
      (5) Therapy: treatments, medications, diet, activity, personal health habits
      (6) Prevention of complications
      (7) Skills (e.g., insulin administration and pulse taking)
      (8) Community resources
   c. Determine methods.
      (1) Individual or group
         (a) Use an individual method when you are assessing patient's knowledge, when family members or friends try to dominate teaching sessions, when the information you will teach provokes anxiety or is considered a topic not generally discussed in public.
         (b) Individual methods include programmed instruction, reading materials, audiovisual aids, and one-to-one instruction.
         (c) Group sessions lessen feelings of alienation and being "different"; learners learn from other learners.
         (d) Patient-operated groups and self-help groups offer the benefit of encouraging patients to share coping techniques and useful hints.
         (e) Group teaching saves time and money.
         (f) Family members gain support from health professionals and other patients and their families.
         (g) Combinations may be helpful to meet the patient's individual needs.
      (2) Teaching methods: The teacher of adults is a facilitator more than a teacher; use various methods.
         (a) Lecture
            (i) May be in group session, on videotape, or on closed-circuit television
            (ii) Is usually no longer than 20 minutes
            (iii) Includes introduction to establish the need to know, body to deliver content that needs to be known, and a summary to review what was covered
         (b) Discussion
            (i) Helps the patient to ask any questions about information that is in doubt
            (ii) Guides the nurse to assess what the patient needs to know more about
         (c) Audiovisual media
            (i) Includes visual and auditory stimulation to teach content
         (d) Printed materials
            (i) May be used in place of other techniques but should include a discussion with the nurses after reading for clarification of content
            (ii) May be used as a supplement to other methods
            (iii) Useful as an aid to review at a later date
            (iv) Should be written at approximately fourth-grade level; picture books may be especially helpful in multilanguage areas

(e) Explanations
 (i) Give only as much information as requested.
 (ii) Ask for feedback.
(f) Exploration: encourage patient to answer own questions.
(g) Demonstration and return demonstration
 (i) Used when the patient must learn a new skill
 (ii) Describe what you are going to do, and then do it while the patient observes; then talk to patient through the process while he or she does it; finally, have the patient perform the skill while he or she tells you how to do it
(h) Role playing
 (i) Provides practice in a safe setting
 (ii) Useful to see how others might respond

3. Implement
 a. Assign one person to teach the patient to minimize confusion, contradiction, and incompleteness.
 b. Schedule teaching sessions according to the patient's receptiveness; let the patient set the pace and choose topics of most interest first.
 c. Provide ideal setting: control the environment.
 d. Know your subject area: be competent and confident.
 e. Speak the patient's language: minimize use of medical terminology.
 f. Consider your presentation style.
  (1) Keep the presentations of material short.
  (2) Place key points up front.
  (3) Use verbal headings.
  (4) Summarize at the end.
  (5) Obtain feedback and request questions.
 g. Include "why" where appropriate.
 h. Use visual aids.
 i. Remember that successful learning takes time and reinforcement.
 j. Provide a means for the patient to learn more such as written information for reading and review, resource groups, and outpatient program.
 k. Coordinate education through written teaching plans, patient care conferences, and documentation.
  (1) Written teaching plans should include the following:
   (a) Objectives
   (b) Content
   (c) Teaching methods
   (d) Methods of evaluation
  (2) Documentation should include the following:
   (a) Objectives
   (b) Content outline
   (c) Method used
   (d) Evaluation of learning
    (i) How was learning evaluated
    (ii) Evaluation of learning
    (iii) Objective met
    (iv) Objective partially met—needs reinforcement
    (v) Objective not met—needs repeat teaching
   (e) Comments
   (f) Signature

4. Evaluate learning using any of the following methods:
 a. Written tests
 b. Oral evaluation
 c. Return demonstration
 d. Analysis of physical findings (e.g., serum glucose and weight)
 e. Follow-up questionnaire

Education for Low-Literacy Individuals

1. Definition: adults with poorly developed skills in reading, writing, listening, and speaking
2. Assessing literacy level
 a. Individuals reading at a fifth-grade or higher level are considered literate; hand printing instructions and asking the patient to read them back to you is a nonthreatening way to assess reading ability.
 b. Incongruent behavior may signal a literacy problem; be alert for behavior that does not match the reported level of understanding.
 c. Low-literacy materials are preferred for the low-literacy individuals.
3. Teaching strategies for low-literacy patients
 a. Identify and eliminate or minimize stress, anxiety, or other distractions before teaching.
 b. Correct misconceptions that affect learning.
 c. Personalize the health message and explain the need for the information.
 d. Relate information to patient's past experiences and actively involve the patient and family in discussions.
 e. Consider qualities of poor readers and use teaching strategies that are helpful (Table 12-11)

Table 12-11 Qualities of Poor Readers and Appropriate Teaching Strategies

Qualities of Poor Readers	Teaching Strategies
Take words literally	Explain the meaning of all words
Read slowly; miss meaning	Use common words and examples
Skip over uncommon words	Use examples; review content frequently
Miss content	Describe content first; use verbal heading and visuals
Tire quickly	Use short segments

LEARNING ACTIVITIES

1. **DIRECTIONS:** Complete the following crossword puzzle.

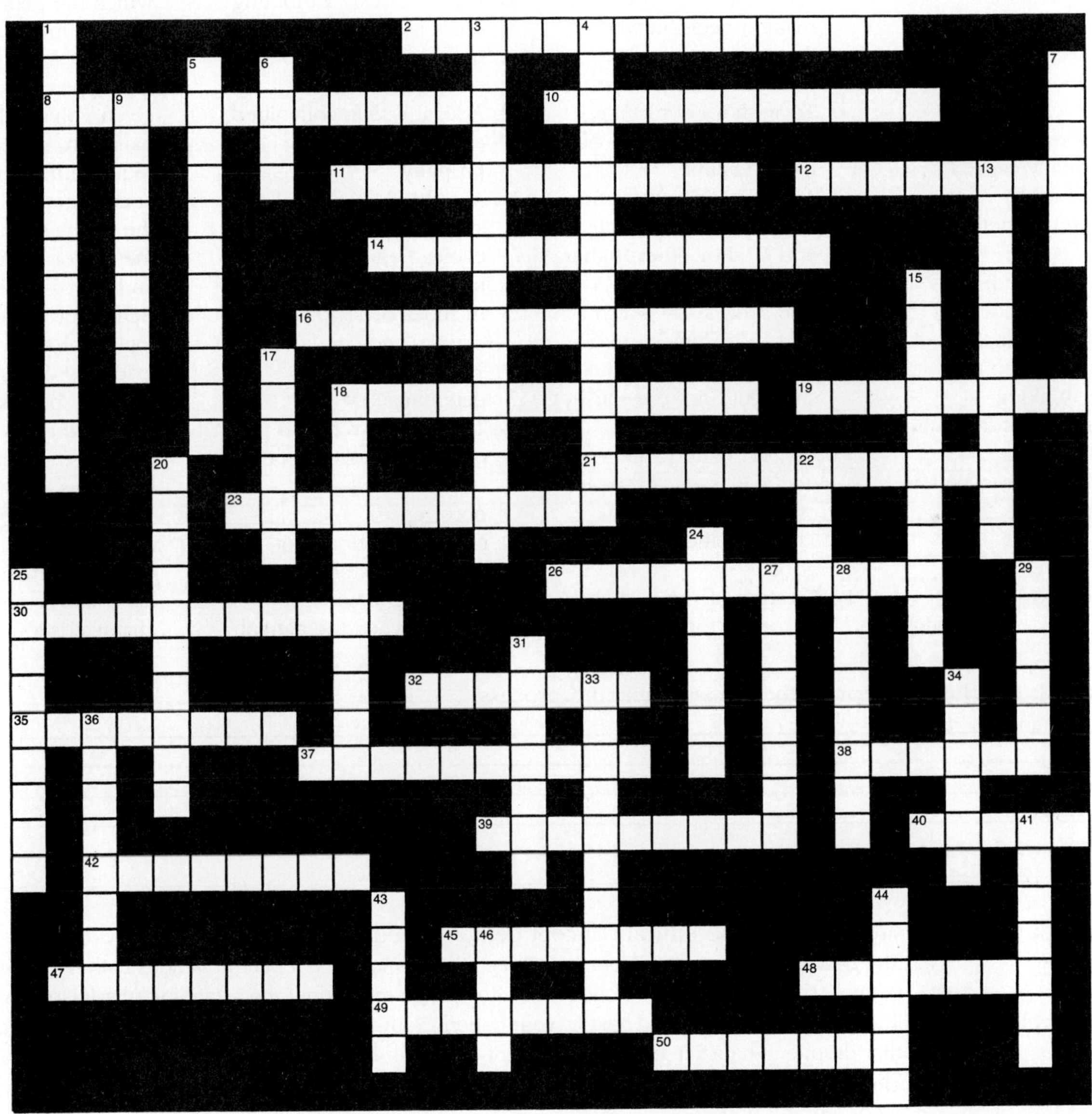

Across

2. Answerability or responsibility
8. Working together
10. A statutory right of a defined group
11. A basic human phenomenon that helps create meaning in the world
12. The obligation to tell the truth
14. Perceived lack of control over the outcome of a specific situation or problem
16. The ethical approach that asserts that actions are right or wrong based on the greatest good for the greatest number
18. Use of scents for therapeutic purposes
19. The obligation to be faithful to agreements and responsibilities accepted
21. The process of seeking, giving, and receiving help
23. Unintentional tort
26. Directing energy from unacceptable drives into socially acceptable behavior
30. Involves use of conscious mental effort to control involuntary body function, such as blood pressure, heart rate, and respiratory rate
32. Nursing care delivery system in which one nurse has accountability for the patient's care during the entire hospitalization
35. This type of thinking is controlled, purposeful, and goal-directed reasoning
37. Ethical approach that asserts that actions are right or wrong based on a set of morals or rules
38. Systems of valued behaviors and beliefs that govern proper conduct
39. Ethical approach that asserts that actions are right or wrong based on consequences

40. Type of charges that could be filed if a nurse unintentionally causes a patient's death
42. Specific unified system of an expression of the belief in and reverence for a supernatural power accepted as the creator and governor of the universe
45. Type of charges that would be filed if a nurse intentionally caused a patient's death
47. Working on another's behalf
48. Learned, shared, and transmitted values, beliefs, and practices of a particular group that guides thinking
49. The process of facilitating learning
50. The obligation to be fair to all persons

Down

1. The process by which an individual or group takes on the behaviors and practices of the dominant culture
3. The obligation to respect privileged information
4. The obligation to do no harm
5. To assist an individual to make a decision when that person does not have the data or expertise
6. To wish for something with the expectation of its fulfillment
7. An intimate conversation between an individual and God or other Higher Being
9. The process by which a person becomes capable of doing something he or she could not previously do
13. Assault, battery, and defamation are examples of this type of tort
15. The obligation to do good
17. Treating obvious reality factors as though they do not exist because they are consciously intolerable
18. Insertion of needles into specific points in the body for therapeutic purposes
20. Unconsciously attributing one's own unacceptable qualities and emotions to others
22. A legal wrong committed against a person or property
24. An ethical ____ is a situation that requires a choice between two undesirable alternatives
25. Includes behavior, criteria, and condition
27. The right to self-determination
28. This type of report is completed for errors or other unusual occurrences
29. Mental, emotional, or physical tension
31. This type of consent applies when the patient cannot give consent but treatment is needed immediately
33. Going back to an earlier level of emotional development
34. An acute state of stress in which the person feels overwhelmed by stressors
36. This type of consent is given voluntarily after the patient has been given required information
41. Focusing and directing the imagination through the use of specific words and suggestions
43. Belief not based on logical proof or material evidence
44. Personal beliefs about the truth and the worth of thoughts, objects, and behaviors
46. A group of persons related by common descent of heredity who have similar physical characteristics

2. DIRECTIONS: List the six steps of the decision-making process.

a. ____________________
b. ____________________
c. ____________________
d. ____________________
e. ____________________
f. ____________________

3. DIRECTIONS: Match the situation with the ethical concept demonstrated. More than one may be listed.

___ 1. Veracity
___ 2. Confidentiality
___ 3. Autonomy
___ 4. Nonmaleficence
___ 5. Fidelity
___ 6. Justice
___ 7. Advocacy

a. The new surgical resident has made three attempts to place a central venous catheter in an elderly patient. The nurse insists that no more attempts be made until the attending physician is present.
b. There is a code in the bed next to your patient. Your patient asks you if the patient died. You reply that despite exhaustive efforts, the patient did die (but you do not disclose the patient's name).
c. The patient has decided that he does not want to be intubated again. You ensure that his wishes are recorded and honored.
d. The nurse explains to the patient that care still be will provided despite the fact that he has no health insurance.
e. The nurse's next-door neighbor is in the hospital. She visits him, but she does not read his chart.
f. The nurse begins on time, takes only the allotted time for lunch, and leaves after completion of work and report.
g. The confused patient keeps reaching for his endotracheal tube. The nurse applies soft restraints to prevent self-extubation.

4. DIRECTIONS: Match the ethical approach to the statement that best describes a "right" decision using the approach.

___ 1. Utilitarianism
___ 2. Egoism
___ 3. Deontology
___ 4. Paternalism
___ 5. Social contract
___ 6. Natural law
___ 7. Teleology

a. When it results in the most good for the most people
b. When it results in a positive outcome
c. When it is the best thing in the opinion of the decision maker
d. When it provides significant benefit to the decision maker
e. When it is in accordance with human nature
f. When it is inherently right morally
g. When some rights must be lost for the best of society.

5. DIRECTIONS: Match the level of Maslow's hierarchy of needs to the example.

___ 1. Physiologic
___ 2. Safety and security
___ 3. Love and belonging
___ 4. Esteem and recognition
___ 5. Self-actualization

a. Developing an innovative way to improve patient care
b. Being able to take a lunch break
c. CCRN on your nametag
d. Being invited to socialize after work
e. Lighting and guards in the parking garage

6. DIRECTIONS: List eight complementary therapies that are helpful to patients with stress, anxiety, or pain.

a. ____________________
b. ____________________
c. ____________________
d. ____________________
e. ____________________
f. ____________________
g. ____________________
h. ____________________

7. DIRECTIONS: List five of the most important needs of families as identified by Leske.

a. ____________________
b. ____________________
c. ____________________
d. ____________________
e. ____________________

8. DIRECTIONS: List five of the essential elements of collaboration.

a. ____________________
b. ____________________
c. ____________________
d. ____________________
e. ____________________

9. DIRECTIONS: Describe a change model and how you might use it to make a change that you feel is needed on your unit.

____
____
____

10. DIRECTIONS: Identify the following as T (true) or F (false).

a. ___ The nurses' own values and beliefs will not affect their sensitivities with their patients.
b. ___ Pain is influenced by culture.
c. ___ Race is not a factor in drug absorption and action.
d. ___ It is never appropriate for a nurse to pray with a patient; the nurse should call the chaplain.
e. ___ Decisions concerning medical care should be made by the physician alone.
f. ___ Physical care should always take precedence over psychosocial and spiritual care.
g. ___ Inability to speak English is an indication of ignorance.

11. DIRECTIONS: Match the religion with the implication.

___ 1. Islam (Muslim)
___ 2. Catholicism
___ 3. Judaism
___ 4. Hinduism
___ 5. Christian Scientist
___ 6. Seventh-Day Adventist
___ 7. Jehovah's Witnesses

a. Provide kosher diet as requested
b. Opposed to blood transfusions
c. Provide same-sex caregivers
d. Medical care may be refused; prayer is used as the primary treatment of illness
e. The patient must have been baptized before death
f. Procedures may be refused between dusk on Friday to dusk on Saturday
g. The patient's head is turned to the right after death

12. Directions: Complete the following crossword puzzle regarding clinical inquiry.

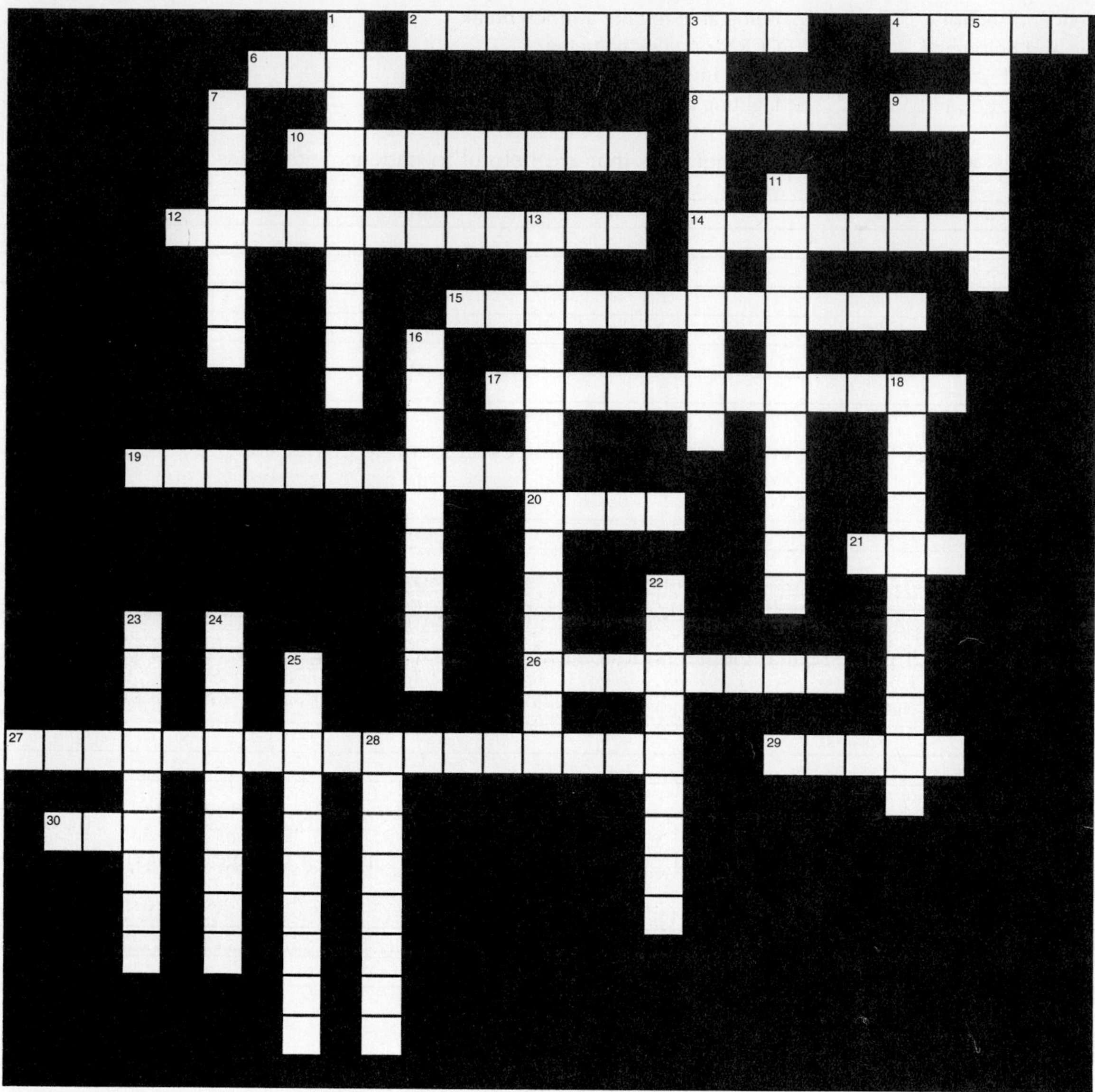

Across

2. The fifth point on the ACE Star Model
4. Quality, quantity, and consistency are used to _____ the evidence
6. Format for posing clinical questions (abbreviation)
8. Process for rapid cycle change (abbreviation)
9. The integration of best evidence, clinician expertise, patient values, and circumstances (abbreviation)
10. A reference point against which performance can be compared
12. Type of research that controls study variables as much as possible and has objective and measurable data collection
14. A concept examined in a research study
15. Type of research that uses randomization and a control group to test the effects of an intervention
17. Statistical technique for conducting quantitative systematic reviews
19. Type of research that takes place in the individual's natural setting with emphasis on understanding human experience
20. A collection of essential nursing information for comparison across patient populations (abbreviation)
21. A statement designed to assist the clinician in making decisions about the appropriate health care for specific clinical situations (abbreviation)
26. Type of consent that must be obtained before inclusion as a subject in a study
27. Quantitative research design that does not use a control group or randomization
29. One way to eliminate the gap between research and practice is to establish _____ appointment between academic and clinical facilities
30. The gold standard of evidence (abbreviation)

Down

1. This method is a systematic approach to solving problems that controls variables and biases
3. Quality _____ emphasizes innovation
5. Type of research to solve a particular problem
7. A goal for fostering evidence-based practice is to create a spirit of _____
11. The third point on the ACE Star Model

13. The fourth point on the ACE Star Model
16. The second point on the ACE Star Model is the ____ of evidence
18. Type of variable that is the presumed cause
22. The first point on the ACE Star Model is discovery of _____
23. Nurse ____ indicators are those indicators that capture care or its outcomes most affected by nursing care
24. The type of variable that is the response or outcome the researcher would like to explain or predict
25. Statement that predicts a relationship among two or more variables
28. The kind of evidence that is "best" if it is available

13. DIRECTIONS: List five ways to share research findings with colleagues.

a. ______________________________
b. ______________________________
c. ______________________________
d. ______________________________
e. ______________________________

14. DIRECTIONS: List five qualities of an adult learner.

a. ______________________________
b. ______________________________
c. ______________________________
d. ______________________________
e. ______________________________

LEARNING ACTIVITIES ANSWERS

1.

1 ACCULTURATION
2 ACCOUNTABILITY
3 CONFIDENTIALITY
4 NONMALFICENCE
5 PATERNALISM
6 HOPE
7 PRAYER
8 COLLABORATION
9 LEARNING
10 ENTITLEMENT
11 SPIRITUALITY
12 VERACITY
13 INTENTIONAL
14 POWERLESSNESS
15 BENEFICENCE
16 UTILITARIANISM
17 DENIAL
18 AROMATHERAPY
18 ACUPUNCTURE
19 FIDELITY
20 PROJECTION
21 CONSULTATION
22 TORT
23 MALPRACTICE
24 DILRMAA
25 OBJECTIVE
26 SUBLIMATION
27 AUTONOMY
28 INCIDENT
29 STRESS
30 BIOFEEDBACK
31 IMPLIED
32 PRIMARY
33 REGRESSION
34 CRISIS
35 CRITICAL
36 INFORMED
37 DEONTOLOGY
38 ETHICS
39 TELEOLOGY
40 CIVIL
41 IMAGERY
42 RELIGION
43 FAITH
44 VALUES
45 CRIMINAL
46 RACE
47 ADVOCACY
48 CULTURE
49 TEACHING
50 JUSTICE

2. a. Information, collection, and problem identification
b. Identification of possible solutions or actions
c. Analysis of the possible consequences of each solution or action
d. Selection of the best possible solution or action for implementation
e. Implementation of the solution or action
f. Evaluation of the results

3. b 1.
b, e 2.
c 3.
g 4.
f 5.
d 6.
a 7.

4. a 1. Utilitarianism
d 2. Egoism
f 3. Deontology
c 4. Paternalism
g 5. Social contract
e 6. Natural law
b 7. Teleology

5. b 1.
e 2.
d 3.
c 4.
a 5.

6. Any eight of the following:
- Progressive muscle relaxation
- Breathing
- Meditation
- Comeditation
- Guided imagery
- Massage
- Hypnosis
- Biofeedback
- Therapeutic (or healing) touch
- Purposeful touch
- Music therapy
- Aromatherapy
- Pet therapy
- Humor
- Acupuncture

7. Any five of the following:
- To have questions answered honestly
- To be assured that the best care possible is being given to the patient
- To know the prognosis
- To feel there is hope
- To know specific facts about the patient's progress
- To be called at home about changes in the patient's condition
- To know how the patient is being treated medically
- To feel hospital personnel care about the patient
- To receive information about the patient daily
- To have understandable explanations
- To know exactly what is being done for the patient
- To know why things were done for the patient
- To see the patient frequently
- To talk to the doctor every day
- To be told about transfer plans

8. Any five of the following:
- Communication
- Trust
- Respect
- Understanding and acceptance of team members' roles
- Competence
- Shared responsibility and accountability
- Shared goal setting
- Flexibility
- Administrative support

9. You could have chosen any of the change models in Table 12-6 and described how you would implement each aspect of the model to change practice.

10. a. False
b. True
c. False
d. False
e. False
f. False
g. False

11. g. Islam (Muslim)
e. Catholicism
a. Judaism
c. Hinduism
d. Christian Scientist
f. Seventh-Day Adventist
b. Jehovah's Witnesses

12.

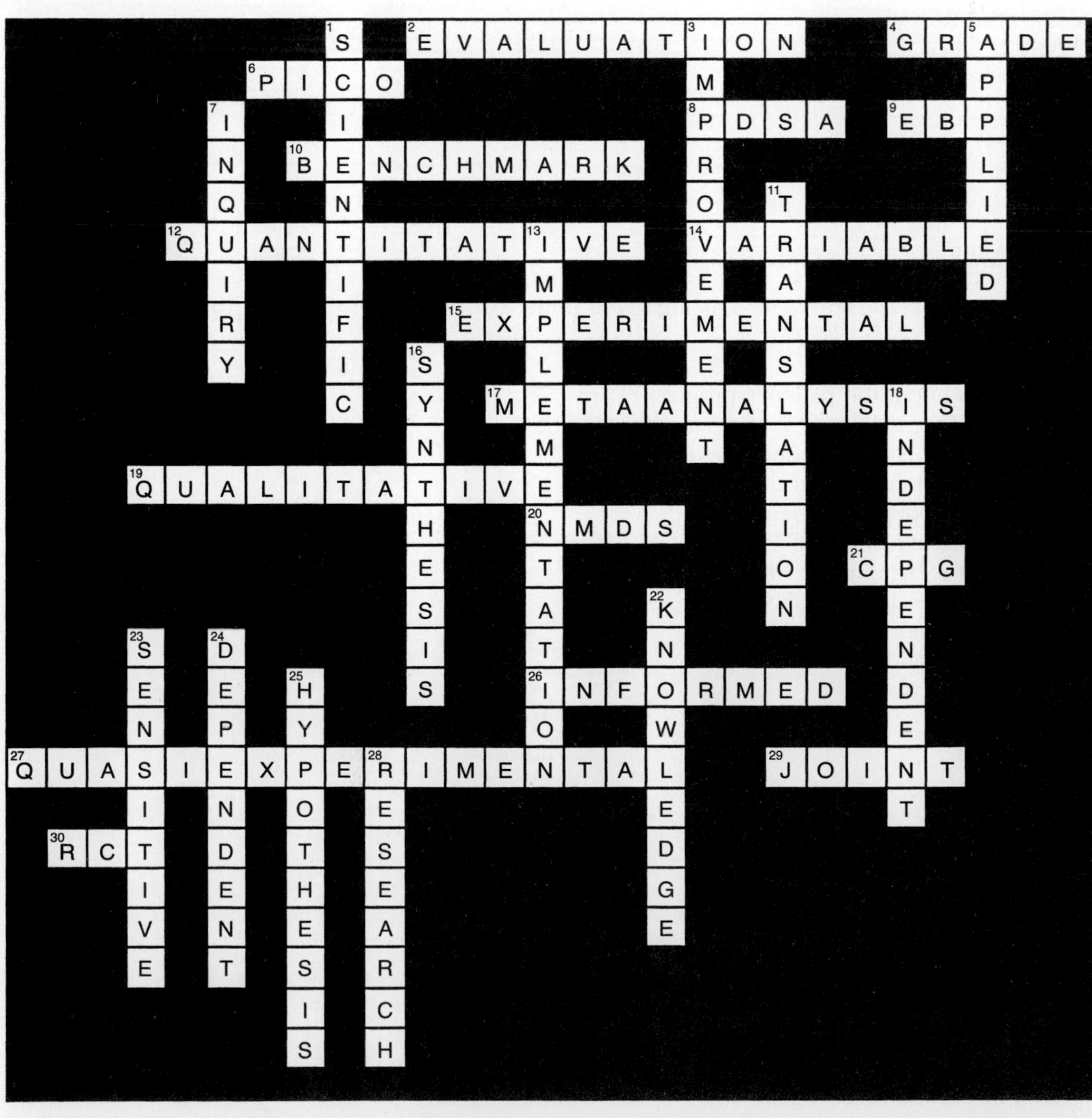

13. • Bulletin boards for current articles
• Journal clubs
• Patient care conferences
• Protocol and procedure development
• Care paths

14. Any of the following:
Goal oriented
Less flexible
Requires longer time in the performance of learning tasks
Impatient in the pursuit of objectives
Finds little use for isolated facts
Strives for recognition and success
Has multiple responsibilities, all of which draw upon his or her time
Experienced in the "school of life"
Requires a more constant and ideal learning environment
Usually comes to the teaching program on a voluntary basis
Wishes to be involved in mutual planning of learning experiences
Likes to participate in diagnosing needs for learning, formulating learning objectives, and evaluating learning
Expects a climate of mutual respect, trust, and collaboration that supports learning

References

Alfaro-LeFevre, R. (2003). *Critical thinking in nursing: A practical approach* (3rd ed.). Philadelphia: W. B. Saunders Company.

American Association of Critical-Care Nurses. (2004). *The 4 A's to rise above moral distress.* Aliso Viejo, CA: Author.

American Association of Critical-Care Nurses. (2005a). *AACN standards for establishing and sustaining healthy work environments.* Retrieved August 5, 2006, from http://www.aacn.org/aacn/pubpolcy.nsf/Files/HWEStandards/$file/HWEStandards.pdf

American Association of Critical-Care Nurses. (2005b). *Critical care nursing fact sheet.* Retrieved August 1, 2006, from http://www.aacn.org/AACN/practice.nsf/ad0ca3b3bdb4f33288256981006fa692/818297476d23f9628825692900802d92?OpenDocument

American Association of Critical-Care Nurses. (2005c). *Role of the critical care nurse.* Retrieved July 29, 2006, from http://www.aacn.org/AACN/pubpolcy.nsf/64c71bdeda6f392a882567310071cbf2/4b9dd3eb98c7a273882566090004b13f?OpenDocument

American Association of Critical-Care Nurses. (2006). *AACN fact sheet.* Retrieved August 1, 2006, from http://www.aacn.org/AACN/mrkt.nsf/vwdoc/AACNFactSheet?opendocument

AACN Certification Corporation. (2005). *The AACN Synergy model for patient care.* Retrieved March 15, 2007, from http://www.certcorp.org/certcorp/certcorp.nsf/vwdoc/SynModel?opendocument#Nurse%20Characte

American Hospital Association. (2003). *The patient care partnership: Understanding expectations, rights and responsibilities.* Retrieved August 3, 2006, from http://www.aha.org/aha/ptcommunication/content/pcp_english_030730.pdf

American Nurses Association. (1995). *The ANA basic guide to safe delegation.* Washington, DC: Author.

American Nurses Association. (1999). *Nursing-sensitive quality indicators for acute care settings and ANA's safety & quality initiative.* Retrieved August 2, 2006, from http://www.nursingworld.org/readroom/fssafe99.htm

American Nurses Association. (2006). *What do nurses do?* Retrieved August 1, 2006, from http://www.nursingworld.org/nursecareer/#do

Berwick, D. M. (2003). Disseminating innovations in health care. *Journal of American Medical Association, 289*(15), 1969-1975.

Berwick, D. M., & Kotagal, M. (2004). Restricted visiting hours in ICUs: Time for change. *Journal of the American Medical Association, 292*(6), 736-737.

Ciliska, D. K., Pinelli, J., DiCenso, A., & Cullum, N. (2001). Resources to enhance evidence-based nursing practice. *AACN Clinical Issues, 12*(4), 520-528.

Cohen, E. L., & Cesta, T. G. (2001). *Nursing case management: From essentials to advanced practice applications* (3rd ed.). St. Louis: Mosby.

Curley, M. A. Q. (1998). Patient-nurse synergy: optimizing patients' outcomes. *American Journal of Critical Care, 7*(1), 64-72.

Curtin, L. (1982). Ethics in nursing administration. In A. Marriner (Ed.), *Contemporary nursing management.* St. Louis: C. V. Mosby.

Dracup, K., & Bryan-Brown, C. W. (1999). Empathy: A challenge for critical care. *American Journal of Critical Care, 8*(4), 204-205.

Environmental Protection Agency. (1974). *Information on levels of environmental noise requisite to protect public health and welfare with an adequate margin of safety.* Retrieved August 3, 2006, from http://www.nonoise.org/library/levels74/ levels74.htm

Erikson, E. (1968). *Identity, youth and crisis.* New York: W. W. Norton.

Gonzalez, C. E., Carroll, D. L., Elliott, J. S., Fitzgerald, P. A., & Vallent, H. J. (2004). Visiting preferences of patients in the intensive care unit and in a complex care medical unit. *American Journal of Critical Care, 13*(3), 194-198.

Gordon, S. (2006). What do nurses really do? [Electronic Version]. *Topics in Advanced Practice Nursing eJournal,* 6. Retrieved August 1, 2006 from http://www.medscape.com/viewarticle/520714_print

Gray, J. A. M. (1997). *Evidence-based healthcare: How to make health policy and management decisions*. London: Churchill Livingstone.

Havelock, R. (1973). *The change agent's guide to innovation in education*. Englewood Cliffs, NJ: Educational Technology Publications.

Henneman, E. A., & Cardin, S. (2002). Family-centered critical care: A practical approach to making it happen. *Critical Care Nurse, 22*(6), 12-19.

Institute for Healthcare Improvement. (nd). *How to improve: Improvement methods*. Retrieved August 5, 2006, from http://www.ihi.org/IHI/Topics/Improvement/Improvement Methods/HowToImprove/

Jackson, M., Ignatavicius, D. D., & Case, B. (2006). *Conversations in critical thinking and clinical judgment*. Boston: Jones and Bartlett.

Johnson, S. A., & Romanello, M. L. (2005). Generational diversity: Teaching and learning approaches. *Nurse Educator, 30*(5), 212-216.

Kotter, J. P., & Cohen, D. S. (2002). *The heart of change: Real-life stories of how people change their organizations*. Boston: Harvard Business School Publishing.

Kübler-Ross, E. (1969). *On death and dying*. New York: Macmillan.

Leske, J. (1991). Overview of family needs after critical illness: from assessment to intervention. *AACN Clinical Issues in Critical Care Nursing, 2*, 220.

Lewin, K. (1951). *Field theory in social sciences*. New York: Harper.

Lippitt, R., Watson, J., & Westley, B. (1958). *The dynamics of planned change*. New York: Harcourt, Brace and Company.

Mangurten, J. A., Scott, S. H., Guzzetta, C. E., Sperry, J. S., Vinson, L. A., Hicks, B. A., et al. (2005). Family presence: Making room. *American Journal of Nursing, 105*(5), 40-49.

Marquis, B. L., & Huston, C. J. (2006). *Leadership roles and management functions in nursing: Theory and application* (5th ed.). Philadelphia: Lippincott.

Maslow, A. (1968). *Toward a psychology of being* (2nd ed.). Princeton, MA: Van Nostrand.

McCaffery, M. (1968). *Nursing practice theories related to cognition, bodily pain and main environment interactions*. Los Angeles: University of California, Los Angeles.

McCaffery, M. (2002). Teaching your patient to use a pain rating scale. *Nursing2002, 32*(8), 17.

Melnyk, B. M., & Fineout-Overholt, E. (2002). Putting research into practice. *Reflections on Nursing Leadership, 28*(2), 22-25.

Nolan, T. W. (1998). Understanding medical systems. *Annals of Internal Medicine, 128*(4), 293-298.

Prochaska, J. M. (2000). A transtheoretical model for assessing organizational change: A study of family service agencies' movement to time-limited therapy. *Family in Society: The Journal of Contemporary Human Services, 81*(1), 76-85.

Prochaska, J. M., Prochaska, J. O., & Levesque, D. A. (2001). A transtheoretical approach to changing organizations. *Administration and Policy in Mental Health, 28*(4), 247-261.

Rogers, E. M. (1995). *Diffusion of innovations* (4th ed.). New York: Free Press.

Sackett, D. L., Straus, S. E., Richardson, W. S., Rosenberg, W., & Haynes, R. B. (2000). *Evidence-based medicine: How to practice and teach EBM* (2nd ed.). Edinburgh: Churchill Livingstone.

Sommers, M. S. (1994). The near-death experience following multiple trauma. *Critical Care Nurse, 14*(4), 62.

Stevens, K. R. (2005). *ACE Star Model of Knowledge Transformation*. Retrieved August 6, 2006, from http://www.acestar.uthscsa.edu/Learn_model.htm

Tamburri, L. M., DiBrienza, R., Zozula, R., & Redeker, N. (2004). Nocturnal care interactions with patients in critical care units. *American Journal of Critical Care, 13*(2), 102-115.

U.S. Department of Health and Human Services, Health Resources and Services Administration. (2001). *Cultural competence works*. Retrieved August 4, 2006, from ftp://ftp.hrsa.gov/financeMC/cultural-competence.pdf

Yoder-Wise, P. (2003). *Leading and managing in nursing* (3rd ed.). St. Louis: Mosby.

Bibliography

Acton, G. J. (2001). Meta-analysis: A tool for evidence-based practice. *AACN Clinical Issues, 12*(4), 539-545.

AGREE Collaboration. (2001). *Appraisal of Guidelines for Research & Evaluation (AGREE) Instrument*. Retrieved December 8, 2004, from http://www.agreecollaboration.org

Alspach, G. (2004). Communicating health information: An epidemic of the incomprehensible. *Critical Care Nurse, 24*(4), 8-13.

Alspach, G. (2006). Extending the Synergy Model to preceptorship. *Critical Care Nurse, 26*(2), 10-14.

American Association of Critical-Care Nurses. (2005c). *Standards for acute and critical care nursing practice*. Retrieved August 1, 2006, from http://www.aacn.org/AACN/practice.nsf/ad0ca3b3bdb4f33288256981006fa692/5e3c9805e57b3b0888256a6b00791f35?OpenDocument

American Nurses Association. (2001). *Code of ethics for nurses with interpretative statements*. Washington, DC: American Nurses Publishing.

Annis, T. D. (2002). The interdisciplinary team across the continuum of care. *Critical Care Nurse, 22*(5), 76-79.

Bally, K., Campbell, D., Chesnick, K., & Tranmer, J. E. (2003). Effects of patient-controlled music therapy during coronary angiography on procedural pain and anxiety distress syndrome. *Critical Care Nurse, 23*(2), 50-58.

Barnsteiner, J., & Prevost, S. (2002). How to implement evidence-based practice: Some tried and true pointers. *Reflections on Nursing Leadership, 28*(2), 18-21.

Barnum, B. S. (2002). *The new healers: Minds and hands in complementary medicine*. Long Branch, NJ: Vista Publishing.

Benner, P. (2002). Creating compassionate institutions that foster agency and respect. *American Journal of Critical Care, 11*(2), 164-104.

Benner, P. (2003). Enhancing patient advocacy and social ethics. *American Journal of Critical Care, 12*(4), 374-375.

Benner, P. (2004). Relational ethics of comfort, touch, and solace—Endangered arts? *American Journal of Critical Care, 13*(4), 346-349.

Benner, P., Kerchner, S., Corless, I. B., & Davies, B. (2003). Attending death as a human passage: Core nursing principles for end-of-life care. *American Journal of Critical Care, 12*(6), 558-561.

Billings, D., & Kowalski, K. (2004). Teaching learners from varied generations. *Journal of Continuing Education in Nursing, 35*(3), 104-105.

Brown, S., & Bachtel, G. (2000). Enhancing self-esteem among cardiac patients. *Dimensions of Critical Care Nursing, 19*(5), 50-54.

Burns, N., & Grove, S. V. (2003). *Understanding nursing research.* Philadelphia: W. B. Saunders.

Clausing, S. L., Kurtz, D. L., Prendeville, J., & Walt, J. L. (2003). Generational diversity—The Nexters. *AORN Journal, 78*(3), 373-379.

Cmiel, C. A., Karr, D. M., Gasser, D. M., Oliphant, L. M., & Neveau, A. J. (2004). Noise control: A nursing team's approach to sleep promotion. *American Journal of Nursing, 104*(2), 40-49.

Cooke, H. (2000). *When someone dies: A practical guide to holistic care at the end of life.* Oxford, England: Butterworth Heinemann.

Cullen, L., Titler, M., & Drahozal, R. (2003). Family and pet visitation in the critical care unit. *Critical Care Nurse,* 23(5), 62-66.

Daly, B. J. (2006). End-of-life decision making, organ donation, and critical care nurses. *Critical Care Nurse, 26*(2), 78-86.

Damboise, C., & Cardin, S. (2003). Family-centered critical care: How one unit implemented a plan. *American Journal of Nursing, 103*(6), 56AA-56EE.

Day, L. (2006). Advocacy, agency, and collaboration. *American Journal of Critical Care, 15*(4), 428-430.

Dlugacz, Y. D., Stier, L., Lustbader, D., Jacobs, M. C., Hussain, E., & Greenwood, A. (2002). Expanding a performance improvement initiative in critical care from hospital to system. *Journal on Quality Improvement, 28*(8), 419-434.

Ecklund, M. M., & Stamps, D. C. (2002). Promoting synergy in progressive care. *Critical Care Nurse, 22*(4), 60-67.

Egan, K. A., & Arnold, R. L. (2003). Grief and bereavement care. *American Journal of Nursing, 103*(9), 42-53.

Erhrle, R. (2006). Timely referral of potential organ donors. *Critical Care Nurse, 26*(2), 88-93.

Ersek, M. (2004). The continuing challenge of assisted death. *Journal of Hospice and Palliative Nursing, 6*(1), 46-59.

Fain, J. A. (2004). *Reading, understanding, and applying nursing research.* Philadelphia: F. A. Davis.

Felgen, J. A. (2003). Caring: Core value, currency, and commodity. ... Is it time to get tough about "soft"? *Nursing Administration Quarterly, 27*(3), 208-214.

Flowers, D. L. (2004). Culturally competent nursing care: A challenge for the 21st century. *Critical Care Nurse, 24*(4), 48-52.

Funnell, M. M. (2004). Patient empowerment. *Critical Care Nursing Quarterly, 27*(2), 201-204.

Gerteis, M., Edgman-Levitan, S., Daley, J., & Debanco, T. L. (1993). *Through the patient's eyes: Understanding and promoting patient-centered care.* San Francisco: Jossey-Bass.

Guzzetta, C. E. (2004). Critical care research: Weaving a body-mind-spirit tapestry. *American Journal of Critical Care, 13*(4), 320-327.

Hardin, S., & Hussey, L. (2001). Clinical inquiry. *Critical Care Nurse, 21*(2), 88-91.

Hayes, C. (2000). Strengthening nurses' moral agency. *Critical Care Nurse, 20*(5), 90-94.

Hedges, C. (2006). If you build it, will they come? Generating interest in nursing research. *AACN Advanced Critical Care, 17*(2), 226-229.

Herr, K., Coyne, P. J., Key, T., Manworren, R., McCaffery, M., Merkel, S., et al. (2006). Pain assessment in the nonverbal patient: Position statement with clinical practice recommendations. *Pain Management in Nursing, 7*(2), 44-52.

Institute for Healthcare Improvement. (2004). *PDSA worksheet.* Retrieved August 5, 2006, from http://www.ihi.org/NR/rdonlyres/8C03F6DC-8EEC-4297-AF91-BD4E7436F043/656/PDSAWorksheet2.pdf

Jezewski, M. A., Meeker, M. A., & Robillard, I. (2005). What is needed to assist patients with advance directives from the perspective of emergency nurses. *Journal of Emergency Nursing, 31*(2), 150-155.

Kerfoot, K. (2002). The leader as synergist. *Critical Care Nurse, 22*(2), 126-129.

Kinney, M., Dunbar, S., Brooks-Brunn, J. A., Molter, N., & Vitello-Cicciu, J. (1998). *AACN clinical reference for critical care nursing* (4th ed.). St. Louis: Mosby.

Kirchhoff, K. T., Foth, K. T., Lues, S. N., & Gilbertson-White, S. H. (2004). Documentation on withdrawal of life support in adult patients in the intensive care unit. *American Journal of Critical Care, 13*(4), 328-334.

Kruse, J. A., Fink, M. P., & Carlson, R. W. (2003). *Saunders manual of critical care.* Philadelphia: Saunders.

Kuebler, K. K., Berry, P. H., & Heidrich, D. E. (2002). *End of life care: Clinical practice guidelines.* Philadelphia: W. B. Saunders.

Lancaster, J. (1999). Managing change. In J. Lancaster (Ed.), *Nursing issues in leading and managing change* (pp. 149-169). St. Louis: Mosby.

Langley, G. L., Nolan, K. M., Nolan, T. W., Norman, C. L., & Provost, L. P. (1996). *The improvement guide: A practical approach to enhancing organizational performance.* San Francisco: Jossey-Bass.

Leske, J. S. (2003). Comparison of family stresses, strengths, and outcomes after trauma and surgery. *AACN Clinical Issues, 14*(1), 33-41.

Lindquist, R., Tracy, M. F., Savik, K., & Watanuki, S. (2005). Regional use of complementary and alternative therapies by critical care nurses. *Critical Care Nurse, 25*(2), 63-75.

LoBiondo-Wood, G., & Haber, J. (2002). *Nursing research: Methods, critical appraisal, and utilization.* St. Louis: Mosby.

Loxton, M. H. (2003). Patient education: The nurse as source of actionable information [Electronic Version]. *Topics in Advanced Practice Nursing eJournal,* 3. Retrieved August 2, 2006 from http://www.medscape.com/viewarticle/453348_print

Markey, D. W. (2001). Applying the Synergy Model: Clinical strategies. *Critical Care Nurse, 21*(3), 72-76.

Martin, C. A. (2003). Transcend generational timelines. *Nursing Management, 34*(4), 24-28.

Mauk, K. L., & Schmidt, N. K. (2004). *Spirtual care in nursing practice.* Philadelphia: Lippincott Williams & Wilkins.

McCaughan, D., Thompson, C., Cullum, N., Sheldon, T. A., & Thompson, D. R. (2002). Acute care nurses' perceptions of barriers to using research information in clinical decision-making. *Journal of Advanced Nursing, 39*(1), 46-60.

Monsivais, D., & Reynolds, A. (2003). Developing and evaluating patient education materials. *Journal of Continuing Education in Nursing, 34*(4), 172-176.

Norton, S. A., Tilden, V. P., Tolle, S. W., Nelson, C. A., & Eggman, S. T. (2003). Life support withdrawal: Communication and conflict. *American Journal of Critical Care, 12*(6), 548-555.

O'Brien, M. E. (1999). *Spirituality in nursing: Standing on holy ground.* Boston: Jones and Bartlett.

Payen, J.-F., Bru, O., Bosson, J.-L., Lagrasta, A., Novel, E., Deschaux, I., et al. (2001). Assessing pain in critically ill sedated patients by using a behavioral pain score. *Critical Care Medicine, 29*(12), 2258-2263.

Pitorak, E. F. (2003). Care at the time of death. *American Journal of Nursing, 103*(7), 42-53.

Polit, D. F., Beck, C. T., & Hungler, B. P. (2001). *Essentials of nursing research* (5th ed.). Philadelphia: Lippincott.

Pope, B. B. (2002). The synergy match-up. *Nursing Management, 33*(5), 38-41.

Puntillo, K. A., Miaskowski, C., Kehrle, K., Stannard, D., Gleeson, S., & Nye, P. (1997). Relationship between behavioral and physiological indicators of pain, critical care patients' self-reports of pain, and opioid administration. *Critical Care Medicine, 25,* 1159-1166.

Renn, C. L., & Dorsey, S. G. (2005). The physiology and processing of pain: A review. *AACN Clinical Issues, 16*(3), 227-290.

Rich, K. (2004). An overview of clinical trials. *Journal of Vascular Nursing, 22*(1), 32-34.

Robinson, C. A. (2001). Magnet nursing services recognition: Transforming the critical care environment. *AACN Clinical Issues, 12*(3), 411-423.

Rosswurm, M. A., & Larrabee, J. H. (1999). A model for change to evidence-based practice. *Image: Journal of Nursing Scholarship, 31*(4), 317-322.

Rushton, C. (2006). Defining and addressing moral distress. *AACN Advanced Critical Care, 17*(2), 161-168.

Scherer, Y., Jezewski, M. A., Graves, B., Wu, Y.-W. B., & Bu, X. (2006). Advance directives and end-of-life decision making: Survey of critical care nurses' knowledge, attitude, and experience. *Critical Care Nurse, 26*(4), 30-40.

Scott, L. D., Rogers, A. E., Hwang, W. T., & Zhang, Y. (2006). Effects of critical care nurses' work hours on vigilance and patients' safety. *American Journal of Critical Care, 15*(1), 30-37.

Shafer, T. J., Wagner, D., Chessare, J., Zampiello, F. A., McBride, V., & Perdue, J. (2006). Organ donation breakthrough collaborative: Increasing organ donation through system redesign. *Critical Care Nurse, 26*(2), 33-49.

Smith, A. R. (2006). Using the Synergy Model to provide spiritual nursing care in critical care settings. *Critical Care Nurse, 26*(4), 41-47.

Smith, L. S. (2003). Help! My patient's illiterate. *Nursing2003, 33*(11), 32hn36-32hn38.

Spector, R. E. (2000). *Cultural diversity in health & illness.* Upper Saddle River, NJ: Prentice Hall Health.

Stetler, C. B. (2001). Updating the Stetler model of research utilization to facilitate evidence-based practice. *Nursing Outlook, 49*(6), 272-279.

Stone, P. W., Larson, E. L., Mooney-Kane, C., Smolowitz, J., Lin, S. X., & Dick, A. W. (2006). Organizational climate and intensive care unit nurses' intention to leave. *Critical Care Medicine, 34*(7), 1907-1912.

Straus, S. E., Richardson, W. S., Glasziou, P., & Haynes, R. B. (2005). *Evidence based medicine* (3rd ed.). London: Churchill Livingstone.

Titler, M. G., & Everett, L. Q. (2001). Translating research into practice. *Critical Care Nursing Clinics of North America, 13*(4), 587-602.

Titler, M. G., Kleiber, C., Steelman, V. J., Rakel, B. A., Budreau, G., Everett, L. Q., et al. (2001). The Iowa model of evidence-based practice to promote quality care. *Critical Care Nursing Clinics of North America, 13*(4), 497-509.

Tracy, M. F., & Ceronsky, C. (2001). Creating a collaborative environment to care for complex patients and families. *AACN Clinical Issues, 12*(3), 383-400.

Tran, M. N. (2003). Take benchmarking to the next level. *Nursing Management, 34*(1), 18-24.

Trinkoff, A., Geiger-Brown, J., Brady, B., Lipscomb, J., & Muntaner, C. (2006). How long and how much are nurses now working? *American Journal of Nursing, 106*(4), 60-72.

Tuttas, C. A. (2002). The facts of end-of-life care. *Journal of Nursing Care Quality, 16*(2), 10-16.

Urden, L., Stacy, K., & Lough, M. (2006). *Thelan's critical care nursing: Diagnosis and management* (5th ed.). St. Louis: Mosby.

Wagner, J. M. (2004). Lived experience of critically ill patients' family members during cardiopulmonary resuscitation. *American Journal of Critical Care, 13*(5), 416-420.

Wheelan, S. A., Burchill, C. N., & Tilin, F. (2003). The link between teamwork and patients' outcomes in intensive care units. *American Journal of Critical Care, 12*(6), 527-534.

Whitman, G. R., Kim, Y., Davidson, L. J., Wolf, G. A., & Wang, S.-L. (2002). Measuring nurse-sensitive patient outcomes across speciality units. *Outcomes Management, 6*(4), 152-158.

Wilkin, K., & Slevin, E. (2004). The meaning of caring to nurses: An investigation into the nature of caring work in an intensive care unit. *Journal of Clinical Nursing, 13,* 50-59.

Williams, J. K., & Cooksey, M. M. (2004). Navigating the difficulties of delegation. *Nursing2004, 34*(9), 32hn12.

Zink, S., & Wertlieb, S. (2006). A study of the presumptive approach to consent for organ donation: A new solution to an old problem. *Critical Care Nurse, 26*(2), 129-136.

Critical Care Pharmacology

CHAPTER 13

NOTE: Pharmacology is not a separate section on the CCRN® examination blueprint. Questions related to pharmacology will be integrated into the appropriate section where the medication is indicated for treatment of a specific condition. The intention of this chapter is not to discuss every drug that might be administered to a critically ill patient but rather to provide a review of issues that are most likely to be seen on the CCRN® examination.

Introduction to Critical Care Pharmacology

Definitions (Lehne, 2007)

1. Drug: a chemical that can produce a biologic response in a living organism; drugs modify existing functions but do not produce new functions
   a. Three most important characteristics of a drug
      (1) Effectiveness: the drug elicits the desired responses
      (2) Safety: the drug does not produce harmful effects
      (3) Selectivity: the drug elicits only the desired response
   b. Other desirable properties
      (1) Reversibility
      (2) Predictability
      (3) Ease of administration
      (4) Absence of drug interactions
      (5) Low cost
      (6) Chemical stability
      (7) Simple generic name
2. Pharmacology: the study of drugs and their interactions with living systems
3. Clinical pharmacology: the study of drugs in humans
4. Pharmacotherapeutics: the use of drugs to diagnose, prevent, or treat disease

Drug Action: Consists of Three Phases

1. Pharmaceutic phase: only applies to drugs administered via the gastrointestinal (GI) tract
   a. Disintegration: breakdown of a tablet or capsule into smaller particles
      (1) Enteric-coated tablets or capsules and sustained-release capsules should not be crushed.
   b. Dissolution: dissolving of the smaller particles in the GI fluid
      (1) Drugs in liquid form are already in solution.
      (2) Drugs are disintegrated faster in the acid environment of the stomach.
      (3) Food in the GI tract may interfere with dissolution, though some drugs (e.g., gastric irritants) should be given with food.
2. Pharmacokinetic phase
   a. Absorption: the movement of drug particles from the site of administration into the blood
      (1) Aspects of absorption
         (a) Rate determines how soon the effects will occur.
         (b) Amount determines how intense the effects will be.
      (2) Processes
         (a) Passive absorption: primarily diffusion
         (b) Active absorption: requires a carrier and energy
         (c) Pinocytosis: cells carry drugs across their membrane by engulfing the drug particles
      (3) Factors affecting drug absorption
         (a) Surface area: the larger the surface area, the faster absorption will be
         (b) Local conditions at site of absorption (e.g., perfusion and temperature)
         (c) Drug solubility
            (i) The more soluble the drug, the more rapidly it will be absorbed, so oral solutions are absorbed more rapidly than capsules, tablets, or caplets.
            (ii) Lipid-soluble drugs are absorbed more rapidly because they can more readily cross the membranes separating them from the blood.

(d) Additional variables affecting absorption related to the route of administration
   (i) Oral or nasogastric
      a) Gastric pH
      b) GI motility
      c) Perfusion
      d) Presence of other medications or food in GI tract
   (ii) Intramuscular: muscle mass; pH of the medication
   (iii) Subcutaneous: pH of medication
   (iv) Transdermal: surface area
   (v) Inhalation: surface area
   (vi) Transtracheal: surface area
   (vii) Rectal: surface area
   (viii) Intravenous (IV): no absorption required
(e) pH
   (i) Acidic drugs tend to dissociate less in an acid medium and are absorbed better in the stomach.
   (ii) Alkaline drugs tend to dissociate less in an alkaline medium and are absorbed better in the intestine.
(f) Drug concentrations or preparations
   (i) High concentrations or dosages are more rapidly absorbed.
   (ii) Some preparations (e.g., SR, XL, CD, ER) are developed for delayed absorption.

(4) Bioavailability: percentage of the administered drug dose that reaches the systemic circulation; factors affecting bioavailability include the following:
   (a) Route
      (i) IV: 100%
      (ii) Oral: less than 100%; if the drug goes to the liver first (hepatic first pass), bioavailability is only 20% to 40%, so oral dose will be 3 to 5 times the IV dose
   (b) Drug form (i.e., tablet, capsule, sustained-release tablet or capsule, liquid, transdermal patch, suppository, inhalation, or instillation down endotracheal tube)
   (c) GI motility and surface area and function of mucosa
   (d) Food and other drugs in GI tract
   (e) Changes in liver metabolism

b. Distribution: the movement of drugs throughout the body
   (1) Factors affecting distribution
      (a) Relative rate of perfusion, which determines the rate that drugs are delivered to a particular tissue
      (b) Ability to leave the vascular system and enter the tissues
         (i) Permeability: physical-chemical properties of the drug
            a) Fat-soluble medications readily penetrate fat tissue and are widely distributed.
               i) Drugs must be lipid soluble to cross the blood-brain barrier.
            b) Non–fat-soluble medications will have less tissue penetration.
         (ii) Binding of a drug to plasma proteins
            a) Decreases movement of drug into the tissues because plasma proteins, given their large size, stay in the vascular bed
            b) Decreases the concentration of free drug in circulation and prevents the drug from reaching its site of action in full concentration
               i) As the free drug is eliminated from the body, more drug can be dissociated from the protein to replace what is lost.
            c) Consider the following:
               i) The length of time to reduce toxic drug levels to subtoxic is longer in plasma protein–bound drugs.
               ii) Malnutrition increases free blood levels because less plasma protein is available for binding.
               iii) The addition of another plasma protein–bound drug increases free plasma levels.
               iv) Plasma protein–bound drugs are not dialyzable.
      (c) Ability to enter cells: affected by same factors as for leaving the vascular system

c. Biotransformation (previously referred to as metabolism)
   (1) Chemical alterations are produced by enzyme systems in the blood and in all body cells, especially the liver.
      (a) Conversion of drugs into products that are generally less active and more easily excreted than the original form; some drugs are converted to active and inactive metabolites
      (b) Conversion of fat-soluble drugs to water-soluble for excretion by the kidneys
   (2) The half-life of a drug is the time it takes for one half of the drug concentration to be eliminated; half-life is affected by the following:
      (a) Chemical properties of the drug
      (b) Hepatic disease
      (c) Severe cardiovascular disease because liver engorgement and hypoperfusion may occur
      (d) Renal disease because active metabolites must be excreted to eliminate the drug's effect
   (3) Factors affecting drug biotransformation

d. Excretion (also referred to as elimination)
 (1) Routes of excretion
  (a) Renal system: renal excretion affected by the following factors
   (i) Glomerular filtration rate; best evaluated by creatinine clearance
   (ii) Urine pH
   (iii) Protein-binding: drug must be free to be excreted
  (b) Lungs
  (c) Biliary system
  (d) Skin
3. Pharmacodynamic phase
 a. Drug response
  (1) Primary physiologic effect: desirable
  (2) Secondary physiologic effect: may be desirable or undesirable
  (3) Onset of action: time it takes to reach the minimum effective concentration
  (4) Peak action: time when the drug reaches its high blood concentration
  (5) Duration of action: length of time that the drug has a pharmacologic effect
  (6) Therapeutic index: ratio that measures the effective dose in 50% of persons or animals and the lethal dose in 50% of animals; measures the margin of safety of a drug
   (a) Low therapeutic index: narrow margin of safety
   (b) High therapeutic index: wide margin of safety
  (7) Peak drug level: the highest plasma concentration of the drug at a specific time
  (8) Trough drug level: the lowest plasma concentration of a drug; measures the rate at which the drug is eliminated
 b. Variables affecting drug action
  (1) Age: the very young and the very old are more likely to have pronounced or prolonged drug action
  (2) Body mass
   (a) High amount of body muscle increases required dosage, whereas low amount of body muscle decreases required dosage
   (b) High amount of body fat allows more fat storage and prolongs drug action
  (3) Gender
   (a) Females are usually lower in body weight but higher fat proportion and therefore require lower drug dosages
  (4) Genetics (i.e., pharmacogenetics): drug actions may be enhanced or diminished by hereditary factors
   (a) Hypertensive blacks do not respond well to beta-blockers or angiotensin-converting enzyme (ACE) inhibitors, whereas the response to thiazide diuretics is more effective in blacks than in whites.
   (b) Asian Americans have an exaggerated response to stimulants (e.g., caffeine) and beta-blockers.
   (c) Idiosyncratic responses (e.g., malignant hyperthermia) have genetic predisposition.
  (5) Environmental milieu: temperature; metabolic rate; hypoxia
  (6) Time of administration: presence or absence of food in the stomach; biologic rhythms
  (7) Pathologic states: pain; anxiety; fever; infection; circulatory, hepatic, and renal dysfunction
  (8) Psychological factors: faith in the effects of the drug; placebo effect
  (9) Tolerance: decreased physiologic response to the repeated administration of a drug
   (a) Cross-tolerance: occurs with pharmacologically similar drugs and drugs that act at the same receptor sites
   (b) Tachyphylaxis: rapidly developing tolerance that occurs after repeated administration of a drug
  (10) Cumulative effects: when the body cannot metabolize one dose of a drug before another dose is administered
  (11) Drug dependence: physical or psychological dependence
  (12) Summation, additive effect, synergism: combined effect of two drugs acting simultaneously is equal to or greater than the effect of each agent given alone
  (13) Drug antagonism: effect of two drugs is less than the sum of the drugs acting separately
  (14) Drug interaction: results from the concurrent administration of two or more drugs
 c. Side effects: a nearly avoidable secondary drug effect produced at therapeutic doses
 d. Adverse drug events: more serious than side effects
  (1) Iatrogenic diseases
   (a) Blood dyscrasia
   (b) Hepatotoxicity
   (c) Nephrotoxicity
   (d) Dermatologic conditions (e.g., toxic epidermitis necrosis)
  (2) Drug allergies: may range from rash to anaphylaxis
 e. Toxic effects: adverse drug effects caused by drug overdosage or drug accumulation

Drug Safety

1. Definitions
 a. Error: "the failure of a planned action to be completed as intended or the use of a wrong plan to achieve an aim" (Kohn, Corrigan, & Donaldson, 2000)
 b. Medication error: "any preventable event that may cause or lead to inappropriate medication use or patient harm while the medication is in the control of the health care professional, patient, or consumer" (American Society of Health-System Pharmacists, 1998)

c. Adverse drug events (ADEs): events when the patient is harmed by a drug; more encompassing term than medication errors because it includes harm as a result of an error and adverse effects of drugs such as rash, anaphylaxis, nephrotoxicity, hepatotoxicity, or blood dyscrasias; about one third of ADEs are associated with medication errors and, therefore, are considered preventable (Bates et al., 1995)
d. Potential ADE: a medication error that was caught before it reached the patient but could have harmed the patient if the drug had actually been administered; frequently referred to as near misses, near hits, or good catches
e. Harm: "death or temporary or permanent impairment of body function/structure requiring intervention. Intervention may include monitoring the patient's condition, change in therapy, or active medical or surgical treatment" (National Coordinating Council for Medication Error and Prevention, 2004).
f. High-alert medications (Box 13-1): "medications that bear a heightened risk of causing significant patient harm when they are used in error" (Institute for Safe Medication Practices, 2005); note that although errors may or may not be more common with these drugs, the consequences of an error with these medications are clearly more devastating to patients

BOX 13-1 High-Alert Medication Infusions Frequently Administered in Critical Care Areas

Classes/Categories of Medications

Adrenergic agonists (e.g., epinephrine, norepinephrine, dopamine, and dobutamine)
Adrenergic antagonists (e.g., esmolol)
Anesthetic agents (e.g., propofol)
Anticoagulants (e.g., heparin, bivalirudin, argatroban, and lepirudin)
Antidysrhythmic agents (e.g., amiodarone and lidocaine)
Antineoplastic agents
Dextrose, hypertonic, 20% or greater
Electrolyte solutions (e.g., potassium chloride, potassium phosphate, magnesium sulfate, and hypertonic sodium chloride)
Fibrinolytic agents (e.g., streptokinase, anistreplase, alteplase, and tenecteplase)
GP IIb/IIIa inhibitors (e.g., eptifibatide)
Inotropic agents (e.g., milrinone)
Liposomal forms of drugs (e.g., liposomal amphotericin B)
Moderate sedation agents (e.g., midazolam, lorazepam, and diazepam)
Narcotics/opiates
Neuromuscular blocking agencies (MNBAs) (e.g., atracurium, vecuronium, cisatracurium, and pancuronium)
Total parenteral nutrition solutions
Vasodilators (e.g., nitroglycerin, nitroprusside, and nesiritide)

Modified from Institute for Safe Medication Practices. (2005). *ISMP's list of high-alert medications.* Retrieved August 10, 2006, http://www.ismp.org/Tools/highalertmedications.pdf

2. Prevention of errors
   a. Individual responsibility
      (1) Ten rights
         (a) Right patient: use two patient identifiers (neither patient's room number nor bed number)
         (b) Right drug
         (c) Right dose
         (d) Right time
         (e) Right route
         (f) Right reason
         (g) Patient's right to education
         (h) Patient's right to refuse
         (i) Patient evaluation: clarify titration parameters
         (j) Right documentation
      (2) Reporting of errors and near hits so that system analysis can occur and prevent future errors
   b. Systems thinking
      (1) Nonpunitive culture
      (2) Adherence to policies, procedures, protocols
         (a) Avoidance of unapproved abbreviations, trailing zeros
         (b) Avoidance of verbal orders; if necessary, a verbal repeat should be used for confirmation
         (c) Label with drug being administered
            (i) Bag
            (ii) Pump chamber (using channel labels on infusion pump if available)
            (iii) Tubing
      (3) Use of information
         (a) Patient information (e.g., laboratory values and vital signs); electronic patient record is preferred because the record is available to more than one health care professional simultaneously
         (b) Drug information: use up-to-date medication references such as *Micromedex, Epocrates,* and drug books that are updated annually
      (4) Use of technology
         (a) Automated dispensing devices
         (b) Bar code point of care (BPOC)
         (c) Computerized provider order entry (CPOE)
         (d) "Smart" pumps with guardrails to alert the nurse of too high or too low of a dose
      (5) Standardization
         (a) Restriction of formulary (i.e., do you really need to have three glycoprotein [GP] IIb/IIIa inhibitors or will one or two suffice?)
         (b) Standardization of infusion concentrations (i.e., avoid double, triple, or quadruple concentration)
         (c) Standardization of equipment (e.g., infusion pumps)
      (6) Pharmacist
         (a) Review of all prescriptions
         (b) Presence on unit and on rounds

(7) Medication reconciliation
(8) Environment control
(a) Adequate lighting
(b) Noise reduction
(c) Distraction avoidance
(d) Clean, clutter-free, organized space for preparation of medications
(9) Teamwork
(a) Clarification of any unclear prescription
(b) Use of independent double-checks of drug, dose, calculation, patient identity, infusion rate, and appropriate line for all high-alert medications (Box 13-1)
(i) "Check this *with* me" is unacceptable because it causes confirmation error (i.e., you see what you expect to see)
(ii) Also applies to dose changes of these high-alert drugs
(c) Use of time-out if there is a question about the safety of the drug for this patient, at this time, at this dose, by this route; never administer a drug that is unsafe
(d) Documentation and communication of changes in patient response or adverse drug events

c. Recommended process for safe IV infusion of high-alert medications (Figure 13-1)

Drug Calculations in Critical Care Areas

Note that you will only be allowed a simple function calculator for the CCRN® examination.

1. Most drugs prescribed for critically ill patients are administered by body weight
2. Common formulae used for calculation of IV infusions (Table 13-1)

Autonomic Nervous System

Many Critical Care Drugs Work by Stimulating or Blocking One of the Branches of the Autonomic Nervous System

Sympathomimetic Drugs

Also referred to as adrenergic drugs.

1. Receptors of the SNS
   a. Alpha: constriction of blood vessels
   b. $Beta_1$: increase in heart rate (HR), contractility, and conductivity
   c. $Beta_2$: dilation of bronchi, dilation of blood vessels
   d. Dopaminergic: dilation of mesenteric and renal blood vessels
2. Sympathomimetic (also referred to as adrenergic) drugs stimulate SNS (Table 13-2)
   a. Respiratory selective beta stimulants (e.g., albuterol [Proventil]) stimulate predominantly $beta_2$ receptors, so they cause less tachycardia and hypertension.

Sympatholytic Drugs

Also referred to as adrenergic-blocking drugs, sympatholytic drugs block or inhibit the SNS.

1. Alpha-blockers: prevent vasoconstriction rather than cause a direct vasodilation; used as antihypertensives

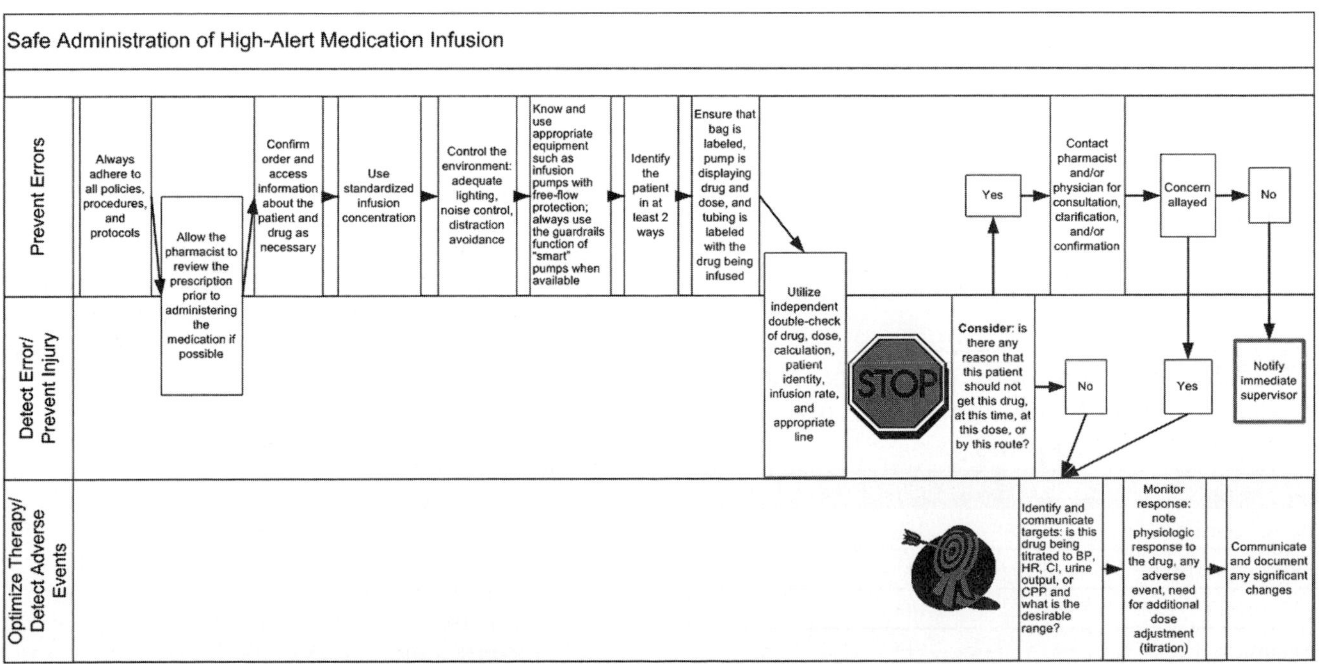

Copyright Robin Donohoe Dennison; permissions should be directed to robin@robindennison.com

Figure 13-1 Flowchart for safe IV infusion of high-alert medications.

Table 13-1 Drug Calculation Formulae

Calculation	Formula
To calculate mcg/kg/min if you know the rate of the infusion	$\frac{(\text{mcg/mL}) \times (\text{mL/hr})}{(60 \text{ min/hr}) \times (\text{kg of body mass})}$
To calculate rate in mL/hr if you know the dose in mcg/kg/min	$\frac{(\text{dose in mcg/kg/min}) \times (60 \text{ min/hr}) \times (\text{weight in kg})}{\text{mcg/mL of the solution}}$
To calculate mg/min if you know the rate of the infusion	$\frac{(\text{mg/mL}) \times (\text{mL/hr})}{(60 \text{ min/hr})}$
To calculate rate in mL/hr if you know the dose in mg/min	$\frac{(\text{dose in mg/min}) \times (60 \text{ min/hr})}{\text{mg/mL of the solution}}$
To calculate mcg/min if you know the rate of the infusion	$\frac{(\text{mcg/mL}) \times (\text{mL/hr})}{(60 \text{ min/hr})}$
To calculate rate in mL/hr if you know the dose in mcg/min	$\frac{(\text{dose in mcg/min}) \times (60 \text{ min/hr})}{\text{mcg/mL of the solution}}$

2. Beta-blockers: decrease HR, contractility, and conductivity and prevent vasodilation and bronchodilation
   a. Cardioselective beta-blockers (e.g., metoprolol [Lopressor]) block predominantly $beta_1$ receptors, so they are less likely to cause bronchospasm in patients with history of asthma or chronic obstructive pulmonary disease (COPD).

Parasympathomimetic Drugs

Also referred to as cholinergic drugs, parasympathomimetic drugs stimulate the peripheral nervous system (PNS).

1. Example: pyridostigmine (Mestinon)
2. These drugs increase the amount of acetylcholine at the neuromuscular junction and are used for myasthenia gravis; they are also used as an antagonist to nondepolarizing muscle relaxants

Parasympatholytics Drugs

Also referred to as anticholinergic drugs, parasympatholytic drugs inhibit the PNS

1. Example: atropine
2. Note that the effects of blocking PNS are similar to the effects of stimulating the SNS

Table 13-2 Sympathomimetic Drugs and Their Effect on Sympathetic Nervous System Receptors

Drug	Alpha	$Beta_1$	$Beta_2$
Phenylephrine	++++	0	0
Norepinephrine	++++	++	0
Epinephrine	++++	++++	++
Dopamine	+++	+++	+
Dobutamine	+	++++	++
Isoproterenol	0	++++	++++

Determinants of Cardiac Output (Heart Rate × Stroke Volume)

Goal

A common goal with critically ill patients is to increase cardiac output (CO) and/or minimize oxygen (O_2) consumption; Figure 2-55 illustrates therapeutic manipulations to optimize CO and vital organ perfusion and/or minimize myocardial O_2 consumption.

Terms Used to Describe Cardiac Drug Effects; May Be Positive or Negative

1. Inotropic: effect on contractility
2. Chronotropic: effect on HR
3. Dromotropic: effect on conductivity

Inotropic Agents

Indications

1. Decreased CO caused by decreased myocardial contractility
2. Heart failure
   a. Acute left ventricular systolic dysfunction
   b. Chronic left ventricular systolic dysfunction: may be used while awaiting cardiac transplantation or to improve quality of life but not used as often as they were in the past because they have been shown to actually increase mortality by increasing myocardial O_2 consumption

Types of Inotropes and Specific Actions and Indications

1. Cardiac glycosides (e.g., digoxin [Lanoxin])
   a. Actions
      (1) Increases force and velocity of myocardial contraction
      (2) Decreases sinus node firing rate
      (3) Increases the refractory period of the atrioventricular (AV) node
      (4) Decreases atrial automaticity
      (5) Increases ventricular automaticity

(6) Increases glomerular filtration rate (GFR) and urine output
b. Indications
(1) Chronic left ventricular systolic failure
(2) Atrial dysrhythmias especially in the presence of heart failure
2. Sympathomimetics (i.e., adrenergic) agents (e.g., dobutamine [Dobutrex] and dopamine [Intropin])
a. Actions: stimulation of $beta_1$ receptors
(1) Increase myocardial contractility
(2) Increases HR (dopamine more than dobutamine)
(3) Dopamine causes vasoconstriction, whereas dobutamine causes vasodilation
(4) Note dose-dependency of dopamine
(a) 2 to 5 mcg/kg/min: beta receptor stimulation
(b) 5 to 10 mcg/kg/min: alpha and beta receptor stimulation
(c) Greater than 10 mcg/kg/min: alpha receptor stimulation with tachycardia
(d) Note that what was previously thought of as "renal dopamine" is now thought to be due primarily to the inotropic effects of dopamine and dobutamine actually increases glomerular filtration rate (GFR) more than dopamine does
b. Indications
(1) Acute left ventricular failure
(2) Low CO states
(3) Vasogenic shock states: dopamine greater than 5 mcg/kg/min
3. Phosphodiesterase (PDE) inhibitors (e.g., inamrinone [Inocor] and milrinone [Primacor])
a. Actions
(1) Inhibits PDE III in cardiac and vascular smooth muscle
(a) Increased myocardial contractility by increasing cyclic adenosine monophosphate levels and promoting calcium influx (cAMP)
(b) Vasodilation by directly acting on the vascular smooth muscle and the coronary arteries
(i) Dilation of arteries and veins
(ii) Dilation of renal arteries unpredictable
(c) No significant change in myocardial O_2 consumption
(2) Inamrinone has more vasodilation and less inotropic effect than milrinone; milrinone causes less thrombocytopenia than inamrinone
(3) Long half-life complicates titration
b. Indications
(1) Short-term treatment of heart failure that has not improved with conventional therapy
(2) Pharmacologic bridge to cardiac transplantation
(3) Low CO after cardiac surgery
(4) May be used with dobutamine or digoxin; synergistic effect with these other inotropic agents
4. Hemodynamic effects of inotropic agents (Tables 13-3 and 13-4)

Vasodilators

Action: Vasodilation (Table 13-5)

1. Venous vasodilators reduce *pre*load because veins are *before* the heart.
2. Arterial vasodilators reduce *after*load because arteries are *after* the heart.

Indications

1. Hypertension
2. Heart failure
3. Cardiogenic shock
a. Inotropic agents are likely to be required to support blood pressure (BP).
b. An intraaortic balloon pump may be required to reduce afterload in patients who are significantly hypotensive.
4. Coronary artery disease: angina; myocardial infarction
5. Peripheral vascular disease

Types of Vasodilators and Specific Actions and Indications

1. Hydralazine
a. Action: directly dilates arterial system, decreasing afterload
b. Indication: hypertension
2. Nitroglycerin
a. Action: relaxes vascular smooth muscles
(1) Dilates primarily venous system, decreasing preload

Table 13-3 Hemodynamic Effects of Inotropic Agents

Drug	CO/CI	MAP	PAOP	SVR	Heart Rate
Digoxin	↑	⇔	⇔	⇔	↓
Dobutamine	↑	↑	↓	↓	⇔ or ↑
Dopamine	↑	↑	↑	↑	↑
Inamrinone/milrinone	↑	⇔	↓	↓	⇔

CO/CI, Cardiac output/cardiac index; *MAP,* mean arterial pressure; *PAOP,* pulmonary artery occlusive pressure; *SVR,* systemic vascular resistance.

Table 13-4 **Selected Inotropic Agents**

Drug	Administration	Adverse Effects	Nursing Implications
Digitalis (digoxin [Lanoxin], digitoxin, lanatoside C)	• IV, PO • Digitalizing dose: 0.75-1.5 mg dose over 24 hours, usually in four doses of 0.25 mg • Administer IV dose over 5 minutes • Maintenance dose: 0.125-0.5 mg qd • Therapeutic blood level: 0.5-2 ng/mL	• Toxic effects ○ Anorexia, nausea, vomiting, diarrhea ○ Fatigue, muscle weakness ○ Agitation ○ Hallucinations ○ Visual disturbances ○ SA and AV blocks ○ Junctional and ventricular dysrhythmias • Treatment of toxicity ○ Discontinue drug ○ Correct hypoxemia, ischemia, acid-base or electrolyte imbalance — Correction of hypokalemia is recommended before Digibind administration ○ Treat tachydysrhythmias as prescribed: usually lidocaine ○ Treat bradydysrhythmias as prescribed: usually atropine or pacemaker ○ Administer digoxin immune FAB [Digibind] as prescribed for life-threatening dysrhythmias or blocks ○ Average dose is 400-800 mg over 30 minutes or IV bolus if cardiac arrest ○ Administered through in-line filter ○ Reversal of digitalis toxicity occurs within 30-60 minutes, but digoxin levels remain elevated	• Monitor apical HR, ECG, and serum electrolytes, especially potassium, calcium, and magnesium. • Note contraindications: known hypersensitivity, sick sinus syndrome, SA or AV block, ventricular tachycardia, hypertrophic cardiomyopathy, and WPW syndrome. • Use cautiously in patients with acute MI, hypothyroidism, liver disease, renal disease, and in older adults. • Assess patient for clinical indications of digitalis toxicity. • Withhold for 1-2 days before elective electrical cardioversion.
Dopamine hydrochloride (Intropin)	• IV infusion: mix 400 mg in 250 mL (1600 mcg/mL) and infuse at 0.5-20 mcg/kg/min depending on desired effect • Maximum: 20 mcg/kg/min • Administer through central venous catheter if possible; if administered peripherally, use a large vein • Do not administer with alkaline solutions	• Tachycardia • Ventricular ectopy • Hypertension or hypotension • Nausea, vomiting • Dyspnea • Headache • Palpitations • Chest pain in patients with CAD • Tissue necrosis with high dosages or extravasation	• Monitor HR, BP, ECG, PAP, PAOP, SVR, CI, and urine output. • Note contraindications: known hypersensitivity, uncorrected tachydysrhythmias, ventricular fibrillation, pheochromocytoma, hypertrophic cardiomyopathy and patients receiving MAO inhibitors. • Use cautiously in peripheral vascular disease. • Consider the cause of hypotension instead of automatically initiating dopamine to increase the blood pressure; *improve perfusion* by treating the cause of hypotension (e.g., volume replacement, inotropes, or preload or afterload reduction). • Provide volume expansion during weaning; taper gradually to wean. • Do not administer drug if it is discolored. • Prevent extravasation because necrosis may occur; treat extravasation with phentolamine (Regitine).

Table 13-4 Selected Inotropic Agents—cont'd

Drug	Administration	Adverse Effects	Nursing Implications
Dobutamine hydrochloride (Dobutrex)	• IV infusion; mix 250 mg in 250 mL (1000 mcg/mL) and infuse at 2-40 mcg/kg/min • Maximum: 40 mcg/kg/min • Administer though central venous catheter if possible; if administered peripherally, use a large vein • Do not administer with alkaline solutions	• Tachycardia • Ventricular ectopy • Hypertension or hypotension • Nausea, vomiting • Dyspnea • Headache • Anxiety • Paresthesia • Palpitations • Chest pain	• Monitor BP, HR, ECG, PAP, PAOP, SVR, and CI. • Note contraindications: known hypersensitivity and hypertrophic cardiomyopathy. • Use cautiously in patients with hypertension or ventricular dysrhythmias. • Note that the increase in heart rate is less than with dopamine. • Use with nitroprusside as prescribed in cardiogenic shock; dobutamine increases contractility and decreases preload (and to a lesser degree afterload), and nitroprusside decreases afterload and preload.
Inamrinone (Inocor) (Note change in generic name to avoid confusion between previously named amrinone and amiodarone)	• IV injection: 0.75 mg/kg over 2-3 minutes; may repeat in 30 minutes • IV infusion: mix 500 mg in 500 mL (1000 mcg/mL) and infuse at 5-15 mcg/kg/min • Maximum: 10 mg/kg/day • Do not reconstitute with dextrose	• Ventricular dysrhythmias • Hypotension • Anorexia, nausea, vomiting, abdominal pain, diarrhea • Increased liver enzymes, hepatotoxicity • Hypokalemia • Tremor	• Monitor heart rate, BP, ECG, PAP, PAOP, CI, SVR, platelet counts, liver function studies, electrolytes (especially potassium), BUN, and creatinine. • Platelet count below 150,000/mm^3 usually requires dosage reduction • Platelet count below 100,000/mm^3 usually requires discontinuance.
Milrinone (Primacor)	• IV injection: 50 mcg/kg over 10 minutes • IV infusion: mix 30 mg in 250 mL (120 mcg/mL); usual dose 0.375 to 0.75 mcg/kg/min (less if renal insufficiency)	• Thrombocytopenia (inamrinone more than milrinone) • Chest pain • Hypersensitivity reactions • Headache • Burning at injection site • Fever • Blurred vision (milrinone)	• Note contraindications: known hypersensitivity to this drug or bisulfites (preservative), severe aortic or pulmonic valvular disease, hypertrophic cardiomyopathy, and ventricular dysrhythmias. • Use cautiously in renal disease, liver disease, atrial dysrhythmias, and in older adults. • Use cautiously in acute MI because myocardial oxygen consumption is increased. • Correct hypokalemia and hypovolemia before or during amrinone use. • Use cautiously in acute MI because myocardial oxygen consumption is increased. • Note that milrinone is more frequently prescribed than amrinone because of the greater incidence of thrombocytopenia with amrinone.

AV, Atrioventricular, *BP,* blood pressure; *BUN,* blood urea nitrogen; *CAD,* coronary artery disease; *CI,* cardiac index; *ECG,* electrocardiogram; *HR,* heart rate; *IV,* intravenous; *MAO,* monoamine oxidase; *MI,* myocardial infarction; *PAP,* pulmonary artery pressure; *PAOP,* pulmonary artery occlusive pressure; *PO,* oral; *SA,* sinoatrial; *SVR,* systemic vascular resistance; *WPW,* Wolff-Parkinson-White.

(2) Dilates arterial system at higher doses, decreasing afterload
(3) Relieves vasospasm
(4) Redistributes blood flow in the heart, improving myocardial O_2 consumption

b. Indications
(1) Coronary artery disease
(a) Angina
(i) Acute
(ii) Prophylactic use before activities that may cause angina
(b) Myocardial infarction
(2) Coronary artery spasm
(3) Acute left ventricular failure

3. Nitroprusside
a. Action: relaxes vascular smooth muscles
(1) Dilates arterial system at higher doses, decreasing afterload
(2) Dilates venous system, decreasing preload

b. Indications
(1) Hypertension
(2) Acute left ventricular failure

Table 13-5 Vasoactive Effects of Selected Drugs

Drug	Arteries	Veins
Fenoldopam mesylate (Corlopam)	Yes	No
Hydralazine (Apresoline)	Yes	No
Milrinone (Primacor)	Yes	Yes
Minoxidil (Loniten)	Yes	No
Morphine sulfate	No	Yes
Nicardipine (Cardene)	Yes	Yes
Nifedipine (Procardia)	Yes	Yes
Nitroglycerin (Tridil)	Only if greater than 1 mcg/kg/min	Yes
Nitroprusside (Nipride)	Yes	Yes
Phentolamine (Regitine)	Yes	Yes
Prazosin (Minipress)	Yes	Yes

(3) Cardiogenic shock
(4) Acute aortic dissection
(5) BP control during and after vascular surgery

4. Nesiritide (Natrecor)
   a. Action: acts as endogenous human B-type natriuretic peptide
      (1) Dilates arteries and reduces systemic vascular resistance (SVR)
      (2) Dilates veins and reduces pulmonary artery occlusive pressure (PAOP)
      (3) Decreases aldosterone and norepinephrine levels
      (4) Inhibits renin-angiotensin-aldosterone system and endothelin pathways, prompting the release of fluid and sodium from the body
   b. Indication: decompensated heart failure in persons who have dyspnea at rest or with minimal activities and clinical evidence of fluid overload
      (1) Systolic and diastolic dysfunction
      (2) Decompensation is defined as sustained deterioration in function of at least one New York Heart Association (NYHA) class, usually associated with evidence of total body salt and water overload
5. Fenoldopam mesylate (Corlopam)
   a. Actions
      (1) Dilates arterial system, decreasing afterload
      (2) Stimulates dopaminergic receptors, causing diuresis
   b. Indications
      (1) Hypertension
      (2) Renal protection when patient is receiving nephrotoxic dyes
6. Calcium channel blockers
   a. Action: block calcium flow through cardiac and smooth muscle cells (Table 13-6)
   b. Indications
      (1) Hypertension
      (2) Hypertrophic cardiomyopathy
      (3) Angina, especially when caused by vasospasm
      (4) Raynaud's disease
      (5) Atrial dysrhythmias (verapamil and diltiazem)
   c. Types of calcium channel blockers and specific actions
      (1) Dihydropyridine type: nifedipine (Procardia), nicardipine (Cardene), amlodipine (Norvasc), felodipine (Plendil), isradipine (DynaCirc)
      (2) Diphenylalkylamine type: diltiazem (Cardizem)
      (3) Benzothiazepine type: verapamil (Calan)

Table 13-6 Effects of Calcium Channel Blockers

Type of Calcium Channel Blocker	Coronary Arterial Dilation	Peripheral Arterial Dilation	Atrioventricular Nodal Depression	Sinoatrial Nodal Depression	Effect on Left Ventricular Contractility
Dihydropyridine type (e.g., nifedipine)	+	+++	0	0	0
Diphenylalkylamine type (i.e., diltiazem)	+	++	↓	↓	↓
Benzothiazepine type (i.e., verapamil)	+	+	↓	↓	↓↓

7. ACE inhibitors (e.g., captopril [Capoten], enalapril [Vasotec], benazepril [Lotensin], fosinopril [Monopril], lisinopril [Prinivil, Zestril], moexipril [Univasc], perindopril [Aceon], quinapril [Accupril], ramipril [Altace], and trandolapril [Mavik]) and angiotensin II blockers (e.g., losartan [Cozaar], valsartan [Diovan], irbesartan [Avapro], telmisartan [Micardis], and candesartan [Atacand])
   a. Actions
      (1) Vasodilation
         (a) ACE inhibitors block the conversion of angiotensin I to angiotensin II.
            (i) Interfere with the breakdown of bradykinin and, therefore, frequently cause cough
         (b) Angiotensin II blockers (or angiotensin receptor blockers) block angiotensin II.
      (2) Diuresis by inhibition of aldosterone
         (a) Decrease retention of sodium and water
         (b) Retention of potassium
      (3) Preserve renal function in diabetic patients
   b. Indications
      (1) Hypertension
      (2) Heart failure: systolic dysfunction
      (3) Myocardial infarction (MI) to prevent remodeling
         (a) Anterior MI
         (b) Large inferior MI
         (c) Presence of indications of heart failure
      (4) Diabetic nephropathy
8. Sympathetic blockers
   a. Selective alpha-blockers: doxazosin (Cardura), prazosin (Minipress), terazosin (Hytrin), phentolamine (Regitine)
   b. Alpha and beta-blockers: labetalol (Normodyne), carvedilol (Coreg); both of these are alpha- and beta- (noncardioselective) blockers
      (1) Actions
         (a) Blocks response to alpha and beta stimulation
         (b) Causes decrease in SVR and BP without reflex tachycardia
         (c) Causes decrease in HR
      (2) Indications
         (a) Hypertension
         (b) Angina
         (c) NYHD Class II or III heart failure (carvedilol)

Table 13-7 Selected Vasodilators

Drug	Administration	Adverse Effects	Nursing Implications
Hydralazine (Apresoline)	• PO: 10-50 mg every 6-8 hours • IV injection: 5-20 mg over 3-5 minutes every 4-6 hours • Maximum: 400 mg/day	• Tachycardia • Orthostatic hypotension • Anorexia, nausea, vomiting, diarrhea • Sodium retention • Weight gain • Palpitations • Flushing • Headache • Tremors • Dizziness • Lupuslike syndrome • Exacerbation of HF or chest pain • Leukopenia, agranulocytosis	• Monitor HR, BP, and ECG • Note contraindications: known hypersensitivity to hydralazine, coronary artery disease, mitral valve disease, and severe aortic stenosis. • Use cautiously in renal disease and cerebrovascular disease. • Administer beta-blockers as prescribed for reflex tachycardia because it may cause myocardial ischemia.
Nitrates (nitroglycerin [Tridil], isosorbide dinitrate [Isordil])	• Sublingual: 0.3-0.4 mg at 5-minute intervals to a maximum of three tablets or metered-dose sprays • PO (isosorbide): 5-40 mg every 6 hours • Transdermal: 1-4 inches every 8 hours • IV infusion: mix 50 mg in 250 mL (200 mcg/mL); initial dose 5-10 mcg/min, increase by 5-10 mcg/min every 5 minutes until desired results are achieved (e.g., control of chest pain and preload reduction)	• Tachycardia or bradycardia • Hypotension or hypertension • Palpitations • Weakness • Apprehension • Flushing • Dizziness • Syncope • Headache • Methemoglobinemia with resultant reduction in Sao_2, and Spo_2, tissue oxygen delivery	• Monitor HR, BP, and urine output. • Monitor RAP, PAP, PAOP, SVR, and CI by hemodynamic monitoring if nitroglycerin is being administered IV and pulmonary artery catheter has been inserted. • Note contraindications: known hypersensitivity, anemia, intracranial hypertension, cerebral hemorrhage, hypertrophic cardiomyopathy, right ventricular infarction, and ingestion of sildenafil (Viagra), vardenafil (Levitra), or tadalif (Cialis) within the last 24 hours. • Use cautiously in hypotension; IV nitroglycerin is titratable and preferred in acute situations. • Decrease nitrate tolerance by scheduling oral nitrates with nitrate-free period at night and by removing transdermal nitrates at night.

Continued

Table 13-7 **Selected Vasodilators—cont'd**

Drug	Administration	Adverse Effects	Nursing Implications
	• Maximum: 400 mcg/min • Administer in glass bottle and via non–PVC tubing		• Administer aspirin or acetaminophen for headache—usually dose-related. • Teach patient to protect tablets from light and moisture and to replace them every 3 months. • Teach patient to limit NTG to 3 tablets every 5 minutes and, if no relief is obtained, to go to the ED • Teach patient to apply nitroglycerin paste to any relatively hairless area between the knees and shoulders and to rotate sites to prevent maceration. • Note that patients receiving IV NTG and heparin IV concurrently require more heparin to achieve therapeutic aPTT; monitor aPTT closely with NTG dosage changes or discontinuance.
Nitroprusside (Nipride)	• IV infusion: mix 50 mg in 250 mL (200 mcg/mL) and infuse at 0.5-10 mcg/kg/min • Maximum: 10 mcg/kg/min • Protect from light by wrapping aluminum foil around bag or bottle; it is not necessary to wrap foil around tubing, but avoid exposure of tubing to direct sunlight	• Nausea, vomiting, abdominal pain • Headache • Tinnitus • Dizziness • Diaphoresis • Apprehension • Hypotension • Tachycardia • Palpitations • Coronary artery steal causing myocardial ischemia and chest pain • Intrapulmonary shunt causing hypoxemia (referred to as nitroprusside-induced intrapulmonary shunt) • Methemoglobinemia with resultant reduction in Sa_{O_2}, Sp_{O_2}, and tissue oxygen delivery • Thiocyanate toxicity	• Monitor HR, BP, urine output, and neurologic status. • Note contraindication: known hypersensitivity. • Use cautiously in liver disease, renal disease, anemia, hypovolemia, hypothyroidism, and in older adults. • Discard solution after 24 hours. • Use foil on bottle to protect it from light. • Discard solution if dark brown, blue, green, or red. • Monitor patient for thiocyanate toxicity. ◦ Thiocyanate levels should be determined daily if drug is used longer than 72 hours. ◦ Signs of thiocyanate toxicity are metabolic acidosis, confusion, hyperreflexia, and seizures. ◦ Treatment includes amyl nitrate, sodium nitrate, and/or sodium thiosulfate. ◦ Simultaneous infusion with thiosulfate with nitroprusside may prevent thiocyanate toxicity.
Nesiritide (Natrecor)	• IV injection: mix 1.5 mg in 250 mL of sodium chloride (6 mcg/mL) and administer 2 mcg/kg over 1 minute followed by IV infusion • IV infusion: 0.01 mcg/kg/min for up to 48 hours; may be titrated up to 0.03 mcg/kg/min	• Hypotension • Headache • Back pain • Nausea • Dizziness • Anxiety • Ventricular dysrhythmias	• Monitor HR, BP, urine output, and neurologic status. • Note contraindications: shock; systolic BP less than 90 mm Hg, significant valvular stenosis, restrictive or obstructive cardiomyopathy, constrictive pericarditis, and tamponade. • Use caution when the patient is receiving other drugs that cause hypotension (e.g., ACE inhibitors)
Fenoldopam mesylate (Corlopam)	• IV infusion: mix 10 mg in 250 mL (40 mcg/mL); usual dose is 0.03-0.3 mcg/kg/min • Maximum: 1.7 mcg/kg/min	• Tachycardia, hypotension • Ventricular dysrhythmias • Dizziness • Anxiety • Headache	• Monitor HR, BP, urine output, and neurologic status. • Note contraindications: known hypersensitivity to fenoldopam or sulfite, and intracranial hypertension. • Use caution in patients with glaucoma or ocular hypertension and in patients taking

Table 13-7 Selected Vasodilators—cont'd

Drug	Administration	Adverse Effects	Nursing Implications
		• Flushing • Nausea, vomiting, abdominal pain • Hypokalemia • Increased intraocular pressure • Increased intracranial pressure	other drugs that may cause hypotension (e.g., beta-blockers).
Nifedipine (Procardia)	• PO immediate release: 10-30 mg tid or qid; maximum 180 mg/24 hour • Not FDA approved for sublingual use and *not* recommended for sublingual use (causes precipitous drop in BP that may cause organ hypoperfusion) • PO sustained release: 30-120 mg/daily	• Tachycardia • Dysrhythmias • Hypotension • Nausea, vomiting, heartburn • Diarrhea or constipation • Headache • Flushing • Fatigue • Dizziness • Rash • Pedal edema • Hypokalemia	• Monitor HR, BP, and potassium. • Note contraindications: known hypersensitivity, and severe aortic stenosis. • Use caution in HF, sick sinus syndrome, second- or third-degree AV block, systolic BP less than 90 mm Hg, liver disease, renal insufficiency or failure, and in the elderly.
Nicardipine (Cardene)	• PO: 20 mg tid initially; may be increased to 20-40 mg tid after 3 days if tolerated well • IV infusion: mix 25 mg in 240 mL (0.1 mg/mL) and infuse at 5 mg/hr (50 mL/hr); may be increased by 2.5 mg/hr (25 mL/hour) every 5 minutes until desired BP reduction is achieved. • Do not mix in lactated Ringer's solution • Maximum: 15 mg/hr	• Tachycardia • Hypotension • Nausea, vomiting, heartburn • Flushing • Headache • Chest pain • Heart failure • Hepatitis • Renal failure • Local irritation at injection site	• Monitor HR and BP. • Note contraindications: known hypersensitivity, sick sinus syndrome, second- or third -degree AV block, systolic BP less than 90 mm Hg, and severe aortic stenosis. • Use caution in HF, hypotension, liver disease, renal insufficiency or failure, and in the elderly.
Captopril (Capoten)	• PO: 6.25-150 mg every 8-12 hours • Administer 1 hour before meals • Maximum: 450 mg/day • Other ACE inhibitors: ○ Enalapril (Vasotec) – PO: 5-40 mg daily – IV injection: 0.625 mg every 6 hours ○ Lisinopril (Zestril): 10-80 mg PO daily ○ Ramipril (Altace): 1.25-20 mg PO daily ○ Benazepril (Lotensin): 10-40 mg PO daily in one or two equally divided doses ○ Quinapril (Accupril): 5-80 mg PO daily ○ Fosinopril (Monopril): 10-80 mg PO daily	• Tachycardia • Hypotension especially after first dose • Anorexia • Fatigue • Headache • Loss of taste • Rash, angioedema • Dizziness • Photosensitivity • Proteinuria, nephrotic syndrome, renal failure • Pancytopenia • Hyperkalemia • Bronchospasm • Cough	• Monitor HR, BP, urine output, protein in urine, serum potassium, and WBC • Check periodically for proteinuria. • Monitor WBC and differential counts before treatment and periodically during treatment. • Note contraindications: known hypersensitivity, AV block, and hypotension. • Use cautiously in renal disease, lupus, scleroderma, hypovolemia, leukemia, diabetes mellitus, thyroid disease, COPD, asthma, hyperkalemia, and in patients taking drugs that may affect WBC counts or immune response. • Monitor for allergic reaction: rash, fever, pruritus, and urticaria; antihistamines may be used; discontinuance may be necessary. • Administer thiazide diuretics as prescribed; these drugs frequently are given together. • Angiotensin II blocker (e.g., losartan [Cozaar] or valsartan [Diovan]) may be prescribed if cough develops.

Continued

Table 13-7 Selected Vasodilators—cont'd

Drug	Administration	Adverse Effects	Nursing Implications
Labetalol hydrochloride (Normodyne, Trandate)	• PO: 100-400 mg every 12 hours • IV injection: 20 mg over 2 minutes, may repeat 40 mg every 10 minutes • IV infusion: mix 300 mg in 250 mL for a total volume of 300 mg in 300 mL (1 mg/mL); usual dose is 2 mg/min until satisfactory response is achieved • Maximum: 300 mg	• Bradycardia • Orthostatic hypotension • Ventricular dysrhythmias • AV blocks • HF • Nausea, vomiting, diarrhea • Dizziness • Lethargy • Hypoglycemia without symptoms in type 1 DM	• Monitor HR, BP, ECG, breath sounds, and daily weight. • Note contraindications: known hypersensitivity, shock, second- or third-degree AV block, sinus bradycardia, sick sinus syndrome, NYHA Class IV HF, and asthma. • Use cautiously in diabetes mellitus, renal disease, hepatic disease, thyroid disease, COPD, CAD, bronchospasm, and peripheral vascular disease. • Keep patient supine for 3 hours after IV administration (labetalol). • Do not discontinue suddenly.
Carvedilol (Coreg)	• PO: 6.25 mg bid initially; after 7-14 days, if tolerated well, may be increased to 12.5 bid; after 7-14 days, if tolerated well, may be increased to 25 mg bid • Maximum: 50 mg/day	• Hyperglycemia in type 2 DM • Agranulocytosis, thrombocytopenia • Bronchospasm in patients with COPD or asthma	

ACE, Angiotensin-converting enzyme; *aPTT,* activated partial thromboplastin time; *AV,* atrioventricular; *BP,* blood pressure; *CAD,* coronary artery disease; *CI,* cardiac index; *COPD,* chronic obstructive pulmonary disease; *DM,* diabetes milletus; *ECG,* electrocardiogram; *ED,* emergency department; *FDA,* Food and Drug Administration; *HR,* heart rate; *IV,* intravenous; *NTG,* nitroglycerine; *NYHA,* New York Heart Association; *PAOP,* pulmonary artery occlusive presssure; *PAP,* pulmonary artery pressure; *PO,* oral; *PVC,* polyvinyl chloride; *RAP,* right atrial pressure; *Sao_2,* arterial oxygen saturation; *Spo_2,* oxygen saturation by pulse oximetry; *SVR,* systemic vascular resistance; *WBC,* white blood cell.

Vasopressors

Action: Vasoconstriction

Indications

1. Severe hypotension
   a. Note that it is always important to determine the reason for hypotension rather than simply start vasopressor therapy.
   b. Focus on restoration of perfusion rather than just a blood pressure.
2. Vasogenic shock: vasopressors are indicated to make dilated vessels normal size rather than to make normal size vessels small (which would decrease perfusion).

Types of Vasopressors and Specific Actions and Indications

See Table 13-2.

1. Phenylephrine (Neo-Synephrine)
   a. Action: stimulates alpha receptors
      (1) Causes vasoconstriction and increases BP but does not cause tachycardia
      (2) Increases aortic root pressure and coronary artery perfusion pressure
   b. Indications
      (1) Vasogenic shock especially when tachycardia is detrimental
2. Norepinephrine (Levophed)
   a. Action: stimulates alpha and beta receptors
      (1) Causes vasoconstriction and increases BP with minimal tachycardia
      (2) Increases aortic root pressure and coronary artery perfusion pressure
   b. Indications
      (1) Vasogenic shock especially when tachycardia is detrimental
3. Epinephrine
   a. Action: stimulates alpha and beta receptors
      (1) Causes vasoconstriction and increases BP with minimal tachycardia
      (2) Increases HR, myocardial contractility
      (3) Increases aortic root pressure and coronary artery perfusion pressure
      (4) Acts as a histamine antagonist in anaphylaxis
   b. Indications
      (1) Cardiac arrest
         (a) Asystole
         (b) Ventricular fibrillation (VF)
         (c) Pulseless electrical activity (PEA)
      (2) Asthma
      (3) Anaphylaxis
      (4) Vasogenic shock
4. Vasopressin (Pitressin): antidiuretic hormone
   a. Action
      (1) Reduces portal venous pressure through vasoconstriction

(2) Increases water reabsorption in the renal tubule
(3) Causes contraction of coronary, splanchnic, GI, pancreatic, skin, and muscular vascular beds

b. Indications
(1) Cardiac arrest: alternative to epinephrine with longer half-life
(2) Upper GI hemorrhage
(3) Diabetes insipidus
(4) Vasogenic shock

5. Dopamine (see Inotropic Agents; Table 13-8)

Table 13-8 Selected Vasopressors

Drug	Administration	Adverse Effects	Nursing Implications
Phenylephrine (Neo-Synephrine)	• IV infusion: mix 30 mg in 500 mL (60 mcg/mL); usual dose is 2-10 mcg/kg/min	• Reflex bradycardia • Ventricular dysrhythmias • Hypertension • Nausea, vomiting • Paresthesia • Palpitations • Anxiety • Restlessness • Headache • Tremor • Chest pain	• Monitor BP, heart rate, and ECG • Note contraindications: known hypersensitivity, ventricular fibrillation, tachydysrhythmias, pheochromocytoma, and narrow-angle glaucoma. • Use cautiously in older adults and those with hyperthyroidism, CAD, hypertension, psychoneurosis, diabetes mellitus, and peripheral vascular disease. • Prevent extravasation because necrosis may occur; treat with phentolamine (Regitine). • Treat reflex bradycardia with atropine. • Discard drug if discolored or precipitate is present.
Norepinephrine bitartrate (Levophed)	• IV infusion: mix 4 mg in 250 mL (16 mcg/mL) and infuse at 0.5-30 mcg/min; titrate to BP response • Maximum: 30 mcg/min • Administer through central venous catheter if possible; if administered peripherally, use a large vein • Do not administer with alkaline solutions	• Bradycardia • Ventricular dysrhythmias • Hypertension • Anxiety • Headache • Tremor • Chest pain • Dizziness • Metabolic (lactic) acidosis • Severe vasoconstriction may cause renal or mesenteric necrosis • Local necrosis with high dosages or if infusion infiltrates	• Monitor heart rate, BP, ECG, urine output, and neurologic status. • Note contraindications: known hypersensitivity, ventricular fibrillation, tachydysrhythmias, pheochromocytoma, and narrow-angle glaucoma. • Use cautiously in peripheral vascular disease, hyperthyroidism, CAD, hypertension, psychoneurosis, diabetes, in patients receiving MAO inhibitors or tricyclic antidepressants, and in older adults. • Note that this drug may cause a fluid shift from intravascular to interstitial space, causing depletion of intravascular volume. • Do not use discolored solution. • Prevent extravasation because necrosis may occur; treat with phentolamine (Regitine).
Epinephrine hydrochloride (Adrenalin)	• Cardiac arrest ○ IV injection: 1 mg; may repeat at 3- to 5-minute intervals ○ IV infusion: mix 1 mg in 250 mL (4 mcg/mL) and infuse at 2-10 mcg/min; titrate to desired effect ○ Administer through central venous catheter if possible; if administered peripherally, use a large vein ○ Do not administer with alkaline solutions • Asthma or anaphylaxis ○ Subcutaneous 0.1-0.5 mg, or 0.1-0.25 mg IV	• Tachycardia • Dysrhythmias • Palpitations • Anxiety • Restlessness • Headache • Dizziness • Tremor • Cerebral hemorrhage • Chest pain • Hyperglycemia	• Monitor BP, heart rate, and ECG • Note contraindications: glaucoma, organic brain damage, or cardiomegaly. • Use cautiously in older adults and those with hyperthyroidism, chest pain, hypertension, psychoneurosis, and diabetes mellitus. • Prevent extravasation because necrosis may occur; treat with phentolamine (Regitine). • Discard drug if discolored or precipitate is present.

Continued

Table 13-8 Selected Vasopressors—cont'd

Drug	Administration	Adverse Effects	Nursing Implications

Vasopressin (Pitressin)	• For cardiac arrest
	  ○ IV injection: 40 units (if no response, epinephrine may be used after 10-20 minutes)
	• For GI hemorrhage
	  ○ IV infusion: mix 100 units/100 mL (1 unit/mL) and administer at 0.1-0.8 unit/min (concurrent nitroglycerin administration is recommended with doses higher than 0.4 unit/min)
	  ○ Maximum: 1 unit/min
	• For diabetes insipidus
	  ○ Aqueous vasopressin 5-10 units subcutaneous 2 to 3 times daily or 3 units/hr IV
	  ○ Vasopressin in oil 5 mg deep IM
	  ○ Lypressin or desmopressin (DDAVP) given by nasal spray
	• For vasogenic shock
	  ○ IV infusion: 0.01 to 0.04 unit/min
		• Bradycardia
		• Hypertension
		• Fever
		• Water intoxication (e.g., SIADH), hyponatremia
		• Nausea, abdominal cramps
		• Tremor
		• Headache
		• Seizures
		• Coma
		• Constriction of cardiac arteries, resulting in chest pain and myocardial ischemia
			• Monitor heart rate, BP, daily weight, and serum sodium.
			• Note contraindications: known hypersensitivity and nephritis.
			• Use cautiously in coronary artery disease.
			• Administer NTG as prescribed concurrently with IV vasopressin infusion to prevent potential complications related to cardiac ischemia.
			• Prevent extravasation because necrosis may occur; treat with phentolamine (Regitine).

Antidysrhythmic Agents

Action: Prevent or Treat Dysrhythmias

Indication: Dysrhythmias, Particularly When Symptomatic

Types of Antidysrhythmics and Specific Actions and Indications

Figure 13-2 shows how the classes of the Vaughan-Williams classification system affect the action potential.

1. Class I antidysrhythmic agents block the influx of sodium into the cell during phase 0 (depolarization)
   a. Class IA (e.g., quinidine [Quinidex, Cardioquin], procainamide [Pronestyl], and disopyramide [Norpace])
      (1) Actions
         (a) Block sodium influx during phase 0, which depresses the rate of depolarization
         (b) Prolongs repolarization and action potential and lengthens refractory period
         (c) Decreases contractility (negative inotrope)
      (2) Indications
         (a) Supraventricular dysrhythmias
         (b) Ventricular dysrhythmias
   b. Class IB (e.g., lidocaine [Xylocaine], tocainide [Tonocard], and mexiletine [Mexitil])
      (1) Actions
         (a) Blocks sodium influx during phase 0, which depresses the rate of depolarization
         (b) Shortens repolarization and action potential duration
         (c) Suppresses ventricular automaticity in ischemic tissue
      (2) Indication: ventricular dysrhythmias
   c. Class IC (e.g., flecainide [Tambocor] and propafenone [Rythmol])
      (1) Actions
         (a) Blocks sodium influx during phase 0, which depresses the rate of depolarization
         (b) Does not change repolarization and action potential duration
      (2) Indication: life-threatening or refractory ventricular dysrhythmias
2. Class II antidysrhythmic agents (e.g., propranolol [Inderal], esmolol [Brevibloc], acebutolol [Sectral], and sotalol [Betapace]; note that sotalol has Class II and Class III characteristics)
   a. Actions: block the beta receptors
      (1) Depresses sinoatrial (SA) node automaticity
      (2) Increases refractory period of atrial and AV junctional tissue to slow conduction

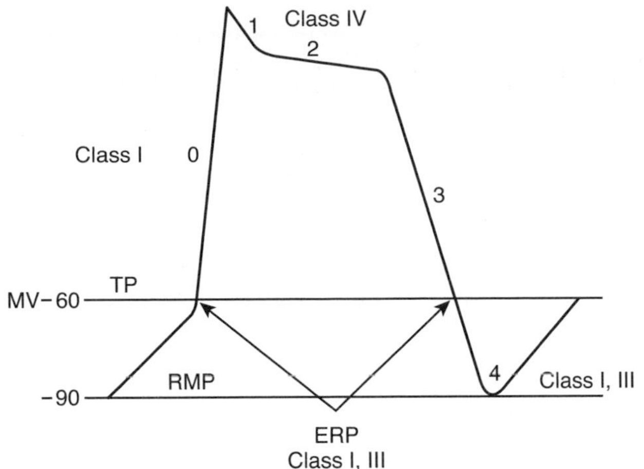

Figure 13-2 Effects of antidysrhythmic agents on the action potential. *TP*, threshold potential; *RMP*, resting membrane potential; *ERP*, effective refractory period.

(3) Shortens action potential duration
(4) Decreases myocardial contractility
(5) Blocks sympathetic nervous system beta receptors (Box 13-2)
(a) Noncardioselective beta-blockers block $beta_1$ and $beta_2$ receptors.
(b) Cardioselective beta-blockers block predominantly $beta_2$ receptors
(6) Decreases myocardial O_2 consumption

b. Indications
(1) Dysrhythmias (particularly when caused by SNS stimulation): supraventricular and ventricular
(2) Other nondysrhythmia indications for beta-blockers
(a) Hypertension
(b) Heart failure (NYHA Class II or III)
(c) Coronary artery disease
(i) Acute MI
(ii) Angina
(iii) Primary and secondary prophylaxis to prevent MI
(d) Pheochromocytoma
(e) Hyperthyroid crisis
(f) Hypertrophic cardiomyopathy
(g) Intraoperative or postoperative tachycardia and/or hypertension (esmolol)

3. Class III antidysrhythmic agents (e.g., amiodarone [Cordarone], sotalol [Betapace], ibutilide [Corvert], and dofetilide [Tikosyn])
a. Actions
(1) Blocks potassium movement during phase III
(2) Increases action potential duration
(3) Prolongs effective refractory period
(4) Slows conduction through accessory pathways
b. Indications
(1) Amiodarone
(a) Life-threatening or refractory ventricular dysrhythmias
(b) Refractory supraventricular dysrhythmias especially those caused by Wolff-Parkinson-White (WPW) syndrome

BOX 13-2 Beta-Blockers Categorized as Noncardioselective or Cardioselective

Noncardioselective
Propranolol (Inderal)
Nadolol (Corgard)
Timolol (Blocadren)
Pindolol (Visken)
Carteolol (Cartrol)
Penbutolol (Levatol)
Labetalol (Normodyne; alpha and beta receptors)
Carvedilol (Coreg; alpha and beta receptors)

Cardioselective
Acebutolol (Sectral)
Atenolol (Tenormin)
Metoprolol (Lopressor)
Esmolol (Brevibloc)
Betaxolol (Kerlone)
Bisoprolol (Zebeta)

(2) Sotalol: life-threatening or refractory ventricular dysrhythmias
(3) Ibutilide or dofetilide: recent onset atrial fibrillation or atrial flutter

4. Class IV antidysrhythmic agents (e.g., verapamil [Calan, Isoptin] and diltiazem [Cardizem])
a. Actions
(1) Blocks the efflux calcium movement during phase II (plateau) to prolong the action potential and, therefore, refractory periods
(2) Depresses automaticity in the SA and AV nodes
(3) Prolongs the conduction time in the AV junction and increases the refractory period at the AV junction
(4) Decreases contractility (negative inotrope)
b. Indications
(1) Supraventricular dysrhythmias with rapid ventricular response rate
(2) Other nondysrhythmia indications for beta-blockers
(a) Hypertension
(b) Coronary artery disease: angina
(c) Hypertrophic cardiomyopathy

5. Miscellaneous: some drugs do not fit in the categories of the Vaughan-Williams classification system
a. Digoxin (see Inotropic Agents)
b. Adenosine (Adenocard)
(1) Actions
(a) Blocks reentry mechanism
(b) Shortens action potential of atrial tissue with little or no effect on action potential of ventricle
(c) Prolongs AV nodal refractory period
(d) Decreases SA node automaticity and slows sinus rate
(2) Indications
(a) Supraventricular tachycardias (SVTs) including those associated with Wolff-Parkinson-White (WPW) syndrome

(b) Wide QRS complex tachycardia of unknown origin
(c) Note that adenosine is not effective in atrial fibrillation or atrial flutter but may slow rate so that fibrillatory or flutter waves can be identified

c. Atropine
(1) Action
(a) Blocks parasympathetic nervous system effects to increase SA node firing rate and to improve AV nodal conduction
(b) Relaxes smooth muscle; prevents bronchospasm
(c) Decreases GI and tracheobronchial secretions
(2) Indications
(a) Symptomatic sinus bradycardia
(b) Asystole
(c) Nondysrhythmia indications
(i) Preoperative preparation for surgery
(ii) Anticholinesterase insecticide (organophosphate) poisoning
(iii) Bronchospasm, asthma (e.g., ipratropium [Atrovent])

d. Isoproterenol
(1) Actions: stimulates beta receptors
(a) Increases HR, myocardial contractility, and conductivity
(b) Relaxes smooth muscle
(i) Peripheral vasodilation
(ii) Bronchodilation
(2) Indications
(a) Torsades de pointes
(b) Bradycardia in a patient after cardiac transplant because denervated heart does not respond to atropine

Text continued on p. 811

Table 13-9 Selected Antidysrhythmic Agents

Drug	Administration	Adverse Effects	Nursing Implications
CLASS IA			
Quinidine sulfate	• PO, IM: 200-400 mg every 4-6 hours ◦ Give PO dose with food • Therapeutic blood level: 2-6 mcg/mL	• Dysrhythmias including torsades de pointes • Hypotension • Anorexia, nausea, vomiting, diarrhea • Hepatotoxicity • Rash • Fever • Vertigo, light-headedness • Headache • Tinnitus • Blurred vision • HF • Hemolytic anemia, thrombocytopenia, agranulocytosis	• Monitor HR, BP, and ECG ◦ Report hypotension and widening of QRS complex greater than 25% or prolongation of QT interval to more than half of RR interval. • Note contraindications: known hypersensitivity, blood dyscrasia, AV block, and myasthenia gravis. • Use cautiously in renal disease, liver disease, HF, respiratory distress, potassium imbalance, and in patients taking digitalis. ◦ Drug may precipitate digitalis toxicity in patients receiving digitalis. ◦ Dose should be decreased in HF and liver disease. • Instruct patient to report skin rash, fever, unusual bleeding, bruising, ringing in ears, or visual disturbances
Procainamide hydrochloride (Pronestyl)	• PO 0.5-1 g every 4-6 hours • IM 250-500 mg every 4-6 hours • IV injection: 50-100 mg every 5 minutes ◦ Stop injections and start maintenance infusion when suppression of dysrhythmia, widening of QRS complex by 50%; hypotension, or a total of 17 mg/kg occur • IV infusion: mix 2 g in 500 mL (4 mg/mL) and infuse at 1-4 mg/min • Therapeutic blood level: 3-10 mcg/mL	• Bradycardia • Hypotension • AV block • Dysrhythmias including torsades de pointes • Anorexia, nausea, vomiting, abdominal pain, diarrhea • Hepatic dysfunction • Bitter taste • Rash, urticaria • Fever • Mental depression • Hallucinations • Seizures • Bone marrow depression, thrombocytopenia • Worsening HF • Lupuslike syndrome	• Monitor BP, HR, and ECG ◦ ECG effects include increased PR interval, QRS complex width, and QT interval. • Note contraindications: known hypersensitivity, myasthenia gravis, and AV block. • Use cautiously in renal disease, liver disease, HF, respiratory depression, and in patients receiving digitalis. • Administer PO drug with food. • Instruct patient to report fever, rash, muscle pain, bruising or bleeding, diarrhea, and chest pain.

Table 13-9 Selected Antidysrhythmic Agents—cont'd

Drug	Administration	Adverse Effects	Nursing Implications
CLASS IB			
Lidocaine hydrochloride (Xylocaine)	• IV injection: ○ VF: 1.5 mg/kg repeated every 3-5 minutes ○ VT: 1 mg/kg repeated every 5-10 minutes ○ Maximum: 3 mg/kg • IV infusion: mix 2 g in 500 mL (4 mg/mL) and infuse at 1-4 mg/min • Therapeutic blood level: 2-5 mcg/mL	• Hypotension • SA arrest • AV block • Nausea, vomiting • Tremors • Restlessness • Light-headedness • Anaphylaxis *Clinical indications of toxicity (in relative order of occurrence)* • Perioral paresthesias • Feelings of dissociation • Dizziness • Drowsiness • Euphoria • Mild agitation • Dysarthria • Hearing impairment • Disorientation • Confusion • Muscle twitching • Seizures • Respiratory arrest	• Monitor BP, HR, and ECG • Note contraindications: known hypersensitivity, AV block, supraventricular dysrhythmias, and sick sinus syndrome. • Use cautiously in liver disease, HF, respiratory depression, malignant hyperthermia, and in older adults. • Note that toxicity incidence is increased if patient has HF or liver disease, has low lean body mass or is elderly, or is concurrently taking cimetidine (Tagamet) or a beta-blocker. • Note that the prophylactic administration of lidocaine after MI is no longer recommended; while the incidence of ventricular fibrillation is decreased, the incidence of asystole is increased.
Tocainide (Tonocard)	• PO: initial dose of 600 mg; then 400 mg bid or tid; maximum 2400 mg/day	• Proarrhythmia including PVCs, ventricular tachycardia, torsades de pointes, PACs, supraventricular tachycardia, bradycardia, SA block or arrest, AV block, bundle branch block • Hypotension • Palpitations • Anorexia, nausea, vomiting, diarrhea, abdominal pain • Chest pain • Diaphoresis • Pulmonary fibrosis (dyspnea, cough, wheezing) • Mood changes • Headache • Dizziness • Paresthesias, tremors • Confusion • Diplopia, blurred vision • Seizures • Coma • Rash • Fever, chills • Thrombocytopenia, aplastic anemia, agranulocytosis	• Monitor HR, BP, and ECG • Note contraindications: second- or third-degree block or sick sinus syndrome without pacemaker and patients with a history of allergic reactions to local amide-type anesthetics. • Use cautiously in older adults and patients with heart failure. • Administer with meals to decrease GI adverse effects. • Note that risk of toxicity is greater if patient is concurrently receiving cimetidine (Tagamet) or a beta-blocker. • Note that dosage is adjusted in heart failure or liver disease. • Instruct patient to report dyspnea or cough (may indicate pulmonary fibrosis) or excessive bruising (may indicate thrombocytopenia) or frequent or unresponsive infection (may indicate agranulocytosis).

Continued

Table 13-9 Selected Antidysrhythmic Agents—cont'd

Drug	Administration	Adverse Effects	Nursing Implications
Mexiletine (Mexitil)	• PO: initial dose of 200-400 mg followed by 200-400 bid, tid, or qid; maximum 1200 mg/day	• Proarrhythmia including PVCs, ventricular tachycardia, torsades de pointes, PACs, supraventricular tachycardia, bradycardia, AV block, bundle branch block • Hypotension • Nausea, vomiting • Diarrhea or constipation • Elevated liver enzymes • Palpitations • Chest pain • Dyspnea • Headache • Paresthesia, tremors, nystagmus, ataxia, dysarthria • Tinnitus • Blurred vision • Dizziness • Drowsiness, insomnia • Confusion • Seizures	• Monitor HR, BP, and ECG • Note contraindications: second- or third-degree block or sick sinus syndrome without pacemaker, and cardiogenic shock. • Administer with meals to decrease GI adverse effects. • Note that risk of toxicity is greater if patient is concurrently receiving cimetidine (Tagamet) or a beta blocker. • Dosage is adjusted in heart failure and liver disease. • Monitor closely for clinical indications of toxicity: tremor, dizziness, ataxia, and nystagmus.
CLASS IC			
Flecainide (Tambocor)	• PO: 50-200 mg twice daily; maximum dose 400 mg/day	• Proarrhythmia including PVCs, ventricular tachycardia, torsades de pointes, PACs, supraventricular tachycardia, bradycardia, SA block or arrest, AV block, bundle branch block • Nausea, vomiting, abdominal pain, constipation • Dyspnea • Chest pain • Headache • Drowsiness • Dizziness • Blurred vision • Tremor • Dry mouth	• Monitor HR, BP, and ECG ○ Report widening of QRS complex of greater than 25%. • Monitor patient closely for heart failure. • Note contraindications: known hypersensitivity, second- or third-degree AV block, and cardiogenic shock. • Use cautiously in heart failure, SA or bifascicular blocks or sick sinus syndrome without a pacemaker, renal disease, liver disease, and myasthenia gravis. • Use cautiously in patient also receiving another negative inotropic agent (e.g., verapamil, procainamide, or a beta-blocker). • Correct electrolyte imbalance before therapy if possible.
Propafenone (Rythmol)	• PO: 150-300 mg tid; maximum 900 mg/day	• Proarrhythmia including PVCs, ventricular tachycardia, torsades de pointes, PACs, supraventricular tachycardia, bradycardia, SA block or arrest, AV block, bundle branch block • AV block • Nausea, vomiting, constipation • Heart failure • Dyspnea, bronchospasm • Dizziness	• Monitor HR, BP, ECG ○ Report widening of QRS complex of greater than 25%. • Monitor patient closely for clinical indications of heart failure. • Note contraindications: heart failure, cardiogenicshock; SA, AV, or bifascicular blocks or sick sinus syndrome without a pacemaker; myasthenia gravis; COPD; and hypotension. • Use cautiously in patients with renal or liver disease; dosage may be adjusted. • Use cautiously if the patient also is receiving another negative inotropic agent (e.g., verapamil, procainamide, or a beta-blocker).

Table 13-9 Selected Antidysrhythmic Agents—cont'd

Drug	Administration	Adverse Effects	Nursing Implications
		• Diplopia • Paresthesia • Headache • Bitter or metallic taste • Leukopenia, agranulocytosis, thrombocytopenia, anemia • Bruising	• Use cautiously in patients receiving digitalis because this drug can increase the plasma concentration. • Use cautiously in patients receiving oral anticoagulants because propafenone can increase the plasma concentration. • Administer with food to diminish GI adverse effects. • Correct electrolytes before therapy. • Instruct patient to report recurrent or persistent infection.
CLASS II			
Propranolol (Inderal)	• PO: 10-80 mg tid or qid • IV injection: 0.1 mg/kg in three divided doses at rate not to exceed 1 mg/min • IV infusion: mix 20 mg in 250 mL (0.08 mg/mL); usual dose is 3-8 mg/hr • Therapeutic blood level: 0.04-0.9 mcg/mL	• Bradycardia • AV block • Hypotension • Nausea, vomiting, diarrhea • Fatigue, lethargy • Rash • Syncope • HF • Bronchospasm, especially in patients with asthma • Mental depression • Hyperglycemia in type 2 DM • Asymptomatic hypoglycemia in type 1 DM • Impotence • Emotional lability • Insomnia • Agranulocytosis, thrombocytopenia	• Monitor HR, BP, and ECG • Monitor patient for clinical indications of heart failure. • Note contraindications: known hypersensitivity, sinus bradycardia, AV block greater than first degree, HF, shock, asthma, and Raynaud's syndrome. • Use cautiously in diabetes mellitus, renal disease, hyperthyroidism, COPD, liver disease, myasthenia gravis, peripheral vascular disease, and hypotension. ○ Drug may potentiate the hypoglycemic effects of insulin and prevents sympathetic symptoms of hypoglycemia. • Note that this drug limits cardiac reserve and exercise capacity because the heart rate cannot increase. • Note that this drug masks sympathetic clinical indications of shock because the receptors are blocked.

Esmolol (Brevibloc)	• IV injection: loading dose of 500 mcg/kg over 1 minute followed by maintenance dose of 50 mcg/kg/min for 4 minutes
	  ○ If desired effect does not occur, repeat the loading dose of 500 mcg/kg over 1 minute and follow with a dose increased by 50 mcg/kg/min for 4 minutes (e.g., 500 + 100, 500 + 150, 500 + 200)
	• IV infusion: when desired effect is achieved, no additional loading doses are needed and the maintenance dose is increased by 50 mcg/kg/min and maintained
		• Bradycardia
		• Hypotension
		• AV block
		• Nausea, vomiting
		• Fatigue, lethargy
		• HF
		• Bronchospasm, especially in patients with asthma
		• Urinary retention
		• Inflammation and induration at injection site
			• Monitor HR, BP, and ECG
			• Monitor patient for clinical indications of heart failure.
			• Note contraindications: known hypersensitivity, bradycardia, AV block greater than first degree, HF, shock, and asthma.
			• Use cautiously in diabetes mellitus, renal disease, hyperthyroidism, COPD, liver disease, myasthenia gravis, peripheral vascular disease, and hypotension.
			  ○ Drug may potentiate the hypoglycemic effects of insulin and prevents sympathetic symptoms of hypoglycemia; it masks sympathetic clinical indications of shock because the receptors are blocked.

Continued

Table 13-9 Selected Antidysrhythmic Agents—cont'd

Drug	Administration	Adverse Effects	Nursing Implications
Metoprolol (Lopressor)	• PO: 100-450 mg daily in one or two doses • IV injection: 5 mg IV slowly at 5 minute intervals to a total of 15 mg	• Bradycardia • AV block • Hypotension • Nausea, vomiting, diarrhea, constipation • Fatigue, lethargy • Rash • Syncope • HF • Dyspnea, wheezing • Mental depression • Hyperglycemia in type 2 DM • Asymptomatic hypoglycemia in type 1 DM • Impotence • Emotional lability • Agranulocytosis, thrombocytopenia	• Monitor HR, BP, and ECG • Monitor patient for clinical indications of heart failure. • Note contraindications: known hypersensitivity, sinus bradycardia, AV block greater than first degree, HF, shock, asthma, and Raynaud's syndrome. • Use cautiously in diabetes mellitus, renal disease, hyperthyroidism, COPD, liver disease, myasthenia gravis, peripheral vascular disease, and hypotension. ○ Drug may potentiate the hypoglycemic effects of insulin and prevents sympathetic symptoms of hypoglycemia. • Note that this drug limits cardiac reserve and exercise capacity because the heart rate cannot increase. • Note that this drug masks sympathetic clinical indications of shock because the receptors are blocked.
Sotalol (Betapace) (NOTE: Class II and III)	• PO: initial 80 mg bid followed by 160-320 mg/daily divided into two to three doses	• Proarrhythmia including torsades de pointes, sinus bradycardia; second- or third-degree AV block • Heart failure • Hypotension • Dyspnea • Bronchospasm (especially in patients with history of asthma) • Headache	• Monitor HR, BP, and ECG ○ Report prolongation of QT interval to more than half of RR interval or hypotension. ○ Monitor serum glucose in patients with DM. • Monitor patient closely for clinical indications of heart failure. • Note contraindications: second- or third-degree AV block and SA block without pacemaker. • Do not administer concurrently or within 4 hours of Class IA antiarrhythmics or other Class III antiarrhythmics; do not administer with other drugs that prolong the QT interval such as phenothiazines and tricyclic antidepressants. • Correct electrolytes before therapy. • Warn patient not to discontinue drug abruptly.
CLASS III			
Amiodarone hydrochloride (Cordarone)	• PO: loading dose of 800-1600 mg/day for 1-3 weeks; then 600-800 mg/day for 1 month; then 200-800 mg daily • IV injection (loading dose): 150 mg over 10 minutes followed by • IV infusion: mix 900 mg in 500 mL (1.8 mg/mL); usual dose is 1 mg/min for the next 6 hours followed by 0.5 mg/min ○ Use central venous catheter if more concentrated solution is used ○ Use solutions diluted in PVC containers within 2 hours and solutions diluted in glass or polyolefin containers within 24 hours	• Hypotension • Proarrhythmia including PVCs, ventricular tachycardia, torsades de pointes, PACs, supraventricular tachycardia, bradycardia, SA block or arrest, AV block, and bundle branch block • HF • Nausea, vomiting • Dizziness • Headache • Fatigue, malaise, muscle weakness • Corneal microdeposits • Rash, photosensitivity • Altered liver enzymes, hepatotoxicity • Hyperthyroidism, hypothyroidism	• Monitor HR, BP, ECG and depth, breath sounds, electrolytes, liver function studies, thyroid function studies, pulmonary function studies, chest x-ray, and neurologic symptoms. ○ Monitor patient for clinical indications of heart failure and pulmonary fibrosis. • Note contraindications: known hypersensitivity, marked sinus bradycardia, second- or third-degree AV block unless functioning pacemaker, and cardiogenic shock. • Use cautiously in patients with sinus node disease, conduction disturbances, severely depressed ventricular function, and marked cardiomegaly. • Do not confuse amiodarone (an antidysrhythmicagent) with amrinone (an inotropic agent). • Advise methylcellulose ophthalmic solution and annual eye examinations for patients on long-term therapy. • Advise use of SPF 15 sunscreen and sunglasses for patients on long-term therapy.

Table 13-9 Selected Antidysrhythmic Agents—cont'd

Drug	Administration	Adverse Effects	Nursing Implications
	○ Administer through PVC tubing because dosing has taken into account adsorption to tubing • Therapeutic blood level: 1.5-2.5 mcg/mL	• Blue-gray skin discoloration • Tremors, peripheral neuropathies, extrapyramidal symptoms • Cough, progressive dyspnea, pulmonary fibrosis	• Monitor for drug interactions: interacts with digitalis, anticoagulants, beta-blockers, calcium channel blockers, phenytoin, and Class I antidysrhythmic agents. ○ If used concurrently with digitalis, monitor patient closely for indications of digitalis toxicity. • Administer oral drug with food to decrease GI adverse effects.
Ibutilide (Corvert)	• IV infusion: mix 1 mg in 50 mL and infuse over 10 minutes for patients weighing more than 60 kg (0.01 mg/kg in patients weighing less than 60 kg); may be repeated after 10 minutes if needed • Discontinue if atrial fibrillation or flutter terminates, a new dysrhythmia occurs, or prolongation of the QT interval occurs	• Proarrhythmia including PVCs, ventricular tachycardia, torsades de pointes, PACs, supraventricular tachycardia, bradycardia, AV block, bundle branch block • Hypotension	• Monitor HR, BP, and ECG ○ Report widening of QRS complex by greater than 25% or prolongation of QT interval to more than half of RR interval or hypotension. • Correct electrolyte imbalances (especially hypokalemia) before initiating ibutilide therapy. • Administer anticoagulants for 2-3 weeks as prescribed for patients with atrial fibrillation of more than 2 to 3 days' duration. • Note contraindications: patients with second- or third-degree AV block, SA block without pacemaker, hypersensitivity to ibutilide, or congenital or acquired long QT syndrome and patients receiving verapamil or drugs that prolong the QT interval. • Use cautiously in patients receiving digitalis because this drug may mask the cardiotoxicity associated with excessive digoxin levels. • Do not administer concurrently or within 4 hours of Class IA antiarrhythmics or other Class III antiarrhythmics; do not administer with other drugs that prolong the QT interval such as phenothiazines and tricyclic antidepressants.
Dofetilide (Tikosyn)	• PO: 500 mcg twice daily ○ Initiation of this oral therapy requires hospitalization for monitoring of QT interval while dosage is adjusted ○ Dosage also is adjusted according to creatinine clearance	• Proarrhythmia including PVCs, ventricular tachycardia, torsades de pointes, PACs, supraventricular tachycardia, bradycardia, AV block, bundle branch block • Hypotension • Nausea • Syncope • Chest pain	• Monitor HR, BP, and ECG ○ Report widening of QRS complex by greater than 25% or prolongation of QT interval to more than half of RR interval or hypotension. • Correct electrolyte imbalances (especially hypokalemia or hypomagnesemia) before initiating dofetilide. • Note contraindications: patients with second- or third-degree AV block, SA block without pacemaker, or hypersensitivity to dofetilide and patients receiving verapamil or drugs that prolong the QT interval. • Do not administer concurrently or within 4 hours of Class IA antiarrhythmics or other Class III antiarrhythmics; do not administer with other drugs that prolong the QT interval such as phenothiazines and tricyclic antidepressants.
CLASS IV Verapamil (Calan)	• PO: 40-120 mg every 6 hours • IV injection: 0.075-0.15 mg/kg (5-10 mg); may be repeated in 15-30 minutes at 5-10 mg	• Bradycardia • AV block • Hypotension • Nausea • Constipation or diarrhea • Elevated liver enzymes • Headache	• Monitor HR, BP, ECG, liver function studies, breath sounds, and heart sounds. • Note contraindications: known hypersensitivity, AV block, sick sinus syndrome, WPW syndrome advanced HF, and cardiogenic shock. • Use cautiously in HF, hypotension, liver disease, and renal disease and in patients receiving digitalis or beta-blockers.

Continued

Table 13-9 Selected Antidysrhythmic Agents—cont'd

Drug	Administration	Adverse Effects	Nursing Implications
	◦ Maximum: 20 mg • IV infusion: mix 50 mg in 250 mL (200 mcg/mL); usual dose is 1-5 mcg/kg/min • Therapeutic blood level: 0.1-0.15 mcg/mL	• Dizziness • Heart failure	• Do not give concurrently with IV beta-blockers. • Administer calcium (500 mg to 1 g IV over 10 minutes) as prescribed before IV verapamil to prevent hypotension.
Diltiazem (Cardizem)	• PO: 30-60 mg every 6 hours • IV injection: 0.15-0.25 mg/kg (20 mg average) over 2 minutes, may be repeated in 15 minutes at 0.35 mg/kg (25 mg average) over 2 Minutes • IV infusion: mix 125 mg in 100 mL for a total volume of 125 mL (1 mg/mL) and infuse at 5-15 mg/hr	• Bradycardia • Dysrhythmias • AV block • Hypotension • Nausea • Headache • Flushing • Fatigue • Drowsiness • Edema • Rash • Renal failure • Transient elevation in liver enzymes	• Monitor HR, BP, and ECG. • Note contraindications: known hypersensitivity, severe hypotension, second- or third-degree AV block, SSS, WPW syndrome, acute MI, and pulmonary edema. • Use cautiously in HF, hypotension, liver disease, renal disease, and in older adults.
MISCELLANEOUS			
Digitalis (Digoxin; See Table 13-4)			
Adenosine (Adenocard)	• IV injection: 6 mg IV; must be given within 6 seconds; repeat at 12 mg IV if conversion is not achieved within 1-2 minutes; 12-mg dose may be repeated once ◦ Must be administered as quickly as possible (referred to as IV "slam") because of very short half-life (10 seconds); administer as quickly as possible into NS flush or insert Y connector into line to push NS flush as quickly as possible and push adenosine as quickly as possible	• Transient dysrhythmias at the time of conversion (including short asystolic pause) ◦ Pause may be prolonged especially in patients with sick sinus syndrome • Hypotension if large doses are used • Nausea • Facial flushing • Headache • Dyspnea • Bronchospasm • Chest pressure • Recurrence of dysrhythmias	• Monitor HR, BP, ECG, BP and depth, and breath sounds. • Note contraindications: known hypersensitivity, second- or third-degree AV block, sick sinus syndrome, and ventricular dysrhythmias. • Use cautiously in patients with asthma or older adults. • Decrease initial dosage as prescribed in patients receiving dipyridamole (Persantine), diazepam (Valium), phenobarbital, or carbamazepine (Tegretol); initial dose may be prescribed as 3 mg. • Increase initial dosage as prescribed if patient is receiving aminophylline or another xanthine; initial dose may be prescribed as 12 mg. • Store at room temperature; solution must be clear at time of use.
Atropine sulfate Ipratropium (Atrovent)	• IV injection: 0.5-2 mg (0.5 mg given as initial dose in sinus bradycardia, 1 mg given as initial dose in asystole, 2 mg given as initial dose in organophosphate poisoning); repeated as needed at 3- to 5-minute intervals ◦ Maximum: 0.04 mg/kg (usually approximately 3 mg) • Nebulizer: 0.025 mg/kg diluted with 3-5 mL of normal saline every 6-8 hours • Handheld inhaler: two puffs every 6-8 hours	• Tachycardia, palpitations • Bradycardia if given slowly or in dose of less than 0.5 mg • Hypotension • Dry mouth • Blurred vision, dilated pupils • Urinary retention • Constipation, paralytic ileus • Headache • Dizziness • Restlessness • Increased myocardial oxygen consumption and chest pain in patients with CAD	• Monitor HR, BP, ECG, urine output, and bowel sounds. • Note contraindications: known hypersensitivity to belladonna, glaucoma, GI obstruction, myasthenia gravis, thyrotoxicosis, ulcerative colitis, prostatic hypertrophy, and tachydysrhythmias. • Use cautiously in renal disease, HF, hyperthyroidism, hepatic disease, and hypertension. • Use cautiously in acute MI: do not administer atropine for bradycardia unless the patient is symptomatic; increasing heart rate increases myocardial oxygen consumption and can increase infarction size. • Do not use pupils as a reflection of brain status after atropine administration: pupils will be dilated and nonreactive.

Table 13-9 Selected Antidysrhythmic Agents—cont'd

Drug	Administration	Adverse Effects	Nursing Implications
		NOTE: Ipratropium (by inhalation) causes virtually no systemic adverse effects.	• Use hard candy to help alleviate side effect of dry mouth unless contraindicated.
Isoproterenol (Isuprel)	• Mix 1 mg in 250 mL (4 mcg/mL); infuse at 2-20 mcg/min	• Tachycardia, palpitations • Hypotension • Ventricular dysrhythmias • Chest pain • Flushing • Headache • Nausea, vomiting • Anxiety, tremor • Hyperglycemia	• Monitor BP, heart rate, ECG • Note contraindications: tachydysrhythmias, digitalis toxicity, angina, narrow-angle glaucoma. • Use cautiously in older adults and those with hyperthyroidism, chest pain, hypertension, psychoneurosis, and diabetes mellitus.

AV, Atrioventricular; *BP,* blood pressure; *CAD,* coronary artery disease; *COPD,* chronic obstructive pulmonary disease; *DM,* diabetes mellitus; *ECG,* electrocardiogram; *GI,* gastrointestinal; *HR,* heart rate; *IV,* intravenous; *MI,* myocardial infarction; *NS,* normal saline; *PAC,* premature atrial contraction; *PO,* oral; *PVC,* premature ventricular contraction; *SA,* sinoatrial; *SPF,* skin protection factor; *SSS,* sick sinus syndrome; *WPW,* Wolff-Parkinson-White.

Drugs Affecting Clotting

Platelet Aggregation Inhibitors

1. Although many drugs inhibit platelet aggregation as an adverse effect (e.g., nonsteroidal antiinflammatory agents and quinidine), others (Box 13-3) are prescribed for the specific purpose of impairing platelet aggregation to prevent the development of the platelet plug and indication of the intrinsic pathway.
2. Actions
   a. Inhibits platelet aggregation and platelet-mediated thrombosis
      (1) Quality: inhibit platelet aggregation; though this effect has traditionally been thought to last as long as the platelet lives (9 to 12 days), evidence now suggests that the effect decreases after 24 hours
      (2) Quantity: may decrease the number of platelets, though this is an undesirable effect
         (a) Referred to as thrombotic thrombocytopenic purpura; treated by discontinuance of the offending drug and may require administration of platelets

BOX 13-3 Drugs Used to Decrease Platelet Aggregation

- Aspirin
- Cilostazol (Pletal)
- Clopidogrel (Plavix)
- Dextran 40 (LMD)
- Dipyridamole
- Dipyridamole and aspirin (Aggrenox)
- GP IIb/IIIa platelet receptor blockers (e.g., abciximab [ReoPro], eptifibatide [Integrilin], tirofiban HCl [Aggrastat])
- Heparin
- Ticlopidine (Ticlid)

         (b) Monitor for and report petechiae, ecchymosis, or bleeding
   b. Aspirin blocks synthesis of thromboxane A_2, inhibiting platelet aggregation
   c. Ticlopidine and clopidogrel block adenosine diphosphate from binding to its receptor, inhibiting platelet aggregation
   d. GP IIb/IIIa inhibitors block the GP IIb/IIIa platelet receptor; this interrupts the final common pathway for platelet aggregation by interfering with platelet aggregation via fibrinogen, von Willebrand's factor, and fibronectin
      (1) Differences between these agents
         (a) Half-life
            (i) Abciximab: 10 to 30 minutes
            (ii) Tirofiban: 120 minutes
            (iii) Eptifibatide: 150 minutes
         (b) Duration of platelet inhibition
            (i) Abciximab causes the most significant and prolonged (i.e., usually 18 to 36 hours but may be up to a week) reduction in platelet aggregation
            (ii) Tirofiban and eptifibatide: 1 to 2 hours after cessation of infusion
         (c) Effect of renal insufficiency on dosing
            (i) Abciximab may be used with no adjustment.
            (ii) Tirofiban requires dosage adjustment.
            (iii) Eptifibatide is contraindicated if serum creatinine is 4 mg/dL or higher and requires dosage adjustment if serum creatinine is greater than 2 mg/dL.
3. Indications
   a. Oral agents
      (1) Carotid artery disease for stroke prophylaxis (especially clopidogrel [Plavix], aspirin, or dipyridamole and aspirin [Aggrenox])

 (2) Peripheral arterial disease (especially cilostazol [Pletal])
 (3) After vascular surgery (especially dextran 40)
 (4) Maintenance of coronary artery stent patency (especially clopidogrel [Plavix] or aspirin)
 (5) Acute coronary syndrome with or without myocardial infarction (especially aspirin)
 b. IV agents: GP IIb/IIIa platelet receptor blockers (e.g., abciximab [ReoPro], eptifibatide [Integrilin], and tirofiban hydrochloride [HCL] [Aggrastat])
 (1) Acute coronary syndrome (ACS) with or without percutaneous coronary intervention (PCI); note that abciximab is only used for ACS if PCI is planned within 24 hours
 (2) PCI when risk for thrombosis is high (i.e., coronary artery stent placement)
4. Evaluation of effect: bleeding time
5. Reversal agent: no specific reversal agent; platelet transfusion may be indicated

Anticoagulants

1. Indirect thrombin inhibitors (e.g., unfractionated heparin [UFH] or low-molecular-weight heparin [LMWH])
 a. Action: accelerates the formation of the antithrombin III–thrombin complex, which deactivates thrombin and prevents the conversion of fibrinogen to fibrin
 (1) Prevents extension of existing clots
 (2) Decreases platelet aggregation
 (3) Note that there is an unpredictable dose-response relationship, though prediction of response is improved with weight dosing
 b. Indications
 (1) Acute coronary syndrome (UFH or LMWH)
 (2) Prevention or treatment of deep venous thrombosis (DVT) (UFH or LMWH)
 (3) Pulmonary embolism (UFH or LMWH)
 (4) Peripheral arterial emboli (UFH)
 (5) Transient ischemic attack or ischemic stroke (UFH)
 (6) Disseminated intravascular coagulation with clinical evidence of thromboembolism (UFH)
 (7) Maintenance of arterial patency after PCI or fibrinolytic therapy (UFH)
 (8) Maintenance of arterial line patency (UFH)
 c. Differences between UFH and LMWH
 (1) LMWH is more potent at inactivating factor Xa than inactivating thrombin.
 (2) LMWH has a longer half-life: 4 to 6 hours compared with 1 to 2 hours for UFH.
 (3) LMWH has 90% bioavailability, whereas UFH has only 30% bioavailability, which allows a more predictable anticoagulant response for LMWH.
 (4) Less risk of heparin-induced thrombocytopenia (HIT) with LMWH than UFH.
 (5) Cost of LMWH is greater, but there is not a need for ongoing laboratory monitoring.
 d. Evaluation of effect
 (1) UHF: activated partial thromboplastin time (aPTT), activated clotting time (ACT)
 (2) LMWH: monitoring of coagulation parameters is not required but may prolong prothrombin time (PT) and aPTT
 e. Reversal agent: protamine
 (1) One mg of protamine neutralizes approximately 100 units of heparin.
 (2) Administer protamine slowly to avoid hypotension.
2. Direct thrombin inhibitors (lepirudin [Refludan], argatroban [Acova], and bivalirudin [Angiomax])
 a. Action: inhibit thrombin activity (Note that there is a predictable dose-response relationship.)
 b. Indications
 (1) HIT and associated thromboembolic complications (specifically lepirudin and argatroban)
 (2) Patient with acute coronary syndrome undergoing PCI (specifically bivalirudin)
 (3) Being evaluated for use in ischemic stroke, disseminated intravascular coagulopathy, and MI
 c. Evaluation of effect: aPTT, ACT
 d. Reversal agent: none
3. Oral anticoagulants (e.g., warfarin [Coumadin])
 a. Actions: limits the availability of vitamin K, which is necessary for the formation of factors II (prothrombin), VII, IX, and X, along with the anticoagulant proteins C and S
 (1) Prevents development of a clot
 (2) Prevents extension of an existing clot and secondary thromboembolic complications
 b. Indications
 (1) DVT
 (2) Valvular heart disease
 (3) Arial dysrhythmias
 (4) After valve replacement
 c. Evaluation of effect: PT, international normalized ratio (Table 13-10)
 d. Reversal agent: vitamin K

Table 13-10 Recommended International Normalized Ratio for Selected Indications

Indication	INR
Prophylaxis for venous thrombosis	2.0-3.0
Treatment of venous thrombosis	2.0-3.0
Treatment of pulmonary embolism	2.0-3.0
Prevention of systemic embolism	2.0-3.0
Tissue heart valves	
Acute MI	
Valvular heart disease	
Atrial fibrillation	
Mechanical prosthetic valves	2.5-3.5

Fibrinolytic Agents

1. Action: activation of plasminogen to accelerate clot lysis
   a. Recombinant plasminogen activators (e.g., alteplase [Activase], reteplase [Retavase], and tenecteplase [TNKase])
      (1) Activate plasminogen to plasmin, the active agent that degrades the fibrin clot (i.e., speeds up the normal process to allow early reperfusion)
      (2) Causes clot-specific lysis to reestablish flow
   b. Streptokinase (Streptase)
      (1) Activates plasminogen systemically and converts it to plasmin, which then degrades fibrin clots, fibrinogen, and other plasma proteins
      (2) Causes systemic lytic state
   c. Comparison of agents (Table 13-11)
2. Table indications
   a. Myocardial infarction (within 6 hours or still having ischemic chest pain)
      (1) The goal is to have fibrinolytic agents initiated within 30 minutes of the patient's arrival to the emergency department because time is muscle.
         (a) Door
         (b) Data
         (c) Decision
         (d) Drug
      (2) Note that primary PCI is preferred if a cardiac catheterization laboratory and an interventional cardiologist are available; the goal is to have the catheter passing the stenosis within 60 to 90 minutes.
   b. Ischemic stroke (within 3 hours): it is necessary to perform a computed tomography (CT) scan to rule out hemorrhagic stroke and have that CT scan interpreted within the 3-hour window before administering the fibrinolytic agent
   c. Massive pulmonary embolism: as indicated by acute right ventricular failure, refractory hypoxemia, and/or hemodynamic instability
   d. Acute arterial occlusion: typically administered intraarterially

Antisepsis Drug (Drotrecogin Alfa [Activated; Xigris])

1. Actions
   a. Exerts an antithrombotic effect by inhibiting factors Va and VIIIa.
   b. Exerts an indirect profibrinolytic activity through inhibition of plasminogen activator inhibitor-1 and limiting generation of activated thrombin-activatable-fibrinolysis-inhibitor
   c. Exerts an antiinflammatory effect by inhibition of human tumor necrosis factor production by monocytes, by blocking leukocyte adhesion to selectins, and by limiting the thrombin-induced inflammatory responses within the microvascular endothelium
2. Indications: severe sepsis (sepsis associated with acute organ dysfunction) in patients who have a high risk of death (e.g., acute physiology and chronic health evaluation [APACHE] II score greater than 25); the criteria used in the clinical trials include the following:
   a. Suspected or proven infection
   b. Evidence of three of the systemic inflammatory response syndrome criteria
      (1) Tachycardia (greater than 90 beats/min)
      (2) Hyperpnea (respiratory rate greater than 20 breaths/min or $Paco_2$ less than 32 mm Hg)
      (3) Hyperthermia (temperature above 38°C or 100.4°F) or hypothermia (temperature below 36°C or 96.8°F); hypothermia is more common in elderly patients
      (4) White blood cell count (WBC) greater than 12,000 cells/mm^3 or less than 4000 cells/mm^3 or more than 10% bands

Table 13-11 Comparison of Fibrinolytic Agents

	Streptokinase	Recombinant Fibrinolytics
Half-life	20 minutes, but effects last 48-72 hours because of fibrinogen depletion	~5 minutes for alteplase ~15 minutes for reteplase ~20 minutes for tenecteplase
90-minute expected reperfusion rate	50%-60%	70%-85%
Fibrin specificity	No	Yes
Anticoagulant effect	Yes; depletes fibrinogen for up to 72 hours; aspirin is given, but heparin is not recommended	No; aspirin and heparin are required to prevent reocclusion
Allergic reactions	Yes	No
Hypotensive effects	++	+
Contraindications	Prior streptokinase or streptococcal infection within 6-9 months (some references say up to 5 years)	None specific to rt-PA or r-PA
Cost	+	+++++

c. Presence of at least one organ failure within a 24-hour period
   (1) Cardiovascular: hypotension with a systolic BP of less than 90 mm Hg or mean arterial pressure (MAP) of 70 mm Hg for at least an hour despite adequate fluid resuscitation or intravascular volume status or the need for vasopressors to maintain a systolic BP of 90 mm Hg or MAP of 70 mm Hg
   (2) Renal: oliguria for 1 hour despite adequate fluid administration
   (3) Pulmonary: hypoxemia defined as a Pao_2/FIo_2 (fraction of inspired O_2) ratio of less than 250
   (4) Hematologic: platelet count less than 80,000/mm^3 or a 50% decrease in the platelet count from the highest value recorded over the previous 3 days
   (5) Unexplained metabolic acidosis (Table 13-12)

Text continued on p. 821

Table 13-12 Selected Drugs That Affect Clotting

Drug	Administration	Adverse Effects	Nursing Implications
Abciximab (ReoPro)	• IV injection: 0.25 mg/kg administered between 10 minutes and 1 hour before the start of the percutaneous coronary intervention (PCI) followed by infusion • IV infusion: 0.125 mcg/kg/min (10 mcg/min maximum) for 12 hours	• Bleeding ○ Intracranial hemorrhage ○ Hematuria ○ Hematemesis ○ Bleeding at sheath site or other puncture point • Thrombocytopenia • Hypotension • Bradycardia • Nausea, vomiting, abdominal pain • Chest pain • Back pain • Headache • Pain at injection site • Allergic reaction, anaphylaxis (especially with repeat administration)	• Monitor PT, aPTT, or ACT, and platelet count. • Administer with aspirin and heparin therapy as prescribed. • Note contraindications: patients with active internal bleeding, clinically significant bleeding in the GI or GU tract within the last 6 weeks, bleeding diathesis, history of CVA within the last 2 years or CVA with significant residual neurologic deficit, intracranial neoplasm, aneurysm, AV malformation, severe uncontrolled hypertension, use of oral anticoagulants within 7 days unless prothrombin time is less than 1.2 × control, thrombocytopenia, presumed or documented history of vasculitis, major surgery or trauma within the last 6 weeks, pericarditis, and known hypersensitivity to abciximab or murine proteins. • Use cautiously in patients who weigh less than 75 kg, patients older than 65 years of age, patients with a history of GI disease, and patients receiving thrombolytics. • Do not administer with dextran. • Monitor oral secretions, sputum, vomitus, NG aspirate, stool, and urine for blood. • Limit venipuncture and urinary catheterization as much as possible; use IV catheter with saline lock for blood sampling; avoid noncompressible IV sites. • Avoid nasotracheal and nasogastric tubes if possible. • Avoid automatic BP cuffs. • Administer platelets as prescribed for thrombocytopenia. • Store drug refrigerated, do not shake (should be clear), and administer through a filter.
Eptifibatide (Integrilin)	For acute coronary syndrome • IV injection: 180 mcg/kg over 1-2 minutes followed by: ○ IV infusion: 2 mcg/kg/min for up to 72 hours; decreased to 0.5 mcg/kg/min during PCI and continued for 24 hours after PCI	• Bleeding ○ Intracranial hemorrhage ○ Hematuria ○ Hematemesis ○ Bleeding at sheath site • Hypotension	• Monitor PT, aPTT, or ACT, and platelet count. • Note contraindications: active internal bleeding, clinically significant bleeding in the GI or GU tract within the last 6 weeks, bleeding diathesis, history of CVA within the last 2 years or CVA with significant residual neurologic deficit, intracranial neoplasm, aneurysm, or AV malformation, severe uncontrolled hypertension, use of oral

Table 13-12	Selected Drugs That Affect Clotting—cont'd		
Drug	**Administration**	**Adverse Effects**	**Nursing Implications**
	For PCI without acute coronary syndrome • IV injection: 135 mcg/kg over 1-2 minutes before procedure followed by: • IV infusion: 0.5 mcg/kg/min for 24 hours		anticoagulants within 7 days unless prothrombin time is less than 1.2 × control, thrombocytopenia, presumed or documented history of vasculitis, major surgery or trauma within the last 6 weeks, pericarditis, known hypersensitivity to eptifibatide, renal failure, and thrombocytopenia. • Administer drug with aspirin and heparin therapy as prescribed. • Monitor oral secretions, sputum, vomitus, NG aspirate, stool, and urine for blood. • Limit venipuncture and urinary catheterization as much as possible; use IV catheter with saline lock for blood sampling; avoid noncompressible IV sites. • Avoid nasotracheal and nasogastric tubes if possible. • Avoid automatic BP cuffs. • Administer platelets as prescribed for thrombocytopenia. • Store drug refrigerated.
Tirofiban HCl (Aggrastat)	• IV infusion: premixed as 25 mg in 500 mL; usual dose is 0.4 mcg/kg/min for 30 minutes and then continued at 0.1 mcg/kg/min (dosage is decreased in renal failure)	• Bleeding ○ Intracranial hemorrhage ○ Hematuria ○ Hematemesis ○ Bleeding at sheath site • Hypotension • Bradycardia • Pelvic pain	• Monitor PT, aPTT, or ACT, and platelet count. • Note contraindications: active internal bleeding, clinically significant bleeding in the GI or GU tract within the last 6 weeks, bleeding diathesis, history of CVA within the last 2 years or CVA with significant residual neurologic deficit, intracranial neoplasm, aneurysm, or AV malformation, severe uncontrolled hypertension, use of oral anticoagulants within 7 days unless prothrombin time is less than 1.2 × control, thrombocytopenia, presumed or documented history of vasculitis, major surgery or trauma within the last month, pericarditis, and known hypersensitivity to tirofiban. • Use cautiously in patients who weigh less than 75 kg, patients older than 65 years of age, patients with a history of GI disease, patients receiving thrombolytics, and patients with thrombocytopenia. • Administer drug with aspirin and heparin therapy as prescribed. • Limit venipuncture and urinary catheterization as much as possible, use IV catheter with saline lock for blood sampling, avoid noncompressible IV sites. • Monitor oral secretions, sputum, vomitus, NG aspirate, stool, and urine for blood.
Unfractionated heparin (UFH)	• Subcutaneous: usually prophylactic, dose is 5000 units every 12 hours (also called mini-heparin) • IV injection: usually 80 units/kg (maximum 10,000 units) followed by infusion (only 60 units/kg recommended if patient is receiving fibrinolytic agents or GP IIb/IIIa inhibitors) • IV infusion: mix 25,000 units in 500 mL (50 units/mL) and infuse at 18 units/kg/hr	• Hemorrhage with excessive aPTT • Hypertension or hypotension • Hypersensitivity reaction including bronchospasm • Fever • Hepatitis • Hyperkalemia especially in patients with renal failure • Thrombocytopenia	• Monitor aPTT and platelet count, and monitor patient for signs of hemorrhage. ○ Note petechiae and request platelet count if petechiae are noted; heparin usually is discontinued if platelet count is less than 100,000/mm^3. – Administer lepirudin (Refludan) or argatroban as prescribed for HITT. • Note contraindications: known hypersensitivity, active bleeding, blood dyscrasias (except DIC), suspected intracranial hemorrhage, severe hypertension, peptic ulcer disease, open wounds, recent surgery, endocarditis, shock, and threatened abortion.

Continued

Table 13-12 Selected Drugs That Affect Clotting—cont'd

Drug	Administration	Adverse Effects	Nursing Implications
	(maximum 1000 units/hr; only 12 units/kg recommended if patient is receiving fibrinolytic agents or GP IIb/IIIa inhibitors); dose is adjusted to achieve aPTT of 1.5-2.5 times the laboratory control • NOTE: The trend in IV weight-dosed heparin is to decrease the amount of heparin (60 units/kg for injection followed by 12 units/kg/hr for infusion) and desirable aPTT (45-60 seconds) • Maximum: 40,000 units/day	(caused by immune response referred to as HITT)	• Use cautiously in alcoholism, liver disease, and renal disease and in older adults. • Monitor oral secretions, sputum, vomitus, NG aspirate, stool, and urine for blood. • Ensure that protamine sulfate (antidote) is available. • Avoid IM, arterial, or venous punctures if at all possible. • Hold pressure for longer than usual if punctures are necessary. • Do not discontinue drug suddenly: warfarin usually will have already been started and the PT will be within therapeutic range before heparin is discontinued. • Do not aspirate before subcutaneous administration, and do not massage after administration. • Note that NTG interacts with heparin, causing more heparin to be required to achieve therapeutic aPTT; monitor aPTT closely with significant NTG dosage changes or discontinuance.
Low-molecular-weight heparin	Enoxaparin (Lovenox) • SC: 30 mg bid Dalteparin sodium (Fragmin) • SC: 2,500 units daily starting 1-2 hours before surgery and repeated daily for 5-10 days postoperatively Ardeparin (Normiflo) • SC: 50 antifactor Xa units/kg every 12 hours beginning the evening before surgery and continued until the patient is ambulatory Tinzaparin sodium (Innohep) • SC: 175 antifactor Xa units/kg daily for approximately 6 days or until adequate anticoagulation with warfarin	• Bleeding • Epidural or spinal hematoma (especially when used with patients with epidural or spinal anesthesia) • Fever • Elevation of liver enzymes • Thrombocytopenia • Chest pain	• Note that LMW heparin does not require routine laboratory monitoring because it does not usually alter PT or aPTT. • Note that contraindications and cautions are as for heparin. • Obtain baseline platelet count; monitor patient for petechiae. • Monitor oral secretions, sputum, vomitus, NG aspirate, stool, and urine for blood. • Ensure that protamine sulfate (antidote) is available. • Avoid IM, arterial, or venous punctures if at all possible. • Hold pressure for longer than usual if punctures are necessary. • Administer deep subcutaneously but avoid IM injection.

Lepirudin (Refludan)	• IV injection: 0.4 mg/kg (maximum 44 mg) administered over 15-20 seconds followed by IV infusion
	• IV infusion: 0.15 mg/kg/hr (maximum 16.5 mg/kg/hr) for 2-10 days
	• Reduce dosage in renal or hepatic disease
		• Bleeding
		• Anemia
		• Abnormal liver function studies
		• Skin reactions
			• Monitor PT, aPTT, and CBC, and monitor patient for signs of bleeding.
			• Note that contraindications and cautions are as for heparin.
			• Obtain baseline platelet count and aPTT; monitor aPTT every 4 hours.
			  ○ Anticoagulant effects may increase as the duration of therapy increases.
			  ○ Anticoagulant effects are increased in patients receiving platelet aggregation inhibitors, fibrinolytic agents, or other anticoagulants.
			• Monitor oral secretions, sputum, vomitus, NG aspirate, stool, and urine for blood.
			• Avoid IM, arterial, or venous punctures if at all possible.

Table 13-12 Selected Drugs That Affect Clotting—cont'd

Drug	Administration	Adverse Effects	Nursing Implications
			• Hold pressure for longer than usual if punctures are necessary. • Gradually reduce the lepirudin dosage to reach an aPTT ratio just above 1.5 before initiating oral anticoagulant therapy.
Argatroban (Acova)	• IV infusion: mix 250 mg in 250 mL of normal saline (1 mg/mL); administer initially at 2 mcg/kg/min; no loading dose is given • Maximum: 10 mcg/kg/min • Reduce dosage in hepatic disease; start at 0.5 mcg/kg/min	• Bleeding: gastrointestinal, genitourinary, intracranial • Allergic reaction • Dyspnea • Hypotension • Fever • Diarrhea • Sepsis • Cardiac arrest	• Monitor PT, aPTT, and CBC, and monitor patient for signs of bleeding. • Note that contraindications and cautions are as for heparin. • Obtain baseline platelet count and aPTT; monitor aPTT every 4 hours. ○ Anticoagulant effects are increased in patients receiving platelet aggregation inhibitors, fibrinolytic agents, or other anticoagulants. • Monitor oral secretions, sputum, vomitus, NG aspirate, stool, and urine for blood. • Avoid IM, arterial, or venous punctures if at all possible. • Hold pressure for longer than usual if punctures are necessary. • Protect infusion from direct sunlight.
Bivalirudin (Angiomax)	• IV injection: 0.75 to 1 mg/kgfollowed by IV infusion • IV infusion: mix 250 mg in 250 mL of normal saline (1 mg/mL) and infuse at 1.75 to 2.5 mg/kg/hr for 4 hours, and then decrease infusion to 0.2 mg/kg/hr for an additional 14 to 20 hours if needed	• Bleeding • Back pain • Generalized pain • Headache • Nausea • Hypotension	• Monitor PT, aPTT, and CBC, and monitor patient for signs of bleeding. • Note that contraindications and cautions are as for heparin. • Obtain baseline platelet count and aPTT; monitor aPTT every 4 hours; ACT also may be used. ○ Anticoagulant effects are increased in patients receiving platelet aggregation inhibitors, fibrinolytic agents, or other anticoagulants. • Monitor oral secretions, sputum, vomitus, NG aspirate, stool, and urine for blood. • Avoid IM, arterial, or venous punctures if at all possible. • Hold pressure for longer than usual if punctures are necessary. • Protect infusion from direct sunlight.
Warfarin (Coumadin, Panwarfin)	• PO: 2-10 mg daily depending on PT and INR ○ INR 2.0-3.0 – MI – DVT prophylaxis or treatment – Pulmonary embolus – Valvular heart disease atrial fibrillation – Tissue heart valve ○ INR 2.5-3.5 ○ Mechanical heart valve	• Hemorrhage with excessive PT • Agranulocytosis, leukopenia • Hepatitis • Diarrhea • Fever • Rash • Skin necrosis: occurs during the first several days of warfarin therapy; lesions occur on extremities, breasts, trunk, and penis • Cholesterol microemboli causing purple toe syndrome	• Monitor PT and monitor patient for signs of hemorrhage. • Note contraindications: known hypersensitivity, bleeding disorders, leukemia, peptic ulcer disease, liver disease, severe hypertension, endocarditis, acute nephritis, blood dyscrasias, eclampsia, suspected intracranial hemorrhage, open wounds, recent surgery, and threatened abortion. • Use cautiously in alcoholism, pregnancy, lactation, during menses, and during use of any drainage tube and in older adults or in any patient in whom slight bleeding is dangerous. • Ensure that vitamin K (AquaMEPHYTON) is available. • Avoid IM, arterial, or venous punctures if at all possible. • Hold pressure for longer than usual if punctures are necessary.

Continued

Table 13-12 Selected Drugs That Affect Clotting—cont'd

Drug	Administration	Adverse Effects	Nursing Implications
			• Monitor oral secretions, sputum, vomitus, NG aspirate, stool, and urine for blood. • Do not discontinue drug suddenly. • Teach patient to avoid trauma and increased amounts of vitamin K (green leafy vegetables) and how to monitor for bleeding. • Teach the patient to report fever or rash; this usually necessitates discontinuance.
Recombinant plasminogen activator; (r-PA) reteplase (Retavase)	• IV injection of 10 units over 2 minutes initially followed by 10 units over 2 minutes after 30 minutes • Heparin is administered concurrently	• Severe, spontaneous bleeding including potential cerebral, retroperitoneal, GU, GI bleeding, and surface bleeding • Reperfusion dysrhythmias	• Monitor aPTT, PT, thrombin time, and neurologic status, and monitor patient for signs of hemorrhage. • Note contraindications: active bleeding; history of cerebral hemorrhage, intracranial neoplasm, and AV malformation or aneurysm; recent (within 2 months) intracranial or intraspinal surgery or trauma; known bleeding disorder; severe uncontrolled hypertension; and prolonged CPR. • Use cautiously in recent (within 10 days) major surgery, GI, GU bleeding, or trauma; hypertension with SBP greater than 180 mm Hg or DBP greater than 110 mm Hg; high likelihood of thrombus of the left side of the heart; acute pericarditis; significant liver dysfunction; pregnancy; retinopathy; septic thrombophlebitis; advanced age (greater than 70-75 years); patients taking oral anticoagulants; any condition in which bleeding constitutes a significant hazard or would be particularly difficult to manage because of its location. • Identify indications of reperfusion in MI: ○ Cessation of pain ○ ST segments descending back to baseline ○ Reperfusion dysrhythmias (ventricular ectopy including PVCs, VT or VF, accelerated idioventricular rhythm, junctional escape rhythms, or bradycardia) ○ Early CK peak • Limit venipuncture and urinary catheterization as much as possible; use IV catheter with saline lock for blood sampling; avoid noncompressible IV sites. • Avoid nasotracheal and nasogastric tubes if possible. • Avoid automatic BP cuffs. • Administer all drugs through existing IVs started before initiation of thrombolytic therapy or by mouth. • Monitor oral secretions, sputum, vomitus, NG aspirate, stool, and urine for blood. • Bleeding precautions are maintained for 12-24 hours.
Recombinant tissue plasminogen activator; (rt-PA) alteplase (Activase)	For acute MI • IV injection: 15 mg followed by: • IV infusion: 0.75 mg/kg (not to exceed 50 mg) over next 30 minutes, followed by 0.5 mg/kg (not to exceed 35 mg) over the next 60 minutes	• Severe, spontaneous bleeding including potential cerebral, retroperitoneal, GU, GI bleeding, surface bleeding • Reperfusion dysrhythmias	• Monitor aPTT, PT, thrombin time, fibrinogen, and neurologic status, and monitor patient for signs of hemorrhage. • Note contraindications: active bleeding; history of cerebral hemorrhage, intracranial neoplasm, and AV malformation or aneurysm; recent (within 2 months) intracranial or intraspinal surgery or trauma; known bleeding disorder; severe uncontrolled hypertension; and prolonged CPR.

Table 13-12 Selected Drugs That Affect Clotting—cont'd

Drug	Administration	Adverse Effects	Nursing Implications
	• Heparin started within 1 hour of initial dose For ischemic stroke • Total dose: 0.9 mg/kg with maximum dose of less than or equal to 90 mg • IV injection: 10% of this total dose over 1 minute followed by: • IV infusion: remaining 90% of this total dose administer over 60 minutes • Anticoagulants and platelet aggregation inhibitors are not used for at least 24 hours For acute pulmonary embolism • IV infusion: 100 mg at 50 mg/hr for 2 hours For acute arterial occlusion • 0.05 to 0.1 mg/kg/hr by local intraarterial infusion • Reconstitution in sterile water only		• Use cautiously in recent (within 10 days) major surgery, GI, GU bleeding, or trauma; hypertension with SBP greater than 180 mm Hg or DBP greater than 110 mm Hg; high likelihood of thrombus of the left side of the heart; acute pericarditis; significant liver dysfunction; pregnancy; retinopathy; septic thrombophlebitis; advanced age (greater than 70-75 years); patients receiving oral anticoagulants; and any condition in which bleeding constitutes a significant hazard or would be particularly difficult to manage because of its location. • Monitor patient for indications of reperfusion in MI: ○ Cessation of pain ○ ST segments descending back to baseline ○ Reperfusion dysrhythmias (ventricular ectopy including PVCs, VT or VF, accelerated idioventricular rhythm, junctional escape rhythms, and bradycardia) ○ Early CK peak • Note that signs of reperfusion are much more subtle in PE and thrombotic stroke. • Limit venipuncture and urinary catheterization as much as possible; use IV catheter with saline lock for blood sampling; avoid noncompressible IV sites. • Administer all drugs through existing IVs started before initiation of thrombolytic therapy or by mouth. • Avoid nasotracheal and nasogastric tubes if possible. • Avoid automatic BP cuffs. • Monitor oral secretions, sputum, vomitus, NG aspirate, stool, and urine for blood. • Bleeding precautions are maintained for 12-24 hours.
Recombinant tissue plasminogen activator; (rt-PA) tenecteplase (TNKase)	• IV injection over 5 seconds: ○ Less than 60 kg: 30 mg ○ At least 60 but less than 70 kg: 35 mg ○ At least 70 but less than 80 kg: 40 mg ○ At least 80 but less than 90 kg: 45 mg ○ Greater than 90 kg: 50 mg • Heparin is administered concurrently	• Severe, spontaneous bleeding including potential cerebral, retroperitoneal, GU, and GI bleeding and surface bleeding • Reperfusion dysrhythmias	• Monitor aPTT, PT, thrombin time, and neurologic status, and monitor patient for signs of hemorrhage. • Note contraindications: active bleeding; history of cerebral hemorrhage, intracranial neoplasm, and AV malformation or aneurysm; recent (within 2 months) intracranial or intraspinal surgery or trauma; known bleeding disorder; severe uncontrolled hypertension; and prolonged CPR. • Use cautiously in recent (within 10 days) major surgery, GI, GU bleeding, or trauma; hypertension with SBP greater than 180 mm Hg or DBP greater than 110 mm Hg; high likelihood of thrombus of the left side of the heart; acute pericarditis; significant liver dysfunction; pregnancy; retinopathy; septic thrombophlebitis; advanced age (greater than 70-75 years); patients receiving oral anticoagulants; and any condition in which bleeding constitutes a significant hazard or would be particularly difficult to manage because of its location.

Continued

Table 13-12 Selected Drugs That Affect Clotting—cont'd

Drug	Administration	Adverse Effects	Nursing Implications
			• Identify indications of reperfusion in MI: ○ Cessation of pain ○ ST segments descending back to baseline ○ Reperfusion dysrhythmias (ventricular ectopy including PVCs, VT or VF, accelerated idioventricular rhythm, junctional escape rhythms, and bradycardia) ○ Early CK peak • Limit venipuncture and urinary catheterization as much as possible; use intravenous catheter with saline lock for blood sampling; avoid noncompressible intravenous sites. • Avoid nasotracheal and nasogastric tubes if possible. • Avoid automatic BP cuffs. • Administer all drugs through existing IVs started before initiation of thrombolytic therapy or by mouth. • Monitor oral secretions, sputum, vomitus, NG aspirate, stool, and urine for blood. • Bleeding precautions are maintained for 12-24 hours.
Streptokinase (Streptase)	IV: mix 1.5 million units in 250 mL (6000 units/mL) • For acute MI usual loading dose is 750,000 units IV injection followed by 750,000 units IV infusion over next hour • For PE and arterial thromboembolism, usual loading dose is 250,000 units over 30 minutes followed by 100,000 units/hr for up to 72 hours	• Allergic reaction (angioneurotic edema, pruritus, bronchospasm, dyspnea, hypotension, cyanosis, seizures, loss of consciousness) • Severe spontaneous bleeding • Cerebral, retroperitoneal, GU, GI, surface bleeding • Reperfusion dysrhythmias	• Monitor aPTT, PT, thrombin time, and neurologic status; monitor patient for signs of hemorrhage. • Note contraindications: patients who have had recent streptococcal infection or have used streptokinase within 6 months to 5 years. • Note that indications in MI, contraindications, cautions, and signs of reperfusion after use for MI are as for tPA. • Administer diphenhydramine (Benadryl) and hydrocortisone sodium succinate (Solu-Cortef) if chance of allergic reaction. • Limit venipuncture and urinary catheterization as much as possible; use IV catheter with saline lock for blood sampling; avoid noncompressible sites. • Administer all drugs through existing IVs started before initiation of thrombolytic therapy or by mouth. • Avoid nasotracheal and nasogastric tubes if possible. • Avoid automatic BP cuffs. • Monitor oral secretions, sputum, vomitus, NG aspirate, stool, and urine for blood. • Maintain bleeding precautions for 48-72 hours because of fibrinogen depletion seen with streptokinase therapy.
Drotrecogin alfa (activated; Xigris)	• IV infusion: mix 20 mg in 100 mL (0.2 mg/mL) and administer at 24 mcg/kg/hr for 96 hours via a dedicated IV catheter or lumen • No titration necessary • Complete each infusion within 12 hours of preparation;	• Bleeding (should clinically important bleeding occur, stop drug immediately)	• Monitor HR, BP, temperature, and clinical indications of bleeding. • Note contraindications: ○ Active internal bleeding ○ Recent (within 3 months) hemorrhagic stroke ○ Recent (within 2 months) intracranial or intraspinal surgery or severe head injury ○ Trauma with an increased risk of life-threatening bleeding

Table 13-12 Selected Drugs That Affect Clotting—cont'd

Drug	Administration	Adverse Effects	Nursing Implications
	no antibacterial preservatives have been added • Avoid exposure to heat and/or direct sunlight • Store in refrigerator • No dosage adjustment required for age, gender, or hepatic or renal dysfunction • Discontinue 2 hours before invasive surgical procedures with an inherent risk of bleeding		○ Presence of an epidural catheter ○ Intracranial neoplasm or mass lesion or evidence of cerebral herniation ○ Known contraindications in patients with known hypersensitivity to drotrecogin alfa • Use caution in patients with the following (predispose to bleeding): ○ Concurrent therapeutic heparin use (greater than or equal to 15 units/kg/hr) ○ Platelet count less than 30,000 × 10^6/L, even if platelet count is increased after transfusion ○ Prothrombin time: INR greater than 3.0 ○ Recent (within 6 weeks) GI bleeding ○ Recent (within 3 days) administration of fibrinolytic therapy ○ Recent (within 7 days) administration of oral anticoagulants or glycoprotein IIb/IIIa inhibitors ○ Recent (within 7 days) administration of aspirin greater than 650 mg/day or other platelet inhibitors ○ Recent (within 3 months) ischemic stroke ○ Intracranial AVM or aneurysm ○ Known bleeding diathesis ○ Chronic severe hepatic disease ○ Any other condition in which bleeding constitutes a significant hazard or would be particularly difficult to manage because of its location • Monitoring: Drug may variably prolong the aPTT, so aPTT cannot be used to assess the status of coagulopathy during Xigris infusion. • Protect infusion from direct sunlight.

ACT, Activated clotting time; *aPTT,* activated partial thromboplastin time; *AV,* atrioventricular; *AVM,* arteriovenous malformation; *BP,* blood pressure; *CBC,* complete blood count; *CK,* creatine kinase; *CPR,* cardiopulmonary resuscitation; *CVA,* cerebrovascular accident; *DBP,* diastolic blood pressure; *DIC,* disseminated intravascular coagulation; *DVT,* deep vein thrombosis; *GI,* gastrointestinal; *GP,* glycoprotein; *GU,* genitourinary; *HCl,* hydrochloride; *HIT,* heparin-induced thrombocytopenia; *HR,* heart rate; *IM,* intramuscular; *INR,* international normalized ratio; *IV,* intravenous; *LMW,* low molecular weight; *MI,* myocardial infarction; *NG,* nasogastric; *NTG,* nitroglycerin; *PCI,* percutaneous coronary intervention; *PCTA,* percutaneous transluminal coronary angioplasty; *PE,* pulmonary embolism; *PO,* oral; *PT,* prothrombin time; *PVC,* premature ventricular contractions; *SBP,* systolic blood pressure; *SC,* subcutaneous; *tPA,* tissue plasminogen activator; *VF,* ventricular fibrillation; *VT,* ventricular tachycardia.

Respiratory Drugs

Bronchodilators

1. Action: smooth muscle relaxation and bronchodilation
2. Indications
   a. Asthma (i.e., reactive airway disease)
   b. Acute bronchospasm related to anaphylaxis
   c. Pulmonary hypertension (specifically xanthines)
3. Types of bronchodilators and specific actions
   a. Sympathomimetics ($beta_2$ stimulants; e.g., epinephrine, isoproterenol [Isuprel], albuterol [Proventil], isoetharine [Bronkosol], metaproterenol [Alupent], terbutaline sulfate [Brethine], and salmeterol [Serevent])
   b. Anticholinergics (e.g., ipratropium [Atrovent])
   c. Xanthines (e.g., aminophylline, oxtriphylline [Choledyl], and theophylline [Theo-Dur]); additional effects include the following:
      (1) Relaxes smooth muscle of pulmonary vessels and decreases pulmonary vascular resistance
      (2) Increases cardiac contractility causing increased CO and GFR
      (3) Inhibits histamine and slow-reacting substance of anaphylaxis
   d. Electrolytes (e.g., magnesium)

Pulmonary Vasodilators

1. Action: relax the smooth muscle of the pulmonary vascular system
2. Indications
   a. Primary pulmonary hypertension
   b. Secondary pulmonary hypertension

(1) Remember that the most common cause of secondary pulmonary hypertension is hypoxemia; O_2 is the first treatment.
(2) Secondary pulmonary hypertension caused by left ventricular failure requires treatment of the heart failure.

3. Types of pulmonary vasodilators (Table 13-13)
   a. Xanthines: oral or IV
   b. Nitric oxide: administered by inhalation so that only vessels to ventilated alveoli are dilated
   c. Epoprostenol (prostacyclin, Flolan): IV
   d. Bosentan (Tracleer): oral

Sedatives

Actions

1. Reduces anxiety, agitation, and skeletal muscle tension
2. Causes sedation or hypnosis
3. Provides conscious or unconscious sedation
4. Inhibits the stress response
5. Potentiates analgesia
6. Decreases O_2 requirements
7. Reduces unnecessary recall (provides amnesia; especially benzodiazepines)

Table 13-13 Selected Respiratory Drugs

Drug	Administration	Adverse Effects	Nursing Implications
Epinephrine (see Table 13-8) Isoproterenol (Isuprel; see Table 13-9)			
Albuterol (Proventil, Ventolin)	• PO: 2-4 mg every 6-8 hours • Handheld inhaler: one to two inhalations every 4-6 hours • Nebulizer: 0.5 mL (2.5 mg) in 3-5 mL of normal saline over 10-15 minutes every 6 hours	• Tachycardia • Palpitations • Nausea, vomiting • Anxiety • Tremor • Headache	• Monitor HR, BP, and breath sounds. • Note contraindications: known hypersensitivity, glaucoma, and tachydysrhythmias; do not give with MAO inhibitors. • Use cautiously in older adults and patients with diabetes mellitus, hypertension, hyperthyroidism, cardiac disease, seizure disorder, and prostatic hypertrophy. • Do not administer with beta-blockers (they block the effect).
Metaproterenol (Alupent, Metaprel)	• PO: 20 mg every 6-8 hours • Handheld inhaler: two to three inhalations every 3-4 hours • Nebulizer: 0.2-0.3 mL of undiluted 5% solution or 2.5 mL of a 6% solution every 6-8 hours	• Tachycardia • Palpitations • Nausea, vomiting • Anxiety • Tremor • Headache	• Monitor HR, BP, and breath sounds. • Note contraindications: known hypersensitivity, glaucoma, and tachydysrhythmias; do not give with MAO inhibitors. • Use cautiously in older adults and patients with DM, hypertension, hyperthyroidism, cardiac disease, seizure disorder, and prostatic hypertrophy. • Do not administer with beta-blockers (they block the effect).

Aminophylline (theophylline [Elixophyllin, Quibron]; Oxtriphylline [Choledyl]; theophylline, ephedrine hydrochloride, phenobarbital [Tedral])	• PO: 250-500 mg every 6-8 hours
	• IV: loading dose of 5-6 mg/kg (250-500 mg) over 20 minutes followed by infusion
	• IV infusion: mix 500 mg in 250 mL (2 mg/mL) and infuse at 0.1-0.9 mg/kg/hr
	  ◦ HF, liver disease: – 0.1-0.2 mg/kg/hr
	  ◦ COPD: ~0.3 mg/kg/hr
	  ◦ Smokers: ~0.8 mg/kg/hr
	• Therapeutic blood level: 10-20 mcg/mL
		• Tachycardia
		• Hypotension
		• Palpitations
		• Anxiety
		• Restlessness
		• Insomnia
		• Dizziness
		• Tremors
		• Headache
		  ◦ Signs of toxicity
		  ◦ Anorexia, nausea, vomiting
		  ◦ Ventricular dysrhythmias
		  ◦ Agitation, seizures
			• Monitor HR, BP, ECG, respiratory rate and rhythm, breath sounds, urine output, and fluid status.
			• Note contraindications: known sensitivity and cardiac dysrhythmias.
			• Use cautiously in older adults and patients with acute MI, HF, hypertension, hepatic disease, acute peptic ulcer, hyperthyroidism, and DM.
			• Administer oral drug with meals to decrease GI adverse effects.

BP, Blood pressure; *COPD,* chronic obstructive pulmonary disease; *DM,* diabetes mellitus; *ECG,* electrocardiogram; *HR,* heart rate; *IV,* intravenous; *GI,* gastrointestinal; *HF,* heart failure; *MAO,* monoamine oxidase; *MI,* myocardial infarction; *PO,* oral.

Indications

1. Sedation in critical care
2. Preoperative anxiety
3. Minor surgical or nonsurgical procedures (e.g., cardioversion)
4. Use of neuromuscular blocking agents (NMBAs)
5. Mechanical ventilation
6. Alcohol withdrawal
7. Seizures
8. Intracranial hypertension (especially pentobarbital)
9. Terminal care

Assessment of Degree of Sedation

1. Ramsay sedation scale (Table 13-14)
2. Sedation-agitation scale (Table 13-15)
3. Motor activity assessment scale (Table 13-16)
4. Bispectral index (BIS) monitoring
   a. An electroencephalogram (EEG) parameter developed specifically to measure patient's response to sedation and anesthesia
   b. Method
      (1) A sensor pad is placed on the patient's forehead to detect electrical activity in the brain.
      (2) The EEG signals are transmitted to the BIS module, and they are processed to provide a measure of level of consciousness.
      (3) Changes reflect changes in the effects of sedative and anesthetic agents.
   c. Evaluation: usual goal is a BIS between 60 and 70
      (1) Value of close to 100 corresponds to a fully awake state.
      (2) Value of greater than 80 corresponds to anxiolysis with response to normal voice.
      (3) Value of 60 to 80 corresponds to a light hypnotic state with response to loud commands or gentle shaking.
      (4) Value of 40 to 60 corresponds to a deep level of sedation; person is unresponsive to verbal stimuli.
      (5) Value of 40 or less corresponds to a deep hypnotic state or barbiturate coma.
      (6) Value of 0 corresponds to a flat line EEG.

Table 13-14 Ramsay Sedation Scale

Score	Description
1	Anxious, agitated or restless, or both
2	Cooperative, oriented, tranquil
3	Responding to commands only
4	Asleep but with brisk response to light glabellar tap or loud auditory stimulus
5	Asleep with sluggish response to light glabellar tap or loud auditory stimulus
6	Asleep, unresponsive

From Ramsay, M., Savege, T., Simpson, B., & Goodwin, R. (1974). Controlled sedation with alphaxalone-alphadolone. *British Medical Journal, 2*, 656.

Types of Sedatives

See Tables 13-17 and 13-18.

1. Benzodiazepines (e.g., diazepam [Valium], lorazepam [Ativan], and midazolam [Versed])
   a. Midazolam is the benzodiazepine of choice for short-term (less than 24 hours) sedation of critically ill patients.

Table 13-15 Sedation-Agitation Scale

Score	Definition	Description
7	Dangerous agitation	Pulling at ET tube, trying to remove catheters, climbing over bed rail, striking at staff, thrashing side to side
6	Very agitated	Does not calm despite frequent verbal reminding of limits; requires physical restraints, biting ET tube
5	Agitated	Anxious or mildly agitated, attempting to sit up, calms down to verbal instructions
4	Calm and cooperative	Calm, wakes easily, follows commands
3	Sedated	Difficult to rouse, awakens to verbal stimuli or gently shaking but drifts off again, follows simple commands
2	Very sedated	Arouses to physical stimuli but does not communicate or follow commands, may move spontaneously
1	Unarousable	Minimal or no response to noxious stimuli, does not communicate or follow commands

From Riker, R., Picard, J., & Fraser, G. (1999). Prospective evaluation of the Sedation-Agitation Scale for adult critically ill patients. *Critical Care Medicine, 27*, 1325.
ET, Endotracheal.

Table 13-16 Motor Activity Assessment Scale

Score	Definition
0	Unresponsiveness
1	Responsive only to noxious stimuli
2	Responsive to touch
3	Calm and cooperative
4	Restless and cooperative
5	Agitated
6	Dangerously agitated

From Devlin, J. W., Boleski, G., Mlynarek, M., Nerenz, D. R., Peterson, E., Jankowski, M., et al. (1999). Motor activity assessment scale: A valid and reliable sedation scale for use with mechanically ventilated patients in an adult surgical intensive care unit. *Critical Care Medicine, 27*(7), 1271-1275.

Table 13-17 Comparison of Selected Sedative Agents

	Propofol (Diprivan)	Midazolam (Versed)	Lorazepam (Ativan)	Diazepam (Valium)	Dexmedetomidine (Precedex)
Elimination half-life	1-8 hours	1-12 hours	10-20 hours	20-80 hours	2 hours
Onset	1 minute	2-5 minutes	5-20 minutes	2-5 minutes	2-6 minutes
Active metabolites	No	Yes	No	Yes	No
Continuous infusion	Yes	Yes	Yes	No	Yes

Table 13-18 Selected Sedative Agents

Drug	Administration	Adverse Effects	Nursing Implications
Diazepam (Valium) and other benzodiazepines	Diazepam (Valium) • PO: 2-10 mg every 6-8 hours • IV injection: 1-15 mg at rate no faster than 2 mg/min; may repeat every 2-4 hours • Maximum: 60 mg • Do not mix with any other drugs or dextrose solution *Other benzodiazepines* Lorazepam (Ativan) • PO: 2-6 mg/day in divided doses • IV injection: 1-4 mg slowly every 2-4 hours • IV infusion: 1-10 mg/hr adjusted to desirable sedation level Alprazolam (Xanax) • PO: 0.25-0.5 mg 3 times daily	• Tachycardia • Hypotension (IV) • Nausea, vomiting • Urinary retention • Drowsiness • Dizziness, ataxia • Blurred vision • Slurred speech • Confusion • Respiratory depression (IV) • Drug dependence may occur	• Monitor heart rate, BP, ECG, and respiratory rate and depth. • Note contraindications: known hypersensitivity, glaucoma, and psychosis. • Use cautiously in liver disease and renal disease and in older adults. • Use large veins for IV injection. • Administer flumazenil (Romazicon), a benzodiazepine antagonist, if necessary and prescribed.
Midazolam hydrochloride (Versed)	• IM injection: 0.07-0.35 mg/kg • IV infusion: 0.15-0.35 mg/kg • IV injection: mix 150 mg in 250 mL (0.6 mg/mL); usual dose is 0.05-0.25 mg/kg/hr	• Bradycardia • Dysrhythmias • Hypotension • Nausea, vomiting, hiccups • Headache • Agitation • Bronchospasm • Respiratory depression, apnea • Pain and tenderness at injection site	• Monitor BP, HR, and respiratory rate and depth. • Note contraindications: known hypersensitivity, shock, coma, acute alcohol intoxication, and glaucoma. • Use cautiously in COPD, HF, and renal failure and in older adults and debilitated persons. • Use large muscle mass if drug is given IM, use large vein if drug is given IV, avoid infiltration. • Administer flumazenil (Romazicon), a benzodiazepine antagonist, if necessary and prescribed.
Propofol (Diprivan)	• IV injection: 5 mcg/kg initially and then increase dose by 5-10 mcg/kg/min every 5-10 minutes until level of sedation is reached; followed by IV infusion • IV infusion: premixed in 10 mg/mL concentration; infuse 5 to 50 mcg/kg/min	• Bradycardia • Hypotension • Decreased cardiac output • Nausea, vomiting • Headache • Twitching • Rash • Green urine	• Monitor heart rate, BP, ECG, and respiratory rate. • Note that this drug allows for faster weaning process and faster time to extubation than neuromuscular paralytic agents. • Note contraindications: known hypersensitivity to propofol or lipid emulsion, hyperlipidemia and disorders of lipid metabolism, and intracranial hypertension.

Table 13-18 Selected Sedative Agents—cont'd

Drug	Administration	Adverse Effects	Nursing Implications
	• Maximum: 150 mcg/kg/min • Use strict aseptic technique; discard tubing and unused solution at least every 12 hours	• Respiratory depression • Reactions such as agitation, hyperactivity, and combativeness may occur • Burning/pain at injection site • Hypertriglyceridemia with prolonged infusion • Metabolic acidosis with prolonged infusion • Pancreatitis • Sepsis	• Use cautiously in respiratory depression, dysrhythmias, pancreatitis, hypotension, hypovolemia, and in older adults. • Correct hypovolemia before administration of propofol. • Administer drug with analgesics if needed because this drug provides no analgesia. • Wean by reducing the rate by 5-10 mcg/kg/minevery 10-15 minutes; stop when patient reaches baseline consciousness and orientation.
Dexmedetomidine HCl (Precedex)	• IV injection: 1 mcg/kg over 10 minutes followed by IV infusion • IV infusion: 0.2-0.7 mcg/kg/hr titrated to patient response for up to 24 hours	• Hypotension or hypertension • Bradycardia or tachycardia • Dysrhythmia especially atrial fibrillation • Nausea, vomiting • Fever • Hypoxia • Anemia	• Monitor heart rate, BP, Sao_2. • Arousability and alertness with stimulation does not necessarily indicate lack of efficacy in the absence of other clinical findings. • Use caution in patients with advanced heart block. • Coadministration with other anesthetics, sedatives, hypnotics, and opioids is likely to lead to enhancement of the effects of those drugs. • Avoid contact of dexmedetomidine with rubber because it may interact with natural rubber.
Pentobarbital (Nembutal)	For intracranial hypertension • IV injection: 3 mg/kg IV slowly • IV infusion: mix 2 g in 500 mL (4 mg/mL); usual dose is 1-3 mg/kg/hr For status epilepticus • IV injection: 2-8 mg/kg IV slowly • IV infusion: mix 2 g in 500 mL (4 mg/mL); usual dose is 1-3 mg/kg • Therapeutic blood level: 25-40 mg/dL	• Bradycardia • Hypotension • Rash • Agranulocytosis, thrombocytopenia, anemia • Myocardial depression; may induce HF • Respiratory depression	• Monitor heart rate, BP, respiratory rate, and neurologic status. ○ Note that ICP monitoring is recommended because the most important indicator of neurologic status (LOC) is eliminated by induced coma. ○ Monitor patient for clinical indications of heart failure. • Note contraindications: known hypersensitivity, respiratory depression, liver failure, and renal failure. • Use cautiously in anemia, liver disease, renal disease, hypertension, and in older adults.

BP, Blood pressure; *COPD,* chronic obstructive pulmonary disease; *ECG,* electrocardiogram; *HCl,* hydrochloride; *HF,* heart failure; *HR,* heart rate; *ICP,* intracranial pressure; *IM,* intramuscular; *IV,* intravenous; *LOC,* level of consciousness; *PO,* oral; Sao_2, arterial oxygen saturation.

b. Lorazepam is the benzodiazepine of choice for long-term (more than 24 hours) sedation of critically ill patients.

2. Sedative-hypnotics (e.g., propofol [Diprivan])
   a. Provides advantage of reversibility to allow for short-term breathing trial daily for patients on mechanical ventilation (i.e., "sedation vacation")
3. Alpha$_2$-adrenoceptor agonist (e.g., dexmedetomidine [Precedex])
4. Nursing management principles of sedation (Park et al., 2001)
   a. Always treat pain first.
   b. Ensure patient safety.
   c. Talk to the patient, assess orientation, and reorient as required.

d. Identify and treat cause of agitation (e.g., pain, anxiety, sleep deprivation, and alcohol or drug withdrawal).
e. Complement medication use with provision of comfort and control of environment.
f. Determine the need for sedation.
g. Select and treat to a target level of sedation; use the smallest effective dose of drug.
h. Continually reassess the need for analgesics and sedatives.

Neuromuscular Blocking Agents

Actions

1. Block the transmission of nerve impulses at the skeletal neuromuscular junction.
2. Cause paralysis of all striated muscle.
3. Do not affect consciousness or cerebration or relieve pain.

Indications

1. Patient-ventilator asynchrony
   a. High-frequency ventilation
   b. Pressure-controlled inverse-ratio ventilation
2. Poor lung/chest wall compliance
3. Poor gas exchange
4. Increased intracranial pressure
5. Tetanus
6. Need to decrease O_2 consumption
7. Need to facilitate procedures (e.g., intubation)
8. Need to eliminate shivering

Assessment of Degree of Neuromuscular Blockade

1. Use of a peripheral nerve stimulation device to evaluate train-of-four (Figure 13-3)
   a. Method
      (1) Attach leads over the ulnar nerve at the wrist.
      (2) Attach peripheral nerve stimulator to leads (remember: negative is black; positive is red).
      (3) Evaluate voltage required before paralysis if possible.
         (a) Turn voltage dial to 2 to start; increase voltage as necessary.
         (b) Turn unit on and push train-of-four button.
         (c) Look for thumb twitch, eyelid twitch, foot dorsiflexion, or plantar flexion of great toe.
         (d) Increase voltage if necessary.
   b. Evaluation
      (1) Desired response is one or two twitches out of four stimuli if the patient is receiving the adequate dose for neuromuscular blockade.
      (2) Underparalysis
         (a) Three or four responses of four stimuli indicates underparalysis.
         (b) Dosage should be increased.
      (3) Overparalysis
         (a) No response even with the voltage at maximum indicates overparalysis.
         (b) Dosage should be decreased.

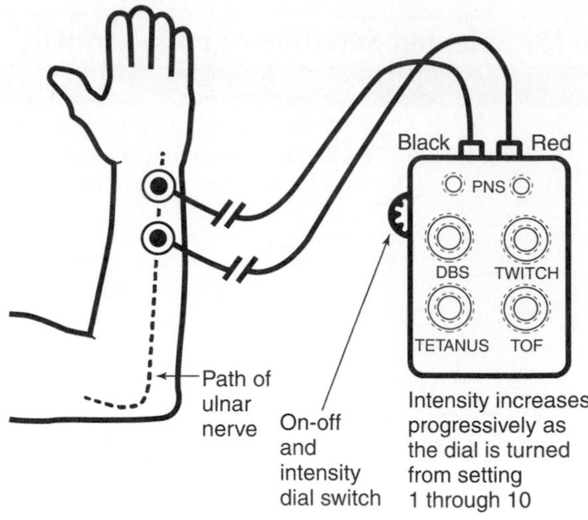

Figure 13-3 Peripheral nerve stimulator. Note placement of electrodes along ulnar nerve. If train-of-four is used, one or two twitches of the thumb is a desirable result. Absence of any thumb twitch indicates overparalysis (reduce dosage of paralytic agent). Three or four twitches of the thumb indicates underparalysis (increase dosage of paralytic agent). (Urden, L., Stacy, K., & Lough, M. [2006]. *Thelan's critical care nursing: Diagnosis and management* [5th ed.]. St. Louis: Mosby.)

Types of Neuromuscular Blockers and Duration of Action

1. Depolarizing
   a. Succinylcholine (Anectine): 8-10 minutes
2. Nondepolarizing
   a. Mivacurium (Mivacron):15-30 minutes
   b. Rocuronium (Zemuron): 20-30 minutes
   c. Atracurium (Tracrium): 20-35 minutes
   d. Vecuronium (Norcuron): 25-30 minutes
   e. Cisatracurium (Nimbex): 30-50 minutes
   f. Tubocurarine (Tubocuraine): 30-100 minutes
   g. Pancuronium (Pavulon): 60-75 minutes
   h. Pipecuronium (Arduan): 60-140 minutes
   i. Doxacurium (Nuromax): 100-150 minutes

Nursing Management Principles of Neuromuscular Blockade

1. Give sedative and/or analgesics concurrently with paralytic agents (Table 13-19).
   a. Clinical signs of inadequate sedation in a patient receiving NMBAs
      (1) Hypertension
      (2) Tachycardia
      (3) Diaphoresis
      (4) Lacrimation
2. Explain the situation to the patient before paralysis.
3. Protect the patient's corneas, skin, and joints; DVT prophylaxis is indicated.
4. Evaluate dose by evaluating train-of-four and adjust accordingly.

Analgesics

Action

Analgesics modify pain perception and reaction.

Table 13-19 Selected Neuromuscular Blocking Agents

Drug	Administration	Adverse Effects	Nursing Implications
Atracurium (Tracrium)	• IV injection: 0.2-0.5 mg/kg followed by IV infusion of 4-12 mcg/kg/min Other neuromuscular blockers • Pancuronium (Pavulon): IV injection 0.1-0.2 mg/kg initially followed by 1-2 mcg/kg/min • Cisatracurium (Nimbex): IV injection 0.1-0.2 mg/kg followed by IV infusion of 1-3 mcg/kg/min • Doxacurium (Nuromax): IV injection of 0.05-0.1 mg/kg; IV infusion is not typical • Mivacurium (Mivacron): IV injection 0.1-0.25 mg/kg followed by IV infusion of 8-10 mcg/kg/min • Pipecuronium (Arduan): IV injection 0.1-0.2 mg/kg followed by IV infusion of 0.5-2 mcg/kg/min • Rocuronium (Zemuron): IV injection 0.6-1.2 mg/kg followed by IV infusion of 10-12 mcg/kg/min • Vecuronium bromide (Norcuron): IV injection 0.08-0.1 mg/kg followed by IV infusion of 1-2 mcg/kg/min	• Bradycardia or tachycardia • Hypertension or hypotension • Bronchospasm, wheezing • Laryngospasm, stridor • Residual muscle weakness • Prolonged use may make weaning difficult because of muscle reconditioning	• Monitor HR, BP, serum electrolytes (especially potassium and magnesium), inspiratory effort, and nerve stimulation. • Use this drug only with intubated patients. • Note contraindication: known hypersensitivity. • Use cautiously in CAD, renal disease, electrolyte imbalance, neuromuscular disease, and pulmonary disease. • Store drug in refrigerator. • Inform patient that paralysis is temporary, and always give analgesic and/or sedative concurrently. • Provide eye care with artificial tears or Lacrilube to prevent corneal abrasion because the patient cannot blink. • Evaluate dose by using peripheral nerve stimulation train-of-four; one to two twitches out of four indicates sufficient but not excessive dose; if no twitches out of four, decrease dose; if three to four twitches, increase dose.

BP, Blood pressure; *CAD,* coronary artery disease; *HR,* heart rate; *IV,* intravenous.

Indications: Pain

Types of Analgesics

See Table 13-20.

1. Agonists
   a. Codeine
   b. Morphine
   c. Oxycodone
   d. Oxymorphone (Numorphan)
   e. Meperidine (Demerol): repeated use is avoided because of accumulation of metabolite normeperidine, especially in elderly patients or patients with renal insufficiency
2. Partial agonist: buprenorphine (Buprenex)
3. Mixed agonist-antagonist
   a. Pentazocine (Talwin)
   b. Nalbuphine (Nubain)
   c. Butorphanol (Stadol)
4. Nonnarcotics
   a. Aspirin
   b. Acetaminophen (Tylenol)
   c. Ketorolac (Toradol)
   d. Ibuprofen (Motrin)

Diuretics

Action

Diuretics promote excretion of fluid and sodium.

Indications

1. Hypertension
2. Heart failure
3. Edema
   a. Pulmonary (usually a loop diuretic)
   b. Cerebral (usually mannitol)
   c. Peripheral
4. Drug toxicity (forced diuresis; usually mannitol)
5. Renal pigments (e.g., hemoglobinuria and myoglobinuria; usually mannitol)

Types of Diuretics and Specific Actions

See Table 13-21.

1. Thiazide diuretics
   a. Examples
      (1) Hydrochlorothiazide (HydroDIURIL)
      (2) Chlorthalidone (Hygroton, Thalitone)
      (3) Chlorothiazide (Diuril)

Table 13-20 Selected Analgesics

Drug	Administration	Adverse Effects	Nursing Implications
Opiates	Morphine • PO: 10-30 mg every 4 hours • IM injection: 4-15 mg every 4 hours • IV injection: 10 mg of MS in 9 mL of saline for total volume of 10 mL and concentration of 1 mg/mL; titration for pain • IV infusion: mix 200 mg in 250 mL (0.8 mg/mL) and titrate for pain management; usual dose 0.05-0.3 mg/kg/hr Fentanyl • IV injection: 50-400 mcg over 2-5 minutes; may repeat 25 mcg every 5 minutes with maximum of 500 mcg within 4-hour period • IV infusion: 0.5-2 mcg/kg/min Hydromorphone (Dilaudid) (especially if renal insufficiency) • IV injection: 1-3 mg every 2-4 hours	• Bradycardia • Orthostatic hypotension • Anorexia, nausea, vomiting • Constipation • Urinary retention • Rash • Euphoria • Drowsiness, confusion • Dizziness • CNS depression • Respiratory depression • Drug tolerance • Physical dependence	• Monitor BP, HR, respiratory rate and depth, urine output, and patient evaluation of pain. • Note contraindications: known hypersensitivity, hemorrhage, asthma, and increased intracranial pressure. • Use cautiously in liver disease, renal disease, head injury, respiratory depression, prostatic hypertrophy, and addictive personality. • Note that maximal respiratory depression occurs within 7 minutes after IV dose. • Administer naloxone (Narcan) as indicated and prescribed for opiate overdosage.

BP, Blood pressure; *CNS,* central nervous system; *IM,* intramuscular; *IV,* intravenous; *HR,* heart rate, *MS,* morphine sulfate; *PO,* oral.

Table 13-21 Selected Diuretics

Drug	Administration	Adverse Effects	Nursing Implications

Furosemide (Lasix)	• PO: 20-80 mg daily
	• IV injection: 20-120 mg; administer at rate not to exceed 20 mg/min; if initial dose is ineffective, the next dose is usually double the original dose
	• IV infusion: mix 250 mg in 250 mL (1 mg/mL); usual dose is 0.1-0.75 mg/kg/hr; not to exceed 4 mg/min
	• Maximum: 1 g/day
	• Do not mix with acidic solutions
	Other loop diuretics
	• Torsemide (Demadex): 5-20 mg daily PO or IV (over 2 minutes); may be titrated to desired effect, but single dose should not exceed 200 mg
	• Bumetanide (Bumex): 0.5-1 mg IV; may be repeated at 2- to 3-hour intervals
		• Hypotension
		• Hypovolemia
		• Nausea, vomiting, abdominal pain
		• Rash
		• Electrolyte imbalance: hypocalcemia, hypokalemia, hypomagnesemia, hyponatremia
		• Acid-base imbalance: hypochloremic alkalosis
		• Increased uric acid and BUN
		• Renal failure
		• Hyperglycemia
		• Photosensitivity
		• Thrombocytopenia, agranulocytosis, leukopenia, neutropenia, anemia
		• Transient deafness (with rapid IV injection)
			• Monitor heart rate, BP, urine output, serum electrolytes, BUN, creatinine, uric acid, CBC, and daily weights.
			  ○ Monitor patients also taking digitalis for clinical indications of digitalis toxicity.
			  ○ Monitor serum glucose in patients with DM.
			  ○ Monitor for clinical indications of gout.
			• Note contraindications: known hypersensitivity to sulfonamides, anuria, hypovolemia, and electrolyte depletion.
			  ○ Sulfonamide-sensitive patients may have allergic reaction to these drugs (furosemide, bumetanide, torsemide) because they are sulfa-derivatives.
			• Use cautiously in diabetes mellitus, dehydration, severe renal disease, gout, and hepatic disease.
			• Do not administer if yellow or if precipitate is present.
			• Teach patient about potassium-rich foods.

Mannitol (Osmitrol)	• IV infusion: 1-2 g/kg over 30-60 minutes; average dose 50-100 g • Use in-line filter when administering mannitol	• Tachycardia • Nausea, vomiting • Fluid and electrolyte imbalance • Pulmonary edema • Thirst • Phlebitis	• Monitor BP, heart rate, urine output, serum osmolality, serum electrolytes, BUN, uric acid, and daily weights. • Note contraindications: known hypersensitivity, active intracranial bleeding, anuria, and severe dehydration.

Table 13-21 Selected Diuretics—cont'd

Drug	Administration	Adverse Effects	Nursing Implications
		• Seizures • Rebound cerebral edema 8-12 hours after diuresis	• Use cautiously in severe renal failure, HF, and dehydration. • Check bottle or ampule for crystallization: discard and replace if crystalized. • Monitor patient closely for rebound effect: return of clinical indications of intracranial hypertension 8-12 hours after mannitol administration.

BP, Blood pressure; *BUN,* blood urea nitrogen; *CBC,* complete blood count; *DM,* diabetes mellitus; *HF,* heart failure; *HR,* heart rate; *IV,* intravenous.

(4) Polythiazide (Renese)
(5) Indapamide (Lozol)
(6) Metolazone (Mykrox, Zaroxolyn)

b. Actions
(1) Inhibit sodium reabsorption in the ascending loop of Henle and the early distal tubule
(2) Decrease water reabsorption

c. Potential adverse effects
(1) Hyponatremia
(2) Hypokalemia
(3) Hypercalcemia
(4) Hypomagnesemia
(5) Hypovolemia
(6) Hyperglycemia
(7) Hyperuricemia
(8) Increased blood urea nitrogen (BUN)
(9) Hepatitis
(10) Anemia, thrombocytopenia, neutropenia

2. Loop diuretics: used most often in critical care because of their potency
a. Examples
(1) Furosemide (Lasix)
(2) Ethacrynic acid (Edecrin)
(3) Bumetanide (Bumex)
(4) Torsemide (Demadex)

b. Actions
(1) Inhibit sodium reabsorption in the ascending loop of Henle
(2) Decrease water reabsorption

c. Potential adverse effects
(1) Hyponatremia
(2) Hypokalemia
(3) Hypocalcemia
(4) Hypomagnesemia
(5) Hypochloremic alkalosis
(6) Hypovolemia
(7) Hyperglycemia
(8) Hyperuricemia
(9) Increased BUN
(10) Hearing loss
(11) Thrombocytopenia, agranulocytosis, leukopenia, anemia

3. Osmotic diuretics
a. Example: mannitol (Osmitrol)

b. Actions
(1) Expand intravascular volume and increase GFR
(2) Increase osmolality of the tubular fluid leading to decreased absorption of sodium and water

c. Potential adverse effects
(1) Hyponatremia
(2) Hypokalemia
(3) Hypocalcemia
(4) Hypomagnesemia
(5) Initial intravascular hypervolemia followed by hypovolemia
(6) Increased intravascular volume may cause pulmonary edema in patients with poor cardiac function
(7) Hyperglycemia
(8) Hyperuricemia
(9) Increased BUN
(10) Confusion

d. Aldosterone antagonists (frequently referred to as potassium-sparing diuretics)
(1) Examples
(a) Spironolactone (Aldactone)
(b) Triamterene (Dyrenium)
(c) Amiloride (Midamor)
(2) Actions
(a) Act as an aldosterone-antagonist
(b) Block sodium and potassium exchange mechanism in the distal tubule, causing loss of sodium and water and retention of potassium
(3) Potential adverse effects
(a) Hyponatremia
(b) Hyperkalemia
(c) Hypocalcemia
(d) Hypomagnesemia
(e) Hypovolemia
(f) Hyperchloremic metabolic acidosis

e. Carbonic anhydrase inhibitors
(1) Examples: acetazolamide (Diamox)

(2) Actions
(a) Block the action of carbonic anhydrase in the proximal tubule, preventing bicarbonate and sodium reabsorption
(b) Cause increased water loss and a decrease in serum pH; may be used to treat metabolic alkalosis
(3) Potential adverse effects
(a) Hyponatremia
(b) Hypokalemia
(c) Hypocalcemia
(d) Hypomagnesemia
(e) Hypovolemia
(f) Hyperchloremic metabolic acidosis
(g) Thrombocytopenia, agranulocytosis, leukopenia, anemia

Gastrointestinal Drugs

Drugs Used to Decrease Gastric Acidity and/or Protect Gastric Mucosa

1. Indications: prevention or treatment of peptic ulcer
2. Types of agents and specific actions (Table 13-22)
a. Antacids
(1) Examples
(a) Aluminum-magnesium complex (Riopan)
(b) Magnesium hydroxide and aluminum hydroxide (Maalox, Mylanta)
(c) Calcium carbonate (Tums)
(2) Actions
(a) Buffers gastric acid
(b) Increases pH to decrease the activity of pepsin
b. Histamine (H_2) receptor antagonists
(1) Examples
(a) Cimetidine (Tagamet)
(b) Ranitidine (Zantac)
(c) Famotidine (Pepcid)
(d) Nizatidine (Axid)
(2) Action: blocks the action of histamine on parietal cells to inhibit volume and concentration of gastric secretions

Table 13-22 Selected Gastrointestinal Drugs

Drug	Administration	Adverse Effects	Nursing Implications
Ranitidine (Zantac)	• PO: 150 mg twice daily with 300 mg at bedtime • IM: 50 mg every 6-8 hours • IV injection: 50 mg in 20 mL slowly every 6-8 hours or 50 mg in 100 mL over 15-20 minutes • IV infusion: mix 300 mg in 250 mL (1.2 mg/mL); usual dose 6.25-12.5 mg/hr	• Dizziness • Elevated liver enzymes, hepatotoxicity • Headache • Malaise	• Monitor HR, BP, liver enzymes, and gastric pH. ○ pH is maintained 3.5 or greater. • Note contraindication: known hypersensitivity. • Use cautiously in liver disease and renal disease.
Pantoprazole sodium (Protonix)	• IV injection: 40 or 80 mg over 2 minutes; may also be diluted in 100 mL and infused over 15 minutes	• Headache • Diarrhea, abdominal pain, flatulence • Rash • Hyperglycemia	• Monitor patient for GI complaints and/or bleeding and monitor serum glucose. • Note contraindication: known hypersensitivity.
Vasopressin (see Table 13-8)			
Octreotide acetate (Sandostatin)	• SC: 50-150 mcg bid or tid • IV injection (for GI bleeding): 50 mcg followed by IV infusion • IV infusion (for GI bleeding): 50 mcg/hr for 1-5 days	• Anorexia, nausea, vomiting • Abdominal pain • Diarrhea, constipation, steatorrhea • Abdominal bloating, flatulence • Increase in liver enzymes • Anxiety • Dizziness • Drowsiness • Heartburn • Hypoglycemia or hyperglycemia • Rectal spasm	• Monitor patient for GI complaints and/or bleeding and monitor serum glucose. • Note contraindication: known hypersensitivity. • Note that this drug is tolerated better than vasopressin for GI bleeding especially in patients with CAD • Do not administer if precipitation or discoloration occurs.

BP, Blood pressure; *CAD,* coronary artery disease; *GI,* gastrointestinal; *HR,* heart rate, *IM,* intramuscular; *IV,* intravenous; *PO,* oral; *SC,* subcutaneous.

c. Proton pump inhibitors
   (1) Examples
      (a) Omeprazole (Prilosec)
      (b) Lansoprazole (Prevacid)
      (c) Pantoprazole sodium (Protonix)
   (2) Action: inactivate hydrogen pump, causing prevention of the formation of hydrochloric acid by parietal cells
d. Mucosal protectant (prostaglandin E_1 analog)
   (1) Example: misoprostol (Cytotec)
   (2) Actions
      (a) Enhances the body's normal gastric mucosal protective mechanisms
      (b) Increases mucosal blood flow
      (c) Decreases gastric acid secretion
e. Mucosal protectant
   (1) Example: sucralfate (Carafate)
   (2) Actions
      (a) Combines with gastric acid and forms an adhesive protective coating over an ulcer crater
      (b) Adsorbs pepsin

Agents Used for Gastrointestinal Hemorrhage

1. Vasopressin (see Table 13-8)
2. Octreotide acetate (Sandostatin)
   a. Actions
      (1) Suppresses secretion of serotonin, gastroenteropancreatic peptides, and growth hormones
      (2) Decreases splanchnic blood flow
      (3) Stimulates fluid and electrolyte absorption from GI tract and prolongs GI transmit time
   b. Indications
      (1) Severe diarrhea associated with carcinoid tumors or vasoactive intestinal peptide tumors
      (2) GI bleeding (off-label)
      (3) GI or pancreatic fistula (off-label)
      (4) After partial pancreatectomy (Whipple procedure; off-label)

Anticonvulsants

See Table 13-23.

Actions

1. Thought to stabilize neurons
2. Decreases sodium influx during action potential of cardiac muscle

Indications: Seizures or Potential for Seizures

Table 13-23 Selected Anticonvulsant Agents

Drug	Administration	Adverse Effects	Nursing Implications
Phenytoin sodium (Dilantin) Fosphenytoin sodium (Cerebyx)	Phenytoin sodium • PO: 300 mg daily • IV loading dose: 15-20 mg/kg at a rate no faster than 50 mg/min • Do not mix with any other drugs or dextrose; flush tubing thoroughly with saline before and after administration • Therapeutic blood level: 10-18 mcg/mL Fosphenytoin sodium • IV loading dose: 15-20 mg phenytoin equivalents (PE) • IV infusion: 4-6 mg PE/kg per 24 hours	• Hypotension if given too rapidly IV • Nausea, vomiting • Headache • Confusion • Nystagmus, diplopia • Dizziness, ataxia • Skin eruptions • Gingival hyperplasia • Slurred speech • Blood dyscrasias • Toxic hepatitis • Lymphadenopathy	• Monitor BP, heart rate, respiratory rate and depth, and response to therapy. • Note contraindications: known hypersensitivity, psychosis, bradycardia, SA or AV block, and sick sinus syndrome. • Use cautiously in allergy, liver disease, and renal disease. • Less hypotension and dysrhythmia potential with fosphenytoin sodium.

AV, Atrioventricular; *BP,* blood pressure; *IV,* intravenous; *PO,* oral; *SA,* sinoatrial.

LEARNING ACTIVITIES

1. Directions: Complete this crossword puzzle dealing with critical care pharmacology. Use only generic names.

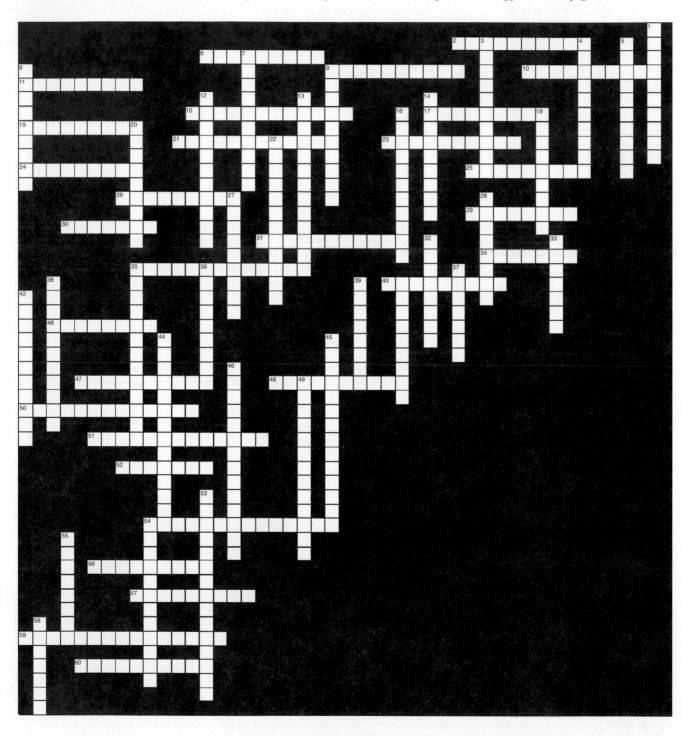

Across

2. An arterial dilator with dopaminergic stimulation used to improve renal flow
6. This electrolyte is used in torsades de pointes
9. A Class IC antidysrhythmic agent used for refractory ventricular dysrhythmias
10. The sympathomimetic inotropic agent used most frequently in cardiogenic shock
11. A GP IIb/IIIa inhibitor frequently used after PCIs
15. An IV pulmonary vasodilator used in pulmonary hypertension
17. An IV Class III antidysrhythmic agent used for acute onset atrial fibrillation
19. An inhaled bronchodilator that is more $beta_2$ specific than isoproterenol
21. A tissue plasminogen activator with a longer half-life; given as a single bolus
23. A drug used for GI hemorrhage and pancreatitis
24. A tissue plasminogen activator with short half life; given as a bolus followed by an infusion
25. A Class IV antidysrhythmic agent; frequently used in SVT
26. An ACE inhibitor; may cause rash or cough
29. A sympathomimetic with dose-dependent effects
30. A cardioselective beta-blocker with short half-life; given by IV infusion
31. A hormone used in pulseless ventricular tachycardia (VT) or VF as an alternative to epinephrine; longer half-life than epinephrine
34. A parenteral indirect thrombin inhibitor
35. A predominantly arterial vasodilator that may cause thiocyanate toxicity
40. A nucleoside used to break reentrant mechanism in paroxysmal supraventricular tachycardia
43. An IV sedative with short half-life; suspended in 10% lipids
47. A short-acting nondepolarizing NMBA
48. A phosphodiesterase inhibitor that may cause thrombocytopenia
50. A pure beta stimulant; may be used in torsades de pointes
51. An alpha-selective sympathomimetic
52. An electrolyte used in hyperkalemia, hypermagnesemia, hypocalcemia, and calcium channel blocker toxicity
54. A drug used in peripheral arterial disease to increase the flexibility of the red blood cells
56. A Class IB antidysrhythmic agent; monitor for indications of toxicity such as paresthesia, confusion, and seizures
57. A short-acting benzodiazepine that causes amnesia
59. An IV agent for short-term sedation (less than 24 hours); patient can be extubated while receiving this drug
60. An alpha- and beta-blocker used in heart failure

Down

1. An oral Class III antidysrhythmic agent used for new onset atrial fibrillation; requires hospitalization and ECG monitoring during initiation of therapy
3. A calcium channel blocker frequently used in variant angina
4. A cardioselective beta-blocker; used for secondary prevention of acute MI
5. A Class III antidysrhythmic agent; first-line antidysrhythmic agent for pulseless VT or VF
7. A beta-type natriuretic hormone used in heart failure
8. An angiotensin receptor blocker used for hypertension
9. A loop diuretic; rapid administration may cause temporary deafness
12. A sympathomimetic used in pulseless VT, VF, asystole, and PEA
13. A corticosteroid that may be used to reduce cerebral edema associated with brain tumor
14. A phosphodiesterase inhibitor; more potent and with fewer side effects than amrinone
16. A calcium channel blocker used for hypertension; available for IV use
18. An ACE inhibitor available in IV form
20. An alpha- and beta-blocker; used for hypertension
22. An alpha-blocker; frequently used for sympathomimetic drug infiltration to prevent tissue necrosis
27. A direct thrombin inhibitor that may be used for heparin-induced thrombosis and thrombocytopenia (HITT)
28. An analgesic of choice in acute MI; venous vasodilator
32. An osmotic diuretic frequently used for intracranial hypertension
33. A cardiac glycoside; decreases ventricular response rate in atrial fibrillation and flutter
35. A predominantly venous nitrate-type vasodilator
36. An electrolyte; usually included in postoperative fluid replacement
37. A platelet aggregation inhibitor used for primary and secondary prevention of MI
38. A noncardioselective beta-blocker
39. An oral agent that interferes with the production of prothrombin
41. A Class IV antidysrhythmic agent that decreases contractility less than verapamil
42. An arterial dilator administered by IV injection; used in hypertension especially if related to pregnancy
44. An aldosterone antagonist that may be used in heart failure
45. A corticosteroid indicated in sepsis when steroid depletion occurs
46. An alpha-dominant sympathomimetic
49. A xanthine bronchodilator
53. A recombinant activated protein C; used in severe sepsis (two words)
54. A Class IA antidysrhythmic agent; may cause prolongation of the QT interval and torsades de pointes
55. A benzodiazepine anxiolytic
58. A low-molecular-weight form used as a platelet aggregation inhibitor especially after vascular surgery

2. **Directions:** Complete the following calculations.

a.

Drug: dobutamine
Dose: 5 mcg/kg/min
Concentration: 500 mg/500 mL
Patient's weight: 80 kg
Rate: _____

b.

Drug: sodium nitroprusside
Dose: _____
Concentration: 50 mg/250 mL
Patient's weight: 70 kg
Rate: 45 mL/hr

c.

Drug: dopamine
Dose: _____
Concentration: 400 mg/250 mL
Patient's weight: 70 kg
Rate: 14 mL/hr

d.

Drug: nitroglycerin
Dose: 50 mcg/min
Concentration: 50 mg/500 mL
Rate: _____

e.

Drug: lidocaine
Dose: 3 mg/min
Concentration: 2 g/500 mL
Rate: _____

LEARNING ACTIVITIES ANSWERS

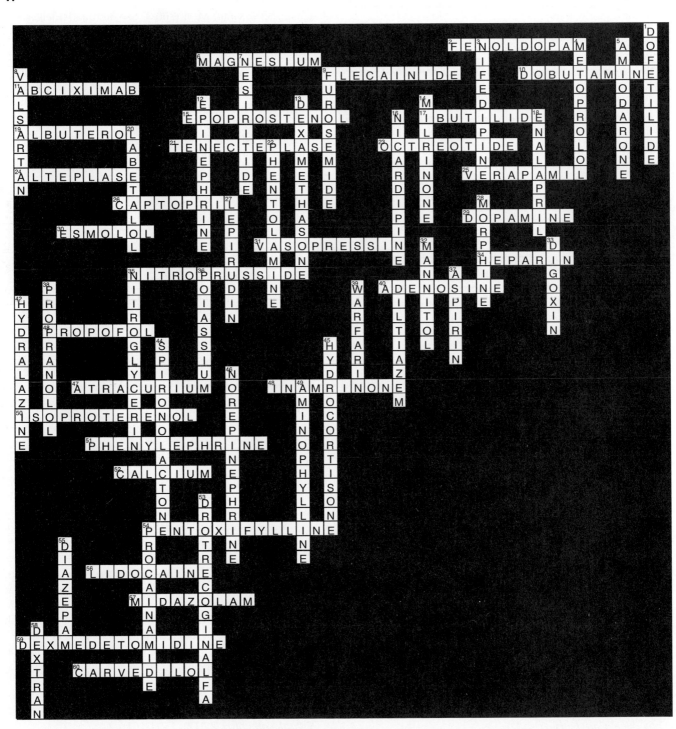

1.

1 DOFETILIDE
2 FENOLDOPAM
3 NIFEDIPINE
4 METOPROLOL
5 AMIODARONE
6 MAGNESIUM
7 NESIRITIDE
8 VALSARTAN
9 FLECAINIDE
10 DOBUTAMINE
11 ABCIXIMAB
12 EPINEPHRINE
13 DEXAMETHASONE
14 MILRINONE
15 EPOPROSTENOL
16 NICARDIPINE
17 IBUTILIDE
18 ENALAPRIL
19 ALBUTEROL
20 LABETALOL
21 TENECTEPLASE
22 PHENTOLAMINE
23 OCTREOTIDE
24 ALTEPLASE
25 VERAPAMIL
26 CAPTOPRIL
27 LEPIRUDIN
28 MORPHINE
29 DOPAMINE
30 ESMOLOL
31 VASOPRESSIN
32 MANNITOL
33 DIGOXIN
34 HEPARIN
35 NITROGLYCERIN
36 POTASSIUM
37 ASPIRIN
38 PROPRANOLOL
39 WARFARIN
40 ADENOSINE
DILTIAZEM
42 HYDRALAZINE
43 PROPOFOL
44 SPIRONOLACTONE
45 HYDROCORTISONE
46 NOREPINEPHRINE
47 ATRACURIUM
48 INAMRINONE
49 AMINOPHYLLINE
50 ISOPROTERENOL
51 PHENYLEPHRINE
52 CALCIUM
53 DROTRECOGIN ALFA
54 PENTOXIFYLLINE
PROCAINAMIDE
55 DIAZEPAM
56 LIDOCAINE
57 MIDAZOLAM
58 DEXTRAN
59 DEXMEDETOMIDINE
60 CARVEDILOL

2. a. 24 mL/hr
b. 2 mcg/kg/min
c. 5 mcg/kg/min
d. 30 mL/hr
e. 45 mL/hr

References

American Society of Health-System Pharmacists. (1998). Suggested definitions and relationships among medication misadventures, medication errors, adverse drug events, and adverse drug reactions. *American Journal of Health-System Pharmacy,* 55, 165-166.

Bates, D. W., Boyle, D. L., Vander Vliet, M. B., Schneider, J., & Leape, L. (1995). Relationship between medication errors and adverse drug events. *Journal of General Internal Medicine,* 10, 199-205.

Institute for Safe Medication Practices. (2005). ISMP's list of high-alert medications. Retrieved August 10, 2006, from http://www.ismp.org/Tools/highalertmedications.pdf

Kohn, L. T., Corrigan, J. M., & Donaldson, M. S. (Eds.). (2000). To err is human. *Building a safer health system.* Washington, DC: National Academy Press.

National Coordinating Council for Medication Error and Prevention. (2004). NCC MERP taxonomy of medication errors. Retrieved November 26, 2004, from http://www.nccmerp.org/pdf/taxo2001-07-31.pdf

Park, G., Coursin, D., Ely, E. W., England, M., Fraser, G. L., Mantz, J., et al. (2001). Balancing sedation and analgesia in the critically ill. *Critical Care Clinics, 17,* 1015-1027.

Bibliography

Albright, T. N., Zimmerman, M. A., & Selzman, C. H. (2002). Vasopressin in the cardiac surgery intensive care unit. *American Journal of Critical Care, 11*(4), 326-332.

American Heart Association. (2005). Part 7.3: Management of symptomatic bradycardia and tachycardia. *Circulation, 112*(24 suppl), IV67-IV77.

American Heart Association. (2005). Part 7.4: Monitoring and medications. *Circulation, 112*(24 suppl), IV78-IV83.

Arbour, R. (2000). Sedation and pain management in critically ill adults. *Critical Care Nurse, 20*(5), 39.

Arbour, R. (2003). A continuous quality improvement approach to improving clinical practice in the areas of sedation, analgesia, and neuromuscular blockade. *Journal of Continuing Education in Nursing, 34*(2), 64-71.

Arbour, R. (2004). Using bispectral index monitoring to detect potential breakthrough awareness and limit duration of neuromuscular blockade. *American Journal of Critical Care, 13*(1), 66-73.

Archer-Chicko, C. (2000). Continuous intravenous prostacyclin for advanced primary pulmonary hypertension. *Dimensions of Critical Care Nursing, 19*(2), 14-21.

Argo, A. L., Cox, K. K., & Kelly, W. N. (2000). The ten most common lethal medication errors in hospital patients. *Hospital Pharmacy, 35*(5), 470-474.

Armitage, G., & Knapman, H. (2003). Adverse events in drug administration: A literature review. *Journal of Nursing Management, 11,* 130-140.

Bakris, G. (2003). *The implications of JNC 7 for antihypertensive treatment protocols.* Retrieved July 27, 2003, from http://www.medscape.com/viewprogram/2513_pnt

Barber, J. M. (2003). Pharmacologic management of integrative brain failure. *Critical Care Nursing Quarterly, 26*(3), 192-207.

Barkman, A., & Pooler, C. (2001). Carvedilol: A countermeasure to heart failure. *Dimensions of Critical Care Nursing, 20*(5), 11.

Bateman, S., & Grap, M. J. (2003). Sedation and analgesia in the mechanically ventilated patient. *American Journal of Nursing, 103*(5), 64AA-64HH.

Bates, D. W., Rothschild, J. M., & Keohane, C. (2003, November). *Intravenous medication safety errors.* Paper presented at the Infusion Safety: Addressing Harm with High-Risk Drug Administration, San Diego, CA.

Bernard, G. R., Vincent, J.-L., Laterre, P.-F., LaRosa, S. P., Dhainaut, J.-F., Lopez-Rodriguez, A., et al. (2001). Efficacy and safety of recombinant human activated protein C for severe sepsis. *New England Journal of Medicine, 344*(10), 699-709.

Cleveland, K. W. (2003). Argatroban: A new treatment option for heparin-induced thrombocytopenia. *Critical Care Nurse, 23*(6), 61-66.

Crouch, M. A., Limon, L., & Cassano, A. T. (2003). Clinical relevance and management of drug-related QT interval prolongation. *Pharmacotherapy, 23*(7), 881-908.

Cuddy, P. G. (2000). Monitoring drug therapy in the intensive care unit. *Critical Care Nursing Quarterly, 22*(4), 14-22.

De Jong, M., & Sabadlie-Garretson, W. (2001). Tenecteplase: a promising new fibrinolytic agent. *Dimensions of Critical Care Nursing, 20*(6), 19.

de Wit, M., & Epstein, S. K. (2003). Administration of sedatives and level of sedation: Comparative evaluation via the sedation-agitation scale and the bispectral index. *American Journal of Critical Care, 12*(4), 343-348.

Dennison, R. D. (2005). Creating an organizational culture for medication safety. *Nursing Clinics of North America, 40*(1), 1-23.

Devlin, J. W., Boleski, G., Mlynarek, M., Nerenz, D. R., Peterson, E., Jankowski, M., et al. (1999). Motor activity assessment scale: A valid and reliable sedation scale for use with mechanically ventilated patients in an adult surgical intensive care unit. *Critical Care Medicine, 27*(7), 1271-1275.

Dina, R., & Jafari, M. (2000). Angiotensin II-receptor antagonists: an overview. *American Journal of Health-System Pharmacy, 57*(13), 1231.

Donnelly, J., & Lynch-Smith, D. (2004). Analgesia and sedation protocols. *American Journal of Nursing, 104*(5), 72EE-72HH.

Donovan, P. (2001). Heparin-induced thrombocytopenia: strategies for identification and treatment. *Clinician Reviews, 11*(2), 93.

Erstad, B. L., Jordan, C. J., & Thomas, M. C. (2002). Key articles and guidelines relative to intensive care unit pharmacology. *Pharmacotherapy, 22*(12), 1594-1610.

Fiorini, D. M. (2001). The use of low-molecular-weight heparin in acute coronary syndromes. *AACN Clinical Issues, 12*(1), 53-61.

Futterman, L., & Lemberg, L. (2004). The resurrection of spironolactone on its golden anniversary. *American Journal of Critical Care, 13*(2), 162-165.

Gahart, B., & Nazareno, A. (2007). *2007 Intravenous medications* (23rd ed.). St. Louis: Mosby.

Harrington, C. (2003). Managing hypertension in patients with stroke: Are you prepared for labetalol infusion? *Critical Care Nurse, 23*(3), 30-38.

Jones, S. K. (2003). An algorithm for train-of-four monitoring in patients receiving continuous neuromuscular blocking agents. *Dimensions of Critical Care Nursing, 22*(2), 50-59.

Kajs-Wyllie, M. (1999). Antihypertensive treatment for the neurologic patient: A nursing challenge. *Journal of Neuroscience Nursing, 31*(3), 142.

Kayser, S. R. (2002). The use of nesiritide in the management of acute decompensated heart failure. *Progress in Cardiovascular Nursing, 17*(2), 89-95.

Kee, J. L., Hayes, E. R., & McCuistion, L. E. (2006). *Pharmacology: A nursing process approach* (5th ed.). St. Louis: Elsevier.

Knight, D. (2003). Which heparin is best? *American Journal of Nursing, 103*(12), 81.

Kost, M. (2004). *Moderate sedation/analgesia: Core competencies for practice* (2nd ed.). Philadelphia: W. B. Saunders.

Kruse, J. A., Fink, M. P., & Carlson, R. W. (2003). *Saunders manual of critical care*. Philadelphia: Saunders.

Kuhn, M. A. (2002). Herbal remedies: Drug-herb interactions. *Critical Care Nurse, 22*(2), 22-34.

Lehne, R. (2007). *Pharmacology for nursing care* (6th ed.). Philadelphia: Saunders.

Luer, J. (2002). Sedation and neuromuscular blockade in patients with acute respiratory failure. *Critical Care Nurse, 22*(5), 70-75.

MacCallum, E. (2000). The role of beta-blockers in the management of patients with heart failure. *Dimensions of Critical Care Nursing, 20*(1), 24.

McIntyre, K. M. (2004). Vasopressin in asystolic cardiac arrest. *New England Journal of Medicine, 350*(2), 179-181.

McKenry, L. M., Tessier, E., & Hogan, M. (2006). *Mosby's pharmacology in nursing* (22nd ed.). St. Louis: Mosy.

Miano, T. A. (2006). Evolving role of vasopressin in the treatment of cardiac arrest. *Pharmacotherapy, 26*(6), 828-839.

Munoz, C., & Hilgenberg, C. (2005). Ethnopharmacology. *American Journal of Nursing, 105*(8), 40-49.

Murphy, J. (2003). Pharmacological treatment of acute ischemic stroke. *Critical Care Nursing Quarterly, 26*(4), 276-282.

Nasraway, Jr., S. A., Wu, E. C., Kelleher, R. M., Yasuda, C. M., & Donnelly, A. M. (2002). How reliable is the bispectral index in critically ill patients? A prospective, comparable, single-blinded observer study. *Critical Care Medicine, 30*(7), 1483-1487.

Navuluri, R. (2001). Anticoagulant therapy. *American Journal of Nursing, 101*(11), 24A-24D.

Navuluri, R. (2001). Antiplatelet and fibrinolytic therapy. *American Journal of Nursing, 101*(10), 24A.

Navuluri, R. (2001). Nursing implications of anticoagulant therapy. *American Journal of Nursing, 101*(11), 24A-24C.

Olsen, D. M., Cheek, D. J., & Morgenlander, J. C. (2004). The impact of bispectral index monitoring on rates of propofol administration. *AACN Clinical Issues, 15*(1), 63-73.

O'Malley, P. (2005). Ethnic pharmacology: Science, research, race, and market share. *Clinical Nurse Specialist, 19*(6), 291-293.

Pape, T. M. (2003). Applying airline safety practices to medication administration. *MedSurg Nursing, 12*(2), 77-94.

Park, G., Coursin, D., Ely, E. W., England, M., Fraser, G. L., Mantz, J., et al. (2001). Balancing sedation and analgesia in the critically ill. *Critical Care Clinics, 17*, 1015-1027.

Porter, B. (2002). The role of the advanced practice nurse in anticoagulation. *AACN Clinical Issues, 13*(2), 221-233.

Powers, J., & Jacobi, J. (2003). Treatment of severe sepsis. *Clinical Nurse Specialist, 17*(3), 128-130.

Prows, C. A., & Prows, D. R. (2004). Medication selection by genotype. *American Journal of Nursing, 104*(5), 60-71.

Ramsay, M., Savege, T., Simpson, B., & Goodwin, R. (1974). Controlled sedation with alphaxalone-alphadolone. *British Medical Journal, 2*, 656.

Reeder, S., & Hoffmann, R. (2001). Beta-blocker therapy for hypertension. *Dimensions of Critical Care Nursing, 20*(2), 2.

Riker, R., Picard, J., & Fraser, G. (1999). Prospective evaluation of the Sedation-Agitation Scale for adult critically ill patients. *Critical Care Medicine, 27*, 1325.

Sabo, J. A., & Nord, P. (2000). Intravenous epoprostenol. *Critical Care Nurse, 20*(6), 31-40.

Salmaan, K., Devlin, J. W., Piekos, K. A., & Racine, E. (2001). Recombinant human activated protein C, drotrecogin alfa (activated): A novel therapy for severe sepsis. *Pharmacotherapy, 21*(11), 1389-1402.

Sica, D. (2001). Clinical pharmacology of the angiotensin receptor antagonists. *Journal of Clinical Hypertension, 3*(1), 45-49.

Spruill, W. J., Wade, W. E., Huckaby, W. G., & Leslie, R. B. (2001). Achievement of anticoagulation by using a weight-based heparin dosing protocol for obese and nonobese patients. *American Journal of Health-System Pharmacy, 58*(22), 2143-2146.

Togger, D. A., & Brenner, P. S. (2001). Metered dose inhalers. *American Journal of Nursing, 101*(10), 26-32.

Urden, L., Stacy, K., & Lough, M. (2006). *Thelan's critical care nursing: Diagnosis and management* (5th ed.). St. Louis: Mosby.

Vance, D. L. (2001). Treating acute ischemic stroke with intravenous alteplase. *Critical Care Nurse, 21*(4), 25-34.

Verma, A. K., Levine, M., Shalansky, S. J., Carter, C. J., & Kelton, J. G. (2003). Frequency of heparin-induced thrombocytopenia in critical care patients. *Pharmacotherapy, 23*(6), 745-753.

Warkentin, T. E., & Greinacher, A. (Eds.). (2001). *Heparin-induced thrombocytopenia* (2nd ed.). New York: Marcel Dekker.

Wenzel, V., Krismer, A. C., Arntz, H. R., Sitter, H., Stadlbauer, K. H., & Lindner, K. H. (2004). A comparison of vasopressin and epinephrine for out-of-hospital cardiopulmonary resuscitation. *New England Journal of Medicine, 350*(2), 105-113.

Selected Nursing Diagnoses Commonly Seen in Critically Ill Patients

APPENDIX A

Nursing Diagnosis	Defining Characteristics	Nursing Interventions	Expected Outcomes
ACTIVITY INTOLERANCE related to: • Changes in HR, rhythm, or conduction • Inability to increase HR in response to exercise • Effects of drugs (e.g., beta-blockers) • Imbalance between oxygen supply and demand • Hypoxemia • Dyspnea • Anemia • Weakness, fatigue • Uremia • Osteomalacia; osteoporosis • Pain: chest pain, leg pain • Fluid and electrolyte imbalance • Immobility • Malnutrition • Obesity	• Verbal report of dyspnea, pain, weakness, fatigue, or syncope • Abnormal physiologic response to exercise ○ Tachycardia or dysrhythmia ○ Hypotension ○ Tachypnea or dyspnea ○ Arterial blood gas changes: hypoxemia and/or hypercapnia during exercise ○ Breath sound changes with exercise: crackles; rhonchi; wheezes • Clinical indications of anemia: chest pain; syncope; hypotension; dyspnea • Lack of desire to engage in physical activity • Radiologic evidence of demineralization • Bone pain, pathologic fractures	• Monitor for changes in defining characteristics ○ Monitor ECG during exercise if indicated ○ Monitor Spo_2 during physical activity if indicated • Explain all procedures thoroughly to decrease anxiety • Assess need for ambulation aids (e.g., cane, walker) • Assess muscle tone and strength daily • Teach relaxation techniques • Teach patient to monitor physiologic response (e.g., pulse rate, shortness of breath) to activity • Monitor the patient's participation in activities of daily living (e.g., bathing, eating); assist with activities of daily living if appropriate • Perform passive ROM exercises during bedrest • Encourage active ROM exercises when tolerated; instruct patient how to avoid Valsalva maneuver • Assist with postural changes gradually; monitor HR and BP response to postural changes as indicated • Collaborate with physical, occupational, and/or recreational therapy to plan and monitor an activity program ○ Focus on what the patient can do rather than on deficits	• Patient reports increased ability to perform daily activities without pain, dyspnea, weakness, fatigue, or syncope • Absence of abnormal responses to exercise • HR within 20 beats/min of patient's normal • ECG rhythm: normal sinus rhythm or patient's usual rhythm (e.g., chronic atrial fibrillation) without ventricular ectopy • BP within 20 mm Hg of patient's normal • RR less than 24/min • Sao_2, Spo_2 greater than 90% • $Paco_2$ 35-45 mm Hg or within 5 mm Hg of patient's normal • Participation in activities (e.g., active ROM, ambulation, resistive exercises)

Continued

Nursing Diagnosis	Defining Characteristics	Nursing Interventions	Expected Outcomes
		○ Encourage participation in graded exercise program ○ Schedule activities (e.g., active ROM, ambulation) when energy levels are highest ○ Avoid activity after meals ○ Group activities to provide rest periods — Plan rest periods before and after activity — Plan rest periods after meals — Provide positive reinforcement for participation in graded activity ○ Administer analgesics before activity as indicated ○ Administer oxygen during activity as indicated **Coronary artery disease or heart failure** • Assist the patient to identify activities that cause chest pain or dyspnea; encourage avoidance of these activities or slowing the pace of these activities • Teach the patient how to use NTG prophylactically before activities likely to cause chest pain **Pulmonary disease** • Assist the patient to identify activities that cause dyspnea; encourage avoidance of these activities or slowing the pace of these activities • Encourage the use of relaxation techniques before exercise • Teach the patient how to cough effectively; encourage airway clearance techniques before exercise • Administer oxygen before and during exercise if Spo_2 if less than 90% or patient is dyspneic during activity **Anemia** • Administer erythropoietin and/or blood and blood products as prescribed **Renal failure** • Restrict dietary phosphorus; administer phosphate-binding gels as prescribed • Administer large doses of vitamin D, dihydrotachysterol, or 1,25-vitamin D as prescribed ○ Dihydrotachysterol does not require 1-hydroxylation by the kidney ○ 1,25-vitamin D is a completely activated form of vitamin D	

Nursing Diagnosis	Defining Characteristics	Nursing Interventions	Expected Outcomes
		• Administer calcium supplements with vitamin D preparations • Evaluate and encourage compliance to prevent secondary hyperparathyroidism	
AIRWAY CLEARANCE, INEFFECTIVE related to: • Altered level of consciousness • Airway obstruction • Artificial airway • Decreased energy/fatigue • Increased amount or viscosity of mucus • Ineffective cough • Tracheobronchial infection • Tracheobronchial trauma • Mucosal swelling and/or bronchospasm • Neuromuscular or impairment • Perceptual/cognitive impairment • Smoking: ineffective cilia • Thoracic, abdominal, or flank pain	• Tachycardia • Tachypnea • Dyspnea • Cough • Cyanosis (depending on hemoglobin level) • Clinical indicators of respiratory distress • Clinical indicators of hypoxemia/hypoxia • Clinical indicators of hypercapnia • Fever • Adventitious breath sounds (e.g., crackles, rhonchi, wheezes) • ABG changes ○ Decreased Sao_2, Pao_2 ○ $Paco_2$ may be decreased or increased depending on ventilation status • May have abnormal chest x-ray	• Monitor for changes in defining characteristics • Monitor oxygenation and ventilation ○ Bedside ventilatory parameters: tidal volume; vital capacity; maximal inspiratory pressure ○ ABGs ○ Pulse oximetry ○ Capnography • Assess ability to clear secretions • Maintain a patent airway ○ Ensure proper positioning of head and neck (e.g., sniffing position) ○ Encourage deep breathing and sustained inspiratory maneuvers ○ Utilize chest physiotherapy to mobilize secretions if indicated and not contraindicated — Postural drainage — Percussion — Vibration ○ Encourage coughing if rhonchi are audible — Instruct and supervise controlled coughing ○ Suction only if coughing is ineffective in clearing secretions or patient if too fatigued to cough — ET tubes hold the epiglottis open and prevent effective coughing — Utilize techniques to prevent complications of suctioning ○ Encourage rest periods between coughing sessions and chest physiotherapy ○ Utilize artificial airways if necessary — Secure tube with tape, ties, or stabilization devices designed for ET tubes — Restrain patient's wrists if necessary to prevent self-extubation — Maintain cuff inflation to prevent drainage of upper airway secretions into lungs if ET tube or tracheostomy tube utilized • Assess color, consistency, amount, and odor of mucus ○ Obtain sputum for culture and sensitivity if indicated	• Patient able to cough effectively to clear airways • Sputum: thin, clear • Vital capacity of at least 10 mL/kg and maximal inspiratory pressure of at least −20 cm H_2O • Breath sounds clear and equal bilaterally • Pao_2 of at least 60 mm Hg; Sao_2 of at least 90%; Svo_2 greater than 60% • $Paco_2$ 35-45 mm Hg or within 5 mm Hg of the patient's normal

Continued

Nursing Diagnosis	Defining Characteristics	Nursing Interventions	Expected Outcomes
		• Assess of indications of pulmonary infection: fever; tachycardia; tachypnea; yellow, green, or brown sputum; rhonchi on auscultation; abnormal chest x-rays • Encourage noncaffeinated oral fluids to thin secretions ○ 2-3 L of fluid/24 hr unless contraindicated by cardiac or renal disease • Adequate humidification provided via mask, humidifier, nebulizer in patients with artificial airways • Administer oxygen if patient is hypoxemic; oxygen must be humidified if greater than 3 L/min or if artificial airway • Position the patient for optimal chest excursion and optimal coughing: high-Fowler's position with knees drawn up; reposition at least every 2 hr • Administer pharmacologic therapies as prescribed: expectorants, mucolytics, antibiotics • Teach patient abdominal muscle-tightening exercises and diaphragmatic breathing if muscle weakness if a factor • Teach family assisted coughing techniques if indicated (e.g., cervical or high thoracic level spinal cord injury) • Teach and provide incisional splinting if thoracic pain is a factor	
ANXIETY related to: • Acute change in health status • Unfamiliar environment • Recommended life style changes • Altered body image • Change in self-concept • Change in role in family • Threat of death • Social isolation • Hemorrhage • Pain • Fear of unknown • Financial concerns	• Patient verbalizes anxiety, apprehension, nervousness, uncertainty, fear, worry, inability to cope, feeling of impending doom • Tachycardia, palpitations • Mild hypertension • Tachypnea • Restlessness, fidgeting • Diaphoresis • Anorexia, nausea, vomiting, and/or diarrhea • Dry mouth • Increased muscle tension • Poor eye contact • Inability to concentrate • Concentration on self; narrow focus of attention • Wrinkled brow, worried facial expression • Crying • Tremor, trembling, shakiness • Expresses feelings of helplessness, inadequacy, regret, concern	• Monitor for changes in defining characteristics • Establish rapport; give patient undivided attention; listen to patient • Consider individuality of this patient; treat the patient as a person • Identify prior coping strategies; assist the patient to utilize coping mechanisms that have been helpful (e.g., prayer, family, relaxation techniques, breathing techniques) • Explain all procedures, the reasons for them, and their importance in a simple, concise, reassuring manner • Explain critical care unit environment including noises, visiting policy, meal times, what is scheduled today • Provide opportunity for patient to verbalize feelings, concerns, fears, anxieties	• Patient verbalizes absence of anxiety • Absence of nonverbal indicators of anxiety • Patient able to verbalize fears, concerns, anxieties

Nursing Diagnosis	Defining Characteristics	Nursing Interventions	Expected Outcomes
	• Withdrawal • Verbalization of inability to cope • Inability to solve problem effectively • Inability to meet role expectations • Inappropriate or ineffective use of defense mechanisms • Verbal manipulation • Excessive food intake, alcohol consumption, smoking • Digestive, bowel disturbance • Chronic fatigue or sleep pattern disturbance	• Talk and reassure patient in a calm, firm voice; be unhurried; maintain calm, confident attitude • Provide for comfort: decrease stimuli, adjust room temperature, allow for rest periods, treat pain • Allow patient to make decisions regarding environment and self-care activities • Teach and encourage utilization of relaxation techniques • Identify coping mechanisms that have been used by the patient in other anxiety-provoking situations; encourage use of effective coping mechanisms • Assist the patient to develop anxiety-reducing skills (e.g., relaxation, deep breathing, imagery, positive self-statements) • Administer minor tranquilizers as prescribed and indicated • Provide diversionary activities (e.g., music, television, books) • Allow visitation by family/ significant other and encourage their participation in care ○ Evaluate patient's physiologic and psychological response to visitation; utilize this assessment in decision-making regarding frequency and duration of visits ○ Allow private family time daily • Answer questions simply and concisely; begin teaching about disease process, treatments, recommended life style changes when the patient indicates readiness to learn • Assess usual roles and discuss feelings about changes in role performance • Refer for rehabilitation as appropriate	
ASPIRATION, RISK FOR related to: • Decreased level of consciousness • Oropharyngeal airway in conscious patient • Presence of ET tube (splints epiglottis open) • Facial/oral/neck surgery or trauma • Wired jaws • Impaired gag and/or cough reflex	• Tachycardia • Tachypnea • Dyspnea • Cough • Fever • Breath sound changes: diminished breath sounds; presence of adventitious sounds (e.g., crackles, rhonchi, wheezes) • ABG changes: hypoxemia with hypocapnia • Abnormal chest x-ray	• Monitor for changes in defining characteristics • Assess gag and cough reflex; assess ability to swallow • Keep suction equipment available • Position unconscious patients on their side • Offer foods with consistency that patient can swallow; cut food into small pieces; soft and semiliquid foods may be easier for the patient to swallow than liquids • Encourage the patient to chew thoroughly and eat slowly; discourage talking while eating	• Absence of dyspnea, cough, tachypnea, tachycardia, or fever • Breath sounds clear and equal • Normal ABGs and chest x-ray

Continued

Nursing Diagnosis	Defining Characteristics	Nursing Interventions	Expected Outcomes
• Impaired swallowing • Increased gastric volume or retention • Increased intra-abdominal pressure • GI tubes, especially large bore NG tubes • Decreased gastric motility • Enteral feedings		• Maintain upright position for 30-45 min after feeding • Administer antacids, proton pump inhibitors, and/or histamine$_2$ receptor antagonists as prescribed to decrease the acidity of gastric contents in patients at high risk of aspiration **NG suction** • Maintain NG or orogastric suction as prescribed ○ Use appropriate suction — Nonvented tubes should be on intermittent low suction — Vented tubes should be on continuous low suction — Reposition tube as needed to maintain drainage **Enteral nutrition** • Check placement of tube before use; chest x-ray is required for small-lumen feeding tube • Elevate HOB 30 degrees during and after intermittent enteral feedings; keep HOB elevated at all times if continuous enteral feedings are used • Utilize small-lumen feeding tubes, which cause less gastroesophageal incompetence than do larger-lumen NG tubes; percutaneous gastroscopy or jejunostomy tubes also help to prevent aspiration • Check for gastric retention before intermittent enteral feedings and at least every 4 hr if receiving continuous enteral feedings; hold feeding for 1 hr if greater than 100 mL is aspirated • Administer metoclopramide HCl (Reglan) as prescribed to promote gastric motility **ET tube** • Keep ET or tracheostomy tube cuff inflated utilizing minimal occlusive volume or minimal leak technique; tracheal pressure should be between 20 and 25 mm Hg (25-35 cm H_2O) to prevent aspiration of subglottic secretions while avoiding tracheal ischemia • Do not routinely deflate cuff as upper airway secretions are allowed to fall down into airway	
BODY IMAGE, DISTURBED related to: • Change in body function and/or appearance	• Missing body part • Not touching or looking at body part • Hiding or overexposing body part	• Monitor for changes in defining characteristics • Assess patient's prehospital perception of body image • Listen to patient's verbalization of alterations in body image	• Patient looks at and touches affected body part or area • Patient participates in care of affected body part or area

Nursing Diagnosis	Defining Characteristics	Nursing Interventions	Expected Outcomes
	• Refusal to verify actual change • Preoccupation with change or loss • Personalization of part or loss by name • Depersonalization of part or loss by impersonal pronouns • Verbalization of negative feelings about body • Verbalization about change in lifestyle • Focus on past strength, function, or appearance	• Assess perceived impact of change on ADLs, social behavior, personal relationships, occupation, and recreation • Use simple explanations when describing patient's illness, surgery, treatments, progress, status • Provide information regarding healing status of body part • Assist the patient to identify actual changes and establish realistic goals • Encourage physical mobility and activity • Encourage diversionary activities • Encourage the patient to participate in his own care and ADLs • Refer patient to appropriate support groups	• Patient sets realistic goals regarding changes in lifestyle, return to work, etc. • Patient participates in self-care and physical activity
BREATHING PATTERN, INEFFECTIVE related to: • Anxiety • Airway or tracheobronchial obstruction • Abdominal distention • Barotrauma • CNS depression (e.g., opiates, head injury) • Increased work of breathing • Decreased compliance • Increased airway resistance • Decreased energy/fatigue • Immobility • Morbid obesity • Muscle deconditioning • Neuromuscular or musculoskeletal impairment • Thoracic or abdominal pain • Ventilator malfunction	• Tachycardia • Tachypnea • Dyspnea • Cough • Prolonged expiratory time • Diminished chest excursion • Asymmetric chest excursion • Clinical indicators of respiratory distress • Clinical indicators of hypoxemia/hypoxia • Clinical indicators of hypercapnia • Breath sound changes: diminished and/or unequal breath sounds; crackles; wheezes • Decreased tidal volume and vital capacity • ABG changes ○ Decreased Sao_2, Pao_2 ○ $Paco_2$ may be decreased or increased depending on ventilation status • May have abnormal chest x-ray	• Monitor for changes in defining characteristics • Monitor oxygenation and ventilation ○ Bedside ventilatory parameters: tidal volume; vital capacity; maximal inspiratory pressure ○ Arterial blood gases ○ Pulse oximetry ○ Capnography • Position for optimal ventilation and optimal ventilation-perfusion matching ○ Elevate HOB 30-45 degrees for optimal chest excursion ○ Prone and semiprone positions may also be used to improve ventilation ○ Turn every 2 hr; if unilateral lung condition, turn from good lung down to back (except patients after pneumonectomy, who should be turned from operative side to back) • Encourage deep breathing every 2 hr; incentive spirometry may also be helpful • Utilize chest physiotherapy as indicated • Administer oxygen if patient is hypoxemic to maintain Sao_2 95% or greater unless contraindication; if patient has chronic hypercapnia, maintain Sao_2 90%-92% • Encourage coughing if rhonchi are audible • Suction patient if coughing is inadequate	• HR less than 120/min or within 20 beats/min of patient's normal • RR rate less than 24/min • Absence of subjective reports of dyspnea • Absence of intercostal retractions or use of accessory muscles • Chest excursion of at least 3 cm • Clear and equal breath sounds • Symmetrical breath sounds • Tidal volume at least 5 mL/kg; vital capacity at least 10 mL/kg • Pao_2 of at least 60 mm Hg; Sao_2 or Spo_2 of at least 90% • $Paco_2$ 35-45 mm Hg with pH between 7.35 and 7.45

Continued

Nursing Diagnosis	Defining Characteristics	Nursing Interventions	Expected Outcomes
		• Encourage rest periods between coughing sessions and chest physiotherapy • Administer pharmacologic therapies as prescribed ○ Bronchodilators for bronchospasm ○ Expectorants and mucolytics for excess mucus ○ Antibiotics for infection ○ Analgesics for pain ○ Sedatives should be avoided if possible • Keep artificial airways and manual resuscitation bag readily available • Institute mechanical ventilation as indicated by inadequate ventilation (elevated $Paco_2$ with respiratory acidosis) ○ Assess ability to breathe in "synch" with ventilator ○ Sedate as necessary • Maintain nutritional status and prevent muscle wasting by providing appropriate meals and/or supplements ○ Provide high-protein, high-calorie meals and supplements; avoid high carbohydrates in patients with acute respiratory failure or while weaning because CHO metabolism increases CO_2 production • Assess and maintain functioning of chest tubes if appropriate **If esophageal-gastric balloon tamponade** • Keep scissors at the bedside in patients with Sengstaken-Blakemore (or Minnesota or Linton) tube in place; if tube accidentally becomes displaced upward blocking the airway, cut across all lumina and remove tube • Keep an extra tube in the room for immediate replacement if needed to control bleeding • Always electively deflate the esophageal balloon before the gastric balloon	
CO, DECREASED related to: • Increased or decreased HR; dysrhythmias • Decreased or increased preload • Decreased contractility	• Clinical indications of sympathetic nervous system innervation initially ○ Tachycardia ○ Tachypnea ○ BP changes: narrowed pulse pressure ○ Increased SVR	• Monitor for changes in defining characteristics • Obtain baseline vital signs and monitor as indicated • Monitor ECG for dysrhythmias • Assess for chest pain • Auscultate heart and lung sounds • Monitor intake and output and daily weights	• Alert and oriented • HR 60-100 beats/min • MAP greater than 70 mm Hg • CI 2.5-4.0 L/min/m² • PAOP 18 mm Hg or less • Urine output greater than 0.5 mL/kg/hr

Nursing Diagnosis	Defining Characteristics	Nursing Interventions	Expected Outcomes
• Increased afterload • Drug effects • Vasodilation causing a relative hypovolemia • Structural or valvular defects	• Clinical indications of hypoperfusion eventually ○ Chest pain ○ Dysrhythmias ○ Hypotension ○ Cool or cold, clammy skin ○ Decreased bowel sounds ○ Decreased urine output ○ Elevation in BUN, creatinine ○ Syncope, vertigo ○ Changes in level of consciousness: restlessness → confusion → lethargy → coma • Clinical indications of LVF ○ Dyspnea, orthopnea ○ S_3 ○ Crackles ○ Increased PAP, PAOP • Clinical indications of RVF ○ Jugular venous distention ○ Peripheral edema ○ Hepatomegaly ○ Fatigue, weakness ○ Weight gain ○ Increased RAP • Changes in hemodynamic parameter ○ Decreased CO and CI ○ Decreased or increased PAOP: decreased if hypovolemia or vasodilation; increased if heart failure ○ Decreased Svo_2 • Metabolic acidosis; elevated serum lactate levels	• Assess ABGs as indicated • Initiate IV therapy with prescribed fluid at prescribed rate • Assist with insertion of hemodynamic monitoring catheters ○ Provide standardized care for monitoring and maintaining hemodynamic monitoring catheters • Affirm or establish airway; intubation may be necessary • Evaluate adequacy of oxygenation (Sao_2, Spo_2, Pao_2); administer oxygen therapy as prescribed and indicated to maintain Spo_2 greater than 95% unless contraindicated • Evaluate adequacy of ventilation ($Paco_2$); intubation and mechanical ventilation may be necessary • Insert a urinary catheter as prescribed; monitor hourly urine output • Administer fluids, inotropes, and/or vasodilators as indicated and prescribed; monitor for effectiveness and adverse effects, diuretics or venous vasodialators may also be indicated if preload (PAOP) increased • Assist with insertion of IABP if indicated ○ Provide standardized care for monitoring, maintaining, and timing of the IABP • Establish and maintain position of comfort • Maintain environment conducive to rest and sleep • Assess for and treat anxiety • Minimize excessive nonmeaningful stimuli • Allow patient to rest between nursing activities • Administer stool softeners as prescribed • Encourage patient to turn and breathe deeply • Keep patient warm to prevent vasoconstriction and shivering • Assist with ADLs • Provide nutrition appropriate to needs and digestive capabilities ○ Low sodium ○ Low cholesterol and saturated fat ○ High fiber ○ High potassium if patient receiving potassium-wasting diuretics	

Continued

Nursing Diagnosis	Defining Characteristics	Nursing Interventions	Expected Outcomes
COMMUNICATION, VERBAL, IMPAIRED related to: • Artificial airway • Aphasia	• Inability to speak • Difficulty expressing thoughts, needs, desires	• Monitor for changes in defining characteristics • Emphasize temporary nature of loss of ability to speak • Establish acceptable method of communication ○ Picture communication board ○ Alphabet board ○ Felt-tip pen or marker and paper — Pencils and ballpoint pens require more pressure ○ Magic slate ○ Lip reading is usually not an acceptable method especially if oral tube is in place • Use short, simple questions that elicit "yes" or "no" answers • Use nonverbal communication (e.g., facial expressions, gestures, pointing) • Be calm and unhurried • Allow time for communication; be patient • Minimize distractions • Utilize family and significant others to assist with communication	• Patient, nurse, and significant others are satisfied with ability to communicate • Patient able to communicate needs and desires
CONSTIPATION related to: • Inactivity, immobility • Emotional stress • Drug effect (e.g., opiates) • Electrolyte imbalance • Inadequate dentition • Inadequate fiber intake • Decreased GI motility • Inadequate fluid intake • Hemorrhoids • Chronic enema or laxative use • Lack of privacy	• Change in bowel pattern • Decreased frequency or amount of stool • Dry, hard, formed stool and/or oozing liquid stool • Pain with defecation • Straining at stool • Anorexia, nausea, vomiting, abdominal distention, abdominal pain • Change in bowel sounds • Palpable mass in LLQ • Blood on stool or toilet tissue • Feeling of pressure in rectum or abdominal fullness	• Monitor for changes in defining characteristics • Discuss usual pattern of bowel elimination • Evaluate usual dietary habits, eating habits, eating schedule, liquid intake, activity, medications • Inspect the color, consistency, amount of stool • Auscultate bowel sounds • Examine abdomen for distention, palpable masses • Encourage fluids unless contraindication; fruit juices and warm fluids are especially helpful • Collaborate with physician and dietician regarding patient's diet ○ Encourage dietary fiber unless contraindicated ○ Teach patient about foods high in fiber • Encourage physical activity as tolerated • Provide privacy for the patient at the time of day that bowel elimination usually occurs • Digitally remove fecal impaction if necessary • Administer pharmacologic agents as prescribed ○ Stool softeners ○ Chemical irritants ○ Bulk fiber ○ Suppositories ○ Oil retention enema	• Normal amount and frequency of stool • Absence of abdominal pain or pain with stool • Absence of blood with stool • Absence of abdominal mass

Nursing Diagnosis	Defining Characteristics	Nursing Interventions	Expected Outcomes
COPING, INDIVIDUAL AND FAMILY, INEFFECTIVE related to: • Overwhelming disease process • Dependence on technology • Situational crisis • Disruption of usual family functions and roles	• Patient and/or significant others verbalize anxiety, apprehension, nervousness, uncertainty, fear, worry, grief, hopelessness, powerlessness, isolation • Patient and/or significant others express inability to cope • Patient and/or significant others demonstrate nonverbal indicators of anxiety • Hesitancy of significant others to spend time with critically ill patient or inappropriate behavior when visiting • Misinterpretation of information • Inability to make decisions • Lack of cooperation among family members • Inappropriate emotional outbursts • Arguments among family members; arguments with patient • Inability to respond to each other's feelings and support each other	• Monitor for changes in defining characteristics • Recognize common causes of stress in patient ◦ Sudden, unexpected change in health status ◦ Body image changes (e.g., incision, wounds, loss of limb, skin color, vascular access) ◦ Fear of unknown ◦ Long-term hospitalization ◦ Role changes ◦ Sexuality changes ◦ Fear of death • Establish rapport; give patient undivided attention; LISTEN to patient • Consider individuality of this patient; treat the patient as a person • Identify patient's perception of the situation; identify significant other's assessment of the situation • Assess past and current coping mechanisms; support effective copying mechanisms • Explain all procedures, the reasons for them, and their importance in a simple, concise, reassuring manner • Provide honest and accurate information • Provide opportunity for patient to verbalize feelings, concerns, fears, anxieties • Talk and reassure patient in a calm, firm voice; be unhurried; maintain calm, confident attitude • Provide for comfort: decrease stimuli, adjust room temperature, allow for rest periods • Teach and encourage utilization of relaxation techniques • Allow patient to make decisions regarding environment and self-care activities • Encourage the patient to participate in self-care activity if they are able; praise efforts • Allow visitation by family/significant other and encourage their participation in care • Encourage family and significant other's participation in care • Observe family and significant others for signs of fatigue and need for emotional or spiritual support; utilize psychiatric liaison nurse, psychologists, social workers, and chaplain	• Patient and/or significant others express fears and concerns • Patient and/or significant others able to participate in decision-making and care • Patient and/or significant others able to utilize psychosocial support

Continued

Nursing Diagnosis	Defining Characteristics	Nursing Interventions	Expected Outcomes
		• Assess usual roles and discuss feelings about changes in role performance • Promote hope and positive attitude • Identify and encourage utilization of community resources and support groups	
DIARRHEA related to: • Anxiety • Viral, bacterial, parasitic infection • Antibiotics causing change in normal intestinal flora ○ *Clostridium difficile* • Adverse drug effects • Enteral feedings ○ Hyperosmolality ○ Bolus feeding ○ Bacterial contamination ○ Lactose intolerance ○ Low-fiber enteral formula • Increased GI motility ○ Inflammatory bowel disease ○ Irritable bowel syndrome ○ GI bleeding • Lactose intolerance • Excessive intake of fruit, fruit juice, vegetables, whole grains	• Change in bowel pattern • Increased frequency or amount of stool • Liquid or semiliquid stool • Abdominal pain or cramping • Change in bowel sounds • Urgency • Weight loss • Dehydration	• Monitor for changes in defining characteristics • Inspect the color, consistency, amount of stool • Examine abdomen for distention • Auscultate bowel sounds • Encourage fluids; avoid fruit juices • Provide perianal care with each diarrheal stool • Collaborate with physician and dietician regarding patient's diet ○ Small, soft feedings ○ Yogurt and/or acidophilus ○ Avoidance of fruit and vegetables ○ Whole grain fiber may be helpful • Collaborate with physician and dietician regarding patient's enteral feedings ○ Provide isotonic feeding ○ Deliver feedings slowly or continuously with an infusion pump ○ Deliver feeding at room temperature ○ Prevent bacterial contamination by allowing feeding to hang at room temperature no longer than 4 hr (unless prepared under aseptic conditions) ○ Use fiber additives or high-fiber formula ○ Use lactose-free formula if indicated • Provide rest to decrease bowel motility • Provide privacy for the patient • Administer pharmacologic agents as prescribed ○ Antidiarrheals ○ Antispasmodics ○ Fluid and electrolyte replacement • Collect stool specimen for *C. difficile* toxin; if positive, administer antibiotic as prescribed (usually metronidazole [Flagyl] or vancomycin)	• Normal amount and frequency of stool • Absence of abdominal pain or cramping • No clinical indications of dehydration

Nursing Diagnosis	Defining Characteristics	Nursing Interventions	Expected Outcomes

FLUID VOLUME, DECREASED related to:
• Inadequate fluid intake or fluid restriction
• Inadequate fluid replacement
• Fluid loss (e.g., diaphoresis, vomiting, gastric suction, diarrhea, diuresis, draining wounds)
• Increased insensible loss caused by hyperventilation, fever
• Fluid sequestration (e.g., ascites, pleural effusion, pericardial effusion)
• Blood loss (e.g., trauma, coagulopathy)
• Blood sequestration (e.g., hemothorax, intra-abdominal, retroperitoneal)
• Decreased ADH or aldosterone synthesis, secretion, or effect
	• Orthostatic changes in HR and BP
	• Tachycardia
	• Hypotension
	• Increased body temperature
	• Decreased right atrial pressure, PAOP
	• Decreased CO and CI
	• Decrease in urine output (oliguria)
	• Increase in urine concentration
	• Weight loss
	• Peripheral pulses 1+/3+ in quality
	• Decreased skin turgor
	• Dry skin, dry, sticky mucous membranes and tongue and longitudinal furrowing of the tongue
	• Weakness and/or fatigue
	• Change in level of consciousness
	• Hemoconcentration: increased serum sodium; increased hematocrit; increased serum osmolality; hematocrit will be decreased if blood is lost
	• Increased blood urea nitrogen (BUN)
	• Thirst (polydipsia)
		• Monitor for changes in defining characteristics
		• Weigh daily with same scale and at same time of day (1 kg = 1 L)
		• Record accurate intake and output hourly
		• Assist with insertion of CVP, PA, or arterial catheter as indicated
		  ○ Provide standardized care for monitoring and maintaining hemodynamic monitoring catheters
		• Assess renal function: urine volume; urine creatinine clearance; serum creatinine, BUN nitrogen
		  ○ Insert urinary catheter and monitor urine output hourly
		• Administer oral fluids as tolerated
		  ○ Keep water pitcher within reach; keep fluids of choice available
		• Assist patient with diet and fluids
		• Administer parenteral fluids as prescribed
		  ○ Volume: based on patient losses including insensible losses in the calculation; frequently administered on a milliliter for milliliter loss basis
		    — Monitor closely for clinical indications of fluid overload (e.g., tachycardia, tachypnea, dyspnea, S_3, crackles)
		  ○ Solution: based on patient losses and serum osmolality and serum sodium
		    — Type and crossmatch for multiple units of blood for patients actively bleeding
		  ○ Monitor response to fluid and/or blood replacement
		  ○ Administer appropriate electrolyte replacement as prescribed
		• Administer antiemetics or antidiarrheals as indicated and prescribed
		• Administer prescribed pharmacologic agents for endocrine dysfunction (e.g., DI, DKA)
		  ○ Hormone replacement
		  ○ Agents that stimulate secretion of a hormone
		  ○ Agents that increase the effect of a hormone at its target organ
			• HR and BP within 10% of patient baseline
			• Normothermia
			• Right atrial pressure: 2-6 mm Hg
			• PAOP: 8-12 mm Hg
			• CI 2.5-4.0 L/min/m^2
			• Normalization of urine output (usually 0.5 mL/kg/hr)
			• Normalization in urine concentration: specific gravity 1.005-1.030; urine osmolality 50-1200 mOsm/kg as appropriate for serum osmolality
			• Weight normalization in relation to patient's usual body weight
			• Peripheral pulses 2+/3+ in quality
			• Normal skin turgor, moist skin, mucous membranes, intact skin and mucous membranes
			• Alert and oriented to person, place, and date
			• Normal serum sodium: 136-145 mEq/L
			• Normal hematocrit: 40%-52% for male patients; 35%-47% for female patients
			• Serum osmolality: 280-295 mOsm/kg

Continued

Nursing Diagnosis	Defining Characteristics	Nursing Interventions	Expected Outcomes

		• Maintain skin and mucous membrane integrity
		  ○ Careful assessment of skin and mucous membranes
		  ○ Turn at least every 2 hr
		  ○ Provide mouth care every 4 hr	

FLUID VOLUME, EXCESS related to:
• Excessive fluid intake or replacement
• Excessive sodium intake or replacement
• Inadequate renal perfusion or function
• Sodium and/or water retention
• Increased ADH or aldosterone synthesis, secretion, or effect
• Stress
• Decreased CO
	• Tachycardia
	• Hypertension or hypotension
	• Increased right atrial pressure, PAOP
	• Abnormal CO and CI
	• Change in urine output
	• Change in urine concentration
	• Weight gain
	• Edema, ascites, pericardial or pleural effusion, and/or anasarca
	• Jugular venous distention, positive hepatojugular reflux
	• Peripheral pulses 3+/3+ in quality
	• S_3
	• Dyspnea, orthopnea, tachypnea
	• Breath sound changes: crackles
	• Anorexia, nausea, vomiting, abdominal pain
	• Weakness, fatigue
	• Restlessness, anxiety
	• Change in level of consciousness
	• Seizures
	• Hemodilution: decreased serum sodium; decreased hematocrit; decreased serum osmolality
		• Monitor for changes in defining characteristics
		• Record accurate intake and output hourly and weights daily
		• Assess renal function: urine volume; urine creatinine clearance; serum creatinine, BUN
		• Monitor closely for clinical indications of pulmonary edema and/or cerebral edema
		• Restrict fluids and/or sodium depending on serum sodium and serum osmolality; include oral fluids, parenteral fluids, irrigation fluids, ice chips, CO injectates, medication volumes
		  ○ For accuracy in intravenous infusion volumes
		    — Use volumetric infusion pump
		    — Use decanting method in which volume equal to the volume of medication to be added if removed before addition of medication
		• Administer diuretics as prescribed and monitor urinary output response; do not administer diuretics to anuric patients
		• Administer parenteral fluids carefully as prescribed: use minidrip and/or volumetric pump
		  ○ Volume: based on patient losses including insensible losses in the calculation; frequently administered on a milliliter for milliliter loss basis
		  ○ Solution: based on patient losses and serum osmolality and serum sodium
		• Monitor serum electrolytes and administer appropriate electrolyte replacement as prescribed
		  ○ Severe hyponatremia may be treated with hypertonic (3%) saline
		    — Institute seizure precautions for serum sodium level 125 mEq/L or less
		  ○ Potassium replacement may be required
		• Prepare patient for hemodialysis if necessary (pulmonary edema is an indication for emergency dialysis in a patient with renal failure)
			• Normalization of urine output (usually 0.5 mL/kg/hr)
			• Normalization in urine concentration: specific gravity 1.005-1.030; urine osmolality 50-1200 mOsm/kg as appropriate for serum osmolality
			• Weight normalization
			• Absence of edema, ascites, pericardial or pleural effusion, and/or anasarca
			• Absence of jugular venous distention, positive hepatojugular reflux
			• Peripheral pulses 2+/3+ in quality
			• Absence of S_3
			• Absence of dyspnea, orthopnea, tachypnea
			• Absence of crackles
			• Absence of anorexia, nausea, vomiting, abdominal pain
			• Alert and oriented to person, place, and date
			• Absence of seizures
			• Normal serum sodium: 136-145 mEq/L
			• Normal hematocrit: 40%-52% for male patients; 35%-47% for female patients
			• BP within 10% of patient baseline
			• Right atrial pressure: 2-6 mm Hg
			• PAOP: 8-12 mm Hg
			• CI 2.5-4.0 L/min/m^2

Nursing Diagnosis	Defining Characteristics	Nursing Interventions	Expected Outcomes
		• Administer prescribed pharmacologic agents for endocrine dysfunction (e.g., SIADH) ○ Agents that inhibit secretion of a hormone ○ Agents that decrease the effect of a hormone at its target organ • Maintain skin and mucous membrane integrity ○ Careful assessment of skin and mucous membranes ○ Turn at least every 2 hr ○ Provide mouth care every 4 hr	
GAS EXCHANGE, IMPAIRED related to: • Decreased driving pressure of oxygen ○ Decreased inspired oxygen content (e.g., smoke) ○ Decreased barometric pressure (high altitude) • Alveolar hypoventilation • Increased alveolar dead space • Shunt • Ventilation-perfusion mismatch • Alveolar-capillary membrane changes • Decreased hemoglobin and/or abnormal hemoglobin • Decreased 2,3-DPG levels	• Tachycardia • Dysrhythmias • Mild hypertension • Tachypnea • Dyspnea, orthopnea • Use of accessory muscles • Cyanosis (depending on hemoglobin level) • Cough: sputum may be pink tinged and frothy in pulmonary edema • Breath sound changes: diminished intensity of breath sounds; presence of adventitious sound (e.g., crackles) • Decreased exercise capacity, fatigue • Neurologic changes: restlessness → confusion → lethargy • Pulmonary hypertension ○ Pam greater than 20 mm Hg ○ Pad more than 5 mm Hg greater than PAOP ○ PVR greater than 250 dyne/sec/cm^{-5} • Decreased Spo_2 • ABG changes ○ Decreased Sao_2, Pao_2 ○ $Paco_2$ may be decreased or increased depending on ventilation status • Elevated serum arterial lactate levels • May have abnormal chest x-ray	• Monitor for changes in defining characteristics • Assess respiratory effort, rate, depth, rhythm, and use of accessory muscles • Assess breath sounds as indicated • Assess pulse oximetry and arterial blood gases as indicated • Monitor pH and serum arterial lactate levels • Assess patient for chest pain; administer analgesics as indicated and prescribed • Monitor hemoglobin and CO ○ Administer blood as prescribed for anemia ○ Administer fluids replacement as prescribed for hypovolemia ○ Administer inotropes, venous vasodilators, diuretics as prescribed for heart failure ○ Monitor for effectiveness and adverse effects • Position for optimal ventilation and optimal ventilation-perfusion matching ○ Elevate HOB 30-45 degrees for optimal chest excursion ○ Prone and semiprone positions may also be used to improve ventilation ○ Turn every 2 hr; if unilateral lung condition, turn from good lung down to back (except patients after pneumonectomy, who should be turned from operative side to back) • Administer oxygen at 2-6 L/min to maintain Spo_2 of 95% or greater if patient is hypoxemic; if patient has chronic hypercapnia, administer oxygen to maintain Spo_2 at 90%-92%	• Alert and oriented • Absence of dyspnea, orthopnea, use of accessory muscles, cough • RR less than 24/min • Clear and equal breath sounds • Absence of crackles, rhonchi • Skin color normal for race; absence of cyanosis • Absence of dysrhythmias • BP and HR within 10% of patient's normal levels • Pao_2 greater than 60 mm Hg; Sao_2 greater than 90% • $Paco_2$ 35-45 mm Hg or at patient's normal level

Continued

Nursing Diagnosis	Defining Characteristics	Nursing Interventions	Expected Outcomes
		• Keep artificial airways and manual resuscitation bag readily available; intubation and mechanical ventilation may be necessary • Encourage the patient to turn and breathe deeply; encourage the patient to cough if rhonchi are audible • Suction only if coughing is ineffective in clearing secretions (e.g., ET tube) or patient is too fatigued to Cough • Instruct and assist in splinting for deep breathing and coughing • Encourage rest periods between coughing sessions and chest physiotherapy • Utilize techniques to prevent complications of suctioning • Encourage noncaffeinated oral fluids to thin secretions ○ 2-3 L of fluid/24 hr unless contraindicated by cardiac or renal disease • Provide humidification of inspired air and therapeutic oxygen • Keep room cool and comfortable • Provide calm and quiet environment • Identify and treat anxiety • Assist in insertion of chest tube and institution water seal drainage system if necessary for pneumothorax or hemothorax	
INFECTION, RISK FOR related to: • Artificial airway • Decreased activity of the Kupffer cells • Decreased function of immune system • Decreased number or function in of leukocytes • Exposure to unusually virulent (e.g., hospital-acquired) organism • Humidifiers and nebulizers • Hyperglycemia • Immunodeficiency • Impaired or absent protective reflexes • Inadequate primary defenses • Increased amounts of circulating corticosteroids	• Tachycardia • Fever • Leukocytosis (especially with increased neutrophils with increased bands) • Redness, warmth, induration, purulent drainage at catheter insertion site or surgical wound • Positive blood, sputum, urine, or wound cultures • Cloudy, foul-smelling urine • Crackles, abnormal chest x-ray • Yellow, brown, or green sputum; may be foul smelling	• Monitor for changes in defining characteristics • Practice handwashing for at least 15 sec using mechanical friction and soap and water before catheter insertion, catheter manipulation, blood sampling, dressing changes • Utilize universal precautions ○ Wear gloves for suctioning, oral care, repositioning of ET tube, IV care, indwelling urinary bladder catheter care, wound care, and for any other procedure that involves contact with body fluids, secretions or blood ○ Utilize disposable gowns situations when clothing may be contaminated by body fluids ○ Utilize eye protection during tracheobronchial suctioning or any other time when spraying of secretions may occur	• Normothermia • WBC less than 11,000 mm^3 • Absence of clinical indications of local infection: redness; swelling; purulent drainage from IV sites, wounds, incision lines • Urine clear and faintly ammonia scented • Clear lung sounds • Chest x-ray: absence of changes indicative of pneumonia, atelectasis • Negative culture if obtained

Nursing Diagnosis	Defining Characteristics	Nursing Interventions	Expected Outcomes
• Intestinal perforation • Invasive procedures and/or catheters • Loss of normal flora • Malnutrition • Side effects of drugs • Surgical procedures • Translocation of GI bacteria to blood or lymph • Uremic toxins		• Avoid invasive procedures is possible; discontinue invasive catheters as soon as possible • Utilize aseptic techniques to protect from cross-contamination and nosocomial infection • Monitor environment, visitors, personnel caring for patient for possible contamination sources • Change catheters, tubings, dressings at regular intervals; meticulous aseptic technique when caring for invasive lines ○ Handle all IV lines aseptically ○ Secure catheters to prevent catheter movement and vein irritation ○ Maintain an occlusive, sterile dressing on invasive lines; change at least every 48-72 hr and more often if soiled ○ Change IV tubing every 48-72 hr or per hospital policy ○ Eliminate all nonessential stopcocks; cover stopcock ports with occlusive covers ○ Remove and replace catheters inserted in an emergency, without proper asepsis as soon as possible under aseptic conditions ○ Inspect skin for redness, localized warmth, or drainage from incisions, venous catheter sites, arterial catheter sites ○ Remove and culture catheters at any sign of infection • Avoid indwelling urinary catheter is possible; straight catheterization intermittently is usually preferable unless hourly urine output monitoring is necessary • Ensure maintenance of a closed drainage system if indwelling urinary catheter is used; empty collection bag at least every 8 hr and measure carefully; observe urinary drainage for color, odor, and sediment • Provide meticulous skin care to avoid breaks in skin integrity; apply lotion to dry skin • Provide aseptic vascular access care; monitor for redness, induration, purulent drainage • Keep nails clipped short to decrease scratching trauma; pruritus is a serious problem in renal failure	

Continued

Nursing Diagnosis	Defining Characteristics	Nursing Interventions	Expected Outcomes
		• Provide meticulous pulmonary care: encourage deep breathing; incentive spirometry; coughing or suctioning if needed; monitor sputum production and appearance ◦ Encourage patient to cough if rhonchi are audible ◦ Observe and record amount and character of sputum; culture as indicated ◦ Provide oral hygiene every 4-8 hr ◦ Provide stoma care every 8 hr; change gauze dressing more often if copious secretions are present ◦ Maintain sterile technique in suctioning ET tubes or tracheostomy tubes; aseptic technique for oropharyngeal or nasopharyngeal airways ◦ Empty humidifier condensation into water trap; not back into humidifier reservoir ◦ Change ventilator tubing circuit every 48 hr or as per hospital policy • Utilize appropriate isolation techniques for patients with positive hepatitis antigen: private room; separate hemodialysis machine if on dialysis; caution with all body secretions • Obtain culture and sensitivity studies of purulent drainage, malodorous and/or cloudy urine, malodorous or discolored sputum as indicated; blood cultures are indicated for temperatures higher than 101°F or 39°C • Evaluate nutritional status and provide appropriate nutritional support and vitamin supplementation • Assess for early clinical indications of sepsis (e.g., cognitive changes, tachycardia, tachypnea, fever) • Assess for hemodynamic monitoring for changes of septic shock (e.g., decreased SVR, increased CO/CI, increased Svo_2) • Administer antibiotics as prescribed ◦ Administer antibiotics on time to ensure maintenance of therapeutic blood levels ◦ Monitor peak and tough levels and for clinical indications of toxicity ◦ Monitor creatinine clearance as indicated; especially when giving aminoglycoside antibiotics	

Nursing Diagnosis	Defining Characteristics	Nursing Interventions	Expected Outcomes
INJURY, RISK FOR related to: • Altered cerebral function ○ CNS infection or malignancy ○ Inadequate cerebral perfusion or oxygenation ○ Increased ammonia levels ○ HIV encephalopathy ○ Hypoglycemia • Seizures • ET intubation • Intravenous and/or arterial catheters • Microshock • Stress ulcer • Vascular access • Increased intrathoracic pressure • Inadequate blink reflex	• Disorientation • Impaired judgment • Sensory-perceptual deterioration • Patient reaching for ET tube • Clinical manifestations of air embolism ○ Respiratory distress ○ Hypotension ○ Change in level of consciousness • Clinical manifestations of venous thrombosis ○ Edema ○ Erythema ○ Ipsilateral swelling of arm, neck, face ○ Pain at site • Clinical manifestations of arterial thrombosis ○ Pain of limb distal to puncture and occlusion ○ Pallor ○ Pulselessness and decreased capillary refill rate ○ Motor and/or sensory changes ○ Coolness or coldness • Dysrhythmias caused by microshock • Stress caused by critical care environment and critical illness and/or administration of corticosteroids • Presence of vascular access • History of emphysema, congenital blebs or use of large tidal volumes or levels of PEEP • Use of muscle paralytic agents • Absence of blink reflex	• Monitor for changes in defining characteristics **Altered cerebral function** • Maintain a quiet environment to reduce environmental stimuli ○ Dim lights ○ Minimize noise • Reorient patient often: have clock, calendar, family pictures in room • Keep needed items (e.g., call light) placed within easy reach • Provide simple, brief explanations • Provide consistency in caregiver assignment • Caution visitors to avoid stress provoking discussion • Maintain side rails up and bed in low position • Monitor closely for clinical indications of hypoglycemia especially during peak times of insulin effect, if meals are missed, or if exertion is increased • Reduce and maintain BUN less than 100 mg/dL by dialysis, prevention of constipation, dehydration, and GI bleeding **Seizures** • Initiate seizure precautions if indicated ○ Instituted if serum sodium less than 125 mEq/L or if patient has a history of or predisposition to seizures ○ Includes close observation, padded side rails, supplemental oxygen, oral airway at bedside • Prophylactic anticonvulsants may be prescribed **Intubation** • Restrain only as necessary for patient protection • Reorient patient frequently and inform of purpose of tube, why patient cannot speak, etc. **Intravenous and/or arterial catheters** • Use Luer-Lok connections on all intravenous and intra-arterial catheters • Instruct patient to hold breath during tubing changes on central venous catheter • Monitor for clinical manifestations of venous thrombosis; catheter should be removed as soon as possible • Monitor for clinical manifestations of arterial thrombosis; catheter should be removed immediately	• Absence of injury • Patient does not self-extubate • Absence of clinical manifestations of air embolism • Absence of clinical manifestations of venous thrombosis • Absence of clinical manifestations of arterial thrombosis • Absence of dysrhythmias caused by microshock • Negative guaiac stools and vomitus • Patient does not develop pneumothorax, pneumomediastinum, or subcutaneous emphysema • Absence of corneal abrasion

Continued

Nursing Diagnosis	Defining Characteristics	Nursing Interventions	Expected Outcomes
		Microshock • Recognize patients at risk of microshock (e.g., patients with intracardiac catheter, pacemaker leads • Do not touch a piece of electrical equipment at the same time as you touch the patient • Touch the side rail before you touch the patient to discharge static electricity • Report 60-cycle interference or any piece of malfunctioning equipment to the biomedical department immediately • Ensure proper grounding of all electrical equipment **Stress ulcer** • Assess gastric pH; monitor gastric aspirate and/or stools for occult blood • Monitor bowel habits; observe for tarry or bloody stools • Provide oral or enteral feedings to decrease gastric acidity and protect the gastric mucosa; antacids, proton pump inhibitors, and/or histamine receptor antagonists may be prescribed to decrease the acidity of gastric contents (maintain pH 3.5-5.0); sucralfate (Carafate) may be used as a mucosal barrier **Potential for barotrauma** • Monitor peak inflation pressure and compliance • Monitor for clinical indications of pneumothorax: sudden increase in peak inflation pressure, diminished breath sounds on affected side, hypoxemia • Assist with emergency decompression with needle tap and/or insertion of chest tube as requested **Vascular access** • Assess external vascular access connections to ensure that they are tightly connected • Perform frequent neurovascular assessments of limb with vascular access **Inadequate blink reflex** • Instill artificial tears or Lacrilube as indicated	
INTRACRANIAL ADAPTIVE CAPACITY, DECREASED related to: • Cerebral edema	• Change in level of consciousness • Pupillary change ○ Oval pupil ○ Unequal pupil ○ Nonreactive pupil(s)	• Monitor for changes in defining characteristics • Assist with insertion of ICP monitoring device and measure ICP and calculate CPP if indicated	• Alert and oriented to person, place, and date • Pupils round, equal, and reactive to light • Eupnea

Nursing Diagnosis	Defining Characteristics	Nursing Interventions	Expected Outcomes

• Cerebral hemorrhage
• Intracranial hematoma
• Cerebral vasodilation caused by sensory hypercapnia, hypoxemia, vasodilators
• Hydrocephalus
• Intracranial mass (e.g., tumor, abscess, or other space-occupying lesions)
	• Papilledema
	• Respiratory pattern change
	• Motor changes
	• Sensory changes
	• Vital sign changes
	  ○ Increased systolic BP
	  ○ Decreased diastolic BP
	  ○ Bradycardia
	• Headache
	• Visual changes
	• Seizures
	• Vomiting
	• Pathologic reflexes (e.g., Babinski reflex, grasp reflex)
	• Glasgow Coma Scale less than 13
	• ICP greater than15 mm Hg
	• CPP less than 60 mm Hg
	• Decreased brain compliance as evidenced during volume pressure response testing
		• Maintain patent airway and ventilation
		• Elevate HOB 30 degrees
		• Keep head in neutral alignment; avoid pillow or allow only small pillow
		• Prevent compression of the jugular veins by head position, cervical collar, tracheostomy ties, etc.
		• Avoid hip flexion
		• Teach patient how to avoid Valsalva maneuver
		  ○ Teach patient to cough with mouth open if coughing is necessary
		  ○ Teach patient to avoid straining, bending, sneezing
		  ○ Administer stool softeners and antiemetics as prescribed
		• Avoid activities that increase ICP if possible; if an activity that increases ICP is necessary, allow time between multiples activities that increase ICP
		• Reorient patient frequently to person, place, date, and time
		• Explain procedures thoroughly
		• Monitor for clinical indications of infection; administer antibiotics as prescribed
		• Maintain normothermia with antipyretics, cooling blanket
		• Administer prescribed pharmaceutical agents (e.g., mannitol [Osmitrol], barbiturates) to decrease intracranial hypertension
		• Drain CSF via ventriculostomy if indicated and intraventricular catheter in place
		• Prepare patient for surgery for evacuation of clot, drainage of abscess, etc. as requested
			• Able to move all extremities spontaneously and/or on verbal request
			• Absence of sensory deficits
			• Vital signs within normal range or within 10% of patient's normal
			• Glasgow Coma Scale of 15
			• ICP 15 mm Hg or less
			• CPP greater than 60-70 mm Hg

NUTRITION: IMBALANCED, LESS THAN BODY REQUIREMENTS related to:
• Inability to obtain or prepare adequate amount or quality of food
  ○ Poverty
  ○ Disability or chronic illness
• Inability to ingest food
  ○ Food restriction (e.g., nothing by mouth)
  ○ Anorexia
	• Patient verbalizes complaints of anorexia, nausea, vomiting, diarrhea, dysphagia, sore mouth
	• Apathy
	• Fatigue, weakness
	• Headache
	• Poor muscle tone
	• Evidence of delayed wound healing
	• Unplanned weight loss of 20% within 6 months
	• Daily caloric intake less than estimated nutritional requirements
	• Decreased serum total protein, albumin, transferrin, folic acid, total lymphocytes
		• Monitor for changes in defining characteristics
		  ○ Weigh daily at same time on same scale
		  ○ Record daily food intake and calorie count
		• Evaluate bowel sounds and appropriateness to feed
		• Assess adequate dentition; assess fit of dentures; request dental consultation if necessary
		• Administer antiemetics as prescribed for nausea, especially before meals
		• Utilize prescribed drugs for oral infections
		  ○ Nystatin or clotrimazole (Mycelex) are frequently used for oral candidiasis (thrush)
			• Caloric intake equals estimated nutritional requirements
			• Cessation of weight loss and gradual weight gain
			• Normal muscle tone and strength
			• Evidence of wound healing
			• Serum albumin greater than 3.5 g/dL
			• Total lymphocytes greater than 1500/mm^3
			• Negative serum ketones and urine ketones
			• Normal serum total protein and albumin

Continued

Nursing Diagnosis	Defining Characteristics	Nursing Interventions	Expected Outcomes
○ Altered sense of taste ○ Nausea, vomiting ○ Abdominal pain ○ Alcoholism ○ Gingivitis ○ Stomatitis ○ Esophagitis ○ Dysphagia • Unwillingness to ingest food ○ Eating disorders ○ Dislike for dietary restrictions ○ Depression • Inability to digest food ○ Altered digestive enzymes • Inability to absorb or metabolize food ○ Insulin deficiency: absolute or relative ○ Increase in gastric or intestinal mobility • Increase in metabolic requirements causing a relative deficiency of nutrients ○ Burns ○ Sepsis ○ Hyperthyroidism • Adverse drug effects	• Diminished skinfold and arm circumference measurement • Elevated serum ketones and urine ketones • Absence of response to skin antigen testing	○ Acyclovir (Zovirax) is frequently used for oral herpes infections ○ Viscous lidocaine may be utilized before meals with patients with stomatitis • Utilize appetite-enhancing methods ○ Remove any noxious stimuli (e.g., emesis pan, bedpan) ○ Oral hygiene before meals ○ Small servings ○ Attractive presentation ○ Comfortable environment: lighting; temperature; family present if possible • Collaborate with physician, dietician, and pharmacist to estimate patient's metabolic needs and establish a plan for meeting these needs ○ Provide sufficient calories and nutrients — Oral feedings • Provide small, frequent feedings and dietary supplements as indicated • Identify and provide patient's food preferences unless contraindicated by dietary restrictions — Enteral feedings — Parenteral feedings if GI tract cannot be utilized ○ Maintain protein intake of approximately 1 g/kg of ideal body weight/24 hr; more will be needed in patients with protein malnutrition for repletion — If protein is restricted, ensure that protein is of high biological value (i.e., contains essential amino acids); egg white has all eight essential amino acids ○ Provide CHO and calories in sufficient amounts so that protein is not utilized for energy needs ○ Maintain caloric intake of approximately 50 kcal/kg of ideal body weight/24 hr; more will be needed for repletion or if patient is hypermetabolic (e.g., sepsis) — Provide CHOs and calories in sufficient amounts so that protein is not utilized for energy needs; 30% of nonprotein calories are usually in the form of fat (e.g., intralipid)	• Patient verbalizes understanding of dietary guidelines and intention to follow guidelines

Nursing Diagnosis	Defining Characteristics	Nursing Interventions	Expected Outcomes
		• Acute respiratory failure: CHOs may be decreased and fats increased in patients especially during weaning from mechanical ventilator because CHO metabolism produces more CO_2 than fat metabolism • Diabetes mellitus: 60% of calories are usually provided in the form of CHO with the remainder provided as 20% protein and 20% fat ○ Administer vitamin and iron supplements • Maintain nutrient and/or electrolyte restrictions as indicated • Administer insulin as prescribed • Provide rest periods before and after meals • Consult psychological or social services if needed ○ Meals-on-wheels referral may be needed at time of discharge due to fatigue and decreased energy	
PAIN related to: • Biological injury • Chemical injury • Physical injury • Psychological factors	• Verbal complaints of pain • Tense, guarded posture • Sympathetic responses: tachycardia; mild hypertension; tachypnea; pupillary dilation; diaphoresis • Grimacing, moaning, crying, restlessness, withdrawal • Impaired concentration, irritability • Knees flexed to relieve pain in peritoneal irritation • Tense, guarded posture • Rebound tenderness may be present	• Monitor for changes in defining characteristics • Observe patient for verbal and nonverbal expression of pain or discomfort • Assess pain: PQRST ○ P: provocation, palliation ○ Q: quality ○ R: region, radiation ○ S: severity ○ T: timing • Utilize nonpharmacologic approaches ○ Place patient in position of comfort ○ Relaxation techniques including imagery ○ Distraction • Administer analgesics as prescribed ○ Narcotics (e.g., morphine) — Intravenous: intermittent; basal continuous dose — Epidural: basal continuous dose; intermittent bolus — Oral: absorption is affected by GI perfusion; infrequently used in critical care situations ○ Non-narcotics: NSAIDs are particularly helpful for surgical and inflammatory pain ○ Local anesthetics (e.g., bupivacaine [Marcaine]) — Interpleural — Intercostal	• Patient verbalizes relief of pain • Absence of nonverbal indicators of pain • BP and HR within 10% of patient's normal levels **If chest pain** • Absence of ST-T wave changes • Absence of dysrhythmias

Continued

Nursing Diagnosis	Defining Characteristics	Nursing Interventions	Expected Outcomes
		• Provide environment conducive to rest whenever possible ○ Comfortable temperature ○ Dim lighting ○ Quiet or relaxing music • Prepare patient for procedures to be preformed and any anticipated pain • Instruct patient to inform nurse of any new pain **Chest pain** • Obtain baseline vital signs and monitor as indicated • Obtain multiple lead ECG with each episode of chest pain ○ Assess ECG for: — ST-T wave changes — Conduction defects ○ Monitor continuous ECG for rate, rhythm, and dysrhythmias • Monitor for accompanying signs/symptoms • Obtain cardiac enzymes and isoenzymes as indicated • Initiate IV infusion and administer solution at prescribed rate or to keep vein open • Administer oxygen at 5 L/min via nasal cannula unless contraindicated • Administer antianginal agents (e.g., NTG) or analgesic (e.g., morphine) as prescribed • Remain with patient during chest pain • Report persistent chest pain, significant changes in BP, HR or rhythm, RR and rhythm to physician **Abdominal pain** • Assess for changes in bowel sounds, abdominal distention, rebound tenderness • Maintain gastric suction and nothing-by-mouth status as indicated • Prepare patient for procedures to be preformed and any anticipated pain **Headache** • Do not give narcotics if there are clinical indications of intracranial hypertension; nonnarcotic analgesics are usually used	
PROTECTION, INEFFECTIVE related to electrolyte imbalance caused by: • Acid-base imbalance • Acute pancreatitis	• Clinical manifestations of hyponatremia ○ Anorexia ○ Nausea/vomiting ○ Muscle cramps and twitching ○ Hypotension	• Monitor for changes in defining characteristics • Identify cause or causes of electrolyte balance • Monitor serum electrolyte values • Monitor ECG for indications of electrolyte imbalance	• Absence of clinical manifestations of electrolyte imbalance • Absence of laboratory indicators of electrolyte imbalance

Nursing Diagnosis	Defining Characteristics	Nursing Interventions	Expected Outcomes
• ADH deficiency or excess • Decreased electrolyte excretion • Dietary restrictions • Diuretic therapy • Excessive intake • Gastric or intestinal suction • Hemorrhage • Increased insensible losses due to increased ventilatory rate, fever • Increased secretion of ADH • Insulin deficiency • Therapeutic dietary restrictions • Vomiting	◦ Seizures ◦ Coma • Clinical manifestations of hypernatremia ◦ Low grade fever ◦ Dry, sticky mucous membranes ◦ CNS irritability: restlessness, agitation ◦ Muscle cramps, increased deep tendon reflexes ◦ Seizures • Clinical manifestations of hyperkalemia ◦ Nausea, vomiting, intestinal colic, diarrhea ◦ Muscle weakness progressing to flaccid paralysis ◦ Increased deep tendon reflexes ◦ Lethargy, mental confusion ◦ ECG changes: tall, peaked T waves, asystole ◦ Respiratory muscle weakness, respiratory distress or arrest • Clinical manifestations of hypokalemia ◦ Anorexia, nausea, vomiting ◦ Decreased bowel motility ◦ Muscle cramps, muscle weakness progressing to flaccid paralysis ◦ Mental apathy, confusion, drowsiness ◦ Dysrhythmias • Clinical manifestations of hypomagnesemia ◦ Hyperactive deep tendon reflexes ◦ Circumoral paresthesia ◦ Carpopedal spasm ◦ Seizures ◦ Dysrhythmias • Clinical manifestations of hypocalcemia ◦ Hyperactive deep tendon reflexes ◦ Circumoral paresthesia ◦ Carpopedal spasm ◦ Laryngospasm ◦ Dysrhythmias ◦ Seizures • Clinical manifestations of hypophosphatemia ◦ Anorexia, nausea, vomiting ◦ Malaise, fatigue	• Initiate IV infusion and administer solution as prescribed • Initiate electrolyte replacement as indicated and prescribed ◦ Intravenous replacement ◦ Dietary replacement • Restrict dietary and drug intake of elevated electrolytes as indicated • Administer other drug therapies as prescribed (e.g., glucose and insulin for critical hyperkalemia) • Identify cause or causes of electrolyte balance • Monitor serum electrolyte values • Monitor ECG for indications of electrolyte imbalance • Initiate IV infusion and administer solution as prescribed • Initiate electrolyte replacement as indicated and prescribed ◦ Intravenous replacement ◦ Dietary replacement	

Continued

Nursing Diagnosis	Defining Characteristics	Nursing Interventions	Expected Outcomes
	○ Muscle weakness especially respiratory muscles ○ Dysrhythmias • Laboratory indicators of electrolyte imbalance (e.g., serum electrolyte lower or higher than laboratory-defined normal values)		
PROTECTION, INEFFECTIVE related to: • Congenital clotting abnormality (e.g., hemophilia) • Fibrinolytic, anticoagulant, platelet aggregation inhibitor therapy • Inadequate intake or absorption of vitamin K • Decreased fibrinogen production (e.g., liver disease) • Decreased production of clotting factors	• Increased PT, aPTT, bleeding times; decreased platelet count • Petechiae, bruising	• Monitor clotting parameters and bleeding times • Detect bleeding ○ Monitor for oral, nasal, scleral, rectal, or vaginal bleeding ○ Monitor for petechiae, ecchymosis, hematoma, bleeding from puncture points, catheter insertion sites, wounds ○ Monitor gastric aspirate and/or stools for occult blood ○ Monitor bowel habits; observe for tarry or bloody stools ○ Monitor for joint or bone pain ○ Monitor for changes in neurologic status • Prevent bleeding ○ Keep nails cut short to prevent scratches that may bleed ○ Administer antipruritics as prescribed ○ Encourage use of soft toothbrush ○ Encourage avoidance of blade razor ○ Avoid unnecessary injections and blood sampling — If arterial puncture is necessary: hold pressure for 10-15 min — If venous puncture is necessary: hold pressure for 5 min ○ Suction only if necessary ○ Avoid use of noninvasive BP cuffs ○ Avoid aspirin and aspirin-containing drugs unless specifically prescribed ○ Assess gastric pH; antacids, histamine$_2$ receptor antagonists, proton pump inhibitors, or mucosal barriers may be prescribed to decrease the acidity of gastric contents ○ Have vitamin K and/or protamine available for reversal of anticoagulants	• Absence of bleeding from surface wounds, body systems • PT, aPTT, bleeding time within normal limits or within therapeutic range if drugs are being given to affect these parameters
SKIN INTEGRITY, IMPAIRED related to: • Dry skin • Edema	• Breaks in skin or mucous membranes • Reddened excoriated skin • Edematous skin	• Monitor for changes in defining characteristics • Turn patient or assist patient in turning at least every 2 hr	• Skin is clean, dry, intact • Absence of reddened areas or breaks in skin or mucous membranes

Nursing Diagnosis	Defining Characteristics	Nursing Interventions	Expected Outcomes
• Diaphoresis • Dermatitis • Skin lesions • Pruritus • Prolonged skin contact with body secretions ○ Incontinence ○ Diarrhea ○ Fistula ○ Stoma • Adhesives • Surgical procedures • Invasive procedures and catheters • Bacterial or fungal infections • Immobility • Malnutrition • Age • Pronounced body prominences • Radiation therapy • Hypothermia or hyperthermia	• Incisions or other wounds	• Inspect skin for erythema or prolonged blanching with each position change • Use turning sheets to turn patient rather than letting them scoot • Position with pillows to relieve pressure • Keep HOB elevated no more than 30 degrees to prevent shearing forces • Keep linens dry and wrinkle free • Special beds may be necessary for patients with increased risk of skin breakdown (e.g., malnutrition, incontinence) • Limit time sitting in chair to 2 hr at a time • Keep skin clean and dry • Apply water-soluble lubricant to each nostril every 8 hr for patients with NG tube • Clean rectal area after each episode of diarrhea using a mild soap • Avoid tape and adhesives if possible • Keep edematous limbs elevated • Administer medications for itching (e.g., antihistamines) as prescribed • Administer topical antibiotics as prescribed • Provide active and/or passive ROM exercises • Collaborate with physician and dietician to provide adequate nutritional support ○ High-protein unless contraindicated ○ Enough CHOs that the protein will not be used for energy ○ Monitor serum total protein, serum albumin, and serum transferrin levels for improvement in nutritional status • Provide standardized care for monitoring and maintaining intravenous and arterial catheters • Apply gentle consistent pressure to bleeding sites • Limit injections, invasive procedures if possible • Avoid rectal temperatures, tubes • Provide oral hygiene every 4 hr • Avoid drying solutions (e.g., alcohol-containing mouthwashes, lemon and glycerin swabs) • Moisturize lips with lubricant	• Absence of redness, induration at intravenous or intra-arterial catheter sites • Indicators of adequate healing of surgical incisions or wounds • Decrease in clinical indications of inflammation (redness, swelling, warmth, pain)

Continued

Nursing Diagnosis	Defining Characteristics	Nursing Interventions	Expected Outcomes
SLEEP PATTERN, DISTURBED related to: • Noise • Unfamiliar surrounding • Discomfort with room temperature, humidity, lighting, odor • Frequent awakenings by health care professionals • Physical restraint • Immobility • Lack of privacy • Absence of sleep partner • Nocturia • Pain • Dyspnea • Nausea, vomiting, dyspepsia • Disturbance of circadian rhythm • Daylight/darkness exposure • Anxiety, fear • Thinking about home, health, problems • Depression • Loneliness • Drug effect	• Inability to go to sleep • Frequent awakenings • Early awakening • Verbalization of difficulty falling asleep • Verbalization of not feeling rested • Decreased proportion of REM sleep	• Monitor for changes in defining characteristics • Provide daytime activities (e.g., ROM, ambulation) as tolerated • Encourage the patient to discuss fears and concerns • Maintain light-dark patterns and wake-sleep patterns; discourage excessive sleep during the day • Assess the patient's usual presleep nighttime rituals; assist the patient to perform these rituals (e.g., assist with mouth care, washing of face and hands, beverage at bedside) • Avoid stimulants close to bedtime (e.g., caffeine-containing beverages, chocolate) • Avoid heavy meal before sleep; a small snack may be helpful • Provide back rub at bedtime if desired • Provide relaxing music if desired • Assist the patient to a position of comfort • Allow the patient's spouse to sleep in the patient's room if possible? • Ensure comfort ○ Room temperature and bed coverings ○ Lighting ○ Elimination of offensive odors ○ Elimination of unnecessary noise (e.g., decrease volume of alarms, close door, ask staff to lower voices) • Administer pharmacologic agents as prescribed ○ Anxiolytics ○ Sedatives ○ Hypnotics ○ Analgesics • Avoid interrupting the patient's sleep unless absolutely necessary (e.g., omit vital sign measurement during sleep if possible, schedule medications before sleep)	• Patient verbalizes satisfaction with amount and quality of sleep
THERMOREGULATION, INEFFECTIVE related to: • Brain or spinal cord injury • Aging • Thyroid disorder • Trauma • Illness • Fluctuating environmental temperature	• Fluctuations in body temperature higher or lower than the normal range • Warm or cool skin • Flushed or pale skin • Piloerection • Shivering • Decreased capillary refill (more than 3 sec)	• Monitor for changes in defining characteristics • Monitor body temperature at least every 4 hr; more often if significant abnormalities noted • Monitor for clinical indications of infection as a possible cause of hyperthermia • Regulate room temperature **For hypothermia** • Provide warm fluids and food • Apply warmed blankets	• Normal body temperature • Patient verbalizes comfort with temperature • Normal skin color and temperature • No piloerection or shivering • Normal capillary refill (less than 3 sec)

Nursing Diagnosis	Defining Characteristics	Nursing Interventions	Expected Outcomes
		• Use radiant heat lamps (especially helpful in patients with burns) • Place warming blanket on bed; place sheet between patient and blanket • Infuse warm IV fluids, assist with peritoneal lavage with warm fluid, irrigate bladder with warm fluid, and warm inhaled air for severe hypothermia **For hyperthermia** • Remove excess bedding • Place cooling blanket on bed; place sheet between patient and blanket • Use fans to circulate air • Sponge patient with tepid water if necessary • Place ice bags to axilla and groin • Administer antipyretics as prescribed; may be helpful depending on cause of hyperthermia • Administer meperidine (Demerol) as prescribed for shivering	
THOUGHT PROCESSES, DISTURBED related to: • Sensory overload (of nonmeaningful stimuli) • Sensory deprivation (of meaningful stimuli) • Sleep deprivation • "ICU psychosis" • CNS injury • Organic mental disorder • Drug ingestion • Uremia • GI hemorrhage • Hepatic encephalopathy	• Disorientation to person, place and/or time • Confusion regarding purpose of hospitalization, confinement • Sleep disturbances • Agitation, anxiety, irritability • Hallucinations	• Monitor for changes in defining characteristics • Use the patient's name when speaking to him or her • Speak slowly and clearly • Reorient patient to person, place, time verbally frequently; have clock, calendar in room • Be respectful when correcting the patient's misperceptions • Maintain light-dark patterns using windows and lighting • Eliminate as much nonmeaningful visual, auditory, and tactile stimulation as possible • Allow family visitation as indicated; encourage the family to bring in familiar objects (e.g., photos) • Eliminate invasive and intrusive procedures if possible • Protect from self-injury through use of side rails; restraints only as needed for self-protection **Renal failure** • Restrict protein intake but provide adequate calories so that protein is not utilized for energy (catabolism increases BUN) • Institute dialysis as prescribed to keep BUN less than 100 mg/dL **GI hemorrhage** • Check stools and NG aspirate for occult blood; blood (being primarily protein) metabolism increases BUN and ammonia	• Patient alert and oriented • Absence of agitation, irritability • Patient verbalizes absence of anxiety; absence of nonverbal indicators of anxiety • Absence of injury

Continued

Nursing Diagnosis	Defining Characteristics	Nursing Interventions	Expected Outcomes
		• Treat GI bleeding by irrigating until clear with room temperature saline • Administer antacids and histamine receptor antagonists as prescribed • Administer osmotic laxative (e.g., sorbitol) as prescribed • Prevent constipation **Hepatic encephalopathy** • Restrict protein intake but provide adequate calories so that protein is not utilized for energy • Administer neomycin as prescribed to decrease bacterial action in intestine • Administer osmotic laxative (e.g., sorbitol) as prescribed • Prevent constipation	
TISSUE PERFUSION, IMPAIRED related to: • Arterial thrombus, embolism, spasm, hemorrhage • Decreased CO • Inadequate hemoglobin • Vasopressor therapy • Intra-arterial catheter or sheath • Fracture or circumferential burn • Poor positioning and arterial compression	• Myocardial ○ Chest pain ○ Tachycardia, hypotension ○ ST-T wave changes on ECG ○ Decreased CO/CI • Cerebral ○ Change in level of consciousness: restlessness → confusion → lethargy → coma ○ Syncope ○ Pupillary changes ○ Motor or sensory changes ○ Aphasia ○ Altered thought processes • Pulmonary ○ Dyspnea ○ Hemoptysis ○ Pleuritic pain ○ Pleural friction rub ○ Decreased Sao_2, Spo_2, Pao_2 • Renal ○ Decrease in urine output ○ Hematuria ○ Pyuria ○ Flank pain ○ Changes in BUN, creatinine • Splenic ○ LUQ pain radiating to left shoulder ○ Abdominal rigidity • Mesenteric ○ Abdominal pain ○ Watery, bloody diarrhea • Peripheral ○ Pain and/or intermittent claudication ○ Pale and/or cyanotic extremities ○ Diminished or absent peripheral pulses	• Monitor for changes in defining characteristics • Decrease oxygen requirements by limiting activity, anxiety, pain ○ Administer analgesics as indicated and prescribed ○ Identify and treat anxiety • Initiate IV infusion in a nonischemic limb and administer solution as prescribed ○ Crystalloids (e.g., normal saline, lactated ringers) ○ Colloids (e.g., albumin, dextran 70, hetastarch) ○ Blood and blood products (e.g., packed red blood cells) — Blood and/or blood products are indicated by symptoms such as hypotension, chest pain, syncope, dyspnea not simply by as certain hematocrit level • Assess cause of anemia (e.g., actual blood loss versus suppression of erythropoietin as in renal failure) ○ Administer recombinant erythropoietin (Epogen) as ordered for the anemia caused by erythropoietin deficiency in chronic renal failure; iron, folic acid, pyridoxine, and vitamin B_{12} may by indicated in anemia seen in chronic renal failure • Affirm or establish airway; intubation may be necessary • Administer oxygen therapy as indicated and prescribed; mechanical ventilation and PEEP may be necessary • Insert a urinary catheter if indicated and prescribed and monitor urine output hourly	• Cardiac ○ Absence of chest pain ○ Tachycardia, hypotension ○ ST-T wave changes • Cerebral ○ Patient alert and oriented ○ Absence of pupil changes, motor or sensory changes, speech changes • Pulmonary ○ Absence of dyspnea, hemoptysis, pleuritic pain, pleural friction rub • Renal ○ Urine output greater than 0.5 mL/kg/hr ○ Normal BUN and creatinine ○ Absence of hematuria, pyuria, flank pain • Splenic ○ Absence of LUQ pain, abdominal rigidity • Mesenteric ○ Absence of abdominal pain ○ Bloody diarrhea • Peripheral ○ Absence of limb pain, diminished pulses, pallor, motor or sensory changes, coolness or coldness

Nursing Diagnosis	Defining Characteristics	Nursing Interventions	Expected Outcomes
	○ Motor or sensory changes ○ Cool or cold extremities ○ Decreased capillary refill (more than 3 sec) ○ Dry, thick, brittle nails ○ Hair loss ○ Bruits ○ Ulcerations ○ Poor healing of wounds	**Myocardial** • Assist with insertion of pulmonary artery catheter and measure hemodynamic parameter if indicated • Administer fibrinolytics, anticoagulants, and/or platelet aggregation inhibitors as prescribed • Prepare patient for PCI or CABG as requested • Administer inotropes (e.g., dobutamine), vasodilators (e.g., nitrates) as prescribed • Assist with insertion of IABP, LVAD, RVAD or bi-VAD as requested **Cerebral** • Assist with insertion of ICP monitoring device and measure ICP and calculate CPP if indicated • Prepare patient for surgery if indicated • Maintain patent airway and ventilation • Elevate HOB 30 degrees; keep head aligned with body; prevent compression of the jugular veins by head position, cervical collar, tracheostomy ties, etc. • Teach patient how to avoid Valsalva maneuver • Avoid activities that increase ICP if possible; if activity is necessary, allow time between multiples activities that increase ICP **Pulmonary** • Prevention • Establish and maintain position of comfort • Encourage patient to turn and breathe deeply • Perform passive ROM or encourage active ROM • Encourage patient to move toes, dorsiflex and hyperextend feet, bend legs at knees • Apply antiembolic stockings or sequential compression devices • Administer low-molecular-weight heparin subcutaneously as prescribed • Treatment • Administer oxygen to maintain Spo_2 at 95% or greater unless contraindicated • Administer heparin by IV infusion as prescribed • Administer fibrinolytics as prescribed • Prepare patient for embolectomy if requested	

Continued

Nursing Diagnosis	Defining Characteristics	Nursing Interventions	Expected Outcomes
		Renal, mesenteric, splenic • Ensure adequate hydration • Monitor for clinical indications of bowel perforation • Prepare patient for angioplasty or surgical procedure as requested **Peripheral** • Eliminate/minimize vasoconstrictive activities and agents ○ Smoking ○ Stress ○ Vasoconstrictive agents (e.g., phenylephrine, norepinephrine, dopamine) • Decrease oxygen requirements by limiting activity, anxiety, pain • Keep patient warm with extremities flat; avoid bending of limb at a cannulation, injury, or surgical site • Assist with removal of IABP or sheath as requested • Assist with intra-arterial fibrinolytic or prepare patient for embolectomy or surgical procedure as requested • Assist with escharotomy (circumferential burn) or fasciotomy (compartment syndrome)	
VENTILATORY WEANING RESPONSE, DYSFUNCTIONAL related to: • History of mechanical ventilation of more than 1 week • Pain or discomfort • Muscle weakness • Malnutrition • Anemia • Ineffective airway clearance • Inappropriate pacing of diminished ventilator support • Adverse environment • Decreased motivation • Fear, anxiety • Hopelessness, powerlessness • Sleep pattern disturbance • Knowledge deficit of weaning process • History of multiple unsuccessful weaning attempts	Responds to weaning attempts with: • Tachycardia • Tachypnea • Hypertension • Restlessness • Anxiety • Agitation • Dyspnea • Increased concentration on breathing • Inability to cooperate • Diaphoresis • Accessory muscle use • Paradoxical abdominal breathing • Inability to breathe in "synch" with ventilator • Decreased level of consciousness • Diminished breath sounds • Decreased Spo_2 • ABG changes • Decreased Sao_2, Pao_2 • Increased $Paco_2$ • Respiratory acidosis	• Monitor for changes in defining characteristics • Ensure adequate nutritional status, hemodynamics, and psychological readiness • CHOs may need to be decreased with equivalent calories supplies in the form of fats because CHO metabolism increases CO_2 production ○ Enterally: Pulmocare ○ Parenterally: substitute increased lipids for decrease in CHO • Establish a plan for weaning with other members of the health care team; involve the patient in planning • Convey confidence in patient's ability to succeed • Time weaning efforts when the patient is rested and support staff is available (e.g., anesthesia, respiratory therapy) • Administer oxygen as prescribed • Suction airway as indicated • Administer analgesics as prescribed and indicated • Control the environment: quiet, cool room • Supply positive reinforcement and reassurance	• Successful weaning from mechanical ventilation with: ○ HR, BP, RR within normal range ○ ABGs within normal limits or patient's normal

Nursing Diagnosis	Defining Characteristics	Nursing Interventions	Expected Outcomes
• Patient-perceived inefficacy about the ability to wean		• Stay with patient during weaning attempts or as ventilator settings are changed; touch the patient, hold their hand • Maintain a calm, confident attitude • Increase or decrease family visitation depending on their effect on the weaning process	

ABG, Arterial blood gas; *ADH,* antidiuretic hormone; *ADLs,* activities of daily living; *aPTT,* activated partial thromboplastin time; *bi-VAD,* bilateral ventricular assist device; *BP,* blood pressure; *BUN,* blood urea nitrogen; *CABG,* coronary artery bypass grafting; *CHO,* carbohydrate; *CI,* cardiac index; *CNS,* central nervous system; *CO,* cardiac output; CO_2, carbon dioxide; *CPP,* cerebral perfusion pressure; *CSF,* cerebrospinal fluid; *CVP,* central venous pressure; *DI,* diabetes insipidus; *DKA,* diabetic ketoacidosis; *2,3-DPG,* 2,3-diphosphoglycerate; *ECG,* electrocardiogram; *ET,* endotracheal; *GI,* gastrointestinal; *HIV,* human immunovirus; *HOB,* head of bed; *HR,* heart rate; *IABP,* intra-aortic balloon pump; *ICP,* intracranial pressure; *ICU,* intensive care unit; *IV,* intravenous; *LLQ,* left lower quadrant; *LUQ,* left upper quadrant; *LVAD,* left ventricular assist device; *LVF,* left ventricular failure; *MAP,* mean arterial pressure; *NG,* nasogastric; *NSAID,* nonsteroidal anti-inflammatory drug; *NTG,* nitroglycerin; *PA,* pulmonary artery; $Paco_2$, arterial partial pressure of carbon dioxide; PaO_2, arterial partial pressure of oxygen; *PAOP,* pulmonary artery occlusive pressure; *PAP,* pulmonary artery pressure; *PCI,* percutaneous coronary intervention; *PEEP,* positive end-expiratory pressure; *PT,* prothrombin time; *RAP,* right atrial pressure; *ROM,* range of motion; *RR,* respiratory rate; *RVAD,* right ventricular assist device; *RVF,* right ventricular failure; Sao_2, arterial oxygen saturation; *SIADH,* syndrome of inappropriate antidiuretic hormone; Spo_2, oxygen saturation measured with pulse oximetry; Svo_2, venous oxygen saturation; *SVR,* systemic vascular resistance; *WBC, white blood cell count.*

Common Abbreviations and Acronyms Used in Critical Care Nursing

APPENDIX B

2,3-DPG	2,3-diphosphoglyceric acid
A	Alveolar (e.g., PAO_2)
a	Arterial (e.g., Pao_2)
A_2	Aortic (first) component of S_2
AAA	Abdominal aortic aneurysm
AACN	American Association of Critical-Care Nurses
AAL	Anterior axillary line
ABG	Arterial blood gas
ABI	Ankle-brachial index
AC	Assist-control
ACC	American College of Cardiology
ACE	Angiotensin-converting enzyme
ACLS	Advanced cardiac life support
ACS	Acute coronary syndrome
ACT	Activated clotting time
ACTH	Adrenocorticotropic hormone
ADA	American Diabetes Association
ADH	Antidiuretic hormone
ADL	Activities of daily living
ADP	Adenosine diphosphate
AED	Automated external defibrillator
AF	Atrial fibrillation
AHA	American Heart Association
AHA	American Hospital Association
AHRQ	Agency for Healthcare Research and Quality
AICD	Automatic implantable cardiac defibrillator
AIDS	Acquired immunodeficiency syndrome
AIVR	Accelerated idioventricular rhythm

ALI	Acute lung injury
ALS	Amyotrophic lateral sclerosis
ALT	Alanine aminotransferase
ANA	Antinuclear antibody
ANA	American Nurses Association
ANCC	American Nurses Certification Corporation
ANF	Atrial natriuretic factor
ANS	Autonomic nervous system
APRV	Airway pressure release ventilation
aPTT	Activated partial thromboplastin time
AR	Aortic regurgitation
ARB	Angiotensin receptor blocker
ARDS	Acute respiratory distress syndrome
ARF	Acute respiratory failure
AS	Aortic stenosis
ASA	Acetylsalicylic acid (aspirin)
AST	Aspartate aminotransferase
ATN	Acute tubular necrosis
ATP	Adenosine triphosphate
AV	Atrioventricular
AVM	Arteriovenous malformation
BA	Bronchoalveolar lavage
BBB	Bundle branch block
Bi-PAP	Positive airway pressure on both inspiration and expiration
BIS	Bispectral index
Bi-VAD	Biventricular assist device
BLS	Basic life support
BMI	Body mass index
BNP	Brain-type natriuretic peptide
BP	Blood pressure
BPOC	Bar-code point of care
BSA	Body surface area
BUN	Blood urea nitrogen
C	Celsius (also referred to as centigrade)
CABG	Coronary artery bypass graft
CAD	Coronary artery disease
Cao_2	Oxygen content in arterial blood
CAP	Community-acquired pneumonia
CAPP	Coronary artery perfusion pressure
CASS	Continuous aspiration of subglottic secretions
CAVH	Continuous arteriovenous hemofiltration
CAVHD	Continuous arteriovenous hemodialysis
CBC	Complete blood count
CBF	Cerebral blood flow
CCO	Continuous cardiac output
CCU	Critical care unit

CDC	Centers for Disease Control and Prevention
CEA	Carcinoembryonic antigen
CHB	Complete heart block
CHO	Carbohydrate
CHP	Capillary hydrostatic pressure
CI	Cardiac index
CK	Creatinine kinase
CK-MB	Creatinine kinase-myocardial band
cm	Centimeter
CMV	Cytomegalovirus
CNS	Central nervous system
CO	Cardiac output
CO_2	Carbon dioxide
COP	Colloidal oncotic pressure
COPD	Chronic obstructive pulmonary disease
CPAP	Continuous positive airway pressure
CPD	Citrate phosphate dextrose
CPOE	Computerized provider order entry
CPP	Cerebral perfusion pressure
CPR	Cardiopulmonary resuscitation
CRRT	Continuous renal replacement therapy
CSF	Cerebrospinal fluid
CSWS	Cerebral salt wasting syndrome
CT	Computed tomography
cTnI	Cardiac troponin I
cTnT	Cardiac troponin T
CVA	Costovertebral angle
CVA	Cerebrovascular accident
Cvo_2	Oxygen content in venous blood
CVP	Central venous pressure
CVVHD	Continuous venovenous hemodialysis
D_5LR	5% dextrose in lactated ringer's
D_5NS	5% dextrose in normal saline
D_5W	5% dextrose in water
DAI	Diffuse axonal injury
DBP	Diastolic blood pressure
DCA	Directional coronary atherectomy
DCD	Deceased after cardiac death
DHA	Docosahexanoic acid
DI	Diabetes insipidus
DIC	Disseminated intravascular coagulation
DKA	Diabetic ketoacidosis
dL	Deciliter
DM	Diabetes mellitus
DNA	Deoxyribonucleic acid
DNR	Do not resuscitate

DO_2	Oxygen delivery to the tissues
DO_2I	Delivery of oxygen to the tissue index
DPL	Diagnostic peritoneal lavage
DTR	Deep tendon reflexes
DVT	Deep vein thrombosis
EBP	Evidence-based practice
$ECCO_2OR$	Extracorporeal carbon dioxide removal
ECF	Extracellular fluid
ECG	Electrocardiogram (frequently abbreviated EKG)
ECMO	Extracorporeal membrane oxygenator
ED	Emergency department
EDH	Epidural hematoma
EECP	Enhanced external counterpulsation
EEG	Electroencephalogram
EF	Ejection fraction
ELCA	Excimer laser coronary arthrectomy
ELISA	Enzyme linked immunosorbent assay
EMG	Electromyogram
EMI	Electromagnetic interference
ENG	Electronystagmography
EPA	Eicosapentaenoic acid
EPA	Environmental Protection Agency
EPS	Electrophysiology studies
ERCP	Endoscopic retrograde cholangiopancreatography
ERV	Expiratory reserve volume
ESR	Erythrocyte sedimentation rate
ET	Endotracheal
ETC	Esophageal tracheal Combitube
EVG	Endovascular graft
F	Fahrenheit
f	Frequency of ventilation
FAST	Focused abdominal sonography for trauma
FDA	Food and Drug Administration
FEV	Forced expiratory capacity
FFA	Free fatty acid
FFP	Fresh frozen plasma
FiO_2	Fraction of inspired oxygen
FRC	Functional residual capacity
FSP	Fibrin split products (also referred to as fibrin degradation products)
FT_c	Flow time corrected
FVC	Forced vital capacity
g	Gram
GALT	Gut-associated lymphoid tissue
GCS	Glasgow Coma Scale
GERD	Gastroesophageal reflux disease

GFR	Glomerular filtration rate
GI	Gastrointestinal
GIK	Glucose-insulin-potassium
GP	Glycoprotein
GU	Genitourinary
H^+	Hydrogen ion
H_2O	Water
HAART	Highly active antiretroviral therapy
HAP	Hospital-acquired pneumonia
HBV	Hepatitis B virus
HCO_3	Bicarbonate
Hct	Hematocrit
HDL	High-density lipoproteins
HF	Heart failure
HFV	High-frequency ventilation
Hg	Mercury
Hgb	Hemoglobin
HHNK	Hyperglycemic hyperosmolar nonketotic (condition or coma)
HITT	Heparin-induced thrombosis and thrombocytopenia; also referred to as heparin-associated thrombosis and thrombocytopenia (HATT) or white clot syndrome
HIV	Human immunodeficiency virus
HLA	Human leukocyte antigen
HOB	Head of bed
HR	Heart rate
HRT	Hormone replacement therapy
I:E	Inspiration: expiration
IABP	Intra-aortic balloon pump
IAP	Intra-abdominal pressure
IBW	Ideal body weight
IC	Inspiratory capacity
ICH	Intracranial hematoma
ICOP	Interstitial colloidal oncotic pressure
ICP	Intracranial pressure
ICS	Intercostal space
ICU	Intensive care unit
IFD	Intermittent flush device
Ig	Immunoglobulin
IHD	Inflammatory heart disease
IHP	Interstitial hydrostatic pressure
IHSS	Idiopathic hypertrophic subaortic stenosis
IL	Interleukin
ILV	Independent lung ventilation
IM	Intramuscular
IMV	Intermittent mandatory ventilation
INR	International normalized ratio

INVOS	In-vivo optical spectroscopy
IPPB	Intermittent positive pressure breathing
IRA	Infarct-related artery
IRV	Inspiratory reserve volume
IRV	Inverse ratio ventilation
ISMP	Institute for Safe Medication Practices
ITP	Idiopathic thrombocytopenic purpura
IU	International units
IV	Intravenous
IVP	Intravenous pyelogram
IVUS	Intravascular ultrasound
JCAHO	Joint Commission on Accreditation of Healthcare Organizations (now The Joint Commission [TJC])
JVD	Jugular venous distention
kg	Kilogram
KS	Kaposi's sarcoma
KUB	Kidneys, ureters, bladder (same as flat plate of abdomen)
L	Liter
LA	Left atrium
LAAL	Left anterior axillary line
LAD	Left anterior descending (artery)
LAD	Left axis deviation
LAH	Left anterior hemibundle
LAP	Left atrial pressure
LBB	Left bundle branch
LBBB	Left bundle branch block
LCA	Left circumflex artery
LDH	Lactate dehydrogenase
LDL	Low-density lipoproteins
LES	Lower esophageal sphincter
LICS	Left intercostal space
LLQ	Left lower quadrant
LMA	Laryngeal mask airway
LMAL	Left midaxillary line
LMCL	Left midclavicular line
LMN	Lower motor neuron
LMWH	Low-molecular-weight heparin
LOC	Level of consciousness
LP	Lumbar puncture
LPAL	Left posterior axillary line
LPH	Left posterior hemibundle
LR	Lactated Ringer's (solution)
LSB	Left sternal border
LUQ	Left upper quadrant
LV	Left ventricle
LVAD	Left ventricular assist device

LVEDP	Left ventricular end-diastolic pressure
LVEDV	Left ventricular end-diastolic volume
LVF	Left ventricular failure
LVH	Left ventricular hypertrophy
LVMI	Left ventricular myocardial infarction
LVSWI	Left ventricular stroke work index
M_1	Mitral (first) component of S_1
mA	Milliampere (unit of measurement for electrical current)
MAL	Midaxillary line
MALT	Mucosa-associated lymphoid tissue
MAO	Monoamide oxidase (as in MAO inhibitors)
MAP	Mean arterial pressure
mcg	Microgram (unit of measurement for weight)
MCL	Midclavicular line
MCT	Medium-chain triglycerides
MDF	Myocardial depressant factor
MDMA	Methylenedioxymethamphetamine (i.e., Ecstasy)
mEq	Milliequivalent (unit of measurement for solutes in solution)
mg	Milligram (unit of measurement for weight)
MI	Myocardial infarction
MIC	Minimum inhibitory concentration
MIDCABG	Minimally invasive coronary artery bypass graft
MIP	Maximal inspiratory pressure (or force) (also referred to as negative inspiratory pressure [or force])
mL	Milliliter (unit of measurement for volume)
mm	Millimeter (unit of measurement for length)
mm Hg	Millimeters of mercury
MODS	Multiple organ dysfunction syndrome
mOsm/kg	Milliosmols per kilogram (unit of measure for osmolality)
MR	Mitral regurgitation
MRA	Magnetic resonance angiography
MRI	Magnetic resonance imaging
MS	Mitral stenosis
MSL	Midsternal line
MUGA	Multiple-gated acquisition scan
MV	Mechanical ventilation
MVA	Motor vehicle accident
MVO_2	Myocardial oxygen consumption
MVP	Mitral valve prolapse
NAC	N-acetylcysteine
NDE	Near-death experience
NDNQI	National Database of Nursing Quality Indicators
NG	Nasogastric
NIBP	Noninvasive blood pressure
NIF	Negative inspiratory force
NIHSS	National Institutes of Health Stroke Scale

NK	Natural killer
NNRTI	Non-nucleoside reverse transcriptase inhibitor
NO	Nitric oxide
NPO	Nothing by mouth
NRTI	Nucleoside analogue reverse transcriptase inhibitor
NS	Normal saline
NSAID	Nonsteroidal antiinflammatory drug
NSR	Normal sinus rhythm
NTG	Nitroglycerin
NTP	Nitroprusside
NtRTI	Nucleotide reverse transcriptase inhibitor
NYHA	New York Heart Association
O_2	Oxygen
O_2EI	Oxygen extraction index
O_2ER	Oxygen extraction ratio
OPG	Oculoplethysmography
P_2	Pulmonic (second) component of S_2
PA	Pulmonary artery
PAC	Premature atrial contraction
$Paco_2$	Partial pressure of carbon dioxide in arterial blood
PAd	Pulmonary artery diastolic pressure
PAL	Posterior axillary line
PAm	Pulmonary artery pressure mean
Pao_2	Pressure of oxygen in arterial blood
PAO_2	Pressure of oxygen in the alveolus
PAOP	Pulmonary artery occlusive pressure (previously referred to as pulmonary capillary wedge pressure or pulmonary artery wedge pressure)
PAP	Pulmonary artery pressure
PAs	Pulmonary artery systolic pressure
PAT	Paroxysmal atrial tachycardia
PC/IRV	Pressure controlled/inverse ratio ventilation
PCA	Patient-controlled analgesia
PCI	Percutaneous coronary intervention
PCP	Phencyclidine
PCP	*Pneumocystis carinii* pneumonia
PCR	Polymerase chain reaction
PCV	Pressure-controlled ventilation
PD	Postural drainage
PDE	Phosphodiesterase
PDF	Probability density function
PDSA	Plan-Do-Study-Act
PE	Pulmonary embolism
PEA	Pulseless electrical activity
$PECO_2$	Partial pressure of carbon dioxide in exhaled air
PEEP	Positive end-expiratory pressure

PEFR	Peak expiratory flow rate
PEG	Percutaneous endoscopic gastrostomy
PEJ	Percutaneous endoscopic jejunostomy
PET	Positron emission tomography
P_{ETCO_2}	Partial pressure of carbon dioxide in end-tidal air
PFC	Perfluorocarbon
pH	Hydrogen ion concentration
pHi	Intramucosal pH
PICC	Percutaneously inserted central catheter
PIP	Peak inspiratory pressure
PJC	Premature junctional contraction
PMI	Point of maximal impulse
PML	Progressive multifocal leukoencephalopathy
PMN	Polymorphonuclear leukocyte
PMR	Papillary muscle rupture
PMR	Progressive muscle relaxation
PND	Paroxysmal nocturnal dyspnea
PNS	Parasympathetic nervous system
PO	orally
PPD	Purified protein derivative
PPF	Plasma protein fraction
PPI	Proton pump inhibitor
PPN	Peripheral parenteral nutrition
PRVC	Pressure-regulated volume-controlled (mode of mechanical ventilation)
PSB	Protected specimen brush
PSV	Pressure support ventilation
PSVT	Paroxysmal supraventricular tachycardia
PT	Physical therapy
PT	Prothrombin time
PTCA	Percutaneous transluminal coronary angioplasty
P_{TCO_2}	Transcutaneous partial pressure of oxygen
PTFE	Polytetrafluoroethylene
PTMR	Percutaneous transmyocardial revascularization
PTT	Partial prothrombin time
PV	Peak velocity
PVC	Polyvinyl chloride
PVC	Premature ventricular contraction
PVR	Pulmonary vascular resistance
PVRI	Pulmonary vascular resistance index
Q	Perfusion
QI	Quality improvement
QM	Quality management
QT_c	QT interval corrected for rate
RA	Right atrium
RAA	Renin-angiotensin-aldosterone

RAAL	Right anterior axillary line
RAD	Right axis deviation
RAP	Right atrial pressure
RAS	Reticular activating system
RBB	Right bundle branch
RBBB	Right bundle branch block
RBC	Red blood cell
RCA	Right coronary artery
REF	Right (ventricular) ejection fraction
REM	Rapid eye movement
RHD	Rheumatic heart disease
RICS	Right intercostal space
RLQ	Right lower quadrant
RMAL	Right midaxillary line
RMCL	Right midclavicular line
RN	Registered nurse
RNA	Ribonucleic acid
ROM	Range of motion
r-PA	Recombinant plasminogen activator
RPAL	Right posterior axillary line
RQ	Respiratory quotient
RR	Respiratory rate
RSB	Right sternal border
RSBI	Rapid shallow breathing index
RSV	Respiratory syncytium virus
r-PA	Recombinant plasminogen activator
rt-PA	Recombinant tissue plasminogen activator
RUQ	Right upper quadrant
RV	Residual volume
RV	Right ventricle
RVAD	Right ventricular assist device
RVEDP	Right ventricular end-diastolic pressure
RVEDV	Right ventricular end-diastolic volume
RVESV	Right ventricular end-systolic volume
RVF	Right ventricular failure
RVH	Right ventricular hypertrophy
RVMI	Right ventricular myocardial infarction
RVSWI	Right ventricular stroke work index
RYGB	Roux-Y gastric bypass
SA	Sinoatrial
SAED	Semiautomatic external defibrillator
SAH	Subarachnoid hemorrhage
Sao_2	Oxygen saturation of arterial blood
SARS	Severe acute respiratory syndrome
SC	Subcutaneous
SCI	Spinal cord injury

SCUF	Slow continuous ultrafiltration
$ScvO_2$	Oxygen saturation of central venous blood
SDD	Selective decontamination of digestive tract
SDH	Subdural hematoma
SIADH	Syndrome of inappropriate antidiuretic hormone
SIMV	Synchronized intermittent mandatory ventilation
SIRS	Systemic inflammatory response syndrome
Sjo_2	Oxygen saturation of jugular venous blood
SK	Streptokinase
SLE	Systemic lupus erythematosus
SNS	Sympathetic nervous system
SPECT	Single photon emission computed tomography
Spo_2	Oxygen saturation in plasma (e.g. Pulse oximetry)
SRS-A	Slow reacting substance of anaphylaxis
SV	Stroke volume
SI	Stroke index
Svo_2	Oxygen saturation of mixed venous blood
SVR	Systemic vascular resistance
SVRI	Systemic vascular resistance index
SVT	Supraventricular tachycardia
T	Temperature
T_1	Tricuspid (second) component of S_1
TAA	Thoracic aortic aneurysm
TB	Tuberculosis
TBI	Toe-brachial index
TCA	Tricyclic antidepressants
$TcPo_2$	Transcutaneous carbon dioxide pressure
TEC	Transluminal extraction catheter
TENS	Transcutaneous electrical nerve stimulation
TIA	Transient ischemic attack
TIBC	Total iron-binding capacity
TIPS	Transjugular intrahepatic portosystemic shunt
TLC	Total lung capacity
TLC	Total lymphocyte count
TMP-SMX	trimethoprim-sulfamethoxazole
TNA	Total nutrient admixture
TNF	Tumor necrosis factor
TPN	Total parenteral nutrition
TTP	Thrombotic thrombocytopenia purpura
UAP	Unlicensed assistive personnel
UES	Upper esophageal sphincter
UFH	Unfractionated heparin
UMN	Upper motor neuron
UTI	Urinary tract infection
V	Ventilation
V/Q	Ventilation/perfusion ratio (also ventilation/perfusion)

V_A	Alveolar minute ventilation
VAC	Vacuum-assisted closure
VAD	Ventricular assist device
VAP	Ventilator-associated pneumonia
VAPSV	Volume-assured pressure support ventilation
VBG	Vertical banded gastroplasty
VC	Vital capacity
V_D	Anatomical deadspace
V_E	Minute ventilation
VF	Ventricular fibrillation
VILI	Ventilator-induced lung injury
VO_2	Oxygen consumption by the tissues
VO_2I	Consumption of oxygen by the tissue index
VPR	Volume pressure response
VSD	Ventricular septal defect
VT	Ventricular tachycardia
V_T	Tidal volume
WBC	White blood cell
WPW	Wolff-Parkinson-White syndrome

Normal Laboratory Values

APPENDIX C

Blood

Chemistries

Sodium:	136-145 mEq/L
Potassium:	3.5-5.5 mEq/L
Chloride:	96-106 mEq/L
Calcium:	8.5-10.5 mg/dL
Phosphorus:	3.0-4.5 mg/dL
Magnesium:	1.5-2.2 mEq/L or 1.8-2.4 mg/dL
Carbon dioxide (CO_2):	23-30 mEq/L
Glucose:	70-110 mg/dL
Blood urea nitrogen (BUN):	5-20 mg/dL
Creatinine:	0.7-1.5 mg/dL
Uric acid:	3-7 mg/dL
Osmolality:	280-295 mOsm/kg
Lactate:	Less than 1 mmol/L
Gastrin:	Less than 200 ng/L
Pepsinogen:	200-425 units/mL
Ammonia:	15-110 mOsm/dL
Iron:	50-150 mcg/dL
Iron-binding capacity:	250-410 mcg/dL
Carcinoembryonic antigen (CEA):	Less than 2 ng/mL
Homocysteine:	Less than 15 μmol/L
C-reactive protein:	Less than 1 mg/dL
Brain-type natriuretic peptide (BNP):	Less than 100 pg/mL
Bilirubin	
Total:	0.3-1.3 mg/dL
Direct:	0.1-0.3 mg/dL
Indirect:	0.1-1.0 mg/dL

Proteins

Total protein:	6-8 g/dL
C-reactive protein:	less than 0.8 mg/dL
Albumin:	3.5-4.5 g/dL
Prealbumin:	15-35 mg/dL
Transferrin:	250-300 mg/dL
Globulin:	2.3-3.5 g/dL
Albumin/globulin ratio (A/G):	1.5/1-2.5/1
Fibrinogen:	200-400 mg/dL or 2-4 g/L

Lipids

Cholesterol:	150-200 mg/dL
Triglycerides:	40-150 mg/dL
Lipoprotein-cholesterol fractionation	
High-density lipoprotein (HDL):	29-77 mg/dL
Low-density lipoprotein (LDL):	62-130 mg/dL

Enzymes

Total creatine kinase (CK):	normal 55-170 units/L for male patients; 30-135 units/L for female patients
CK-MB:	0% of total CK
Lactate dehydrogenase (LDH):	90-200 units/L
LDH-1:	17%-25% of total LDH
Alanine aminotransferase (ALT):	5-36 units/mL (formerly called SGPT)
Aspartate amino-transferase (AST):	15-45 units/mL (formerly called SGOT)
Gamma-glutamyl transferase (GGT):	5-38 units/L
Alkaline phosphatase:	30-85 units/L
Amylase:	56-190 units/L
Lipase:	0-1.5 units/mL

Muscle Proteins

Myoglobin:	Normal, less than 110 ng/mL
Troponin I:	Normal, less than 1.5 ng/mL
Troponin T:	Normal, less than 0.1 ng/mL

Arterial Blood Gases

pH:	Normal, 7.35-7.45
$Paco_2$:	Normal, 35-45 mm Hg
Bicarbonate (HCO_3):	Normal, 22-26 mEq/L
Base excess:	−2-+2
Pao_2:	Normal, 80-100 mm Hg
Sao_2:	Greater than 95%

Hematology

Red blood cells (RBCs):	4.4-5.9 × 10^6/mL for male patients; 3.8-5.2 × 10^6/mL for female patients; red cell indices include the following
Mean corpuscular volume (MCV):	80-100 μm^3
Mean corpuscular hemoglobin (MCH):	27-31 pg
Mean corpuscular hemoglobin concentration (MCHC):	32-36 g/dL
Reticulocyte count:	0.5-1.5% of RBCs
Erythrocyte sedimentation rate (ESR or sed rate):	1-15 mm/hr for male patients, 1-20 mm/hr for female patients
Hematocrit:	40%-52% for male patients; 35%-47% for female patients
Hemoglobin:	13-18 g/dL for male patients; 12-16 g/dL for female patients
Platelets:	150,000-400,000/mm^3
White blood cells (WBCs):	3500-11,000 mm^3
Differential	
Neutrophils:	40%-80%
Eosinophils:	0%-5%
Basophils:	0%-2%
Monocytes:	3%-8%
Lymphocytes:	10%-40%
Immune profile	
CD4 cell count:	800 cells/mm^3; varies with age
CD4/CD8 ratio:	Helper cells: suppressor/cytotoxic cells ratio: 1.8
Human immunodeficiency virus (HIV) antibody screening:	negative

Clotting Profile

Prothrombin time (PT):	12-15 sec
Activated partial thromboplastin time (aPTT):	25-38 sec
Partial thromboplastin time (PTT):	60-90 sec
Activated clotting time (ACT):	70-120 sec
Thrombin time:	10-15 sec
Bleeding time:	1-9.5 min
Lee White clotting time:	6-12 min
International normalized ratio (INR):	Less than 2.0
Platelets:	150,000-400,000/mm^3
Fibrinogen:	200-400 mg/dL or 2-4 g/L
Fibrin split products (FSPs) (also referred to as fibrin degradation products (FDPs):	0-10 mcg/dL
D-dimer:	Normal, less than 250 ng/mL

Hormones

Thyroid-stimulating hormone (TSH):	Normal, 2-10 milliunits/L
Triiodothyronine (T_3):	0.2-0.3 mcg/dL
Thyroxine (T_4):	6-12 mcg/dL
Adrenocorticotropic hormone (ACTH):	15-100 pg/mL in AM, 10-50 pg/mL in PM
Cortisol:	6-28 mcg/dL at 8 AM, 4-12 mcg/dL at 4 PM; 2-12 mcg/dL at 8 PM
Antidiuretic hormone (ADH):	1-5 pg/mL

Toxicology

Alcohol:	0 mg/dL
Dilantin:	Therapeutic 10-20 mcg/mL
Digoxin:	Therapeutic 0.5-2.0 ng/mL
Lidocaine:	Therapeutic 1.5-5.0 mcg/mL
Phenobarbital:	Therapeutic 10-40 mcg/mL
Theophylline:	Therapeutic 10-20 ng/dL

Urine

Glucose:	Negative
Ketones:	Negative
Protein:	0-8 mg/dL; less than 150 mg/24-hr urine output
Amylase:	3-21 units/hour
Bilirubin:	Negative
Bilinogen:	0.3-3.5 mg/dL
RBCs:	0-2/low-power field
WBCs:	0-4/low-power field
Hemoglobin/myoglobin:	Negative
Bilirubin:	None
Specific gravity:	1.005-1.030
Osmolality:	50-1200 mOsm/L
Creatinine clearance:	85-135 mL/min
Culture and sensitivity:	No bacteria present; if bacteria are present appropriate antibiotic therapy is identified
pH:	4.0-8.0 with average of 6.0
Spot urine electrolytes	
Sodium:	40-220 mEq/L/day
Potassium:	25-120 mEq/L/day
Chloride:	110-250 mEq/day

Hormone metabolites

17-hydroxycorticosteroids:	4.5-10 mg/24 hr for male patients, 2.5-10 mg/24 hr for female patients
17-ketosteroids:	8-15 mg/24 hr for male patients, 6-12 mg/24 hr for female patients

Stool

Fecal occult blood test:	Negative
Ova, parasites, blood (OPB):	Negative
Fecal fat:	5 g/24 hr
Urobilinogen:	0-4 mg/day
Culture:	Intestinal flora
Assay for *Clostridium difficile* toxin A or B:	Normal is negative; positive if diarrhea is caused *C. difficile*

Note: Values may vary depending on the laboratory.

Formulae Significant to Critical Care Nursing

APPENDIX D

General

Conversion

To convert pounds to kilograms	1 lb = .45 kg
To convert inches to centimeters	1 in = 2.54 cm
To convert mm Hg to cm H_2O	1 mm Hg = 1.36 cm H_2O
To convert Fahrenheit to Celsius	(°F-32) ÷ 1.8

Drug Administration

To calculate mcg/kg/min if you know the rate of the infusion	$\frac{(\text{mcg/mL}) \times (\text{mL/hr})}{(60\ \text{min/hr}) \times (\text{kg body weight})}$
To calculate rate in mL/hr if you know the dose in mcg/kg/min	$\frac{(\text{dose in mcg/kg/min}) \times (60\ \text{min/hr}) \times (\text{wt in kg})}{\text{mcg/mL of the solution}}$
To calculate mg/min if you know the rate of the infusion	$\frac{(\text{mg/mL}) \times (\text{mL/hr})}{(60\ \text{min/hr})}$
To calculate rate in mL/hr if you know the dose in mg/min	$\frac{(\text{dose in mg/min}) \times (60\ \text{min/hr})}{\text{mg/mL of the solution}}$
To calculate mcg/min if you know the rate of the infusion	$\frac{(\text{mcg/mL}) \times (\text{mL/hr})}{(60\ \text{min/hr})}$
To calculate rate in mL/hr if you know the dose in mcg/min	$\frac{(\text{dose in mcg/min}) \times (60\ \text{min/hr})}{\text{mcg/mL of the solution}}$

Cardiovascular

Parameter	Method of Calculation	Normal
Mean arterial pressure (MAP)	[BP systolic + (BP diastolic × 2)] ÷ 3	70-105 mm Hg (Normal systolic BP 90-140 mm Hg; normal diastolic BP 60-90 mm Hg)
Cardiac index (CI)	CO ÷ BSA	2.5-4.0 L/min/m^2
Stroke volume (SV)	CO ÷ HR	60-120 mL/beat
Stroke index (SI)	SV ÷ BSA	30-65 mL/m^2/beat
Systemic vascular resistance (SVR)	[(MAP − RAP) × 80] ÷ CO	900-1,400 dyne/sec/cm^{-5}
Systemic vascular resistance index (SVRI)	[(MAP − RAP) × 80] ÷ CI	1,700-2,600 dyne/sec/cm^{-5}/m^2

Continued

Parameter	Method of Calculation	Normal
Pulmonary vascular resistance (PVR)	[(PAm − PAOP) × 80] ÷ CO	100-250 dyne/sec/cm^{-5}
Pulmonary vascular resistance index (PVRI)	[(PAm − PAOP) × 80] ÷ CI	225-315 dyne/sec/cm^{-5}/m^2
Left ventricular stroke work index (LVSWI)	[SI × (MAP − PAOP)] × 0.0136	45-65 g · m/m^2
Right ventricular stroke work index (RVSWI)	[SI × (PAm − RAP)] × 0.0136	5-12 g · m/m^2
Coronary artery perfusion pressure (CAPP)	Diastolic BP − PAOP	60-80 mm Hg
Right ventricular end-diastolic volume index (RVEDVI)	RVEDV ÷ BSA	60-100 mL/m^2
Right ventricular end-systolic volume index (RVESVI)	RVESV ÷ BSA	30-60 mL/m^2
Arterial oxygen content (Cao_2)	1.34 × Hgb × Sao_2	18-20 mL/dL
Venous oxygen content (Cvo_2)	1.34 × Hgb × Svo_2	12-16 mL/dL
Oxygen delivery (Do_2)	CO × Cao_2 × 10	900-1,100 mL/min
Oxygen delivery index (Do_2I)	CI × Cao_2 × 10	550-650 mL/min/m^2
Oxygen consumption (Vo_2)	CO × Hgb × 13.4 × (Sao_2 − Svo_2)	200-300 mL/min
Oxygen consumption index (Vo_2I)	CI × Hgb × 13.4 × (Sao_2 − Svo_2)	110-160 mL/min/m^2
Oxygen extraction ratio (O_2ER)	Cao_2 − Cvo_2/Cao_2	22%-30%
Oxygen extraction index (O_2EI)	Sao_2 − Svo_2/Sao_2	20%-27%
Coronary artery perfusion pressure (CAPP)	Diastolic BP − PAOP	60-80 mm Hg
Corrected QT	QT ÷ √RR	0.35-0.43 sec

Pulmonary

Parameter	Method of Calculation	Normal
Static compliance	$\frac{\text{Tidal volume}}{\text{Plateau pressure} - \text{PEEP}}$	50-100 mL/cm H_2O
Dynamic compliance	$\frac{\text{Tidal volume}}{\text{Peak pressure} - \text{PEEP}}$	35-55 mL/cm H_2O
a/A ratio	(Pao_2/PAO_2) Note: PAO_2 is calculated as: Fio_2 (760 − 47) − ($Paco_2$/0.8) Note: Fio_2: fraction of inspired oxygen (written as a decimal) Pb: barometric pressure (760 mm Hg at sea level, adjust for higher altitudes) $Paco_2$: arterial carbon dioxide tension 47 is the pressure of water vapor at sea level and is subtracted from barometric pressure; 0.8 is the usual respiratory quotient	normal greater than 0.8 moderately abnormal 0.5-0.8 significantly abnormal 0.25-0.5 critically abnormal less than 0.25
A:a gradient	PAO_2 − Pao_2	Less than 10 mm Hg Note: A:a gradient × 0.05 = approximate % shunt
Pao_2/Fio_2 ratio	$\frac{Pao_2}{Fio_2 \text{ (decimal)}}$	Greater than 300 300 = approximately 15% shunt 200 = approximately 20% shunt
Respiratory index	$\frac{PAO_2 - Pao_2}{Pao_2}$	Less than 1.0

Neurologic

Parameter	Method of Calculation	Normal
Cerebral perfusion pressure (CPP)	MAP − intracranial pressure ICP	60-100 mm Hg

Nutrition

Parameter	Method of Calculation	Normal
Body mass index (BMI)	Wt (kg)/Ht (m) × Ht (m)	Optimal: 20-25 Obesity: greater than 25 Underweight: less than 20

Fluid, Electrolyte, Acid-Base

Parameter	Method of Calculation	Normal
Serum osmolality	$(2 \times \text{Na}) + \frac{\text{BUN}}{2.6} + \frac{\text{glucose}}{18}$	280-295 mOsm/L
Anion gap	$(\text{Na} + \text{K}) - (\text{Cl} + \text{HCO}_3)$	5-15

BP, Blood pressure; *BSA*, body surface area; *BUN*, blood urea nitrogen; *Cao*$_2$, arterial oxygen content; *Cl*, chloride; *Co*, cardiac output; *Cvo*$_2$, venous oxygen content; *Fio*$_2$, fraction of inspired oxygen; *HCO*$_3$, bicarbonate; *Hgb*, hemoglobin; *HR*, heart rate; *Ht*, height; *ICP*, intracranial pressure; *K*, potassium; *MAP*, mean arterial pressure; *Na*, sodium; *Paco*$_2$, arterial partial pressure of carbon dioxide; *PAm*, mean pulmonary artery pressure; *Pao*$_2$, arterial partial pressure of oxygen; *PAO*$_2$, alveolar partial pressure of oxygen; *PAOP*, pulmonary artery occlusive pressure; *PEEP*, positive end-expiratory pressure; *RAP*, right atrial pressure; *RVEDV*, right ventricular end-diastolic volume; *RVESV*, right ventricular end-systolic volume; *Sao*$_2$, arterial oxygen saturation; *SI*, stroke index; *Svo*$_2$, venous oxygen saturation; *Wt*, weight.

Index

Page numbers followed by *f* indicate figure(s); *b*, boxes; *t*, table(s).

J

K